KU-017-473

OXFORD MEDICAL PUBLICATIONS

Effective Care in Pregnancy and Childbirth

EDITORS

Iain Chalmers MB BS, MSc, DCH, FFCM, FRCOG
Director, National Perinatal Epidemiology Unit, Oxford

Murray Enkin MD, FRCS(C), FACOG
Professor Emeritus,
Departments of Obstetrics and Gynaecology, and Clinical Epidemiology and Biostatistics,
McMaster University

Marc J. N. C. Keirse MD, DPhil, DPH
Professor of Obstetrics,
Leiden University and
Visiting Professor of Obstetrics,
University of Leuven

Effective Care in Pregnancy and Childbirth

VOLUME 1: PREGNANCY

PARTS I–V

Edited by

IAIN CHALMERS MURRAY ENKIN

MARC J. N. C. KEIRSE

Foreword by

ARCHIE COCHRANE

Oxford · New York · Toronto
OXFORD UNIVERSITY PRESS

Oxford University Press, Walton Street, Oxford OX2 6DP
Oxford New York Toronto
Delhi Bombay Calcutta Madras Karachi
Petaling Jaya Singapore Hong Kong Tokyo
Nairobi Dar es Salaam Cape Town
Melbourne Auckland
and associated companies in
Berlin Ibadan

Oxford is a trade mark of Oxford University Press

Published in the United States
by Oxford University Press, New York

First published 1989
Reprinted (with corrections) 1991

British Library Cataloguing in Publication Data
Effective care in pregnancy and childbirth
1. Pregnant women. Medical care.
I. Chalmers, Iain. II. Enkin, Murray. III. Keirse Marc J. N. C.
618.2'4
ISBN 0–19–261558–0 v.1.
ISBN 0–19–261880–6 v. 2.

Library of Congress Cataloging in Publication Data
(Data available)

Set by Latimer Trend & Company Limited, Plymouth
Printed and bound by Bookcraft (Bath) Ltd.

This book is dedicated to
Jan Chalmers, Eleanor Enkin, and Nelly Keirse,
and to
Anne B. M. Anderson, MD, PhD, FRCOG
10 February 1937—11 February 1983

Foreword

Archie Cochrane
Formerly Director, MRC Epidemiological Research Unit, Cardiff

In 1979, while reviewing the vital importance of randomized controlled trials for evaluating the effectiveness of the treatments we impose upon our patients, I suggested that every medical specialty should compile a list of all the randomized controlled trials within its field, to be available for those who wish to know which of the treatments used were effective.

I went on to discuss which specialties had made the best use, and which had made the worst use of randomized trials. While I had little difficulty in deciding which specialty (at the time) had made the best use of trials, I had some difficulty in deciding which one was worst. Surgery, cardiology, and psychiatry were close runners up, but I finally chose obstetrics as the specialty most deserving of the 'wooden spoon'. I think that I made a reasonable defence of my choice.

That, however, was nearly a decade ago, and a great deal has happened since. There has been a marked increase in the use of randomized trials in the world of obstetrics. Moreover, the systematic review of the randomized trials of obstetric practice that is presented in this book is a new achievement. It represents a real milestone in the history of randomized trials and in the evaluation of care, and I hope that it will be widely copied by other medical specialties. I now have no hesitation whatsoever in withdrawing the slur of the wooden spoon from obstetrics, and I feel honoured by being associated, even in an indirect way, with such an important publication.

Rhoose Farm House,
Rhoose,
South Glamorgan.
July 1987

Preface

Care during pregnancy and childbirth should be effective. While no one is likely to disagree with this principle, marked disagreement exists as to what constitutes effective care. The disagreement arises from differences of opinion both about the objectives of care, and about the best means of achieving them.

The objectives of care, or the relative emphases placed on particular objectives, depend on what individuals or communities think is most important. This may range from enjoyment of the experience of childbirth, to shaving another fraction of a percentage point off the perinatal mortality rate, regardless of the costs. This diversity has resulted in widely differing recommendations for care during pregnancy and childbirth.

Differing views about the objectives of care also help to explain the disparate indicators used to assess the effects of care. Some people rate women's satisfaction with the care that they have received as the most important measure of its effectiveness; others seem to regard indirect measures of the baby's well-being, such as fetal heart rate tracings or estimates of the acid-base status of umbilical cord blood, as more important.

In preparing this book, we have not attempted to assess the desirability of different objectives of care during pregnancy and childbirth. These will always remain a matter for individual judgement, and they are unlikely to be influenced by the kind of evidence reviewed in the chapters that follow. What we have tried to do, however, is to give systematic attention to the second reason for disagreements about what constitutes effective care—the differences of opinion about how to attain the various objectives considered to be important.

These differences of opinion are manifested in dramatic variations in the patterns of care from country to country, from community to community, from institution to institution, and from one caregiver to another. The variations exist throughout the various phases of care during pregnancy and childbirth. A variety of methods are used to assess the risk status of the mother and the well-being of the fetus. Strongly held opinions differ as to whether pregnant women should take iron or vitamin supplements routinely during pregnancy; whether the cervix should be examined each time a woman attends for antenatal care; and whether all women should have an ultrasound examination. There is disagreement about whether women who have an uncomplicated twin pregnancy, or who develop non-albuminuric hypertension, should be hospitalized for bed rest. There is no agreement about the place of external version for breech presentation, cervical cerclage for 'incompetent cervix', corticosteroids for fetal lung maturation, or betamimetics for inhibition of preterm labour. Some people believe that women should not be permitted to eat or drink once labour has started, and that intravenous fluids should be administered routinely; others believe that such restriction is not warranted. There is no consensus about many of the suggested indications for caesarean section and operative vaginal delivery, or about the relative merits of forceps delivery and vacuum extraction. People disagree as to when and how an episiotomy should be performed, and about the best method and suture material to use for its repair. Professionals often present women experiencing difficulties with breastfeeding with conflicting advice about how to overcome these problems. The list of examples that could be cited is endless.

A number of factors may explain these variations in the patterns of care. Some relate to differences in the needs of childbearing women and their babies. Others reflect differences in culture, tradition, status, and fashion; differences in the availability of buildings, personnel, hospital beds, and equipment; differences in the need to provide opportunities for clinicians in training to gain experience; differences in the extent to which malpractice litigation is feared; differences in the extent to which doctors are paid on a 'piecework' basis; and differences in commercial pressures from drug and equipment manufacturers and others.

The focus of this book, however, relates to another important, but rather different determinant of variations in practice. This is the collective uncertainty that exists among those who provide care about the effectiveness and safety of many of the elements of care given during pregnancy and childbirth. A vast amount of data is available to address this collective uncertainty. Unfortunately, these data are widely scattered, and must be collated and analysed before they can be useful. This collation and analysis is the task that we have set for ourselves and our collaborators. It constitutes the research on which this book is based.

It has been a difficult but rewarding process. First, we carried out a systematic search of the literature for those studies that would be least likely to be misleading. These, along with data from unpublished studies that were kindly made available to us by clinicians and researchers throughout the world, were brought together, and they form the core of the evidence presented in this book. These controlled evaluations were always reviewed before weaker forms of evidence were considered.

Throughout the book we have tried to ensure that each chapter ends with a clear statement of the authors' conclusions about the implications of the evidence reviewed, both for current practice and for future research. There is still scope for considerable disagreement about many of the conclusions that we and our collaborators have reached, however. While we have made great efforts to ensure that the data presented are comprehensive and accurate, it is likely that some important studies have been overlooked, and that errors and misinterpretations have crept in. We invite readers to bring these to our attention for inclusion or correction in later editions. We shall ensure that those who help us in this way are appropriately acknowledged.

I. C.
M. E.
M. J. N. C. K.

Acknowledgements

Primary credit for this book must go to the women and investigators who participated in and conducted the controlled trials of care in pregnancy and childbirth on which so much of the evidence presented in the book is based. We wish to begin our acknowledgements by expressing our gratitude to these tens of thousands of unnamed people, and to Archie Cochrane, who first drew our attention to the particular importance of their contributions to an understanding of the effects of care during pregnancy and childbirth.

Most of our editorial work has been based at the *National Perinatal Epidemiology Unit*. We are greatly indebted to those who carried the main workload, namely, Philippa Claiden, Frances Grant, Jini Hetherington, Myrna Holmes, Sally Hunt, Emily Oakley, Janelle Rogers, Mark Starr, and Mary Tinker. In addition, we are grateful to Peter Applegarth, Hazel Ashurst, Sarah Ayers, Chris Catton, Lesley Mierh, Malcolm Newdick, Lynda Pilcher, Sylvia Russell, Ralph Targett, and Kathy Worton for help of various kinds in Oxford. Our editorial work in Canada, The Netherlands, and Italy was supported by Paulette Morley at *McMaster University*; Barry d'Arnaud, Hanneke Ensink-Wittenberg, Nelly Keirse, Liesbeth Olthof, and Jaco Stouten at *Leiden University*; and Roberto and Gianna Celli, Susan Garfield, and Ken Warren at the *Rockefeller Foundation*'s *Study Centre at Bellagio*. We are greatly indebted to all these people. Our editorial task has been made easier by the trust placed in us by *Oxford University Press*; this has been manifested in the support we have received from Alison Langton, Richard Charkin, and Adam Hodgkin, and the excellent assistance we have received from Eric Buckley, Ian Hall, John Harrison, Phil Russell, and Pete Russell.

Some individuals were of enormous help to us because of the general guidance and other kinds of help that they provided. In particular, we thank Susan Boron, Mike Bracken, Hamish Chalmers, Tom Chalmers, John Collins, Diana Elbourne, Ruth Evans, Bob Fraser, Jo Garcia, Adrian Grant, Muir Gray, Gordon Guyatt, Ellen Hodnett, Frank Hytten, Brigitte Jordan, Karyn Kaufman, John Kennell, Marshall Klaus, Irvine Loudon, Jerry Lucey, Henry McQuay, Ann Oakley, Andy Oxman, Richard Peto, Mary Renfrew, Martin Richards, David Sackett, Roberta Shaw, Madeleine Shearer, Alec Turnbull, Jack Sinclair, and Andre Van Assche.

We are grateful to the Department of Health (England), the Department of Obstetrics and Gynaecology at McMaster University, and the Department of Obstetrics, Gynaecology and Reproduction at Leiden University for granting us time to work on this project. Data collection for the Oxford Database of Perinatal Trials, which has played such an important role in our work, was supported by funds provided by the World Health Organization. The Rockefeller Foundation provided us with important help by granting us time and facilities to work together as scholars in residence at their study centre in the Villa Serbelloni, and by a grant towards our travel and communication expenses during the final year of work on the book.

It is difficult to conceive how the book could have been completed without the many forms of editorial assistance provided by Eleanor Enkin. We are profoundly grateful to her for the patient help that she gave to each and all of us over a period of more than five years.

Finally, we owe an enormous debt to our families. Two of us have been guilty of gross dereliction of paternal duties over a period when our children had a right to expect more of our attention than they received: we acknowledge with gratitude the understanding and tolerance shown to us by Hamish and Theo Chalmers, and Koen and Anne Keirse. We wish we could find adequate words to express our love and gratitude to Jan Chalmers, Eleanor Enkin, and Nelly Keirse; we know how much they sacrificed over the many years during which we have been so deeply involved with this project. In short, our work could not have been completed without the unwavering support provided by our families in so many different ways; we are profoundly grateful to them.

Acknowledgement of help in preparing specific chapters

Both the authors and the editors express their gratitude to those individuals who have provided help in preparing specific chapters. For *Chapter 1:* Doug Altman, Hazel Ashurst, Jesse Berlin, Mike Bracken, Tom Chalmers, Rory Collins, Adrian Grant, Gord Guyatt, Austin Bradford Hill, Frank Hytten, Carol Lefebvre, Irvine Loudon, Jerry Lucey, Klim McPherson, Richard Peto, Andy Oxman, Jean Robinson, Jack Sinclair, and Elizabeth Wilson; for *Chapter 2:* Doug Altman, Jesse Berlin, Mike Bracken, Tom Chalmers, Rory Collins, Lisa Curtice, Salim Daya, Kay Dickersin,

Mike Drummond, Harold Gamsu, Jo Garcia, Gord Guyatt, Jim Julian, Alison Macfarlane, Klim McPherson, Pat Mohide, Fred Mosteller, Miranda Mugford, Arne Ohlsson, Andy Oxman, Richard Peto, Martin Richards, Joyce Roberts, Rob Roberts, Peter Sandercock, Bill Silverman, John Simes, Barbara Stocking, Dave Streiner, Donna Stroup, Steve Thacker, and Elizabeth Wilson; for *Chapter 3:* Dave Sackett; for *Chapter 4:* Meg Stacey and Phil Strong; for *Chapter 5:* Jonathan Lomas; for *Chapter 7:* Elisabeth Bing, Margot Edwards, Judith Ellis, Judith Flanagan, Jeffrey Gould, Doris Haire, Lester Hazell, Brigitte Jordan, Marshall Klaus, Judith Lumley, Niles Newton, Miriam Orleans, Diana Petitti, Elizabeth Shearer, Thomas Shearer, Penny Simkin, and Diony Young; for *Chapter 8:* Ann Oakley; for *Chapter 9:* Ned Divelbiss, John Rapson, R. Sheldon Jones, Delbert W. Jones, and C. A. DeVries; for *Chapter 10:* Susan Bradley, Carolyn Dereky, Josephine Golden, Keith Jacka, Ann Thomson and the Department of Health (England); for *Chapter 11:* Michael Bull, Diana Elbourne, Maurie Gelfand, Emily Hamilton, Sara Lazzam, Aidan Macfarlane, and Alec Turnbull; for *Chapter 14:* Michael Bracken, Ann Cartwright, and Monique Kaminski; for *Chapter 15:* José Belizán, Béatrice Blondel, Robert Bryce, Judy Dance, Sandra Elliott, Henry Heins, John Kelly, John Kennell, Marshall Klaus, Michael Kramer, Charles Larson, Tessa Leverton, Alice Lovell, Stephen Ng, David Olds, Margaret Reid, Alan Rothberg, David Rush, Mary Sexton, Brenda Spencer, Nadine Spira, Fiona Stanley, Anita Stevens, and José Villar; for *Chapter 18:* Frank Hytten, Dawn James, Ian MacGillivray, David Rush, Angus Thomson, and Nancy Stewart; for *Chapter 19:* J. Foulkes, Leela Iyengar, J. Metz, J. Rolshau, G. Tchernia, and K. Trigg; for *Chapter 20:* Kay Heeren; for *Chapter 22:* Godelieve Nasuy-Stroobant; for *Chapter 23:* Anne Lynette Noble and the Spastics Society; for *Chapter 24:* Jos Schot-van Blarkom; for *Chapter 27:* Margaret McNay and Charles Whitfield; for *Chapter 28:* Lil Valentin and Tom Weber; for *Chapter 29:* Fondation Erasme, Christine Gervy, and William Spellacy; for *Chapter 33:* Jon Godwin and Jos Schot-van Blarkom; for *Chapter 35:* J. Stam-Rietkerken; for *Chapter 36:* Patrick Mohide and David Sackett; for *Chapter 37:* Glenda Chaplin and Pauline Ruddiforth; for *Chapter 38:* Jayne Berrier, Ragu Nagalingam, Dinah Reitman, Scott Rubin, and Martha Ziegenfus; for *Chapter 39:* Hazel Ashurst, Margaret Black, and David Scott; for *Chapter 40:* Malcolm Macnaughton, Emile Papiernik, and Rob Rush; for *Chapter 41:* R. Liddicoate, G.K. Nelson, and Rashmi Varma; for *Chapter 44:* Tom Barden, Andrew Calder, Curtis Cetrulo, Cees de Vos, Calvin Hobel, Jørgen Falck Larsen, Kenneth Leveno, Frederico Mariona, A. Martin, Naren Patel, A. Scommegna, Christopher Thomasson, Alec Turnbull, Rashmi Varma, Nicholas Wald and S. Wonnacott; for *Chapter 45:* Anne Anderson, Harold Gamsu, Mont Liggins, and John Morrison; for *Chapter 46:* Tor Bjerkedal and staff at the Medical Birth Registry of Norway, Anders Ericson and staff at the Medical Birth Registry of Sweden, and the National Institutes of Health (Contract No. NO1-HD-8–2826); for *Chapter 47:* Per Bergsjø, Andrew Curtain, Donald Dyson, George Henry, Peter Lenehan, Dermot MacDonald, Denis Martin, and Malcolm Pearce; for *Chapter 48:* S.M. van Mechelen, M.A.M. Taverne, and N. Touber; for *Chapter 49:* Ellen Hodnett, John Kennell, and Marshall Klaus; for *Chapter 50:* Louise Hanvey; for *Chapter 51:* Sarah Ayers, and Ann Thomson, Editor of Midwifery; for *Chapter 52:* Selwyn Crawford, John Evans, and Michael Rosen; for *Chapter 54:* Dermot MacDonald; for *Chapter 55:* Rose Conklin and Janet Regas; for *Chapter 56:* Kathy Gotshall and Kay Heeren; for *Chapter 57:* Therese K. Abboud, E. Abbouleish, P.D. Challen, Paula Elliot, Michael Finster, Klas-Henry Hokegard, Helge Jenssen, D.H. Morison, Kari G. Smedstad, J. Scanlon, and M.E. Tunstall; for *Chapters 61–63:* Benny Andreasson, Richard Beard, John Beazley, Per Bergsjø, Paul Bernstein, Gérard Bréart, Katarina Bremme, Marc Bygdeman, Dominique Cabrol, Andrew Calder, Ian Craft, Dennis Davey, Günvör Ekman, Murdo Elder, Max Elstein, Emanuel Friedman, Mohsen Iskander, Aksel Lange, Ian Lange, Russell Laros, Anthony Letchworth, J.R. Leiberman, William LeMaire, Mont Liggins, Gert Lykkesfeldt, Ian MacKenzie, Alastair MacLennan, Callum Macnaughton, John MacVicar, F. Maillard, Denis Martin, Ed Mason, William Naismith, Walter Parewijck, Shan Ratnam, Jacques Rioux, Charles Rodeck, Yehia Saleh, H. Sande, William Spellacy, Philip Steer, Claude Sureau, Michel Thiery, Gareth Thomas, John Tylleskär, Ulf Ulmsten, Dirk Wildemeersch, H.P. Zahradnik, and Frank Zlatnik; for *Chapter 64:* Harriet McGory; for *Chapter 66:* M.E. Carpenter, Patricia Crowley, Elizabeth Fern, Adrian Grant, Donna Jean Van Lier, Mim Orleans, Mary Renfrew, and Michael Turner; for *Chapter 67:* Tricia Aldrick, Doreen Daley, Emanuel Friedman, Neville Hacker, Joanna Harding, Michael Newton, Frances Potter, and Gordon Stirrat; for *Chapter 68:* A.D.G. Roberts; for *Chapter 69:* Geoffrey M. Anderson, Klim McPherson, Karel Stembera, and Ralph Targett; for *Chapter 70:* Geoffrey M. Anderson, Janet Barnsley, Jonathan Lomas, Betsy MacKinnon, Lynda Marsh, and Eugene Vayda and members of the Planning Committee, National Consensus Conference on aspects of Caesarean Birth; for *Chapter 71:* A.H. Lasbury, Avon Simpson, and Michel Thiery; for *Chapter 72:* Ros Osmond; for *Chapter 74:* Inge van Kamp, Harry Kragt, Margot van de Bor, Pauline Verloove-Vanhorick, and Robert Verwey; for *Chapter 75:* Hope Perryman and John C. Sinclair; for *Chapter*

76: Diane Moore; for *Chapter 78:* Karyn Kaufman and Robin Whyte; for *Chapter 79:* Henry McQuay; for *Chapter 80:* Chloe Fisher, Wendy Nicholson, Sylvia Slaven, Michael Woolridge, and Churchill Livingstone Ltd for permission to reproduce Figure 1; and Chloe Fisher and Felicity King for permission to reproduce Figure 2; for *Chapter 82:* Anna Mattei and Maria Nigro; for *Chapter 83:* J. Karsdon; for *Chapter 84:* Ann Lynette Noble and the Spastics Society; for *Chapter 85:* S. Iles, and patients and staff of the Maternity Unit at the John Radcliffe Hospital, Oxford; for *Chapter 86:* Judy Moss and Livio Lanceri; and for *Chapter 89:* all contact authors of previous chapters, Muir Gray, Denise Winn, and Elizabeth Wilson and her colleagues at the Department of Health (England).

Acknowledgement of information provided about unpublished trials

Many individuals and organizations helped us to obtain information about unpublished trials. We are greatly indebted to colleagues in many countries for helping us to survey over 40 000 obstetricians and paediatricians. They include Per Bergsjø, Hans Bossart, Gérard Bréart, Bob Bryce, E. Cserhati, Gabriel Duc, Joachim Dudenhausen, Per Finne, Col Fisher, Nils Hahnemann, Justus Hofmeyr, Peter Husslein, Pentti Jouppila, Ingemar Kjellmar, László Lampé, Mont Liggins, Jerold Lucey, Patrick Mohide, Fred Paccaud, E.T. Rippmann, Alan Rothberg, R. Tambyraja, and Michel Tournaire. In addition to these named individuals we were assisted by officers and staff of the American College of Obstetricians and Gynecologists, the American Pediatric Society, the British Paediatric Association, Ross Laboratories, the Royal Australian College of Obstetricians and Gynaecologists, the Royal College of Obstetricians and Gynaecologists, the Society of Obstetricians and Gynaecologists of Canada, and the Society for Paediatric Research. Some of the financial support for our survey was provided by NCHSR/HCTA Grant No. RO1 HS 05523–02.

Many obstetricians, paediatricians and others responded to our letters requesting information about perinatal trials that had not been published. We are grateful to all of them, even though some of the information that they provided could not be incorporated in the final manuscript of this edition of this book. The trials notified to us by neonatalogists are being reviewed by our colleagues Jack Sinclair and Jerry Lucey as they and their collaborators prepare the sequel to this book—*Effective Care of the Newborn Infant.* Obstetricians, midwives and others who provided information about trials relevant to the topics covered in the present book include Ursula Ackermann-Liebrich, Susan Alberstein, Jo Alexander, Omar Althabe, Erol Amon, Felicity Ashworth, Ove Axelsson, Jeanne Ballard, Cecily Begley, José Belizán, Saul Bender, Erik Bendvold, Robin Bell, Per Bergsjø, Anne Bird, Sharon Birk, Béatrice Blondel, Saul Bloomfield, Peter Boylan, Gérard Bréart, Bob Bryce, Colin Bullough, Shannon Burke, Tom Burling, Dominique Cabrol, Andrew Calder, Doris Campbell, Linda Cardozo, Lieve Christiaens, Sheila Cohen, P.J. Collipp, David Conway, Selwyn Crawford, Robert Creasy, Caroline Crowther, Andrew Cseizel, Michael Dalmat, Sanjay Datta, Dennis Davey, Robert Davey, Ted Daw, Yusoff Dawood, Andrew Dawson, Peter Dear, Michael de Swiet, Johannes Dietl, Jim Dornan, Sheila Dubois, D.L. Dunlop, R.G. Farquarson, Neil Finer, Orvar Finnström, Alan Fleming, Charles Flowers, Michael Foley, Robert Fraser, Jonathan Gardosi, Tom Garite, S. George, Robert Goodlin, Ian Gross, Leif Hagglund, Greta Hally, John Hamerton, Ann Hamilton, Mary Hannah, Lorne Hanson, Ulf Hanson, Denis Hawkins, Brenda Henson, Lawrence Hester, Justus Hofmeyr, David Hollander, Cas Holleboom, Mary Holohan, Alan Hughes, Samuel Hughes, Henk Huisjes, David Hunter, Ingemar Ingemarsson, David James, D. Janssens, Simon Jenkinson, Mary Johnston, Frank Johnstone, Ed Kass, John Kelly, Julian Kenyon, Abubakr Kiwanuka, Arnold Klopper, T.A. Kuit, Marie Laga, Ronald Lamont, László Lampé, Justin Lavin, Christopher Lennox, Peter Lewis, Tom Lind, Abby Lippman, R.M. Liston, Luciano Lizzi, Mike Lobb, Robert Lorenz, Richard Lowensohn, Richard Lilford, Yuen Lin, Judith Lumley, Christine MacArthur, Dermot MacDonald, Hamish MacDonald, Alastair MacLennan, Gertie Marx, Dudley Mathews, Hugo Mendoza, Ernesto Meriggi, Jack Metz, Tony Milner, George Mitchell, Richard Molina, John Morrison, Richard Morton, Jean-Marie Moutquin, John Murphy, John Newnham, Niles Newton, Stephen Ng, Hein Odendaal, George O'Neil, Camillo Orlandi, Mogens Osler, Meg Ounsted, John Owen, Emile Papiernik, W. Parewijck, Laura Pello, Nilo Pereira Luz, C. J. Pickles, Anthony Reading, George Rhoads, A.M. Richards, Jeffrey Robinson, Roberto Romero, Irl Rosner, Alan Rothberg, Håkan Rydhstrøm, Saroj Saigal, Nigel Saunders, Harold Schulman, Neils Jørgen Secher, Elisabeth Serle, K. Sankaran, Jerry Shime, Kirk Shy, Jennifer Sleep, Karen Smedstad, Norman Smith, Philip Smith, Jean Sorrells-Jones, Bonny Specker, William Spellacy, Fiona Stanley, Philip Steer, Anita Stevens, Ann Tabor, William Tarnow-Mordi, G. Tchernia, Michel Thiery, A.C. Thomsen, Jim Thornton, Greg Tricklebank, Reginald Tsang, Michael Turner, Sheila Tyrrell, Ulf Ulmsten, Henry Van Kets, José Villár, Nick Wald, Ulla Waldenstrom, Roland Waner, P.J.M. Watney, Selman Welt, Michael Whitfield, Klas Wichman, Beth Wilson, Berndt Wittmann, Richard Windsor, Olavi Ylikorkala, Christos Zoupas.

Contents

VOLUME 2: CHILDBIRTH

VI Care during labour

VII Initiating labour

VIII Care during delivery

IX Care of the mother and newborn infant

X Promoting effective care during pregnancy and childbirth

Contributors

Sophie Alexander MD. Obstetrician, École de Santé Publique, Université Libre de Bruxelles, Campus Erasme CP 590/5, 808 route de Lennik, 1070 Brussels, Belgium.

Douglas Altman BSc. Head, Medical Statistics Laboratory, Imperial Cancer Research Fund, P O Box 123, Lincoln's Inn Fields, London WC2A 3PX, UK.

Jill Astbury BA, MEd, PhD. Lecturer, Key Centre for Women's Health in Society, Department of Community Medicine, University of Melbourne, Parkville 3052, Australia.

Cornelia J. Baines MD, MSc. Associate Professor, Dept Preventive Medicine & Biostatistics, University of Toronto, Toronto, Ontario, Canada M5S 1A8.

Leiv S. Bakketeig MD. Head, Department of Epidemiology, National Institute of Public Health, Geitmyrsveien, N-0462 Oslo 4, Norway.

David Banta MD, MPH, MS. Professor of Technology Assessment, Department of Health Economics, University of Limburg, P O Box 616, 6200 MD Maastricht, The Netherlands.

Jack Bennebroek Gravenhorst MD. Professor of Obstetrics and Gynaecology, Leiden University, University Hospital, Rijnsburgerweg 10, 2333 AA Leiden, The Netherlands.

Howard M. Berger MD, MRCP, BSc. Senior Lecturer, Department of Neonatology, University of Leiden, University Hospital, Rijnsburgerweg 10, 2333 AA Leiden, The Netherlands.

Per Bergsjø MD, PhD. Professor and Head of Department of Obstetrics and Gynaecology, University of Bergen, Kvinneklinikken, Haukeland Sykehus, N-5021, Bergen, Norway.

Eve Blair PhD. Research Officer, NH and MRC Research Unit in Epidemiology and Preventive Medicine, University Department of Medicine, The Queen Elizabeth II Medical Centre, University of Western Australia, Nedlands, Perth, Western Australia 6009, Australia.

Béatrice Blondel BA, MA, PhD. Chargée de Recherches, Groupe de Recherches Épidémiologiques sur la Mère et l'Enfant, INSERM Unité 149, 16 Avenue Paul-Vaillant-Couturier, 94807 Villejuif, France.

Martin Bobrow DSc, MB BCh, FRCP, MRCPath. Prince Philip Professor of Paediatric Research, University of London, Paediatric Research Unit, Division of Medical and Molecular Biology, United Medical and Dental Schools of Guy's and St Thomas' Hospitals, 8th Floor, Guy's Tower, Guy's Hospital, London Bridge, London SE1 9RT, UK.

Michael Bracken PhD, MPH, MPhil, BSc, FACE. Professor of Epidemiology, and Obstetrics and Gynaecology, Department of Epidemiology and Public Health, Yale University Medical School, 60 College Street, New Haven, Connecticut 06510, USA.

Ian Brown MB BS, FRCOG. Honorary Lecturer, Department of Obstetrics and Gynaecology, University of Zimbabwe, Harare Maternity Hospital, P O Box ST14, Southerton, Harare, Zimbabwe.

Robert Bryce MB BS, MSc, MRCOG, FRACOG. Senior Research Officer, NH and MRC Unit in Epidemiology and Preventive Medicine, University Department of Medicine, The Queen Elizabeth II Medical Centre, University of Western Australia, Nedlands, Perth, Western Australia 6009, Australia.

Pierre Buekens MD. Obstetrician, Université Libre de Bruxelles, École de Santé Publique, Campus Erasme CP 590/5, 808 route de Lennik, 1070 Bruxelles, Belgium.

Hubert Campbell MA, MB BS, FRCP, FFCM, FSS. Emeritus Professor of Medical Statistics, University of Wales College of Medicine, Pwll Coch Uchaf, Druidstone Road, Cardiff CF3 9XE, UK.

Iain Chalmers MB BS, MSc, DCH, FFCM, FRCOG. Director, National Perinatal Epidemiology Unit, Radcliffe Infirmary, Oxford OX2 6HE, UK.

Thomas Chalmers MD. Distinguished Physician, Veterans Administration; Lecturer, Harvard School of Public Health; President and Dean Emeritus, Mt Sinai Medical Center, New York. Technology Assessment Group, Harvard University School of Public Health, 677 Huntington Avenue, Boston, Massachusetts 02115, USA.

Rory Collins MB BS, MSc. British Heart Foundation Senior Research Fellow, University of Oxford, Clinical Trials Service Unit, Radcliffe Infirmary, Oxford OX2 6HE, UK.

Patricia Crowley MB BCh, DCH, MRCOG, MRCPI. Senior Lecturer, Department of Obstetrics and Gynaecology, University College Dublin, Coombe Lying-in Hospital, Dolphins Barn, Dublin 8, Republic of Ireland.

Caroline Crowther MD ChB, DCH, MRCOG, FRACOG. Senior Lecturer in Obstetrics and Gynaecology, University of Adelaide, Department of Obstetrics, Queen Victoria Hospital, Rose Park, South Australia 5067, Australia.

Michael Daker PhD. Senior Lecturer in Cytogenetics, University of London, Paediatric Research Unit, Division of Medical and Molecular Biology, United Medical and Dental Schools of Guy's and St Thomas' Hospitals, 8th Floor, Guy's Tower, Guy's Hospital, London Bridge, London SE1 9RT, UK.

Kay Dickersin MA PhD. Assistant Professor, Department of Ophthalmology, University of Maryland School of Medicine, 22 South Greene St, Baltimore, Maryland 21201, USA.

Michael Drummond BSc, MCom, DPhil. Director, Health Services Management Centre, University of Birmingham, Park House, 40 Edgbaston Park Road, Birmingham B15 2RT, UK.

Diana Elbourne BSc, MSc, PhD. Social Statistician, National Perinatal Epidemiology Unit, Radcliffe Infirmary, Oxford OX2 6HE, UK.

Eleanor Enkin BHSc. Honorary Research Assistant, National Perinatal Epidemiology Unit, 47 Bowman Street, Hamilton, Ontario, Canada L8S 2T5.

Murray Enkin MD, FRCS(C), FACOG. Professor Emeritus, Departments of Obstetrics and Gynaecology, and Clinical Epidemiology and Biostatistics, McMaster University, 1200 Main Street West, Hamilton, Ontario, Canada L8N 3Z5.

Gillian C. Forrest MB BS, MRCPsych, MRCGP. Consultant Child Psychiatrist, The Park Hospital for Children, Old Road, Headington, Oxford OX3 7LQ, UK.

Robert Fraser MD, MRCOG, DCH. Senior Lecturer/Honorary Consultant, Department of Obstetrics and Gynaecology, University of Sheffield, Clinical Sciences Centre, Northern General Hospital, Herries Road, Sheffield S5 7AU, UK.

Jo Garcia BA, MSc. Social Scientist, National Perinatal Epidemiology Unit, Radcliffe Infirmary, Oxford OX2 6HE, UK.

Sally Garforth BNurs, SCM. Formerly Research Midwife, National Perinatal Epidemiology Unit, 15 Clifton Park Road, Caversham, Reading RG4 7PD, UK.

Peter A. Goldstein BA. Medical Student, Mt Sinai School of Medicine of the City University of New York (CUNY), Clinical Trials Unit, Mt Sinai Medical Center, One Gustave Levy Place, New York, NY 10029, USA.

Adrian Grant DM, MSc, MRCOG. Epidemiologist, National Perinatal Epidemiology Unit, Radcliffe Infirmary, Oxford OX2 6HE, UK.

John Grant MB ChB, MRCP, MRCOG. Consultant Obstetrician and Gynaecologist, Bellshill Maternity Hospital, North Road, Bellshill NL4 3JN, UK.

Jane Green BA, BM BCh, DPhil. Honorary Research Associate, National Perinatal Epidemiology Unit, Radcliffe Infirmary, Oxford OX2 6HE, UK.

Elina Hemminki MD. Assistant Professor, Department of Public Health, University of Helsinki, Haartmaninkatu 3, 00290 Helsinki, Finland.

Jini Hetherington. Unit Administrator, National Perinatal Epidemiology Unit, Radcliffe Infirmary, Oxford OX2 6HE, UK.

G. Justus Hofmeyr MB BCh, MRCOG. Professor and Head, Department of Obstetrics and Gynaecology, Coronation Hospital and University of the Witwatersrand Medical School, York Road, Parktown 2193, South Africa.

David J. S. Hunter MB ChB, FRCOG, FRCS(C). Professor, Department of Obstetetrics and Gynaecology, McMaster University, 1200 Main Street West, Hamilton, Ontario, Canada L8N 3Z5.

Frank Hytten MD, PhD, FRCOG. Editor Emeritus, British Journal of Obstetrics and Gynaecology, 27 Sussex Place, Regent's Park, London NW1 4RG, UK.

Sally Inch SRN, SCM. Midwife, Oxfordshire Health Authority, 3 Willow Close, Garsington, Oxford OX9 9AN, UK.

Claire Johnson. Medical Student, University of Oxford, Green College, 43 Woodstock Road, Oxford OX2 6HG, UK.

Humphrey H. H. Kanhai MD. Senior Lecturer, Leiden University, Department of Obstetrics, University Hospital, Rijnsburgerweg 10, 2333 AA Leiden, The Netherlands.

Marc J. N. C. Keirse MD, DPhil, DPH. Professor of Obstetrics, Leiden University, and Visiting Professor, University of Leuven, Belgium; Leiden University Hospital, Rijnsburgerweg 10, 2333 AA Leiden, The Netherlands.

James King MB BS, FRCS, FRCOG, FRACOG. Medical Superintendent, Mater Mothers' Hospital, South Brisbane, Queensland 4101, Australia.

Sheila Kitzinger MLitt. Standlake Manor, Standlake, nr Witney, Oxon OX8 7RH, UK.

Michael Klein MD, CCFP, FCFP, ABFP, FCPS, FAAP. Professor Family Medicine, Chief and Director, The Herzl Family Practice Centre, McGill University School of Medicine, 5750 Côte de Neiges, Montreal PQ, Canada H3S 1Y7.

Alessandro Liberati MD. Chief, Clinical Epidemiology Unit, Mario Negri Institute, Istituto Mario Negri, Via Eritrea 62, 20157 Milano, Italy.

Jonathan Lomas MA. Associate Professor; Associate Coordinator, Centre for Health Economics and Policy Analysis, Department of Clinical Epidemiology and Biostatistics, McMaster University, 1200 Main Street West, Hamilton, Ontario, Canada L8N 3Z5.

Judith Lumley MA, MB BS, PhD. Senior Lecturer, Monash University, Department of Paediatrics, Queen Victoria Children's Hospital, Monash Medical Centre, 246 Clayton Road, Clayton, Victoria 3168, Australia.

Sally MacIntyre BA, MSc, PhD. Director, Medical Research Council Medical Sociology Unit, University of Glasgow, 6 Lilybank Gardens, Glasgow G12 8QQ, UK.

Kassam Mahomed MB ChB, MRCOG. Lecturer, Department of Obstetrics and Gynaecology, University of Zimbabwe, Harare Maternity Hospital, P O Box ST14, Southerton, Harare, Zimbabwe.

Patrick Mohide MD, FRCS(C), MSc. Associate Professor, Department of Obstetrics and Gynaecology, McMaster University, 1200 Main Street West, Hamilton, Ontario, Canada L8N 3Z5.

Miranda Mugford BA. Economist, National Perinatal Epidemiology Unit, Radcliffe Infirmary, Oxford OX2 6HE, UK.

Cornelis Naaktgeboren PhD. Former leader, Research Group for Comparative Obstetrics, University of Amsterdam, Dorpsweg K157, 1676 GK Twisk, The Netherlands.

James Neilson BSc, MD, MRCOG. Senior Lecturer, Department of Obstetrics and Gynaecology, University of Edinburgh, Centre for Reproductive Biology, 37 Chalmers Street, Edinburgh EH3 9EW, UK.

Ann Oakley MA PhD. Deputy Director, Thomas Coram Research Unit, 41 Brunswick Square, London WC1N 1AZ, UK.

Arne Ohlsson MD, FRCP(C). Staff Neonatologist, Regional Perinatal Unit, University of Toronto, Women's College Hospital, 76 Grenville Street, Toronto, Ontario, Canada M5S 1B2.

A. Carla C. van Oppen. Staff Obstetrician, Department of Obstetrics, Leiden University Hospital, Rijnsburgerweg 10, 2333 AA Leiden, The Netherlands.

Fabio Parazzini MD. Researcher, Epidemiology Unit, Mario Negri Institute, Istituto Mario Negri, Via Eritrea 62, 20157 Milano, Italy.

John Parboosingh MB ChB, BSc, FRCOG, FRCP(C). Professor, Department of Obstetrics and Gynaecology, University of Calgary, Foothills Hospital, 1403 – 29th Street NW, Calgary, Alberta, Canada T2N 2T9.

James F. Pearson MD, FRCOG. Reader in Obstetrics and Gynaecology, University of Wales College of Medicine, Department of Obstetrics and Gynaecology, University Hospital of Wales, Heath Park, Cardiff CF4 4XN, UK.

Maureen Porter BSc, MSc, PhD. Honorary Research Fellow, Department of Sociology, Edward Wright Building, University of Aberdeen, Old Aberdeen AB9 2ZE, UK.

Shirley Post MHA. Formerly Executive Director, Canadian Institute of Child Health, Suite 105, 17 York Street, Ottawa, Ontario, Canada K1N 5S7.

Walter J. Prendiville MRCOG, MAO, FRACOG. Senior Lecturer, Department of Obstetrics and Gynaecology, University of Western Australia, King Edward Memorial Hospital, Subiaco, Western Australia 6008, Australia.

Gareth Rees MB BCh, FFARCS. Consultant Anaesthetist, Department of Anaesthetics, University Hospital of Wales, Heath Park, Cardiff CF4 4XN, UK.

Margaret Reid MA, PhD. Lecturer, Department of Community Medicine and Social and Economic Research, University of Glasgow, 2 Lilybank Gardens, Glasgow G12 8QQ, UK.

Joan Reisch PhD. Associate Professor of Family Practice and Community Medicine, Department of Paediatrics, University of Texas, Southwestern Medical Center, 5323 Harry Hines Blvd, Dallas, Texas 75235-9063, USA.

Mary J. Renfrew BSc, RGN, SCM, PhD. Midwife Researcher, National Perinatal Epidemiology Unit, Radcliffe Infirmary, Oxford OX2 6HE, UK.

Joyce Roberts CNM, PhD. Director, Graduate Nurse-Midwifery Program; Professor, School of Nursing; Associate Professor, School of Medicine. Department of Obstetrics and Gynaecology, School of Nursing C-288, University of Colorado Health Sciences Center, 4200 East Ninth Avenue, Denver, Colorado 80262, USA.

Jane Robinson MA, PhD, AIPM, RGN, ONC, RHV, HVT, Cert Ed. Director, Nursing Policy Studies Centre, University of Warwick, Coventry, Warwickshire CV4 7AL, UK.

Sarah Robinson BSc. Senior Research Fellow, Nursing Research Unit, Department of Nursing Studies,

King's College, University of London, Coleridge Building, 552 King's Road, London SW10 0UA, UK.

Patrizia Romito PhD. Researcher, Istituto di Puericultura, Ospedale Burlo Garofalo, Via dell' Istria 65/1, I-34100 Trieste, Italy.

Janet Rush RN, BScN, MHSc. Assistant Clinical Professor, Department of Nursing, McMaster University and Patient Care Coordinator, Chedoke McMaster Hospitals, Department of Nursing, 1200 Main Street West, Hamilton, Ontario, Canada L8N 3Z5.

David Rush MD. Head of Epidemiology Program, Human Nutrition Research Center on Aging, Tufts University, 711 Washington Street, Boston, Massachusetts 02111, USA.

Henry S. Sacks PhD, MD. Director, Clinical Trials Unit/Associate Professor, Department of Medicine and Biomathematics, Mt Sinai Medical Center, One Gustave Levy Place, New York, NY 10029, USA.

Marie-Josèphe Saurel-Cubizolles BA, MA, PhD. Chargée de Recherches, Groupe de Recherches Epidémiologiqes sur la Mère et l'Enfant (INSERM Unité 149), 16 Avenue Paul-Vaillant-Couturier, 94807 Villejuif, France.

Madeleine Shearer Editor, *Birth*, 110 El Camino Real, Berkeley, California 94705, USA.

William Silverman MD. 90 La Cuesta Drive, Greenbrae, California 94904, USA.

Penny Simkin BA, PT. Childbirth Educator, Consultant in Family Centred Maternity Care, 1100 23rd Avenue East, Seattle, Washington 98112, USA.

Jennifer Sleep BA. District Research Co-ordinator, West Berkshire Health Authority, Department of Midwifery, Royal Berkshire Hospital, Craven Road, Reading RG1 5AN, UK.

Fiona Smaill MB ChB, FRACP, FRCP(C). Assistant Professor, Infectious Disease and Microbiology, Department of Microbiology, McMaster University, 1200 Main Street West, Hamilton, Ontario, Canada L8N 3Z5.

Fiona Stanley MD, MSc, MFCM. Director, Western Australian Research Institute for Child Health, Princess Margaret Hospital, Subiaco, Perth 6008, Western Australia.

Rosalind Stanwell-Smith MB BCh, MRCOG, MFCM. Specialist in Community Medicine, Bristol and Weston Health Authority, 10 Marlborough Street, Bristol BS1 3NP, UK.

Michel Thiery MD, PhD, FRCOG. Professor and Chairman, Department of Obstetrics, University Hospital, De Pintelaan 135, B-900 Gent, Belgium.

Mary Ellen Thomson PhD, MSc, BSc. Manager of Research Projects, Research and Evaluation, Ministry of Health, 1515 Blanchard Street, Victoria, British Columbia, Canada V8W 3C8.

Gianni Tognoni MD. Chief, Laboratory of Clinical Pharmacology, Istituto Mario Negri, Via Eritrea 62, 20157 Milano, Italy.

Pieter Treffers MD. Professor of Obstetrics and Gynaecology, University of Amsterdam, Meibergdreet 9, 1105 Amsterdam Zuidoost, The Netherlands.

Jon E. Tyson MD. Associate Professor of Pediatrics and Obstetrics/Gynecology, University of Texas, Southwestern Medical Center, 5323 Harry Hines Blvd, Dallas, Texas 75235-9063, USA.

Aldo Vacca MB BS, DGO, MRCOG, FRACOG. Director of Obstetrics and Gynaecology, Mater Mothers' Hospital, South Brisbane, Queensland 4101, Australia.

Raymond G. De Vries BA, MA, PhD. Associate Professor, Department of Sociology, St Olaf College, Northfield, Minnesota 55057, USA.

Henk C. S. Wallenburg MD, PhD. Director of Obstetrics, Department of Obstetrics and Gynaecology, Erasmus University Medical School EE 2283, P O Box 1738, 3000 DR Rotterdam, The Netherlands.

Elaine Wang MD, CM, MSc, FRCP(C). Assistant Professor, Pediatrics, University of Toronto, Department of Infectious Diseases, Hospital for Sick Children, 555 University Avenue, Toronto, Canada M5G 1X8.

Robert Watson MB ChB, MRCOG. Consultant Obstetrician and Gynaecologist, Department of Obstetrics and Gynaecology, Barnsley District General Hospital, Gawber Road, Barnsley, S Yorks S75 2EP, UK.

Ruta Westreich MA. Staff Psychologist, Institute of Community and Family Psychiatry, Jewish General Hospital, 5750 Côte de Neiges, Montreal PQ, Canada H3T 1E2.

Flavia Zanaboni MD. Resident, Third Obstetric Gynecology Clinic, University of Milan, Istituto Provinciale Maternita Infanzio, Via M Melloni, 20188 Milano, Italy.

Luke Zander MB BChir, DCH, DObstRCOG, FRCGP. Senior Lecturer, Department of General Practice, United Medical and Dental Schools of Guy's and St Thomas', Lambeth Road Group Practice, 80 Kennington Road, London SE11 6SP, UK.

Part I

Evaluation of care during pregnancy and childbirth

1 Evaluating the effects of care during pregnancy and childbirth

Iain Chalmers

1 Introduction

'No species of fallibility is more important or less understood than fallibility in medical practice. The physician's propensity for damaging error is widely denied, perhaps because it is so intensely feared'

Gorowitz and MacIntyre 1976

'Is the application of the numerical method to the subject matter of medicine a trivial and time wasting ingenuity, as some hold; or is it an important stage in the development of our art, as others proclaim?'

Major Greenwood 1921, cited in Schoolman 1982

Judgements about the effects of care during pregnancy and childbirth, as in other areas, are neither value-free nor situation-free; different observers see different problems, and often reach different conclusions (Susser 1984). Whatever their frame of reference, however, those who make these judgements need to give careful consideration to the strengths and weaknesses of the various kinds of evidence on which they base their conclusions. This is necessary because the development of care during pregnancy and childbirth has witnessed not only important advances, but also some tragic disasters (Silverman 1980): those who provide care owe it to their clients to consider carefully how best to maximize the former and minimize the latter. False conclusions about the effects of care result in some women and babies being denied effective forms of care during pregnancy and childbirth, and others being offered care which is either ineffective, or actually harmful.

Many of the judgements about the value and safety of existing forms of obstetric care continue to be based on evidence that is likely to be invalid (Chalmers and Richards 1977; Cochrane 1979). Similarly, the introduction of new forms of care is not accompanied by the kind of careful evaluation that history suggests would be a responsible and ethical way to proceed (Tyson *et al.* 1983; Chalmers 1987). This is regrettable, not only because, in dealing with large numbers of basically healthy people, there is considerable potential for doing more harm than good on a very large scale; but also because the available evidence suggests that only a minority of innovations in health care turn out to be superior to existing practices (Gilbert *et al.* 1977; Barral 1986; Buyse 1987).

What kind of evidence, then, should be considered in any attempt to assess the effects of care during pregnancy and childbirth? Different people will answer this question in different ways. Because so much is at stake, however, everyone should be required to be explicit about their reasons for favouring some forms of evidence over others. As already explained in the Preface of this book, most of its contents are based on a systematic analysis of evidence which is relevant in assessing the effects of care. In this opening chapter, the rationale for the 'hierarchy of evidence' used by contributors to this book has been explained and, whenever possible, justified with empirical evidence. The essence of the rationale for the hierarchy that has been adopted is the need, when comparing alternative forms of care, to minimize the chances that one will be misled either by systematic errors of one kind or another (biases), or by random errors (the play of chance).

After using this hierarchy to review factors that should be taken into account in assessing the 'internal validity' of reported evaluations of care, the chapter ends with a discussion of the more difficult subject of the 'external validity' of formal comparisons of alternative forms of care, that is, the extent to which the results of research may be relevant in guiding everyday clinical practice. This important issue is also considered in Chapter 2, which describes the materials and methods that have been used to assemble evidence about the effects of care during pregnancy and childbirth.

2 What is the role of studies without formal controls?

2.1 Clinical impressions

> 'In my indictment of the statistician, I would argue that he may tend to be a trifle too scornful of the clinical judgement, the clinical impression. Such judgements are, I believe, in essence, statistical. The clinician is attempting to make a comparison between the situation that faces him at the moment and a mentally recorded but otherwise untabulated past experience'
>
> Austin Bradford Hill 1952

> 'There are lies, damned lies, and clinical impressions'
>
> Sam Shuster 1972

In the quotations with which this section begins, Austin Bradford Hill—the medical statistician who introduced the randomized controlled trial to medical research—is careful to remind us of the importance of taking seriously informal impressions concerning the effects of care. By contrast, Sam Shuster—a clinician—warns us that these impressions can be seriously misleading. Both Bradford Hill and Shuster are right, of course: informal evaluation of care based on impressions, and formal evaluation based on well-controlled comparisons of alternative forms of care, both play essential roles in the promotion of more effective care during pregnancy and childbirth.

Two anecdotes may help to illustrate the strengths and dangers of impressions about the effects of care. During the 1960s, an obstetrician interested in the physiology of parturition had the impression that lambs whose mothers had been given corticosteroids to initiate labour showed signs of respiratory distress less often than might have been expected (Liggins 1969). Further observations made in the context of controlled experiments in sheep confirmed that lambs born after maternally-administered corticosteroids were indeed less likely than control lambs to develop respiratory distress. Together with a paediatric colleague, the obstetrician went on to conduct further well-controlled investigations in humans, and demonstrated that antenatal administration of corticosteroids prior to preterm delivery resulted in an important reduction of neonatal morbidity (Liggins and Howie 1972). Because of the possibility that there might be long term adverse consequences of fetal exposure to corticosteroids, long term follow-up of the steroid-exposed and control babies was conducted; so far no adverse effects have been detected (MacArthur *et al.* 1982).

The second anecdote refers to another obstetrician who, in the early 1950s, encountered a number of research reports from prestigious institutions in the United States in which the clinical investigators had concluded that diethylstilboestrol (DES) was an effective drug for the 'support of placental function'. Consulted by a woman who had had two previous stillbirths, the obstetrician prescribed the drug from early pregnancy onwards. The pregnancy ended with the birth of a liveborn child, as did a subsequent pregnancy similarly managed. Reasoning that the woman's 'natural' capacity for successful childbearing may have improved over this time, the obstetrician withheld medication during the woman's fifth pregnancy: the baby died *in utero* from 'placental insufficiency'. During her sixth and final pregnancy, the obstetrician and the woman were in no doubt that prescription of diethylstilboestrol should be resumed: the pregnancy ended with the birth of another liveborn child. The impression gained of the apparent effects of diethylstilboestrol (three livebirths following treatment with diethylstilboestrol, and three intrauterine deaths when the drug had not been used) led both the obstetrician and the woman to infer that it was a useful drug (personal communication).

As these two anecdotes illustrate, impressions about the effects of care are sometimes right, and sometimes wrong. In the first, an informal impression initiated a series of well-designed investigations and a discovery which must rate as one of the most important ever made in obstetrics (see Chapter 45). In the second case the impression left on the obstetrician and the mother was never substantiated in the properly controlled studies that were being conducted and reported during the years over which the woman was receiving care (see Chapter 38). Tragically, this evidence was widely ignored, for not only was diethylstilboestrol ineffective, it was actually harmful. The drug caused a variety of abnormalities, including cancer, in many of the children of the millions of women who had taken it during pregnancy (Grant and Chalmers 1985).

The costs of not assessing the validity of informal impressions about the effects of care using more formal evaluations can be high, both because effective forms of care are not recognized as promptly as possible, and also because forms of care that are ineffective or positively harmful are not detected efficiently. Clinical practice should not be based solely on clinical impressions about the value of forms of care that are potentially harmful or costly (and this probably includes most innovations in care). As McCormick (1976) has put it, 'Impressions about the quantifiable are no substitute for measurement. "In my experience" is no substitute for a controlled trial'.

2.2 Cases and case series without formal controls

'Therapeutic reports with controls tend to have no enthusiasm, and reports with enthusiasm tend to have no controls'
David Sackett 1986

Sometimes the outcome of current forms of care can be predicted with such certainty that past experience provides a valid basis for interpreting current observations. In these circumstances it may be justified to make causal inferences and recommendations for practice on the basis of observations that a new form of care prevents the predicted outcome in individual cases, or in uncontrolled case series (Bradford Hill 1952). More widespread adoption of the lower segment operation for caesarean section on the basis of the uncontrolled case series reported by Kehrer in 1882, for example, might have prevented many maternal deaths between that time and the 'rediscovery' of the operation by Munro Kerr nearly 40 years later (see Chapter 70).

Similarly, if a particular form of care is associated with an abnormal outcome that has not been observed before, observations without formal controls may be an adequate basis for abandoning the form of care in question. The observation of babies with a bizarre embryopathy associated with administration of large doses of vitamin A during pregnancy (Lammer *et al.* 1985), for example, is an adequate basis for warning women about the probable teratogenic potential of the vitamin.

The circumstances in which case reports and uncontrolled case series provide a secure basis for evaluating the effects of care are rare, however, particularly because they appear to be very prone to selective reporting (see Section 7, below). There are several examples of this kind of publication bias where the reported enthusiasm for treatments has been shown to be inversely related to the number of patients studied (Chalmers TC *et al.* 1965; Benhamou *et al.* 1972; Chalmers TC 1984; Berlin *et al.* 1987).

There are few formal assessments of how often conclusions based on analyses of single cases and uncontrolled case series turn out to be incorrect in the light of the results of subsequent, controlled analyses. The results of one such assessment, however, suggest that the rate of false inferences may be as high as 50 per cent (Venning 1982). As long as the limitations of these reports as a basis for causal inference are acknowledged, this need not necessarily be interpreted as a problem. Given their poor validity overall, however, the main role of individual case reports and uncontrolled case series should be to stimulate the controlled investigations that will distinguish the true from the false leads.

Unfortunately, although past experience suggests that caution is appropriate in interpreting the results of uncontrolled case series, it is often not exercised. Investigators discussing the implications of their use of maternal hyperoxygenation in 5 pregnancies in which severe fetal growth retardation had been diagnosed, for example, referred to 'the benefit (*sic*) of maternal oxygen therapy' (which they reported was being investigated in a prospective double-blind trial) (Nicolaides *et al.* 1987). In the light of wording such as this, it is not surprising that television and press reports of the study referred to maternal hyperoxygenation as 'a new treatment that can prevent stillbirth' which future mothers might be able to have 'in the comfort of their own homes, using oxygen cylinders' (Steven 1987). Whether or not maternal hyperoxygenation does more good than harm remains to be seen; but the unintended consequences of manipulating the blood gas levels of immature human beings (Silverman 1980) suggest that in this field more than most, studies with proper controls are required to assess the value, if any, of the treatment.

3 In studies with formal controls, how were the comparison groups derived?

> 'Daniel purposed in his heart that he would not defile himself with the king's food, nor with the wine which he drank . . . Then said Daniel to the steward: "Let them give us pulse to eat, and water to drink. Then let our countenances be looked upon before thee, and the countenances of the youths that eat of the king's food" . . . And at the end of ten days their countenances appeared fairer, and they were fatter in flesh than all the youths that did eat the king's food.'
>
> Daniel 1:11–15, cited in Bloom 1986

It is not a new idea that judgements about the effects of care should be supported by comparisons between the experiences of people who have received a particular form of care with those of 'controls' who have received either an alternative form of care, or no care at all. The principle underlying this practice is that uncontrolled observations of events following a particular form of care usually leave questions unanswered about what might have happened if a different form of care (or no care at all) had been provided (Feinstein 1985).

Controlled comparisons of groups of people who received alternative forms of care will strengthen inferences that any differences observed reflect the relative effects of the alternative forms of care. The strength of these inferences depends on the extent to which it is justified to assume that people who received the alternative forms of care were comparable in every respect that matters. The challenge is thus to select comparison groups that are comparable 'in every respect that matters'.

3.1 Historical controls

One approach to the selection of controls involves making comparisons between people who have received a relatively recently introduced form of care with other people who were cared for in a different way during an earlier era. Use of such 'historical controls' sometimes leads to inferences about the effects of care which are later supported by the results of comparative studies in which it is more certain that 'like is being compared with like'. For example, the introduction of oxytocic drugs was followed by a reduced risk of maternal death from postpartum haemorrhage. The inference that these drugs had contributed to the reduced risk was subsequently supported by the results of well-controlled studies (Prendiville *et al.* 1988).

The results of well-controlled studies do not always support the inferences prompted by analyses using historical controls, however. For example, 5 studies using historical controls suggested that administration of diethylstilboestrol during pregnancy led to a dramatic decrease in the risks of miscarriage and stillbirth, whereas 3 well-controlled evaluations failed to detect any beneficial effects of the drug (Table 1.1).

Stringent criteria have been proposed for reducing the biases to which comparisons using historical controls appear to be prone (Pocock 1976). Such criteria are necessary but not sufficient to ensure that bias has been controlled effectively, however. In 1 of the 5 studies of diethylstilboestrol using historical controls, for example, an attempt was made to adjust statistically for differences between the characteristics of women who had, and had not received the drug. The resulting analysis still suggested a dramatic benefit of the drug (Table 1.1).

Table 1.1 Differences in livebirth rates in diethylstilboestrol (DES)-treated and control groups in studies using either historical or randomized controls (Sacks *et al.* 1982)

Type of controls (Number of studies)	Proportion (%) of livebirths in:	
	DES-treated groups	Control groups
Historical		
analysis unadjusted (n = 4)	85	56
analysis adjusted (n = 1)	45	8
Randomized (n = 3)	87	87

The most telling evidence of the inadequacy of statistical adjustment for imbalances in the characteristics of groups compared in studies using historical controls comes from comparisons made between apparently identically defined and identically treated groups of patients assembled at different points in time. These have shown that it is not unusual to observe statistically significant changes in prognosis over time (usually improvements) within what is, on the face of it, a homogeneous category of patients (Pocock 1977). These differences can be of the same order as those observed in studies using historical controls and certainly large enough to result in misleading inferences about the effects of care (Schneiderman 1966; Farewell and D'Angio 1981; Micciolo *et al.* 1985). For example, Diehl and Perry (1986) matched 43 groups of cancer patients who had served as controls in studies using historical controls, with 43 groups of similar patients who had served as controls in randomized treatment comparisons. In 16 of these matched pairs the absolute differences in survival rates ranged between 11 and 30 per cent; in 2 pairs it was greater than 30 per cent.

The most useful role for treatment comparisons using historical controls may be as 'screening tests' for promising new forms of care. It is rare for the results of published studies using historical controls to suggest that new forms of care are ineffective when studies using less biased control groups suggest that they are effective (Sacks *et al.* 1982, 1983). Inferences based solely on studies using historical controls thus tend to lead either to conclusions that new forms of care are effective when less biased comparisons suggest that they are not, or to overestimates of the size of any real advantages of the new treatment compared with the old (Sacks *et al.* 1982, 1983). Even when substantial differences in outcome following treatment compared with the past are observed, these may simply be a reflection of changes in other, undocumented factors that have modified the outcome over the period of time during which the comparison groups have received care, and not the documented factors on which attention has been focused (Christie 1979; Doll and Peto 1980).

Without unbiased comparisons between different forms of care there is, unfortunately, no way of knowing which of the studies using historical controls provide a reliable basis for causal inferences about the effects of care. Even among those who have defended the use of historical controls there is an implied assumption that the results of studies using randomized controls provide the 'Gold Standard' against which the validity of studies using historical controls should be judged (Gehan 1982, 1986). Unfortunately, this Gold Standard can only be applied in retrospect. Attempts to support the use of historical controls by citing instances where they have generated results that were subsequently confirmed by studies using randomized controls are thus of little practical relevance. New treatments that are useful must be distinguished prospectively, not retrospectively, from those that are useless or harmful.

If studies using historical controls are used as a basis for selecting from alternative forms of care, it is inevitable that some people will receive care which is ineffective or actually harmful. Furthermore, continued investigation of these false leads may result in delay in evaluating forms of care that really are useful. The available estimates suggest that somewhere between 40 and 60 per cent of studies using historical controls will lead to an incorrect inference that a new form of care is effective when it is not (Sacks *et al.* 1982, 1983). These considerations have probably been important in the relative and absolute decline in the number of studies using historical controls. For example, in the early 1970s, studies using historical controls accounted for about 1 in 5 of the studies evaluating the effects of therapy reported in the *New England Journal of Medicine*; by the end of the decade, reports of such studies had virtually disappeared (Chalmers TC and Schroeder 1979).

3.2 Case-control studies

Although case-control studies have sometimes been used to evaluate the effectiveness of medical care (see, for example, Horwitz and Feinstein 1981), their role in the evaluation of care during pregnancy and childbirth has principally been to explore the extent to which certain 'adverse outcomes' can be attributed to particular forms of care. The underlying principle is straightforward: groups of people who have, and who have not, experienced the 'outcome' concerned are assembled; then the frequencies with which each has received the form of care in question are compared. This approach is particularly valuable when the 'outcome' is either very infrequent or cannot be ascertained for some months or years after the form of care in question has been received.

The relationship between vaginal adenocarcinoma in young women and prior intrauterine exposure to diethylstilboestrol provides an example. After the mother of a patient with vaginal cancer had suggested that her daughter's malignancy might be related to the hormone she had taken during pregnancy (cited in Ulfelder 1980), and questioning of other mothers of cases had revealed that they too had taken diethylstilboestrol (Colton and Greenberg 1982), a case-control study was set up to test the resulting hypothesis more formally. Herbst and his colleagues (1971) identified a total of 8 cases. For each case they chose as controls 4 girls without vaginal cancer who had been born in the same hospital within 5 days of the case. By interviewing and examining the medical records of cases and controls, details were collected about a variety of factors (for example, maternal drinking and smoking, X-ray exposure, and bleeding in pregnancy) that might have been implicated in the aetiology of the tumours. Most factors were found to be equally common in cases and controls. Previous pregnancy loss and bleeding in early pregnancy were both more common in the cases. It was exposure to synthetic oestrogens in pregnancy, however, that differed most strikingly between the two groups. The mothers of 7 of the 8 cases, compared with none of the mothers of the 32 controls, had been prescribed diethylstilboestrol in the 1st trimester of pregnancy (Table 1.2). These findings were soon replicated in other case-control studies (Greenwald *et al.* 1971).

Case-control studies have been used to explore the relationship between a wide variety of unwanted out-

Table 1.2 Case-control comparison showing the frequency of fetal exposure to diethylstilboestrol in 8 cases of vaginal adenocarcinoma, compared with 32 controls matched for age and place of birth (Herbst *et al.* 1971)

	Fetal exposure to diethylstilboestrol		
	Exposed	Not exposed	Total
Cases of vaginal adenocarcinoma	7	1	8
Controls	0	32	32
Total	7	33	40

comes of pregnancy and antecedent forms of care during pregnancy and childbirth. The adverse outcomes studied include various congenital abnormalities, stillbirths and infant deaths, low birthweight, neonatal jaundice, neonatal convulsions, cerebral palsy, and childhood cancers. The forms of care examined include drugs, X-rays and ultrasound, amniocentesis, induction of labour, caesarean section, and the kind of instrument used for assisted vaginal delivery. Case-control studies have also been used to explore the consequences of suboptimal obstetric care, as judged by a variety of criteria derived from clinical consensus (Niswander *et al.* 1984). Thus, fetuses whose deaths have been ascribed to asphyxia or trauma, and babies born at term who have experienced very early neonatal seizures, have been shown in case-control studies to have been more likely to have received suboptimal obstetric care than controls, both during pregnancy, and in reaction to fetal distress during labour (Table 1.3).

Although case-control studies may sometimes offer the only practicable research strategy for evaluating some aspects of care during pregnancy and childbirth, they are known to be subject to biases of various kinds (Sackett 1979). These must inevitably restrict the value of the case-control approach as a basis for making causal inferences about the effects of care. To take the examples cited above, was the crucial difference between cases of vaginal adenocarcinoma and controls, in fact, not the fetal exposure to diethylstilboestrol, but the maternal history of previous pregnancy loss or bleeding in early pregnancy? Was the crucial difference between cases of very early neonatal seizures in babies born at term and controls not the quality of intrapartum care, but a greater likelihood of antecedent hydramnios and some other, unrecognized fetal abnormality (Minchom *et al.* 1987)?

Attempts to address questions like these can be made by using controls that have been matched for factors that are likely to be important confounders of the comparisons (like date and hospital of birth in the diethylstilboestrol example). Alternatively, one can try to take account of such factors by statistical adjustments

Table 1.3 Case-control comparisons showing the frequency of suboptimal care during pregnancy and in reaction to fetal distress during labour among cases of fetal death ascribed to asphyxia or trauma, very early neonatal seizures in babies born at term, and among controls; and relative risks (and approximate 95 per cent confidence intervals) for suboptimal obstetric care (Niswander *et al.* 1984)

Quality of care	Fetal deaths	Neonatal seizures	Controls
In pregnancy			
Suboptimal	8	5	17
Satisfactory	45	31	355
Relative risk (95% CI)	3.7 (1.6–8.6)	3.4 (1.2–9.2)	
For fetal distress			
Suboptimal	1	3	5
Satisfactory	4	33	361
Relative risk (95% CI)	18.0 (0.3–1500)	6.6 (1.8–23.9)	

in the analysis (like adjustments for 'clinical complexity' in the case of the relationship between neonatal seizures and suboptimal obstetric care). Because case-control studies sometimes represent the most valid available method for testing hypotheses about long-term effects of care, it is important that they should be designed as carefully as possible so that biases are reduced to a minimum (Horwitz and Feinstein 1979; Feinstein and Horwitz 1982). Because it can never be known with any certainty how successful these measures to reduce selection and other biases in case-control studies have been, however, causal inferences based upon them are often insecure.

Like the results of studies using historical controls, the results of case-control studies are sometimes supported and sometimes not supported by the results of studies which are less subject to bias. For example, the inference that diethylstilboestrol causes vaginal cancer is supported by the results of follow-up studies of women entered as fetuses into randomized controlled trials of diethylstilboestrol: although no cases of vaginal cancer have been observed in the relatively small samples studied in the trials, women who were exposed to the drug *in utero* have been found to be far more likely than controls to have vaginal adenosis and other abnormalities of the genital tract (Grant and Chalmers 1985). Similarly, the inference that suboptimal clinical response to fetal distress in labour predisposes to very early neonatal seizures in infants born at term is supported by the results of a randomized comparison of intensive and less intensive methods of fetal monitoring during labour. This study was large enough to show that the more intensive method of monitoring resulted in a reduced risk of neonatal seizures (MacDonald *et al.* 1985).

On other occasions, the inferences based on case-control studies are not supported by the results of studies that are less subject to bias. For example, a belief based on observations made both in case-control comparisons and non-randomized cohort studies (see Section 3.3, below) that folate deficiency during pregnancy was responsible for an increased risk of placental abruption (Hibbard and Jeffcoate 1966; Martin *et al.* 1967; Streiff and Little 1967) has not been supported by the results of studies of folate supplementation using randomized controls (see Chapter 19). In many instances, however, there are simply no unbiased comparisons available against which to assess the likely validity of causal inferences derived from case-control comparisons, and so it is not possible to estimate how often inferences based on such studies are likely to be misleading.

In summary, although case-control studies are subject to a variety of biases, there are circumstances in which they may represent the only available formal approach for assessing some of the potential effects of care. In these circumstances, consistent findings from a number of well-designed case-control studies may provide the most secure evidence that is ever likely to be available. For example, the belief that the antinauseant Debendox (Bendectin) is *not* a teratogen is supported by the results of several case-control studies (see Chapter 32).

3.3 Non-randomized concurrent controls

A common approach to controlled evaluation of care involves comparison of two or more 'cohorts' of individuals who happen to have received alternative forms of care concurrently. Often the comparison groups have been derived from individuals receiving care within a particular institution. More than a century ago, Ignaz Semmelweiss used such a study design to compare the effects of medical care and midwifery care within a large maternity hospital in Vienna (Semmelweiss 1861). The two wards in the hospital were on intake for admissions on different days of the week. One ward was staffed by medical students and physicians; the other by midwifery students and midwives. Between 1841 and 1846, 1,989 (9.9 per cent) of the 20,042 women admitted to the medical ward died, compared with only 691 (3.4 per cent) of the 17,791 women admitted to the midwifery ward (Semmelweiss 1861). This striking difference in the overall maternal mortality rate reflected the different rates of maternal death from puerperal infection in the two wards.

These findings were of profound importance for the development of care during childbirth. Before making causal inferences about the effects of care on the basis of the results of such studies, however, people must convince both themselves and others that like has been compared with like. Semmelweiss's inference that medical care during childbirth increased the risk of maternal death compared with midwifery care was strengthened by the fact that the groups of women that he had compared were indeed likely to be comparable at the time that they had been admitted to the hospital: their assignment to either medical or midwifery care had been determined by something very close to chance—the day of the week on which they happened to be admitted.

Often it is less certain that the groups compared are comparable. For example, it is not clear whether members of the Faith Assembly—who reject all professional care during pregnancy and childbirth—are comparable with other residents of Indiana (Kaunitz *et al.* 1984). The demographic information available on the two groups suggests that, if anything, they should be at lower obstetric risk than other residents of the state. Yet they experience substantially higher maternal and fetal mortality rates (Table 1.4). This observation seems most likely to reflect their rejection of professional care, an interpretation supported by associations observed in studies that have investigated the relationships between the outcome of pregnancy and the staff and facilities available for care (Bakketeig *et al.* 1978; Paneth *et al.* 1982; Stilwell *et al.* 1988). It should be noted, however, that such relationships have not always been found when they have been sought (Eksmyr 1985; Reznik *et al.* 1987).

Table 1.4 Perinatal and maternal mortality in a religious group avoiding obstetric care (Faith Assembly, Indiana), and in controls (other residents of Indiana), 1975–82 (Kaunitz *et al.* 1984)

	Faith Assembly members	Other Indiana residents	Rel. risk (95% CI)
Total number of births	355	681,142	
Maternal mortality rate (/100,000 live births)	872	9	92 (19–280)
Stillbirth rate (/1000 births)	32	9	3.6 (1.8–6.3)
Neonatal mortality rate (/1000 live births)	17	9	1.9 (0.7–4.2)

Not infrequently, it is quite clear that the groups compared in non-randomized cohort studies were not comparable in important respects. Table 1.5, for example, shows the lack of comparability of study groups in 5 reported comparisons of women and babies deli-

Table 1.5 Lack of comparability of study groups in 5 studies comparing cohorts of women and babies delivered by vacuum extraction with non-randomized, concurrent cohorts of women and babies delivered with forceps

Study, and descriptive characteristic	Vacuum extraction Frequency (%)	Forceps delivery Frequency (%)
Nyirjesy *et al.* (1963)		
Cervix not fully dilated	28	1
Occiput lateral or posterior	34	7
Shenker and Serr (1967)		
Head above spines	41	0
Gries *et al.* (1981)		
Mid-cavity procedures	80	44
Wider *et al.* (1967)		
No previous experience of operator with instrument	99	72
Punnonen *et al.* (1986)		
Performed by doctor in training	84	34

vered by vacuum extraction, and women and babies delivered with forceps. In each case, the prognostic variables tabulated suggest that the vacuum extraction group was at higher prior risk of difficult delivery than the forceps group. The differences in outcome observed in these studies may thus either reflect these differences in the characteristics of the comparison groups, or other, unrecognized differences; or differences in the relative merits of the two instruments. In fact, less biased comparisons of the two instruments suggest that the inferences based on the results of most of the studies represented in Table 1.5 are incorrect (see Chapter 71).

There are a number of ways in which bias can affect comparisons between non-randomized, concurrent cohorts receiving different forms of care (Sackett 1979). For example, there have been many such comparisons made between extremely preterm, low birthweight infants delivered by caesarean section, with other babies delivered vaginally. In most reports of such comparisons, infant outcome has been better in the group delivered by caesarean section. In the light of these observations, people have often concluded that operative delivery is the preferred method of care in these circumstances. In very few of these non-randomized, concurrent comparisons, however, has it been adequately acknowledged that the two groups of babies compared may not have been at comparable prior risk of death and morbidity (see Chapter 74). For example, caesarean section is less likely to be used to deliver babies whose chances of survival are judged to be minimal anyway; vaginal delivery, on the other hand, is more likely to have occurred when labour has been precipitate, in itself a risk marker for poor outcome. These and other factors of probable prognostic importance thus introduce bias into comparisons of the two methods of delivery. Very much the same kind of selection biases have confounded comparisons of fetuses that were, and were not, monitored with electronic fetal heart rate monitoring during labour (Grant 1985a), and babies delivered at home and in hospital (Campbell and Macfarlane 1986).

Occasionally, as was the case for Semmelweiss, the opportunity to exploit a more satisfactorily controlled 'natural experiment' occurs. For example, women who are referred by general practitioners for specialist obstetric care within the British National Health Service are involved in a process in which chance plays a large part. As a result, fairly comparable groups of women end up receiving obstetric care which may differ substantially because the specialists to whom they have been referred differ in their opinions about the relative merits of alternative forms of care. Table 1.6 shows contrasts in the type of care offered by two obstetric teams that worked in the same hospital and provided care for women who were known to be comparable in many important respects (Chalmers I *et al.* 1976a). Table 1.7 shows that there were no striking differences in the risks of perinatal morbidity and mortality experienced by babies under the care of the two teams: if anything, there was a tendency for the babies cared for by the more 'active' team to fare somewhat worse. As Table 1.8 shows, however, the women cared for by the two obstetric teams, although comparable (as predicted) in many respects, did differ in some respects that may have been important. The possibility that these differences were important in influencing outcome was investigated in further analyses. These analyses supported the inferences based on the unadjusted comparisons (Chalmers I *et al.*

Table 1.6 Contrasts in obstetric care provided by two obstetric teams working in the same hospital (Chalmers I *et al.* 1976a)

	'Active' team (n = 5227)		'Conservative' team (n = 4680)	
	No.	(%)	No.	(%)
Induction of labour (with amniotomy & oxytocin)	1406	(26.9)	431	(9.2)
Urinary oestrogen assay	858	(16.4)	422	(9.0)
Ultrasonography	505	(9.7)	6	(0.1)
Abdominal radiography	1018	(19.5)	471	(10.1)

Table 1.7 Perinatal morbidity and mortality among babies delivered under the care of two obstetric teams with contrasting approaches to care working in the same hospital (Chalmers I *et al.* 1976a)

	'Active' team (n = 5227)		'Conservative' team (n = 4680)	
No. (%) cases of fetal distress	930	(17.8)	847	(18.1)
No. (%) babies with Apgar score < 4	267	(5.1)	192	(4.1)
No. perinatal deaths (rate/1000 total births)	170	(32.5)	120	(25.6)

1976a,b), and they are also in line with the results of subsequently conducted randomized comparisons of active induction policies (see Chapter 47). Nevertheless, differences such as those observed, or other, undocumented differences between comparison groups in studies using non-randomized, concurrent controls, can and do result in imbalances. Differences in the distribution of important prognostic factors in comparison groups result in biased estimates of the relative effects of the forms of care compared.

Computerized databases, such as the one used to conduct the studies presented in Tables 1.6–1.8, are becoming increasingly available and they offer the possibility of conducting more sophisticated analyses of studies which compare non-randomized, concurrent cohorts receiving different forms of care (Jennett *et al.* 1977; Bates *et al.* 1977; Mullen *et al.* 1980; Knaus *et al.* 1982; Wennberg *et al.* 1987). An example of the more sophisticated type of analysis made possible by such a

Table 1.8 Known contrasts in the characteristics of women attended by two obstetric teams working in the same hospital (Chalmers I *et al.* 1976a)

	'Active' team (n = 5227)		'Conservative' team (n = 4680)	
	No.	(%)	No.	(%)
Rhesus iso-immunization	183	(3.5)	471	(1.0)
Cardiac disease	152	(2.9)	75	(1.6)
Pyelonephritis	308	(5.9)	187	(4.0)
Diabetes/pre-diabetes	53	(1.0)	19	(0.4)
Non-albuminuric hypertension	1260	(24.1)	651	(13.9)

database is provided by a study assessing the relative merits of different modes of delivery for babies presenting by the breech. Rosen and Chik (1984) used detailed descriptive information (about the mothers and babies who had received care) to adjust statistically for differences in factors of probable prognostic importance between the two groups compared (caesarean and vaginal delivery, respectively). Crude comparisons suggested an advantage of caesarean section over vaginal delivery for breech presentation; but this 'advantage' melted away after information describing the characteristics of women and babies was used to adjust statistically for the imbalances in prognostic factors that existed between the two comparison groups.

An eloquent illustration of the way in which unrecognized bias may lead to incorrect causal inferences is provided by an analysis based on data from a well-designed randomized comparison of the effects of a cholesterol-lowering drug (clofibrate) and placebo on the risk of death within five years following myocardial infarction (Coronary Drug Project Research Group 1980). The analysis showed that the mortality rate was significantly greater among patients who had not complied fully in taking their tablets regularly, than it was among those who had complied fully, *regardless of whether they had been prescribed active or placebo tablets* (Table 1.9). The investigators attempted, but failed, to explain this dramatic difference in mortality between compliers and non-compliers by statistical adjustments using data describing each patient in terms of 40 risk markers (age, electrocardiographic patterns, transaminase levels, and so on) that are known to be associated with an increased risk of early death following myocardial infarction (Table 1.9). The explanation for the difference in mortality between compliers and non-compliers must thus be ascribed to other, as yet unrecognized factors that are associated both with an individual's propensity to comply with medical instructions (even if these only involve instructions to take an inactive tablet), and with an increased risk of premature death after myocardial infarction.

The use of databases to evaluate the effects of care during pregnancy and childbirth seems bound to increase, both as the databases themselves multiply, and as their contents become ever more detailed. As later chapters in this book make clear, the accuracy of perinatal risk assessment leaves much to be desired (see, in particular, Chapter 22). Important biases in comparing alternative forms of care may well persist therefore, even after making statistical adjustments using the kind of descriptive information that is likely to be available. Bias from unrecorded and often unrecognized risk factors will thus continue to undermine confidence in causal inferences based on comparisons of different forms of care using non-randomized, concurrent controls (Grant 1985b).

Table 1.9 Numbers of patients, unadjusted mortality rates (%), and mortality rates (%) adjusted for 40 baseline risk markers, 5 years after myocardial infarction among patients assigned to take clofibrate or placebo, by compliance in taking medication (Coronary Drug Project Research Group 1980)

Compliance	Clofibrate (n = 1065)			Placebo (n = 2695)		
	No. patients	Unadjusted death rate (%)	Adjusted death rate (%)	No. patients	Unadjusted death rate (%)	Adjusted death rate (%)
Good compliance	708	15.0	15.7	1813	15.1	16.4
Poor compliance	357	24.6	22.5	882	28.2	25.8
Difference in mortality rates between good and poor compliers		$p<0.0001$			$p = 4.7 \times 10^{-16}$	

Carefully conducted studies involving comparisons of very large, non-randomized cohorts receiving alternative forms of care for the same condition may be helpful for identifying forms of care which are *unlikely* to differ substantially in their effects. The potential of such analyses will improve if risk markers can be identified which make it possible to estimate prognosis in individual patients with a degree of accuracy that approaches certainty (Knaus *et al.* 1985; Murray 1986). As investigators using such databases have warned, however, comparisons which suggest differential effects of alternative forms of care can not be assumed to be unbiased (Mullen *et al.* 1980; Lee *et al.* 1980). Indeed, depending on the choice of variables used to make the statistical adjustments for imbalances, the likelihood of bias may increase rather than decrease after adjustment (Detre *et al.* 1981).

3.4 Randomized controls

3.4.1 Rationale

The recognition that casting lots (randomization) is a fair and valid way of generating truly comparable comparison groups to evaluate the effects of alternative forms of care is not new. In 1662, a physician questioning the orthodox medical practice of bloodletting proposed that the effectiveness of this treatment should be evaluated as follows: 'Let us take out of the hospitals 200 or 500 people that have fevers . . . Let us cast lots, that one half of them may fall to my share, and the other to yours. I will cure them without bloodletting; but you do as ye know . . . We shall see how many funerals both of us shall have.' (Van Helmont 1662, cited in Bloom 1986). The more general use of randomization as a method adopted by human societies to guide choices in circumstances in which there is uncertainty is at least as old as recorded history (Silverman 1985). Very recently, for example, it was used in California and Pennsylvania in the military draft lottery. (Incidentally, an analysis of the 'natural experiment' that this democratic approach to risk-sharing produced showed that drafted men were statistically significantly more likely than undrafted controls to die from suicide and motor vehicle accidents, and other causes of death not directly related to military action [Hearst *et al.* 1986].)

The preceding discussion of studies that use non-randomized controls to evaluate alternative forms of care has made repeated reference to the susceptibility of such studies to biases of various kinds (Sackett 1979). The most important of these are the selection biases which result in people at different prior risk of the outcome of interest differentially receiving one or other of the alternative forms of care being compared. The judgement that selection bias can lead to incorrect causal inferences about the effects of care has been supported above by showing that the results of studies using non-randomized controls are frequently in conflict with those derived from randomized studies which control for selection bias. Because such bias may result from unrecognized as well as recognized characteristics of the individuals compared, it is important to realize that randomization (allowing the play of chance to decide which of the alternative forms of care a particular woman or baby should receive) is the *only* known way to control for *unknown* selection biases. As Peto (1987) has put it, 'unless you randomize, you cannot *know* that you have avoided bias and no-one else will know that you have avoided it'.

It is also important to be clear that although randomization achieves the crucial objective of abolishing selection bias in generating two or more comparison groups of individuals, it does not guarantee, nor does it need to guarantee, that the resulting groups will be exactly matched in respect of all baseline characteristics (Altman 1985). What randomization does guarantee is that comparison of the randomized groups will be unbiased, despite any imbalances. This is because the statistical test procedures used in making these comparisons take into account the risk that such chance imbalances may have affected the study results (Whiting-O'Keefe 1982; Meier 1983).

The logic underlying the use of randomization, both to distribute known and unknown risks and benefits fairly, and to create comparable groups of patients for the comparison of alternative forms of care, has great force once it has been clearly perceived. As Hooke (1983) has put it, 'there is a logic in the planning of experiments and in the analysis of their results that all intelligent people can grasp'.

All of the main features of good study design and the strengths and limitations of treatment evaluation using randomized controls were clearly described by Bradford Hill more than a generation ago (Bradford Hill 1952). Since then, the principles have been reiterated on many occasions (see, for example, Mainland 1960; Frederickson 1968; Cochrane 1972; Chalmers TC 1975a; Peto *et al.* 1976, 1977; Byar *et al.* 1976; Cochrane 1979; Silverman 1985), and the actual methods have been elaborated in great detail (see, for example, Pocock 1983; Meinert 1986; Gardner and Altman 1989). Indeed, the randomized controlled trial has become widely accepted as the methodological Gold Standard for comparing alternative forms of care. This has been reflected in a growth in the numbers of published reports of randomized controlled trials, a growth to which those evaluating care during pregnancy, childbirth, and early infancy have contributed (Chalmers I and Sinclair 1984; Chalmers I *et al.* 1986; Chalmers I 1988; Fig. 1.1, and Table 1.10). To use the terminology of the philosopher of science Thomas Kuhn, the randomized trial has emerged as a new 'paradigm' (Hill 1983).

It is important to be clear that the strength of studies using randomized controls is not that the successful identification of beneficial or harmful forms of care is impossible without them. As the examples cited earlier have made clear, it is possible to identify many of the most dramatic advances in care (handwashing for the prevention of puerperal sepsis, for example), as well as some of the most dramatic hazards (phocomelia resulting from thalidomide, for example), using study designs with non-randomized controls. Such dramatic effects of care are relatively rare, however. Furthermore, an increasing proportion of comparisons seems likely to involve assessments of the relative merits of two 'active' forms of care, comparisons in which dramatic differences are usually implausible. Reliable detection of the moderate differential effects of alternative forms of care which are both plausible and important thus requires avoidance of the moderate biases that are inevitable in studies using non-randomized controls (Peto 1987).

3.4.2 Unit of randomization

Randomization—the casting of lots—to decide which of two or more alternative forms of care should be offered usually involves randomized assignment of the individual participants because this is the most certain way of abolishing selection bias. Nevertheless, other units of randomization are sometimes used (Armitage 1982). Randomizing the sequential order of different treatments given to each individual is one example of a unit of randomization other than the individuals themselves (Hills and Armitage 1979; Vere 1979; Guyatt *et al.* 1986). This 'crossover' design has its origins in the physiological research of Claude Bernard and involves deciding, at random, whether to give or withhold an experimental treatment during each one of a sequence of consecutive time periods. The interpretation of such

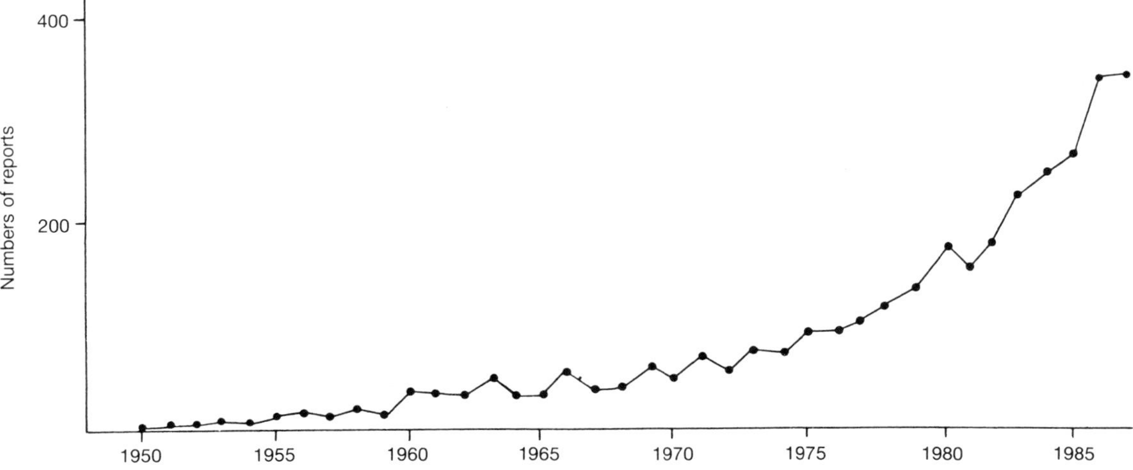

Fig. 1.1 Annual numbers of published reports of perinatal trials which have compared alternative care strategies after random or quasi-random allocation of participants, 1950–87 (Source: *Oxford Database of Perinatal Trials*)

Table 1.10 Randomized controlled trials in perinatal medicine as a proportion of all publications in selected obstetric, paediatric, and anaesthetic journals, 1966–88

		1966–70	1971–75	1976–80	1981–85	1986–88
Obstetric journals (*Acta Obstet Gynecol Scand, Am J Obstet Gynecol, Austral NZ J Obstet Gynaecol, Br J Obstet Gynaecol, Obstet Gynecol*)	Total no. publications*	5567	5778	6201	7351	4727
	No. perinatal trials†	95	95	187	210	143
	Trial publication rate (%)	(1.7)	(1.6)	(3.0)	(2.9)	(3.0)
Paediatric journals (*Acta Paediatr Scand, Am J Dis Child, Arch Dis Childhood, J Pediatr, Pediatrics*)	Total no. publications*	5627	8031	8713	9255	5502
	No. perinatal trials†	51	83	136	233	137
	Trial publication rate (%)	(0.9)	(1.0)	(1.6)	(2.5)	(2.5)
Anaesthetic journals (*Acta Anaesth Scand Anaesthesia, Anesth Analg, Anesthesiology, Br J Anaesth*)	Total no. publications*	2990	4283	4736	6469	4747
	No. perinatal trials†	15	32	38	113	137
	Trial publication rate (%)	(0.5)	(0.8)	(0.8)	(1.8)	(2.9)

*Indexed by National Library of Medicine.
†Indexed by Oxford Database of Perinatal Trials.

'crossover' trials is not straightforward because the assumptions of independence between the treatment and control periods may not be justified (Hills and Armitage 1979; Vere 1979). But quite apart from this concern, any potential offered by crossover trials lies in assessing the effects of treatment in chronic, stable conditions. These circumstances rarely apply during pregnancy and childbirth. One example of such a trial assessed the value of offering dilute hydrochloric acid to women whose symptoms of heartburn had not responded to sodium bicarbonate, and vice versa (Atlay *et al.* 1978). The trial showed that heartburn that does not respond to alkalis usually responds to acid, and vice versa (see Chapter 32).

Any move away from the randomization of individuals risks the possibility that 'like will not be compared with like'. There are some circumstances, however, in which the undoubted strength of randomizing individuals may be outweighed by the difficulties it causes in other respects. For instance, in a controlled trial to assess the value of formal fetal movement counting (see Chapter 28), the investigators felt that the inevitable contacts (in antenatal clinics and elsewhere) between women assigned to the counting group and controls would gradually result in a blurring of the two policies ('contamination'), with the result that any real effects of the counting policy might be obscured. Obstetricians (or hospitals) were therefore matched in pairs on the basis of similarities between the women coming to them for care, and similarities in their clinical practice. These 'clusters' (consisting of an obstetrician or hospital, together with all the women who subsequently received care under their supervision) were then randomly assigned either to a policy of formal fetal movement counting, or to a control group that did not institute the policy.

Because the effects of surgical and other procedures may be intimately linked to the level of the operator's skill, experience with, and enthusiasm for a particular procedure (Fielding *et al.* 1978; Whiting-O'Keefe *et al.* 1984), operators, rather than patients, have sometimes been proposed as the units of randomization (Van der Linden 1980; Rudicel and Esdaile 1985). This proposal arose because of the conflicting results obtained in two trials in which patients with acute cholecystitis were randomly assigned to either early or delayed cholecystectomy. One trial suggested that early surgery was preferable to delayed surgery, the other suggested the reverse. In both trials, however, the better treatment was the one that had been the standard procedure used in the centre concerned prior to the randomized comparison (Van der Linden and Sunzel 1970; Lahtinen *et al.* 1978).

The extent to which it is justified to generalize the rationale for randomizing the operator from this specific example is unknown. There are a number of examples of studies in which evidence of an operator effect has been sought, but not found (see, for example, Sleep *et al.* 1984; EC–IC Bypass Study Group 1985; Tabor *et al.* 1986). Indeed, the advantages of a new technique may actually outweigh the theoretical advantages of greater experience with an older technique: randomized comparisons of vacuum extraction with forceps delivery, for example, have consistently shown less maternal trauma associated with vacuum extraction, in spite of the fact that the operators who took part in these trials were more familiar with forceps delivery than with vacuum extraction (see Chapter 71).

The most appropriate unit of randomization in trials of surgical and other procedures requiring technical expertise thus remains a matter of dispute (*Lancet* 1980, 1986). Inferences about the relative merits of alternative operations based on comparisons of people randomized to different surgeons because the latter happen to have developed skills in one or other of the particular procedures have to be tempered by a recognition that the surgeons, and those working with them, may well differ in other important respects. In other words, it is not simply the alternative operations that are being compared. Similarly, when group (cluster) randomization is used, it cannot be assumed that the individuals forming the groups are comparable in the way that such an assumption would be justified if they had been randomized as individuals.

In summary, randomization of units other than individuals may leave selection bias less well-controlled. Furthermore, for a given number of individuals involved in a comparison of randomized clusters, a trial will have somewhat less statistical 'power' (see Sections 5.1 and 5.2, below) to rule out chance differences. For these reasons, comparisons based on randomization of individuals are preferable in principle, even if practical considerations may sometimes lead to the adoption of other units of randomization.

4 Was systematic error (bias) minimized in comparisons between alternative forms of care?

It is probably because the randomized trial, if well-designed and well-executed, represents such a powerful method for making unbiased comparisons between different treatments that the quality of trial reports has been a subject of interest and concern for nearly three decades (Mahon and Daniel 1964; Reiffenstein *et al.* 1968; Mosteller *et al.* 1980; Hemminki 1982a; DerSimonian *et al.* 1982; Lavori *et al.* 1983; Zelen 1983; Emerson *et al.* 1984; Williamson *et al.* 1986; Reitman *et al.* 1987). Because the quality of studies purporting to be randomized trials is very variable, schemes have been developed for assessing their methodological quality formally (see, for example, Chalmers TC *et al.* 1981; Tyson *et al.* 1983). In this section, some of the most important features of a well-designed and well-conducted randomized trial are considered.

4.1 Was bias avoided during the assignment of participants to alternative forms of care?

Studies that purport to have assigned individuals to alternative forms of care at random may have become subject to selection biases if precautions have not been taken to secure true randomization. Such precautions might involve, for example, arranging for allocation to be assigned from a central co-ordinating office and only after an eligible participant has been registered in the trial. Failure to make secure arrangements for randomization increases the likelihood that potential participants in a 'randomized' comparison will be entered selectively, depending on prior knowledge of the group to which they have been allocated, or, alternatively, selectively 'withdrawn' before entry has been registered formally. Table 1.11 displays data that show how failure to secure the randomization procedure against tampering of this kind is associated with important imbalances between the comparison groups in terms of known prognostic variables. These tendencies will be reflected both in the reported differences in the outcomes of care, and in the inferences drawn from the results. Although conscious or unconscious breaching of random assignment may not introduce as much bias as is common in studies which have made no attempt to use randomized controls (Table 1.11), bias in treatment assignment can sometimes be a more important deter-

Table 1.11 Imbalance of prognostic variables, proportion of prognostic variables favouring experimental group, frequency of statistically significant differences ($p < 0.05$), and authors' conclusions about the effects of the experimental treatment, by method of treatment assignment (Chalmers TC *et al.* 1983)

	'Randomization'		Non-random assignment
	Cheating difficult ($n = 57$) %	Cheating easy ($n = 45$) %	($n = 43$) %
Proportion of studies with 1+ variable imbalanced ($p < 0.05$)	14.0	26.7	58.1
Proportion of prognostic variables favouring experimental group	56.1	77.6	81.4
Proportion of studies with $p < 0.05$ difference	8.8	24.4	58.1
Proportion of studies in which authors strongly favoured experimental treatment	29.8	31.1	55.8

minant of outcome than the effects of the forms of care being compared (Chalmers TC *et al.* 1983).

This form of selection bias is certainly an issue in 'randomized controlled trials' of alternative forms of care during pregnancy and childbirth: in one recently published 'randomized' study in which different methods of inducing labour were compared, there was a less than one in a billion likelihood that the reported differences in the prior characteristics of the groups compared were simply a reflection of chance, as they should have been if proper randomization had been performed (Keirse 1988)!

4.2 Was bias minimized in the way in which alternative forms of care were delivered and received?

The mere expectation among those administering or receiving care that it will have particular effects may result in the implicit prophecy being fulfilled (*Lancet* 1972). When the effects are pleasant or beneficial in some other way, this phenomenon is referred to as the 'placebo effect' (literally, 'I will please'); when the effects are unpleasant or unwanted, the phenomenon is referred to as 'symptom anticipation' or 'symptom suggestion' (Melmed *et al.* 1986). Such effects, which are associated with a wide range of interventions, cannot be explained on a pharmacological or physical basis.

Hammar and his colleagues have demonstrated the placebo effect nicely in two randomized trials involving pregnant women with leg cramps (Table 1.12). In the first of their two trials (Hammar *et al.* 1981), an oral calcium preparation containing calcium gluconate, calcium lactate, and calcium carbonate was significantly more effective than no treatment in relieving leg cramps; in the second randomized trial (Hammar *et al.* 1987), by contrast, no difference could be detected between the effects of the same calcium preparation and a placebo. This suggests either that the apparently beneficial effect of calcium in the first trial was a placebo effect of taking a tablet rather than not taking a tablet; or that the substance used for the placebo control in the second trial (ascorbic acid) was as effective as calcium in relieving leg cramps during pregnancy; or that the two forms of tablet, while having no pharmacological effect, had equivalent placebo effects. (No advantage of calcium compared with a placebo of unspecified composition was detected in the only other trial of calcium for leg cramps in pregnancy [Odendaal 1974; see Chapter 32].)

In a classic paper reviewing the effectiveness of placebo treatment, Beecher (1955) estimated that about 30 per cent of patients with a variety of symptoms ranging from coughs and colds to severe post-operative wound pain would obtain relief from inert tablets or injections. He also drew attention to the very important fact that the total 'drug' effect of a pharmacologically-active preparation comprises its 'active' effect *plus* its placebo effect. Indeed, a drug's placebo effect may, in some circumstances, be so powerful that its pharmacological effects are overridden. Wolf (1959), for example, reported the case of a woman with hyperemesis gravidarum who was able to obtain relief from the emetic drug ipecacuanha!

The strength of the psychological effect can be influenced by the appearance of the inert substance or drug. Capsules, in general, are more effective than tablets; an injection works better than either, and an injection that stings is more effective than a painless one (Evans 1974). The colour of the tablet or capsule can also be important (Shapira *et al.* 1970; Blackwell *et al.* 1972; Blum 1986): in one experiment, for example, the same inert substance tended to be sedative if given in blue capsules and stimulant if given in pink capsules (Blackwell *et al.* 1972). Furthermore, a single, inert substance, uniformly prepared and presented, can mediate effects psychologically in opposite directions if those prescribing it have different beliefs about its effectiveness (Wolf 1950, 1959; Uhlenhuth *et al.* 1959; Gracely *et al.* 1985).

As shown in Table 1.13, however, pharmacologically-inert tablets are not by any means always effective in relieving symptoms (Thomas 1978). Furthermore, they may have adverse effects ranging from dry mouth, nausea, and headache, to weakness, palpitation, and anaphylactoid shock (Beecher 1955; Wolf 1959; Loftus and Fries 1979). This 'dark side of the placebo effect' (Loftus and Fries 1979) was illustrated in a placebo-controlled trial of drugs for angina: patients who had

Table 1.12 Effects of calcium tablets in relieving leg cramps during pregnancy in two randomized trials, one in which no placebo was used, the other placebo-controlled

	Proportion of women obtaining relief					
	Calcium Nos.	(%)	No treatment Nos.	(%)	Placebo Nos.	(%)
Hammar *et al.* (1981)	19/21	(90.5)	2/21	(9.5)	—	(—)
Hammar *et al.* (1987)	19/30	(63.3)	—	(—)	22/30	(73.3)

Table 1.13 Frequency (%) of symptomatic improvement following either 'diagnosis' with prescription of a pharmacologically inert preparation, or 'reassurance' with no prescription, in two randomized control trials involving patients presenting in general practice with symptoms, but no abnormal physical signs and in whom no definite diagnosis could be made

	Prescription of inert preparation	No prescription of inert preparation
	Proportion improved	Proportion improved
Thomas (1978)	55/100	61/100
Thomas (1987)	53/100	50/100

been told there was a possibility of gastrointestinal side-effects were between two and three times more likely to experience these problems than patients who had not been given this information during the informed consent procedure (Table 1.14; Cairns *et al.* 1985).

Psychological effects of care are not only mediated by inert tablets, capsules, and other 'medicines'. The decision to use or not to use diagnostic tests can have psychologically-mediated consequences. Among patients with non-specific chest pain, for example, it was found that a group who had routine electrocardiograms and estimates of serum creatine phosphokinase experienced significantly greater short term improvement in symptoms than randomized controls who had no diagnostic testing (Sox *et al.* 1981). Furthermore, the available evidence suggests that the more expensive to the patient the ('inert') intervention, the more effective it is likely to be (Brody 1980). Surgical operations can also have beneficial psychological effects on symptoms, and mock (placebo) operations have occasionally been used to control for this effect (Beecher 1961). Although the use of mock operations may seem to be carrying the evaluation of clinical practice to unnecessary extremes, it has led to the abandonment of some useless operations earlier than might have been the case had less rigorous methods of research been used (Table 1.15).

Table 1.14 The effect of symptom suggestion: prevalence of gastrointestinal side-effects in patients who were warned and others who were not warned that they might experience them (Cairns *et al.* 1985)

	Warned about side-effects (n = 399)	Not warned about side-effects (n = 156)
No. (%) of patients who experienced side-effects	175 (43.8)	25 (16.0)

Although psychological effects of care are often perceived as a bother by researchers, they are measurable and often clinically important. Ideally then, any formal evaluation of a particular type of care should be designed to distinguish its psychological effects from its pharmacological or physical effects. Both wanted and unwanted effects can be mediated through either of these mechanisms. Unfortunately, examples of research designed in this way are rare (see, for example, Timm 1979). Sometimes previous research may have indicated that the particular kind of care being evaluated is unlikely to have any important psychologically-mediated effect on the condition or conditions of interest; in these circumstances, there might be less need to control for psychological effects of care when assessing pharmacological or physical effects (Khurmi *et al.* 1986). Often, however, in an attempt to control for psychological effects, those conducting formal evaluations of care wish to try to keep both providers and recipients of care masked to the identity of the particular form of care offered.

Table 1.15 Frequency (%) of improvement in angina following actual and sham internal mammary artery ligation in two trials (cited in Beecher 1961)

	Artery ligated		Artery not ligated	
	No.	%	No.	%
Trial 1	10/13	(76.9)	5/5	(100.0)
Trial 2	3/8	(37.5)	4/9	(44.4)

Identifying psychologically-mediated effects of care can be an objective worth pursuing. It is important to know when a form of care has no pharmacologically- or physically-mediated effects. Even if it has beneficial psychologically-mediated effects, it may be possible to achieve these more safely and economically by other means. But it has to be acknowledged that blinding (masking) those providing and those receiving care to the identity of the particular form of care being given within a comparative trial is frequently impossible, particularly with surgical operations and other non-pharmacological forms of care. Published assessments of the extent to which attempts to achieve masking have been successful in drug trials (in which it is most likely to be achieved) are not common. The available evidence suggests that even determined efforts to achieve masking may only be partly successful (see, for examples, Chalmers TC 1975b; Vere and Chaput de Saintonge 1976; Brownell and Stunkard 1982; Byington *et al.* 1985). Obviously, this is not necessarily an argument for abandoning attempts to mask the identity of the actual forms of care compared in trials (any more than the knowledge that a determined cheat can corrupt arrangements for random assignment is a reason for abandoning attempts to abolish selection bias). It does mean, however, that it will often be difficult to disentangle psychological from pharmacological and physical effects of care.

Another reason for trying to ensure that those providing care remain unaware of which one of the alternative forms of care being compared they are administering, is to reduce the extent to which they may be prompted to adjust their care in other ways in the light of this knowledge. This phenomenon, termed 'co-intervention', may make the results of the trial somewhat more difficult to interpret. In the randomized trials of cervical cerclage, for example, there was a tendency for women assigned to cerclage to be prescribed tocolytic drugs more frequently than controls (see Chapter 40).

Attempts to mask those providing and receiving care are particularly likely to be worthwhile when one or more of the forms of care being compared seems likely (or is known) to have psychologically-mediated effects on one or more of the outcomes of interest, or when co-interventions seem likely to cause confusion. But the effort made to achieve masking in other circumstances may not be repaid by more valid results than would have been obtained by simpler study designs. In an investigation which spanned nine different subject areas, a comparison of the results of placebo-controlled randomized trials with those in which masking had not been used, it was not possible to detect any material difference between the estimates of treatment effects on either 'hard' or 'soft' endpoints (Reitman *et al.* 1988).

4.3 Was bias minimized when the outcomes of care were assessed?

Perception (observation) of the outcomes of interest in a comparison of two or more forms of care can be affected by knowledge of which particular form of care has been received by a particular individual in whom the outcomes are sought. When the outcomes in question are self-reported symptoms this amounts to one and the same thing, hence the use of placebo controls, as discussed in the previous section. In addition to controlling for psychological effects of care, however, there are other circumstances in which observation of the postulated outcomes of care may be biased if the observer knows which form of care was actually received. These biases may occur, for example, if the people providing care consciously or unconsciously believe that one or other of the forms of care being compared is either superior or inferior. In these circumstances they may tend to record the outcomes of care in ways that confirm their expectations. For example, how should one interpret the observation in an unblinded randomized trial of abdominal decompression, conducted in the centre that pioneered this form of obstetric care, that serious hypertension was less common in the decompressed group than in the control group (see Chapter 41)? It may be that this form of care does indeed have such an effect, but 'observer biases' obviously have the potential for prompting misleading inferences about the effects of this and other forms of care.

Protection against observer biases is obviously most secure when the outcome in question is quite unambiguous ('hard'); death is the obvious example. The chances of observer biases among those providing or receiving care affecting observations of 'softer' outcomes will obviously be reduced, and sometimes abolished, by masking using placebos; but as explained earlier, this may frequently prove impossible. A precaution which is often more practical is to make arrangements for outcomes to be assessed by observers who are neither providers nor recipients of care, and who can therefore be more easily kept in ignorance of the form of care received by the individuals in whom judgements about outcomes have to be made. The neonatal neurological status of infants born during a randomized comparison of alternative methods of intrapartum fetal heart rate monitoring, for example, was assessed by a paediatrician who was kept unaware of the assigned method of monitoring (MacDonald *et al.* 1985). Similarly, in a randomized comparison of liberal and restricted use of episiotomy, the midwives who assessed the perineal trauma 10 days after delivery were unaware of whether the mother had been allocated to liberal or restricted use of episiotomy (Sleep *et al.* 1984).

4.4 Was bias avoided by ensuring that all the people who were randomized appeared in the analysis?

Even after ensuring complete control of selection bias by meticulous attention to the procedure for random assignment of individuals to alternative forms of care, selection bias may be introduced into studies using randomized controls (or concurrent non-randomized controls, for that matter) by biased withdrawal or drop-out of individuals after the form of care has been assigned (Sackett and Gent 1979; *Lancet* 1987). Because withdrawal and drop-out may be prompted either by knowledge of the assigned form of care, or by some effect of the care itself, these losses from the randomized groups may occur in a biased way.

These considerations underlie recommendations that the *primary* analysis of a study that has been designed to abolish selection bias by using randomized controls should be based on data relating to *all* the eligible individuals who were randomly assigned to one or other of the alternative forms of care, regardless of whether or not they went on to receive the assigned form of care (Bradford Hill 1971; Peto *et al.* 1976, 1977; Gail 1985). This so-called 'intention to treat' analysis is the only analysis that can confidently be assumed to be free from selection bias. If decisions to withdraw participants have been taken in ignorance of the group to which they were assigned, and if it is possible to be confident that the reason for withdrawal or drop-out has nothing to do with the assigned form of care, an unbiased comparison between randomized groups that have experienced attrition for either of these reasons may be valid, particularly if the documented proportions of withdrawals and drop-outs, and the reasons for them, are similar in the comparison groups.

Secondary analyses, for example, those restricted to individuals within the randomized groups who actually received the form of care assigned, may be informative, particularly in addressing questions about whether a particular form of care *can* work in *ideal* circumstances, as opposed to questions about whether the form of care *does* work in *typical* circumstances (Schwartz *et al.* 1970; Sackett and Gent 1979). But bias may also render such analyses misleading.

Table 1.16 provides an illustrative example. In a randomized comparison of two policies for managing the perineum during childbirth, women who were expected to have a spontaneous vaginal delivery were randomly allocated either to a policy of using episiotomy (to avoid a perineal tear), or to a policy of avoiding episiotomy (Sleep *et al.* 1984). This resulted in 51 per cent of the first group and 10 per cent of the second group actually having an episiotomy. The analysis based on comparisons of all the women in these two randomized cohorts (the 'intention to treat' analysis) achieved comparability between the two comparison groups in respect of variables of prognostic importance for discomfort after childbirth (Sleep *et al.* 1984), one of which (primiparity) is tabulated in Table 1.16 (i). Table 1.16 (ii) illustrates the effect of basing the analysis on women who actually had an episiotomy in the 'use episiotomy' group, and those who did not have one in the 'avoid episiotomy' group (that is, after withdrawing 'non-compliers' in an attempt to achieve a 'cleaner' comparison). Imbalance, and thus selection bias, in the prognostic variable shown (primiparity) results from excluding these women. This bias results in confounding of the comparison of outcome: whereas the 'intention to treat' analysis did not suggest that postpartum perineal discomfort was associated with more frequent use of episiotomy, the comparison of women who did and did not have an episiotomy suggests that the operation predisposes to postpartum discomfort.

Sometimes it may be possible to judge the direction of the likely bias introduced in secondary analyses conducted after exclusions have been made from the randomized cohorts, and thus make allowance for the biases introduced. There are no grounds for great confidence in such judgements, however. In half of a group of studies analysed using both of the two approaches outlined above, differences in outcome between treatment and control groups were greater when the 'intention to treat' (primary) approach was used; in the remaining studies, differences in outcome between the two groups were more marked when based on secondary analyses conducted after excluding withdrawals and drop-outs, thus leading to an overestimate of treatment differences (Bhaskar *et al.* 1986).

The effect of analysing by 'intention to treat',

Table 1.16 (i) 'Intention to treat' analysis* compared with (ii) analysis after withdrawal of 'non-compliers'†, showing introduction of selection bias (imbalance in prognostic variable) and confounding of comparison of outcome (prevalence of perineal pain postpartum)

	Policies compared	
	Use episiotomy to avoid tear	Avoid episiotomy
(i) *Analysis based on all women randomized*	(*n* = 502)	(*n* = 498)
Primigravidae (%)	43.6	40.4
Prevalence (%) of pain 10 days postpartum	22.6	22.6
(ii) *Analysis based only on those having, and not having, episiotomy*	(*n* = 257)	(*n* = 447)
Primigravidae (%)	57.2	36.9
Prevalence (%) of pain 10 days postpartum	32.2	19.9

*Data from Sleep *et al.* (1984)
†Unpublished data provided by Adrian Grant and Hazel Ashurst

although generating inferences that are both unbiased and likely to be of greater relevance to typical circumstances, is conservative and probably tends to minimize and even obscure differences between different forms of care (*Lancet* 1987). The larger the size of the study, the less of a problem this will present (Peto *et al.* 1976). In practice, because studies are almost always smaller than one would like, it is increasingly common practice to report primary ('intention to treat') analyses based on all eligible participants randomized, *and* secondary, exploratory analyses, conducted after excluding participants who did not receive the assigned form of care. This approach provides the data necessary to make causal inferences that take into account the dangers both of selection bias and of overlooking real, but diluted differential treatment effects of alternative forms of care (Sackett and Gent 1979).

5 Was random error (the play of chance) controlled sufficiently?

5.1 Sample size

> 'The least excusable of unnecessary suffering is that on women—and particularly on mothers of young children . . . What serious study has ever been made bearing upon the harm or harmlessness of the variety of procedures, or concerning the failure or effectiveness of each? To achieve this there is a need for collective experimentation, since no one man is likely to have a large experience'
>
> R. L. Dickinson 1920

More than half a century ago the President of the American Gynecological Society recognized that meaningful assessment of the effects of alternative forms of care could only be achieved through widespread collaboration, because of the misleading way that the play of chance can affect the pattern of rare adverse outcomes witnessed by individual clinicians. He probably also had in mind that 'collective experimentation' would lead to inferences about the effects of care that were not only less subject to random errors resulting from the play of chance, but also more confidently generalizable than inferences based on experiments conducted on a more restricted basis (see next section).

Although properly randomized controlled trials that have been correctly designed and analysed will control for *systematic errors* resulting from the biases discussed in the previous section, the results of such trials may still be misleading because of *random errors* resulting from the play of chance. Random errors are reduced by increasing the size of the study sample.

Tests of statistical significance are used to assess the likelihood that the observed differences between alternative forms of care may simply be a reflection of random errors (chance). These tests are used to prevent people inferring that a real difference exists when it does not—sometimes referred to as a Type I error. Unfortunately, differences between alternative forms of care that are not statistically significant tend to be dismissed as simply being a reflection of the play of chance when this inference is not justified. This mistake is sometimes referred to as a Type II error (Freiman *et al.* 1978; Reed and Slaichert 1981; Hall 1982; Altman 1983; Makuch and Johnson 1986). In 67 of 71 randomized controlled trials in which the investigators had concluded that there were no differential effects of the forms of care compared because the results of significance tests had yielded values of p greater than 0.1, there was a greater than 10 per cent chance that a real difference of as much as 25 per cent in the effectiveness of the treatments compared had been missed (Freiman *et al.* 1978). Furthermore, these differences tended to be in favour of the newer of the forms of care being compared. This low statistical 'power' of many randomized controlled trials to control for random errors thus too often leads to the opposite problem to that caused by the systematic errors (biases) in non-randomized comparative studies: real advances in care tend not to be recognized for what they are (Sacks *et al.* 1983).

There is, however, a second way in which random error can be misleading (Bulpitt 1987). If, after applying a test of statistical significance to the observed differences in outcome associated with alternative forms of care, chance is rejected as an explanation of the differences observed, the magnitude of the observed differences will tend to overestimate the extent of the true differences in small trials. Small trials with results which suggest spectacular and implausible differences between alternative forms of care such as these can be misleading, either because they lead to an overestimate of a true difference between different forms of care, or because they suggest that there is a difference when, in reality, there is none. This would not be a problem if the results of all small trials were reported. As it is, trials in which dramatic, statistically significant differences have been observed are more likely to be reported in print than trials in which the differences observed have been more modest (and plausible), and not 'statistically significant' (see Section 7.2, below).

The way in which random error can prompt the two kinds of false inference outlined above can be illustrated using the results of randomized trials in which intensive intrapartum fetal monitoring (with continuous heart rate recording and acid–base assessment when indicated) has been compared with standard fetal monitoring (with intermittent auscultation of the fetal heart). In both the two small randomized comparisons of these alternative forms of care (Renou *et al.* 1976; Haverkamp *et al.* 1979), all six cases of neonatal seizures were observed among the babies who had received standard fetal monitoring, thus suggesting a protective effect of more intensive monitoring in this respect (Chalmers I 1979). Applying tests of statistical significance to these differences, however, makes it clear that the observed differences could easily be explained by the play of chance; thus the two monitoring policies could not be judged with any confidence to have differential effects (Table 1.17a). Only in a trial in which the same general pattern of seizures was observed among a far larger number of babies was it possible to reject chance as a likely explanation for the observed differences between the two policies (Table 1.17b). The conclusion is that using the more intensive method of fetal monitoring does indeed lead to a reduction in the risk of neonatal seizures to a level of about half that experienced by babies monitored using the standard method (see Chapter 54).

Table 1.17 Distribution of cases of neonatal seizures in two small ($n = 350$; $n = 462$) and one large ($n = 13{,}084$) randomized comparisons of intensive and standard fetal monitoring during labour

	Method of fetal monitoring		p
	Intensive	Standard	
(a) *Small trials*			
Renou *et al.* (1976)	0/175	4/175	Not signif.
Haverkamp *et al.* (1979)	0/230	2/232	Not signif.
(b) *Large trial*			
MacDonald *et al.* (1985)	12/6530	27/6554	< 0.025

This example illustrates only the first of the two ways in which random errors can be misleading. This, and the second way discussed above, can be illustrated by a *post hoc* analysis of the data derived from 4 consecutive recruitment phases in the large trial cited above—as if the 4 phases had, instead, been 4 independently conducted trials, each with quarter the sample size of the large trial (Table 1.18). The differences in seizure rates in each of these 4 comparisons point consistently to a protective effect of the more intensive method of fetal monitoring. In the first 3 comparisons, however, these differences, after testing for statistical significance, would have been ascribed to chance. In the fourth comparison, by contrast, the dramatic difference in the same direction would have been judged to have been unlikely to reflect the play of chance (random error), but the strength of the protective effect of intensive fetal monitoring would have been grossly overestimated. The available evidence (see Section 7.2, below) suggests that had the fourth comparison been a small trial it would have been more likely to have appeared in print than the first three.

Table 1.18 Distribution of 39 cases of neonatal seizures in a large ($n = 13{,}084$) randomized comparison of intensive and standard fetal monitoring during labour, analysed (after completion) in four successive recruitment phases (data made available by Adrian Grant)

Recruitment phase	Method of fetal monitoring		p
	Intensive	Standard	
First	5	9	Not signif.
Second	3	4	Not signif.
Third	3	5	Not signif.
Fourth	1	9	< 0.025

The message is clear: random errors will be reduced as samples yielding larger numbers of the outcomes of interest are studied. This can be achieved both by conducting larger randomized trials than has been usual in the past (Yusuf *et al.* 1984), and by incorporating all the available data from broadly similar trials within a particular field of enquiry in systematic overviews (meta-analyses)—as has been done in the preparation of this book (see Chapter 2).

5.2 Confidence intervals

'The accept/reject philosophy of significance testing based on the "magical" $p = 0.05$ barrier remains dominant in the minds of many non-statisticians'

Stuart Pocock 1985

'In clinical matters, the null hypothesis of "no difference" is a probability theorist's abstraction. (Clinical) decision makers need to know if a difference makes any difference'

William Silverman 1987

One of the factors that predisposes to incorrect inferences resulting from random errors is the widespread use of particular p values (often 0.05) to dichotomize studies into those that are interpreted as providing evidence that there are real differences between the alternative forms of care compared ($p < 0.05$), and those which are deemed to provide evidence that they have equivalent effects ($p > 0.05$). Presenting the actual p value is more sensible than this 'all or nothing' approach. In addition or instead, however, confidence intervals can be presented to indicate the range within which the true difference between alternative forms of care is likely to lie (Wulff 1973; Rothman 1978). The implication of significance testing—that there is always either a difference or no difference between alternative forms of care—is patently unrealistic; alternative treatments are always likely to have differential effects, even if these differences are, for all practical purposes, sometimes trivial.

It is not surprising that confidence intervals provide more information than *p* values, if only because a confidence interval is defined by two numbers rather than the single number that denotes a *p* value (Rothman 1986). Since Wulff (1973) pointed out the advantages of estimating the differential effects of alternative forms of care using confidence intervals rather than testing the null hypothesis using tests of statistical significance to generate *p* values, support for estimation of effects using confidence intervals has become very widespread (Rothman 1978; Detsky and Sackett 1985; Pocock 1985; Gardner and Altman 1986; Simon 1986; Bulpitt 1987).

The advantages of using confidence intervals for estimation can be illustrated using the data derived from one of the two small trials and the large trial comparing intensive and standard forms of fetal monitoring during labour, already referred to above. As previously noted, in the small trial, significance testing and the *p* value obtained (>0.1) encourage an assumption that the two policies are equivalent: the difference in the estimated seizure rates associated with the two policies can easily be dismissed as simply a reflection of random error (chance). Calculation of the 95 per cent confidence interval of the relative effects of the two policies on seizure risk (0.01–2.18), however, reveals that the differences observed are compatible both with virtual abolition of the risk of seizures by using the more intensive method of monitoring, and also with a doubling of the risk (Table 1.19a): in other words, there is a 95 per cent chance that the true difference lies somewhere in between these two very wide limits (Gardner and Altman 1986).

Clearly, the information derived from this small trial is not very helpful because it does not even indicate the direction of any differential effect of the two methods of fetal monitoring, let alone its magnitude. The results of the larger trial, because they are less subject to random error (the play of chance), are more helpful (Table 1.19b). The *p* value (<0.025) derived from using a test of statistical significance suggests that the observed reduction in seizure risk associated with the more intensive method of monitoring is unlikely to be due to chance. Because it does not include 1, the 95 per cent confidence interval (0.25–0.87) of the estimate of the differential effects of the two policies (the odds ratio, see Chapter 2) confirms that the observed difference is unlikely to be due to chance; but in addition, it provides the potentially important information that the more intensive method of monitoring is likely to lead to a *reduction* in seizure risk, and that the magnitude of the 'true' reduction is likely to lie somewhere between about 13 and about 75 per cent.

The advantages of estimations using confidence intervals rather than (or in addition to) testing the null hypothesis with tests of statistical significance have led to the adoption of the former when the results of comparisons of alternative forms of care have been presented in subsequent chapters in this book (see Chapter 2).

6 Were the number and nature of the comparisons made prespecified?

Munchausen's statistical grid

'Recently the Baron's statistical writings have come to light, and with them a statistical device, Munchausen's statistical grid. The great virtue of this device is that it can resurrect a significant result from any foundering therapeutic trial. First the patients in the trial are allocated to five classes (for example, age groups). Then the five classes are divided by sex, to make ten subgroups. The experimenter declares a probability of $P = 0.05$—that is, one in twenty—to be significant, and now there is a fifty–fifty chance that one of the subgroups will produce the desired result. Should the experimenter still have bad luck, subdividing the classes along some other line—for example, Scandinavian and non-

Table 1.19 Distribution of neonatal seizures in a small ($n = 462$) and a large ($n = 13{,}084$) randomized comparison of intensive and standard fetal monitoring during labour, *p*-values, and 95 per cent confidence intervals of odds ratios

	Method of fetal monitoring		*p*	95% conf. int. of odds ratio
	Intensive	Standard		
(a) *Small trial*				
Haverkamp *et al.* (1979)	0/230	2/232	Not signif.	0.01–2.18
(b) *Large trial*				
MacDonald *et al.* (1985)	12/6530	27/6554	< 0.025	0.25–0.87

Scandinavian patients—provides a second chance of winning; it should give twenty subclasses and considerably improve the chances of a significant result'

Graham Martin 1984

Because information derived from groups of individuals has to be used in making treatment decisions about individuals, there is an understandable tendency to explore the results of controlled trials in the hope that it will be possible to identify particular subcategories of individuals showing better than average or worse than average responses to one or other of the forms of care being compared. As Baron Munchausen's statistical grid illustrates, these multiple comparisons may lead to conclusions that differences exist when they do not. For every 20 comparisons so made, one can be expected to be statistically significant simply because of the play of chance. A similar problem results from repeated 'peeking' as the data accumulates in a trial, and so statistical guidelines exist for progressively adjusting the level of confidence that it is reasonable to place on any differences observed (McPherson 1982; Benichou and Chastang 1986).

The key issue as far as subgroup analyses are concerned is whether or not they were prespecified prior to analysing the results of the trial. If there was some *prior* reason for expecting differential responses to a particular form of care among different subgroups of the individuals who have participated, this should have been built into the plan of the investigation. Randomized trials mounted to evaluate the effect of an antioestrogen drug (tamoxiphen) in the treatment of breast cancer, for example, sought (but did not find) evidence that the drug was more effective in the control of tumours in which oestrogen receptors had been detected (Early Breast Cancer Trialists Collaborative Group 1988).

Confident inferences that a particular form of care has opposite effects in particular subcategories of individuals are very rare (Chalmers TC and Buyse 1988). Any real differences that do exist between subcategories are far more likely to be differences in the magnitude rather than the direction of the effect. Nevertheless, there are some circumstances in which it is conceivable that an intervention may have effects in the opposite direction in different individuals. Cervical cerclage, for example, may reduce the risk of 2nd-trimester miscarriage or preterm delivery in women who are at increased risk of these outcomes because of cervical incompetence. Used in women without this condition, however, it is conceivable that this operation, involving manipulation of the cervix, might actually cause the uterus to contract and lead to the very outcomes it is intended to prevent. As with other hypotheses about differential effects of particular forms of care in particular subgroups of individuals, this hypothesis of a differential effect of cervical cerclage depending on the prior risk of cervical incompetence should be stated clearly and tested prospectively in randomized trials of cervical cerclage.

The search for differential effects of care among subcategories of individuals which have *not* been specified prior to inspecting the results of the treatment comparisons is, however, a totally different kind of activity. 'Fishing expeditions' or 'data dredges', as these activities are sometimes called, certainly increase the likelihood that 'differential effects' will be observed; but it will not be possible to distinguish with any confidence those that are real and those that are due to chance (Peto 1982). This problem cannot be better illustrated than by reference to the inferences drawn from controlled trials to evaluate the effects of administering corticosteroids to enhance fetal maturation prior to preterm delivery. Data dredging and subgroup analysis of the controlled trials in this field have led people to infer that this form of care only confers benefit on black, female fetuses, born within a particular range of gestational age and at least 24 hours after the drug has been administered (see, for example, Roberton 1982, 1986). None of these inferences are justified by the available evidence (see Chapter 45).

The dangers of data-dependent dredges for subcategories of individuals who show differential responses to particular forms of care is well-illustrated by a subgroup analysis based on the results of a recent trial concerned with the used of beta-blockade in the treatment of acute myocardial infarction (Table 1.20): the analysis showed that almost all of the observed benefit of treatment was explained by the responses of people who were born under the astrological sign of Scorpio. Although there may be some people who will interpret this observation as evidence of a real subgroup effect, most people will probably agree with the investigators that it would be unwise to conclude that beta-blockers should only be given to those heart attack victims whose birthdays fall between 24 October and 22 November (Collins *et al.* 1987)!

When the results of controlled trials are reported,

Table 1.20 Subgroup analysis by astrological birth sign in a randomized trial of over 16,000 patients with suspected acute myocardial infarction (Collins *et al.* 1987)

Astrological birth sign	Percentage reduction in odds of death (SE)	2-sided p value
Scorpio	− 48 (23)	< 0.04
All others	− 12 (8)	Not signif.
Overall	− 15 (7)	< 0.05

data-derived hypotheses about possible effects of care should be identified by the investigators so that this information can be taken into account by those who have to make decisions about clinical care (Smith *et al.* 1987). For example, in the large randomized comparison of intensive and standard intrapartum fetal monitoring to which reference has already been made above (MacDonald *et al.* 1985), the most striking differences in seizure rates in the two groups were within the subgroups of infants born following relatively prolonged labour. Because it had not been predicted prior to the trial that these babies would show a particularly marked differential response to the two methods of intrapartum monitoring compared, this observation serves only to generate, but not to test the hypothesis that a differential effect exists. The difference observed must be considered in the light of data derived from other trials in order to assess whether it is likely to be true, or simply a result of the play of chance. If the evidence derived from a number of similar trials all points in the same direction in respect of an observed, but unpredicted association, this consistency will tend to support the conclusion that it reflects a differential effect of the alternative forms of care compared, and not simply chance (see Chapter 2).

7 Are the studies identified representative of all relevant studies?

'Many excellent notions or experiments are, by sober and modest men, suppressed'

Sir Robert Boyle, 1661; cited in Hall 1965

7.1 Citation bias

All the considerations about study design discussed so far are relevant in evaluating the 'internal validity' of a particular study, that is the extent to which systematic error (bias) and random error (the play of chance) have been minimized. Although there may be some circumstances in which it may be reasonable to base decisions about clinical practice on the results of a single, large trial (Johnson 1985), it is usually important to consider the results of any particular trial in the context of the results of other, similar studies (see Chapter 2). This is not as straightforward a process as it may seem.

If searches of the literature for studies relevant to the review of a particular topic are conducted in an informal way, it is quite likely that they will yield samples of published reports that are both incomplete and unrepresentative (biased). Reviewers who base their searches for relevant studies on the reports cited in any relevant publications that are already available to them, for example, may find themselves guided to an unrepresentative sample of studies (Christensen-Szalanski and Beach 1984; Cooper 1986). Gøtzsche (1987) has shown that published reports of trials of drugs tend to cite as references an unrepresentative sample of previous reports that have evaluated the drugs in question: previously published reports which have shown positive features of the drug are more likely to be cited than those which have cast doubt on its value or safety. Selective citation can also occur as a result of a conscious or unconscious tendency for reviewers to include data that agree with, or reinforce, their preconceptions.

A more systematic approach to the identification of relevant reports can be pursued using one or more of the available bibliographic sources (John 1985; Snow 1985; Haynes *et al.* 1986; Menke and McClead 1987). Unfortunately, the available evidence suggests that use of these sources to identify reports of randomized controlled trials is likely to yield less than half of the relevant studies (Dickersin *et al.* 1985; Poynard and Conn 1985; Bernstein 1988; Hewitt *et al.* 1988). Furthermore, the fraction of controlled trials identified in this way may be an unrepresentative sample of the totality of relevant published reports. In a review of trials relevant to two therapeutic issues in the cancer field, Simes (1987) found that trials in which statistically significant differences had been observed were more likely to have been published in the more widely read journals.

7.2 Publication bias

In addition to these factors leading to citation bias, however, there is a tendency among investigators, peer reviewers, and journal editors to allow the direction and statistical significance of research findings to influence decisions regarding submission and publication. As the quotation with which this section opens makes clear, this departure from good scientific practice has been recognized since the dawn of the scientific era. During the last 30 years it has been documented empirically in a variety of disciplines (Sterling 1959; Smart 1964; Chalmers TC *et al.* 1965; Greenwald 1975; Mahoney 1977; Smith 1980; Hemminki 1980; White 1982; Devine and Cook 1983; Simes 1986; Davidson 1986; Simes 1987; Sommer 1987; Dickersin *et al.* 1987; Vandenbroucke 1988; Begg and Berlin 1988). The bias sometimes results in observed differences between study groups *not* being reported, for example, when side-effects of new drugs are concerned (Hemminki 1980). More usually, if comparisons have yielded differences that are in a particular direction and statistically significant, research is *more* likely to be reported in print. Publication bias thus tends to promote conclusions that an association exists when in fact it does not, or that the association is stronger than it is in reality (Kurosawa 1984). Simes (1987), for example, has shown how an analysis of the results of trials reported in print leads to the conclusion that combination chemotherapy is statistically significantly superior to a single alkylating agent in the treatment of advanced ovarian cancer. Extending the analysis to include the results of trials of comparable methodological quality that have not been published, however, resulted in disappearance of the statistically significant advantage of combination chemotherapy. Peto (1978) and Moertel (1984) have come to similar conclusions in respect of 5-fluorouracil as an adjuvant therapy for colon cancer.

A problem that is related to result-dependent selective publication of whole studies is result-dependent reporting of some outcomes but not others in studies that are published. The selective presentation of data relating to some rather than all outcomes assessed in a trial does not necessarily imply, as has been suggested (Sacks *et al.* 1987), that some outcomes have not been found acceptable by peer reviewers. The problem arises because results relating to particular outcomes may be included in manuscripts submitted for publication and in published reports because the direction or magnitude of a difference was perceived to be 'interesting', both by those reporting the study and by referees and editors. Conversely, 'uninteresting' results may be selectively excluded from manuscripts, or pruned out by journal editors who are unaware of the bias which they are thereby introducing (Chalmers I 1985a,b).

As indicated in the previous section, consistency of evidence derived from a number of independent but similar trials will tend to strengthen inferences about the differential effects of alternative forms of care, even if these have not been predicted prior to examining the data. There is obviously a danger, however, that selective reporting of outcomes may result in biased estimates of the effects of care.

When publication or reporting bias leads to incorrect conclusions about the safety and efficacy of some forms of care, it raises not only scientific, but also ethical concerns because it will tend to result in people receiving forms of care that are either ineffective or actually harmful. Investigators, those who commission and fund research, and journal editors must share the blame for this state of affairs (Begg and Berlin 1989). A comparison of the characteristics of published and unpublished clinical trials reported to Dickersin and her colleagues (1987) in a survey of clinical investigators confirmed that trials yielding results which favoured new therapies were more likely to be reported in print than those which showed either no clear trend, or favoured standard therapy or placebo (Table 1.21). An additional finding of the survey was that non-publication was primarily a result of failure to write-up and submit the results of trials that had shown no statistically significant advantage of the new therapy, rather than because there had been editorial rejection of submitted manuscripts. Although investigators appear to be mainly to blame for this kind of misconduct in medical research (Chalmers I 1989), some journal editors contribute to the problem by actively discouraging the submission of 'negative' studies (Chalmers I 1985b).

Table 1.21 Investigators' reports of trend of results of published randomized controlled trials, and completed but unpublished randomized controlled trials, in a survey of investigators known to have co-authored at least one published report of a randomized controlled trial (Dickersin *et al.* 1987)

Trend	Published RCTs (n = 767) %	Completed, unpublished RCTs (n = 178) %
Favours new therapy, $p < 0.05$	55.1	14.6
Favours new therapy, $p > 0.05$	16.0	22.5
No clear trend	22.2	44.4
Favours standard therapy, $p > 0.05$	3.3	12.9
Favours standard therapy, $p < 0.05$	3.4	5.6

The problem of publication bias will only be addressed satisfactorily by prospective registration of clinical trials at inception (Schoolman 1979; Simes 1986; Simes 1987; Dickersin 1988; Meinert 1988; Hetherington *et al.* 1989), combined with the adoption of editorial policies designed to minimize it (Walster and Cleary 1970; Feige 1975; Lane and Dunlap 1978; Chalmers I and Sinclair 1984; Rahimtoola 1985; Newcombe 1987; Piantadosi and Byar 1988). The problem presented by selective reporting of some outcomes and not others (depending on what was found) is a more difficult issue to tackle systematically. Its solution lies primarily in more open and honest exchange of information among clinical researchers.

8 Are the results of formal comparisons of alternative forms of care generalizable?

8.1 Characteristics of the recipients of care

Even if it is possible to be reasonably certain that a particular study is both '*internally valid*' (systematic and random error have been controlled) and *representative* of all relevant studies, questions may remain about its '*external validity*'; that is, the extent to which it is possible to generalize the results of the study (Kramer and Shapiro 1984; Chalmers TC 1988). Generalizability may be compromised either by differences between participants in trials and people receiving care outside the context of trials, or by differences in the nature of care given within trials and that provided outside trials.

Sometimes the limited generalizability of the study

may be relatively clear: To return to an example raised earlier, it would seem inadvisable to extrapolate the results of a randomized trial of cervical cerclage in which the participating women had been at *lower* than average risk of 2nd-trimester miscarriage and preterm delivery to women who are at very high risk of these adverse outcomes of pregnancy (and far more likely to have cervical incompetence). On other occasions, too, the differences between the population in the trial and that to which extrapolation of the results is being considered may be sufficient to justify reservations about their generalizability: the results of trials assessing the value of prescribing prophylactic folic acid for pregnant women in developing countries, for example, may well not be relevant in relatively well-nourished populations (see Chapter 19).

More usually, it will not be possible to conclude with any confidence that the results of controlled trials are *inapplicable* in practice. Furthermore, there is a distinct danger that concern about differences between the characteristics of participants in trials and clients receiving care outside the context of trials will be used as an argument for dismissing valid evidence about the effects of care. If women and babies are to derive any benefit from the results of internally valid research evaluating care, then a leap of faith from this evidence to practice has to be made at some point (see Section 4 of Chapter 2).

Sometimes the generalizability of the results of formal comparisons of alternative forms of care is called into question because not all individuals eligible for the particular forms of care were recruited into the studies upon which inferences have been based (Wilhelmsen *et al.* 1976; Feinstein 1983; Charlson and Horwitz 1984). Such objections are obviously flawed: no formal comparison of alternative forms of care can ever include *all* the human beings who meet the eligibility criteria. In spite of the fact that participants in trials can never be assumed to be a random sample of some hypothetical population, the experiences of trial participants have often been widely accepted as generalizable.

It is important to recognize that the assumptions underlying these objections are usually based on speculation and not evidence. For example, it was suggested by some neurosurgeons that, because some eligible patients had not been entered into a randomized evaluation of anastomosis of the external carotid with the internal carotid artery (EC–IC Bypass Study Group 1985), the conclusions reached by the study were of questionable relevance in actual practice (Sundt 1987; Goldring *et al.* 1987; Dudley 1987). As others (including other surgeons) pointed out in response to these suggestions, the onus is on those who speculate about the possible consequences of less than total recruitment of eligible patients in unbiased, formal comparisons to demonstrate (in further, properly controlled comparisons) that inclusion of a greater proportion of all eligible patients, or different kinds of patients, leads to different inferences about the effectiveness of the procedure (Barnett *et al.* 1987; Warlow and Peto 1987; Bamford 1987; Baum 1987; Chalmers TC *et al.* 1987). This duty to substantiate opinion with evidence should be taken particularly seriously by those who wish to persuade others that a particular form of care should be used when the results of the only unbiased assessments available suggest that it is ineffective (as is the case in respect of the operation of external carotid–internal carotid arterial anastomosis) (Robin 1987).

None of the above implies that the participants in a formal, controlled comparison of alternative forms of care are necessarily identical or almost identical to those who receive the same, alternative forms of care outside the context of the controlled trial: it is clear that their characteristics do indeed sometimes differ systematically (see, for example, Wilhelmsen *et al.* 1976; Charlson and Horwitz 1984; Edlund *et al.* 1985). This is not the key issue, however. The crucial issue is whether the unbiased estimates of the *differential effects* of the alternative forms of care which were derived from the experience of those who participated in the trial apply among those who did not participate in it. As already discussed in Section 6, above, confident inferences that a particular form of care has *opposite* effects in particular subcategories of individuals are very rarely justified. Any real differences in the effects of care that do exist as between participants and non-participants in a controlled trial are therefore far more likely to be differences in magnitude than differences in the direction of any effect. The judgement must then be made more in terms of whether the estimated magnitude of the differential effect in a particular patient or group of patients is sufficient to warrant modification of usual clinical practice.

There is a second way in which this difference in the magnitude of effect may be mediated by differences between participants in trials and people receiving care outside trials, and thus sometimes compromise the generalizability of the results of an internally valid study. This is through differences in the level of compliance with treatment within trials compared with outside the context of trials. Compliance with some forms of prescribed treatment (drugs, for example), is known to be quite poor (Haynes *et al.* 1979). Compliance with prescribed treatment among those receiving care may be better than usual within controlled trials. Participation in the trial may change behaviour in other ways, for example, by improving self-care and use of the health services, and this may result in the people in the control group experiencing better outcomes than might be expected in a similar, but non-participant group in the general population (Kramer and Shapiro 1984). However, other aspects of randomized trials (the uncertainty engendered by randomization, for example) may actually discourage compliance (Kramer and Shapiro 1984). In summary, if compliance with prescribed care among participants in a controlled trial has been unusually good, the trial results will tend to overestimate the differential effects of the alternative forms of care as used in everyday practice. If, on the other hand, people in the control group have modified their behaviour in ways that are atypical but predispose to improved outcome, or if compliance within the trial in general has been worse than can be expected in everyday practice, the study may underestimate real, differential effects of the alternative forms of care.

8.2 Characteristics of the care provided

8.2.1 Efficacy versus effectiveness

In addition to differences between those receiving care in the context of controlled trials and those receiving care outside trials, and in the extent to which they comply with prescribed treatment, there may also be differences in the nature of the care provided. These may also raise questions about the external validity of internally valid studies.

The care provided within the context of formal, randomized trials may differ in a variety of ways from the care given in the less formal circumstances of usual clinical practice. Indeed, the design of trials may reflect an emphasis on one of two broad objectives (Schwartz *et al.* 1970; Sackett 1980). In the first of these two kinds of study—the 'explanatory' trial—the main question addressed is '*Can* this treatment work?'. In the second type of study—the 'pragmatic trial'—the main question addressed is '*Does* this treatment work?'. Using an alternative terminology, explanatory trials aim to assess the 'efficacy' of a particular form of care when it is provided in ideal circumstances; pragmatic trials aim to assess the 'effectiveness' of the same form of care, as it is used in circumstances that are closer to everyday practice.

Each of these approaches has its strengths and limitations (Sackett 1980). It is obviously important to know whether a form of care *can* work and it will sometimes be worth going to great lengths to try to create the circumstances which are likely to maximize the chances of its effects being detected. In practice, this may involve selecting those individuals thought most likely to benefit from the form of care concerned; 'blinding' (masking) both those giving and those receiving care so that interpretation of the comparisons made is not complicated by trying to assess the independent effects of co-interventions; ensuring maximum compliance both among those delivering the care and those receiving it; possibly allowing individualization of drug dosage in an attempt to maximize beneficial effects and minimize side-effects; and, sometimes, excluding non-compliers from the analysis (with the inevitable consequent risk of introducing bias (see Section 4.4, above)).

If such an 'explanatory' trial yields results suggesting that a particular form of care is efficacious, the extent to which the results are applicable in usual clinical practice will depend on the extent to which it is possible to create the circumstances necessary for the form of care concerned to be implemented more widely. For example, in two trials of routine, two-stage ultrasonography during pregnancy mounted concurrently in adjacent populations in Norway (Eik-Nes *et al.* 1984; Bakketeig *et al.* 1984), beneficial effects were detected in one but not in the other. A possible explanation for the differences in the estimated effects is that the ultrasonographers serving one of the two populations were relatively experienced, while those serving the other population were relatively inexperienced. The trial using experienced ultrasonographers might thus be characterised as an 'explanatory' (or 'efficacy') trial, and the trial using less experienced ultrasonographers as a 'pragmatic', (or 'effectiveness') trial. Because it is important to distinguish efficacy from effectiveness, the results of both explanatory and pragmatic trials are useful, particularly when considered in conjunction with each other. In the instance cited above, the results of the two trials taken together suggest first, that important beneficial effects of routine ultrasonography may await discovery (see Chapter 27), and second, that quality control of routinely performed ultrasonography may be crucial if its potential benefits are to be realized in practice. Taken together in this way, the results of both of the trials provide evidence that is relevant in guiding everyday clinical practice.

Related considerations apply in connection with the evaluation of other technical innovations in care. Controlled evaluations of newly introduced technical procedures are not infrequently dismissed because of fears among the innovators that the procedures concerned will be discredited prematurely because they have been evaluated too early in their evolution, and during a period over which operators are learning to use them (Hemminki 1982b). Formal evaluation in these circumstances, however, allows some estimate of the human 'costs', in terms of morbidity and mortality, of this learning process.

Most controlled trials, including the two trials of ultrasound used as illustrations above, do not fall neatly into one or other of the two categories of trials—explanatory and pragmatic—identified above. But the distinction first proposed by Schwartz and his colleagues (1970) can be helpful in provoking the kind of questions that are relevant in considering the applicability of the results of particular controlled trials in everyday clinical practice. This may apply particularly in circumstances in which technical skills are an important determinant of the effects of care. It is certain that real and important differences in the skills of individual clinicians exist. Such differences may well explain, for example, why some individual accoucheurs are particularly successful in helping women to achieve a vaginal delivery without perineal or vaginal trauma; why different surgeons have different rates of infection following caesarean section; and why there is sometimes agreement among both professionals and clients that a particular individual is, quite simply, a very skilled and effective clinician (Luborsky *et al.* 1985). Indeed, controlled trials sometimes generate evidence that confirms that these factors can be influential; but as noted earlier (see Section 3.4.2), differences attributable to experience are not always detected when sought (Sleep *et al.* 1984; Tabor *et al.* 1986).

Judgements about the applicability of the results of controlled comparisons of forms of care which involve technical skills may well be less secure than judgements based on controlled trials of drugs. This should not be regarded as a licence to abandon or dismiss attempts to mount properly controlled evaluations of these forms of care, as some surgeons have implied (Love 1975; Bonchek 1979; 1982; Dudley 1985). Because surgeons, like other caregivers, may do more harm than good in their efforts to help patients, they have a responsibility to produce credible evidence to reassure others that the care they are offering is effective and reasonably safe (Spodick 1971, 1973, 1975; Bryce *et al.* 1983; Chalmers I 1986c; Gray *et al.*, in press). If, as some have suggested, certain forms of surgical and other types of care are too complex to permit formal evaluation using techniques to reduce bias, then the advocates of such care should be clear about the implications. As one surgeon has noted, except in situations in which prognosis can be predicted with great confidence, there are some expensive and complex technologies which, by their very nature, do not lend themselves to scientific evaluation. For this reason they have as much justification in their use as osteopathy or homeopathy for the same disease processes (Baum 1987).

The curious double standard whereby stringent requirements exist in most developed countries for unbiased assessment of the efficacy and safety of new drugs, but not for non-drug forms of care, has no rational basis. Evidence that repairing perineal trauma using a new form of suture material (glycerol-impregnated catgut) can result in a doubling of the prevalence of pain during intercourse as long as 3 years after it has been used (Grant *et al.* 1989), for example, is testimony to the disturbing consequences of continued acquiescence in the double standard whereby drugs must be evaluated carefully, but other forms of intervention are accepted into clinical practice without good evidence showing that they are more likely to do good than harm (Chalmers I 1986a).

8.2.2 Psychological aspects

> 'If you can believe fervently in your treatment, even though controlled tests show that it is quite useless, then your results are much better, your patients are much better, and your income is much better too. I believe this accounts for the remarkable success of some of the less gifted, but more credulous members of our profession, and also for the violent dislike of statistics and controlled tests which fashionable and successful doctors are accustomed to display'
>
> Richard Asher 1972

Aspects of the style and content of interactions between those providing and those receiving care can affect the outcome of care (Luborsky *et al.* 1985). Because the style and content of these interactions may be different within the context of a randomized trial from interactions in everyday practice, these differences may compromise the extent to which the results of some trials can be generalized. In some circumstances, and for some outcomes, a feeling of 'specialness' may result from participation in a formal study. This may have beneficial psychological effects, and these, in turn, may be reflected in improved outcome of treatment expressed in terms of 'physical' outcomes (Kramer and Shapiro 1984).

The differences in the way that those providing and those receiving care interact within as compared with outside the context of randomized trials may, however, differ as a result of externally imposed requirements concerning the nature and content of the interaction. Professionals involved in formal, controlled comparisons of alternative forms of care are often required by research ethics committees to admit their uncertainty about the effects of treatment to patients, and to provide them with uniform, detailed, and unsolicited information about the alternative forms of care concerned, including details of possible side-effects. Clinicians offering identical forms of care outside the context of formal, randomized comparisons are not usually subject to such restrictions. The operation of this irrational double standard (Baum 1986; King 1986; Chalmers I and Silverman 1987) may result in the psychological effects of care within randomized controlled comparisons being atypical, and thus less generalizable than they might otherwise be.

The first way in which psychological effects of care may operate reflects differing expectations among those seeking care (Bradley 1988). While some people will wish to be provided with detailed information about the uncertainties surrounding the beneficial and adverse effects of alternative forms of care, others may welcome and benefit from a relatively 'paternalist' approach in which the professional is confident and reassuring (Brewin 1985; King 1986). Caregivers are very properly wary of externally imposed requirements for delivering care in ways that do not allow for this variation (Jones 1981; Gillon 1985). They will wish to maximize the placebo effects of care and avoid symptom suggestion whenever possible; these objectives will be achieved using different approaches for different individuals.

For many individuals receiving care the confident professional certainty which is typical of everyday practice constitutes a more effective form of care than the explicit admission of professional uncertainty that is often required of those who are providing care within the context of formal, randomized comparisons. Explicit admission of professional uncertainty has been shown to have the capacity for reducing the placebo effectiveness of inert tablets, capsules, and injections (Beecher 1955; Wolf 1959; Dahan *et al.* 1986) and of at least some forms of surgery that have no known potential for physically-mediated beneficial effects (Beecher 1955; Wolf 1959). In a randomized comparison conducted in a general practice setting, for example, patients presenting with symptoms but no abnormal physical signs, in whom no firm diagnosis could be made, were more satisfied with care and more likely to experience symptomatic improvement following a 'positive' consultation (with a confident assurance that the symptoms would disappear in a few days), than control patients were after a more 'neutral' style of consultation (in which the doctor admitted that he could not be certain what was wrong or whether his prescribed treatment would have any effects) (Thomas 1987; Table 1.22). In another controlled trial, involving women undergoing termination of pregnancy, it was found that, compared with an 'egalitarian' style of consultation, a 'paternalistic' approach not only prompted women to have greater confidence in the physician, but also resulted in them experiencing less discomfort during the procedure (LeBaron *et al.* 1985). Other evidence confirms the importance of psychological and educational factors in mediating the effects of care (Devine and Cook 1983).

Table 1.22 The placebo effect of a confident practitioner: frequency of patient satisfaction and symptomatic improvement following 'positive' and 'neutral' styles of consultation for patients presenting with symptoms, but no abnormal physical signs, and in whom no definite diagnosis could be made (Thomas 1987)

	Style of consultation	
	'Positive' (n = 100)	'Neutral' (n = 100)
Proportion (%) of patients who felt that they had been helped a lot by the doctor	55	23
Proportion (%) of patients whose symptoms had disappeared 2 weeks after the consultation	64	39

The second way in which psychological effects of care may differ within the context of trials is through symptom suggestion. This may result from the common requirement that clinicians providing care within the context of randomized controlled trials should provide fuller unsolicited information about the possible side-effects of the forms of care involved. This can have adverse effects (associated with both 'active' and 'inert' treatments) because of symptom suggestion (Brownell and Stunkard 1982; Cairns *et al.* 1985; see Table 1.14). The consequence of symptom suggestion affecting controls taking placebos will be that comparisons between the actively-treated and placebo-treated groups will tend to *underestimate* the true rate of side-effects attributable to the active treatment, thus compromising the generalizability of the study findings.

In summary, the atypical requirements for consent to treatment that are required only when care is being provided within the context of randomized trials may reduce beneficial placebo effects and increase adverse effects resulting from symptom suggestion. This will mean that the observed differences between alternative forms of care studied will tend to underestimate the differences that may actually exist when the same forms of care are used in everyday clinical practice. The fact that the beneficial psychological effects of individualized care can almost certainly be pursued more effectively outside the context of formal trials may well account for some of the different impressions that exist about the effectiveness of particular forms of care. Those who have the impression that a particular form of care is beneficial (particularly if they are enthusiasts) when no supportive evidence is available from controlled trials may be detecting the (real) placebo effects of the form of care in question. If this impression of benefit is not shared by other, more sceptical people, this may be because, 'in their hands', there are no psychologically-mediated beneficial effects, and possibly some psychologically-mediated adverse effects.

9 Conclusions

'Many physicians attack experimentation, believing that medicine should be a science of observation; but physicians make therapeutic observations daily on their patients so this inconsistency cannot stand careful thought. Medicine by its nature is an experimental science, but it must apply the experimental method systematically'

Claude Bernard 1865

'In the 36 years that have passed since the end of the Second World War, the clinical trial has come to play a progressively larger part in medical practice ... That this has happened is due not only to the growing influence of science on medicine . . . but also to the realization that every time a doctor treats a patient, whether by giving him a drug, operating on him, or modifying his way of life by putting him in bed or changing his diet, he is performing an experiment. And if the medical profession is a scientific one it should plan that experiment and record its results in such a way as to make it possible for something to be learnt that will contribute to the improvement of treatment in the future'

Richard Doll 1982

In this chapter, the different kinds of evidence on which judgements about the effects of care are often based have been arranged in a hierarchy. The rationale for this hierarchy has been supported, not just by theoretical considerations, but with empirical evidence. The hierarchy reflects a belief that the main challenge facing those who wish to evaluate the effects of care during pregnancy and childbirth is to minimize the likelihood that they will be misled by systematic errors (biases) and random errors (the play of chance). The consequences of being misled in this way are that some women and babies will be denied effective care, while others will receive care that is ineffective or actually harmful.

In the hierarchy proposed, evidence derived from comparisons of people who happened, for one reason or another, to have received one or other of alternative forms of care (observational evidence), has been distinguished from evidence derived from comparisons of people who have been randomized in prospectively planned trials to alternative forms of care (experimental evidence). The crucial distinction between these two kinds of evidence has been noted by those who provide care during pregnancy and childbirth (see, for example, Malpas 1953; Friedman 1961; Kerr 1975; Pontonnier and Grandjean 1975; Bryce and Enkin 1985; Macdonald 1987; Lilford 1987); by clinical researchers (see, for example, Chalmers I and Richards 1977; Chalmers I 1980; Grimes 1986; Lumley 1987; Bracken 1987); and recently, by representatives of the women who use the maternity services (see, for example, Beech 1986, 1987; Somorjay 1987).

The separation of evidence derived from experiments from evidence derived from observations made outside the context of experiments is the most relevant step in any consideration of how to reduce bias in assessing the effects of care. Clinical impressions, uncontrolled case series, and studies using non-randomized controls so frequently lead to biased estimates of the differences between alternative forms of care that they should usually be seen as 'screening tests' for identifying forms of care that *may* be valuable. When evidence from such studies does suggest that one form of care may be superior to another, it should not be used as a basis for clinical practice unless it has been validated in prospective comparisons of the forms of care in question, with randomization used to eliminate selection bias, and other precautions taken to control other biases.

Although otherwise well-designed randomized trials may offer protection against the possibility of being misled by bias (systematic error), too often they provide little protection against being misled by the play of chance (random error). One consequence of this problem is that forms of care that do, in fact, have differential effects of practical importance are deemed to be equivalent. This problem can be addressed by increasing the size of the sample studied and estimating the range of differential effects within which the true difference is likely to lie. Random error, combined with publication bias, also tends to lead to overestimates of the differential effects of alternative forms of care; this problem can only be satisfactorily addressed by ensuring that all well-conducted studies are published, regardless of the differences observed.

The results of studies in which systematic and random errors have been controlled effectively should usually provide the most secure basis for maximizing benefits and minimizing risks when selecting from alternative forms of care in everyday practice. Nevertheless, either because of differences in the characteristics of those receiving care, or differences in the nature of the care itself, or both, there are circumstances in which the results of formal comparisons of care may not be generalizable in this way. In particular, beneficial, psychologically-mediated effects of care may well be more common, and harmful psychological effects less common, in normal clinical practice than in formal comparisons of alternative forms of care.

Consistent with the hierarchy of evidence outlined in this chapter, the approach used throughout this book is that, within each of the subject areas considered, evidence from any and all of the available randomized controlled trials has been considered before observational data have been reviewed. For some aspects of practice (the effects of prophylactic administration of antibiotics in association with caesarean section for example), a considerable amount of experimentally-derived evidence is available. In other areas (the routine use of ultrasound, for example), the available experimentally-derived data are inadequate to support strong inferences about the effects of care. In still other fields, not only are there no data available from controlled trials to guide decisions about care, but it is unlikely that there ever will be (the treatment of massive placental abruption is an example). The strengths of the conclusions about the effects of particular forms of care will thus reflect the strength of the evidence available, as judged by the hierarchy set out above.

Finally, it is worth noting that, although the hierarchy of evidence for assessing the effects of care which has been set out in this chapter and applied throughout this book has been accepted and translated into practice in many medical specialties, it continues to be viewed with scepticism by some authorities within obstetrics (Noller and Melton 1985). A recent example is provided by the authoritarian reaction of the editor of one leading obstetric journal to the results of a formal assessment of the methodological quality of studies evaluating the effects of obstetric and neonatal paediatric care (see Shearer 1984; Chalmers I 1986b).

One characteristic of a well-designed enquiry into the effects of clinical practice is that it is basically anti-authoritarian. Not surprisingly therefore, authorities may use one or more of a variety of strategies to discredit studies that yield results that challenge their certainties about the effects of particular forms of care (Chalmers TC 1974; Spodick 1982; McIntyre and Popper 1983; Spodick 1983; Chalmers I 1983). The interests of authorities are obviously served best when there is a complete absence of any relevant evidence. In these circumstances (which unfortunately apply in respect of many elements of care during pregnancy and childbirth) unsubstantiated opinions reign supreme as the determinants of practice. Authorities are also served well by circumstances in which there is a predominance of data derived using research designs that are relatively weak: the inherent difficulties in controlling for biases and thus interpreting the meaning of the associations observed often seem to result in everyone's (often incompatible) certainties remaining intact. By contrast, it is less easy for authorities to defend their certainties when the evidence that challenges them has been derived from unbiased comparisons of alternative forms of care. It is probably worth noting at the outset that the evidence used to prepare this book has helped to shatter some of the most fondly cherished certainties of its editors and their collaborators!

References

Altman DG (1983). Size of clinical trials. Br Med J, 286: 1842–1843.

Altman DG (1985). Comparability of randomised groups. Statistician, 34: 125–136.

Armitage P (1982). The role of randomization in clinical trials. Stat Med, 1: 345–352.

Asher R (1972). Talking Sense. London: Pitman Medical.

Atlay RD, Weekes ARL, Entwistle GD, Parkinson DJ (1978). Treating heartburn in pregnancy: Comparison of acid and alkali mixtures. Br Med J, 2: 919–920.

Bakketeig LS, Hoffman HJ, Sternthal PM (1978). Obstetric service and perinatal mortality in Norway. Acta Obstet Gynecol Scand Suppl, 77.

Bakketeig LS, Jacobsen G, Brodtkorb CJ, Eriksen BC, Eik-Nes SH, Ulstein MK, Balstad P, Jorgensen NP (1984). Randomised controlled trial of ultrasonographic screening in pregnancy. Lancet, 2: 207–210.

Bamford J (1987). Extracranial–intracranial bypass, one; clinical trials, nil. Br Med J, 295: 211–212.

Barnett HJM, Sackett D, Taylor DW, Haynes B, Peerless SJ, Meissner I, Hachinski V, Fox A (1987). Are the results of the extracranial–intracranial bypass trial generalizable? New Engl Med J, 316: 820–824.

Barral E (1986). Douze ans de résultats de la recherche pharmaceutique dans le monde (1975–1986). Prospective et santé 36: 90.

Bates D, Caronna JJ, Cartlidge NEF, Knill-Jones RP, Levy DE, Shaw DA, Plum F (1977). A prospective study of non-traumatic coma: Methods and results in 310 patients. Ann Neurol, 2: 211–220.

Baum M (1986). Do we need informed consent? Lancet, 2: 911–912.

Baum M (1987). Endoscopic coagulation of upper gastrointestinal haemorrhage, one; randomised clinical trials, two. Br Med J, 295: 212.

Beech BL (1986). Consumer view of randomised trials of chorionic villus sampling. Lancet, 1: 1157.

Beech BL (1987). Who's Having Your Baby? London: Camden Press.

Beecher HK (1955). The powerful placebo. JAMA, 159: 1602–1606.

Beecher HK (1961). Surgery as placebo. JAMA, 176: 1102–1107.

Begg CB, Berlin JA (1988). Publication bias: A problem in interpreting medical data. J R Stat Soc (Series A), 151: 419–463.

Begg CB, Berlin JA (1989). Publication bias and dissemination of clinical research. J Natl Cancer Inst, 81: 107–115.

Benhamou JP, Rueff B, Sicot C (1972). Severe hepatic failure: A critical study of current therapy. In: Liver and Drugs. Orlandi F, Jezequel AM (eds). New York: Academic Press, pp 213–228.

Benichou J, Chastang C (1986). Practicability of sequential methods in randomized clinical trials with a censored response criterion. Rev Epidémiol Santé Publique, 34: 196–208.

Berlin JA, Begg CB, Louis TA (1987). Assessing the magnitude of publication bias in clinical trials. Controlled Clin Trials, 8: 180–183.

Bernstein F (1988). The retrieval of randomized clinical trials in liver diseases from the medical literature: Manual versus MEDLARS searches. Controlled Clin Trials, 9: 23–31.

Bhaskar R, Reitman D, Sacks HS, Smith H, Chalmers TC (1986). Loss of patients in clinical trials that measure long-term survival following myocardial infarction. Controlled Clin Trials, 7: 143–148.

Blackwell B, Bloomfield SS, Buncher CR (1972). Demonstration to medical students of placebo responses and non-drug factors. Lancet, 1: 1279–1282.

Bloom BS (1986). Controlled studies in measuring the efficacy of medical care: A historical perspective. Int J Techn Assess Health Care, 2: 299–310.

Blum AL (1986). Why do dyspeptic patients prefer one liquid antacid to another? Eur J Clin Invest, 16: 515–518.

Bonchek LI (1979). Are randomized trials appropriate for evaluating new operations? New Engl Med J, 301: 44–45.

Bonchek LI (1982). The role of the randomized clinical trial in the evaluation of new operations. Surg Clin North Am, 62: 761–769.

Bracken MB (1987). Clinical trials and the acceptance of uncertainty. Br Med J, 294: 1111–1112.

Bradford Hill A (1952). The clinical trial. New Engl Med J, 247: 113–119.

Bradford Hill A (1971). Principles of Medical Statistics (9th edn). London: Lancet.

Bradley C (1988). Clinical trials – time for a paradigm shift? Diabetic Medicine 5: 107–109.

Brewin T (1985). Truth, trust and paternalism. Lancet, 2: 490–492.

Brody H (1980). Placebos and the Philosophy of Medicine. Chicago: University of Chicago Press.

Brownell KD, Stunkard AJ (1982). The double-blind in danger: Untoward consequences of informed consent. Am J Psychiatry, 139: 1487–1489.

Bryce RL, Enkin MW (1985). Six myths about controlled trials in perinatal medicine. Am J Obstet Gynecol, 151: 707–710.

Bryce R, Fuller P, Mohide P (1983). Clinical trial of chorion biopsy. Can Med Assoc J, 63: 349–357.

Bulpitt CJ (1987). Confidence intervals. Lancet, 2: 494–497.

Buyse M (1987). In: Clinical Trial Size—The Perfect, the Practicable and the Present. Haybittle J (ed). London: Medical Research Council/Cancer Research Campaign, p 5.

Byar DP, Simon RM, Friedewald WT, Schlesselman JJ, DeMets DL, Ellenberg JH, Gail MH, Ware JH (1976). Randomized controlled trials: Perspectives on some recent ideas. New Engl J Med, 295: 74–80.

Byington RP, Curb JD, Mattson ME (1985). Assessment of double-blindness at the conclusion of the beta-blocker heart attack trial. JAMA, 253: 1733–1736.

Cairns JA, Gent M, Singer J, Finnie KJ, Froggatt GM, Holder DA, Jablonsky G, Kostuk WJ, Melendez LJ, Myers MG, Sackett DL, Sealey BJ, Tanser PH (1985). Aspirin, sulfinpyrazone, or both in unstable angina. New Engl Med J, 313: 1369–1375.

Campbell R, Macfarlane AM (1986). Place of delivery: A review. Br J Obstet Gynaecol, 93: 675–683.

Chalmers I (1979). Randomized controlled trials of intrapartum fetal monitoring, 1973–1977. In: Perinatal Medicine. Thalhammer O, Baumgarten K, Pollak A (eds). Stuttgart: Georg Thieme, pp 260–265.

Chalmers I (1980). An introduction to perinatal audit and surveillance. In: Perinatal Audit and Surveillance. Chalmers I, McIlwaine G (eds). London: Royal College of Obstetricians and Gynaecologists, pp 7–16.

Chalmers I (1983). Scientific inquiry and authoritarianism in perinatal care and education. Birth, 10: 151–166.

Chalmers I (1985a). Proposal to outlaw the term 'negative trial'. Br Med J, 290: 1002.

Chalmers I (1985b). Biased touching of the editorial tiller. Arch Dis Childhood, 60: 394.

Chalmers I (1986a). Minimising harm and maximising benefit during innovation in health care: Controlled or uncontrolled experimentation? Birth, 13: 155–164.

Chalmers I (1986b). Editors, peers and the process of scientific review. In: Gynaecology and Obstetrics. Thomsen K, Ludwig H (eds). Proceedings of the XIth World Congress. Berlin: Springer, pp 59–61.

Chalmers I (1986c). Minimizing harm and maximizing benefit during innovation in health care: Controlled or uncontrolled experimentation? Birth, 13: 155–164.

Chalmers I (ed) (1988). The Oxford Database of Perinatal Trials. Oxford: Oxford University Press.

Chalmers I (1989). Misconduct in medical research. Br Med J, 298: 256.

Chalmers I, Richards MPM (1977). Intervention and causal inference in obstetric practice. In: Benefits and Hazards of the New Obstetrics. Chard T, Richards MPM (eds). Clinics in Developmental Medicine, No. 64. London: Spastics International Medical Publications, Heinemann Medical Books, pp 34–61.

Chalmers I, Silverman WA (1987). Professional and public double standards on clinical experimentation. Controlled Clin Trials, 8: 388–391.

Chalmers I, Sinclair JC (1984). Is it time for a change of emphasis in perinatal research? Early Hum Dev, 10: 171–191.

Chalmers I, Lawson JG, Turnbull AC (1976a). Evaluation of different approaches to obstetric care I. Br J Obstet Gynaecol, 83: 921–929.

Chalmers I, Lawson JG, Turnbull AC (1976b). Evaluation of different approaches to obstetric care II. Br J Obstet Gynaecol, 83: 930–933.

Chalmers I, Hetherington J, Newdick M, Mutch L, Grant A, Enkin M, Enkin E, Dickersin K (1986). The Oxford Database of Perinatal Trials: Developing a register of published reports of controlled trials. Controlled Clin Trials, 7: 306–324.

Chalmers TC (1974). The impact of controlled trials on the practice of medicine. Mt Sinai J Med (NY), 41: 753–759.

Chalmers TC (1975a). Randomization of the first patient. Med Clin North Am, 59: 1035–1038.

Chalmers TC (1975b). Effects of ascorbic acid on the common cold. Am J Med, 58: 532–536.

Chalmers TC (1984). The need for randomized control trials. J Clin Apheresis, 2: 105–111.

Chalmers TC, Buyse ME (1988). Meta-analysis. In: Data Analysis for Clinical Medicine: The Quantitative Approach to Patient Care in Gastroenterology. Chalmers TC (ed). Rome: International Unviversity Press. pp. 75–84.

Chalmers TC, Schroeder B (1979). Controls in journal articles. New Engl Med J, 301: 1293.

Chalmers TC, Koff RS, Grady GF (1965). A note on fatality in serum hepatitis. Gastroenterology, 49: 22–26.

Chalmers TC, Smith H, Blackburn B, Silverman B, Schroeder B, Reitman D, Ambroz A (1981). A method for assessing the quality of a randomized control trial. Controlled Clin Trials, 2: 31–49.

Chalmers TC, Celano P, Sacks HS, Smith H (1983). Bias in treatment assignment in controlled clinical trials. New Engl Med J, 309: 1358–1361.

Chalmers TC, Meier P, Plum F (1987). The EC–IC Bypass Study. New Engl Med J, 317: 1030–1031.

Charlson ME, Horwitz RI (1984). Applying the results of randomised trials to clinical practice: Impact of losses before randomisation. Br Med J, 289: 1281–1284.

Christensen-Szalanski JJJ, Beach LR (1984). The citation

bias: Fad and fashion in the judgement and decision literature. Am Psychol, 39: 75–78.
Christie D (1979). Before-and-after comparisons: A cautionary tale. Br Med J, 2: 1629–1630.
Cochrane AL (1972). Effectiveness and Efficiency. London: Nuffield Provincial Hospitals Trust.
Cochrane AL (1979). 1931–1971: A critical review with particular reference to the medical profession. In: Medicines for the Year 2000. Teeling-Smith G (ed). London: Office of Health Economics, pp 1–11.
Collins R, Gray R, Godwin J, Peto R (1987). Avoidance of large biases and large random errors in the assessment of moderate treatment effects: The need for systematic overviews. Stat Med, 6: 245–250.
Colton T, Greenberg ER (1982). Epidemiologic evidence for adverse effects of DES exposure during pregnancy. Am Statistician, 36: 268–272.
Cooper HM (1986). Literature-searching strategies of integrative research reviewers. Knowledge: Creation, Diffusion, Utilization, 8: 372–383.
Coronary Drug Project Research Group (1980). Influence of adherence to treatment and response of cholesterol on mortality in the coronary drug project. New Engl Med J, 303: 1038–1041.
Dahan R, Caulin C, Figea L, Kanis JA, Caulin F, Segrestaa JM (1986). Does informed consent influence therapeutic outcome? A clinical trial of the hypnotic activity of placebo in patients admitted to hospital. Br Med J, 293: 363–364.
Davidson RA (1986). Source of funding and outcome of clinical trials. J Gen Intern Med, 1: 155–158.
DerSimonian R, Charette LJ, McPeek B, Mosteller F (1982). Reporting on methods in clinical trials. New Engl J Med, 306: 1332–1337.
Detre KM, Peduzzi P, Chan Y-K (1981). Clinical judgement and statistics. Circulation, 63: 239–240.
Detsky AS, Sackett DL (1985). When was a 'negative' clinical trial big enough? How many patients you needed depends on what you found. Arch Intern Med, 145: 709–712.
Devine EC, Cook TD (1983). A meta-analytic analysis of effects of psychoeducational interventions on length of postsurgical hospital stay. Nursing Res, 32: 267–274.
Dickersin K (1988). Report from the Panel on the Case for Registers of Clinical Trials at the 8th Annual Meeting of the Society for Clinical Trials. Controlled Clin Trials, 6: 306–317.
Dickersin K, Hewitt P, Mutch L, Chalmers I, Chalmers TC (1985). Comparison of MEDLINE searching with a perinatal clinical trials database. Controlled Clin Trials, 6: 306–317.
Dickersin K, Chan SS, Chalmers TC, Sacks HS, Smith H (1987). Publication bias in randomized control trials. Controlled Clin Trials, 8: 343–353.
Dickinson RL (1920). A program for American gynecology. Am J Obstet Gynecol, 1: 2–10.
Diehl LF, Perry DJ (1986). A comparison of randomized concurrent control groups with matched historical control groups: Are historical controls valid? J Clin Oncol, 4: 1114–1120.
Doll R (1982). Clinical trials: Retrospect and prospect. Stat Med, 1: 337–344.
Doll R, Peto R (1980). Randomised controlled trials and retrospective controls. Br Med J, 1: 44.
Dudley HAF (1985). Trials and tribulations for surgeons. Br J Surg, 72: 255.
Dudley HAF (1987). Extracranial–intracranial bypass, one; clinical trials, nil. Br Med J, 294: 1501–1502.
Early Breast Cancer Trialists Collaborative Group (1988). Effects of adjuvant tamoxiphen and cytotoxic therapy on early mortality in breast cancer: an overview of all 61 randomized trials among 28,896 women. First Report. New Engl J Med, 319: 1681–1692.
EC–IC Bypass Study Group (1985). Failure of extracranial–intracranial arterial bypass to reduce the risk of ischaemic stroke. New Engl Med J, 313: 1191–1200.
Edlund MJ, Craig TJ, Richardson MA (1985). Informed consent as a form of volunteer bias. Am J Psychiatry, 142: 624–627.
Eik-Nes SE, Okland O, Aure JC, Ulstein M (1984). Ultrasound screening in pregnancy: A randomised controlled trial. Lancet, 1: 1347.
Eksmyr R (1985). Geographically defined populations with different organisation of medical care. Comparison of perinatal risks. Acta Paediatr Scand, 74: 855–860.
Emerson JD, McPeek B, Mosteller F (1984). Reporting clinical trials in general surgical journals. Surgery, 95: 572–579.
Evans FJ (1974). The power of a sugar pill. Psychology Today, April: 55–61.
Farewell VT, D'Angio GJ (1981). A simulated study of historical controls using real data. Biometrics, 37: 169–176.
Feige EL (1975). The consequences of journal editorial policies and a suggestion for revision. J Polit Economy, 83: 1291–1296.
Feinstein AR (1983). An additional basic science for clinical medicine: II. The limitations of randomized trials. Ann Intern Med, 99: 544–550.
Feinstein AR (1985). Clinical Epidemiology: The Architecture of Clinical Research. Philadelphia: W B Saunders.
Feinstein AR, Horwitz RI (1982). Double standards, scientific methods, and epidemiologic research. New Engl J Med, 307: 1611–1617.
Fielding LP, Stewart-Brown S, Dudley HAF (1978). Surgeon-related variables and the clinical trial. Lancet, 2: 778–779.
Frederickson DS (1968). The field trial: Some thoughts on the indispensable ordeal. Bull NY Acad Med, 44: 985–993.
Freiman JA, Chalmers TC, Smith H, Kuebler RR (1978). The importance of beta, the type II error and sample size in the design and interpretation of the randomized control trial. New Engl Med J, 299: 690–694.
Friedman EA (1961). The statistical approach to the study of clinical phenomena. Am J Obstet Gynecol, 82: 219–225.
Gail MH (1985). Eligibility exclusions, losses to follow-up, removal of randomized patients, and uncounted events in cancer clinical trials. Cancer Treat Rep, 69: 1107–1112.
Gardner MJ, Altman DG (1986). Confidence intervals rather than P values: Estimation rather than hypothesis testing. Br Med J, 292: 746–750.
Gardner MJ, Altman DG (eds) (1989). Statistics with Confidence. London: British Medical Journal.

Gehan EA (1982). Design of controlled clinical trials: Use of historical controls. Cancer Treat Rep, 66: 1089–1093.

Gehan EA (1986). Randomized or historical control groups in cancer clinical trials: Are historical controls valid? J Clin Oncol, 4: 1024–1025.

Gilbert JP, McPeek B, Mosteller F (1977). Progress in surgery and anesthesia: Benefits and risks of innovative therapy. In: Costs, Risks, and Benefits of Surgery. Bunker JP, Barnes BA, Mosteller F (eds). New York: Oxford University Press, pp 124–169.

Gillon R (1985). Telling the truth and medical ethics. Br Med J, 291: 1556–1557.

Goldring S, Zervas N, Langfitt T (1987). The extracranial–intracranial bypass study: A report of the committee appointed by the American Association of Neurological Surgeons to examine the study. New Engl Med J, 316: 817–820.

Gorowitz S, MacIntyre A (1976). Toward a theory of medical fallibility. J Med Philosophy, 1: 51–71.

Gotzsche PC (1987). Reference bias in reports of drug trials. Br Med J, 295: 654–656.

Gracely RH, Dubner R, Deeter WR, Wolskee PJ (1985). Clinician's expectations influence placebo analgesia. Lancet, 1: 43.

Grant A (1985a). The Dublin Trial of Fetal Heart Rate Monitoring. University of Oxford: DM thesis.

Grant A (1985b). Do computers help or hinder the clinical evaluation of treatments in perinatal medicine? Am J Perinatol, 2: 242–244.

Grant A, Chalmers I (1985). Epidemiology in obstetrics and gynaecology: Some research strategies for investigating aetiology and assessing the effects of clinical practice. In: Scientific Basis of Obstetrics and Gynaecology (3rd edn). Macdonald RR, (ed). London: Churchill Livingstone, pp 49–84.

Grant A, Sleep J, Ashurst H, Spencer J (1989). Dyspareunia associated with the use of glycerol-impregnated catgut to repair perineal trauma—report of a three-year follow-up study. Br J Obstet Gynaecol, 96: 741–743.

Gray DT, Hewitt P, Chalmers TC (in press). The evaluation of surgical therapies. In: Socioeconomics of Surgical Health Care Delivery. Rutkow IM (ed). St Louis: Mosby.

Greenwald AG (1975). Consequences of prejudice against the null hypothesis. Psychol Bull, 82: 1–20.

Greenwald P, Barlow JJ, Nasca PC, Burnett WS (1971). Vaginal cancer after maternal treatment with synthetic estrogens. New Engl Med J, 285: 390–393.

Gries JB, Bienarz J, Scommegna A (1981). Comparison of maternal and fetal effects of vacuum extraction with forceps or caesarean deliveries. Obstet Gynecol, 57: 571–577.

Grimes DA (1986). How can we translate good science into good perinatal care? Birth, 13: 83–87.

Guyatt G, Sackett D, Taylor DW, Chong J, Roberts R, Pugsley S (1986). Determining optimal therapy—randomized trials in individual patients. New Engl Med J, 314: 889–892.

Hall JC (1982). The other side of statistical significance: A review of Type II errors in the Australian medical literature. Austral NZ J Med, 12: 7–9.

Hall MB (1965). Robert Boyle on Natural Philosophy. Bloomington: Indiana University Press, p 121.

Hammar M, Larsson L, Tegler L (1981). Calcium treatment of leg cramps in pregnancy. Acta Obstet Gynecol Scand, 60: 345–347.

Hammar M, Berg G, Solheim F, Larsson L (1987). Calcium and magnesium status in pregnant women. A comparison between treatment with calcium and vitamin C in pregnant women with leg cramps. Int J Vitam Nutr Res, 57: 179–183.

Haverkamp AD, Orleans M, Langendoerfer S, McFee J, Murphy J, Thompson HE (1979). A controlled trial of differential effects of intrapartum monitoring. Am J Obstet Gynecol, 134: 399–412.

Haynes RB, Taylor DW, Sackett DL (1979). Compliance in Health Care. Baltimore: Johns Hopkins.

Haynes RB, McKibbon KA, Fitzgerald D, Guyatt GH, Walker CJ, Sackett DL (1986). How to keep up with the medical literature: IV. Using the literature to solve clinical problems. Ann Intern Med, 105: 636–640.

Hearst N, Newman TB, Hullet SB (1986). Delayed effects of the military draft on mortality: A randomized natural experiment. New Engl Med J, 314: 620–624.

Hemminki E (1980). Study of information submitted by drug companies to licensing authorities. Br Med J, 280: 833–836.

Hemminki E (1982a). Quality of clinical trials—a concern of three decades. Methods Inf Med, 21: 81–85.

Hemminki E (1982b). Problems of clinical trials as evidence of therapeutic effectiveness. Soc Sci Med, 16: 711–712.

Herbst AL, Ulfelder H, Poskanzer DC (1971). Adenocarcinoma of the vagina: Association of maternal stilbestrol therapy with tumour appearance in young women. New Engl Med J, 292: 334–339.

Hetherington J, Chalmers I, Dickersin K, Meinert C (1989). Retrospective or prospective identification of controlled trials: Lessons from a survey of obstetricians and paediatricians. Pediatrics, 84: 374–380.

Hewitt P, Dickersin K, Tingey H, Chalmers TC (1988). Explanation of low retrieval of randomized control trials (RCTs) from MEDLINE. Controlled Clin Trials, 9: 281.

Hibbard BM, Jeffcoate TNA (1966). Abruptio placentae. Obstet Gynecol, 27: 155–167.

Hill GB (1983). Controlled clinical trials—the emergence of a paradigm. Clin Invest Med, 6: 25–32.

Hills M, Armitage P (1979). The two-period cross-over clinical trial. Br J Clin Pharmacol, 8: 7–20.

Hooke R (1983). How to Tell the Liars from the Statisticians. New York: Marcel Dekker.

Horwitz RI, Feinstein AR (1979). Methodologic standards and contradictory results in case-control research. Am J Med, 66: 556–564.

Horwitz RI, Feinstein AR (1981). Improved observational method for studying therapeutic efficacy: Suggestive evidence that lidocaine prophylaxis prevents death in acute myocardial infarction. JAMA, 246: 2455–2459.

Jennett B, Teasdale GM, Braakman R, Minderhoud J, Knill-Jones R (1977). Severe head injuries in three countries. J Neurol Neurosurg Psychiatry, 40: 291–298.

John K (1985). Medical literature searches—how many bibliographic databases are needed for sufficient retrieval in medical topics? Methods Inf Med, 24: 163–165.

Johnson AF (1985). Replication of multicenter clinical trials for efficacy? J Chron Dis, 38: 265–269.

Jones JS (1981). Telling the right patient. Br Med J, 283: 291–292.

Kannry JL, Chalmers TC, Orza M, Reitman D, Brown D (1989). Neglect of aged in clinical trials. Clin. Research (in press).

Kaunitz AM, Spence C, Danielson TS, Rochat RW, Grimes DA (1984). Perinatal and maternal mortality in a religious group avoiding obstetric care. Am J Obstet Gynecol, 150: 826–830.

Keirse MJNC (1988). Amniotomy or oxytocin for induction of labour: Re-analysis of a 'randomized' trial. Acta Obstet Gynecol Scand, 67: 731–735.

Kerr MG (1975). Problems and Perspectives in Reproductive Medicine. Inaugural Lecture No. 61. University of Edinburgh.

Khurmi NS, Bowles MJ, Kohli RS, Raftery EB (1986). Does placebo improve indexes of effort-induced myocardial ischaemia? Am J Cardiol, 57: 907–911.

King J (1986). Informed Consent. IME Bulletin, Suppl No. 3 (December). London: Institute of Medical Ethics.

Knaus WA, Le Gall JR, Wagner DP, Draper EA, Loirat P, Campos RA, Cullen DJ, Kohles MK, Glaser P, Granthil C, Mercier P, Nicolas F, Kikki P, Shin B, Snyder JV, Wattel F, Zimmerman JE (1982). A comparison of intensive care in the USA and France. Lancet, 2: 642–646.

Knaus WA, Draper EA, Wagner DP, Zimmerman JE (1985). Apache II: A severity of disease classification system. Crit Care Med, 13: 818–829.

Kramer MS, Shapiro SH (1984). Scientific challenges in the application of randomized trials. JAMA, 252: 2739–2745.

Kurosawa K (1984). Meta-analysis and selective publication bias. Am Psychol, 39: 73–74.

Lahtinen J, Alhava EM, Aukee S (1978). Early versus delayed operation for acute cholecystitis: A controlled clinical trial. Scand J Gastroenterol, 13: 673–678.

Lammer EJ, Chen DT, Hoar RM, Agnish ND, Benke PJ, Braun JT, Curry CJ, Fernhoff PM, Grix AW, Lott IT, Richard JM, Sun SC (1985). Retinoic embryopathy. New Engl Med J, 313: 837–841.

Lancet (1972). Drug or placebo? Lancet, 2: 122–123.

Lancet (1980). Blindness in surgical trials. Lancet, 1: 1229–1230.

Lancet (1986). The epistemology of surgery. Lancet, 1: 656–657.

Lancet (1987). Drop-outs from clinical trials. Lancet, 2: 892–893.

Lane DM, Dunlap WP (1978). Estimating effect size: Bias resulting from the significance criterion in editorial decisions. Br J Math Stat Psychol, 31: 107–112.

Lavori PW, Louis TA, Bailar JC, Polansky M (1983). Designs for experiments—parallel comparisons of treatment. New Engl J Med, 309: 1291–1299.

LeBaron S, Reyher J, Stack JM (1985). Paternalistic vs egalitarian physician styles: The treatment of patients in crisis. J Family Practice, 21: 56–62.

Lee KL, McNeer F, Starmer F, Harris PJ, Rosati RA (1980). Clinical judgement and statistics: Lessons from a simulated randomized trial in coronary artery disease. Circulation, 63: 508–515.

Liggins GC (1969). Premature delivery of foetal lambs infused with glucocorticoids. J Endocrinol, 45: 515–523.

Liggins GC, Howie RN (1972). A controlled trial of antepartum glucocorticoid treatment for the prevention of respiratory distress syndrome in premature infants. Pediatrics, 50: 515–525.

Lilford RJ (1987). Clinical experimentation in obstetrics. Br Med J, 295: 1298–1300.

Loftus EF, Fries JF (1979). Informed consent may be hazardous to health. Science, 204: 11.

Love JW (1975). Drugs and operations: Some important differences. JAMA, 232: 37–38.

Luborsky L, McLellan T, Woody GE, O'Brien CP (1985). Therapist success and its determinants. Arch Gen Psychiatry, 42: 602–611.

Lumley J (1987). Does this work? Pediatrics, 79: 1040–1044.

MacArthur BA, Howie RN, Dezoete JA, Elkins J (1982). School progress and cognitive development of 6-year-old children whose mothers were treated antenatally with betamethasone. Pediatrics, 70: 99–105.

MacDonald D, Grant A, Sheridan-Pereira M, Boylan P, Chalmers I (1985). The Dublin randomized controlled trial of intrapartum fetal heart rate monitoring. Am J Obstet Gynecol, 152: 524–539.

Macdonald RR (1987). In defence of the obstetrician. Br J Obstet Gynaecol, 94: 833–835.

Mahon WA, Daniel EE (1964). A method for the assessment of reports of drug trials. Can Med Assoc J, 90: 565–569.

Mahoney MJ (1977). Publication prejudices: An experimental study of confirmatory bias in the peer review system. Cogn Ther Res, 1: 161–175.

Mainland D (1960). The clinical trial—some difficulties and suggestions. J Chronic Dis, 11: 484–496.

Makuch RW, Johnson MF (1986). Some issues in the design and interpretation of 'negative' clinical studies. Arch Intern Med, 146: 986–989.

Malpas P (1953). Some aspects of biological causality. J Obstet Gynaecol Br Commnwlth, 60: 384–387.

Martin G (1984). Munchausen's statistical grid, which makes all trials significant. Lancet, 2: 1457.

Martin JD, Davis RE, Stenhouse N (1967). Serum folate and vitamin B_{12} levels in pregnancy with particular reference to uterine bleeding and bacteriuria. J Obstet Gynaecol Br Commnwlth, 74: 697–701.

McCormick JS (1976). The personal doctor 1975. J R Coll Gen Pract, 26: 750–753.

McIntyre N, Popper K (1983). The critical attitude in medicine: The need for a new ethics. Br Med J, 287: 1919–1923.

McPherson K (1982). On choosing the number of interim analyses in clinical trials. Stat Med, 1: 25–36.

Meier P (1983). Statistical analysis of clinical trials. In: Clinical Trials: Issues and Approaches. Shapiro SH, Louis TA (eds). New York: Marcel Dekker, pp 167–169.

Meinert CL (1986). Clinical Trials: Design, Conduct and Analysis. Oxford: Oxford University Press.

Meinert CL (1988). Towards prospective registration of clinical trials. Controlled Clin Trials, 9: 1–5.

Melmed RN, Roth D, Beer G, Edelstein EL (1986). Montaigne's insight: Placebo effect and symptom anticipation are two sides of the same coin. Lancet, 2: 1448–1449.

Menke JA, McClead RE (1987). On-line with Medline: An introduction for the pediatrician. Pediatrics, 80: 605–612.

Micciolo R, Valagussa P, Marubini E (1985). The use of historical controls in breast cancer: An assessment of three consecutive trials. Controlled Clin Trials, 6: 259–270.

Minchom P, Niswander K, Chalmers I, Dauncey M, Newcombe R, Elbourne D, Mutch L, Andrews J, Williams G (1987). Antecedents and outcome of very early neonatal seizures in infants born at or after term. Br J Obstet Gynaecol, 94: 431–439.

Moertel CG (1984). Improving the efficiency of clinical trials: A medical perspective. Stat Med, 3: 455–466.

Mosteller F, Gilbert JP, McPeek B (1980). Reporting standards and research strategies for controlled trials: Agenda for the editor. Controlled Clin Trials, 1: 37–58.

Mullen JL, Buzby GP, Matthews DC, Smale BF, Rosato EF (1980). Reduction of operative morbidity and mortality by combined preoperative and postoperative nutritional support. Ann Surg, 192: 604–613.

Murray GD (1986). Use of an international databank to compare outcome following severe head injury in different centres. Stat Med, 5: 103–112.

Newcombe RG (1987). Towards a reduction in publication bias. Br Med J, 295, 656–659.

Nicolaides KH, Campbell S, Bradley RJ, Bilardo CM, Soothill PW, Gibb D (1987). Maternal oxygen therapy for intrauterine growth retardation. Lancet, 1: 942–945.

Niswander K, Henson G, Elbourne D, Chalmers I, Redman C, Macfarlane JA, Tizard P (1984). Adverse outcome of pregnancy and the quality of obstetric care. Lancet, 2: 827–831.

Noller KL, Melton LJ (1985). Study design in perinatal medicine. Am J Perinatol, 2: 250–255.

Nyirjesy I, Hawks BL, Falls HC, Munsat TI, Pierce WE (1963). A comparative clinical study of the vacuum extractor and forceps. Am J Obstet Gynecol, 85: 1071–1082.

Odendaal H (1974). Evaluation of the aetiology and therapy of leg cramps during pregnancy. S Afr Med J, 48: 780–781.

Paneth N, Kiely JL, Wallenstein S, Marcus M, Pakter J, Susser M (1982). Newborn intensive care and neonatal mortality in low birthweight infants. New Engl Med J, 307: 149–155.

Peto R (1978). Clinical trial methodology. Biomedicine, 28: 24–36.

Peto R (1982). Statistical aspects of cancer trials. In: Treatment of Cancer. Halnan KE (ed). London: Chapman & Hall, pp 867–871.

Peto R (1987). Why do we need systematic overviews of randomized trials? Stat Med, 6: 233–240.

Peto R, Pike MC, Armitage P, Breslow NE, Cox DR, Howard SV, Mantel N, McPherson K, Peto J, Smith PG (1976). Design and analysis of randomized clinical trials requiring prolonged observation of each patient. I: Introduction and design. Br J Cancer, 34: 585–612.

Peto R, Pike MC, Armitage P, Breslow NE, Cox DR, Howard SV, Mantel N, McPherson K, Peto J, Smith PG (1977). Design and analysis of randomized clinical trials requiring prolonged observation of each patient. II: Analysis and examples. Br J Cancer, 35: 1–39.

Piantadosi S, Byar DP (1988). A proposal for registering clinical trials. Controlled Clin Trials, 9: 82–84.

Pocock SJ (1976). The combination of randomized and historical controls in clinical trials. J Chron Dis, 29: 175–188.

Pocock SJ (1977). Randomised clinical trials. Br Med J, 1: 1661.

Pocock SJ (1983). Clinical Trials: A Practical Approach. Chichester: John Wiley.

Pocock SJ (1985). Current issues in the design and interpretation of clinical trials. Br Med J, 290: 39–42.

Pontonnier G, Grandjean H (1975). Les essais thérapeutiques chez la femme enceinte. Anesthésie-Réanimation et Périnatologie, 1: 20–24.

Poynard T, Conn HO (1985). The retrieval of randomized clinical trials in liver disease from the medical literature: A comparison of MEDLARS and manual methods. Controlled Clin Trials, 6: 271–279.

Prendiville W, Elbourne E, Chalmers I (1988). The effects of routine oxytocic administration in the management of the third stage of labour: An overview of the evidence from controlled trials. Br J Obstet Gynaecol, 95: 3–16.

Punnonen R, Aro P, Kuukankorpi A, Pystynen P (1986). Fetal and maternal effects of forceps and vacuum extraction. Br J Obstet Gynaecol, 93: 1132–1135.

Rahimtoola SH (1985). Some unexpected lessons from large multicenter randomized clinical trials. Circulation, 72: 449–455.

Reed JF, Slaichert W (1981). Statistical proof in inconclusive 'negative' trials. Arch Intern Med, 141: 1307–1310.

Reiffenstein RJ, Schiltroth AJ, Todd DM (1968). Current standards in reported drug trials. Can Med Assoc J, 99: 1134–1135.

Reitman D, Sacks HS, Chalmers TC (1987). Technical quality assessment of randomized control trials. Controlled Clin Trials, 8: 282.

Reitman D, Chalmers TC, Nagalingam R, Sacks H (1988). Can efficacy of blinding be documented by meta-analysis? Paper presented to the Society for Clinical Trials, San Diego, 23–26 May.

Renou P, Chang A, Anderson I, Wood C (1976). Controlled trial of fetal intensive care. Am J Obstet Gynecol, 126: 470–476.

Reznik R, Ring I, Fletcher P, Berry G (1987). Mortality from myocardial infarction in different types of hospitals. Br Med J, 294: 1121–1125.

Roberton NRC (1982). Advances in respiratory distress syndrome. Br Med J, 284: 917–918.

Roberton NRC (1986). Textbook of Neonatology. Edinburgh: Churchill Livingstone, pp 289–290.

Robin ED (1987). Saltem plus boni quam mali efficere conare: At least try to do more good than harm. The Pharos, Winter: 40–44.

Rosen MG, Chik L (1984). The effect of delivery route on outcome in breech presentation. Am J Obstet Gynecol, 148: 909–913.

Rothman KJ (1978). A show of confidence. New Engl Med J, 299: 1362–1363.

Rothman KJ (1986). Modern Epidemiology. Boston: Little Brown, p 120.

Rudicel S, Esdaile J (1985). The randomized clinical trial in orthopaedics: Obligation or option? J Bone Joint Surg, 67A: 1284–1293.

Sackett DL (1979). Bias in analytic research. J Chron Dis, 32: 51–63.

Sackett DL (1980). The competing objectives of randomized trials. New Engl J Med, 303: 1059–1060.

Sackett DL (1986). Rules of evidence and clinical recommendations on the use of antithrombotic agents. Chest, 89: 2S-3S.

Sackett DL, Gent M (1979). Controversy in counting and

attributing events in clinical trials. New Engl Med J, 301: 1410–1412.

Sacks HS, Berrier, J, Reitman D, Ancona-Berk VA, Chalmers TC (1987). Meta-analyses of randomized controlled trials. New Engl Med J, 316: 450–455.

Sacks H, Chalmers TC, Smith H (1982). Randomized versus historical controls for clinical trials. Am J Med, 72: 233–240.

Sacks HS, Chalmers TC, Smith H (1983). Sensitivity and specificity of clinical trials: Randomized v historical controls. Arch Intern Med, 143: 753–755.

Schoolman HM (1979). Retrieving information on clinical trial methodology. Clin Pharmacol Ther, 25: 758–760.

Schoolman HM (1982). The clinician and the statistician. Stat Med, 1: 311–316.

Schneiderman MA (1966). Looking backward: Is it worth the crick in the neck? Am J Roentgenol, Radium Ther Nucl Med, 96: 230–235.

Schwartz D, Flamant R, Lellouch J (1970). L'Essai Thérapeutique chez l'Homme. Paris: Flammarion.

Semmelweiss I (1861). The etiology, concept, and prophylaxis of childbed fever. Translated and edited by K. Codell Carter, and republished in 1983 by University of Wisconsin Press: Madison and London, pp 63–64.

Shapira K, McClelland HA, Griffiths NR, Newell DJ (1970). Study on the effects of tablet colour in the treatment of anxiety states. Br Med J, 2: 446–449.

Shearer M (1984). The quality of perinatal studies: A disturbing episode. Birth, 11: 79–80.

Shenker JG, Serr DM (1967). Comparative study of delivery by vacuum extractor and forceps. Am J Obstet Gynecol, 98: 32–39.

Shuster S (1972). Primary cutaneous virilism or ideopathic hirsuties? Br Med J, 2: 285–286.

Silverman WA (1980). Retrolental Fibroplasia: A Modern Parable. London: Academic Press.

Silverman WA (1985). Human Experimentation: A Guided Step into the Unknown. Oxford: Oxford University Press.

Silverman WA (1987). Sample size, representativeness and credibility in pragmatic neonatal trials. Am J Perinatol, 4: 129–130.

Simes RJ (1986). Publication bias: The case for an international registry of clinical trials. J Clin Oncol, 4: 1529–1541.

Simes RJ (1987). Confronting publication bias: A cohort design for meta-analysis. Stat Med, 6: 11–29.

Simon R (1986). Confidence intervals for reporting the results of clinical trials. Ann Intern Med, 105: 429–435.

Sleep J, Grant AM, Garcia J, Elbourne DR, Spencer JAD, Chalmers I (1984). West Berkshire perineal management trial. Br Med J, 289: 587–590.

Smart RG (1964). The importance of negative results in psychological research. Canadian Psychologist, 5: 225–232.

Smith DG, Clemens J, Crede W, Harvey M, Gracely EJ (1987). Impact of multiple comparisons in randomized clinical trials. Am J Med, 83: 545–550.

Smith ML (1980). Publication bias and meta-analysis. Evaluation in Education, 4: 22–24.

Snow B (1985). Database selection in the life sciences. Database, 8: 15–44.

Sommer B (1987). The file drawer effect and publication rates in menstrual cycle research. Psychology of Women Qrtrly, 11: 233–242.

Somorjay L (1987). Letter to the editor. Birth. 14: 109.

Sox HC, Margulies I, Sox CH (1981). Psychologically mediated effects of diagnostic tests. Ann Intern Med, 95: 680–685.

Spodick DH (1971). Revascularization of the heart: Numerators in search of denominators. Am Heart J, 85: 579–583.

Spodick DH (1973). The surgical mystique and the double standard: Controlled trials of medical and surgical therapy for cardiac disease. Am Heart J, 85: 579–583.

Spodick DH (1975). Numerators without denominators: There is no FDA for the surgeon. JAMA, 232: 35–36.

Spodick DH (1982). The randomized controlled clinical trial: Scientific and ethical bases. Am J Med, 73: 420–425.

Spodick DH (1983). Barriers to acceptance of controlled phase III clinical trials: Behavioral factors. Biomed Pharmacother, 37: 60–61.

Sterling TD (1959). Publication decisions and their possible effects on inferences drawn from tests of significance—or vice versa. J Am Stat Assoc, 54: 30–34.

Steven C (1987). Oxygen therapy: Baby lifesaver. The Independent, 29 December.

Stilwell J, Szczepura A, Mugford M (1988). Factors affecting the outcome of maternity care I. Relationship between staffing and perinatal deaths at the hospital of birth. J Epidemiol Community Health, 42: 157–169.

Streiff RR, Little AB (1967). Folic acid deficiency in pregnancy. New Engl J Med, 276: 776–779.

Sundt TM (1987). Was the international randomized trial of extracranial–intracranial arterial bypass representative of the population at risk? New Engl Med J, 316: 814–816.

Susser M (1984). Causal thinking in practice: Strengths and weaknesses of the clinical vantage point. Pediatrics, 74: 842–849.

Tabor A, Philip J, Madsen M, Bang J, Obel EB, Nordgaard-Pedersen B (1986). Randomized controlled trial of genetic amniocentesis in 4606 low-risk women. Lancet, 1: 1287–1293.

Thomas KB (1978). The consultation and the therapeutic illusion. Br Med J, 1: 1327–1328.

Thomas KB (1987). General practice consultations: Is there any point in being positive? Br Med J, 294: 1200–1202.

Timm M (1979). Prenatal education evaluation. Nursing Res, 28: 338–342.

Tyson JE, Furzan JA, Reisch JS, Mize SG (1983). An evaluation of the quality of therapeutic studies in perinatal medicine. J Pediatr, 102: 10–13.

Uhlenhuth EH, Canter A, Neustadt JO, Payson HE (1959). The symptomatic relief of anxiety with mebrobamate, phenobarbital and placebo. Am J Psychiatry, 115: 905–910.

Ulfelder H (1980). The stilbestrol disorders in historical perspective. Cancer, 45: 3008–3011.

Vandenbroucke JP (1988). Passive smoking and lung cancer: A publication bias? Br Med J, 296: 391–392.

Van der Linden W (1980). Pitfalls in randomized surgical trials. Surgery, 87: 258–262.

Van der Linden W, Sunzel H (1970). Early versus delayed operation for acute cholecystitis: A controlled clinical trial. Am J Surg, 120: 6–13.

Venning GR (1982). The validity of anecdotal reports of suspected adverse drug reactions—the problem of false alarms. Br Med J, 284: 249–252.

Vere DW (1979). Validity of cross-over trials. Br J Clin Pharmacol, 8: 5–6.
Vere DW, Chaput de Saintonge DM (1976). Double-blind trials. Lancet, 1: 546.
Walster GW, Cleary TA (1970). A proposal for a new editorial policy in the social sciences. Am Statistician, 24: 16–19.
Warlow C, Peto R (1987). Extracranial-intracranial bypass, one; clinical trials, nil. Br Med J, 295: 211.
Wennberg JE, Roos N, Sola L, Schori A, Jaffe R (1987). Use of claims data systems to evaluate health care outcomes. JAMA, 257: 933–936.
White KR (1982). The relation between socioeconomic status and academic achievement. Psychol Bull, 91: 461–481.
Whiting-O'Keefe QE (1982). Controlled clinical trials. Am J Med, 73: A56.
Whiting-O'Keefe QE, Henke C, Simborg DW (1984). Choosing the correct unit of analysis in medical care experiments. Medical Care, 22: 1101–1114.
Wider JA, Erez S, Steer CM (1967). An evaluation of the vacuum extractor in a series of 201 cases. Am J Obstet Gynecol, 98: 24–31.
Wilhelmsen L, Ljungberg S, Wedel H, Werko L (1976). A comparison between participants and non-participants in a primary preventive trial. J Chron Dis, 29: 331–339.
Williamson JW, Goldschmidt PG, Colton T (1986). The quality of medical literature: An analysis of validation assessments. In: Medical Uses of Statistics. Bailar JC, Mosteller F (eds). Mass: NEJM Books, pp 370–391.
Wolf S (1950). Effects of suggestion and conditioning on action of chemical agents in human subjects—pharmacology of placebos. J Clin Invest, 29: 100–109.
Wolf S (1959). Placebos. In: Research Publications of the Association for Research in Nervous and Mental Disease, U37: 147–161.
Wulff HR (1973). Confidence limits in evaluating controlled therapeutic trials. Lancet, 2: 969–970.
Yusuf S, Collins R, Peto R (1984). Why do we need some large, simple randomized trials? Stat Med, 3: 409–420.
Zelen M (1983). Guidelines for publishing papers on cancer clinical trials: Responsibilities of editors and authors. J Clin Oncol, 1: 164–169.

2 Materials and methods used in synthesizing evidence to evaluate the effects of care during pregnancy and childbirth

Iain Chalmers, Jini Hetherington, Diana Elbourne, Marc J. N. C. Keirse, and Murray Enkin

'If, as is sometimes supposed, science consisted in nothing but the laborious accumulation of facts, it would soon come to a standstill, crushed, as it were, under its own weight. The suggestion of a new idea, or the detection of a law, supersedes much that has previously been a burden on the memory, and by introducing order and coherence facilitates the retention of the remainder in an available form . . . Two processes are thus at work side by side, the reception of new material and the digestion and assimilation of the old; and as both are essential we may spare ourselves the discussion of their relative importance'

Lord Rayleigh 1884

1 Introduction

The quotation with which this chapter opens was cited by Isabella Leitch in a paper in which she went on to stress that a review of research should not only assemble the data on some problem or controversy, but should 'attempt to achieve a synthesis and to formulate a solution' (Leitch 1976). Dr Leitch had an unrivalled ability to assemble, evaluate, and extract the meaning and implications of data (Thomson 1981), an ability epitomized in her and Frank Hytten's classic text on the physiology of pregnancy (Hytten and Leitch 1965).

As noted by Light and Pillemer (1984) at the beginning of an excellent book on 'the science of reviewing research', some scientists have a remarkably casual attitude to the process of synthesizing research evidence. Formal evaluations of the quality of review articles in both the social and medical sciences have confirmed that there are indeed grounds for concern

(Jackson 1980; Cooper 1982; Cooper 1984; Einarson *et al.* 1985; Mulrow 1987; Oxman and Guyatt 1988). A recent analysis of review articles published in four major medical journals, for example, concluded that current medical reviews do not routinely use scientific methods to identify, assess, and synthesize information (Mulrow 1987). As Pillemer (1984) has put it, the usual, informal review is 'subjective, relying on idiosyncratic judgments about such key issues as which studies to include and how to draw overall conclusions. Studies are considered one at a time, with strengths and weaknesses selectively identified and casually discussed. Since the process is informal, it is not surprising that different reviewers often draw very different conclusions from the same set of studies'. In some instances, there is evidence that the conclusions reached by reviewers are based more on factors such as their gender and how they make their living than on the available evidence (Eagly and Carli 1981; Chalmers TC 1982).

Formal reviews of research attempt to bring scientific principles to bear on the review process. To quote Pillemer (1984) again, the basic tenets of formal reviews of research evidence include 'making reviewing practices explicit, and replacing personal decision rules with objective statistical procedures. The reviewer specifies how studies were selected, displays the result summaries on which conclusions are based, and uses integrative techniques consistent with good statistical practice. Different reviewers using the same analysis strategy should come up with the same statistical output. Others may disagree with an analysis, but at least they know what was done.' Acceptance of these principles is beginning to lead to a wider acceptance of the importance of improving the quality of medical research reviews (Morgan 1986; Huth 1987; Sacks *et al.* 1987; L'Abbé *et al.* 1987; Oxman and Guyatt 1988; Mulrow *et al.*, 1988; Thacker 1988; Ellenberg 1988).

One of the most persuasive arguments for conducting formal reviews and syntheses of research results is that it is always difficult, and often impossible, to assimilate and synthesize informally the numerical data generated by a body of independent but related research studies. This limitation of informal reviews has been demonstrated in both observational and experimental studies (Wolf 1986). In an experiment conducted by Cooper and Rosenthal (1980), for example, 32 graduate students and 9 faculty members were randomly assigned to review the same body of research literature, either by using the traditional, informal approach, or by using simple statistical techniques for achieving a quantitative synthesis of the results. Those who used traditional reviewing methods were more likely to overlook a small but significant effect when compared with those who used the formal approach.

Formal, quantitative synthesis of evidence derived from a set of similar, but independent, experiments is not a new way of trying to make sense out of a body of research. It has been used by statisticians for at least half a century (Hedges 1987). Although it is more than 30 years since these methods were first adopted in social, psychological, and medical research (Jones and Fiske 1953; Mosteller and Bush 1954; Beecher 1955), it was not really until the 1970s that they began to be used extensively (Light and Smith 1971). During the 1970s, quantitative synthesis of research results was adopted rapidly by educational and psychological researchers, one of whom named the process 'meta-analysis' (Glass 1976). During the 1980s, meta-analysis has also been rapidly adopted by clinical researchers (Halvorsen 1986; Sacks *et al.* 1987). The authors of a recent review of the subject were able to identify only 17 reports of meta-analyses in the clinical field published prior to 1980, but found that at least 69 had been published between that time and October 1986 (Sacks *et al.* 1987).

The impact of meta-analysis in clinical research is only just beginning to be felt; and, quite properly, questions have been raised about the validity of the approach (Searles 1985; Wachter 1988). Although it is certain that the methods used to conduct formal, quantitative syntheses of research results will be refined and improved, however, it would be wrong to see meta-analysis itself as a fad. As Bangert-Drowns (1986) has put it, meta-analysis is 'rooted in the fundamental values of the scientific enterprise: replicability, quantification, causal and correlational analysis. Valuable information is needlessly scattered in individual studies. The ability . . . to deliver generalizable answers to basic questions of policy is too serious a concern to allow us to treat research integration lightly.'

The process of synthesizing the results of similar but separate randomized trials has been described well by Peto (1987): 'While we cannot assume that different trials are exactly comparable, or that patients in different trials are exactly comparable, it is reasonable to assume that if different trials address related questions then there is going to be some tendency for the answers to come out in the same direction. That tendency may well be obscured in individual trials, or even in some cases reversed, by the play of chance. But elsewhere it may remain, and it is that tendency which the overview is trying to detect. In performing overviews we are not trying to provide exact quantitative estimates of percentage risk reductions in some precisely defined population of patients. We are simply trying to determine whether or not some type of treatment—tested in a wide range of trials—produces any effect on outcome. If it does, then the effect seen in the trials is likely to generalize at least qualitatively to the even more loosely defined range of patients to whom the trial results are likely to be applied in the real world.'

As far as we are aware, the first published report of a

quantitative overview of randomized controlled trials involving care during pregnancy or childbirth was an analysis based on published and unpublished data derived from 4 randomized trials in which different methods of monitoring the fetus during labour had been compared (Chalmers I 1979). The analysis was instructive in at least one respect: the disproportionate distribution of 13 cases of neonatal seizures among the 2000 or so babies who had been entered into the 4 trials before birth was unexpected because it had not previously been detected, and it seemed unlikely to have occurred by chance (Table 2.1a). This observation generated a hypothesis that, compared to intermittent auscultation of the fetal heart, continuous fetal heart monitoring with an option to assess fetal acid–base status using scalp blood sampling led to a reduced risk of subsequent neonatal seizures. This prestated hypothesis was subsequently tested and sustained (Table 2.1b) in a randomized trial involving more than 13,000 women and their babies (MacDonald *et al.* 1985; see Chapter 54). Since the publication of the overview of randomized comparisons of alternative methods of intrapartum fetal monitoring in 1979, several other aspects of care during pregnancy and childbirth have been assessed using this approach (Grant and Mohide 1982; Collins *et al.* 1985; King *et al.* 1985; Thacker 1985; Saunders *et al.* 1985; Grant 1986a,b; Oakley *et al.* 1986; Elbourne *et al.* 1987, 1988; Prendiville *et al.* 1988; King *et al.* 1988; Crowley *et al.* 1990; Goldstein *et al.* 1989; Daya 1989).

Table 2.1 (a) Distribution of 13 cases of neonatal seizures in 2032 babies entered as fetuses in 4 randomized trials comparing different methods of intrapartum fetal monitoring (Chalmers I 1979)

Trial	Continuous EFM + acid–base	Intermittent auscultation	Continuous EFM alone
Haverkamp *et al.* (1976)	—	2/241	2/242
Renou *et al.* (1976)	0/175	4/175	—
Haverkamp *et al.* (1979)	0/230	2/232	2/233
Kelso *et al.* (1978)	—	1/251	0/253

Table 2.1 (b) Distribution of 39 cases of neonatal seizures in 13,084 babies entered as fetuses in a randomized comparison of intermittent auscultation with continuous recording of the fetal heart, with acid–base assessment when indicated, mounted to test hypothesis derived from observations shown in (a), above.

	Continuous EFM + acid–base	Intermittent auscultation	p
MacDonald *et al.* (1985)	12/6530	27/6554	<0.025

In this book we have attempted to extend this work to cover as completely as possible all the randomized controlled trials of care during pregnancy and childbirth. We outlined our strategy for 'achieving a synthesis' of this research more than a decade ago. We chose to concentrate on evidence derived from randomized trials because of the particular strengths of this research design for making unbiased comparisons between alternative forms of care (see Chapter 1). In addition to envisaging a review that concentrated on evidence generated by randomized trials, our outline for this formal review of research evidence also envisaged quantitative syntheses of data derived from similar, but independent, trials. In planning to do this, we hoped that it might sometimes be possible to identify patterns of results which might otherwise have remained obscure (because of the random variation of small numbers), and thus increase the likelihood that relatively small effects of treatment would be detected reliably. Detection of small effects in this way may be dismissed by some people as irrelevant; but as the author of the term 'meta-analysis' has put it, 'by what logic would one *want* to overlook small effects that are actually present but are obscured by uncontrolled error? One may not be satisfied with small effects, but rejecting them as inadequate is different from not seeing them at all. If effects are small, one tries to increase them if one can: or one lives with them if one must.' (Gottman and Glass 1978).

Formal, quantitative syntheses (overviews) of the results of similar, but separate trials in the perinatal field can help to clarify issues that have remained obscure because, in trials with small numbers, the chances of distinguishing random variation from real but moderate treatment effects may be quite low (see Section 5 of Chapter 1). For example, there continues to be disagreement both among obstetricians and among neonatologists about whether or not maternal corticosteroid administration reduces the risk of respiratory distress among infants who deliver before 31 weeks' gestation (see, for example, Roberton 1982). Table 2.2 displays data derived from the 7 trials from which relevant data are available. The table shows that estimates of the effect vary from one trial to another; but it also shows that the data derived from every one of these trials is consistent with the hypothesis that antenatal corticosteroids have a beneficial effect in babies of this gestational age. By synthesizing all the available data in this systematic way, it becomes clear that the protective effect of corticosteroids in very immature babies has tended to be obscured by the random varia-

Table 2.2 Effect of corticosteroids prior to preterm delivery on RDS in babies <31 weeks' gestation

Study	EXPT		CTRL		Odds ratio	Graph of odds ratios and confidence intervals
	n	(%)	*n*	(%)	(95% CI)	0.01 0.1 0.5 1 2 10 100
Liggins and Howie (1972)	10/36	(27.78)	15/26	(57.69)	0.29 (0.11–0.82)	
Taeusch *et al.* (1979)	1/3	(33.33)	4/6	(66.67)	0.30 (0.02–4.18)	
Gamsu (unpub)	4/29	(13.79)	7/39	(17.95)	0.74 (0.20–2.70)	
Collaborative (1981)	6/10	(60.00)	7/16	(43.75)	1.87 (0.40–8.80)	
Morales *et al.* (1986)	17/53	(32.08)	32/52	(61.54)	0.31 (0.14–0.66)	
Papageorgiou *et al.* (1979)	2/5	(40.00)	11/12	(91.67)	0.07 (0.01–0.73)	
Morrison *et al.* (1978)	6/36	(16.67)	11/28	(39.29)	0.32 (0.11–0.97)	
Typical odds ratio (95% confidence interval)					0.38 (0.24–0.60)	

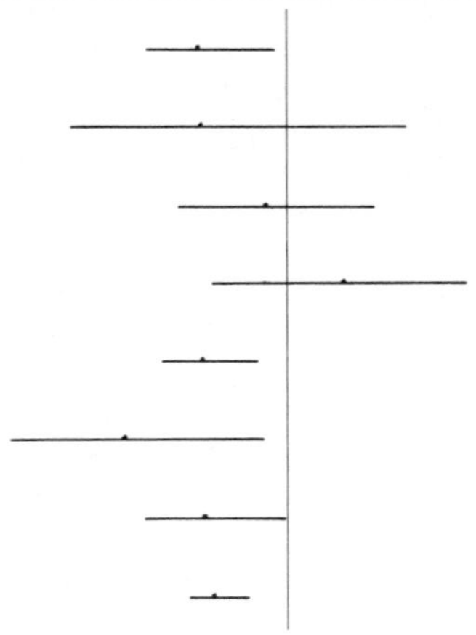

random variation resulting from the small numbers of such babies born in each of the available trials.

The two principal objectives of most of the analyses presented in this book have thus been first, to minimize systematic error (bias) in comparisons of alternative forms of care during pregnancy and childbirth; and second, to minimize random error (the play of chance) and thus increase the likelihood that relatively modest, but potentially important effects of care will not be underestimated (or overestimated). In the sections of this chapter that follow we describe the Materials and Methods that we and our collaborators have used in pursuit of these two objectives, and discuss the interpretation of the trial overviews (meta-analyses) that have resulted.

2 Materials

2.1 Inclusion criteria

For the reasons discussed in Chapter 1, we restricted our systematic search for studies comparing alternative forms of care to those in which the allocation of individuals (mothers or babies) to alternative forms of care had been either by formal random assignment, or by some quasi-random method, such as alternation, case record number, or date of birth (Chalmers I *et al.* 1986). Some commentators have already criticized us for limiting our search to trials in which an effort was made to control selection bias prospectively in this way (Hawkins 1987); in the view of others (Collins, personal communication), we have been too liberal in our inclusion of trials in which treatment allocation could be ascertained prior to inclusion of participants in the study (and which therefore are more likely to have been biased).

We based our decision to identify and retrieve studies in which a process of prospective allocation of individuals to alternative forms of care may have been biased on two considerations. First, we anticipated that some of these trials would be rejected at a later stage in the review process: we felt that a reviewer conducting a focused and systematic analysis could, if necessary, reject reports if they did not meet his or her *prespecified* criteria of methodological adequacy. Second, if we had restricted our consideration to trials in which an apparently secure method of randomization had not only been used, but had also actually been validated as having been secure, we would have ended up with no studies to review at all! Although the actual method of allocation used was sometimes such that it would have been difficult or impossible for those responsible for recruiting participants to know or guess the next treatment in line (for example, when telephone randomization or coded drugs were used), we came across no trial in which there had been any formal assessment of the extent to which treatment allocation was, in fact, predictable among those responsible for recruiting participants.

As Hunter and his colleagues (1982) have pointed out, the assertion of 'methodological inadequacy' always depends on theoretical assumptions about what *might* be true in a study. These assumptions may well be false and are rarely tested in their own right. We have not ignored the likelihood that certain methods of treatment allocation are more likely than others to lead to bias. As discussed in Sections 3.4 and 4.2 of this chapter (see below), the methodological quality of the trials in this and other respects has been formally assessed, and taken into account in the presentation and interpretation of the data.

2.2 Identification of relevant studies

2.2.1 Published reports

If the results of a review of research within a particular field are to be valid, one of the preconditions is that they should have been based on an examination of the results of as high a proportion as possible of all the relevant investigations (see Section 7 of Chapter 1). One of our objectives, therefore, has been to identify as high a proportion as possible of the randomized and quasi-randomized comparisons of alternative forms of care given during pregnancy and childbirth.

A number of search strategies have been used in an attempt to identify as high a proportion as possible of all published reports of randomized controlled trials relevant to this book, and its companion volume on the care of the newborn infant (Sinclair and Bracken, in preparation). These are summarized in Fig. 2.1 and have been described in detail elsewhere (Chalmers I *et al.* 1986). Suffice it to say here that, although we have searched MEDLINE every month since June 1974, the mainstay of our search strategy has been a systematic and ongoing scrutiny of the contents of about 60 journals, beginning with the volumes published in 1950. When it has not been clear in the published report of a study whether or not a controlled trial (as defined above) has been conducted, a letter has been sent to the authors asking them to clarify the method by which they allocated participants to the alternative forms of care compared. Details of eligible trials have then been entered in an electronic database, the *Oxford Database of Perinatal Trials* (Chalmers I *et al.* 1986; Chalmers 1988).

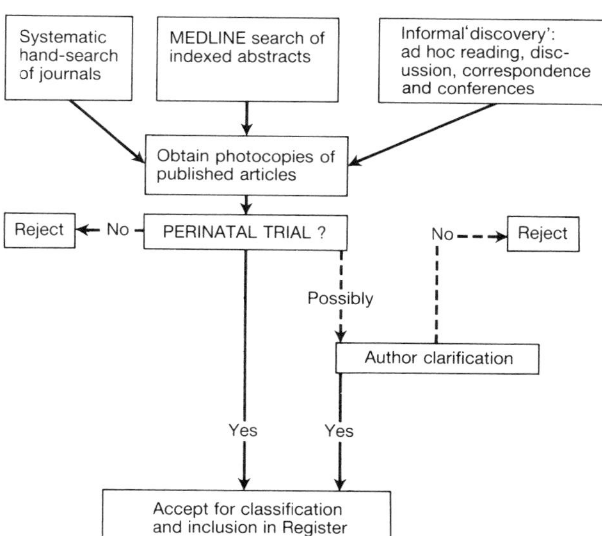

Fig. 2.1 Search strategy for published reports of randomized controlled trials in perinatal medicine

Over 4000 reports of controlled trials published in over 250 journals have been identified in this way (National Perinatal Epidemiology Unit 1985; Chalmers I *et al.* 1986; Chalmers 1988). About two-thirds of this total are reports of obstetric trials and the remainder are mostly reports of trials involving neonates. The latter are currently being analysed and will be published in a sequel to this book entitled *Effective Care of the Newborn Infant* (Sinclair and Bracken, in preparation). Formal comparisons between subject-specific searches of MEDLINE and those using our register of published reports of perinatal trials have shown that more than 85 per cent of all the trial reports identified by the two methods combined can be identified using the *Oxford Database of Perinatal Trials*, compared to less than 50 per cent identified using MEDLINE (Table 2.3). There is no 'Gold Standard' against which to assess what proportions these represent of *all* relevant trials, but omissions have been added to the Database as and when they have been identified.

Table 2.3 Comparison of the yields by subject-specific searching for relevant reports of randomized controlled trials for 5 perinatal topics using MEDLINE, and the Oxford Database of Perinatal Trials (ODPT)

Topic	Total No. of relevant reports identified	No. (%) identified using: MEDLINE	ODPT
Neonatal hyperbilirubinaemia*	96	20 (20.8)	88 (91.7)
Intraventricular haemorrhage*	34	19 (41.2)	29 (85.3)
Progestogens for recurrent miscarriage†	15	6 (40.0)	15 (100.0)
Preterm, prelabour rupture of membranes†	17	8 (47.1)	16 (94.1)
Social support in labour†	4	2 (50.0)	4 (100.0)

* Data published by Dickersin *et al.* 1985
† Data kindly provided by Salim Daya, Arne Ohlsson, and Joy Rogers, October 1987.

2.2.2 Unpublished studies

The problem presented by the tendency among investigators, peer reviewers, and journal editors to allow the direction and statistical significance of research findings to influence decisions regarding submission and publication has been outlined in the previous chapter (see Section 5.2 of Chapter 1). The extent to which this publication bias exists among trials relating to care during pregnancy and childbirth is unknown (Chalmers I 1985a,b); but in any case, it probably varies from topic to topic. In an attempt to minimize the effects of this bias in the reviews prepared for this book, we surveyed over 40,000 obstetricians and paediatricians in 18 countries in an attempt to obtain information about any completed but unpublished controlled trials of which they were aware (Hetherington *et al.* 1989). The survey yielded information about 400 unpublished trials, but the vast majority of these had either been completed quite recently, or were still recruiting or about to begin recruiting. We were notified of only 18 unpublished trials completed more than two or three years previously, a period during which nearly 2000 reports of trials relevant to this book were published.

We are aware of several methodologically sound trials completed during this era which have not yet been reported in print by the investigators responsible for them. Furthermore, the anecdotal information available to us is in line with the research findings cited in the previous chapter (see Chapter 1, Section 5): these unreported studies appear to have yielded results which have been 'disappointing' to the investigators in some way. Conclusions based on published evidence may thus be biased because investigators have withheld unpublished data in this way (Chalmers 1989). Unfortunately, little can be done to reduce this bias in the short term. In the meantime, we remain very grateful to those investigators who did help us to try to overcome this problem by providing information derived from their unpublished studies (Acknowledgements, p xi).

2.3 Obtaining unreported information

A dispute continues about whether, on average, seeking unpublished information from the authors of published reports of trials results in a reduction or an increase in the biases to which trial overviews can be subject (Mosteller 1979; Messer *et al.* 1983; Furberg and Morgan 1987; Sacks *et al.* 1987; Chalmers TC *et al.* 1987b; Peto 1987; Collins *et al.* 1987; Yusuf 1987; L'Abbé *et al.* 1987; Begg and Berlin 1988). Comparisons of overviews in which unreported data have been included with overviews based solely on reported data have shown that conclusions are sometimes similar and that they sometimes differ (Chalmers TC *et al.* 1987b).

It is certainly possible that investigators who are asked for unpublished information about a published study will respond to questions about the methodological rigour with which they conducted their studies in a way which tends to play down any inadequacies. They may even consciously or unconsciously embellish their data in such a way as to encourage unjustified inferences about the effects of a particular form of care. While not unconcerned about the danger of introducing biases by using this approach, however, we have been more concerned about failing to address biases resulting from selective reporting (see Section 5 of Chapter 1), particularly if we could address these by obtaining missing information.

The biases which might result from basing overviews on published, but incomplete data may occur either because a published analysis had not been based on data relating to all participants entered into the trial (see Section 4.4 of Chapter 1), or from selective reporting of some outcome measures and not others (see Section 5.2 of Chapter 1).

As already noted in Section 5.2 of Chapter 1, a 'result-dependent' reporting bias in respect of whole trials is known to exist (Simes 1987; Dickersin *et al.* 1987). We think that unless convincing evidence is produced which suggests otherwise, it should be assumed that bias also influences decisions about which outcomes are reported in published accounts of controlled trials (Furberg and Morgan 1987; Bulpitt 1988).

It was against this background that we encouraged our collaborators to try to obtain missing information from the authors of the trial reports which they were responsible for reviewing. In one instance (see Chapter 38), this advice ran contrary to the known position of the authors on this matter (Sacks *et al.* 1987). The usual approach adopted involved sending dummy tabulations and a covering letter to the authors of the published report, asking them to fill in the blanks with the unpublished information requested. The example of this approach that was sent as guidance to our collaborators has been reproduced as Appendix 2.1.

The experience of others who have tried to obtain unpublished information from authors of published reports has varied. In 1962, for example, Wolins reported writing to 37 authors requesting raw data from studies reported during the two previous years: 21 reported that the data had been lost or destroyed, 5 did not reply, 2 claimed proprietary rights, and 4 sent data too late for them to be used (Wolins 1962). Fortunately, we and others have often received more helpful responses (Chalmers I 1979; Eaton 1984; Thacker 1985; Saunders *et al.* 1985; Peto 1987; Collins *et al.* 1987; King *et al.* 1988; Prendiville *et al.* 1988; Early Breast Cancer Trialists Collaborative Group 1988; see Acknowledgements), and many investigators have been very helpful to us and our collaborators during the preparation of this book (see Acknowledgements, p xi). They have clarified aspects of their study designs and have often been able and willing to provide data that were either not presented at all in the published reports of their trials, or presented in a form (for example, as mean values) which precluded their incorporation in the standard form of overview (based on dichotomized variables) that we adopted (see Sections 3.6 and 3.7 below).

3 Methods

3.1 Provision of bibliographies for chapter authors

We have tried to ensure that references to reports of all controlled trials of probable or possible relevance were available to colleagues who agreed to collaborate on specific chapters in this book. Initially we sent them each a list of 'chapter-specific' references and offered to provide photocopies of any reports which they could not obtain easily. On two further occasions during the following year these initial listings were updated with supplementary listings of references to new accessions to the *Oxford Database of Perinatal Trials*. One year after the initial listings had been sent out, a composite listing of all of the references notified during the course of these three mailings was sent to collaborators for each of the chapters for which they were responsible. Authors were asked to return these composite listings after they had annotated them to show which trials would be referenced in their chapter(s); which trials had been assessed for quality (see Section 3.4, below); which trials had been incorporated in the overviews they had prepared; and which trials would not be discussed in their chapter(s) (giving a brief note of the reasons for this). In addition, we asked our collaborators to notify us of any relevant reports of controlled trials which we had not listed. This request was made so that these references could be added to the *Oxford Database of Perinatal Trials* if they met the accession criteria and had not already been incorporated, or recoded if inaccurate coding had led to their omission from the listings we had provided. Our collaborators also drew our attention to duplicate reporting of the same trial in separate publications. Recognition of duplicate reporting was important, not only to avoid entering data from a particular study more than once into an overview, but also to ensure that all the available data were identified when the results of a particular trial had been reported in more than one publication.

3.2 Grouping studies for overviews (meta-analyses)

Some of the most animated disagreements about the validity of quantitative syntheses of the results of independent studies are fuelled by differences of opinion about which studies are sufficiently alike to be considered for inclusion in a single overview of similar studies. Sometimes criticisms of overviews have been based on a view that it is wrong to combine information from studies that vary in their methodological quality (Eysenck 1978). In addition, some have suggested that differences in either the study populations, the interventions compared, or the outcome measures used in independent studies argue against quantitative syntheses of their results (Goldman and Feinstein 1979; Toth and Horwitz 1983; Horwitz 1987). Others have noted how the conclusions drawn from an overview can be influenced by differences of opinion about which studies to include (Conn and Blitzer 1976; Messer *et al.* 1983; Conn and Poynard 1985).

On the other hand, other commentators have noted that overviews based on data drawn from a variety of contexts provide conclusions that are more robust and therefore more useful for broad policy decisions (Hedges 1988). As Johnson and his colleagues (1982) have put it, 'The more variation in places, people and procedures the research can withstand and still yield the same findings, the more externally valid the findings . . . What practitioners need are validated theories that they can apply conceptually with some confidence, not idiosyncratic operationalizations aimed only at a specific set of circumstances.'

We describe later in this chapter how we have addressed the issue of interpreting overviews when the methodology of the trials included has been of variable quality (see Section 4.2). As far as judgments about the extent to which particular trials are sufficiently similar in other respects to be grouped in an overview, we explicitly left it to chapter authors, most of whom are specialists in the fields that they have reviewed, to make *a priori* judgments about which trials might be grouped together (see Appendix 2.2).

The underlying assumption when trials are grouped in an overview is that, although variations in the way that an intervention is applied may result in effects of different size, and although different populations of trial participants may show differences in the size of the response to the intervention, these differences are likely to be differences in the *extent* of the effect rather than differences in the *direction* of the effect. This does not, of course, mean that a different direction of effect would not occur if a clearly different intervention were to be used, or if the intervention being evaluated were to be used in people for whom there was some prior reason to think that it was inappropriate. In such cases, differences in direction of effect might be anticipated. For instance, cervical cerclage may well be successful in prolonging gestation in women whose obstetrical history is suggestive of cervical incompetence (see Chapter 40), but it is entirely plausible that the operation, when used in women with a negligible risk of preterm delivery, will lead to an increased risk of the very outcome which it is intended to prevent.

There can be no hard and fast rules about which trials are sufficiently similar to be grouped in an overview and some readers may prefer to review different subsets of trials, or to use different endpoints to those chosen and analysed by our collaborators and ourselves. If so, they will often find that the data from each constituent trial have been presented in sufficient detail to enable these further analyses to be performed.

3.3 Control of bias during data collection

A number of writers have drawn attention to the desirability of controlling for observer bias and variability during three stages of data collection for a review of research evidence: during the process of initial selection of studies for inclusion in the review; during assessment of the methodological quality of the studies; and during the process of abstracting data from the reports selected (Rosenthal 1978; Stock *et al.* 1982; Rosenthal 1984; Orwin and Cordray 1985; Louis *et al.* 1985; Light 1987; Sacks *et al.* 1987). TC Chalmers and his colleagues (Chalmers TC *et al.* 1981, 1987a; Sacks *et al.* 1987), for example, suggest differential photocopying of published reports (that is, separating the Materials and Methods sections from the Results sections) so that the quality of the study methods can be scored independently of the quality of the analyses, and in ignorance of the results. They recommend that this should be done independently by at least two assessors who have been blinded both to the identity of the experimental groups, and to the authorship of the report.

Again, although some of our collaborators took these precautions, the resources required to implement them were simply not available to the majority. TC Chalmers and his colleagues (1988) have estimated that an average of about 6 hours per paper is required to blind the copy of the paper; read it; discuss it with co-investigators; and extract the pertinent data (supervisory, secretarial, and analysis time was not included in this estimate). We did ask our collaborators, if at all possible, to make decisions as to whether or not to include a particular trial in an overview after assessing its methodological quality, but before considering its results. We reminded them to be alert to the possibility that their decision to include or exclude a particular trial (or data generated by that trial, see Section 2.3, above) might be influenced by the results rather than the methodological quality of the study in question. We also suggested that they might wish to mention to their readers why they had rejected particular trials, and we encouraged those who wished to publish more detailed accounts of their methodology than we could incorporate in an already very long book to publish their analyses in a fuller form elsewhere (see Appendix 2.2).

3.4 Evaluation of methodological quality of relevant studies

As already noted above, trials that fulfil the methodological criteria for inclusion in our Database (random or quasi-random treatment assignment) have been conducted with varying degrees of methodological rigour (see Section 4 of Chapter 1). When the results of individual trials within the overview appear to conflict, therefore, it is important to consider the extent to which this could be a reflection of bias resulting from methodological weaknesses. In these circumstances, it is obviously appropriate to invest relatively more faith in the results of trials of relatively good methodological quality.

Various approaches have been used for formal assessment of the methodological quality of trial reports (see Chapter 1, Section 4). The scheme proposed and used by TC Chalmers and his colleagues (1981) is probably the most widely known, and it has been adapted and used in the perinatal field by Tyson and his co-workers (1983). Both of these groups have contributed chapters to this book (see Chapters 38 and 75) and they have used their respective quality assessment schemes to evaluate the reports we listed for them. Unfortunately, both these schemes are time-consuming to apply, and we felt it would be unrealistic to require all of our coauthors to adopt this approach in assessing the methodological quality of the studies that they were responsible for reviewing. We had asked some of them to deal with as many as 200 reports of controlled trials, sometimes with little or no technical or secretarial support.

Because of these constraints we drew up a simplified scheme for assessing the methodological quality of the trials reviewed for this book (Prendiville *et al.* 1988). We asked our collaborators to rate the quality of each trial for which they were responsible by concentrating on the three dimensions of trial methodology that we felt were the most important potential sources of significant bias (see Appendix 2.2). These three dimensions were the *control of selection bias at entry* (the quality of the random allocation) (see Section 4.1 of Chapter 1); the *control of selection bias after entry* (the extent to which the primary analysis included every person entered into the randomized cohorts) (see Section 4.4 of Chapter 1); and the *control of bias in assessing outcome(s)* (the extent to which those assessing outcome(s) were kept unaware of the group assignment of the individuals examined) (see Section 4.3 of Chapter 1).

This simplified scheme of quality assessment has been shown to have acceptable replicability between different observers in respect of at least some of the groups of trials reviewed (Prendiville *et al.* 1988; Keirse and van Oppen, unpublished data; Parazzini *et al.*, unpublished data). Although the precise ranking of trials by methodological quality within a particular overview has sometimes varied between independent observers, we have enough experience of the way that the system performs to know that it discriminates satisfactorily between very good trials and trials with potentially important methodological shortcomings. We have decided not to present these quality assessments explicitly in this book, however, because their replicability has not yet been assessed formally on a wide enough scale. Later in this chapter we describe the way in which we have dealt with trials of different quality incorporated within a particular overview (see Section 4.2, below).

3.5 Assembling data for analysis

We asked our collaborators to extract data from each one of a group of similar trials and assemble an array of 'two by two' tables relating to each outcome of interest (see Appendix 2.2). In published trial reports, results are usually reported either as categorical data (number of subjects who either experience, or do not experience, a particular outcome), or as continuous data (with the outcome measure usually being expressed in terms of a mean, often with its standard deviation or standard error, or a median and its range). For example, gestational age at birth may be reported either as the proportion of infants born preterm, or as a mean with its standard deviation or standard error.

We decided to urge our collaborators to concentrate on assembling categorical data. Although comparisons of mean values of continuous variables may increase the chances that statistically significant differences between groups will be detected, the differences in mean values may be clinically irrelevant or, more seriously, may hide differences in rare events that are of great importance. For example, although comparisons of alternative forms of care may yield statistically significant differences in terms of mean gestational ages or mean durations of the second stage of labour, these data are uninformative about the likelihood of either group containing very preterm babies or women who experience a very prolonged second stage of labour. In circumstances in which several cut-off points were available, for example, for doses of anti-Rhesus(D) immunoglobulin administered postpartum, we relied on chapter authors to categorize data in any way that they judged would yield clinically relevant comparisons.

3.6 Statistical methods

As was illustrated by the overview of trials of corticosteroids administered prior to preterm delivery (Table 2.2), the fundamental assumption underlying an overview of more than one trial is that, if the trials concerned have addressed similar questions, then, but for the play of chance, they should yield answers that point in the same direction. This assumption is reflected in the statistical approach we have used (Mantel and Haenszel 1959; Peto *et al.* 1976; Yusuf *et al.* 1985), which has come to be referred to as the Mantel–Haentzel–Peto method (Chalmers TC and Buyse 1988). This method does *not* implicitly assume that the effects on outcome in different trials within an overview of similar trials are of the same size. Nor does it involve comparing participants in one trial with participants in another trial. The only direct comparisons made are between experimental and control participants within the same trial.

The basic principle involved in the method is straightforward. One statistic (and its variance) is calculated from each trial within the overview; these separate statistics are then added together and divided by the sum of their variances, to generate a 'typical' statistic that summarizes the totality of the evidence (see Fig. 2.2).

Trial 1	Difference 1	(experimental vs. control)
Trial 2	Difference 2	(experimental vs. control)
Trial 3	Difference 3	(experimental vs. control)
Grand Total	Difference 1 + Difference 2 + Difference 3	

Note: A test of whether the Grand Total differs significantly from zero entails only comparison of like with like within each separate trial.

The Variance of the Grand Total may be calculated simply by adding the separate variances of the separate differences derived from each trial

Fig. 2.2 Principle of unbiased combination of information from different trials (adapted from Antiplatelet Trialists Collaboration 1988).

Details of the statistical methods are presented in Appendix 2.3. The first step involves calculating, for each trial in the overview, the number of outcomes (for example, cases of respiratory distress syndrome) that would be expected in the experimental group if, in truth, the form of care used (for example, corticosteroid administration prior to preterm delivery) had no effect. This number of *Expected* events (*E*) is then subtracted from the number of events that were actually *Observed* (*O*) in the experimental group. If the form of care in question actually has no effect on the outcome these two numbers would be the same, were it not for the play of chance. If in truth, however, the experimental form of care was *more* effective than the control form of care in reducing the incidence of the outcome in question, fewer outcomes than expected would be observed in the experimental group (subtracting the number Expected from the number Observed would thus yield a negative value). If, on the other hand, the experimental form of care was, in truth, to increase the incidence of the outcome in question, more outcomes than expected would be observed in the experimental group (subtracting the number Expected from the number Observed would thus yield a positive value).

Adding these separate differences (Observed minus Expected) and their variances, derived from each trial, allows the calculation of a statistic (and its variance) that is 'typical' of the differences observed between experimental and control groups in the array of trials within the overview. This can be used not only to test the 'null hypothesis' (that the two forms of care have equivalent effects on the outcome in question), but also to estimate how large, and hence how worthwhile, any differential effects are likely to be. A convenient estimate for the latter purpose in provided by the typical odds ratio and its confidence interval (Yusuf *et al.* 1985). Thus, as shown in Fig. 2.2, the typical odds ratio (and its 95 per cent confidence interval) for respiratory distress syndrome among infants born prior to 31 weeks' gestation after corticosteroid administration is 0.39 (0.24–0.65). The fact that the confidence interval does not include 1 allows rejection of the 'null hypothesis'. In addition, the typical odds ratio of 0.39 allows one to estimate that corticosteroids given prior to preterm delivery result in a 61 per cent reduction in the odds of respiratory distress syndrome in babies born prior to 31 weeks' gestation. As shown by the odds ratios that form the bounds of the 95 per cent confidence interval, however, the true reduction in odds could quite easily be as low as 35 per cent, or as high as 76 per cent.

Because the odds ratio is a less familiar statistic to many people than the relative risk we have discussed their derivation and relationship in Appendix 2.4. The implications of a particular value of the odds ratio in practice are discussed in Section 4.3, below.

A wide choice of statistical methods and statistical descriptors is available for use in overviews (meta-analyses) of controlled trials (Solari and Wheatley 1966; Peto *et al.* 1976; 1977; Elashoff 1978; Hedges and Olkin 1985; Tarone 1981; Fleiss 1981; Hedges 1982, 1983; Yusuf *et al.* 1984, 1985; DerSimonian and Laird 1986; Bailey 1987; Demets 1987; Canner 1987; Buyse and Ryan 1987; Laupacis *et al.* 1988; Berlin *et al.*, in press). Considerable debate exists about the circumstances in which each of these is preferable. As the results of empirical research in this field become available, it is likely that there will be clarification of the validity of the various positions held by different participants in these debates. Readers who wish to use alternative methods of analysis and presentation of the data in this book will usually find that the necessary information has been presented in sufficient detail to allow them to do this.

3.7 Standard format for tabulating results

We considered carefully how best to present the results of the overview analyses in a uniform way throughout the book. We opted for a standard format for tabulating the results which contains both tabular and graphical elements. This standard form of presentation has already been illustrated in Table 2.2. It is illustrated again here using data about the relative effects of vacuum extraction and forceps delivery on the risk of serious maternal trauma (Table 2.4).

The title of each of the standard format tables summarizes the nature of the intervention(s) and the outcome(s) studied. Column 1 identifies each of the trials used in the overview, by the first author's name and the year of publication. Columns 2 and 4 present the numerators (numbers of participants with the outcome of interest) and denominators (total numbers of participants) in the two experimental groups that form the comparison. As the first of these two groups (Column 2) usually relates to the innovative form of care, we have referred to it as the 'experimental group'; the other group (Column 4) has thus been referred to as the 'control group' (control participants have generally received either a more standard form of care, or a placebo, or no active intervention). Columns 3 and 5 present the incidences (or prevalences) of the outcomes in the experimental and control groups, respectively. Columns 6 and 7 of the table present the ratio of the odds of those in the experimental group having the outcome, to the odds of those in the control group having the same outcome, together with the 95 per cent confidence interval of this ratio. These statistics are then presented graphically in the last element of the table, a form of presentation that facilitates a visual assessment of whether or not the results of individual trials are consistent with one another.

Each row of these standardized tables, except for the row at the bottom, relates to an individual trial (identified in Column 1). In the final row, and at the foot of each column, we have presented a 'typical odds ratio', with its 95 per cent confidence interval, derived in the way described in the previous section, and in Appendix 2.3. Sometimes, an overview of the evidence relating to particular forms of care must be based on the results of

Table 2.4 Effect of vacuum extraction vs. forceps delivery on significant maternal injury

Study	EXPT		CTRL		Odds ratio	Graph of odds ratios and confidence intervals
	n	(%)	*n*	(%)	(95% CI)	0.01 0.1 0.5 1 2 10 100
Dell *et al.* (1985)	21/73	(28.77)	22/45	(48.89)	0.42 (0.20–0.91)	
Lasbrey *et al.* (1964)	2/121	(1.65)	10/131	(7.63)	0.27 (0.08–0.86)	
Vacca *et al.* (1983)	17/152	(11.18)	39/152	(25.66)	0.38 (0.21–0.68)	
Typical odds ratio (95% confidence interval)					0.38 (0.24–0.58)	

a single trial. Even though, in these circumstances, the 'typical odds ratio' is that derived from the single trial in question, the standard format for tabulating the overview has been retained. This is to enable the overview to be updated efficiently in future editions of the book, for which additional evidence will be available (see Section 5, below).

4 Interpretation of overviews (meta-analyses)

4.1 Missing data

The steps that we and our collaborators have taken in our attempts to reduce systematic error (bias) and random error (the play of chance) in our overviews of controlled trials have been discussed above. In this section we address two issues that are of relevance in the interpretation of overviews, and then discuss factors which should be considered when judging the implications of overviews for current practice and future research. First, how have we dealt with the problem of missing data? As described in Section 2.3, above, we have made considerable efforts to flush out unpublished studies evaluating the effects of alternative forms of care during pregnancy and childbirth, and we reiterate our gratitude to those investigators who have been kind enough to provide us with relevant information and data (see Acknowledgements, p 000). Nevertheless, it is very likely that we have failed to identify large numbers of unpublished studies, particularly those conducted during the 1960s and 1970s (Hetherington *et al.*, 1989). In the light of the evidence presented in Section 7 of Chapter 1 about publication bias, this must inevitably leave uncertainties about the representativeness of the data we and our collaborators have been able to assemble for analysis.

Some reassurance is provided by the evidence that studies based on relatively small samples not only tend to be methodologically less satisfactory than larger studies (Chalmers TC and Buyse 1988), but also that they are more susceptible to publication bias (Begg and Berlin 1988). If this is the case in the field that we have reviewed, exclusion of such studies from an overview of similar trials will obviously have a less serious impact than the exclusion of methodologically sounder, larger trials.

We have considered using one or other of the statistical techniques (see, for example, Rosenthal 1979) that have sometimes been used to adjust analyses on the assumption that unpublished studies tend to have results suggesting that there are no differences between alternative forms of care (or differences that suggest that the more innovative of the two forms of care is inferior). Such statistical adjustments inevitably involve assumptions that cannot be investigated about the *actual* results of unpublished studies (Hedges 1984). Because of this we prefer to recommend that the confidence intervals surrounding the typical odds ratios based on the actual data that we *have* been able to assemble should be used to indicate the range of uncertainty that exists about the relative merits of alternative forms of care. If, as we have proposed (Hetherington *et al.* 1989), the many arguments in favour of registration of trials at inception become more widely accepted, it should be possible in future to address the problem of publication bias prospectively, as proposed by Simes (1986).

In addition to exercising caution because bias may have resulted from selective publication of whole studies, care should also be taken when assessing the effects of care on particular outcomes for which not all of the relevant identified trials could contribute data. We reiterate our concern that a result-dependent reporting bias may lead to this situation. It was our concern about this potential bias in particular that led us to urge our collaborators to seek unpublished data from investigators. This potential bias could also be addressed in future if registration of trials at inception becomes standard practice.

4.2 Heterogeneity and methodological quality

The fundamental assumption underlying the statistical aggregration used in overviews of trials is that effects are more likely to differ in size than in direction (Peto 1982, 1987; Chalmers TC and Buyse 1988). The overviews presented in this book are syntheses of the results of separate controlled trials that were judged to have been reasonably similar in terms of the characteristics of their participants, the interventions compared, and the outcomes examined (see Section 3.2, above). This implies a prior belief that an analysis of the results of the trials grouped within a particular overview will reveal any tendency that may exist for the effects of care to be operating in one or other direction. If this consistency exists, it is usually reflected in the estimates of the effects of care derived from each of the individual trials in the overview.

In Table 2.2, for example, the point estimates of the effects of corticosteroids on the risk of respiratory distress syndrome in infants born at less than 31 weeks' gestation vary somewhat from trial to trial. Nevertheless, the results of the separate trials in the array show very convincing internal consistency. First, there is a clear tendency for the individual odds ratios derived from each trial to be less than 1; and secondly, the confidence intervals surrounding each of these point estimates all overlap (suggesting that the differences among the point estimates can easily be explained by the play of chance). Similar remarks apply to the data presented in Table 2.4. If trials of adequate methodological quality have generated results with the kind of consistency illustrated in Tables 2.2 and 2.4, reasonable confidence can be placed in inferences about the relative effects of the forms of care compared based on the 'typical odds ratio' and its confidence interval.

Occasionally, however, studies that we or our collaborators had thought were sufficiently similar to include in a single overview have yielded estimates of the effects of care that are not consistent with each other, that is, they are statistically significantly heterogeneous. Because of the very large number of comparisons made during the preparation of analyses for presentation in this book, it is inevitable that some of these unpredicted differences will simply be a reflection of the play of chance (see Chapter 1, Section 5). They should thus be regarded as *generating* hypotheses about possible explanations for the observed variations in trial results. Such hypotheses may relate to variations in the characteristics of study populations, variations in the forms of care compared, or possibly variations in the way that the outcome of care has been assessed. If the hypotheses generated by the data in this way are considered sufficiently important, they should be tested prospectively in future research. Table 2.5 presents an example of the kind of thing we mean: it is not clear why transcutaneous nerve stimulation should apparently increase labour pain in some trials and decrease it in others. These findings are not helpful in guiding current care, but they should provoke more research in an attempt to explain the divergent findings of different trials, and to identify the circumstances (if any) in which transcutaneous nerve stimulation is a useful form of pain relief for women in labour.

Discrepancies in the estimates of effects derived from individual trials may be explained by variations in the methodological quality of the studies included in an overview. Although no relationship has been detected between study quality and the estimate of the magnitude of the difference between the study groups compared in some overviews (Glass and Smith 1978; Redfield and Rousseau 1981), such a relationship does sometimes exist (Glass and Smith 1979; Wortman and Yeaton 1983; Kavale and Forness 1983; Louis *et al.* 1985; Klein *et al.* 1986; Chalmers I 1987; Detsky *et al.* 1987). Although there are exceptions (Devine and Cook 1983), associations between methodological quality of studies and estimates of the size of difference between experimental groups within them usually occur because methodologically inferior studies tend to yield larger differences than those that have employed sounder methods for reducing bias (Williamson *et al.* 1986).

Because of this empirical support for the view that estimates of the size (and sometimes the direction) of effects can be influenced by the methodological quality of the trials incorporated in an overview, we have arranged that, within any particular tabulation, trials have been ranked by our assessment of their methodological quality (see Section 3.4, above). The results of trials judged to have been relatively rigorously conducted have been entered into the array of data before those derived from trials that are methodologically less satisfactory. (When the trials within a particular overview have been judged to be of comparable methodological quality, they have been ranked by year of publication, with the most recently published being entered at the top of the array.)

The most important question bearing on the validity of the data used in an overview is the method of treatment assignment in the primary studies (Sacks *et al.* 1987). Thus, studies in which the people enrolling participants are least likely to discover the assignment (those using telephone randomization, or drugs and placebos coded by a pharmacy) have been entered into the tables above those which have used methods (like sealed, consecutively numbered, opaque envelopes) in which tampering with the method of allocation is more possible. Likewise, these latter studies have been entered into the tables above those in which the method of 'random allocation' was not made explicit, and those that used 'open', quasi-random methods of allocation (such as alternation, or case record number). Trials

Table 2.5 Effect of transcutaneous nerve stimulation in labour on incidence of 'intense pain'

Study	EXPT		CTRL		Odds ratio	Graph of odds ratios and confidence intervals
	n	(%)	*n*	(%)	(95% CI)	0.01 0.1 0.5 1 2 10 100
Harrison *et al.* (1986)	63/64	(98.44)	55/59	(93.22)	3.77 (0.63–22.44)	
Erkkola *et al.* (1980)	43/100	(43.00)	17/100	(17.00)	3.43 (1.87–6.27)	
Nesheim (1981)	10/35	(28.57)	18/35	(51.43)	0.39 (0.15–1.01)	
Bundsen *et al.* (1982)	8/15	(53.33)	5/9	(55.56)	0.92 (0.18–4.65)	
Typical odds ratio (95% confidence interval)					1.82 (1.14–2.91)	

judged to be of similar quality as far as treatment allocation is concerned have been ranked by the extent to which all participants who were randomized appeared in the primary analysis. Trials that were of similar quality in both these respects have been ranked by the extent to which assessment of the main outcomes was made by observers who were unaware of the treatment assignment of the participants they were assessing. When the direction of the treatment effect differs between individual trials ranked in this way, the results of trials presented at the top of the tables are thus less likely to be biased than those appearing at the bottom of the tables.

We hope that this device will help readers to assess the strength of evidence for or against a particular form of care. A couple of examples should help to illustrate the way it can be applied. Table 2.6 shows an array of 5 trials that were conducted to assess the effect of routine administration of an oxytocic drug during the third stage of labour on the risk of postpartum haemorrhage. The trials are of variable quality, and the data derived from them suggest somewhat greater heterogeneity than those shown in Tables 2.2 and 2.4, although not as much as those shown in Table 2.5. The most 'aberrant' results are those derived from a trial that appears at the bottom of the array. Its position at the bottom of the array indicates that the comparison between the experimental and control groups was judged to have been more likely to be biased than in the other trials. In particular, because the process of 'randomization' in this trial could have been violated easily, it seems quite probable that women who were known to be at increased prior risk of postpartum haemorrhage (for example, those who had a postpartum haemorrhage after a previous delivery) may have been selectively withheld from the 'no oxytocic' group. If so, this selection bias at entry would explain why the group of women allocated to prophylactic oxytocic actually experienced a *higher* rate of postpartum haemorrhage than the controls. Apart from the results of this, methodologically weakest of the 5 trials, however, the overview spells out a fairly consistent message. It thus provides strong evidence that routine administration of an oxytocic drug during the third stage of labour reduces the risk of postpartum haemorrhage (Prendiville *et al.* 1988).

Table 2.7 shows the results of 3 trials in which the effectiveness of a calcium preparation for the control of

Table 2.6 Effect of prophylactic oxytocics in third stage of labour on postpartum haemorrhage

Study	EXPT		CTRL		Odds ratio	Graph of odds ratios and confidence intervals
	n	(%)	*n*	(%)	(95% CI)	0.01 0.1 0.5 1 2 10 100
Howard *et al.* (1964)	24/963	(2.49)	25/470	(5.32)	0.43 (0.23–0.78)	
McGinty (1956)	1/150	(0.67)	5/50	(10.00)	0.04 (0.01–0.27)	
Daley (1951)	45/490	(9.18)	80/510	(15.69)	0.55 (0.38–0.80)	
Rooney *et al.* (1985)	34/346	(9.83)	42/278	(15.11)	0.61 (0.38–0.99)	
Friedman (1957)	24/717	(3.35)	2/177	(1.13)	2.19 (0.82–5.83)	
Typical odds ratio (95% confidence interval)					0.57 (0.44–0.73)	

Table 2.7 Effect of calcium for leg cramps in pregnancy on improvement or abolition of leg cramps

Study	EXPT		CTRL		Odds ratio	Graph of odds ratios and confidence intervals
	n	(%)	*n*	(%)	(95% CI)	0.01 0.1 0.5 1 2 10 100
Hammar *et al.* (1987)	11/30	(36.67)	8/30	(26.67)	1.58 (0.54–4.63)	
Odendaal (1974)	16/64	(25.00)	15/65	(23.08)	1.11 (0.50–2.48)	
Hammar *et al.* (1981)	2/21	(9.52)	19/21	(90.48)	0.04 (0.01–0.14)	
Typical odds ratio (95% confidence interval)					0.59 (0.33–1.03)	

leg cramps during pregnancy was assessed. In this example, the results of the trials shown at the bottom of the array (the methodologically least sound of the 3 trials) are again aberrant. This time they suggest that the treatment studied is effective, while evidence from the methodologically sounder trials provide no support for this conclusion. This discrepancy is almost certainly explained by the fact that the trial at the bottom of the array was the only one of the 3 trials in which no placebo control was used. The differences between the experimental and control group in this trial are thus more likely to reflect a non-specific placebo effect than a specific effect of calcium itself. The interpretation of the overview should thus give greater weight to the two methodologically sounder trials. In this case, the conclusion must be that there is currently no good evidence that calcium, *per se*, is effective in the control of leg cramps during pregnancy (see Chapter 32).

Table 2.8 shows a more complex picture derived from the results of trials of phenobarbitone administered prophylactically to very low birthweight infants in an attempt to prevent periventricular haemorrhage. The trials included in this overview are also of heterogeneous methodological quality, but this time the interpretation is not so straightforward. In this array it is the results of the methodologically soundest trial (presented in the first row) which might be seen as aberrant. Clearly, when recommendations for care are made, the results of this trial should carry more weight than either the trial results presented towards the bottom half of the table, or the summary statistic (the typical odds ratio) that these conflicting results have generated. In this particular instance it is clear that prophylactic phenobarbitone should not be given to very low birthweight infants, except in the context of further trials to elucidate its effects more clearly than is possible using the available evidence (Chalmers I 1987).

Lastly, although the tables rank the individual studies within the overview in approximate order of their methodological rigour, they give no indication whether the methodological rigour overall was relatively high, relatively low, or very variable. When all of the trials contributing to an overview are of relatively poor methodological quality, their results might be considered primarily as having implications for future research rather than a basis for making recommendations about practice. In these circumstances we have tried to ensure that this has been made clear in the accompanying text. For example, the results of both of the trials in which routine administration during the third stage of labour of a mixture of oxytocin and ergometrine ('Syntometrine') has been compared with oxytocin alone suggest that the former is a more effective prophylactic against postpartum haemorrhage (Table 2.9). Both of the available trials, however, suffer from methodological limitations, which suggest that their results, although consistent with each other, may be biased. The results of this overview should not, therefore, be interpreted as strong evidence supporting the addition of ergometrine to oxytocin as a routine during the third stage of labour. Rather it should prompt further trials in which more attention is paid to the reduction of bias (Elbourne *et al.* 1988).

Table 2.8 Effect of prophylactic phenobarbitone in very low birthweight infants on severe periventricular haemorrhage

Study	EXPT		CTRL		Odds ratio	Graph of odds ratios and confidence intervals
	n	(%)	*n*	(%)	(95% CI)	0.01 0.1 0.5 1 2 10 100
Kuban *et al.* (1986)	18/145	(12.41)	8/135	(5.93)	2.15 (0.96–4.82)	
Whitelaw *et al.* (1983)	0/30	(0.00)	2/30	(6.67)	0.13 (0.01–2.14)	
Porter et al. (1985)	4/7	(57.14)	4/12	(33.33)	2.52 (0.40–15.85)	
Anwar *et al.* (1986)	14/30	(46.67)	10/28	(35.71)	1.56 (0.55–4.39)	
Donn *et al.* (1981)	2/58	(3.45)	3/64	(4.69)	0.73 (0.12–4.36)	
Bedard *et al.* (1984)	0/21	(0.00)	2/21	(9.52)	0.13 (0.01–2.13)	
Morgan *et al.* (1982)	5/30	(16.67)	9/30	(30.00)	0.48 (0.15–1.57)	
Ruth (1985)	3/25	(12.00)	6/27	(22.22)	0.50 (0.12–2.06)	
Typical odds ratio (95% confidence interval)					1.09 (0.68–1.74)	

Table 2.9 Effect of prophylactic syntometrine vs. oxytocin in third stage of labour on postpartum haemorrhage

Study	EXPT		CTRL		Odds ratio	Graph of odds ratios and confidence intervals
	n	(%)	*n*	(%)	(95% CI)	0.01 0.1 0.5 1 2 10 100
Nieminen and Jarvinen (1963)	5/689	(0.73)	9/689	(1.31)	0.56 (0.20–1.61)	
Dumoulin (1981)	52/1000	(5.20)	74/750	(9.87)	0.50 (0.35–0.72)	
Typical odds ratio (95% confidence interval)					0.50 (0.36–0.71)	

4.3 Implications for practice and future research

'Through seeking we may learn and know things better. But as for certain truth, no man hath known it, for all is but a woven web of guesses'

Xenophanes, sixth century BC

'I am always certain about things that are a matter of opinion'

Charlie ('Peanuts') Brown, twentieth century AD

'Our many errors show that the practice of causal inference . . . remains an art. Although to assist us, we have acquired analytic techniques, statistical methods and conventions, and logical criteria, ultimately the conclusions we reach are a matter of judgement'

Mervyn Susser 1984

Any assessment of the implications of the results of overviews of trials for current practice and future research must inevitably involve a large element of judgement. As with individual trials (see Section 8 of Chapter 1), even if a particular overview appears to have 'internal validity', questions about its 'external validity'—the extent to which the results are applicable in practice—will always remain.

The issue of 'external validity' can be considered at two levels. First, because controlled trials generate evidence about how people respond to particular forms of care *on average*, they may be relevant in guiding the development of the broad policies that are a particularly prominent feature of the care given during pregnancy and childbirth. Thus, for example, there is strong evidence that continuity of personal care, combined with efforts to provide social and psychological support during pregnancy and childbirth, is preferred (on average) by women, and no evidence that it has any associated adverse effects (see Chapters 10, 14, and 49). This evidence should be used to support efforts to ensure that continuity of care and the provision of social and psychological support is pursued as a matter of policy. Similarly, there is strong evidence that, compared with other suture materials, catgut used to repair perineal trauma leads to more short-term perineal discomfort (and long-term perineal discomfort in the case of glycerol impregnated catgut) and that it offers no compensating advantages (see Chapter 68). As a matter of policy, therefore, catgut should be abandoned for suturing perineal trauma.

The second level at which the 'external validity' of the results of an overview might be considered, however, is at the level of decisions about the care of particular individuals. It will sometimes be possible to refine the decisions made about the care of individuals using information derived from controlled trials. This may be possible, for example, if particular individuals and forms of care in everyday practice share characteristics with the participants and forms of care evaluated in particular trials, *and* these trials have yielded estimates of treatment effects that are not subject to unacceptable random error. Similarly, if the individuals encountered in everyday care share characteristics with identifiable subgroups within the available controlled trials, *and* it has been demonstrated with confidence that these subgroups have shown a *prespecified* response to care which differs in either magnitude (or even direction) from the average effect observed in the trial, this too may provide a valid basis for attempts to individualize care. As already discussed above, however, it is usually not possible to make such judgements with any confidence. Indeed, confident predictions about the effects of care on particular individuals are very rarely justified, whether the predictions are based on the results of controlled trials or on some other, less formally derived information (Bradford Hill 1952; Schoolman 1982). As Yusuf and his colleagues (1984) have noted, however, 'it would be unfortunate if desire for perfect knowledge (that is, exactly *who* will benefit from treatment) were to become the enemy of the possible (that is, knowledge of the direction and approximate size of the effects of treatment of wide categories of patients)'.

In assessing the implications for care of the results of overviews of controlled trials (and other kinds of internally valid evidence about the effects of care), there is, of course, a crucially important additional dimension to those noted so far. This relates to judgements about what constitutes a 'benefit from treatment' which is sufficient to outweigh the 'cost of treatment', whether this is assessed in terms of its unwanted physical or psychological effects, its inconvenience, or the resource consequences of using it. The threshold of evidence at which individuals (both those providing and those seeking care) will decide to act on the basis of evidence that is both 'internally valid' and 'externally valid' in a general sense, will vary according to their personal perceptions of the consequences of the action in question (Gillon 1985; Friedman 1986). The greater the risk of doing harm *in their terms*, the higher the threshold for their acceptance of the apparent implications of the data; the larger the estimated magnitude of the benefit *in their terms*, the lower will be the threshold. In other words, different circumstances may provoke different reactions to the same quality of evidence, as common sense would suggest they should.

If, for example, there had been no serious consequences of postpartum haemorrhage within a particular maternity hospital in which oxytocics had not been administered routinely during the third stage of labour, a decision not to introduce such a policy—in spite of good evidence that it would reduce the incidence of postpartum haemorrhage—would be understandable. Similarly, if individual women feel strongly that freedom from as many constraints as possible during labour is more important to them than increasing the chances of their baby *not* having seizures from about 99.7 per cent to 99.9 per cent, it would be very understandable if they rejected the continuous fetal heart rate monitoring combined with fetal acid base assessment which has been shown to achieve this very modest improvement in outcome, in favour of intermittent auscultation (see Chapter 54).

In spite of these reasons for urging caution in assessing the implications of the overviews of trials presented in this book, chapter authors were asked to conclude their contributions with a summary of their perceptions of the implications of their analyses, both for current practice and for future research. If readers are satisfied that particular analyses are likely to be internally and externally valid, and that they may have implications for their particular circumstances, they may wish to make a quantitative assessment of the consequences of adopting (or abandoning) particular forms of care.

A nomogram, shown as Fig. 2.3 in this chapter, but also reproduced as a bookmark, facilitates use of the typical odds ratio and its confidence interval to estimate (across a range of prior risks of the outcome in question) the effects of adopting particular forms of care for individuals or groups of individuals. For example, the overview of trials of routine administration of an oxytocic drug during the third stage of labour provides strong evidence that such a policy reduces the incidence of postpartum haemorrhage: the point estimate of the percentage reduction in the odds of postpartum haemorrhage (the typical odds ratio) is 43 per cent, with a 95 per cent confidence interval ranging from 27 per cent to 56 per cent (Table 2.5). If readers wish to assess what these data may mean in practice, in terms of the reduction in prior risk for a particular woman, or for a particular population, they should draw a line through the estimate of the prior risk (shown on the scale on the left of the nomogram) and the estimate of the typical odds ratio (the scale in the middle of the nomogram) and read off the estimate of the risk following routine use of oxytocics using the scale on the right of the nomogram. Thus, as shown in Fig. 2.3, a prior risk of 10 per cent in a woman, or population of women, in which the policy has not been yet been adopted might, given an odds ratio of 0.57, be reduced to a risk of about 6 per cent associated with adoption of the policy. The odds ratios forming the 95 per cent confidence interval can obviously be used to assess the range within which the true effect is likely to lie. This may be useful if one wishes to estimate the likely maximum or minimum effects of particular forms of care. These estimates may be relevant, for example, when the effects of care are very dependent on strict compliance, either among those providing or among those offered care (see Chapter 1, Section 8.3).

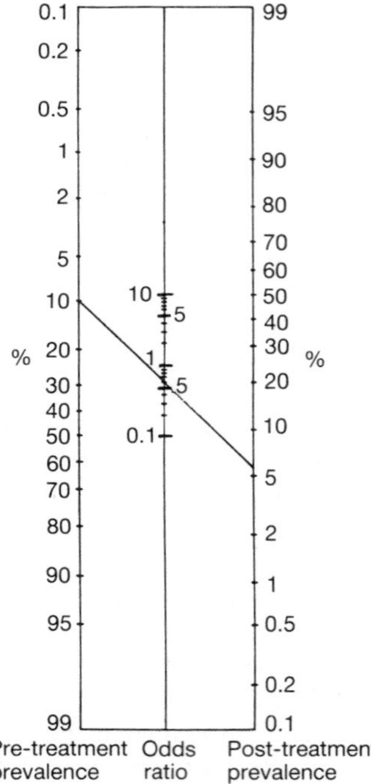

Fig. 2.3 Nomogram for estimating the effect of intervention on the probability of an unwanted outcome, for a given prior probability of the outcome

5 Provisions for updating and amending overviews (meta-analyses) in the light of new data and criticisms

'I shall let the little I have learnt go forth into the day in order that someone better than I may guess the truth, and in his work may prove and rebuke my error. At this I shall rejoice that I was yet a means whereby this truth has come to light'

Albrecht Dürer 1513

We have raised a number of cautions about the interpretation of overviews presented in this book, and readers may sometimes wish to perform alternative analyses, using different materials or different methods. Although we and our collaborators have tried (within the resources available to us) to ensure that bias has been minimized within the analyses presented, we are conscious of the fact that it will be possible to improve many of them. These improvements may result from incorporating data that have not yet been made available to us; by re-analysis of the information to which we have had access, using more thorough blinding during the selection of studies and abstraction of data; by using alternative aggregations of studies; possibly, by using one or other of the alternative statistical methods available; or by some combination of these steps. We urge others to conduct alternative analyses, using alternative materials and methods, so that the stability of the conclusions that we and our collaborators have reached can be assessed.

It is obviously important to amend our analyses efficiently in the light of valid criticisms, and as additional information becomes available. Arrangements have therefore been made for the overviews to be updated on a continuing basis in an electronic publication—the *Oxford Database of Perinatal Trials* (Chalmers I *et al.* 1986; Chalmers I 1988). Readers of this book who have criticisms, comments, or information which may help to improve the quality of the overviews that have been presented in the chapters that follow are invited to communicate with us, or our collaborators. We shall ensure that any assistance we receive in this way will be reflected promptly in the *Oxford Database of Perinatal Trials* and in future editions of this book.

References

Antiplatelet Trialists' Collaboration (1988). Secondary prevention of vascular disease by prolonged antiplatelet treatment. Br Med J, 296: 320–331.

Anwar M, Kadam S, Hiatt IM, Hegyi T (1986). Phenobarbitone prophylaxis of intraventricular haemorrhage. Arch Dis Childhood, 61: 196–197.

Bailey KR (1987). Inter-study differences: How should they influence the interpretation and analysis of results? Stat Med, 6: 351–358.

Bangert-Drowns RL (1986). Review of developments in meta-analytic method. Psychol Bull, 99: 388–399.

Bedard MP, Shankaran S, Slovis TL, Pantoja A, Dayal B, Poland RL (1984). Effect of prophylactic phenobarbital on intra-ventricular haemorrhage in high risk infants. Pediatrics, 73: 435–439.

Beecher HK (1955). The powerful placebo. JAMA, 159: 1602–1606.

Begg CB, Berlin JA (1988). Publication bias: A problem in interpreting medical data. J R Stat Soc (Series A), 151: 419–463.

Berlin JA, Laird NM, Sacks HS, Chalmers TC (in press). A comparison of statistical methods for combining event rates from clinical trials. Stat Med

Bulpitt CJ (1988). Meta-analysis. Lancet, 2: 93–94.

Bundsen P, Ericson K, Peterson LE, Thiringer K (1982). Pain relief in labor by transcutaneous electrical nerve stimulation. Acta Obstet Gynecol Scand, 61: 129–136.

Buyse M, Ryan LM (1987). Issues of efficiency in combining proportions of deaths from several clinical trials. Stat Med, 6: 565–576.

Bradford Hill A (1952). The clinical trial. New Engl J Med, 247: 113–119.

Canner P (1987). An overview of six clinical trials of aspirin in coronary heart disease. Stat Med, 6: 255–263.

Chalmers I (1979). Randomised trials of fetal monitoring 1973–1977. In: Perinatal Medicine. Thalhammer O, Baumgarten K, Pollak A, (eds). Stuttgart: Georg Thieme, pp 260–265.

Chalmers I (1985a). Biased touching of the editorial tiller. Arch Dis Childhood, 60: 394.

Chalmers I (1985b). Proposal to outlaw the term 'negative trial'. Br Med J, 290: 1002.

Chalmers I (1987). The scientific case for greater collaboration in the evaluation of perinatal practice. J Austral Perinat Soc, 3–15.

Chalmers I (ed) (1988). The Oxford Database of Perinatal Trials. Oxford: Oxford University Press.

Chalmers I, Hetherington J, Newdick M, Mutch L, Grant A, Enkin M, Enkin E, Dickersin K (1986). The Oxford Database of Perinatal Trials: Developing a register of published reports of controlled trials. Controlled Clin Trials, 7: 306–325.

Chalmers TC (1982). Informed consent, clinical research and the practice of medicine. Trans Am Clin Climatol Assoc, 94: 204–212.

Chalmers TC, Buyse ME (1988). Meta-analysis. In: Data Analysis for Clinical Medicine in Gastroenterology: The Quantitative Approach to Patient Care. Chalmers TC (ed). Rome: International University Press. pp 75–84.

Chalmers TC, Smith H, Blackburn B, Silverman B, Schroeder B, Reitman D, Ambroz A (1981). A method for assessing the quality of a randomized control trial. Controlled Clin Trials, 2: 31–49.

Chalmers TC, Levin H, Sacks HS, Reitman D, Berrier J, Nagalingam R (1987a). Meta-analysis of clinical trials as a scientific discipline. I: Control of bias and comparison with large co-operative trials. Stat Med, 6: 315–325.

Chalmers TC, Berrier J, Sacks HS, Levin H, Reitman D, Nagalingam R (1987b). Meta-analysis of clinical trials as a scientific discipline. II: Replicate variability and comparison of studies that agree and disagree. Stat Med, 6: 733–744.

Chalmers TC, Berrier J, Hewitt P, Reitman D, Nagalingam R, Sacks H (1988). Logistics of determining rates of rare side effects by meta-analysis. Paper presented at the 9th Annual Meeting of the Society for Clinical Trials, 22–25 May, San Diego.

Collaborative Group on Antenatal Steroid Therapy (1981). Effect of antenatal dexamethasone administration on the prevention of respiratory distress syndrome. Am J Obstet Gynecol, 141: 276–287.

Collins R, Yusuf S, Peto R (1985). Overview of randomised trials of diuretics in pregnancy. Br Med J, 290: 17–23.

Collins R, Gray R, Godwin J, Peto R (1987). Avoidance of large biases in the assessment of moderate treatment effects: The need for systematic overviews. Stat Med, 6: 245–250.

Conn HO, Blitzer BL (1976). Nonassociation of adrenocorticosteroid therapy and peptic ulcer. New Engl J Med, 294: 473–479.

Conn HO, Poynard T (1985). Adrenocorticosteroid administration and peptic ulcer: A critical analysis. J Chron Dis, 38: 457–468.

Cooper HM (1982). Scientific guidelines for conducting integrative research reviews. Rev Educ Res, 52: 291–302.

Cooper HM (1984). The Integrative Research Review. Beverly Hills, CA: Sage Publications.

Cooper HM, Rosenthal R (1980). Statistical versus traditional procedures for summarising research findings. Psychol Bull, 87: 442–449.

Crowley P, Chalmers I, Keirse MJNC (1990). Corticosteroids prior to preterm delivery: An overview of the evidence from controlled trials. Br J Obstet Gynaecol, 97: 11–25.

Daya S (1989). Efficacy of progesterone support for pregnancy in women with recurrent miscarriage: a meta-analysis of the controlled trials. Br J Obset Gynaecol, 96: 275–280.

Daley D (1951). The use of intramuscular ergometrine at the end of the second stage of normal labour. J Obstet Gynaecol Br Commnwlth, 57: 388–397.

Dell DL. Sightler SE, Plauche WC (1985). Soft cup vacuum extraction: a comparison of outlet delivery. Obstet Gynecol, 66: 624–628.

Demets DL (1987). Methods for combining randomized clinical trials: Strengths and limitations. Stat Med, 6: 341–348.

DerSimonian R, Laird N (1986). Meta-analysis in clinical trials. Controlled Clin Trials, 7: 177–188.

Detsky AS, Baker JP, O'Rourke K, Goel V (1987). Perioperative parenteral nutrition: A meta-analysis. Ann Intern Med, 107: 195–203.

Devine EC, Cook TD (1983). A meta-analytic analysis of effects of psychoeducational interventions on length of postsurgical hospital stay. Nursing Res, 32: 267–274.

Dickersin K, Hewitt P, Mutch L, Chalmers I, Chalmers TC (1985). Perusing the literature. Comparison of Medline searching with a perinatal trials database. Controlled Clin Trials, 6: 306–317.

Dickersin K, Chan SS, Chalmers TC, Sacks HS, Smith H (1987). Publication bias in randomized control trials. Controlled Clin Trials, 8: 343–353.

Donn SM, Roloff DW, Goldstein GW (1981). Prevention of intraventricular haemorrhage in preterm infants by phenobarbitone. A controlled trial. Lancet, 2: 215–217.

Dumoulin JG (1981). A re-appraisal of the use of ergometrine. J Obstet Gynaecol. 1: 178–181.

Eagly AH, Carli LL (1981). Sex of researchers and sex-typed communications as determinants of sex differences in influenceability: A meta-analysis of social influence studies. Psychol Bull, 90: 1–20.

Early Breast Cancer Trialists' Collaborative Group (1988). Effects of adjuvant tamoxiphen and cytotoxic therapy on early mortality in breast cancer: an overview of all 61 randomized trials among 28,896 women. First Report. New Engl J Med, 319: 1681–1692.

Einarson TR, McGhan WF, Bootman JL, Sabers DL (1985). Meta-analysis: Quantitative integration of independent research results. Am J Hosp Pharm, 42: 1957–1964.

Elashoff JD (1978). Combining results of clinical trials. Gastroenterology, 75: 1170–1174.

Elbourne D, Richardson M, Chalmers I, Waterhouse I, Holt E (1987). The Newbury Maternity Care Study: A randomized controlled trial to assess a policy of women holding their own obstetric records. Br J Obstet Gynaecol, 94: 612–619.

Elbourne D, Prendiville W, Chalmers I (1988). Choice of oxytocic preparation for routine use in the management of the third stage of labour: An overview of the evidence from controlled trials. Br J Obstet Gynaecol, 95: 17–30.

Ellenberg SS (1988). Meta-analysis: the quantitative approach to research review. Seminars in Oncology, 15: 472–481.

Erkkola R, Pikkola P, Kanto J (1980). Transcutaneous nerve stimulation for pain relief during labour. A controlled study. Ann Chir Gynaecol, 69: 273–277.

Eysenck HJ (1978). An exercise in mega-silliness. Am Psychol, 33: 517.

Fleiss JL (1981). Statistical methods for rates and proportions. New York: John Wiley.

Friedman EA (1957). Comparative clinical evaluation of postpartum oxytocics. Am J Obstet Gynecol, 73: 1306–1313.

Friedman HS (1986). Randomized clinical trials and common sense. Am J Med, 81: 1047.

Furberg CT, Morgan TM (1987). Lessons from overviews of cardiovascular trials. Stat Med, 6: 295–303.

Gillon R (1985). 'Primum non nocere' and the principle of non-maleficence. Br Med J, 291: 130–132.

Glass GV (1976). Primary, secondary and meta-analysis of research. Educational Researcher, 5: 3–8.

Glass GV, Smith ML (1978). Reply to Eysenck. Am Psychol, 33: 517–519.

Glass GV, Smith ML (1979). Meta-analysis of research on class size and achievement. Educational Evaluation and Policy Analysis, 1: 2–16.

Goldman L, Feinstein AR (1979). Anticoagulants and myocardial infarction: The problems of pooling, drowning and floating. Ann Intern Med, 90: 92–94.

Goldstein P, Berrier J, Rosen S, Sacks HC, Chalmers TC (1989). A meta-analysis of randomized control trials of progestational agents in pregnancy. Br J Obstet Gynaecol, 96: 265–267.

Gottman JJ, Glass GV (1978). Analysis of interrupted time series experiments. In: Single Subject Research. TR Kratchowil (ed). New York: Academic Press, pp 197–235.

Grant A (1986a). Controlled trials of routine ultrasound in pregnancy. Birth, 13: 22–28.

Grant A (1986b). Cervical cerclage: Evaluation studies. In: Preterm Birth: New Goals and New Practices in Prenatal Care. Papiernik E, Breart G, Spira N (eds). Paris: INSERM, pp 83–99.

Grant A, Mohide P (1982). Screening and diagnosis in antenatal care. In: Effectiveness and Satisfaction in Antenatal Care. Enkin M, Chalmers I (eds). Clinics in Developmental Medicine Nos. 81/82. London: Spastics International Medical Publications, Heinemann Medical Books, pp 22–59.

Halvorsen KT (1986). Combining results from independent investigations: Meta-analysis in medical research. In: Medical Uses of Statistics. Bailar J, Mosteller F (eds). Mass: NEJM Books, pp 392–416.

Hammar M, Larsson L, Tegler L (1981). Calcium treatment of leg cramps in pregnancy. Acta Obstet Gynecol Scand, 60: 345–347.

Hammar M, Berg G, Solheim F, Larsson L (1987). Calcium and magnesium status in pregnant women. A comparison between treatment with calcium and vitamin C in pregnant women with leg cramps. Int J Vitam Nutr Res, 57: 179–183.

Harrison RF, Woods T, Shore M, Mathews G, Unwin A (1986). Pain relief in labour using transcutaneous electrical nerve stimulation (TENS). A TENS/TENS placebo controlled study in two parity groups. Br J Obstet Gynaecol, 93: 739–746.

Haverkamp AD, Thompson HE, McFee JG, Cetrulo C (1976). The evaluation of fetal heart rate monitoring in high risk pregnancy. Am J Obstet Gynecol, 125: 310–320.

Haverkamp AD, Orleans M, Langendoerfer S, McFee JG, Murphy J (1979). A controlled trial of the differential effects of intrapartum fetal monitoring. Am J Obstet Gynecol, 134: 399–408.

Hawkins D (1987). Book reviews. J Obstet Gynaecol, 8: 97.

Hedges LV (1982). Estimation of effect size from a series of independent experiments. Psychol Bull, 92: 490–499.

Hedges LV (1983). A random effects model for effect sizes. Psychol Bull, 93: 388–395.

Hedges LV (1984). Estimation of effect size under nonrandom sampling: The effects of censoring studies yielding statistically insignificant mean differences. J Educ Stat, 9: 61–85.

Hedges LV (1987). Commentary. Stat Med, 6: 381–385.

Hedges LV (1986). Statistical issues in the meta-analysis of environmental studies. American Statistical Association/Environmental Protection Agency, Office of Policy and Evaluation, Statistical Policy Branch, Washington DC. EPA-230-12-87-032. pp 30–44.

Hedges LV, Olkin I (1985). Statistical Methods for Meta-analysis. London: Academic Press.

Hetherington J, Chalmers I, Dickersin K, Meinert C (1989). Retrospective or prospective identification of controlled trials: Lessons from a survey of obstetricians and paediatricians. Pediatrics, 84: 374–380.

Howard WF, McFadden PR, Keettel WC (1964). Oxytocic drugs in fourth stage of labor. JAMA, 189: 411–413.

Horwitz RI (1987). Complexity and contradiction in clinical trial research. Am J Med, 82: 498–510.

Hunter JE, Schmidt FL, Jackson GB (1982). Meta-analysis: Cumulating Research Findings Across Studies. Beverly Hills, CA: Sage Publications.

Huth EJ (1987). Needed: Review articles with more scientific rigour. Ann Intern Med, 106: 470–471.

Hytten FE, Leitch I (1965). The Physiology of Human Pregnancy. Oxford: Blackwell Scientific Publications.

Jackson GB (1980). Methods for integrative reviews. Rev Educ Res, 50: 438–460.

Johnson DW, Maruyama G, Johnson RT (1982). Separating ideology from currently available data: A reply to Cotton and Cook and McGlynn. Psychol Bull, 92: 186–192.

Jones LV, Fiske DW (1953). Models for testing the significance of combined results. Psychol Bull: 50, 375–382.

Kavale KA, Forness SR (1983). Hyperactivity and diet treatment: A meta-analysis of the Feingold hypothesis. J Learning Disability, 16: 324–330.

Kelso IM, Parsons RJ, Lawrence GF, Arora SS, Edmonds DK, Cooke ID (1978). An assessment of continuous fetal heart rate monitoring in labor. A randomised trial. Am J Obstet Gynecol, 131: 526–532.

King JF, Keirse MJNC, Grant A, Chalmers I (1985). Tocolysis—the case for and against. In: Preterm Labour and its Consequences. Beard RW, Sharp F (eds). London: Royal College of Obstetricians and Gynaecologists, pp 199–208.

King JF, Grant A, Keirse MJNC, Chalmers I (1988). Betamimetics in preterm labour: An overview of the randomized controlled trials. Br J Obstet Gynaecol, 95: 211–222.

Klein S, Simes J, Blackburn GL (1986). Total parenteral nutrition and cancer clinical trials. Cancer, 58: 1378–1386.

Kuban KCK, Krishnamoorthy KS, Brown ER, Teele RL, Baglivo JA, Sullivan KF, Huff KR, White S, Cleveland RH, Allred EN, Spritzer KL, Skouteli HN, Cayea P, Epstein MF (1986). Neonatal intracranial haemorrhage and phenobarbital. Pediatrics, 77: 443–450.

L'Abbé KA, Detsky AS, O'Rourke K (1987). Meta-analysis in clinical research. Ann Intern Med, 107: 224–232.

Lasbrey AH, Orchard CD, Crichton D (1964). A study of the relative merits and scope for vacuum extraction as opposed to forceps delivery. S Afr Med J, 2: 1–3.

Laupacis A, Sackett DL, Roberts RS (1988). An assessment of clinically useful measures of the consequences of treatment. New Engl J Med, 318: 1728–1733.

Leitch I (1976). The collection and dissemination of information on nutrition with special reference to the United Kingdom. Prog Food Nutr Sci, 2: 59.

Light RJ (1987). Accumulating evidence from independent studies: What we can win and what we can lose. Stat Med, 6: 221–228.

Light RJ, Pillemer DB (1984). Summing Up: The Science of Reviewing Research. Cambridge, Mass: Harvard University Press.

Light RJ, Smith PV (1971). Accumulating evidence: Procedures for resolving contradictions among different research studies. Harvard Educ Rev, 41: 429–471.

Liggins GC, Howie RN (1972). A controlled trial of antepartum glucocorticoid treatment for prevention of the respiratory distress syndrome in premature infants. Paediatrics, 10: 515–525.

Louis TA, Fineberg HV, Mosteller F (1985). Findings for

public health from meta-analyses. Ann Rev Public Health, 6: 1–20.

MacDonald D, Grant A, Sheridan-Pereira M, Boylan P, Chalmers I (1985). The Dublin randomized controlled trial of intrapartum fetal heart rate monitoring. Am J Obstet Gynecol, 152: 524–539.

McGinty LB (1956). A study of the vasopresser effects of oxytocics when used intravenously in the third stage of labour. West J Surg, 64: 22–28.

Mantel N, Haenszel W (1959). Statistical aspects of the analysis of data from retrospective studies of disease. J Natl Cancer Inst, 22: 719–748.

Messer J, Reitman D, Sacks HS, Smith H, Chalmers TC (1983). Association of adrenocorticosteroid therapy and peptic-ulcer disease. New Engl J Med, 309: 21–24.

Morales WJ, Diebel ND, Lazar AJ, Zadrozny D (1986). The effect of antenatal dexamethasone administration on the prevention of respiratory distress syndrome in preterm gestations with premature rupture of membranes. Am J Obstet Gynecol, 154: 591–595.

Morgan MEI, Massey RF, Cooke RWI (1982). Does phenobarbitone prevent periventricular hemorrhage in very low-birth-weight babies? A controlled trial. Pediatrics, 70: 186–189.

Morgan PP (1986). Review articles: 2. The literature jungle. Can Med Assoc J, 134: 98–99.

Morrison JC, Whybrew WD, Bucovaz ET, Schneider JM (1978). Injection of corticosteroids into mother to prevent neonatal respiratory distress syndrome. Am J Obstet Gynecol, 131: 358–366.

Mosteller F (1979). Problems of omission in communications. Clin Pharmacol Ther, 25: 761–764.

Mosteller FM, Bush RR (1954). Selected quantitative techniques. In: Handbook of Social Psychology: Vol 1. Theory and Method. G Lindsay (ed). Cambridge, Mass: Addison-Wesley.

Mulrow CD (1987). The medical review article: State of the science. Ann Intern Med, 106, 485–488.

Mulrow CD, Thacker SB, Pugh JA (1988). A proposal for more informative abstracts of review articles. Ann Int Med, 108: 613–615.

National Perinatal Epidemiology Unit (1985). A Classified Bibliography of Controlled Trials in Perinatal Medicine, 1940–1984. Oxford: Oxford University Press.

Nieminen U, Jarvinen P (1963). A comparative study of different medical treatments of the third stage of labour. Ann Chir Gynaecol Fenn, 53: 424–429.

Nesheim BI (1981). The use of transcutaneous nerve stimulation for pain relief during labour. Acta Obstet Gynecol Scand, 60: 13–16.

Oakley A, Elbourne D, Chalmers I (1986). The effects of social interventions in pregnancy. In: Prevention of Preterm Birth: New Goals and New Practices in Prenatal Care. Papiernik E, Breart G, Spira N (eds). Paris: INSERM, pp 329–361.

Odendaal HJ (1974). Evaluation of the aetiology and therapy of leg cramps during pregancy. S Afr Med J, 48: 780–781.

Orwin RG, Cordray DS (1985). Effects of deficient reporting on meta-analysis: A conceptual framework and reanalysis. Psychol Bull, 97: 134–147.

Oxman AD, Guyatt GH (1988). Guidelines for reading literature reviews. Can Med Assoc J, 138: 697–703.

Papageorgiou AN, Desgranges MF, Masson M, Colle E, Shatz R, Gelfand MM (1979). The antenatal use of betamethasone in prevention of respiratory distress syndrome: a controlled double-blind study. Pediatrics, 63: 73–79.

Peto R (1982). Statistical aspects of cancer trials. In: Treatment of Cancer. Halnan KE (ed). London: Chapman & Hall, pp 867–871.

Peto R (1987). Why do we need systematic overviews of randomized trials? Stat Med, 6: 233–240.

Peto R, Pike MC, Armitage P, Breslow NE, Cox DR, Howard SV, Mantel N, McPherson K, Peto J, Smith PG (1976). Design and analysis of randomized clinical trials requiring prolonged observation of each patient. I: Introduction and design. Br J Cancer, 34: 585–612.

Peto R, Pike MC, Armitage P, Breslow NE, Cox DR, Howard SV, Mantel N, McPherson K, Peto J, Smith PG (1977). Design and analysis of randomized clinical trials requiring prolonged observation of each patient. II: Analysis and examples. Br J Cancer, 35: 1–39.

Pillemer DB (1984). Conceptual issues in research synthesis. J Special Educ, 18: 27–40.

Porter FL. Marshall RE, Moore J, Miller RH (1985). Effect of phenobarbital on motor activity and intraventricular hemorrhage in preterm infants with respiratory disease weighing less than 1500 grams. Am J Perinatol, 2: 63–66.

Prendiville W, Elbourne D, Chalmers I (1988). The effects of routine oxytocic administration in the management of the third stage of labour: An overview of the evidence from controlled trials. Br J Obstet Gynaecol, 95: 3–16.

Redfield DL, Rousseau EW (1981). A meta-analysis of experimental research on teacher questioning behaviour. Rev Educ Res, 51: 237–245.

Renou P, Chang A, Anderson I, Wood C (1976). Controlled trial of fetal intensive care. Am J Obstet Gynecol, 126: 470–476.

Roberton NRC (1982). Advances in respiratory distress syndrome. Br Med J, 284: 917–918.

Rooney I, Hughes P, Calder AA (1985). Is routine administration of syntometrine still justified in the management of the third stage of labour? Health Bull, 43: 99–101.

Rosenthal R (1978). How often are our numbers wrong? Am Psychol, 33: 1005–1008.

Rosenthal R (1979). The 'file drawer problem' and tolerance for null results. Psychol Bull, 86: 638–641.

Rosenthal R (1984). The reliability of judgements of quality. In: Meta-analytic Procedures for Social Research. Rosenthal R (ed). Beverly Hills, CA: Sage Publications, pp 55–58.

Ruth V (1985). Brain protection by phenobarbitone in very low birthweight (VLBW) prematures—a controlled trial. Klin Pädiatr, 197: 170–171.

Sacks HS, Berrier J, Reitman D, Ancona-Berk VA, Chalmers TC (1987). Meta-analyses of randomized controlled trials. New Engl J Med, 316: 450–455.

Saunders MC, Dick JS, Brown IMcL, McPherson K, Chalmers I (1985). The effects of hospital admission for bed rest on the duration of twin pregnancy: A randomised trial. Lancet, 2: 793–795.

Schoolman HM (1982). The clinician and the statistician. Stat Med, 1: 311–316.

Searles JS (1985). A methodological and empirical critique of psychotherapy outcome meta-analysis. Behav Res Ther, 23: 453–463.

Simes RJ (1987). Confronting publication bias: A cohort design for meta-analysis. Stat Med, 6: 11–29.

Solari ME, Wheatley D (1966). A method of combining the results of several clinical trials. Clin Trials J, 3: 537–545.

Stock WA, Okun MA, Haring MJ, Miller W, Kinney C, Cuervorst RW (1982). Rigor in data synthesis: A case study of reliability in meta-analysis. Educ Researcher, June-July: 10–14.

Taeusch HW Jr, Frigoletto F, Kitzmiller J, Avery ME, Hehre A, Fromm B, Lawson E, Neff RK (1979). Risk of respiratory distress syndrome after prenatal dexamethasone treatment. Pediatrics, 63: 64–72.

Thacker S (1985). Quality of controlled clinical trials. The case of imaging ultrasound in obstetrics: A review. Br J Obstet Gynaecol, 92: 437–444.

Thacker SB (1988). Meta-analysis: A quantitative approach to research integration JAMA, 259: 1685–1689.

Thomson AM (1981). Isabella Leitch (1890–1980). Br J Nutr, 45: 1–4.

Toth PJ, Horwitz RI (1983). Conflicting clinical trials and the uncertainty of treating mild hypertension. Am J Med, 75: 482–488.

Treadwell M (1982). Letter. J Assoc for Improvements in the Maternity Services, p 15.

Tyson JE, Furzan JA, Reisch JS, Mize SG (1983). An evaluation of the quality of therapeutic studies in perinatal medicine. J Pediatr, 102: 10–13.

Vacca A, Grant AM, Wyatt G, Chalmers I (1983). Portsmouth operative delivery trial: a comparison of vacuum extraction and forceps delivery. Br J Obstet Gynaecol, 90: 1107–1112.

Wachter KW (1988). Disturbed by meta-analysis? Perspective, 16 September: 1407.

Whitelaw A, Placzek M, Dubowitz L, Lary S, Levene M (1983). Phenobarbitone for prevention of periventricular haemorrhage in very low birthweight infants. Lancet, 2: 1168–1170.

Williamson JW, Goldschmidt PG, Colton T (1986). The quality of medical literature. Medical Uses of Statistics. Bailar J, Mosteller F (eds). Mass: NEJM Books, pp 370–391.

Wolf FM (1986). Meta-analysis: Quantitative Methods for Research Synthesis. London: Sage Publications.

Wolins L (1962). Responsibility for raw data. Am Psychol, 17: 657–658.

Wortman PM, Yeaton WH (1983). Synthesis of results in controlled clinical trials of coronary bypass graft surgery. In: Evaluation Studies Review Annual, Vol 8. Light RJ (ed). Beverly Hills, CA: Sage Publications, pp 536–551.

Yusuf S (1987). On obtaining medically meaningful answers from an overview of randomized clinical trials. Stat Med, 6: 281–286.

Yusuf S, Collins R, Peto R (1984). Why do we need some large, simple randomised trials? Stat Med, 3: 409–420.

Yusuf S, Peto R, Lewis T, Collins R, Sleight P (1985). Beta blockade during and after myocardial infarction: An overview of the randomised trials. Prog Cardiovasc Dis, XXVII (5): 336–371.

Appendix 2.1: Example of request to investigator for unpublished information

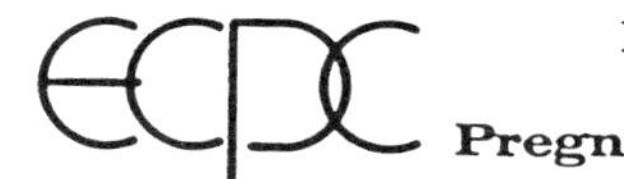

Effective Care in Pregnancy and Childbirth

Publisher

Oxford University Press
attn: Alison Langton
Walton Street
Oxford OX2 6DP
England

Editors

Murray W. Enkin
Dept. Obstetrics
McMaster University
1200 Main Street West
Hamilton
Canada L8N 3Z5
tel. (416) 521-2100

Marc J.N.C. Keirse
Dept. Obstetrics
Leiden University Hospital
Rijnsburgerweg 10
2333 AA Leiden
The Netherlands
tel. (071) 262881

Iain Chalmers
National Perinatal Epidemiology Unit
Radcliffe Infirmary
Oxford OX2 6HE
England
tel. (0865) 816876

* Trial number *

* Author's name *
* Address *
* City *
* Country *

* Date *

Dear * Author *,

As you will undoubtedly know, it is presently not entirely clear which method for induction of labour provides the best results. Relatively few studies have used adequate methodology and those that have, often report outcomes and criteria that are not strictly comparable from one study to another.

For a chapter on induction of labour in the book 'Effective Care in Pregnancy and Childbirth', we have embarked on a meta-analysis of all randomized controlled trials on induction of labour that were judged to have been properly conducted.

Your publication, listed underneath, has been selected for inclusion in our meta-analysis, because it fulfilled a set of quality criteria applied to it.

* full bibliographic reference *

In that meta-analysis we are comparing several items derived from the included studies and, obviously, we wish the data from each of these studies to be as complete and as comparable as possible. Therefore, we should like to enlist your help to provide us with some information, which we could not with certainty extract from your publication.

The items on which additional information is necessary are listed in a separate table. We should be grateful if you could complete the missing information and return the table to us, using the self-adhesive label. Even if you do no longer have the data to complete all of the questions, please say so and complete as much as possible.

We noted that you did not report the results on all of the patients who were entered into your trial. We are concerned that by excluding some cases from the final analysis, you may unintentionally have biased the overall impact of the study. This is particularly important for our meta-analysis, which covers trials with and without exclusions after randomisation.

If possible, we would therefore like to obtain data on all patients entered (including those whom you excluded from your analysis). To allow you to do so, we enclose a separate questionnaire which should only be used for data on the totality of patients entered in the trial. Perhaps it may be difficult to complete all items, but any item that can be completed (and items 1, 6, 12 and 48 in particular) will greatly help us.

We duly realize that we may be demanding a lot of work at the wrong time of the year. Nevertheless, it would be a pity if your contribution to the literature was not given the weight that it deserves in our meta-analysis.

Naturally, we would be most grateful for any additional comments that you may have either about your own study or about our proposed meta-analysis. Perhaps we should mention that, if you wish, we are prepared to send you the penultimate draft of our chapter for your attention and eventual comment.

With anticipated thanks and kind regards.

Yours sincerely,

Carla van Oppen, M.D. Marc J.N.C. Keirse, M.D., D.Phil.

Dear Author,

These are summary sheets of the main data which we have extracted from your paper. As mentioned we would like to obtain information on as many of these items as possible, to allow comparison with other studies. May we please draw your attention to the following points.

Specific Questions:

* Q1 * We have some doubts about the manner in which you allocated women to the different treatment groups. Can you please briefly indicate what system of (random) allocation you have used (for instance, sealed enveloppes, open list of random numbers, etc.)
Allocation by :

* Q2 * Some items such as delivered or not, Caesarean section, etc, are clearly unambiguous but others, such as Apgar scores and morbidity measures, are to some extent subjective assessments. Can you indicate whether or not the persons who assessed these items knew what treatment was being or had been given.

* persons were aware - not aware of treatment given

* Q4 * Your paper does not mention whether you studied normal pregnancies undergoing elective induction of labour, patients with pathology or high risk pregnancy, or both. Please indicate here what your study population consisted of :

* normal pregnancy - at risk / pathology - combination of both

* Q6 * In your paper you have mentioned success and/or failure rates, but you have not clearly stated what you understand by success and failure. Can you please give your definitions here :

MAY WE REQUEST SOME EXTRA ATTENTION TO THE ITEMS WHICH WE HAVE COLOURED BLUE
(this blue will not show up on your copying machine).

Appendix 2.2: Guidelines sent to authors of chapters in which formal overviews of randomized trials may be appropriate

As implied by the title of the book, we wish to document as far as possible the beneficial and adverse effects of the various forms of care available to women and babies during pregnancy, childbirth, and the early postnatal period. In many of the subject areas covered by the book—including those with which you are dealing—relevant and important evidence is available from controlled trials. Because the information derived from these formal human experiments is often of particular value, we wish to encourage contributors to the book to use a standard approach when reviewing and presenting the results of trials. This short paper outlines our suggestions.

1 Identifying relevant trials

We enclose one or more listings of references to published reports of controlled trials which may be relevant in the preparation of your chapter. These listings have been derived from the *Oxford Database of Perinatal Trials* and refer to trials published prior to the end of 1984. Other trials relevant to the subject which you are reviewing may have been published, but classified (or misclassified!) under other headings within the Database. For this reason, a full listing of all the trials contained in the Database will be sent to you later this year. By scanning through this fuller listing you may identify titles which suggest that the reports to which they refer contain data of relevance to your review. You may also come across both published and unpublished reports of relevant trials which have not yet been entered on the Database. We would be very grateful if you would draw Iain Chalmers' attention to these so that they can be registered. Finally, in the summer of 1986, you will be sent a listing of trial reports published during 1985, together with any relevant information we have about unpublished or ongoing trials.

2 Evaluation of the quality of trials

A number of schemes have been proposed during recent years for evaluating the quality of papers reporting controlled trials, and you may wish to consult these. The application of some of these requires a considerable amount of time and effort, and we recognize that it would be unreasonable to expect all of our contributors to follow them in detail. We would, however, ask that you assess each of the controlled trials which is relevant to the subject of your review by systematically asking each of the three following questions:

(i) How were the subjects allocated to the different treatments/policies (control of selection bias at entry)?

The crux of this issue lies in determining whether those enrolling study participants could know which treatment was next in line. Blinding of randomization is assured by assignment by telephone communication (preferably by an individual not involved in the actual treatment), or with indistinguishable drug treatments randomly precoded by a pharmacy. Such trials should be given full credit (***). In some trials, for example, those using sealed envelopes, there is a small but real chance of the next treatment being discovered by those enrolling participants. These studies should be given intermediate credit (**). Trials in which there was no attempt at blinding of the treatment allocation (use of patient record numbers, birth dates, dates of admission, or alternate allocation, etc.) should be given low credit (*).

(ii) Was the primary analysis based on all participants allocated to receive one or other of the alternative treatments (control of selection bias after entry)?

Withdrawal of cases from the trial after treatment allocation, for whatever reason, may tend to introduce selection bias into the comparisons made. Only trials in which the *primary* analysis is based on *all* cases entered should receive full credit (***). Trials in which you judge analyses after withdrawals to be too few to engender any material bias, should, especially if the question was handled carefully, be given intermediate credit (**). Others should be given low credit (*).

(iii) To what extent was the comparison of outcomes in the trial groups likely to have been affected by knowledge of the treatment allocation (control of bias in assessing outcomes)?

Some outcomes in perinatal trials (for example, date of delivery, death, and caesarean section) are unambiguous and unlikely to be subject to observer bias. Others—most measures of morbidity, for example—may be assessed differently if the observer is aware of the trial group to which the participant has been allocated. Trials should only be given full credit (***) if blinding was either of little relevance (because only unambiguous outcomes were compared), or if it was accomplished successfully (as it can be in many placebo-controlled drug trials). Other studies are only partially blindable and these should be given intermediate credit (**). In some trials in which outcomes subject to observer bias have been reported, no attempt will have been made to reduce observer bias: these studies should receive low credit (*).

A table of the following form summarizing your evaluation of each relevant trial should be submitted with your manuscript:

	Selection bias at entry	Analysis bias	Observer bias
Bloggs *et al.* 1985	**	*	**
Smith and Jones 1969	***	***	**
Grimm and Andersen 1975	***	*	*
Starsky and Hutch 1982	**	*	*
Morecambe and Wise 1984	*	*	*

Credit: *** = full; ** = intermediate; * = low

This table and your text should refer to all the relevant trial reports which you examine, even if you decide to exclude some from your formal overview because (as judged by the above criteria) the results might be seriously misleading because of poor methodology. You may wish to mention for your readers the results these trials actually yielded, and why you decided to reject them. If at all possible, your decision as to whether or not to include a particular trial in your formal overview should be based on an assessment (using the above criteria and any others you consider essential) made prior to examining the results of the trial. This last injunction may seem like a 'counsel of perfection'; but be alive to the possibility that your decision to include or exclude a particular trial may be influenced by its results rather than its methodological quality. We may like to think of ourselves as objective scientists, but we should acknowledge that no such beings exist!

3 Obtaining unpublished information from authors of published reports

We have found that it is often necessary to contact the authors of the original publication, either to clarify aspects of their study design, or to obtain data in a form which is not available in the published report itself. This often requires persistence, cajoling, flattery, bribery, blackmail, or other devices! But it has been our experience that these efforts produce dividends sufficiently often for them to be worthwhile. If you feel that any of us (or other contributors to the book) may be able to help (either because of geographical location or because of prior personal contacts), then do not hesitate to let us know.

4 Formal overviews of trials mounted to evaluate similar policies/treatments

Most of the trials you select for review will provide imprecise estimates of treatment differences because of the small size of the samples investigated (have you ever come across a trial that was too big?!). For this reason we wish to encourage you to conduct formal overviews ('meta-analyses') using data derived from all the trials mounted to evaluate similar policies/treatments. (We leave it to you to judge which particular trials can be grouped on the basis of similarity.) You should construct a separate table for each of the outcome variables about which you plan to make inferences, and enter the relevant outcome values from each of the trials for which you have been able to obtain data (either from the published report, or from the authors). If possible, you should try to construct tables referring to *all* cases *entered* into a particular trial, in other words, to overcome the problems which may have been created by withdrawals in the published analysis. You should also aim to fill all the cells, in other words, to obtain comparable information from *all* of the relevant trials.

An example of such a table is given below. From a table like this, it is possible not only to calculate the odds ratios for each trial individually, but also to derive a typical odds ratio using a simple extension of the

Mantel–Haenszel method. We enclose a copy of an article (Yusuf *et al.* 1985) in which this particular methodology is described and justified in detail.

Prevalence of parenchymal haemorrhage in very low birthweight infants after prophylactic administration of phenobarbitone:

Trial	Phenobarbitone group	Control group
Donn *et al.* (1981)	2/58	3/64
Morgan *et al.* (1982)	4/30	8/30
Bedard *et al.* (1984)	0/21	2/21
Whitelaw *et al.* (1983)	0/30	2/30

Please submit tables in the form illustrated above. We will be happy to do the statistical analysis here. We shall be doing this anyway in the course of assembling an electronic database of these overviews from which figures (illustrations) for the book will be produced in a standard format (see Figs 4–6 in article by Yusuf *et al.* 1985). As new trials are published, this electronic database will be updated.

5 Causal inferences based on formal overviews of trials

When conducting your analyses, please make a distinction between hypotheses *tested* by examining the data, as opposed to *hypotheses generated* by examining the data. For example, a review of trials of different methods of intrapartum fetal heart rate monitoring revealed an *unpredicted* distribution of neonatal convulsions which was unlikely to have been due to chance (Chalmers I 1979). This observation *generated* the hypothesis that certain forms of intrapartum fetal monitoring protected against convulsions. The hypothesis was subsequently *tested* (and sustained) in a separate, large trial (MacDonald *et al.* 1985). The combined analyses you conduct will be useful both in testing and generating hypotheses, but the distinction between these two different activities should be clear to readers of your text.

6 Publication of trial overviews

We predict that although doing all that we have asked you to do will involve you in a lot of work, you will find that the end result will be a satisfying and economic summary of the effects of the interventions compared in the trials you have reviewed. You may well decide that you would like to submit your analyses for publication in a journal as a separate paper in addition to submitting them as a chapter to us. This is quite acceptable to us as long as (i) you acknowledge the *Oxford Database of Perinatal Trials* as the source of your listing of relevant trials; (ii) you submit your chapter manuscript to us prior to submitting your journal manuscript; and (iii) no copyright difficulties are created.

If you have any questions or queries on any of the above matters, do not hesitate to let Iain Chalmers know of any ways in which he or anyone else may be able to help you.

Murray Enkin Marc Keirse Iain Chalmers

References

Chalmers I (1979). Randomised controlled trials of fetal monitoring 1973–1977. In: Perinatal Medicine. Thalhammer O, Baumgarten K, Pollak A (eds). Stuttgart: Georg Thieme, pp 260–265.

MacDonald D, Grant A, Sheridan-Pereira M, Boylan P, Chalmers I (1985). The Dublin randomised controlled trial of intrapartum fetal heart rate monitoring. Am J Obstet Gynecol, 152: 524–539.

Yusuf S, Peto R, Lewis T, Collins T, Sleight P (1985). Beta blockade during and after myocardial infarction: An overview of the randomised trials. Prog Cardiovasc Dis, XXVII (5): 336–371.

Appendix 2.3: Statistical methods used to derive typical odds ratio

In the following discussion we follow Yusuf *et al.* (1985). When considering data from a trial grouped in a 2 × 2 table,

	EXPTL group	CTRL group	Totals
Outcome present	a	b	$a + b$
Outcome absent	c	d	$c + d$
Totals	$a + c$	$b + d$	N

a is the OBSERVED number in the experimental group with the specified outcome, and is therefore often given the symbol O. This is contrasted with E, the number that would have been EXPECTED if the treatment made no difference to this outcome. Then

$$E = (a + b)\,(a + c)/N.$$

Under the null hypothesis that treatment has no effect on outcome, $(O - E)$ would have zero expectation, and variance:

$$\mathrm{Var}(O - E) = \frac{E(b + d)\,(1 - (a + b)/N)}{(N - 1)}.$$

If we have i trials ($i = 1,2, \ldots, r$), then likelihood theory shows that the simple unweighted summation

$$\mathrm{GT(grand\ total)} = \sum_i (O_i - E_i),$$

and

$$\mathrm{SIV(sum\ of\ individual\ variances)} = \sum_i \mathrm{Var}(O_i - E_i),$$

can yield an asymptotically efficient test of the null hypothesis, and a simple estimate (the log odds ratio $\beta = \mathrm{GT/SIV}$) of the alternative hypothesis.

Following Cox (1972) and Cox and Oakes (1984), in a single trial, the likelihood is

$$L(\beta) = p_a \exp(a\beta)/\sum p_k \exp(k\beta)$$

where p_k is the null hypothesis probability of k specified outcomes in the experimental group. Taking logs and differentiating at $\beta = 0$ gives

$$dL/d\beta = j - \sum kp_k = (O - E)$$

and

$$d^2L/d\beta^2 = \sum k^2 p_k - (\sum kp_k)^2 = \mathrm{Var}(O - E).$$

If there are i different trials, and $\beta_i = \beta$, the first and second values at $\beta = 0$ are $\sum(O_i - E_i)$ (the slope, s) and $-\sum_i \mathrm{Var}(O_i - E_i)$ (the curvature, c). As s/c is the first Newton–Raphson step from zero towards the maximum likelihood value of β, it estimates the true value of β, with

$$\text{variance} = \mathrm{Var}(s)/c^2 = 1/c.$$

Tests of significance (and confidence intervals) for β are based on the assumption that, under the null hypothesis, β is approximately Normally distributed. Thus the 95% confidence interval for β, the estimated log odds ratio, is given by

$$(s/c \pm 1.96/\sqrt{c})$$

and, for the estimate of the odds ratio, by

$$\text{exponent}(s/c \pm 1.96/\sqrt{c}).$$

If $\beta_i = \beta$, the tests achieve asymptotic efficiency, but they are still valid in the more likely situation of some heterogeneity between different trials.

Example of calculations

An example of the calculation of a typical odds ratio and 95% confidence interval, based on two hypothetical trials, is given below:

Trial 1

	EXPTL group	CTRL group	Totals
Outcome present	75	25	100
Outcome absent	25	75	100
Totals	100	100	200

$$\begin{aligned} E &= (100 \times 100)/200 = 50 \\ O - E &= 75-50 = 25 \\ \mathrm{Var}\,(O - E) &= [50 \times 100 \times (1 - 100/200)] \\ &\quad /(200 - 1) \\ &= 12.5628 \end{aligned}$$

$$\begin{aligned} \underline{\text{Odds ratio estimate}} &= \exp\left[\frac{25}{12.5628}\right] \\ &= \exp[1.99] \\ &= \underline{7.3155} \end{aligned}$$

$$\begin{aligned} \underline{95\%\ \text{confidence interval}} &= \exp[1.99 \pm 1.96/\sqrt{12.5628}] \\ &= \exp[1.99 \pm 1.96/3.544] \\ &= \exp[1.99 \pm 0.553] \\ &= \exp[1.437 \text{ to } 2.543] \\ &= \underline{4.2081 \text{ to } 12.7178} \end{aligned}$$

i.e. Odds ratio (95% CI)
= 7.32 (4.21 to 12.72)

Trial 2

	EXPTL group	CTRL group	Totals
Outcome present	60	40	100
Outcome absent	50	50	100
Totals	110	90	200

$$\begin{aligned} E &= (100 \times 110)/200 = 55 \\ O - E &= 60 - 55 = 5 \\ \mathrm{Var}\,(O - E) &= [55 \times 90 \times (1\text{–}100/200)]/ \\ &\quad (200\text{–}1) \\ &= 12.4372 \end{aligned}$$

$$\begin{aligned} \underline{\text{Odds ratio estimate}} &= \exp\left[\frac{5}{12.4372}\right] \\ &= \exp[0.402] \\ &= \underline{1.4948} \end{aligned}$$

$$\begin{aligned} \underline{95\%\ \text{confidence interval}} &= \exp[0.402 \pm 1.96/\sqrt{12.4372}] \\ &= \exp[0.402 \pm 1.96/3.5266] \\ &= \exp[0.402 \pm 0.5558] \\ &= \exp[-0.1558, 0.9558] \\ &= \underline{0.8557 \text{ to } 2.6008} \end{aligned}$$

i.e. Odds ratio (95% CI)
= 1.49 (0.86 to 2.60)

Typical odds ratio estimate =

$$\exp \frac{[(O-E)_{\text{Trial 1}} + (O-E)_{\text{Trial 2}}]}{[\text{Var}(O-E)_{\text{Trial 1}} + \text{Var}(O-E)_{\text{Trial 2}}]}$$

$$= \exp\frac{[25+5]}{[12.5628+12.4372]}$$

$$= \exp\left[\frac{30}{25}\right]$$

$$= \exp[1.2] = 3.3201$$

95% confidence interval

$$= \exp[1.2 \pm 1.96/\sqrt{25}]$$
$$= \exp[1.2 \pm 0.392]$$
$$= \exp[0.8080 \text{ to } 1.5920]$$
$$= 2.2434 \text{ to } 4.9136$$

i.e. Typical odds ratio (95% CI)
= 3.32 (2.24 to 4.91).

References

Cox DR (1972). Analysis of Binary Data. London: Methuen.
Cox DR, Oakes D (1984). Analysis of Survival Data. London: Chapman & Hall.
Yusuf S, Peto R, Lewis J, Collins T, Sleight P (1985). Beta blockade during and after myocardial infarction: An overview of the randomised trials. Prog Cardiovasc Dis, XXVII (5): 336–371.

Appendix 2.4: The relationship between relative risk and odds ratio

'Risk' and 'odds' are alternative ways of expressing the likelihood that a particular event will or will not occur, but they do so in different ways. Of the two, risk is probably the more familiar concept, except perhaps to gamblers, who may more readily conceptualize likelihood in terms of odds. As noted in Section 3.6 above, we have chosen to present the results of overview analyses in terms of odds ratios. This Appendix outlines the relationship between the odds ratio and the more familiar concept of the relative risk (which is also sometimes referred to as the risk ratio, the rate ratio or the relative probability). Because relative risk is the more familiar of the two concepts, it has been discussed first in each of the comparisons with odds ratio that follow.

If neonatal death occurs in 20 infants *out of a total* number of 100 infants who are born preterm, the *risk* of neonatal death is 20/100 = 0.20. The *odds* of neonatal death, on the other hand, is derived by contrasting the number of infants who die (20) *against* the number who survive the neonatal period (100—20). The odds of neonatal mortality among preterm infants is therefore 20/(100—20) = 0.25. Thus, when expressing the chances of neonatal death as a *risk*, one estimates that, on average, 20 *out of* every 100 infants will die; when expressing the chances as *odds*, one estimates that 20 infants will die *against* (or *for*) every 80 (100—20) who survive. Some examples of the differences between risk and odds as alternative descriptors of likelihood are presented in Table A4.1.

Table A4.1 Examples of the differences between risk and odds as alternative descriptors of likelihood

Number of individuals with outcome	Risk	Odds
2 of 100	2/100 = 0.02	2:98 = 0.02
20 of 100	20/100 = 0.20	20:80 = 0.25
50 of 100	50/100 = 0.50	50:50 = 1.00
80 of 100	80/100 = 0.80	80:20 = 4.00

Since the risk and the odds of an event occurring are interrelated (and indeed are only different methods of expressing the same relationship), it follows that one can be derived from the other. Risk can be converted to odds by dividing risk by 1 minus the risk; odds can be converted to risk, by dividing odds by odds plus 1. That is:

$$(\text{Risk})/(1 - \text{Risk}) = \text{Odds}$$
$$(\text{Odds})/(1 + \text{Odds}) = \text{Risk}$$

The numerical values of risk and odds show little difference when the outcome is relatively rare. However, assuming that odds is *necessarily* an approximation of risk, or vice versa, can be misleading. As Table A4.2 shows, the assumption of equivalence is not justified when the outcomes studied are relatively frequent. Such outcomes include, for example, operative

Table A4.2 Influence of the prevalence of an outcome on relative risk and odds ratio: in all of the examples given in the table it is assumed that the experimental group is exposed to a treatment that will reduce the incidence of an outcome to half its incidence in the untreated (control) group.

Incidence of outcome		Relative risk	Odds ratio
Experimental group	Control group		
2/100	4/100	$\frac{2/100}{4/100} = 0.50$	$\frac{2/98}{4/96} = 0.49$
20/100	40/100	$\frac{20/100}{40/100} = 0.50$	$\frac{20/80}{40/60} = 0.37$
40/100	80/100	$\frac{40/100}{80/100} = 0.50$	$\frac{40/60}{80/20} = 0.17$

delivery, perineal pain following childbirth; or onset of labour during cervical ripening. In the largest reported trial of endocervical prostaglandin gel for cervical ripening, for example, 240 of 416 women went into labour during cervical ripening (Noah *et al.* 1987). These results give a risk of going into labour during cervical ripening of 0.59, but an odds of 1.36.

Risk and odds are both used to express the likelihood that a particular event will occur *within* a particular group of individuals. Risks or odds can also be compared *between* groups, thus expressing the *relative* likelihood that a particular event will occur. These 'relative likelihoods' can be used to summarize the differences between comparison groups in a variety of circumstances. Both forms of statistical expression can be used to summarize the differences in outcome observed in the comparison groups in randomized controlled trials. This is achieved by comparing either the risk or the odds of a particular outcome (for instance, respiratory distress syndrome) in individuals who received one form of care (for instance, prenatal corticosteroids) with the risk or the odds of that outcome in individuals who received some alternative from of care (for instance, placebo). When this relationship is expressed as the ratio of risks it is usually referred to as the *relative risk* (or risk ratio, rate ratio, or relative probability). When the relationship is expressed as a ratio of odds it is referred to as the *odds ratio*.

The association between an outcome and a particular form of care by which it may be influenced can be illustrated in a 2 × 2 table. Figure A4.1 shows that the risk of the outcome can be calculated both for the group that received an innovative form of care (the experimental group) and a group that received a standard form of care (the control group). Likewise odds can be computed for both the experimental group and the control group. The association between the outcome and the forms of care compared in randomized controlled trials can thus be expressed either in terms of *relative risk*, or as an *odds ratio*. The *relative risk* is an expression of the comparison of the risk of a particular outcome in the experimental group *relative to* the risk in the control group; the *odds ratio* is an expression of the comparison of the odds of the outcome in the experimental group with the odds in the control group. The derivation of these two statistics is shown in Fig. A4.1.

From the formulae in Fig. A4.1 it can be appreciated that both the relative risk and the odds ratio will be *less* than 1 when an outcome occurs less frequently in the experimental than in the control group. Likewise, both will be *greater* than 1 if the outcome occurs more frequently in the experimental than in the control group. The *direction* of the relative risk and odds ratio

	Experimental	Control	
Outcome present	a	b	$a+b$
Outcome absent	c	d	$c+d$
	$a+c$	$b+d$	$a+b+c+d$

Risk (exptl) = $\frac{a}{a+c}$ Odds (exptl) = $\frac{a}{c}$

Risk (contl) = $\frac{b}{b+d}$ Odds (contl) = $\frac{b}{d}$

RELATIVE RISK = $\frac{\text{Risk (exptl)}}{\text{Risk (contl)}} = \frac{a/(a+c)}{b/(b+d)}$

ODDS RATIO = $\frac{\text{Odds (exptl)}}{\text{Odds (contl)}} = \frac{a/c}{b/d} = \frac{a \times d}{b \times c}$

Fig. A4.1 A 2 × 2 table showing the relationship between relative risk and odds ratio.

(less than or greater than 1) is always the same. The *extent* to which the odds ratio and relative risk deviate from unity, however, can be quite different. As illustrated in Table A4.2, if the experimental group has received a form of care that reduces the incidence of an outcome to 50 per cent of the level experienced by individuals who did not receive the form of care concerned (the controls), and if the form of care concerned has the same effect (a 50 per cent reduction) irrespective of the baseline risk of the outcome in control individuals, then the relative risk of the outcome in the experimental and control groups is constant at 0.50, irrespective of the risk of death in the untreated individuals. The odds ratio, on the other hand, changes very markedly with changes in the incidence of the outcome in untreated individuals, and ranges from 0.17 to 0.49 in the example shown in Table A4.2. As discussed in Section 4.3 of this chapter, the nomogram presented in Fig. 2.3 (and reproduced as a bookmark) should help readers to estimate the implications, in practice, of an odds ratio of any given value.

Reference

Noah ML, De Coster JM, Fraser TJ, Orr JD (1987). Pre-induction cervical softening with endocervical PGE2 gel. Acta Obstet Gynecol Scand, 66: 3–7.

3 Evaluating diagnosis and screening during pregnancy and childbirth

Patrick Mohide and Adrian Grant

'In dwelling upon the vital importance of sound observation, it must never be lost sight of what observation is for. It is not for the sake of piling up miscellaneous information or curious facts, but for the sake of saving life and increasing comfort . . . It would really seem as if some had considered it (observation) as its own end, as if detection, not cure, was their business'

Florence Nightingale 1860

1 Introduction

As our opening quotation from Florence Nightingale makes clear, 'sound observation' is a necessary but not sufficient criterion for assessing the worth of diagnostic and screening activity in health care. During pregnancy and childbirth, as in other situations, diagnostic and screening procedures do not necessarily lead to improved health of the women and babies to whom they are applied; indeed, they may actually pose threats to their well-being. In this chapter we outline how diagnostic and screening activities can be evaluated systematically to maximize the chance that more good than harm will result from their use in pregnancy and childbirth.

Accurate and prompt diagnosis of problems arising during pregnancy and childbirth can be a crucial element in the provision of effective care. Sometimes the problems will declare themselves with symptoms and signs which result in the pregnant woman herself making the diagnosis. Severe revealed antepartum haemorrhage, for example, is a potentially life-threatening condition which is easily diagnosed with accuracy. It is worth diagnosing promptly because, whatever the origins of the bleeding, there are effective measures (transfusion of blood or plasma expanders) for reducing the threat that it poses to the pregnant woman's life.

Even though some problems will be diagnosed accurately by most women and most of the professionals they consult, the provision of effective care may often depend on refinements in the diagnosis. Thus, although little diagnostic acumen is required to recognize a severe haemorrhage after delivery, accurate diagnosis of the cause of the bleeding (hypotonic uterus, incomplete delivery of the placenta, trauma, or some other problem) requires more experience, and is of obvious importance in selecting effective measures for dealing with the problem.

Some of the problems that complicate pregnancy and childbirth present far more subtle diagnostic challenges than those outlined above. In detecting these, it is not surprising that experience begins to tell. A woman's experience of one or more previous pregnancies, for example, may lead her to recognize departures from normal in her current pregnancy, and to make a diagnosis of twin pregnancy or fetal malpresentation. An experienced clinician may make an accurate diagnosis of abdominal pregnancy based on a pattern of symptoms and clinical signs which less experienced observers might not have perceived so clearly.

The informal weighing and synthesis of factors which lead some experienced individuals to make better predictions than others is clearly an important element in promoting effective care. Unfortunately, this process has proved difficult to document and analyse formally and this has constrained the possibilities for making these skills more widely available to all those who provide care.

2 The statistical approach to diagnosis and screening

Many of the diagnostic judgments made by both experienced and inexperienced individuals will continue to be based on incomplete and imprecise characterization of individual women and babies. Because of this, professionals providing care have tended to categorize individual women as members of *groups* which, in aggregate, are known to be at differing risks of experiencing adverse outcomes of pregnancy; patterns of care which have previously been shown to be effective in reducing the risk of the adverse outcomes in similarly delineated groups are then applied to them.

This systematic way of improving the accuracy of diagnosis and prognosis in individual patients was first suggested more than a hundred years ago by Pierre-Charles-Alexandre Louis (Greenwood 1986). He recognized that with the limited intellectual powers of all human beings, clinicians (experienced and inexperienced) had to address questions about diagnosis, prognosis, and treatment in an informal, but nevertheless essentially statistical way. The problems presented by an individual patient were confronted by drawing on experience derived from seeing similar patients previously. Louis acknowledged that 'No two individuals will have exactly the same symptoms, if we only make a sufficiently long catalogue of symptoms'; but he recognized that 'it might be possible to make a group characterization. To say that symptoms and signs "a", "b", "c" and "d" concur so frequently and when concurring are so frequently precursors of such and such events, that when they have established in an individual, a judgement of diagnosis and prognosis will much more often be right than wrong'. He went on to propose that, to have a valid and efficient system for achieving this objective, one needed to be able to draw on a systematically collected body of accurate observations. The use of this approach does not alter the fact that the groups may often be heterogeneous with respect to characteristics that are important but nevertheless unidentified or undocumented predictors of prognosis.

A century after Louis made his proposals (and put them into effect in respect of patients with gastroenteritis), Alvan Feinstein (1976) noted the lack of progress in implementing them. 'The idea that clinical medicine has no intellectual content, with nothing worthy of science, nothing that can be considered a research challenge, is what has kept the state of clinical practice in its current condition of intellectual decrepitude and servitude throughout the ages ... By ideologically excluding prediction (rather than explanation) from being an important basic scientific challenge, we have excluded the clinician from any kind of scientific activity. The clinician's job is to predict. That's what patients want from him . . . The public expects and wants us to make those predictions with scientific accuracy and confidence.'

In the decade since those words were written there has been progress, both in encouraging a more systematic approach to diagnosis and screening in general (Wald 1984; Sackett *et al.* 1985), and in refining and improving prediction in specific circumstances, such as the use of serum alpha-fetoprotein levels in conjunction with maternal age to refine risk estimates of Down's syndrome (Tabar 1987). Such refinement must continue and every effort should be made to ensure that individual mothers receive care which is appropriate to their individual needs.

It would be a mistake, however, to imagine that any amount of progress in improving diagnostic accuracy will ever lead to a situation in which care can always be individualized with such confidence that the type of care selected and applied will *always* benefit the individual mother and fetus concerned. It will continue to be inevitable that some will receive forms of care from which they cannot benefit and that others will not receive forms of care from which they could have benefited. The challenge is to minimize the occasions on which these situations occur by making intelligent use of the best information available.

In one important way, none of the specific examples given above are typical of the kind of diagnostic problems that cause most difficulty to those providing care during pregnancy and childbirth. Many of the health problems experienced by women and their babies either do not declare themselves at all through symptoms, or do so at a late stage in their development. The delineation of those *asymptomatic* women and babies who are at greater than average risk of experiencing important problems is thus a major objective of care. This *screening*, as opposed to diagnostic, activity rests on the belief that earlier identification and earlier care will have a favourable impact on the natural history of conditions such as pre-eclampsia, preterm labour, fetal growth retardation, urinary tract and other infections, anaemia, treatable fetal malformations, and other fetal problems.

The criterion by which the value of all diagnostic and screening activities must ultimately be assessed is whether or not the individuals to whom they are applied are better off as a result (Davies *et al.* 1977). The activities of diagnosis and screening occupy different parts of a single spectrum, and the distinction between them is not always clear in practice. There are nevertheless fundamental differences in principle which should be recognized. The examples of diagnostic activity outlined above have shown that diagnosis involves people who have already recognized themselves to be at increased risk of some sort of problem for which they seek a solution. Screening activities on the other hand, imply a search by professionals for problems in apparently healthy individuals. The fact that the invitation for screening comes from professionals implies a special responsibility to ensure that more good than harm results. For this reason, criteria have been developed by which the advantages and disadvantages of screening programmes can and should be evaluated (Table 3.1; Wilson and Jungner 1968; Cadman *et al.* 1984).

Table 3.1 Prerequisites of a screening programme

1. The condition sought should be an important health problem.	2. The natural history of the condition, including development from latent to overt stages, should be adequately understood.
3. The condition should have an identifiable latent period or early symptomatic phase during which intervention is possible.	4. A suitable screening test should be available.
5. The test should be acceptable to those tested.	6. There should be a satisfactory diagnostic test with an agreed policy of case definition.
7. There should be an effective management for patients with the recognized condition.	8. The search for the condition should be a continuing process.
9. The resources needed for diagnosis and treatment should be available.	10. The costs incurred as a result of finding cases (which includes both identification and treatment) should be economically balanced in relation to possible expenditure on an alternative programme or on medical care as a whole.

The various screening activities that comprise antenatal care have tended to escape the critical assessment to which most screening programmes have been subjected in recent years (Cochrane 1972). One reason is that antenatal care was established so long ago. This situation is changing and screening during pregnancy and childbirth is now beginning to be assessed more systematically (Wald 1984; see Chapter 22).

3 'Gold' and other standards

Some of the conditions used earlier to illustrate the processes of diagnosis and screening provide obvious 'Gold Standards' (our best measures of the truth) against which to assess the accuracy of the diagnoses made. A woman's diagnosis of multiple pregnancy can be confirmed or rejected by waiting to see how many babies are born; a clinician's diagnosis of an abdominal pregnancy based on clinical observations may or may not be supported by findings at laparotomy.

More often, however, such unequivocal and objective Gold Standards are simply not available for assessing diagnostic accuracy. How, for example, should one assess the accuracy of a diagnosis of preterm labour? If a woman in the 30th week of pregnancy is draining liquor, experiencing painful uterine contractions every 3 minutes, and a vaginal examination reveals that her cervix is effaced and 8 cm dilated, everyone will agree about the diagnosis—and the passage of half an hour or so will likely confirm, in retrospect, the accuracy of that judgement. But what if she is experiencing regular lower abdominal pains but is not draining liquor, and her cervix is uneffaced and only 1cm dilated? In these circumstances there is no Gold Standard against which to assess diagnostic accuracy, so uncertainty and clinical disagreement about the diagnosis is therefore understandable. One has to fall back on assessing the extent to which this constellation of symptoms and signs *predicts* the occurrence of a later event—preterm delivery—which is by no means inevitably associated with the clinical picture described (see Chapter 44).

The quality of *prediction* in antenatal and intrapartum care is a crucial component of the effective care in pregnancy and childbirth. In the second of the two examples given above, clinical symptoms and signs were used to categorize the woman concerned as a member of a group whose fetuses are known from previous observations to be at greater than average risk of experiencing problems—in this case, the problems associated with being born too early in gestation. Clearly, this kind of designation is less than satisfactory; it would obviously be preferable if a more 'diagnostic' judgement identified the woman either as someone who definitely would, or someone who definitely would not go on to deliver her baby preterm. Appropriate care could then be planned and instituted. Unfortunately, however, assessment that has greater diagnostic precision and predictive utility is often not possible, and decisions may have to be taken on the basis of an individual's membership of a group with a known collective risk status.

Identifying and defining such groups is achieved not only by taking symptoms and clinical signs into account, but also by using one or more of a variety of tests in both symptomatic and asymptomatic individuals. The predictive properties of these tests is assessed by comparing test results with whatever appears to come closest to a Gold Standard for the test in question. Of the various conditions which might serve as Gold

Standards against which to assess the predictive ability of various tests of 'fetal well-being', death is the least ambiguous. It is recognizable and clear-cut. But it occurs rarely, so that very large numbers of women and their babies must be studied before the validity of antenatal tests as predictors of death can be properly evaluated. Furthermore, fetal and infant deaths result from a wide variety of pathological processes, many of which remain poorly understood. The predictive qualities of a test may well depend on whether death regardless of cause, or death from a particular cause, is the outcome of interest. Some forms of infant morbidity are as recognizable and clear-cut as death: open neural tube defects are an example. But, like death, they are rare, as are other neonatal conditions that are of particular interest because they are relatively strong predictors of long term impairments (such as prolonged delay in establishing spontaneous respiration or very early neonatal seizures). More frequently occurring conditions, such as low 1- or 5-minute Apgar scores or low cord pH values, are of less value because of their relatively poor or unknown usefulness for predicting health status in childhood.

A commonly used Gold Standard against which the predictive performance of antenatal tests of fetal well-being has been assessed is 'birthweight for gestational age'. This is often assumed to be a good measure of the adequacy of intrauterine growth (growth retardation being arbitrarily defined as weights below the 10th, 5th, or other percentile of weight for any particular gestational age). The assumptions on which these 'growth' standards are based, however, may be quite invalid (see Chapter 26). Cross-sectional data obtained at birth cannot be assumed to reflect longitudinal fetal growth. Such centile charts do not identify as compromised those babies whose intrauterine growth may have been severely retarded, but who happen to weigh more than the 10th percentile on standard 'weight-for-gestational-age' charts.

Sometimes, the attempt to find a Gold Standard against which to assess the validity of a test is dispensed with entirely, and the test in question used as its own Gold Standard (see, for example, Aubry *et al.* 1975); at other times, the results of other tests that are being used in an attempt to identify or predict a condition are used as surrogate measures for the condition itself (see, for example, Brown *et al.* 1976). The practice of giving labels such as 'acute or chronic fetal distress', 'chronic anoxia', or 'placental insufficiency' to the positive results of these tests implies a status and validity that they almost certainly do not possess. Indeed, the expression of the validity of a test in such terms is often self-fulfilling and circular.

The paucity of true Gold Standards (for example, twin birth or perinatal death) for assessing the validity of the diagnostic and screening tests used in pregnancy and childbirth often means that in practice there is no alternative to 'playing the substitution game' (Sackett 1979); that is, using surrogates for adverse outcomes like low birthweight or preterm delivery. But the limitations of doing this should never be forgotten.

4 Characteristics of screening and diagnostic tests

4.1 Reproducibility

Internal validation of a test—assessment of the extent to which the results of repeated measurements agree with each other is obviously less important than external validation of a test—an assessment of the extent to which its results correspond with a Gold Standard. Nevertheless, it is certainly necessary, but not sufficient, that there is good agreement between repeated measurements, that is, good *reproducibility* (sometimes referred to as repeatability, reliability, or consistency). The fact that test results are reproducible does not mean, however, that the test is measuring what it is supposed to be measuring (see next section). Poor reproducibility is worth detecting, however, because it may indicate that steps should be taken to improve the test's performance in this respect.

Repeated measurements using the same test may give varying results for a variety of reasons. First, there may be *inherent variability* in whatever is being tested, such as the degree of wakefulness in an individual fetus whose movements are being counted. A second source of variation may be inherent in the test itself or in its interpretation by an individual clinician (*intra-observer variability*). Finally, there may be differences between different clinicians' interpretations of a test, for example, a fetal heart rate tracing (*inter-observer variability*), (as was found by Trimbos and Keirse (1978) and Beaulieu *et al.* (1982) for cardiotocography), or differences between different pieces of equipment used to perform a test (for example, different electronic fetal heart rate monitoring methods (Keirse *et al.* 1981)). Put another way, the extent to which a test is *reproducible* is affected by variation arising from three major sources: 'the examined', 'the examination', and 'the examiner' (Sackett *et al.* 1985).

Variation *within* a particular observer or piece of equipment is largely random, whereas variation *between* observers or pieces of equipment is largely systematic. Unlike random variation, systematic variation is not reduced by repeated measurement. Sometimes it can be reduced by altering other aspects of the way in which the test is used, for example, by more rigid standardization of the methods with which the test is applied (Trimbos and Keirse 1978). Although the reproducibility of a test is often not assessed systematically, time taken to improve a test's reproducibility may pay dividends in improving its external validity.

Finally, one of the questions rarely addressed is 'What happens to the reproducibility (and other properties) of a test when it is applied, not in a carefully controlled research setting, but in usual clinical practice?'. This issue is of particular concern for tests which incorporate subjective evaluation such as the evaluation of fetal heart rate traces or ultrasound images.

4.2 Sensitivity and specificity

The external validity of a diagnostic or screening test depends on its ability to differentiate those women who have a suspected condition from those who do not. When a Gold Standard exists this process can be conceptualized straightforwardly. The validity of an ultrasound diagnosis of anencephaly, for example, can be assessed by visual examination of the baby after abortion or delivery.

The simplest way of representing the comparison of a test's results with a Gold Standard is with a '2 × 2' table. (Table 3.2). There are several useful ways to assess the important components of the relationship between test results and what the test is purporting to measure or predict. Each is identified by a jargon term which is useful for efficient communication (Haynes 1981). The first two elements of this comparison (sensitivity and specificity) consider how well the test correctly identifies individuals with or without the condition of interest. As shown in the vertical columns of Table 3.2, the Gold Standard indicates that (a + c) individuals actually have the condition; of these, only the a subjects had a positive test result. Thus an index of the test's ability to detect the condition when it is present is the ratio of a to (a + c), usually expressed as a percentage, and referred to as the test's 'sensitivity'. Similarly, the ability of the test to exclude the condition correctly is shown by the ratio of unaffected individuals with a negative test, the d individuals, to all those tested who do not have the condition, the (b + d) individuals; this index d/(b + d) is called 'specificity'. Sensitivity and specificity are considered to be stable properties in most tests: they tend not to vary when the proportions of people with the condition of interest varies, provided that the limits of normality are fixed.

4.3 Normal limits

Approximation to the Gold Standard can also be used to define the normal limits of a test. If, as is the case for nearly all tests, there is an overlap in the range of results for those individuals shown by the Gold Standard to be disease-free and those shown to be diseased, then cut-off points within the distribution of test results can be chosen (see Fig. 3.1). These may be set anywhere between point X, the lowest value for the individuals without the condition, and point Z, the highest value for those with the condition. Notice that the a, b, c, and d in Fig. 3.1 correspond with the a, b, c, d in Table 3.2 and their relationship can be described in the same jargon terms mentioned earlier.

If we want to maximize the number of times that the test result is correct (maximum accuracy), then we set the limit at point Y. In some clinical situations we may wish to be certain of identifying all those with the condition (maximum sensitivity), in which case point Z should be chosen. The price paid for this would be a

Table 3.2 Fourfold table comparing test results

		'Gold Standard' ('the truth')		
		Subjects **have** the condition	Subjects **do not have** the condition	
'Test results' (conclusion drawn from the results of the test)	**Positive** Subjects appear to have the condition	True positives (a)	False positives (b)	a + b
	Negative Subjects appear not to have the condition	(c) False negatives	(d) True negatives	c + d
		a + c	b + d	a + b + c + d

Stable properties: sensitivity: $= a/(a + c)$; specificity $= d/(b + d)$.
Likelihood ratio for positive test $[a/(a + c)]/[b/(b + d)]$
Likelihood ratio for negative test $[c/(a + c)]/[d/(b + d)]$
Frequency-dependent properties: positive predictive value $= a/(a + b)$; negative predictive value $= d/(c + d)$; accuracy: $(a + d)/(a + b + c + d)$; prevalence $= (a + c)/(a + b + c + d)$.

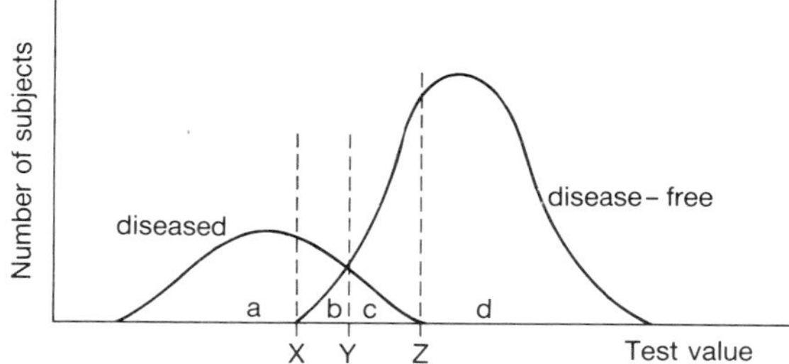

Fig. 3.1 Effect of the choice of a cut-off point on a test's performance: x minimizing false positive results; y minimizing the total false results; and z minimizing false negative results

dramatic increase in the numbers of false positive test results (Table 3.2, cell b: that is, low specificity). Alternatively, we may prefer to minimize the number of false positive test results (high specificity). In this case, point X would be chosen, even though a large proportion of true cases would be missed as a result (low sensitivity).

In this way sensitivity and specificity compete with one another. The cut-off point chosen will determine the way in which borderline results will be classified. This choice must be a value judgment. The dangers of missing the diagnosis in those who actually have the condition c must be weighed against the hazards of falsely labelling people with a condition which in truth they do not have b.

The trade-off can be described graphically on a receiver operating characteristic (ROC) curve (Sackett *et al.* 1985; Richardson *et al.* 1985). Values of sensitivity are plotted against values of 1-specificity for a series of different cut-off points to derive a curve. This method can be used with tests that are based on *continuous* measures, such as blood pressure and haemoglobin, or with tests that have more than two possible *categorical* results, such as antepartum fetal heart rate patterns which can either be interpreted as reactive, equivocal, non-reactive, terminal, or uninterpretable (Rochard *et al.* 1976; Keirse and Trimbos 1980) or scored on a scale of 0 to 10 (Fisher 1976). For example, Keirse and Trimbos (1980, 1981) showed that changing the threshold for 'normal' score from 8 to 6 in their analysis of antenatal cardiotocography, the specificity rose from 88 per cent to 100 per cent, but the sensitivity fell from 75 per cent to 46 per cent. The results of doing this using the data presented by Manning *et al.* (1985) for the prediction of perinatal death by biophysical profile scoring are shown in Fig. 3.2. In this example, the closest cut-off to sensitivity = 1 and specificity = 1 (1-specificity = 0) is at score 6 (abnormal = 0 to 6). This provides the optimal cut-off by minimizing the number of false positive and false negative results.

A much less satisfactory approach to the definition of abnormal individuals than one using a Gold Standard is

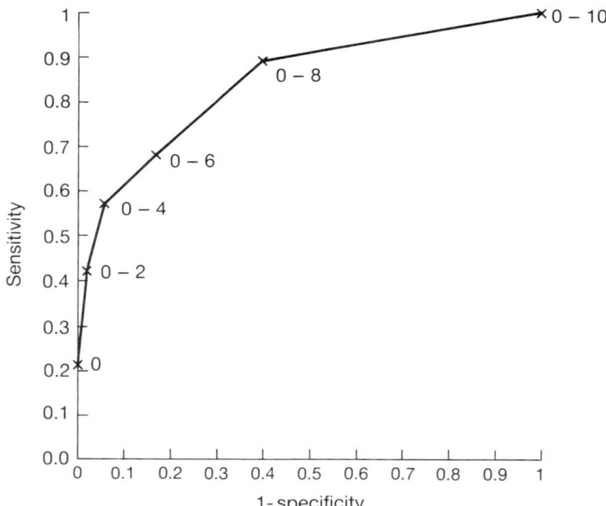

Fig. 3.2 Receiver operating characteristic curve constructed for data of Manning *et al.* (1985)

to use a statistical definition of abnormality based on arbitrarily defined cut-off points at varying distances from the mean or median values of test results. Limits of normality for biochemical placental function tests frequently apply this approach (see Chapter 29). Two standard deviations either side of the mean encompass 95 per cent of its values; abnormals, by definition, lie outside this range. Thus because of normal biological variation, if such a test were to be carried out on 20 pregnant women, on average one abnormal result would be expected to occur by chance. The approach also presupposes that the test values follow a symmetrical (or Gaussian) distribution, though few test results actually do this. While it may be possible to overcome this problem by the use of percentiles, multiples of the median, or statistical transformation, a statistical definition of normality still does not take into account the actual pattern of biological variation, because it assumes a fixed prevalence of disease (in this case 2.5 per cent at both extremes of the distribution).

4.4 Predictive properties

Sensitivity and specificity are not the most useful features of a test in clinical practice, even after normal limits have been defined. A clinician attempting to make a diagnosis is not interested in the academic question: 'If my patient has the condition, how likely is she to have a positive test?' but in the practical question: 'If my patient's test is positive, how likely is it that she really has the condition?' To answer this, referring back to Table 3.2, we must now read horizontally rather than vertically. Of those women with a positive test result (a + b), what proportion actually have the condition of interest? To use the jargon term, we are interested in the 'positive predictive value' of the test: a/(a + b). Conversely, we also want to know, in the case of a negative test result, how confidently we may assume that the condition is not present. This is called the 'negative predictive value', d/(c + d), of the test. Putting them together, the overall 'accuracy' of the test (agreement between the test and the Gold Standard) is expressed as the ratio of true positives and true negatives to the total number of women tested: (a + d)/(a + b + c + d).

Although the sensitivity and specificity of a test usually remain stable, the positive and negative predictive values, and thus the accuracy of the test, fluctuate widely depending on the proportion of women or fetuses who truly have the condition for which they are being tested (Layhew and Goldsmith 1975). This proportion (called the 'prevalence' of the condition) is expressed by the ratio of the number of women (or fetuses) who have the condition to the total number tested, or, by reference to Table 3.2, (a + c)/(a + b + c + d). The prevalence of the condition in the group being tested may have a dramatic effect on the relative sizes of a, b, c, and d, and thus on the predictive value of the test. For this reason it is essential to take account of the clinical context in which a test is to be used when deciding what limits to choose. For example, it can be seen from Fig. 3.1 that it may be wise to choose a less sensitive cut-off point (that is nearer point X) when applying a test to a lower-risk group of women (for instance, when screening for disease) than when the same test is being applied to a group at higher risk (for example, women admitted to hospital because of some abnormality) of whom a large proportion do in fact have the condition.

An understanding of the effect of variations in the prevalence of a condition on the stable and unstable properties of screening and diagnostic tests is central to their rational use. The fact that the same test applied to groups of individuals at different risk will have entirely different predictive properties is not intuitively obvious. Many clinicians are unaware of the important influence of prevalence on the meaning of a test result. This phenomenon is illustrated in Table 3.3. The positive predictive value deteriorates markedly as the true prevalence of the abnormality decreases, as may happen, for example, when a test is applied to a group of women at lower risk. As the prevalence decreases, the proportion of individuals with a positive test result who actually have the disease will fall and the proportion falsely identified as being diseased will rise. Although this striking difference may at first glance seem to violate all reasonable expectations, it is none the less both real and important. It has enormous clinical implications when one considers the many unnecessary interventions that may be prompted on the basis of false positive tests in pregnant women at lower than average risk.

Table 3.3 Impact of prevalence on test performance

	Condition Present	Condition Absent	
Test Positive	180	160	340
Test Negative	20	640	660
	200	800	1000

True prevalence of condition: (200/1000) = 20%.
Positive predictive value of test: (180/340) = 53%.

	Condition Present	Condition Absent	
Test Positive	90	180	270
Test Negative	10	720	730
	100	900	1000

True prevalence of condition: (100/1000) = 10%.
Positive predictive value of test: (90/270) = 33%.

	Condition Present	Condition Absent	
Test Positive	45	190	235
Test Negative	5	760	765
	50	950	1000

True prevalence of condition: (50/1000) = 5%.
Positive predictive value of test: (45/235) = 19%.

Likelihood ratios are the same for all tables above; that is, for a positive test result 4.5 and for a negative test result 0.125.

Fall in positive predictive value when a test with 90% sensitivity and 80% specificity is applied to groups of subjects with decreasing prevalence of a condition.

4.5 Likelihood ratios

While sensitivity, specificity, and predictive values provide helpful information about test properties, they have a number of limitations. As we discussed earlier, predictive values are prevalence-dependent. It is worthless to memorize, and inappropriate to use, the predictive values of a test in providing care to a particular woman unless her chance of having the condition is similar to that of the women in the population from which the original predictive values were derived.

As clinicians do not apply tests to populations but rather to individuals, we shall introduce the more general term '*pretest probability*'. Pretest probability is simply the chance, before the test result is known, that an individual woman (or group of women) has or will develop the condition. Clearly, for groups this is the same as the prevalence of the condition, but for an individual woman this probability must be estimated by considering all relevant information about her before the test result is known.

In fact, clinicians do this all the time in their practice. Consider the following two women whose fetuses are examined using ultrasonography. The first is a woman with an uncomplicated 37-week pregnancy who requests that a biophysical ultrasound examination of her fetus be performed because she is anxious about its well-being. The second woman is a 40-year-old, insulin-dependent diabetic who has noticed some vaginal blood loss and decreased fetal movements. The chance of finding an abnormality in the first woman's fetus is obviously far less than in the second. It might even be possible to make a numerical estimate of this probability. Experienced clinicians, like those to whom we made reference in the introductory section of this chapter, have been shown to be good at making such estimates (Feightner *et al.* 1982; Goldman *et al.* 1981). If a test provides useful additional information, then the risk of abnormality being present should be higher when the test result is positive (abnormal), and lower when it is negative. We thus have new probabilities after the test is performed—'*post-test probabilities*' (which we previously called positive and negative predictive values depending on whether the test results were positive or negative).

Although sensitivity and specificity are relatively stable properties, they cannot be used directly to compute post-test probabilities for positive or negative test results. It is also worrying to note that sensitivity and specificity tend to exaggerate the power of tests, since they include not only the true power of the test to detect abnormal individuals and correctly identify normal individuals, but also the chance predictions that result from random agreement between test results and the target condition. This less than self-evident truth is discussed in more detail later in this chapter.

A third limitation is that sensitivity and specificity also confine us to considering 2 × 2 tables. Many tests provide more than two categories of results. For example, as mentioned above, antenatal cardiotocographs may be classified as reactive, non-reactive, equivocal, unsatisfactory or, alternatively, scored on a scale of 0 to 10 (Keirse and Trimbos 1981; Fischer *et al.* 1976; Kubli *et al.* 1969). We need a stable statistic for each category of possible test result.

There is a simple statistic, which can be used to compute post-test likelihoods (predictive values) for individual women or groups of women, which is stable, reflects only non-random predictive power of a test and can be used for tests with two or more categories of results. This statistic is the *likelihood ratio*. It is used as follows:

$$\text{Pretest likelihood} \times \text{likelihood ratio} = \text{post-test likelihood}$$

The 'likelihood ratio' for a particular test result is a stable predictive property of the test because it combines information from both sensitivity and specificity, and hence is independent of prevalence. The 'pretest likelihood' is derived by clinical estimation (or from the prevalence of the condition in a population of similar women). To use the above expression we need to know two additional things; first, the special way in which pretest and post-test likelihood must be used, and second, how to calculate the likelihood ratio. As this is a stable characteristic of a test, it has to be done only once for each category of test result.

Pretest and post-test likelihoods are expressed as odds, not as probabilities or percentages (see Chapter 2). The basic idea behind a likelihood ratio is simple. It is the ratio of individuals who have a particular test result among those who have the condition, to individuals who have the same test results but do not have the condition. For an abnormal test result in a 2 × 2 table this is sensitivity/(1-specificity).

Examine Table 3.4. Here we have a test for a condition which can have three possible results: abnormal, equivocal, or normal. Let us calculate the likelihood ratio for an 'abnormal' test result (the first row). There are 50 women who have the target condition and an abnormal test result and these represent a correct identification of 50 per cent (50/100) of those who, in fact, have the disease. Ten of 900 women without the disease, or 1.1 per cent of these 900, are incorrectly labelled as abnormal because they have an abnormal test result. The ratio of these two proportions is 50/100 divided by 10/900 or 50 per cent/1.1 per cent

Table 3.4 Tests with different cut-off points

	Disease (or outcome)		
Test result	Present	Absent	Post-test probability
Abnormal	50	10	50/60 = 83%
Equivocal	30	90	30/120 = 25%
Normal	20	800	20/820 = 2.4%
	100	900	1000

Pretest probability of disease = 100/1000 = 10%

0.011) = 45. This is the likelihood ratio for an abnormal test result.

Now try calculating the likelihood ratios for equivocal and normal results. (They are 3 and 0.225 respectively). From these figures it is obvious that these likelihood ratios are thus expressed as odds rather than probabilities. As explained in more detail elsewhere (see Chapter 1) odds and probabilities are two alternative ways of expressing the same information. If an outcome has a 25 per cent (0.25) probability of happening, then it will occur once for every three times that it does not. Its odds are 1:3. The formulae which express the relationship between odds and probability are probability = odds/(1 + odds) and odds = probability/(1-probability). For these formulae to work properly, probability and odds must be expressed as decimal fractions (e.g. 0.5). Odds of 24:3, for instance, become 8:1, or more simply 8. The corresponding probability is 8/(1 + 8) or 0.89.

When the likelihood ratio and pretest probability are known, one can easily calculate the post-test probability with the use of the nomogram shown in Fig. 3.3, and thus avoid the mathematics involved in converting probabilities odds to. First, make an estimate of the probability of the outcome in your patient and line up the points representing pretest likelihood and likelihood ratio in your particular example and use a ruler to read off the post-test likelihood. Remember that this estimate of the post-test likelihood is derived from estimates of pretest likelihood and likelihood ratio. It is therefore only as good as the estimates from which it has been derived.

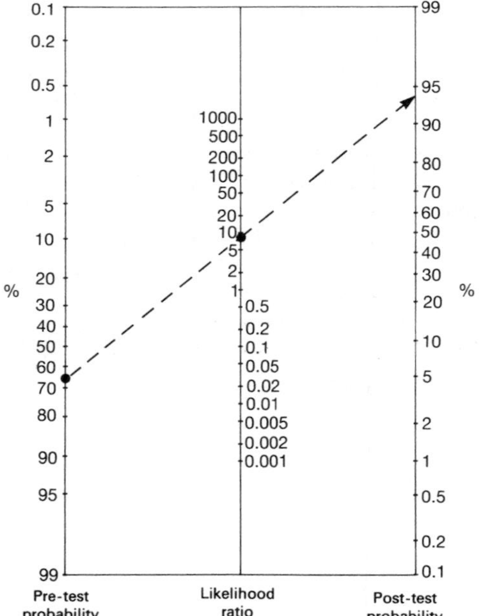

Fig. 3.3 Nomogram

In some circumstances, likelihood ratios can be helpful in expressing the combined results of more than one test performed on the same individual. So far we have discussed the interpretation of a single set of test results. A crude estimate expressing the combination of two test results can be obtained by calculating the product of their individual likelihood ratios. If the two tests were truly independent of one another, the computed ratio would be a good estimate of the combined predictive power of the two tests. Cuckle *et al.* (1987) and Tabor and her colleagues (1987) have recently proposed this method for producing revised estimates of the risk of Down's syndrome based on both maternal age and maternal serum alpha-fetoprotein results. It is important to be clear that the multiplication of likelihood ratios assumes that the tests from which they are derived are truly independent of one another. This is often not the case. For instance, in the presence of meconium, intrapartum fetal heart rate patterns are more likely to be abnormal. This 'concordance' (Sackett *et al.* 1985) will alter the likelihood of acidosis, for instance.

Likelihood ratios constitute a potentially powerful tool in the analysis and interpretation of data from screening and diagnostic tests. As computers begin to play a role in clinical practice and assume the burden of calculating likelihood ratios, the potential of these statistics as practical and useful aids to clinical practice and test evaluation is likely to increase.

5 Practical problems in interpreting and using tests

We have referred on a number of occasions to the quality of the estimates of the various test characteristics discussed in the previous section. A variety of factors may influence this quality and thus the performance of the tests in practice. In this section we review some of these.

5.1 Lack of precision

There has been a tendency to publish and discuss statistics such as sensitivity, specificity, and likelihood ratios without any reference to the degree of confidence that can be placed upon these estimates. In 2 × 2 tables, sensitivity is particularly vulnerable to assumptions of high confidence since it is usually the statistic for which the numerator and denominator are the smallest. In tables with more than 2 rows or columns some cut-off levels of the test result may contain very few cases and some cells may contain no cases at all. This renders the estimate of the likelihood ratio either unreliable (imprecise) or impossible to calculate (when it requires division by zero).

Other issues that are rarely considered are whether the observed result could have been expected on the basis of chance alone and whether any improvement over chance which is provided is statistically or clinically significant. Examine Table 3.5 and the statistics which have been calculated. Although the point estimate of the sensitivity was 0.8, the true value may lie anywhere between 0.51 and 0.98. How much sensitivity could be expected by chance alone? The test categorizes 40 per cent as abnormal. If it did so without any special relationship to the target condition, then 40 per cent of the individuals with the condition would be labelled abnormal and would therefore be 'detected' (an apparent sensitivity of 40 per cent). The observed sensitivity was 80 per cent, but 40 per cent, or half of it, could be due to chance rather than to the test. A similar line of reasoning suggests that, of the estimated 64 per cent specificity, 60 per cent could be credited to chance and only an additional 4 per cent attributed to the power of the test.

In summary, failure to consider the contribution of chance agreement to sensitivity and specificity statistics may lead to overestimation or underestimation of the precision of test statistics. It has been suggested that new chance-corrected statistics, similar to these developed by Cohen (1960), for sensitivity and specificity might be useful (Mohide 1989).

5.2 Potential for bias

We have referred to the fact that sensitivity, specificity, and likelihood ratios are relatively stable test properties in contrast to predictive values (post-test likelihoods) which are unstable. Pretest likelihood (prevalence of the outcome) dramatically influences the latter properties. The implications of this for the usefulness of a test in practice cannot be too strongly stressed. However, the individuals to whom screening and diagnostic testing is applied may differ in more ways than just the frequency of the condition sought. For instance, 'diabetics' in the practice of a community obstetrician may differ from those in a tertiary care centre. It is likely that those seen in the tertiary centre will have more severe abnormalities of blood sugar, more complicating metabolic changes, more vascular complications, and more coincident medical conditions. Women with more severe forms of disease are more likely to have abnormal test results than those with less severe forms. It would be predicted, therefore, that most tests will tend to be more sensitive (as well as more predictive) when applied to specialized clinics than to general obstetrical practice. This difference in sensitivity is, in fact, a direct result of the selection bias which results from referral from primary to secondary or tertiary care (Sackett 1979). To minimize this bias the test should be evaluated in as broad a range of individuals with and without the condition as possible (Ransohoff and Feinstein 1978). Alternatively, the test should be limited in its use to women with a similar spectrum and severity of disease and selected by a similar referral filter.

An additional problem occurs when individuals with diverse pathological problems are grouped indiscriminately together for screening or diagnosis. Just such a situation occurs in antenatal screening. After initial history-taking and physical and laboratory investigation, pregnant women are categorized as at increased or low risk. In different settings, the spectrum of diagnoses in people tested can vary considerably, particularly in 'high risk' groups. It is not surprising therefore that estimates of sensitivity and specificity vary considerably among studies (see Chapters 29 and 30). Where possible, it would be preferable to develop disease-specific estimates for sensitivity and specificity. There is no valid reason, for instance, to presuppose that the same test (such as the biophysical profile) will have the same sensitivity and specificity in women with diabetes, hypertension, or post-term pregnancies. The available evidence suggests that variation by these kinds of subgroups exists as far as antepartum cardiotocography is concerned (Keirse and Trimbos 1980). Another

Table 3.5 Confidence intervals for stable test properties

	Target condition		
Test result	Present	Absent	
Abnormal	8	32	40 (%)
Normal	2	58	60 (%)
	10 (%)	90 (%)	100

Statistic	Estimate	95% Confidence limits* upper	lower
Sensitivity = 8/10	= 0.80	0.98	0.51
Specificity = 58/90	= 0.64	0.74	0.54
LR (abnormal) = (8/10) × (90/32)	= 2.25	2.90	1.17
LR (normal) = (2/10) × (90/58)	= 0.31	0.89	0.04

*Calculations for sensitivity and specificity used the arcsine root-p transformation and for likelihood ratios using the method of Gart.

'spectrum' is advancing gestation, as the fetus ('the observed') undergoes maturational changes that may influence its behaviour and responses to testing. A number of investigators, for example, have noted a strong relationship between gestational age and antenatal screening test results for the contraction stress test (Devoe 1982), fetal heart rate characteristics (Natale *et al.* 1985), biophysical assessments (Nijhuis *et al.* 1986), antenatal cardiotocography (Aladjem *et al.* 1981; Devoe 1982; Druzin *et al.* 1985; Smith *et al.* 1985), and amniotic fluid volume assessment (Bottoms *et al.* 1986). Thus, the spectrum of gestational ages in a study population may have a substantial impact on test properties.

Co-morbidity may also confound the picture, by increasing or decreasing the chance that the target condition will occur. In this context, co-morbidity can be defined as any concurrent but distinct condition affecting the individual tested which is capable of altering either the chance of the detection, or of the occurrence of the condition. In Rhesus isoimmunization, for instance, the likelihood of a Rhesus negative woman becoming sensitized to her Rhesus positive infant is reduced if there is coincident ABO incompatibility (see Chapter 35). Similarly, maternal ingestion of drugs affecting the fetal central nervous system (sedatives, narcotics, antihypertensives) may influence fetal heart rate variability and fetal activity (see Chapter 30).

In addition, biases can operate if the results of the test influence subsequent diagnostic efforts. For instance, in studies to confirm the accuracy of fetal genetic diagnosis in early pregnancy, women with abnormal results may be followed-up more completely than those with normal results. If this is the case, false negatives will be missed, thus producing biased estimates of sensitivity, negative predictive value, and likelihood ratios for negative and positive tests. Biased diagnostic review may occur in cases where knowledge of test results can affect target conditions determined by subjective criteria. For instance, knowledge of a low amniotic fluid lecithin/sphyngomyelin ratio might influence the evaluation of a neonatal chest X-ray.

Another 'bias' that can result in systematic differences among studies and their estimates of sensitivity and specificity has already been alluded to. Studies using the same test to predict or identify a single condition may differ substantially in their computed test statistics if the threshold chosen to distinguish normal from abnormal tests, or to distinguish those with the condition from those without the condition, differs. An abnormal biophysical profile score might be defined as a score of 6 or less, or as a score of 4 or less. Likewise, a low Apgar score to one author might mean less than 8, but to another might mean 5 or less. Lowering the threshold for calling test results abnormal leads to higher estimates of sensitivity and lower estimates of specificity, and vice versa. Lowering the threshold for identification of the target condition will lower the estimates of sensitivity and increase the estimates of specificity. The reverse is also true. These 'threshold biases' may be hidden if definitions of threshold for the test and for the target condition are not clearly stated.

Finally, we must often depend on published reports for evidence as to a test's validity. Sheps (1984) found in a systematic review of the published literature that investigators of new tests were more likely to report high values for both sensitivity and specificity. He expressed the view that 'investigators of new tests may tend to publish their results only if the results are exceptional', that initial and subsequent investigations may be applied to different spectra of patients, and that 'regression to the mean' may occur. These publication biases may go a long way to explain the characteristic cycle of enthusiasm and disappointment associated with many promising new tests.

5.3 Effect of time and intervention

Considerable time may elapse between application of the test and even the short-term outcome measure against which it is being evaluated. For this reason, the status of the infant after birth, for example, may not be a true reflection of the fetal condition at the time when the test was performed. For instance, in attempts to evaluate the correspondence between antenatal cardiotocograph traces and neonatal status, traces obtained nearest to the time of birth have usually been selected for analysis. Although this may seem a reasonable approach, it is likely to overestimate the predictive power of cardiotocography patterns. The clinician is faced with the problem of interpreting tracings deriving from an unknown period of time before delivery and which are thus almost certainly not representative of patterns that would be obtained a short time before birth (Keirse and Trimbos 1981).

In addition, the test and outcome may also be separated by some sort of intervention. Tests aim to detect abnormalities at a time when they can still be favourably affected by management. Paradoxically, although a poor correlation between a positive test result and an adverse outcome can mean a lack of test validity, it can also mean that a valid test prompted an appropriate and successful intervention to prevent the target outcome. Conversely, a good correlation between a positive test result and a bad outcome may suggest the ineffectiveness or harmful effects of the treatment rather than the excellence of the test; that is, the intervention resulting from the test may actually cause the adverse outcome which its use is specifically intended to prevent. A baby born by caesarean section, for example, may be depressed because of, rather than in spite of, the intervention.

It is important to stress that the only way to prevent this distortion of estimates of a test's predictive properties is to ensure that test results are withheld from the clinicians and women, and are not allowed to influence clinical decisions until the test in question has been shown to have predictive properties that are likely to be clinically useful. Sometimes even this may not be enough, when concurrent testing for the same condition with alternative tests continues, leading to treatment that influences the outcomes of interest.

The role of intervention and its effect on the validity of diagnostic tests have been either unappreciated or underestimated in much of the published literature. Let us consider what we would expect to happen in the unusual circumstance of a perfect diagnostic test (no false positives and no false negatives) combined with a totally efficacious therapy (the adverse outcome is prevented in all women), which is applied to all eligible women (perfect compliance). The top part of Table 3.6 shows the results of a hypothetical test when conducted in a blinded fashion without intervention, and shows that it is a perfect test. Now, if the results of this test are released and the efficacious treatment is applied to all women in the top left-hand cell of the table (that is, all women with the condition), then the outcome will be prevented in all of them. Thus, these women would now appear on the right side of the bottom part of Table 3.6 without the outcome. Those with a positive test now all appear to be false positives. Clearly, this is not true and yet, when the test is combined with therapy, the table of results changes in this dramatic manner. In fact, this is what we would hope to see when clinical actions are taken on the basis of test results.

Table 3.6 The perfect test combined with the perfect therapy

Test alone:

Diagnostic test	Target outcome: Present	Target outcome: Absent
Abnormal	TP	O
Normal	O	TN

Test + Therapy:

Diagnostic test	Target outcome: Present	Target outcome: Absent
Abnormal	O	FP
Normal	O	TN

Expected changes in the contents of a hypothetical 2 × 2 table expressing clinical study results as a result of the addition of completely efficacious therapy to a perfectly accurate diagnostic test. (TP = true positives, FP = false positives, TN = true negatives)

Unfortunately, we live in a world of imperfect tests and imperfect interventions. An imperfect test can result in treatment being applied to women with false positive results, who cannot benefit from the intervention, but who will still run the risk of the complications and side-effects that are associated with it. It will also result in intervention being withheld from women who would have benefited from appropriate treatment, but who had false negative results. An intervention may be imperfect either because it is ineffective or because it is less effective than an alternative treatment. Some women with the condition will thus still experience the adverse outcome and, in addition, any risks or complications of the imperfect intervention will be applied to the women with both the true positive and the false positive test results. Table 3.7 shows the net effect of these influences on the contents of the cells of a 2 × 2 table that expresses the results of a clinical study in

Table 3.7 Cell content for imperfect tests and imperfect therapy

Diagnostic test	Target outcome occurs	Target outcome does not occur
Predicts abnormal outcome	*Original Prediction Valid* Rx not efficacious Rx potentially efficacious but too late Poor compliance with Rx (patient, physician, or logistics)	*Original Prediction Valid* Rx efficacious Co-intervention efficacious
	Original Prediction Invalid Rx harmful leading to target outcome Dx test harmful leading to target outcome	*Original Prediction Invalid* Target outcome would not have occurred whether or not Rx applied
Predicts normal outcome	*Original Prediction Valid* Co-intervention produced outcome	*Original Prediction Valid* Rx not applied and target outcome does not occur
	Original Prediction Invalid Rx was not applied to patients who could have benefited	*Original Prediction Invalid* Co-intervention prevented outcome that would have otherwise occurred

When therapy is determined by test results in an environment where more than one test for the target condition is being performed, the relationship between test results and target outcomes can be explained in a number of different ways.

which a diagnostic test is combined with an intervention to prevent or reduce the occurrence of the adverse outcome.

Thus, in studies in which the management plan combines diagnostic tests and interventions (for example, all tests which aim to identify fetal growth retardation), computation of the test's 'positive' properties is likely to be seriously misleading. It is more sensible to compare the outcome of two groups of women, each of which receives a different management plan in a randomized controlled trial (see below). Rates of outcome are then directly comparable between the arms of the study, although it should be recognized that the contributions of the diagnostic test and the therapy will usually be indistinguishable.

If, in such studies, test properties such as sensitivity, specificity, and likelihood ratios are calculated, we propose that they should be described as 'residual'; for example, 'residual positive predictive value'. This will thus identify clearly the predictive power which *remains* after intervention has occurred. If the intervention is beneficial or harmful (that is, alters the rate of the outcome in question) the residual properties should differ significantly from those derived from blinded studies.

6 Benefits and hazards of diagnosis and screening

As was stressed earlier, the ultimate criterion for assessing any test, used either in isolation or as part of a screening programme, is whether, combined with action prompted by the test result, people are better off as a result of being tested. Those most likely to benefit are the individuals identified correctly as either having or not having the unwanted condition. For example, the use of continuous intrapartum fetal heart rate monitoring with assessment of the acid–base status of fetuses with abnormal traces was found to be more effective than intermittent auscultation in detecting and excluding fetal 'asphyxia' (MacDonald *et al.* 1985).

The potential of a test to do harm depends primarily on its capacity for falsely indicating the absence or presence of the condition in question. Women who are falsely labelled as having normal pregnancies may be denied the benefits of potentially efficacious treatment. Women falsely labelled as having abnormal pregnancies will, at the very least, be subjected to further testing; at worst they may suffer unnecessary anxiety (see Chapter 8) and undergo unnecessary and potentially harmful 'treatment' for 'non-disease' (see Chapter 36). For example, in all four randomized controlled trials of antepartum cardiotocography the perinatal death rate was higher in the groups that were tested (see Chapter 30).

Another concern is the frequent assumption that a test that has been shown to be of benefit to women or fetuses at high risk of disease is of benefit to all women or fetuses, regardless of their risk. As we have already pointed out, this assumption is invalid. When the prevalence of the condition decreases in the group of women tested, the positive predictive value of the test diminishes as well. As a consequence, there is a relatively large number of false positives for each true positive and the balance of benefits and risks may actually swing to a net hazard. This phenomenon may go some way towards explaining the conflicting findings of those who have evaluated the validity of serial fundal height measurements in high risk (Quaranta *et al.* 1981) and average risk (Rosenberg *et al.* 1982) populations.

Apart from the repercussions of the test result, the test itself may have either a beneficial or a hazardous effect. For example, mothers viewing their fetuses *in utero* during ultrasound examination in early pregnancy are more likely to act on advice received at the first antenatal visit to reduce either smoking or drinking than are mothers who did not see the screen (Reading *et al.* 1984). Testing by amniocentesis, on the other hand, can cause harm and lead to miscarriage of normal pregnancies and respiratory problems in newborn infants (Tabor *et al.* 1986).

Sometimes the balance of risks and benefits is readily evident; more often it is not. Accurate knowledge about the prevalence of the condition and the positive and negative predictive values of the test, with the likely extent of benefits and hazards that these values imply, may allow a more realistic estimate of the utility of the test. However, relatively small changes in sensitivity and/or specificity may result in major differences in the balance between risks and benefits.

An additional problem is that the benefits are usually measured in a way different from the hazards. Direct comparison is therefore impossible and depends on a subjective assessment of their relative importance. One approach is to convert both benefits and hazards into equivalent units and to give values to both of them and to the cost of the screening process as well (see Chapter 5).

Randomized controlled trials can provide a direct answer to the fundamental question of whether or not women benefit from a particular test programme compared with an alternative form of care (see Chapter 1). In this way, tests and treatment can be assessed together bypassing the need for test validation against a possibly imprecise reference standard. Benefits and hazards are measured directly rather than by inference. As is made clear in other chapters in this book, a number of screening and diagnostic programmes have been evaluated in randomized controlled trials (see Chapter 89).

Much of the methodology for randomized trials of screening and diagnostic technologies has been borrowed from that of randomized trials of therapeutic interventions (see Chapter 2). Some of the design requirements of trials of screening and diagnostic tests, however, present relatively unexplored problems. Test evaluation can be expected to improve as there is progress in dealing with the problems presented by co-intervention (concurrent testing), estimation of expected clinical effects, the reliability of links between test results and subsequent intervention, sample size, and the analysis of the results (Mohide 1989).

7 Conclusions

The purpose of diagnosis and screening in the care of women and their babies during pregnancy and childbirth is to distinguish accurately between those who have problems and those who do not. In the light of the information provided by this process, appropriate care can then be selected and provided. Symptoms and signs may sometimes be such that both the diagnosis and prescription is obvious. On other occasions, these will be more obscure and recognized efficiently only by more experienced observers. Maximizing the accuracy with which less experienced people diagnose problems that are amenable to effective care is obviously a key factor in promoting appropriate and effective care during pregnancy and childbirth.

People have approached this challenge in a variety of ways. These range from reiterating the importance of listening carefully to what every woman says about aspects of her past and present reproductive, medical, and social circumstances (Hall and Chng 1982); through teaching pregnant women to recognize the symptoms and signs of preterm labour (Herron *et al.* 1982); to introducing computers for diagnostic prompting (Morgan *et al.* 1978).

However the challenge of improving the general quality of diagnostic accuracy is addressed, it will inevitably depend on more successful systematization of the information used by successful diagnosticians, whether these are women, clinicians or computers. Diagnostic and screening tests used in the care of women during pregnancy and childbirth should be used with understanding. This means that the inherent variability of the test, the person doing the testing, and the individual being tested should be quantified; abnormal test results should be defined; the validity of the test should be measured against the best or most appropriate Gold Standard available; the effect of prevalence of the condition on the test performance should be understood; the predictive properties of the test in many settings and different types of patients should be evaluated; and the efficacy of the test, together with the care that its results prompt, should be investigated, where appropriate and possible, by randomized controlled trials. Finally, if the test is to be incorporated in a screening programme, all the prerequisites for such a programme should be met before it is widely adopted.

Some may argue that this is a ponderous and impractical approach, likely to obstruct progress and deny effective tests and care to those who might otherwise benefit. Furthermore, they may feel that pre-existing evidence and 'self-evident' notions in the search for disease—and screening for disease in particular—are sufficient reasons to accept or implement the use of a test or programme. The danger of this 'evangelical' (Sackett and Holland 1975) approach is that indiscriminate use of tests, either in isolation or as part of a screening programme, may result in more harm than benefit. The statistically low risk of adverse outcome for the majority of pregnant women makes this consideration particularly pertinent to tests used in pregnancy and childbirth. Careful scientific appraisal rather than expediency is the best safeguard against this happening and the best way of ensuring that, overall, those tested benefit as a result.

References

Aladjem S, Vuolo K, Pazos R, Lueck J (1981). Antepartum fetal testing: Evaluation and redefinition of criteria for clinical interpretation. Seminars Perinatol, 5: 145–154.

Aubry RH, Rounke JE, Cuenca VG, Marshall LD (1975). The random urine estrogen/creatinine ratio. Obstet Gynecol, 46: 64–68.

Beaulieu MD, Fabia J, Leduc B, Brisson J, Bastide A, Blouin D, Gauthier RJ, Lalonde A (1982). The reproducibility of intrapartum cardiotocograms. Can Med Assoc J, 127: 214–216.

Bottoms SF, Welch RA, Zador IE, Sokol RJ (1986). Limitations of using maximum vertical pocket and other sonographic evaluations of amniotic fluid volume to predict fetal growth: Technical or physiologic? Am J Obstet Gynecol, 155: 154–158.

Brown WU, Bell GC, Alper MH (1976). Acidosis, local anesthetics and the newborn. Obstet Gynecol, 48: 27–30.

Cadman D, Chambers LW, Feldman W, Sackett DL (1984). Assessing the effectiveness of community screening programs. JAMA, 251: 1580–1585.

Cochrane AL (1972). Effectiveness and Efficiency. London: Nuffield Provincial Hospitals Trust.

Cohen J (1960). A coefficient of agreement for nominal scales. Educ Psychol Meas, 20: 37–46.

Cuckle HS, Wald NJ, Thompson SG (1987). Estimating a woman's risk of having a pregnancy associated with Down's syndrome using her age and serum alpha-fetoprotein level. Br J Obstet Gynaecol, 94: 387–402.

Davies AC, Chalmers I, Fahmy DR (1977). Predicting fetal death. Br Med J, 1: 443.

Devoe LD (1982). Antepartum fetal heart rate testing in preterm pregnancy. Obstet Gynecol, 60: 431–436.

Druzin ML, Fox A, Kogut E, Carlson C (1985). The relationship of the nonstress test to gestational age. Am J Obstet Gynecol, 153: 386–389.

Feightner JW, Norman GR, Haynes RB (1982). The reliability of likelihood estimates by physicians. Clin Res, 30: 298a.

Feinstein AR (1976). Architecture of clinical research. In: Strategies in Clinical Research. Mead Johnson Symposium on Perinatal and Developmental Medicine, No. 9, pp 10–15.

Fischer WM, Stude I, Brandt H (1976). Ein Vorschlag zur Beurteilung des antepartalen Kardiotokogramms. Z Geburtsh Perinatol, 180: 117–123.

Goldman L, Waternaux C, Garfield F, Cohn PF, Strong R, Barry WH, Cook F, Rosati R, Sherman H (1981). Impact of a cardiology data bank on physician's prognostic estimates. Arch Intern Med, 141: 1631–1634.

Greenwood M (1986). The Medical Dictator and Other Biographical Studies. Cambridge: Keynes Press, p 79.

Hall M, Chng PK (1982). Antenatal care in practice. In: Effectiveness and Satisfaction in Antenatal Care. Clinics in Developmental Medicine Nos. 81/82. Enkin M, Chalmers I (eds). London: Spastics International Medical Publications, Heinemann Medical Books, pp 60–68.

Haynes RB (1981). How to read clinical journals. II. To learn about a diagnostic test. Can Med Assoc J, 124: 703–710.

Herron MA, Katz M, Creasy RK (1982). Evaluation of a preterm birth prevention program: Preliminary report. Obstet Gynecol, 59: 452–456.

Kaar K (1980). Antepartal cardiotocography in the assessment of fetal outcome. Acta Obstet Gynecol Scand (Suppl), 5–56: 94.

Keirse MJNC, Trimbos JB (1980). Assessment of antepartum cardiotocograms in high-risk pregnancy. Br J Obstet Gynaecol, 87: 261–269.

Keirse MJNC, Trimbos JB (1981). Clinical significance of suspicious antepartum cardiotocograms: A study of normal and high-risk pregnancies. Br J Obstet Gynaecol, 88: 739–746.

Keirse MJNC, Trimbos JB, Mallens TEJM, van der Heemst M (1981). Reliability of ultrasound as compared to direct fetal electrocardiography for antepartum cardiotocography. Br J Obstet Gynaecol, 88: 391–394.

Kubli F, Kaeser O, Hinselmann M (1969). Diagnostic management of chronic placental insufficiency In: The Foetoplacental Unit. Pecile A, Finci C (eds). Amsterdam: Excerpta Medica, pp 323–339.

Layhew GS, Goldsmith CH (1975). Generalized Sensitivity–Specificity and Predictive Value Measures of Agreement Statistics. Technical Report 75/1. Hamilton: McMaster University, Department of Applied Mathematics.

MacDonald D, Grant A, Sheridan-Pereira M, Boylan P, Chalmers I (1985). The Dublin randomized controlled trial of intrapartum fetal heart rate monitoring. Am J Obstet Gynecol, 152: 524–539.

Manning FA, Morrison I, Lange IR, Harman CR, Chamberlain PF (1985). Fetal assessment based on fetal biophysical profile scoring: Experience in 12,620 referred high-risk pregnancies. Am J Obstet Gynecol, 151: 343–350.

Mohide PT (1989). The evaluation of diagnostic and screening tests in controlled clinical trials. Masters Thesis in Design, Measurement and Evaluation. Hamilton: McMaster University, Department of Clinical Epidemiology and Biostatistics.

Morgan M, Studney DR, Barnett GO, Winickoff RN (1978). Computerized concurrent review of prenatal care. QRB, 4: 33–36.

Natale R, Naselo-Paterson C, Turliuk R (1985). Longitudinal measurements of fetal breathing, body movements, heart rate, and heart rate accelerations and decelerations at 24 to 32 weeks of gestation. Am J Obstet Gynecol, 151: 256–263.

Nightingale F (1860). Notes on Nursing: What It Is, and What It is Not. New York: Appleton & Co. (published in facsimile of first edition in 1946 by Appleton-Century, xiv, p 140).

Nijhuis JG, Jongsma HW, Crijns IJMJ, de Valk IMGM, var der Velden JWHJ (1986). Effects of maternal glucose ingestion on human fetal breathing movements at weeks 24 and 28 of gestation. Early Hum Dev, 13: 183–188.

Quaranta P, Currell R, Redman CWG, Robinson JS (1981). Prediction of small-for-dates infants by measurement of the symphysial fundal height. Br J Obstet Gynaecol, 88: 115–119.

Ransohoff DF, Feinstein AR (1978). Problems of spectrum and bias in evaluating the efficacy of diagnostic tests. New Engl J Med, 299: 926–930.

Reading AE, Campbell S, Cox DN, Sledmere CM (1984). Health beliefs and health care behaviour in pregnancy. Psychol Med, 12: 379–383.

Richardson DK, Schwartz JS, Weinbaum PJ, Gabbe SG (1985). Diagnostic tests in obstetrics: A method of improved evaluation. Am J Obstet Gynecol, 152: 613–618.

Rochard E, Schifrin BS, Goupil F, Legrand H, Blottiere J, Sureau C (1976). Nonstressed fetal heart rate monitoring in the antepartum period. Am J Obstet Gynecol, 126: 699–706.

Rosenberg K, Grant JM, Hepburn M (1982). Antenatal detection of growth retardation: Actual practice in a large maternity hospital. Br J Obstet Gynaecol, 89: 12–15.

Sackett DL (1979). Bias in analytic research. J Chron Dis, 32: 51–63.

Sackett DL, Holland WW (1975). Controversy in the detection of disease. Lancet, 1: 357–359.

Sackett DL, Haynes RB, Tugwell PX (1985). Clinical Epidemiology: A Basic Science for Clinical Medicine. Toronto: Little Brown.

Sheps SB, Schechter MT (1984). The assessment of diagnostic tests — A survey of current research. JAMA, 252: 2418–2422.

Smith CV, Phelan JP, Paul RH (1985). A prospective analysis of the influence of gestational age on the baseline fetal heart rate and reactivity in a low-risk population. Am J Obstet Gynecol, 153: 780–782.

Tabor A, Madsen M, Obel EB, Philip J, Bang J, Norgaard-Pedersen B (1986). Randomised controlled trial of genetic amniocentesis in 4606 low risk women. Lancet, 1: 1287–1293.

Tabor A, Larsen SO, Nielsen Jan, Nielsen Johannes, Philip J, Pilgaard B, Videbech P, Norgaard-Pedersen B (1987). Screening for Down's syndrome using an iso-risk curve based on maternal age and serum alpha-fetoprotein. Br J Obstet Gynaecol, 94: 636–642.

Trimbos JB, Keirse MJNC (1978). Observer variability in assessment of antepartum cardiotocograms. Br J Obstet Gynaecol, 85: 900–906.

Wald NJ (1984). Antenatal and Neonatal Screening. Oxford: Oxford University Press.

Wilson JMG, Jungner G (1968). Principles and Practice of Screening for Disease. Public Health Paper, No. 34. Geneva: World Health Organization.

4 The role of the social sciences in evaluating perinatal care

Jane Robinson

1 Introduction

No one involved in the provision of health care during the 1980s can have escaped the heavy emphasis on evaluation. Terms such as 'performance indicators', 'value for money', 'diagnosis related groups', and 'consumer satisfaction' have entered the everyday language of the health services in many countries. Within this interest, evaluation of the quality of perinatal care in particular has become a matter of widespread interest, again, on an international scale. The World Health Organization (1985) describes a catalogue of difficulties facing the maternity services, which includes problems ranging from deficient scientific understanding and uncontrolled technological expansion, to widespread uncertainties about the relationship between care and outcome.

The question to be addressed in this chapter is how, in the field of care during pregnancy and childbirth, the social sciences can contribute to this evaluative process. Although the specific examples to which reference will be made in this chapter concern the United Kingdom, trends towards greater evaluative activity in health services and perinatal care are now world-wide. Research into the social aspects of childbearing has proliferated over the past quarter of a century. Grounded in the emergent consumer and women's movements (see Chapter 7), much of this research has achieved a high profile (Macintyre 1980; Butter 1986). Indeed, in many countries it would be true to say that no debate about the quality of perinatal care would now be complete without women's views being expressed.

Yet research that focuses mainly on women's attitudes and experiences can also be misleading. It is defended on the grounds that consumer satisfaction is an important part of quality assurance in health care. Childbirth, it is argued, is a natural process (not a disease) which can, and should, be a joyful and enriching experience. Aspects of the art of care that promote this experience are therefore seen as essential components of effectiveness in policies for childbirth. By extension, obstetric practices that may tend to depersonalize women and dehumanize the experience of pregnancy and childbirth, tend to become severely criticized.

Granting the importance of this focus on the recipients of care, if it is overemphasized there is a very real danger that the professionals working in the maternity services and the dilemmas that they face may receive only marginal attention in social science research. In addition, the equally important need for the social sciences to contribute to the evaluation of the technical quality of care may be overlooked. Social science can, too readily, come to be seen as dealing solely with the woman's point of view. Yet social scientists are, and should be, concerned with far more than that. The social sciences can, and do, play a much broader role in the evaluation of health services, including the maternity services. Professional behaviour, clinical scientific work, and the formulation of policies, are all social activities and thus amenable to social scientific analysis, as Macintyre (1977a) has emphasized in her review of the research issues in the sociology of reproduction.

2 Evaluation

It is important to begin by clearing the ground a little over the problematic notion of 'evaluation'. Vuori (1982) defines evaluation as comprising not only the assessment of the health services currently on offer, but also the process of feeding the results of that initial evaluation back to those who are in a position to influence the direction of future change; further research is then called for to measure any actual change that occurs as a result (see Chapters 5, 87, and 88).

The maternal and child health services in Britain have been among the pioneers in attempting to evaluate the quality of care provided. Possibly because assessment of the 'process' of care has been so difficult they have tended to concentrate on the important, but nevertheless rather narrow, measurement of physical outcome. Indeed, Macintyre (1980) suggests that, prior to 1974, sociologists themselves 'worked mainly in collaboration with obstetricians and within the prevailing paradigms of obstetric and administrative orthodoxy'. Although the limitations of 'audit by death' have been well described (Chalmers 1981), mortality rates have been, and remain, a powerful motivating factor for (and thus focus of) evaluation at both national and local level.

3 Correlations and risk markers

For more than a century, social scientists and epidemiologists have sought to identify, and then explain, the causal mechanisms that lie behind the familiar correlations between death and poverty (Armstrong 1986; Robinson 1986). Increasing refinement in the choice of variables and sophistication in computation techniques has led to the identification of risk markers and the emergence of stereotypes. For infant death, for example, such markers currently include membership of lower social groups, black ethnicity, the extremes of maternal age and parity, and maternal smoking behaviour.

A landmark in this process of identification and explanation was the recognition that the patterns of intermarriage between social groups was highly selective and occurred in a way which tended to maintain the social gradient in mortality risks. Longitudinal studies conducted by Illsley (1955) showed that, among women born into middle class families, those most likely to marry working class men were those of relatively short stature who showed evidence of a nutritional and intellectual status which was below average for their class of origin. Conversely, women born into the working class who, compared with other members of their class, were relatively well-endowed in these respects were found to be more likely to marry middle class men. These observations led to the continuing debate as to whether inequality is inevitable (Brotherston 1978; Chalmers 1985).

The social scientists helped to generate the hypotheses and collect the data that have underscored these debates. It was their questioning of some of the deductions made from these data that fuelled the change of emphasis in their work during the 1970s. From the social construction of a disadvantaged, at risk mother (based on evidence gathered from large scale social surveys) it was not a large step to the recognition that the woman type-cast in this role was not necessarily mistress of her fate, and often needed others to intervene on her behalf. Successive reports on maternal and child health identified the relationship between infant death and socioeconomic disadvantage, but then ignored that association and merely recommended solutions based on improvements in medical care (Butler and Bonham 1963; Butler and Alberman 1969; Chamberlain *et al.* 1975, 1978).

4 Women's views of care

As the death rates at issue fell, however, social scientists began to conduct research that led them to question policies for childbirth that had originated solely from the professional beliefs of obstetricians and paediatricians (Stacey 1987). The social sciences that contributed to this body of evidence were drawn from a range of disciplines—politics, anthropology, sociology, psychology and history—but all came to focus in some way on the unequal personal experiences of pregnant and childbearing women (Graham 1976; Macintyre 1977b; Kitzinger 1978; Llewelyn-Davies 1978; Cartwright 1979; Graham and McKee 1979; Oakley 1979; Lewis 1980; Graham and Oakley 1981; O'Brien 1981). Such work has had and continues to have a huge influence. As has been pointed out previously (Reid 1983), some of the research can be criticized both on methodological grounds and because of the lack of caution with which the results of the research (which was often necessarily based on small and possibly unrepresentative samples) have sometimes been generalized. This said, few would deny its pioneering nature and its crucial role in raising important questions relevant to the evaluation of the maternity services.

Macintyre (1980) suggests that the history of the 1970s needs further analysis, but tentatively concludes that the social movements of that decade, whether they be women's, ecological, consumer, or anti-medicalization, all had substantial influences on social science research into childbearing (see Chapter 5). Another sociologist (Reid 1983) has drawn attention to the bias of several studies of the period. She argues that the researchers themselves, the populations studied, and the reviewers of the research, were all predominantly middle class. As a result, the conclusions drawn from many of the earlier studies about what women in general experienced and wanted did not always agree with the findings of later research, which used samples that were more representative of the working class (Reid *et al* 1983; Robinson 1986, 1989; McIntosh 1987).

5 Views of the service providers

The reasons for the absence of the views of the service providers in the social science literature of this period also needs investigation. Cartwright's (1979) rigorous study of induction of labour was a rare exception. It included data describing the opinions of obstetricians, but even in this study the quotations from individuals were restricted to those from midwives and the mothers. This relative omission may have been due to difficulties experienced by social scientists in gaining research access to professionals, with doctors not perceiving the relevance of such research to their own particular interests. Alternatively, it may have arisen because researchers do not always want to know about the complex and equivocal medical decisions that must sometimes be made. What seems clear, however, is that if future social science work is to progress, then professionals and the nature of their work must be studied more systematically than hitherto.

6 Effects of social research

While I have asserted that studies of childbearing conducted by social scientists have undoubtedly had effects, this does not mean that it is easy to identify a direct relationship between a social science input and a tangible outcome. Yet consciousness has been raised about the issues discussed by social scientists in the light of their research findings. For example, although the Social Services Committee of the House of Commons (1980) continued the pattern of its predecessors in recommending medical rather than social change for childbearing women, there was a new emphasis on humanizing the maternity services. This emphasis on the need to pay attention to the numerous complaints about impersonal care was subsequently reflected in the reports of the Maternity Services Advisory Committee (1984), established by the government in response to some of the recommendations made by the Social Services Committee.

This process of influence is so diffuse that the social sciences rarely receive any credit for promoting it (Miller 1986). Yet it seems that the critical mass of evidence accumulated resulted in feedback that produced a variety of changes. It is not possible to claim, in Vuori's (1982) terms, that the effects of this feedback on the quality of services was *measured*: the process of evaluating the art of care is much more intangible and indirect. Nevertheless, the pattern of incremental change that can be observed in the care of women in pregnancy and childbirth is analagous to that described in social science studies about the ways in which research evidence influences policy (Weiss 1980).

This influence can be detected, for example, in the report of the Royal College of Obstetricians and Gynaecologists (1982) working party on antenatal and intrapartum care. A leading article in the *Lancet* (1982) welcomed the report as having encouraged the incorporation of 'new dimensions in obstetric audit' in its call for 'a flexible attitude on the part of medical and midwifery staff and a willingness to consider alternative approaches to maintain the confidence of pregnant women'. Midwives too, have taken the messages emerging from the social sciences into their reformulated policy objectives. The policy proposals of the Association of Radical Midwives (1986) for the future of the maternity services include, as basic principles, the centrality of the mother, and the need for her to be able and encouraged to exercise informed choice in childbirth.

In a similar way change can be detected in texts for midwifery practice. Ball (1987), for example, incorporates the ideas of Caplan (1961, 1964) and Lazarus (1969) in order to explain for midwives the normal coping and stress patterns which can occur in childbirth, just as they operate in any other major life change. Ball's proposals for flexible support systems in postnatal care are based therefore on specific social science theory and, as such, are themselves amenable to systematic evaluation. Numerous books on childbearing for parents similarly bear the mark of contemporary social science. Kitzinger (1962, 1978) has become a household name, while the *Pregnancy Book* (Health Education Council 1984), which is available throughout the antenatal services, substantially incorporates Graham and McKee's (1979) work on mothers' experience of childbirth.

7 The spectrum of care

Thus far, two stages in the development of social science input into the evaluation of care during pregnancy and childbirth have been described. In the first, survey research identified some of the social factors associated with mortality; in the second, the views and experiences of childbearing women were explored systematically. More recently, however, a third stage can be discerned. Researchers into childbearing have begun the attempt, sometimes in partnership with others, to study aspects of the whole spectrum of care. In Britain, this situation may well have been encouraged by the National Perinatal Epidemiology Unit's (1978) recommendation that local surveys of perinatal deaths should include not only clinical and pathological data for cases and controls derived from geographically defined populations (the clinico-epidemiological perspective), but also information derived from bereaved and control parents, preferably collected in their own homes.

This strategy introduces complex theoretical issues for research designs, which must incorporate perspectives from epidemiology, sociology, and psychology.

Nevertheless, it represents a quantum leap from studies which formerly focused solely on the recipients of care, or which frequently used only one research method. Although as yet few in number, these studies point to possible new forms of collaboration.

Cartwright's (1979) study of induction led the way. She found wide differences between women's views about induction and what obstetricians believed those views to be. Many women did not have the information, or the opportunity, to be involved in making choices. Furthermore, the unmet need for information was found to be greater among working class than among middle class women. Cartwright also noted that the belief held by the majority of obstetricians (and two-thirds of midwives) that the increase in the induction rate to over 30 per cent had contributed to the concurrent fall in the perinatal mortality rate was not supported by evidence. Thus, in this pioneering research, the views of service providers and recipients were not only systematically compared, but the assumptions which underpinned some of them were tested against other findings.

Robinson (1986, 1989), working in a socially deprived area, similarly contrasted assumptions about the problem of perinatal mortality as perceived by health professionals, with those of parents who had lost a baby, and matched control parents. She found a tendency among the doctors to attribute the problems experienced by individuals to various adverse characteristics of the geographical area. In this way abstract concepts (social, ethnic, and marital) were used to explain bad outcomes. Interestingly, this view persisted in spite of the fact that the epidemiological data showed that there were few statistically significant differences in the social and economic characteristics of the parents who lost their babies and those whose babies survived. Both groups shared quite severe social and economic disadvantage. Deficiencies in care and facilities thus tended to be overlooked and explained away by reference to adverse environmental circumstances (Stacey 1987).

Research findings such as these can be very threatening. Yet evidence suggests that evaluative research which involves collaboration between professionals working in the services and researchers drawn from a variety of academic disciplines is not only possible, but can be very fruitful (see, for example, Goldthorp and Richman 1974; Oakley and Chamberlain 1981; Reid *et al.* 1983; Garcia *et al.* 1985). A recent evaluation of antenatal care conducted in Aberdeen, a centre with a strong tradition of multidisciplinary research in obstetrics, serves as an example illustrating the potential which exists. An obstetrician and two sociologists (Hall *et al.* 1985) collaborated in evaluating the introduction of a new system of antenatal care (see Chapter 88). They found (somewhat to their surprise) that it was possible to make quite fundamental alterations in the structure of a service by scheduling fewer routine visits to the hospital during pregnancy. Their research was unable to substantiate several assumptions about the relationship between features of the process of antenatal care and its outcome. They found, for example, that the probability of correctly diagnosing certain pregnancy complications was very low, although it was more likely to be achieved by trained staff in a good centre than by general practitioners, or possibly by midwives. This setting, however, was less likely to meet the women's needs for information, advice, and reassurance; in this respect, the staff in local general practitioner clinics did a better job.

8 Conclusions

There are several implications of the results of this research. One of them is that the objective of accurate and complete diagnosis may need to be pursued separately from the objective of providing the information sought by women using the maternity services. A crucial finding of the research in Aberdeen which could be extrapolated to the evaluation of any aspect of health care, was that in designing an optimum schedule of care in any locality one needs first to disaggregate the aims of care into a number of specific goals; second, to examine whether these aims can be achieved; and third, to explore how, when, where, and by whom they can best be achieved.

Social scientists working in Britain may have been more fortunate than their colleagues in other countries. For more than three decades they have been actively involved in evaluating the care received by women during pregnancy and childbirth, and the results of their research seem to have played a substantial role in determining the direction in which services are being developed. Current research, which brings the insights gained through applying social sciences into conjunction with the insights of health professionals upon the art, technical quality, and structure of care, must surely provide a model for evaluation in the future.

References

Armstrong, D (1986). The invention of infant mortality. Soc Health Illness, 8.3: 211–232.

Association of Radical Midwives (1986). The Vision. The Association, 62 Greetby Hill, Ormskirk, Lancs., L39 2DT.

Ball, J (1987). Reactions to Motherhood: The Role of Postnatal Care. Cambridge: Cambridge University Press.

Brotherston, J (1978). Inequality—is it inevitable? Paper given at DHSS/CPAG Conference. Reaching the Consumer in the Antenatal and Child Health Services. London: Department of Health.

Butler NR, Bonham DG (1963). Perinatal Mortality. The First Report of the 1958 British Perinatal Mortality Survey. Edinburgh and London: E & S Livingstone.

Butler NR, Alberman ED (1969). Perinatal Problems. The Second Report of the 1958 British Perinatal Mortality Survey. Edinburgh and London: E & S Livingstone.

Butter I (1986). The role of women's attitudes in obstetric care. In: Perinatal Care Delivery Systems. Kaminski M, Breart G, Buekens O, Huisjes H, McIlawaine G, Selbman H (eds). Oxford: Oxford University Press.

Caplan G (1961). An Approach to Community Mental Health. London: Tavistock.

Caplan G (1964). Principles of Preventive Psychiatry. London: Tavistock.

Cartwright A (1979). The Dignity of Labour: A Study of Childbearing and Induction. London: Tavistock.

Chalmers I (1981). The limitations of audit by death. In: Changing Patterns of Child-bearing and Child Rearing. Chester R, Diggory P, Sutherland MB (eds). London: Academic Press.

Chalmers I (1985). Short, Black, Baird, Himsworth, and social class differences in fetal and neonatal mortality rates. Br Med J, 291: 231–233.

Chamberlain R, Chamberlain G, Howlett B, Claireaux A (1975). British Births 1970. Vol 1. The First Week of Life. London: Heinemann.

Chamberlain G, Phillips E, Howlett B, Masters K (1978). British Births 1970. Volume 2. Obstetric Care. London: Heinemann.

Garcia J, Anderson J, Vacca A, Elbourne D, Grant A, Chalmers I. (1985). Views of women and their medical and midwifery attendants about instrumental delivery using vacuum extraction and forceps. J Psychosom Obstet Gynaecol, 4: 1–9.

Goldthorp WO, Richman J. (1974). Maternal attitudes to unintended home confinement. A case study of the effects of the hospital strike upon domiciliary confinements. Practitioner, 212: 845–853.

Graham H (1976). Smoking in pregnancy: the attitudes of expectant mothers. Soc Sci Med, 10: 399–405.

Graham H, McKee L (1979). The first months of motherhood. Report on a Health Education Council Project. York University (mimeo).

Graham H, Oakley A (1981). Competing ideologies of reproduction: medical and maternal perspectives on pregnancy. In: Women, Health and Reproduction. Roberts H (ed). London: Routledge & Kegan Paul.

Hall M, Macintyre S, Porter M (1985). Antenatal Care Assessed. Aberdeen: Aberdeen University Press.

Health Education Council (1984). Pregnancy Book: A Guide to becoming Pregnant, being Pregnant and Caring for Your New Born Baby. The Council, 78 New Oxford Street, London WC1A 1AH.

House of Commons (1980). Perinatal and Neonatal Mortality. Second Report from the Social Services Committee. London: Her Majesty's Stationery Office.

Illsley R (1955). Social class selection and social class differences in relation to stillbirths and infant death. Br Med J, 2: 1520.

Kitzinger S (1962). The Experience of Childbirth. London: Victor Gollancz.

Kitzinger S (1978). Women as Mothers. London: Fontana.

Lancet (1982). New dimensions in obstetric audit (Leading article). Lancet, ii: 857–858.

Lazarus RS (1969). Psychological Stress and the Coping Process. New York: McGraw-Hill.

Lewis J (1980). The Politics of Motherhood. London: Croom Helm.

Llewelyn-Davies M (1978). Maternity: Letters from Working Women. Dallas G (ed). London: Virago. (First published 1915.)

Macintyre S (1977a). The management of childbirth: a review of sociological research issues. Soc Sci Med, II: 477–484.

Macintyre S (1977b). Single and Pregnant. London: Croom Helm.

Macintyre S (1980). The sociology of reproduction—review article. Soc Health Illness, 2.2: 215–222.

McIntosh J (1987). Some working class perspectives on childbirth: a study of 80 primigravidae. University of Glasgow: Social Paediatric and Obstretic Research Unit.

Maternity Services Advisory Committee to the Secretaries of State for Social Services and for Wales (1984). Maternity Care in Action. Part II. Care during Childbirth (Intrapartum Care). A guide to good practice and a plan for action. London: Her Majesty's Stationery Office.

Miller R (1986). Selling the sciences. New Society, 78: 1247. 21 November.

National Perinatal Epidemiology Unit. (1978). An Introduction to the NPEU and Annual Report for 1978. Oxford: National Perinatal Epidemiology Unit.

O'Brien M (1981). The Politics of Reproduction. London: Routledge & Kegan Paul.

Oakley A (1979). Becoming a Mother. Oxford: Martin Robertson.

Oakley A, Chamberlain GVP. (1981). Some medical and social factors in postpartum depression. J Obstet Gynaecol, 1: 182–187.

Reid M (1983). A feminist sociological imagination? Reading Ann Oakley—review article. Soc Health Illness, 5.1: 83–94.

Reid M, Gutteridge G, McIlwaine G (1983). A Comparison of the Delivery of Antenatal Care between Hospital and a Peripheral Clinic. Report of the findings submitted to the Health Services Research Committee, SHHD.

Robinson JJA (1986). A Study of the Policy Implications Arising from a Local Survey of Perinatal Mortality. PhD thesis, University of Keele.

Robinson JJA (1989). Perinatal mortality: a report on a research study. Int J Hlth Care Qual Assurance, 2.2: 13–19.

Royal College of Obstetricians and Gynaecologists (1982). Report of the Working Party on Antenatal and Intrapartum Care (Chairman: Prof MC Macnaughton). London: Royal College of Obstetricians and Gynaecologists.

Stacey M (1987). The role of information in the development of social policy. Community Medicine, 9: 216–225.

Vuori HV (1982). Quality Assurance of Health Services: Concepts and Methodology. Public Health in Europe No. 16. Copenhagen: World Health Organization. Regional Office for Europe.

World Health Organization (1985). Having a Baby in Europe. Public Health in Europe No. 16. Copenhagen: WHO Regional Office for Europe.

Weiss CH (1980). Social Science Research and Decision Making. New York: Columbia University Press.

5 The role of economics in the evaluation of care

Miranda Mugford and Michael F. Drummond

1 Introduction

The range of possibilities for health care has been greatly increased by technological advances in medicine. High quality care is expected and demanded by both health care professionals and patients. In almost all countries, however, the resources available for responding to these expectations and demands are becoming increasingly stretched. Post-war demographic changes and changing social structures have led more people to need or seek health care. Given the scarcity of resources—that is, their limited availability when compared to the demands—some tough choices must be made. The key question is how best to choose between the different and competing ways of using the resources that are available.

Obviously, the first consideration must be that the care for which these resources is used is likely to do more good than harm. But additional important considerations must include both the most cost-effective or efficient use of the resources available for maternity care, and the extent to which the society's resources should be allocated to maternity care. In a world where there are many competing uses for the same resources, those wishing to develop health care programmes for pregnant and childbearing women need to demonstrate that allocating more resources to this field would represent good value for society, when compared with the alternative uses that could be made of those resources in other fields.

Given that resources are always scarce in relation to demand, the main purpose of this chapter is twofold: to show why these resources should be used effectively and efficiently; and to suggest ways of assessing whether or not they are being used efficiently. We have taken examples from perinatal research to show how an economic evaluation would have added to the value of the results. The additional information obtained would be useful not only to planners who must decide on the appropriate level of funds for maternity care, but also to professionals within the maternity field who wish to make optimal use of the budgets and resources that are available to them.

We have organized our chapter in the following way. First, we outline some basic concepts of economics in order to de-mystify some of the technical vocabulary and to explain some of the jargon. Second, we describe some of the main methods of economic evaluation, outlining the factors that economists would wish to consider in a comparison of health care programmes and the methods that they use to measure and value these factors. Finally, we discuss some case studies from the perinatal field, both to illustrate specific economic issues, and to demonstrate that undertaking economic analysis alongside clinical and health services research is both appropriate and feasible.

2 Some basic concepts of economics

2.1 Opportunity cost

Economics is not about costs, but about benefits. That is, the costs of using resources (such as trained staff, equipment, or buildings) in a given service are the benefits that would be obtained if the same resources were used in their best alternative use. Although the money paid for these resources might reflect their value in other possible uses, monetary cost is often an inadequate measure of the true economic cost. The use of a given resource (such as an hour of a midwife's time) in one programme automatically means that the use of that resource is denied to any other programme. Hence the economist's notion of *opportunity cost*: the cost of a resource is the benefit forgone from not using it in its best alternative use.

2.2 Utility

When economists refer to benefits, they have in mind the concept of *utility*, the amount of satisfaction gained from consumption of a commodity or a service. It follows, therefore, that when they consider the benefits of health care programmes, they are referring to the improvements in the quality of life that result from the programme. (Health care programmes may also generate other economic benefits, such as resource savings from unnecessary medical care that is averted, or from increases in productivity. These, however, are an incomplete measure of benefit; improvements in quality of life must be considered as well.)

Although evaluative research should take account of the improvements in the quality of life brought about by health care programmes in relation to the resources they consume, both these factors are difficult to measure. The problem for economic analysis is to find a scale or scales of valuation of different health states that will tell us which states are perceived as more desirable for the individuals receiving care. Data derived using these scales can then be combined with clinical outcomes to estimate the overall effect expressed in terms of the differences in 'quality adjusted life years' (QALYs) that result from different programmes or interventions.

In the economy at large, the costs and benefits of activities are made visible through the market system. In the market, consumers make decisions about how much they are willing to pay for goods or services based on the utility they expect to obtain from the various purchases, and on how much money they possess. Although there have been some attempts to estimate directly the consumer's 'willingness-to-pay' in monetary terms for improvements in health (Thompson and Cohen 1981), the market mechanism, in general, either does not apply, or works imperfectly in the health care field. Economists thus have to use other approaches in estimating the benefits of health care programmes. The most promising approach appears to be the valuation of health improvements, not in money terms, but relative to one another. Analysts are beginning to explore how individuals rate states of health on a scale of 'health utilities' (Drummond *et al.* 1987; Williams 1985).

Utility measurement is a growing area of research and policy interest. Research tools for measurement of utility are still being developed, tested, and debated. It will not always be necessary to make full and detailed measurements of both utilities and costs. However, if it has been decided that a given treatment objective *must* be met, one may merely compare options in terms of their relative cost in meeting the chosen objective.

2.3 The margin

Another useful economic concept is that of the *margin*. Few procedures or programmes are totally worthless, but the key question is: *how much* of them should we use? For example, there may be general agreement that certain screening tests should be applied to high risk pregnancies; but should they be applied routinely to all pregnant women? A spectacular example of the importance of marginal analysis can be found in the field of cancer screening. Newhauser and Lewicki (1975) considered a recommendation from the American Cancer Society, in which it was advised that 6 sequential stool tests should be performed on the same population in order to detect asymptomatic cancer of the colon. They pointed out that while the *average* cost per case detected over 6 tests was only $2500, the *marginal* cost of finding an additional case with the 6th test (after previously having done 5) was in excess of $47 million! Such analyses would be particularly useful in the case of the routine and repeated testing that is so common in the care of women during pregnancy and childbirth.

2.4 Types of economic appraisal

The nature and scale of any economic evaluation will vary according to the question that is being asked. While all approaches to some extent involve deriving a balance sheet of the costs and benefits of the different strategies compared, some approaches are more complex than others. *Cost-minimization* analysis is probably the simplest. Either by assuming or demonstrating that the benefits of treatments that are compared are equal, this method merely involves comparing the resource costs without any need to measure benefits. For example, if two prophylactic antibiotic regimens are equally effective in decreasing the risk of infection following caesarean section, one can directly compare the costs of the two regimens. In *cost-effectiveness* analysis, treatments that may have different effects are compared in terms of the relative cost of obtaining a particularly important effect. For example, neonatal intensive care has been evaluated in terms of the cost per year of life gained (Mugford 1988).

More complex methods, which do not assume equivalent benefits from competing treatments, include *cost–benefit* and *cost–utility* analyses, in which benefits are measured either in money terms or calculated in terms of quality adjusted life years. (Further discussion of the different forms of analysis can be found in Drummond *et al.* 1986.)

In the next section we outline how some of these concepts are applied in economic evaluations of choices in health care field.

3 Methods of economic evaluation

There are three main stages of economic evaluation (Drummond 1980). First, the likely costs and benefits must be enumerated; second, they must be measured; and third, they must be expressed in comparable units. Taking each of these stages in turn, we will introduce briefly some of the methodological issues that arise in economic evaluation.

3.1 Enumeration of likely costs and benefits

The economic impact of a health procedure is reflected in the difference it makes to available resources and to overall quality of life. As we need to identify changes in resource use or in benefits that might arise from the use of a particular procedure, we usually measure only those factors that will differ between the options that are compared. These may either be a choice between 'competing' procedures, or a choice between a given procedure and no intervention at all.

Costs and benefits arise from *changes* in uses of a community's resources. These resources include not only physical equipment and buildings, but also the human time, the skill and effort both of health care personnel and of the women giving birth and their families and neighbours.

The range of factors an economist might want to consider are illustrated in Fig. 5.1. The ways in which the health procedure may have an impact can be categorized under the headings of health service resources, family and community resources, and effects on health status.

Health service resources such as medical, nursing, and other staff time, buildings, equipment, drugs, and dressings may be provided by more than one part of the health care sector. Thus, for example, in Britain an evaluation of routine antenatal home visiting would have to take account of both the benefits conferred by such visits and the resources provided by hospitals, the community midwifery service and general practitioners. Concentration on the costs in only one of several sectors can lead to false conclusions. Reduction in the length of postnatal stay in hospital may improve hospital efficiency, but if there is increased work for community midwives or health visitors, this is also part of the health care cost of a policy of early postnatal discharge from hospital.

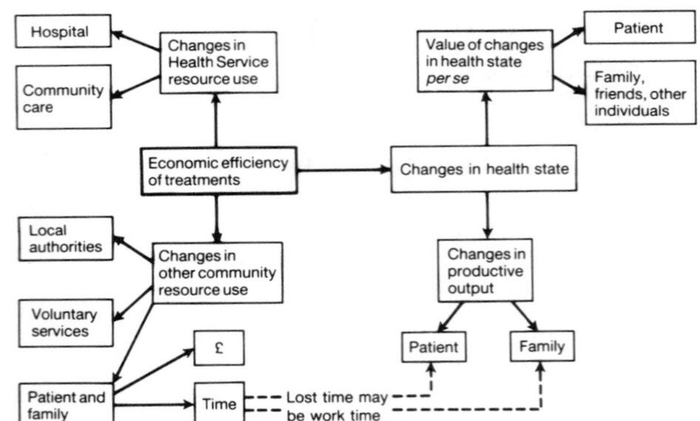

Fig. 5.1 The relevant changes in a comparison of the economic efficiency of treatments/programmes (after Drummond 1980)

An economic comparison of procedures in perinatal care should also consider the effect on the resources of the woman, her family and the community in which she lives. Returning to the example of a policy of early postnatal discharge from hospital, it is likely that more family resources will be needed for informal home care and support for mothers who return home very soon after delivery, but this might be set against the costs of relatives and friends visiting the woman in hospital. In the longer term the effects of a procedure on a family's capacity to work and support itself may be extremely important.

The third category of interest to economists as well as others is how the treatment alternatives affect the quality of life of those receiving care and of those on whom they depend. This corresponds very closely to the sort of measurement that would be considered in clinical evaluation. As this information is needed to provide the basis for quality of life assessment, economists would look for data on the relative valuations made by patients with respect to different physical states of health. For example, Boyle *et al.* (1983) compared the extra costs of establishing a regional neonatal intensive care programme with the extra benefits in terms of improved survival and quality of life. In order to calculate the number of quality adjusted life years (QALYs) gained, they combined assessments of prognosis made by paediatricians with valuations of states of health obtained from members of the general public.

Since resources are used and health effects occur not only at the time of the health intervention but also in the longer term, economic appraisal is not confined to considering the immediate benefits and costs. For example, screening programmes that result in different incidences of a particular impairment can have long term resource consequences; first, because the affected children may have different skills and capacities than unaffected children; second, because they may have different health care, educational and other needs throughout their lives; and third, because their life expectancy may differ. If treatments are compared that may have effects on fertility in the offspring, as in the case of diethylstilboestrol (see Chapter 38), then the long term considerations might be extended to a further generation.

The enumeration of costs and benefits should be undertaken at the earliest possible stage of research. It is likely that much of the detailed measurement can be derived from the clinical and social evaluations, provided that the questions are appropriately framed in the first place.

Finally, it is important to be clear about the perspective from which costs and benefits are being assessed. What is counted as a cost or benefit will depend on whether the viewpoint is that of the hospital, the health care sector, the patient, the government or society as a whole. A medical fee in a private practice setting is a cost to the patient, a benefit to the professional and *may* reflect the costs to society as a whole. Costs to the patient will not usually be considered as costs to the health care sector, but are costs to society. Economists usually agree that the broadest, societal viewpoint should be one of the perspectives to be considered.

3.2 Measurement of costs and benefits

In the above discussion of enumeration we referred both to effects on resources and to effects on health and well-being (utility). In measuring resources, it may be possible to use routine administrative data systems, but there are limitations in this. A hospital accounting system, for example, may be inadequate if all transactions are recorded in financial units alone. For economic evaluation, resources should be measured in physical units initially, as cash values may vary over time and place. Thus, staff time should be measured, rather than the salary bill. (We consider the subject of valuation below.) Depending on the way health care is organized, the accounts of a health care institution may not measure the resources of other health agencies, and certainly do not measure 'out of hospital' costs to individuals. Nevertheless, routine data systems may provide useful information, and should be considered before direct measurement is planned.

Direct observational measurement (by work study or by asking staff or patients to keep diaries) can be very illuminating, but it is costly in research terms. It seems reasonable that such studies should themselves be justified in economic terms: that is, the benefits of more detailed measurement should outweigh the cost of the research.

While recognizing that measurement of the health and social effects of care is also the central concern of others involved in evaluating practice, many economists are interested in measuring these benefits in a way that expresses the relative utilities of the benefits of different options as a single measure. In research that is designed to measure utility (see Drummond *et al.* 1986 for a fuller discussion), assessments are either obtained by interviewing patients, or by interviewing a group of people thought to be representative of the views of society or of those receiving care.

3.3 Expression of costs and benefits in comparable units

When the results of measurement are known, how can they be used to decide on the best use of resources? The choice rests on the relative values that are placed on different resources or outcomes.

If we know that one procedure uses more nursing staff time but less medical staff time to achieve the same outcome of care, then the relative values of medical and nursing time may determine the choice. Money values (but not necessarily market prices) are used as a unit to express opportunity costs of different types of resources. Where there are differences in a large range of resources, there is an increased need for a common accounting unit of value to summarize the difference between the options compared.

In the case of benefits, the economist may choose to leave these in the most convenient natural units (such as years of life gained), or attempt to value them in money terms (Jones-Lee 1976) or as health utilities (Drummond *et al.* 1986). The extent to which valuation of benefits is required depends on the nature of the question being asked. Are we concerned with relative costs of achieving the same unit of output (cost–effectiveness analysis), or with finding the level of provision of care which justifies or is justified by the benefits (cost–benefit or cost–utility analysis)?

The conclusions of such evaluations are considerably affected by taking the timing of costs and benefits into account. It seems to be generally true that present events are valued more highly than those in the future. (This principle is institutionalized in investment appraisal where the current values of future payments are 'discounted' by some amount. Frequently, governments set official discount rates for appraisal of public expenditure projects. The arithmetical procedure is like a compound interest calculation performed in reverse.) In health care evaluation, such calculations can have the most dramatic effects on comparisons of programmes or interventions with different effects on life expectancy and on long term use of resources. The appropriate discount rate is, however, a matter for debate. Where there is debate about how large the discount should be, it can be helpful to take the 'what if?' approach (a sensitivity analysis), applying different rates of discount and seeing if this has any effect on the study conclusions. Sometimes the conclusions will be the same over a wide range of discount rates.

4 Incorporating economic analysis in evaluative research

Economic analysis is not a new phenomenon in the field of pregnancy and childbirth. There have been economic evaluations of screening programmes to detect neural tube defects in early pregnancy (Hagard *et al.* 1976; Henderson 1982; Hibbard *et al.* 1985; Layde *et al.* 1979) and programmes to prevent Rhesus isoimmunization (Torrance and Zipursky 1984). In addition, the relative costs of home and hospital delivery have been compared (Stilwell 1979; Howitz *et al.* 1978). Regional neonatal intensive care services have been evaluated from an economic perspective (eg Pomerance *et al.* 1978; Boyle *et al.* 1983; Newns *et al.* 1984; Sandhu *et al.* 1986) and these studies have been reviewed elsewhere (Mugford 1988). None of the reported studies were linked to controlled trials, although in some instances (Boyle *et al.* 1983) the authors noted that controlled trials had preceded and informed their economic assessment.

Drummond and Stoddart (1984) have argued that economic analyses should be incorporated more frequently into clinical trials, suggesting that this would lead to the production of more rigorous and timely evidence of the costs and benefits of medical practices. They suggested that it would be worth building economic analysis into a trial when large amounts of resources are at stake, when a new technique is likely to become widespread in the near future, or when shortage of resources forces a choice between options for care.

Case studies to illustrate when and how economic measurement was or should have been included in trials are presented in Appendix 5.1. The topics selected are routine ultrasound examination in pregnancy, admission to hospital for antenatal bed rest, prenatal diagnosis using chorion villus sampling, and routine care of the umbilicus in newborn infants.

Large amounts of resources may be at stake, either because the procedures being compared are applied to a large number of women or because there is likely to be a wide difference in cost between the procedures. Even in countries with the lowest birth rates, the care of mothers and babies represents a significant proportion of total health expenditure, because of the large number of routine procedures carried out during normal maternity and neonatal care. Routine rather than selective ultrasound examination, for example, falls into this category, now that in many countries most women are likely to have at least one scan during pregnancy (see Chapters 26 and 27).

Wide differences in costs arise, at least for health care agencies, where women are admitted to hospital for bed rest during pregnancy. Chorion villus sampling for prenatal diagnosis of chromosomal or genetic disorders in the fetus is an example of a new treatment technology that is likely to become widely accepted in clinical practice. Ten years ago the same criterion would have been applied to warrant an economic evaluation of electronic fetal heart monitoring in labour.

Economic evaluation would also be appropriate when resource considerations are prominent. This criterion might apply when it is suggested that resources could be reallocated to better uses by changing or abandoning existing practices, and when a trial is required to ensure that this does not lead to a reduction in the quality of care as judged by clinical and social measures. The effect of routine methods of treatment of the umbilical cord by English community midwives on their workload illustrates this.

5 Conclusions

Any evaluation of health care alternatives should take account of economic factors such as opportunity cost, the margin, and utility as well as the effectiveness. The criteria suggested by Drummond and Stoddart (1984) for choosing aspects of care where economic analysis would be appropriate are useful when applied to trials in the perinatal field. Very few evaluative studies in perinatal medicine have incorporated a formal economic analysis. Analysis of a random sample of trials from the Oxford Database of Perinatal Trials has shown that although economic evaluation would have been useful in up to half of all trials that have taken place, it was not explicitly included in any of the sampled trial reports (Appendix 5.2).

As future trials are planned, it might be a more cost-effective use of research funds to measure economic variables alongside clinical or psychosocial outcomes, rather than to mount independent studies. This change cannot come about until clinical researchers take a broader view of the potential of randomized clinical trials in health care. Rather than simply being a means of answering questions of clinical effectiveness, trials can also be a framework for considering costs and benefits to society. As clinical training does not usually consider the measurement of these aspects of care, it is as important for researchers to work with economists and social scientists as with statisticians when designing clinical trials.

The inclusion of economic analysis in randomized controlled trials might be further encouraged if those commissioning medical research were to require investigation of the relative costs of the treatments alongside the evaluation of effectiveness and acceptability (Drummond and Stoddart 1984). A similar incentive to collaborative research between clinical researchers and economists is created where government health funding is only made available to new projects if data about clinical effectiveness, costs, and acceptability are shown on application for funds. Such a policy was proposed by the New Zealand Labour Party (1978) and is now official policy in New Zealand. The willingness to undertake economic analysis, where appropriate, is also a requirement in research proposals made to the Ministry of Health in Ontario, Canada (1987).

The application of the methods of economics in evaluation of perinatal care cannot overcome the moral dilemmas that arise in choice of treatment or allocation of resources. It does, however, provide a framework within which such factors become less easily avoided, can be more squarely faced, and discussed from the point of view of both care givers and receivers. As the use of resources for health care affects everyone, it could be contended that economics is as much the business of clinicians, midwives, and women who use their services as it is of administrators and academic economists.

Appendix 5.1 Case studies from maternity care

(i) Routine ultrasound imaging in pregnancy

One of many procedures in maternity care that is applied to a large population is routine ultrasound imaging of the fetus during pregnancy. The technique, developed during the 1960s and introduced in obstetric practice during the 1970s, provides a method for identifying problems of fetal growth and development before delivery, and has been widely adopted in addition to routine antenatal examination by a doctor or midwife.

The results of 5 trials have been published (Wladimiroff and Laar 1980; Bennett *et al.* 1982; Neilson *et al.* 1984; Eik-Nes *et al.* 1984; Bakketeig *et al.* 1984). The objectives of these trials were often implicitly rather than explicitly stated. But in all of them a comparison was made between a policy of using ultrasound routinely during pregnancy and a policy in which it was used selectively. The use of ultrasound routinely may: improve the prediction of the expected date of confinement hence reducing the induction rate in pregnancies mistakenly diagnosed as post-term, and improve the management of the truly post-term pregnancy; allow earlier diagnosis of fetal growth retardation, placenta praevia, and twin pregnancies, leading to reduced morbidity and mortality in babies; improve the detection of malformed fetuses, which, if followed by termination of pregnancy, would reduce numbers of births of impaired babies; and alter a woman's feelings about her pregnancy and the fetus she carries (see Chapter 27).

The health resource implications of such a screening programme are mentioned in only 3 of the trial reports, and only 1 (Bakketeig *et al.* 1984) refers explicitly to any cost measurement or economic analysis.

Cost differences that arise between the two strategies of care can be considered under the headings of fixed costs, marginal costs, and costs to the woman and her family. Fixed or less flexible costs might include equipment, trained staff, and clinic accommodation. These data can be collected independently of the trial (unless the staff and equipment are employed exclusively for the trial) as can information about maintenance costs or training costs associated with an ultrasound screening programme. The data that need to be collected during the trial are the costs that are likely to vary with the number of cases treated, and those which are likely to differ between the two types of care offered. Some prior experience is necessary to determine which items would be relevant, either from clinical knowledge or by observation before the trial. Bakketeig *et al.* (1984) included an explicit analysis of costs in which account was taken of the increased use of resources beyond the ultrasound scan procedure itself. It was found that the women allocated to routine scanning had more antenatal hospital admissions and more diagnostic tests performed. These women also spent more time and money because

Table 5.A1 Relevant factors for economic evaluation of ultra-sound screening

Estimated independently of trial
- Equipment
- Staff: numbers and skills
- Buildings: clinic space required
- Other uses of staff, equipment and clinic space

To be estimated during trial
- (1) Health care resources
  - Number of scans: – routine
    - – additional
  - Time per scan
  - Materials used
  - Referrals for specialist care
  - Diagnostic tests recommended
  - Hospital (antenatal) admissions
  - Procedures in labour/delivery
  - Use of neonatal care
- (2) Patient/family factors
  - Travel and waiting time
  - Loss of earnings
  - Satisfaction with care
  - Quality of life (baby)

of their attendance for screening. This would be a less significant cost where ultrasound screening occurs at the same time and place as routine antenatal care. Eik-Nes (1984) did measure hospital bed use and found little difference between the two groups in his trial.

None of the trials attempted to quantify mothers' attitudes to their antenatal care, although there is some evidence to suggest that ultrasound can affect a mother's attitude to her pregnancy positively (Reading *et al.* 1982). If this is the case an economic analysis should take account of such intangible outcomes as the mother's relationship with the infant after it is born, or her sense of loss if the pregnancy ends with the death of the fetus. Such factors would be likely to be reflected in utility measurements, where these are undertaken. For example, women's preferences may be reflected in their willingness to pay for ultrasound examinations. One study in the USA has shown that women would be willing to pay for an ultrasound scan even if there was no clinical benefit (Berwick and Weinstein 1985).

Although the trials were designed to assess the effectiveness of ultrasound for a specific purpose (principally screening for growth retardation and estimation of expected date of delivery), there are other possible uses of ultrasound (including diagnosis of malformations, as an aid in amniocentesis, or for earlier diagnosis of multiple pregnancy or placenta praevia) which only one of these trials addressed. It cannot therefore be assumed that the equipment and staff costs are wholly incurred by the routine screening programme. Thus the marginal cost of the screening programme need not take account of the full capital staffing and running cost of the equipment. Bakketeig and his colleagues (1984), however, estimated that the cost of routine ultrasound scanning for the women in their study was US $250 per case (in 1983) more than it would have been without ultrasound. If such a cost analysis had been included in the other trial reports, it would have allowed a more reasoned comparison between the clinical or psychosocial benefits of routine ultrasound screening, if any, and the substantial health care resources that are being absorbed in the programme.

(ii) Bed rest in hospital during twin pregnancy

Antenatal in-patient care absorbs considerable amounts of health care resources, and thus is an intervention that qualifies for an economic input in any evaluation. It is now more than 30 years since Russell (1952) observed that twins born to middle class women were larger and less likely to die than those born to working class women, and suggested that 'consideration might be given to admitting to hospital all twin mothers at the 30th week, in order, by diet and rest, to tide them over the danger period'. Largely as a result of this recommendation, it became common practice in Britain to admit women with multiple pregnancy to hospital for bed rest (Brown and Dixon 1963).

The fact that, 30 years after Russell made his recommendations, there is still no consensus about the value of hospitalization for bed rest in twin pregnancy (Powers and Miller 1979; Lancet 1981; Grant *et al.* 1982) reflects the dearth of well-controlled studies mounted to evaluate the effects of this policy. In 1979, Powers and Miller noted that, as routine use of ultrasound in early pregnancy became more widespread, a greater proportion of twin gestations would be diagnosed in early pregnancy. They pointed out that, in this rapidly evolving situation, it had become particularly urgent to assess whether hospital bed rest in twin pregnancy prolonged gestation (thus reducing the risks associated with preterm delivery) because this policy has substantial resource implications.

The effects of routine admission to hospital for bed rest in twin pregnancy at the beginning of the 3rd trimester has recently been compared with ambulatory care and selective hospitalization in two controlled trials (Haartikainen-Sorri and Jouppila 1984; Saunders *et al.* 1985). In neither trial was a formal economic evaluation incorporated prospectively. The results of the trials suggest that, if routine bed rest has an effect at all, it is to curtail the duration of gestation. (See Chapter 39.)

In the light of the actual results of these trials, the case for economic analysis from the health service perspective is relatively weak since the cheapest option is also the most effective. However, this was not known before the trials were mounted. The additional costs resulting from hospital admission (hospital costs, diagnostic tests) and differences in family resources used should have been recorded. The authors do give figures for the incremental number of hospital days resulting from the bed rest option, but no financial values were attached to these, or to the other costs associated with each of the two policies compared. A more explicit calculation of the additional costs of bed rest, both to the health service and to the family would reinforce the argument for discontinuing the practice unless further trials show it to be effective in some circumstances. Conversely, if bed rest had proved clinically superior, health service and patients' costs would have been relevant additional factors to have been taken into account.

(iii) Chorion villus sampling for prenatal diagnosis of chromosomal or genetic disorders in the fetus

One of the major problems facing the health care systems of nearly all countries is that new technologies diffuse into the system before their effectiveness, acceptability, safety, and costs have been adequately evaluated. Since clinical trials have an important role in ascertaining effectiveness and safety, they also provide an important vehicle for exploring the economic consequences of new health technologies. The rapidly growing field of fetal diagnosis provides a number of examples of this process, but the recent introduction of a technique called chorion villus sampling illustrates the issues particularly well. Pregnant women who are anxious, either because of their genetic history or because of their age, that they may be carrying a fetus with one or other of a variety of abnormalities are now able to seek reassurance in one of two ways: fetal cells can be examined after obtaining a sampling of liquor by amniocentesis in the 2nd trimester of pregnancy or fetal tissue can be obtained for examination by chorion villus sampling in the 1st trimester. The claims made on behalf of chorion villus sampling stress that it reduces the period of parental anxiety compared with later fetal diagnosis using amniocentesis and that, if termination of pregnancy is required, this can be performed at a stage of gestation when physical and psychological complications are less. Because over 15,000 women a year in England alone are already given information about the normality of their fetuses using amniocentesis, it is clear that it is important to compare this current technique systematically with the proposed new technique (see Chapter 23).

Randomized trials are in progress in Europe and Canada, all of them concentrating primarily on assessing the short term consequences of the two policies in terms of physical risks. In addition, several of the trials will assess the short term psychological consequences and have laid the basis for investigating possible adverse long term physical effects. The protocol for the Canadian trial was exceptional in that plans for an economic analysis were incorporated at the outset (Fuller, personal communication).

Economic considerations are relevant in two main ways. First, the relative costs of chorion villus sampling and amniocentesis need to be compared. Since chorion villus sampling can be performed earlier in pregnancy (at 8–10 weeks) than amniocentesis, it is likely that more procedures in total will be carried out on a given cohort of patients, as some pregnancies will abort spontaneously in the period between 8–10 weeks and 16–20 weeks, when amniocentesis is typically performed. There may also be differences in the costs, both to the health service and to the women, arising from differences in the complication rates of chorion villus sampling and amniocentesis, in the costs of the investigative techniques themselves, and in the cost of management for the pregnancies that require termination.

Secondly, as indicated above, there are likely to be different levels of anxiety associated with the two techniques. For example, chorion villus sampling can provide earlier reassurance to the mother and increase the chances of a safer termination, should this be necessary. On the other hand more women are likely to have to face an explicit decision to abort the fetus after chorion villus sampling, again because some abnormal fetuses would be likely to have aborted spontaneously before amniocentesis can be performed. In addition, if the sensitivity and specificity of the two techniques differ, this will affect the anxiety levels of mothers: false positives and false negatives increase anxiety; true negatives reduce it. That is, in economists' terms, it could be argued that the 'utility' to women (and to their partners) of the two techniques is likely to be a deciding factor. It is for this reason that the Canadian protocol included the plan to measure utility alongside the traditional clinical parameters.

A woman's choice between two methods of prenatal diagnosis would depend on many factors and the relative weight that she attaches to each. These might include the nature of the procedure and the period of waiting for the results, her belief about the efficacy and safety of the procedure, and her beliefs about the potential quality of life for a fetus affected by the condition to be diagnosed. All of these factors might differ with relevant previous knowledge or experience. Recent studies of women's preferences for different hypothetical 'scenarios' (Pauker and Pauker 1977; Bryce *et al.* 1989) represent the very early stages of research that could provide the basis for estimating relative utilities for different options. It may be incorrect to use results derived from small or selected groups as a basis for health policy decisions, and there is continuing debate about whose utilities should provide the baseline for social policy decisions.

(iv) Care of the umbilicus and midwives' workload

This case study illustrates how an evaluation can be prompted by resource constraints. In the United Kingdom, community midwives visit every mother and baby at home after delivery daily at least until the 10th day. After that, they visit at their discretion up to the 28th day after delivery, especially where either mother or baby is not progressing normally, or where advice is needed. Midwives generally regard delayed healing of the umbilicus as a reason to continue visiting after the 10th day (Mugford *et al.* 1986). As previous research has suggested that the treatment of the cord might affect time to healing, there was a possibility that a treatment might be identified which would allow a reduction of community midwifery time required for cord care, allowing this time to be reallocated for other midwifery duties such as antenatal care, breastfeeding support, or care of mothers with puerperal depression. This is important, because at a time when women are discharged increasingly early from hospital after delivery there is growing pressure of work for midwives in the community.

Mugford and colleagues (1986) designed a trial to test the hypothesis 'that one or more methods of cord care is associated with a reduction in the number of home visits by midwives after the statutorily required period of ten days'. Three aspects of cord care were compared in a factorial design: dusting powder, cleansing method, and frequency of application. Clinical outcomes such as time to separation of the umbilical stump, stickiness, or frank infection were also measured. There was a significant difference in the number of home visits made to babies allocated to the different powders; the difference between the groups was enough to account for the work of a whole-time midwife for every 3000–5000 births. Previous studies of cord treatments (Arad *et al.* 1981) have demonstrated an effect on time to cord separation, but have not developed the implications of this further so that the resulting costs can be estimated.

A common theme in the research on the effect of treatment of the umbilicus on time to cord separation or healing has been to suggest that treatments containing antiseptic agents may have a delaying effect on the healing process. None of the studies has demonstrated the benefits of routine antiseptic treatments in reducing the relatively rare occurrence of frank infection.

It has not in the past been the prime concern of hospital control of infection officers to consider the wider cost implications of the policies they recommend. However, the demonstrated costs arising from use of different treatments suggest that, where hospital policy dictates use of the more costly treatment (not just in terms of pharmaceutical prices), the policy should be backed by evidence of effectiveness of the treatment as compared with alternatives that are less costly in 'out of hospital' resources.

Appendix 5.2 Assessment of the proportion of perinatal trials in which economic evaluation would be appropriate

To assess whether the criteria for inclusion of economic measurements proposed by Drummond and Stoddart (1984) are generally workable, and if so, what proportion of perinatal trials might benefit from economic analyses, we studied a random sample of 100 trials drawn from the Oxford Database of Perinatal Trials (Chalmers *et al.* 1986). We then applied the criteria to each of the published reports sampled. In conducting this assessment, it was not our objective to estimate 'between assessor' variability formally (although we found that, in fact, there was no disagreement between the two assessors that could not be resolved easily). Judgements as to whether or not economic analyses should be conducted more widely will tend to reflect the weight which a particular individual attaches to information about resource effects. Our own assessment necessarily reflects the fact that we happen to be well-disposed towards attempts to include economic analyses within controlled trials. Interpreted in this light, the results must be seen as providing only order-of-magnitude rather than precise estimates.

Table 5.A2 Randomized controlled trials in perinatal medicine in which economic measurement would be recommended

Indication for economic measurement	Estimated proportion of trials (per cent)
Large resource implications because large eligible population	35
Large resource implications because large differences in unit cost	30
Imminent diffusion of new technology	11
Cost considerations prompted trial	6
No clear indication for economic analysis	52

(Based on a random sample of 100 trials in the Oxford Database of Perinatal Trials)

There was little difficulty in applying the criteria for including economic measurement in the trial reports we examined. Many procedures fell into more than one category, but this merely reinforced the need for measurement of economic aspects. The 'wide cost difference' category presented the most problems. It is easy to assume that this refers to differences in input costs such as staff time or equipment, but wide cost differences can arise for patients or society as a whole, especially where there are differences in the quality of life associated with or following different treatments. As many of the trials we looked at had neither the statistical power, nor the data derived from long term follow-up, with which to assess these costs, it was impossible to judge whether some trials in our sample might have fallen into the category of 'wide cost differences'.

Table 5.A2 shows that in just over half (52) of the 100 trials sampled it was judged that an economic analysis was not appropriate using the criteria suggested by Drummond and Stoddart (1984). Many of these 52 trials were drug trials in which the costs of the drugs compared were unlikely to differ substantially. There were also trials where the outcomes did not indicate different economic consequences. Economic analyses were judged to have been potentially useful in 48 out of the 100 trials sampled, and some of these met more than one of Drummond and Stoddart's criteria. About a third of the published perinatal trials were concerned with interventions that have large resource implications because (as is often the case in perinatal care) a large population is eligible for the intervention in question. Some of these trials were candidates for economic analysis because the unit costs of the alternative interventions differed widely; we estimated that altogether about one in three perinatal trials could have benefited from economic analyses using this criterion.

In about 1 in 10 of the published trials, economic analysis would have been indicated because the studies involved evaluation of a new technology likely to become widely diffused.

Finally, in 6 of the 100 reports we sampled, cost considerations appeared to have provided the dominant motive for the research, and yet formal economic analysis was not included in the report.

References

Arad I, Eyal F, Fainmesser P (1981). Umbilical care and cord separation. Arch Dis Childhood, 56: 887–888.

Bakketeig LS, Eik-Nes SH, Jacobsen G, Ulstein MK, Brodtkorb CJ, Balstad P, Eriksen BC, Jorgensen NP (1984). Randomised controlled trial of ultrasonographic screening in pregnancy. Lancet, 2: 207–209.

Bennett MJ, Little G, Dewhurst J, Chamberlain G (1982). Predictive value of ultrasound measurement: a randomized controlled trial. Br J Obstet Gynaecol, 89: 338–341.

Berwick DM, Weinstein MC (1985). What do patients value? Willingness to pay for ultrasound in normal pregnancy. Medical Care, 23: 881–893.

Boyle MH, Torrance GW, Sinclair JC, Horwood SP (1983). Economic evaluation of neonatal intensive care for very-low-birthweight infants. New Engl J Med, 308: 1330-1337.

Brown EJ, Dixon HG (1963). Twin pregnancy. J Obstet Gynaecol Br Commnwlth, 70: 251–257.

Bryce R, Bradley MT, McCormick SM (1989). Do women prefer chorionic villus sampling to amniocentesis for prenatal diagnosis? Paed Perinat Epidemiol, 3: 137–145.

Chalmers I, Hetherington J, Newdick M, Mutch LMM, Grant AM, Dickersin K, Enkin E, Enkin M (1986). The Oxford Database of Perinatal Trials: Developing a register of published reports on on controlled trials. Controlled Clinical Trials, 7: 306–324

Drummond MF (1980). Principles of Economic Appraisal in Health Care. Oxford: Clarendon Press.

Drummond MF, Stoddart GL (1984). Economic analysis and clinical trials. Controlled Clinical Trials, 5: 115–128.

Drummond MF, Stoddart GL, Torrance GW (1986). Methods for the Economic Evaluation of Health Care Programmes. Oxford: Oxford University Press.

Eik-Nes SH, Okland O, Aure JC, Ulstein M (1984). Ultrasound screening in pregnancy: a randomised controlled trial. Lancet, 1: 1347.

Fuller PJ (unpublished). The clinical and economic evaluation of prenatal diagnosis comparing chorionic villi sampling and midtrimester amniocentesis. Protocol, Department of Obstetrics, McMaster University, Hamilton, Ontario, Canada.

Grant A, Chalmers I, Enkin M (1982). Screening and diagnostic tests in antenatal care. In: Enkin M, Chalmers I (eds). Effectiveness and Satisfaction in Antenatal Care. London: Spastics International Medical Publications/Heinemann Medical Books.

Haartikainen-Sorri AL, Jouppila P (1984). Is routine hospitalisation needed in antenatal care of twin pregnancy? J Perinat Med, 12: 31–34.

Hagard S, Carter F, Milne RG (1976). Screening for spina bifida cystica. Br J Prev Soc Med, 30: 45–53.

Henderson JB (1982). An economic appraisal of the benefits of screening for open spina bifida. Science and Medicine, 16: 545–560.

Hibbard BM, Roberts CJ, Elder GH, Evans KT, Lawrence KM (1985). Can we afford screening for neural tube defects? The South Wales experience. Br Med J, 290: 293–295.

Howitz P, Ussing J, Fødsel ljemme eller på institution (1978). Ugeskr Laeger, 140: 1569–1573.

Jones-Lee MW (1976). The Value of Life: An Economic Analysis. London: Martin Robertson.

Lancet (1981). Bed rest in obstetrics (editorial). Lancet, 1: 1137–1138.

Layde PM, Allmen SD, Oakley GP (1979). Maternal serum alfa-fetoprotein screening: a cost–benefit analysis. Am J Public Hlth, 69: 566–573.

Mugford M, Somchaiwong M, Waterhouse I (1986). Treatment of umbilical cords. Report of a randomised controlled trial. Midwifery, 2: 177–186.

Mugford M (1988). A review of the economics of care for sick newborn infants. Community Medicine, 10: 99–111.

Neilson JP, Munjanja SP, Whitfield CR (1984). Screening for small for dates fetuses: a controlled trial. Br Med J, 289: 1179–1182.

New Zealand Labour Party (1978). Help Where and When You Need It. New Zealand Labour Party, Auckland, NZ.

Newhauser D, Lewicki AM (1975). What do we gain from the sixth stool guaiac? New Engl J Med, 293: 226–228.

Newns B, Drummond MF, Durbin GM, Colley P (1984). Costs and outcomes in a regional intensive care unit. Arch Dis Childhood, 59: 1064–1067.

Ontario Ministry of Health (1987). Health Research Grants and Awards 1987–88.

Pauker SP, Pauker SG (1977). Prenatal diagnosis: a directive approach to genetic counseling using decision analysis. Yale J Biol Med, 50: 275–289.

Pomerance JJ, Ukrainski GT, Ukra T, Henderson DH, Nash AH, Meredith JL (1978). Cost of living for infants weighing 1000 grams or less at birth. Pediatrics, 61: 908–910.

Powers WF, Miller TC (1979). Bed rest in pregnancy; identification of a critical period and its cost implications. Am J Obstet Gynecol, 134: 23–29.

Reading AD, Campbell S, Cox DN, Sledmore CM (1982). Health beliefs and health care behaviour in pregnancy. Psychosom Med, 12: 379–383.

Russell JK (1952). Maternal and fetal hazards associated with twin pregnancy. J Obstet Gynaecol Br Empire, 59: 208–213.

Sandhu B, Cooke RWI, Stevenson RC, Pharoah POD (1986). Cost of neonatal intensive care for very low birthweight infants. Lancet, i: 600-603.

Saunders MC, Dick JS, Brown IMcL, McPherson K, Chalmers I (1985). The effects of hospitalisation for bed rest on the duration of twin pregnancy: a randomised trial. Lancet, 2: 793–795.

Stilwell JA (1979). Relative costs of home and hospital confinement. Br Med J, 2: 257–259.

Thompson MS, Cohen AB (1981). Decision analysis: electronic fetal monitoring. In: Wartman PM (ed). Methods for Evaluating Health Services. New York: Sage Publications.

Torrance GW, Zipursky A (1984). Cost effectiveness of screening for antepartum Rh immunization. Clinics in Perinatol, 11: 267–281.

Williams A (1985). Economics of coronary artery bypass grafting. Br Med J, 291: 326–329.

Wladimiroff JW, Laar J (1980). Ultrasonic measurement of fetal body sizes, a randomized controlled trial. Acta Obstet Gynaecol Scand, 19: 177–179.

Part II

Social context of care during pregnancy and childbirth

6 Childbirth and society

Sheila Kitzinger

1 Introduction

What in northern industrial cultures are considered 'alternative' forms of care in childbirth are the norm in most countries of the world. This chapter sets out to examine some of the most important patterns of care which are common to different cultures, explores their rationale and social function, and offers an anthropological analysis of some elements in our own culture of childbirth. This may lead us to question some practices, develop more understanding of the needs of childbearing women, and introduce greater flexibility in care.

Birth, like death, is not merely a physiological process, but a social act. Each individual's entry to and exit from the social system is the signal for a realignment of existing relationships and the building of new ones. Birth is a rite of passage which is not only important in the developing consciousness of the woman who becomes a mother, but usually also has special meaning for the father, the extended family of each, and the wider society within which birth takes place.

Beliefs and ceremonies surrounding birth, like those of death, also provide a focus for some of the most significant values in any society. The anthropology of birth is concerned not only with different kinds of behaviour in childbirth, but also with different ways of *thinking*. In looking at the way people are born and how they die we have an opportunity to discover something about the social construction of reality and the dynamics of relationships between human beings in that culture.

All physiological processes are culturally shaped. Eating and drinking, the exit of waste matter from the body, sexual behaviour, the changes involved in puberty and ageing, female biological processes such as menstruation and lactation, and what we do when we belch, cough, fart, or sneeze, are under the direction of cultural imperatives which usually go unquestioned and unchallenged. The result is that we believe our behaviour is 'natural'.

The senses are similarly patterned. The sense of smell, largely incidental to eating, cooking, sexual attraction, and the care of infants in Western culture, is employed in some other cultures—among Malaysian and Mongol peoples, for example, as a greeting which includes the rubbing of noses and a mutual sniffing of cheeks (Argyle 1975). Stance and gesture are also the product of culture. In preliterate societies it is estimated that there are nearly 100 postures which are rarely adopted in the West, including the way in which the Nuer of the Sudan stand for long periods on one leg (Hewes 1957). A simple act like sticking out the tongue may mean a whole range of different things varying between mock terror, embarrassment, polite deference, and provocative contempt, and signify wisdom, negation, the destruction of demons, or that the other person is a fool (Argyle 1975).

In the same way childbirth is never completely 'natural'. It is a cultural artefact. In the processes and events of pregnancy and labour we witness the shaping of nature to social purposes. These are often implicit rather than overt, and can be understood only by revealing the template of values surrounding birth created by that specific culture.

In medieval Europe, for example, birth was seen both as a punishment for the sin of Eve and a religious task obligatory on married women as part of their penance for humanity. Pain was part of this punishment. In the sixteenth century midwives were burned at the stake for relieving labour pain with opium. Even in the nineteenth century anaesthesia was castigated as a 'decoy of Satan' that 'robbed God of the earnest cries which arise in times of trouble for help' (Carter and Duriez 1986). Simpson argued, within the same value framework, that when God removed Adam's rib he caused a deep sleep to fall on him, and that anaesthesia must, therefore, meet with divine approval.

A style of childbirth has been created throughout the West and is being exported to developing countries in the firm conviction that it is the only right one, in which birth is taken outside the home and away from the family and is an event conducted by a team of professionals in an intensive care setting. It has become an *interruption* of normal life rather than an integral part of its flow. Such a system of care may appear to be the only valid one. Our way of looking at birth is 'real', that of other cultures mistaken.

In contemporary Western society the culture pattern imposed on women is predominantly medical. Medicine has taken over from religion the power and authority of the priesthood. Birth is a medical crisis, the termination of a disease called 'pregnancy'. Labour is the sum of the interaction between the 'passage, the powers and the passenger'. The woman has no part in this equation. There is a skeletal framework, uterine contractions, and a fetus. This reproductive mechanism is always at risk of functioning ineffectively. The obstetrician is the senior mechanic and primer of the endocrine pump.

In the context of this biomedical paradigm cultural factors, far from being valued, are perceived as impediments to proper care in childbirth (McClain 1982). This may be partly because medical personnel who work in Third World societies or in large hospitals serving immigrant populations in inner city areas have little opportunity to see normal childbirth and concentrate on dealing with pathology (Newton and Newton 1972).

Where Western caregivers operate within a medical bureaucracy, traditional caregivers function within a system of magic and religion. This is a complex, coordinated set of principles and practices which, combined with empirical knowledge, seeks to restore balance between elements of heat and cold, to free the body of obstacles, or to reconcile human life with spiritual forces. These different systems often interlock or overlap with each other. In Jamaica, for example, concepts of sickness are composed of two in some ways disparate systems, one derived from that of medieval 'humours' and the other clustered around the idea of illness being the result of blockage by objects which, whether by sorcery or other means, are obstructing passages so that body substances can no longer flow. Both these systems combine in the care of women in pregnancy, childbirth, and postpartum and in remedies for reproductive malfunction.

The concept of humours is implicit in the Jamaican herbal pharmacopeia in which substances are categorized according to their heating or cooling properties. Cerasee, for example, is 'hot' and mint and thyme are both 'cold'. A balance must be kept between hot and cold and one of the tasks of the 'nana', the traditional midwife, is to maintain this balance. In many cultures health and disease are seen primarily as the outcome of the interaction between the spiritual and the human. Elements which Western thinking classify as psychological constitute a major theme. Emotional causes of physiological dysfunction and psychological elements in healing skills have paramount importance in most traditional systems. Illness is believed to result from disharmony. The skill of the healer is in restoring harmony between human life and the spiritual world, in the form of gods or ancestors, and between the spirit of the sick person and others in the community.

In childbirth the midwife is traditionally the key person in the exercise of these skills, though there may be other specialists, male priests, sorcerers, and shamans, who can be called on in situations of special danger. Because the midwife is in touch with the spirit world, she cannot be adequately described, as in the phrase used by WHO, merely as a 'traditional birth attendant'. She is expert on birth control and abortion and can bring back to life a baby who is apparently dead. She quenches blood or causes it to flow and fights against the power of monsters and demons. She is a shepherdess between being and non-being, spiritual adviser, mediator between worlds of life and death and orchestrator of female mysteries. The midwife is often one of the most important women in the community, though she may be feared by men and male institutions of power who perceive her as a threat. In Malaysia, for example, the Islamic religious establishment denounces the 'bidan kampungs' because of their dealings with the supernatural, while the medical establishment considers them dangerous and intends to replace them with trained nurses (Laderman 1982).

In many traditional societies, in contrast to our own, childbirth is seen as an expression of health rather than illness. Psychological aspects of the experience and the quality of relationships between those involved are believed to affect the progress of labour. Someone else's anger or envy, unresolved conflict between the father or mother and other members of the community, or the parents' sexual misdemeanours can delay dilatation. Hence the midwife's task includes the diagnosis of what is blocking the progress of birth and advice on how to solve this problem by confession, forgiveness, and reconciliation, by offering sacrifices to the ancestral gods or a gift to someone who has been wronged, or the performance of a psychodrama to dissolve the negative forces which are delaying birth.

In Melanesia for example, when a labour is not going well the woman may be urged to confess any sexual misbehaviour or her husband must seek forgiveness for adultery during the pregnancy (Townsend 1986). Relationships must be put right before the labour can progress.

In Greece anyone who has quarrelled with the woman who is bearing the child must seek her forgiveness. They come forward and beg formal pardon by offering her water to drink out of their hands (Chryssanthopoulou 1984). In other cultures of childbirth powerful emotions of fear, anger, and guilt on the part of the woman in labour are perceived as hazardous to birth-giving. But not only is her own psychological state relevant to the progress of labour. That of all those around her, including the women helping and others in the family and community, may be seen as affecting the birth either positively or negatively. Where there is envy, hatred, or unconfessed sin, for example, there may be a blockage to the unfolding natural processes. Effective uterine action and dilatation—physiological co-ordination—is dependent on social harmony. The elimination of psychosocial stress resulting from conflict in relationships and the fostering of positive relationships is a major element in the support given to the woman in childbirth.

2 Symbols

Symbolic acts of release provide for the labouring woman a potent sign that all will be well. In ancient Greece when a woman began labour she loosened her girdle, first donned at puberty and dedicated to Artemis, untying the ritual knot so that her body might be similarly unloosed (King 1983). A universal symbolic act is the opening of doors and windows, the unstopping of bottles, lifting of lids, scattering of grain, and making water flow in order to help in removing any blockage to birth. Jamaican nanas describe their work as that of freeing the body and combine touch, massage, encouraging words, and advice on breathing with the aim of helping the mother open herself to birth.

For birth to go well in a peasant Greek home today it may be considered wise to unlock doors and cupboards and untie every bond. The husband unknots his tie and unbuttons his clothing. Water may be poured through his sleeve or down the chimney to symbolize the free flowing of life. The child comes to birth as if on the full flood of water (Chryssanthopoulou 1984).

A visual focus provided by an opening flower which gradually spreads its petals in the heat of the room may also be employed. In Greece this flower, which is called the hand of the Mother of God, is put in water where it gradually blossoms. In parts of peasant Italy the flower used is the rose of Jericho. The practice is also common in some areas of southern India, where the unfurling petals symbolize dilatation of the cervix. The labouring woman believes that as the flower unfurls her body is also opening (Kitzinger 1978). Spiritual power can be harnessed and concentrated in an object which symbolically represents creative energy. In Sri Lanka both Muslim and Hindu women wear an object made of iron during labour, for iron is powerful against demons (McGilvray 1982). The wearing of an amulet or lodestone was customary through large parts of Europe until the twentieth century. Among Jews birth amulets which contained Psalm 126, a prayer for deliverance, and the names of the three angels who guard women in childbirth were used (Klein 1987). In England both the Catholic and Reformation churches condemned anything, including 'purses, Measures of our Lady or such other Superstitious Things, to be occupied about the Woman while she laboured, to make her believe to have the better spede by it.' (Forbes 1966.)

Traditionally among native Americans spiritual power has also been sought to aid birth. The Navajo woman wears juniper seed birthing beads. Two straight bands of seeds symbolize the rain and a zigzag strand of bugle beads represents a journey on a road. A horizontal half-circle symbolizes the rainbow's spiritual path which links the child to creative forces (FB Knoki, Navajo traditional midwife, personal communication). Usually a place of refuge and security is made for the labouring woman by those attending her. In some patrilocal societies she returns to her own mother's home to give birth. She may stay there until the baby has been weaned—for two or three years. A special birth hut is customary in some cultures and is used by all women in the village. Whether the woman giving birth is in the home of her origin, the home she has made, a seclusion hut or the local bath-house, she is surrounded by familiar objects and things are done around her which have meaning for her in a specific value system. She understands their significance and they are part of the common fabric of women's lives. Lore and practice which to Western eyes is esoteric is often comfortingly familiar and expected.

In traditional Jewish communities all doors and windows are closed and locked against evil. In eastern Europe incantations to protect the Jewish woman against evil spirits, and particularly Lilith, the winged female demon, were painted on the walls of the birth room and a circle chalked around the bed, while Psalm 121 was recited. The forces of evil could not cross this line (Klein 1987).

The Zulu birth place is a special birth hut prepared by unmarried girls, the floor strewn with dried dung and decorated with woodcarvings, for it is vital that the first thing on which the baby opens its eyes should be beautiful. Traditionally, as in all Zulu dwellings, there is a hole in the roof, and during contractions the labouring women fixes her eyes on the little bit of sky she can see through it, so keeping in contact with the God who dwells in the heavens. It is said of a woman who is giving birth at night that she counts the stars with pain (Kitzinger 1980).

In many societies the birth of a baby symbolizes the regeneration of the community. It is a sacred act. In peasant Greece, for example, 'through childbirth, a woman redeems the fallen state of the male–female relationship' (Hirschon 1978).

The provision of a place of sanctuary, the recreation of harmony, acts of reconciliation and removal of obstacles in order to free the body to give birth—all these find expression through strong symbolic motifs in many different cultures across time and space. In traditional societies such concepts infuse the thinking of the woman in labour and of everyone around her.

Cultural processes which reduce anxiety, explain otherwise preposterous physical sensations, give comfort and enhance psychophysical co-ordination, whether or not they accurately reflect reality in scientific terms, may have a powerful effect on the mind of the woman in childbirth.

In traditional cultures a focus on symbols which have validity for all those participating in the act of birth creates an atmosphere of confidence around the labouring woman. When there is uterine dysfunction and she is exhausted and in pain, this can give her fresh courage and hopes and may have a psychosomatic effect on the progress of labour.

3 Birth as activity

Birth is perceived as activity. Invariably in traditional societies the woman is free to move about and to change position as and when she wishes. A supine position is extremely rare, though women may lie on their sides from time to time, interspersing this with other, upright positions. The midwife and others helping may advise the woman in labour to alter her position or to make a particular pelvic movement. They lend their own bodies to her for physical support and may move with her as she moves in synchronized rocking or circling of the pelvis, and shifting weight between their feet, as if in a dance. The labouring woman may also have support in an upright position from posts, slung hammock, or furniture, or may hold on to a rope, knotted piece of cloth, or kneel, crouch, or squat supported by bricks, stones, a pile of sand, or a birth stool.

The Zulu woman gives birth kneeling or squatting, supported by women on either side. The South American Indian woman often gives birth in her hammock. In Brazil the Kalapano Indian woman sits in her hammock with her legs suspended at either side and holding on to another hammock hung above it. Two helping women sit on each side to support her body, two more to hold her hands and legs, and a fourth cradles her head (Basso 1973). On the Ivory Coast a woman squats with her hands placed on the shoulders of a helper crouching in front of her and another woman behind her to hold her shoulders (Alland 1975). Among the Kwakiutl of British Columbia a helping woman sits on the edge of a shallow pit especially dug and lined with soft cedar bark, her legs stretched across it so that her feet and calves rest on the opposite side. The woman in labour sits facing her on her lap, both legs hanging outside her helper's legs. The two women clasp each other's arms and the midwife crouches behind the woman giving birth, knees pressed against her back during contractions, and her arms around her shoulders. As the baby is born it slips into the cedar bark nest (Niethammer 1977).

In Western culture, in contrast, birth is perceived primarily in terms of the activity of the uterus and the acts of the attendants, rather than of a woman giving birth. She is the object of care and the essential action can proceed without her co-operation, and even in spite of her.

When 'alternative', more 'active' methods are permitted, they are often seen as involving experiment with more or less static postures: with the woman propped up rather than lying flat with her legs in lithotomy stirrups, for example, upright rather than supine, squatting rather than sitting, or using a birth chair in place of the delivery table.

In traditional cultures, however, women change positions frequently and move about in childbirth. They do this spontaneously and if attendants perceive any difficulty, may also be encouraged to make specific movements. Though certain positions may be emphasized in each culture, the labouring woman's movements *between* these postures is probably an important element which has often been overlooked because, in recording cultural variations in childbirth, Western bias has concentrated almost exclusively on fixed delivery positions.

4 Body images

In all societies ideas about health and disease are closely related to concepts of the human body. These are themselves parts of a larger value system. Male and female body concepts, for example, express values about the relative worth of men and women and their major social functions. In Western medicine the male body is accepted as the norm from which the female body deviates. In anatomy and other medical textbooks the male body is virtually always the primary model and the female body is then described in terms of its aberrations from this model.

The value system of which body images form a part is complex and results in some areas being considered clean or pure, others dirty or polluted, some beautiful, others ugly, some being emphasized and adorned, whereas others are ignored or neglected. In Hindu culture the left hand is used for dirty tasks—such as wiping one's bottom, and only the right hand used for eating. Even very young children are taught this distinction between left and right and to put things into their mouths with the right hand only.

Throughout traditional Judaeo-Christian culture, and in some Asian cultures, the body is seen as a container the entrances and exits of which must be kept closed except under special conditions. It is a vessel to be opened only in front of certain people and according to strict rules of conduct (Douglas 1966). Matter issuing from the body is polluted—breath, nasal mucus, saliva, earwax, urine, faeces, blood, sweat, and even personal body heat. (Hence the sense of unease when sitting on a lavatory seat which is still warmed from a previous occupant.) Tears are the one body fluid which is thought to be pure, and Mary Douglas suggests that this is perhaps because they are considered a cerebral fluid.

Female body products are seen as particularly dangerous and threatening to men, and can cause impotence. Thus women's bodies must be kept tightly closed, especially in the presence of the opposite sex. If a man crosses the path of a menstruating woman on his way to the hunting grounds, not only will he fail to kill an animal, but he may be injured. Paradoxically, this negative element of pollution has another and much more positive aspect. It creates and ensures the maintenance of a woman's space. In those societies where women go off to the menstrual seclusion huts every month they know that they have guaranteed time away from the demands made on them by men, and regularly recurring affirmation of the bonds which unite them with other women.

Body concepts like these have a profound effect on behaviour in childbirth. In many traditional societies men dare not risk being present at birth because the power issuing from the female body is so great that it could destroy them. Birth is a matter for women, and almost universally the territory in which birth takes place and the unfolding process is controlled by women. Contemporary Western culture is an exception in that, even when midwives and nurses do most of the work, ultimately birth is usually controlled by men in the person of male obstetricians.

5 The community of women

In nearly every other culture a woman in childbirth is assisted by a community of helping women who are already well known to her. The exceptions are when a woman labours alone or in the company of one other woman and, once labour is established, goes off to the forest or the seashore. World-wide the norm is that of a group of female friends, family members and neighbours, often together with a midwife whose special skills are acknowledged by everyone present and who orchestrates their actions. Birth is a social event.

Margaret Mead says that 20 to 30 women were present during a Samoan labour (Mead 1928). In Aoraucanian childbirth, in Chile, a group of women form a choir who sing to the woman throughout labour (Hilger 1957). It is reported of Australian aborigines (the Aranda) that all women of the camp assemble when a woman goes into labour. An anthropologist describes birth in an Egyptian village with the woman's mother, aunt, cousin, sister, and midwife present. They all 'took turns hugging and kissing her and giving her words of encouragement such as "be strong my love", "I wish it was I who was giving birth", "just a little longer and it will be over my love"' (Morsy in Kay 1982). In India those present may include the woman's mother in law, her husband's sisters and her own mother and sisters, with their small children.

The function of this community of women is not always that of cherishing the woman in labour. It may be rather to assert female solidarity in an atmosphere of festivity. During labour among the Seri Indians of Mexico an anthropologist counted 16 women and children most of whom were sitting around in an aura of fiesta (Moser 1982). A birth among the Gbaya of the Congo is described by another ethnologist who expresses horror at the crowd of women who were 'literally cramming the hut . . . chatting noisily, laughing loudly, feasting, swilling down drink and smoking' (Laman 1957). The most important contribution the group of women make in this case is to reinforce relationships between women by creating and sharing a celebratory experience.

In medieval Europe Church laws proclaimed that it was the duty of every married woman to help other women in childbirth. The 'god sibs' arrived with sustaining foods for the mother, celebratory dishes for after the birth, and strong drink to be consumed throughout, and the men of the household left until it was all over.

In thirteenth- and fourteenth-century paintings of the birth of Mary and of John the Baptist the group of 'god sibs' are depicted surrounding and tending mother and baby. The newly delivered woman is being offered delicacies of many kinds by women who ply her with broth, roast chicken, and sweetmeats. Other women warm the swaddling clothes and wash and care for the child. Such paintings contrast strongly with the birth of Jesus, where the mother is solitary except for the animals and Joseph, the bemused man who is quite clearly out of place. It was not only hardship and poverty, but social isolation and the absence of the tending women, which from a medieval viewpoint distinguished the birth of Jesus from any other birth.

In families of high social status 'god sibs' also testified at the baptism and if the baby died were witnesses as to whether the child had been born alive, and if the mother died also, whether it had died before or after her, thus providing vital testimony affecting inheritance

(Undset 1977). In common usage the term 'god sib' was gradually corrupted to 'gossip'.

As care in childbirth became increasingly professionalized in the twentieth century, family members and women friends lost their function and came to be seen by doctors, and many midwives, as intruders in a medical process that had nothing to do with them. Not only were non-professionals excluded from childbirth, but it was claimed that they had a detrimental effect on the woman's mind in pregnancy. Other women were castigated as spreading 'old wives' tales' and women patients were told by doctors to put their trust only in their medical attendants. In a popular paperback published in 1975 an obstetrician warned the pregnant woman to avoid listening to 'wicked women with their malicious, lying tongues' and dismissed what women said as 'a cartload of rubbish' (Bourne 1975).

In the 1970s women's insistence that they wanted a birth companion with them led to the at first grudging, and later enthusiastic, acceptance of fathers in the delivery room. It seems to be easier to bring fathers under medical control than women friends and relatives. Obstetric staff define the man's role for him, and this task is probably simplified because many men are nervous or reluctant about being present at childbirth. The father's presence has effectively reinforced the ban on women family members and friends being there, often 'because there is no room'. Whereas fathers are welcome if they keep their place, other women usually remain prohibited. In this situation, by gaining the choice of having her male partner with her the labouring women has lost the choice of having women companions.

6 Pain and its meaning

Pain is 'private data' (Engel 1950) and the degree, form of expression and manner in which it is made public depends on the cultural meanings attributed to it. 'Abnormal' is distinguished from 'normal' pain, the pain of injury is treated differently from that of hard work or willingly accepted intense physical activity, and cultural expectations concerning the normality of pain determine whether or not it is perceived as something which requires drugs or other intervention (Zborowski 1952). Each culture has its own language of distress, both verbal and non-verbal. Publicly expressed pain implies a social relationship between the sufferer and those able to give care. People whose pain behaviour fits with generally acceptable values about how those in pain should behave receive most attention (Lewis 1981; Helman 1984).

In many societies birth is seen as a testing time for women, giving proof of their womanhood and marking the transition from child to adult, analogous with a man confronting the challenges which show that he is an adult, whether that involves demonstrating courage in battle, taking his first major decisions in a business venture, or killing his first tiger. In many native American cultures a woman is taught that she must not moan or cry out in labour, but bear pain stoically. Hausa women in Nigeria remain quiet even during difficult birth, whereas neighbouring Yoruba women groan and scream freely. This pattern is not just conformist behaviour or a kind of obligatory performance but an integral part of personality in these cultures which determines emotional responses to pain (LeVine 1973). When women cry out in labour the sounds they make are culturally conditioned. The high pitched 'a'iee, a'iee, a'ieeee' of a Latin American peasant woman is quite different from the 'pene . . . pene . . . pene . . .' of a woman in southern India who is reiterating syllables which she may also employ when working in the fields, and which mean toil. This is different again from the Italian woman's 'mama mia!' or the Caribbean 'Jesus! Jeeesus!'. Many English and American women try to make no noise at all in labour, not only because they wish to be good patients, but to avoid making public that which is private and, if they have been to childbirth classes, to demonstrate that they have learned their lessons well. Thus the very sounds that women make—and whether or not they emit any at all—are patterned by culture.

Labour pain can have negative or positive meaning, depending on the nature of body fantasies, the interaction of the labouring women with those attending her, and her sense of ease or disease in the setting provided for birth. Jamaican peasant women, for example, welcome sacroiliac pain in labour because it indicates that a gate in the lower spine through which the baby must pass to be born is swinging wide open (Kitzinger 1977). In an emotionally unsupportive hospital environment they become distressed at the first signs of the expulsive reflex, however, since—as in many other traditional cultures—they believe that the baby can 'come up out of the belly' and choke them. The involuntary catch in the breath which heralds the active second stage is a sign that this has occurred. Such fantasies of injury turn pain into anguish.

In every society there are cultural stress points, situations which everyone expects to be threatening and in which the labouring woman anticipates pain. In rural Yucatan both labour and delivery are approached with equanimity. But anxiety is expressed during the third stage, since they know that if there is postpartum haemorrhage the woman is far from medical aid (Jordan 1978).

When a woman suffers pain in an alien environment among strangers who make minimal human contact, and when she does not understand what is happening to her or what invasive procedure is likely to occur next, fear, anxiety, and disorientation can intensify pain, produce distress, and inhibit co-ordinated uterine action. This is the birth environment for many women in the contemporary Western hospital. In terms of the transcultural sociology of birth, it is a highly unusual setting, and one unique to modern industrial society.

A woman who finds herself in a situation of acute culture conflict—a peasant woman in a large, urban, high-technology hospital, for example—may either lie uncomprehending and passive or may cling to the reassuring symbols and support provided by religion to help her through the ordeal of giving birth in an alien environment among strangers. Jamaican women take their bibles into the labour wards and shout passages from the psalms (Kitzinger 1978). They clasp each other and rock in unison, calling on the Lord to deliver them, with sounds remarkably similar to those of revivalist Church services in which spirit possession and speaking with tongues is sought. In this way they attempt to incorporate alien hospital practices into peasant culture. When successful, a synthesis is created between birth and ecstatic worship.

In the modern Western hospital most women behave very differently, however. They try to avoid 'making a fuss' and submit to the medical interpretation of childbirth as a high risk process and pathological condition in which they must rely on the skills of professionals and in which religious symbolism would be out of place.

Culture has been defined as 'the process of generating and sustaining systems of meaningful forms (symbols, artefacts, etc.) by means of which humanity transcends the givens of natural existence, bends them to its purpose, controls them in its interest' (Ortner 1974). In traditional cultures the changes which take place in each person's life cycle, the peak experiences and transformations, find expression in rites which signify changes in social status. Biological processes provide images which are expressed in dramatic form to describe the individual's relation to society. Central to this process is a metaphor derived from the great experiences of birth and death, which are archetypes occurring over and over again in all religions and cultures. Birth is the primary symbol for acts of creation and renewal. The medicalization of both birth and death in our own society has, according to Levi-Strauss, emptied birth experiences of 'everything not corresponding to mere physiological processes and rendered them unsuitable to convey other meanings' (Levi-Strauss 1967). This loss of symbolic significance is evidence of a fragmentation of human experience.

7 A way of looking at birth

Complex sociophysiological elements in childbirth like these can not be understood by unidimensional or numerical analysis. To evaluate childbirth as if our Western way of birth were the summit of achievement and all others ways of birth were inferior to our own is analogous with the way in which the Victorians viewed all the institutions of societies other than their own. Nineteenth-century anthropologists classified other cultures in terms of their evolutionary development towards civilization, the culmination of which was the style of living and processes of thinking typical of the Victorian gentleman. It was a linear system of thinking and produced an anthropology which implied that primitive people were astoundingly ignorant, their behaviour brutal, and their thought processes ludicrous.

In the same way, if we view birth in other societies exclusively in terms of perinatal mortality statistics it is impossible to understand the dynamics of human behaviour in childbirth—whether in other cultures or our own. It is necessary to see our own culture, too, in comparative terms, rather than take it as a vantage point.

It was Erving Goffman who first pointed the way to an anthropological analysis of Western social institutions using techniques of participant observation and detailed study of face-to-face interaction (Goffman 1956, 1961, 1971). His now classic study of a psychiatric hospital provides a model for the analysis of any hospital system, whether designed to serve sick people or women having babies.

Social scientists were often hesitant to adopt this kind of model and concentrated instead on analysis of the medical system largely from the angle of the professionals operating that system. They looked at work satisfaction and the hierarchy of power. They were concerned about communication, but often only in terms of whether messages were understood. The joint impact of Goffman's anthropological approach and Ivan Illich's radical challenge to consider the threat implicit in all professionalization of caring skills (Illich 1975) lead students of society to take a new look at our own social institutions, and to start examining them with the same attention to detail that formerly had been applied only to those of traditional societies.

When anthropologists and sociologists began to look at the medical care system of Western society in this way they began to discover remarkable similarities to those of a primitive society. It seemed that many functions previously invested in the priesthood and religious system had been taken over by medicine, including those which control the major life crises of birth and death.

8 Rites of passage

In nearly all societies birth, and the period immediately preceding and following it, is marked by a series of ritual dramatizations of status change which symbolize the woman's social transformation. With the birth of the first baby she changes from a girl into an adult woman and the marriage, often until then friable, or not yet in existence, is cemented. Thus rites of transition are particularly stressed with the birth of the first baby.

Transitional rites function to guard a threshold and to protect and control the behaviour of the individual on the journey between two kinds of social identity. This may be the person who, through death, enters the world of ancestor spirits. Or it may be the young man who, in warrior tribes of East Africa, is initiated into an age-set which will be his major reference point in terms of social identity as he goes through life. Or the adolescent who becomes adult through rites of circumcision, clitoridectomy, scarification, or having teeth knocked out. Or—as in birth—it may be the woman who is becoming a mother, the man socially acknowledged as the father, or the child on the threshold of being a new member of society. While in transition between identities, individuals are in a state of social timelessness and are vulnerable and dangerous to themselves and others. They need to be protected, and others need protecting from them (Leach 1976).

A universal characteristic of transitional rites is the occurrence of specific ceremonial phases, each registering part of the journey on which the individual who is changing status has embarked (Van Gennep 1960). An act of separation segregates the initiate from other people. There follow rites of depersonalization. Once divested of identity, the initiate is expected to assume the behaviour and status of a small child. There is a trial by pain or ordeal by fear, a drama in which the initiated is required to show stamina and courage. Rites of cleansing purge and purify the initiate preparatory to taking on a new identity. As the initiate emerges from the liminal state he or she goes through a ritual act of regeneration and is reborn into a new self, then to be welcomed back into society with ceremonies of reincorporation marked by public acknowledgement of the changed status and by celebration.

In puberty rituals, for example, these elements consist first of separation of the young person from the family. The initiate is often taken into the bush by elders who represent the ancestors. He or she may be required to ritually enact the part of a baby, or sometimes even of a fetus, and is fed and tended as if incapable of caring for himself. Ordinary day-to-day physical functions, such as eating, elimination, cleansing, sleeping, and movement from one place to another are supervised or performed on his behalf by those who control the drama. Ordeals must be endured, such as scarification or whipping. The initiate is ridiculed, humiliated, and exposed to insults and mockery. Throughout this time the initiate is a pupil, and is guided and directed about how to behave in order to be able to take on the new status which is waiting. Then there is an act of rebirth in which physiological symbols of birth often form a part, the boy or girl wriggling out, for example, between the legs of an old man or woman. Finally the novice emerges with a new identity as an adult. Gifts are presented and there is celebration and feasting.

Rituals of this kind function to support and reinforce a social system. As individuals within it change, as children grow up to become adults, for example, and take the place of those who are ageing, their behaviour is canalized so that it conforms to an already established culture pattern. Such rites function, in fact, as powerful agents of social control. In traditional societies ritual also serves another function. It supports the individual through crises. Rites of grieving, for example, allow the expression of mourning in socially acceptable terms, and acknowledge the intensity of personal experience by validating the overwhelming emotions of bereavement.

In Western society we have lost many of these supportive rituals. Instead there is a great deal of ritual, some of it involving flamboyant display, but much of it bureaucratic, which serves to maintain and reinforce the structure and power of large hierarchical institutions, including military, educational, legal, and governmental systems. Hospitals also tend to be institutions of this kind. Hospital patients are at the very bottom of a series of interlocking, overlapping complex hierarchies. They are temporary members of a system which could function very well, and probably better, without them. If they play their parts appropriately and are co-operative patients, they are submissive, passive, and grateful. In her study of medical education in two Boston hospitals, Diana Scully quotes an obstetrician describing a good patient. 'She is', he says, 'someone who understands what I say, listens to what I say, does what I say, believes what I say' (Scully 1980).

The behaviour of, and relationships between, professional caregivers and women in childbirth is regulated by institutionally established protocols which merge with a variety of customs and conventions based on received truths that have only recently come to be questioned or scrutinized. They produce a system of ceremonial procedures enacted from a woman's admission to hospital through her discharge. She is the initiate in a series of rituals which resembles those of puberty rituals in a primitive society.

It is often taken for granted that medical acts must be scientific. This is not so. The use of sterile garments is a case in point. A face mask is ineffective in preventing the passage of bacteria after 15 minutes' use (*Lancet* 1981; Hunter and Williams 1985). But in many delivery rooms masks continue to be used, often for prolonged periods and in a casual manner, being lowered when they become too uncomfortable and then replaced often merely over the mouth. Thus a mask is employed both as a kind of talisman against infection and as a symbol of authority, differentiating staff from patients.

The way in which sterile garments are worn at different levels in the hospital hierarchy also suggests a ceremonial purpose. Roth's study of their use revealed that the higher the individual is in the hospital hierarchy, the fewer sterile garments which are worn (Roth 1957). Those at the bottom of the hierarchy must don protective overshoes, gown, cap, and mask. In the context of childbirth, the father is usually considered the least important member of the labour team and may be required to wear the most protective garments, whereas the obstetrician may wander in his own suit, gown undone.

Ceremonies by which a woman is admitted to hospital for childbirth show many characteristics of transitional rites and incorporate acts of separation, purging, a symbolic return to an infantile state, trial by endurance, and ceremonial re-entry to society in a changed status.

On admission to hospital a woman takes on the identity of a patient, becoming a temporary and low status member of a total institution which regulates every aspect of her conduct and that of the doctors, midwives, and nurses who attend her. Rites reinforce the power of the institution over her most intimate and previously private behaviour: washing, treatment of vaginal bleeding, emptying of bowels and bladder, positions and movements of her body, eating and drinking, sleep, and even the noises she can make without incurring medical intervention.

The 'prepping' ceremony initiates her in her role. From then on, other people decide what is to be done to her and her usual rights as an adult individual are abrogated. Her perineum may be shaved. This practice dates from the nineteenth century. The poor and homeless women, many of them having babies out of wedlock, who were the patients in charity hospitals and workhouse maternity wards, often had lice in their pubic hair. Perineal shaving, however, does not reduce the number of bacteria on the perineum and, in fact may well increase the chances of infection, since surface cells are scraped, creating a port of entry for bacteria (Kantor *et al.* 1965; Long 1967; Romney 1980). Yet the practice persists in some hospitals as a ceremony by which the woman is desexed and returned to the status of a prepubertal child.

The woman may be literally purged from pollution with suppositories or an enema, though it has been shown that routine forced evacuation of the lower bowel is of no physiological benefit (Romney and Gordon 1981).

She is depersonalized through surrender of her own clothing and the donning of hospital garments and plastic identification bracelet, and may be socially isolated from friends and family.

The usual means by which people define their identity are removed, to be replaced by a general anonymity expressed in the words 'dear', 'mother' or terms used to address children.

She is put to bed and may be tethered to machines which record the fetal heart and the rate and strength of contractions. An intravenous drip may be set up which, since she is allowed nothing by mouth, automatically feeds glucose solution into her bloodstream, together with chemical substances which control uterine activity.

Vaginal examinations, artificial rupture of the membranes, and insertion of a urinary catheter reinforce the message that her most intimate body functions, and those of her unborn baby, are under the control of the obstetrician. If she also has an epidural catheter inserted in her back she is trapped in a narrow space from which there can be no escape until after the birth. She is helpless, immobile, and often virtually paraplegic. Like an infant, she depends on those caring for her for the exercise of her most basic physiological functions, and for delivery of the baby by whatever means they consider appropriate.

As delivery approaches she may be covered from the waist down by a sheet, which symbolically represents the surgical nature of the act of birth in Western culture. When the obstetrician isolates the lower half of the patient's body it becomes ritually separated from that part which she is free to control herself and, transformed into the obstetrician's sterile field, is out of bounds to her own touch. This sterile field is not, in fact, sterile because of the juxtaposition of the vagina and anus. It is a convenient fiction by which the genital area is depersonalized and desexed.

Prohibition of any expression of intense feeling contributes further to the desexing of childbirth. The implicit goal for the management of labour is a first stage in which a compliant patient is 'resting quietly' and a second stage in which she is working hard and in which excretory elements are dominant: 'Push, go on push, push like emptying your bowels!' she is instructed, 'Come on, you can do better than that!' In no other spontaneous physiological act would effective function be expected if other people harried and hurried its performance, as is done regularly in childbirth. It would be possible to guarantee pain, distress, and malfunction if the processes of digestion, defecation, going to sleep, and coitus were also made public performances under the direction of strangers who urged one on in a race against time. This dysfunctional behaviour in conducting childbirth can be explained only in terms of its ritual elements.

Finally, immediately prior to delivery, an act of genital mutilation is performed. Episiotomy is a surgical wound which after the birth requires suturing and leaves a scar. There is no good evidence of the value of routine episiotomy (Sleep *et al.* 1984; Kitzinger 1984; Kitzinger and Simkin 1986; Harrison and Brennan 1984). Yet the routine cutting of the woman's perineum continues in many hospitals as part of what can be explained only as a ritualized process to effect safe delivery.

Behaviour in childbirth, far from being biologically dictated, varies as widely as behaviour in other fields of human activity which are more usually associated with the culture process. In childbearing, no less than in art, religion, the beliefs and rituals surrounding death, and marriage and kinship systems, human beings are creatures of their culture. Knowing this, we may be able to stand back and assess hospital practices and the Western culture of childbearing, as if they were those of another society.

Ours is a culture of childbirth which applies diagnostic labels to women from the very beginning of pregnancy. The woman is aware that she is an 'elderly primigravida' a 'grand multigravida', or simply, for one reason or another, 'at risk'. There is evidence that being labelled 'at risk' can have a negative effect on self-perception, relationships, symptoms, and outcomes (Waxler 1981). The question arises as to whether this may not only damage the woman's self-percept, but also have an impact on the whole experience of pregnancy and childbirth, and its outcome.

It is also a culture which is alert to intervene and to practise 'just in case' obstetrics. When research reveals that some procedures are useless or harmful, it is slow to discard what are, in effect, ceremonial rites in the public arena of the delivery room. Many of these ceremonies are so well established that they may not be questioned by professional caregivers, including, in the second stage, the supine position for expulsion, the cheer-leading squad urging the woman on and the practice of routine episiotomy. Others are innovatory high technology ceremonies for which there is no evidence that routine is of any benefit.

The vivid symbols of female creative power which have significance not only for the woman in labour but for all those sharing in the birth experience in traditional societies have been largely replaced by institutional rites which function to assert, reinforce, and maintain medical control over women in childbirth.

Human beings need not be the passive recipients of culture. We have it in our power to create a way of birth which reflects evolving ideals in our social life and which gives conscious expression to those values which are most important to us. Anthropological perspectives on birth can lead us to ask searching questions about the Western way of birth and become more aware of elements in it which are psychosocial as distinct from purely medical.

To see birth as a cultural event raises issues concerning the values of our own society: the status and identity of a woman giving birth and the care given her, the way in which the newborn baby is treated, the quality of relationships between those who share the birth experience and, indeed, about freedom and coercion, power and powerlessness, and the very place of values in a world of facts.

References

Alland A (1975). When the Spider Danced: Notes from an African Village. New York: Doubleday.

Argyle M (1975). Orderly Communication. London: Methuen.

Bourne G (1975). Pregnancy. London: Pan.

Basso EB (1973). The Kalapano Indians of Central Brazil. New York: Holt, Rinehart & Winston.

Carter J, Duriez T (1986). With Child: Birth Through the Ages. Edinburgh: Mainstream.

Chryssanthopoulou V (1984). An Analysis of Rituals Surrounding Birth in Modern Greece. M Phil thesis, Bodleian Library, Oxford.

Douglas M (1966). Purity and Danger: An Analysis of the Concepts of Pollution and Taboo. London: Routledge & Kegan Paul.

Engel GL (1950). 'Psychogenic' pain and the pain-prone patient. Am J Med, 26: 899–909.

Forbes TR (1966). The Midwife and the Witch. Newhaven: Yale University Press.

Goffman E (1956). The Presentation of Self in Everyday Life. Edinburgh: Edinburgh University Press.

Goffman E (1961). Asylums. Garden City, New York: Anchor Books.

Goffman E (1971). Relations in Public. London: Allen Lane.

Harrison RF, Brennan M (1984). Fetal outcome after episiotomy or perineal tear. Paper at the European Congress of Perinatal Medicine, Dublin, Ireland.

Helman C (1984). Culture, Health and Illness. Bristol: Wright.

Hewes G (1957). The anthropology of posture. Scientific American, 196: 123–32.

Hilger MI (1957). Aoraucanian Child Life and its Cultural Background. Washington DC: Smithsonian Institution.

Hirschon R (1978). Open Body/Closed Space: the transformation of female sexuality. In: Defining Females. Ardener S (ed). London: Croom Helm, New York: Halstead.

Hunter MA, Williams D (1985). Mask wearing in the labour ward. Midwives' Chron & Nursing Notes, 98(1164):12–13.

Illich I (1975). Medical Nemesis. London: Calder & Boyars.

Jordan B (1978). Birth in Four Cultures. Quebec: Eden Press.

Kantor H, Rember R, Tabio P, Buchanan R (1965). The value of shaving the pudendal perineal area in delivery preparation. Obstet Gynecol, 25: 509–512.

Kay M (1982) (ed). The Anthropology of Human Birth. Philadelphia: FA Davis.

King H (1983). Bound to bleed: Artemis and Greek women. In: Images of Women in Antiquity. Cameron A and Kuht A. (eds). London: Croom Helm.

Kitzinger S (1977). Education and Counselling for Childbirth. London: Baillière Tindale.

Kitzinger S (1978). Women as Mothers. London: Fontana.

Kitzinger S (1979). Education and Counselling for Childbirth. New York: Schocken.

Kitzinger S (1980). Women as Mothers. New York: Vintage Books.

Kitzinger S (1984). Episiotomy pain. In: Textbook of Pain. Wall PD, Melzack R (eds). London: Churchill Livingstone.

Kitzinger S and Simkin P (1986). Episiotomy and the Second Stage of Labour (2nd edn). Seattle: Pennypress.

Klein M (1987). Be Fruitful and Multiply. Jerusalem: Museum of the Daispora.

Laderman C (1982). Giving birth in a Malay village. In: The Anthropology of Human Birth. Kay M (ed). Philadelphia: FA Davis.

Laman KE (1957). The Kongo. Uppsala.

Lancet (1981). Behind the mask (editorial). Lancet, 1: 8213.

Leach E (1976). Culture and Communication. Cambridge: Cambridge University Press.

LeVine R (1973). Culture, Behavior and Personality. Chicago: Aldine.

Levi-Strauss C (1967). Structural Anthropology. New York: Anchor Books.

Lewis G (1981). Cultural influences on illness behaviour: a medical and anthropological approach. In: The Relevance of Social Science for Medicine. Eisenberg L, Kleinman A (eds). Dordrecht: Reidel.

Long AE (1967). The unshaved perineum at parturition. Am J Obstet Gynecol, 99: 333–336.

McClain C (1982). Toward a comparative framework for the study of childbirth. In: The Anthropology of Human Birth. Kay M (ed). Philadelphia: F A Davis.

McGilvray D (1982). Sexual power and fertility in Sri Lanka: Matticaloa Tamils and Moors. In: Ethnography of Fertility and Childbirth. McCoımack C (ed). London/New York: Academic Press.

Mead M (1928). Coming of Age in Samoa. New York: Morrow.

Morsy SA (1982). Lockmi: an Indian midwife. In: The Anthropology of Human Birth. Kay M (ed). Philadelphia: F A Davis.

Moser MB (1982). Seri: from conception through infancy. In: The Anthropology of Human Birth. Kay M (ed). Philadelphia: F A Davis.

Newton N and Newton M (1972). Modern Perspectives in Psycho-Obstetrics. Edinburgh: Oliver & Boyd.

Niethammer C (1977). Daughters of the Earth. London and New York: Collier Macmillan.

Ortner SB (1974). Is female to male as nature is to culture? In: Woman, Culture and Society. Rosaldo MZ and Lamphere L. (eds). Stanford: Stanford University Press.

Romney ML (1980). Predelivery shaving: an unjustified assault?. J Obstet Gynaecol, 1: 33–35.

Romney ML and Gordon H (1981). Is your enema really necessary? Br Med J, 282: 1268–1271.

Roth JA (1957). Ritual and magic in the control of contagion. Am Soc Rev, 22: 310–314.

Scully D (1980). Men who Control Women's Health. Boston: Houghton Mifflin.

Sleep J, Grant A, Garcia J, Elbourne D, Spencer J, Chalmers I. (1984). West Berkshire perineal management trial. Br Med J, 289: 587–590.

Townsend PK (1986). When birth goes badly: Melanesian cultural responses to complications in childbirth. Paper given at Conference on Medical Anthropology, Cambridge.

Undset S (1977). Kristin Lavransdatter. London: Pan.

Van Gennep A (1960). The Rites of Passage. Chicago: University of Chicago Press.

Waxler NE (1981). The social labelling perspective on illness and medical practice. In: The Relevance of Social Science for Medicine. Eisenberg L, Kleinman A (eds). Dordrecht: Reidel.

Zborowski M (1952). Cultural components in response to pain. J Social Issues, 8: 16–30.

7 Maternity patients' movements in the United States 1820–1985

Madeleine H. Shearer

1 Introduction

'Like thousands of women in America today, I had hoped and prepared for a "natural" birth. And like thousands of others, the birth of my child was a product not of my own efforts but of medical science and all the latest "improvements" that hospitals can provide. Strangers appeared and reappeared to examine me internally. While I focused my total attention on breathing, sedatives were administered without my knowledge or consent. A caudal was inserted incorrectly and later removed because it dripped blood. Labor stopped completely. Pitocin wafers were placed next to my gums . . . After twenty hours of labor and three shifts of hospital attendants, I was finally wheeled into delivery, completely exhausted, frightened, and ready for anything the doctor had to offer to get me out of the experience forever' (Arms 1975a).

'If there's one person who should not be around a laboring woman it's an obstetrician' (Quint 1975).

These quotations from a mother (Arms 1975a) and a doctor (Quint 1975) illustrate the '. . . stunning loss of confidence sustained by medicine during the 1970s' (Starr 1982). Criticism of obstetric care in recent years began with parents and feminists (Karmel 1959; Hazell 1969; Haire 1972; Arms 1975a, 1975b; Rich 1976; Stewart and Stewart 1976; Gaskin 1978). The common themes among these writers were the contrasts between the United States and other countries in the use of heavy medication and forceps and the associated higher maternal and infant mortality. Outside the United States, according to these critics, families were able to stay together more during birth, babies were separated from the family less, and births were more often conducted at home as a normal process.

Close on their heels came books and articles describing the lack of perinatal care for poor women and for normal childbirth (Levy and Marine 1971; Shearer 1977). Critiques of United States obstetric practices were written by sociologists (Shaw 1974; Bean 1977; Ehrenreich and English 1979; Wertz and Wertz 1979), anthropologists (Jordan 1978; Kay 1982), and doctors (Brazelton 1971; Mendelsohn 1979). Some of the most stinging attacks on perinatal practices, especially caesarean section rates when they rose above fifteen per cent, were published by United States government agencies (Marieskind 1979; US Department of Health and Human Services 1980).

During the 1970s patients' protests against obstetric and neonatal care became a popular movement, which was joined by workers in medicine and nursing, public health, government, and the social sciences. Some of these critics were separatists, advocating that women take most of their perinatal care out of the medical system (Howell 1979; Mendelsohn 1979), while some advocated education of patients to enable them to plan births and to make choices from a wide range of obstetric routines and techniques (McKay 1983; Fenlon *et al.* 1979; Simkin *et al.* 1984). Others attacked perinatal care from a position of anti-science fundamentalism (Gaskin 1978; Stewart and Stewart 1976), and a few assailed what they viewed as cruel excesses and the greed of obstetricians and neonatologists (Cohen and Estner 1983; Corea 1979; Stinson and Stinson 1979).

Whatever their stance or occupation, activists in the patients' movement were linked by a common thread: working at a distance from obstetricians and neonatologists for changes in perinatal practices. Working at a distance has sometimes meant practising in competition with medicine, as with midwife attended home birth and homeopathy. More often, however, conflict has mixed with co-operation on both sides. The distance between patients' groups and perinatal caregivers has depended on how willing each was to co-operate with the other.

This chapter will review the story of the shifting ground between patients and perinatal professionals in the United States. Two patients' movements reached sustained national prominence, a century apart. At its height the Popular Health Movement in the 1840s, like the childbirth reform movement in the 1970s, fostered new professions, competition with doctors, groups who publicized medical excesses in childbirth, and educational organizations for patients and perinatal caregivers. These and other players in patients' movements held ever-changing ground, but many of the themes and struggles of the older movement bear striking resemblance to those of today.

2 The first American popular health movement

2.1 The rise of the first American popular health movement: 1820–1850

The protests of the 1970s were not the first such protests against American obstetric care. The earliest evidence of a patients' movement in perinatal care came in Andrew Jackson's populist era as a book, *New Guide to Health* (Thomson 1825). Thomson was a poor New Hampshire farmer whose wife had almost died while six doctors in succession treated her for postpartum convulsions. Mrs Thomson was saved by two women who were root and herb practitioners, but not before she had received the 'heroic' medicine which was in vogue in post-colonial America: repeated bleedings to unconsciousness; disfiguring applications of leeches to the temples and abdomen (and perhaps to the vulva and cervix); blisterings with mustard poultices; dosings with emetics; icepacks; and enemas of calomel, a mercuric salt which was applied until people developed the symptoms of mercury poisoning (Ehrenreich and English 1979).

Thomson wrote of his revelation that healing could be done gently, with simple botanical agents, and by women. He decried the takeover of birth by male doctors, whom he said were motivated primarily by economic gain:

> 'These young, inexperienced doctors ... have little knowledge, except what they get from books, and their practice is to try experiments. . . . The midwife's price was one dollar; when the doctors began to practice midwifery in the country rural areas, their price was three dollars, but they soon after raised it to five; and now they charge twelve to twenty' (Thomson 1825).

By 1839 *New Guide to Health* had sold over 100 000 copies, remarkable at a time in America when many people could not read. Starr (1982) suggests that what Thomson actually sold were franchises to practise his botanical method. Whether motivated by greed or righteousness, Thomson's outrage at the arrogance of the six doctors, their high fees, and the ineffectual misery they caused attracted a large following. As the 1830s closed, Thomsonian botanists were joined by several other healing systems, all popular in the rural areas, the midwest, and southern United States. All of these sects had the support of women. Some had women leaders:

> 'From swapping medical horror stories, women's circles moved on to swapping their own home remedies and from there to seeking more systematic ways to build their knowledge and skills. There were "Ladies' Physiological Societies" where women gathered in privacy to learn about female anatomy and functioning—similar to courses offered . . . today' (Ehrenreich and English 1979).

Indeed, it is accurate to say that the feminist movement in America began as a health movement which advocated less dangerous care than that offered by doctors. Early feminists also adopted the social reform themes of the working-men's movement of the 1820s and 1830s, joining men who protested the exploitive, inhuman conditions in the factories and mills at the start of the industrial revolution.

Also in the 1830s Sylvester Graham (remembered for the Graham cracker, a rolled flatbread made of oat and wheat flour, salt, and molasses) founded the Hygienic movement which called for a diet of fruits, raw vegetables, and whole grains. As testimony to their wide popular support, Thomsonians and Grahamians succeeded in having all restrictive medical licensure laws repealed during the 1840s. However, both groups split up into lay and professional members. They started medical schools, called their graduates 'doctors', and insisted that legislatures license them to practise medicine. Other sects did likewise, including Eclectics, Homeopathists, and Water Cure Practitioners (Shrylock 1966).

In 1848 'regular' doctors regrouped to fight back. They founded the American Medical Association (AMA) which battled to reinstate medical licensing laws. The American Medical Association succeeded, but it took them over 50 years and eventually necessitated their acceptance of some of the 'irregulars'. The AMA Code of Ethics from 1848 exhorted medical doctors to 'unite *tenderness* with *firmness*, and *condescension* with *authority* . . .' (Davis 1855) (emphasis in original text).

Thus, it is evident that populist ideas had not lessened doctors' patrician grandiosity. But they did adopt many of the healthful living principles advocated by the popular health sects. In the 1850s Dolores Burns, founder of the Hygienic Movement, condemned this co-optation in terms familiar to Americans in the maternity patients' movements of the 1980s:

'People learned to bathe, to eat more fruit and vegetables, to ventilate their homes, to get daily exercise, to avail themselves of the benefits of sunshine, to cast off their fears of night air, damp air, cold air, and drafts, to eat less flesh and to adopt better modes of food preparation. It has now been forgotten who promulgated these reforms; the record has been lost of the tremendous opposition to these reforms that the medical profession raised; it is believed that the medical profession was responsible for the decline of disease and death, the decline of the infant death rate, the inauguration of sanitation, and the increased life span' (Burns 1972).

2.2 The fate of the first American popular health movement: 1850–1900

Although elements of the first popular health movement remain today in the form of homeopathy and various natural remedies, the popular health sects declined after 1850, especially in the realm of perinatal care. Why did such widely favoured practitioners with their wholesome, simple health measures fade into obscurity? Many features of their demise have striking parallels in the loss of popularity of the patients' movement of the 1970s.

First, during the 1840s the different sects of the popular health movement divided to compete against each other, as well as with 'regular' medicine, thereby weakening their collective power. By opening medical schools and seeking state licensure the alternative health groups became hard to distinguish from 'regular' doctors. Their philosophies and procedures were easy to adopt, and then to trivialize or transform to fit the goals of 'regular' medicine. Finally, the popular health movement failed to forge alliances with powerful organizations with related goals. For example, after the Civil War (1865) they could have allied themselves with public health, which had entered its 'golden era', enjoying a higher status than medicine due to successes in urban sanitation, improvements in workplace conditions, and immunization against many infectious diseases (Starr 1982).

A second reason that the popular movement in perinatal care faded after 1850 was that 'regular' medicine made important advances. These captured the imagination of the public, and stimulated a flood of charitable donations from wealthy industrialists and civic leaders. The advent of chloroform and ether anaesthetic, Pasteur's identification of the bacterial basis of puerperal fever, and Lister's aseptic surgery technique, were only a few of the solid scientific advances widely publicized in the lay press. After 1863 the Civil War casualties necessitated the building of hospitals, which before then had been warehouses for the disorderly or homeless sick (Starr 1982). In 1873 Johns Hopkins, a Baltimore merchant, died and left seven million dollars to build a hospital and university. This was the largest medical endowment in American history.

'The impulse for founding the early hospitals typically came from physicians who struck up alliances with wealthy and powerful sponsors.... Needing capital and legitimacy, the doctors were obliged to seek out the sponsorship of merchants, bankers, lawyers, and political leaders who could contribute money and lead subscription campaigns ... George Templeton Strong, a Wall Street lawyer active in founding St. Luke's Hospital, noted in his diary in May 1852, after John Jacob Astor had decided to donate $13 000, "If he and Whitney and the other twenty or thirty millionaires of the city would do such things oftener, they would never feel the difference, and in ten years would control the course of things in New York by the public confidence and gratitude they would gain."' (Nevins and Thomas 1952).

Gradually, after the Civil War, people's confidence in 'regular' doctors and hospitals grew in response to news of medical breakthroughs, and the lavish support of medicine by civic leaders. The anti-authoritarian populist period gave way to the conservative Victorian period, which fostered the authority of leaders, and of science.

This was also a period in which the general health of Americans was poorer than at any time before or since. Maternal and infant mortality had risen markedly after 1850 in parallel with industrialization and urbanization; mortality did not begin to decline until around 1900, in parallel with a record low birth rate. Thus, a third reason for the decline in popularity of the less heroic therapies after 1850 was probably that people were actually sicker (Starr 1982). People began to view their illnesses as riskier than having a 'regular' doctor treat them.

Some of the blame for women's worsening reproductive health, as evidenced by rising maternal and infant mortality rates, may be laid to the fashions of the Victorian period. Many well-off women, and even very young girls, wore tight corsets, which in adult women cinched the waist to no more than 18 inches in circumference, compressing the rib cage to the point of deformity, and displacing the abdominal and pelvic organs downward. The social and medical effects of this bizarre dress were widely commented upon; the extreme corseting severely restricted breathing and movement (Jacobi 1972; Stockham 1886). Corseting, being housebound and frail, and a high incidence of depression in middle and upper class women were termed the 'cult of female invalidism' (Jacobi 1972;

Gilman 1973; Stockham 1886). At the same time that many affluent Victorian women were thus enfeebled, large numbers of working class women and even small girls toiled in factories and mills, some perpetually bent over and some partly blinded by ten to twelve hours per day of close work (Wright 1889).

Thus, it is not surprising that many women, both affluent and working class, had real and frightening ailments, nor that they consulted 'regular' doctors if they were able to. Charlotte Perkins Gilman, whose 1878 autobiography was re-issued in 1973, took to her bed with depression for several years. She was among the many who consulted S. Weir Mitchell, the most colourful 'regular' specialist in women's nervous ailments. He prescribed the voguish 'rest cure' which nearly drove Perkins insane:

> 'Live as domestic a life as possible. Have your child with you all the time. (Be it remarked that if I but dressed the baby it left me shaking and crying—certainly far from a healthy companionship for her, to say nothing of the effect on me.) Lie down for an hour after each meal. Have but two hours intellectual life a day. And never touch pen, brush or pencil as long as you live' (Gilman 1973).

Also in pregnancy and birth, middle and upper class women sought 'regular' doctors; from 1850 on, many appear to have demanded maximum treatment and expected maximum effects (Wertz and Wertz 1979; Ehrenreich and English 1979). Fashionable women and a growing women's media were eager for news of painkillers and dramatic medical techniques (Wertz and Wertz 1979).

All manner of women's complaints were treated by removing the ovaries or clitoris (Barker-Benfield 1976). Women would have their uteri 'propped up', even during their teen years, by one of over 200 different mechanical and belt anchored speculae, pessaries, or coil-and-strut devices, to prevent or treat uterine prolapse (Wertz and Wertz 1979). It was also common to treat a variety of women's complaints with acid or caustic injections and hot cauterizations applied through the cervix (Wertz and Wertz 1979; Stockham 1886). Although the bleeding of patients became less popular after 1880 (Stockham 1886), even as late as 1920 doctors occasionally bled pregnant, labouring, and postpartum women for any number of ills, ranging from convulsions to haemorrhage (Siddall 1980). There were several devices for mechanical cervical dilatation in labour (Ashford 1986) and a variety of forceps were commonly used, even by Indian reservation doctors (Engelmann 1883).

Victorian women had many 'ills' but they also sought out 'regular' doctors and hospitals in response to publicity about the conquering of puerperal fever. Routines for douching, enemas, shaving, and scrubbing women before, during, and after birth became selling points for hospitals in their campaigns to attract charitable donations, as well as middle and upper class maternity patients. At Sloan Maternity Hospital in New York City in 1900 each patient:

> '... received an enema immediately upon admission and then a vaginal douche with bichloride of mercury, the favored antiseptic. Nurses then washed the woman's head with kerosene, ether, and ammonia, her nipples and umbilicus with ether; they shaved the pubic hair of charity patients, ... and clipped it for private patients. They gave women in labor an enema every twelve hours and continued to douche the vagina during and after labor with saline solutions to which whiskey or bichloride of mercury was added' (Wertz and Wertz 1979).

Despite such routines hospitals had epidemics of puerperal fever well into the 1930s. At Boston Lying-In Hospital 75 per cent of the maternity patients got puerperal fever in 1883 and 20 per cent died of it (Frederick 1942).

Yet, women and their doctors seemed to be proved correct that women's illnesses were riskier than having a 'regular' doctor treat them: maternal and infant mortality fell around 1900. By 1910 New York City's infant mortality rate had finally declined to the rate it was in 1810 (Bolduen and Winerl 1935). Massachusetts in 1910 achieved an infant mortality rate which was just below that of 1855 (Devitt 1977). Actually, this improvement came at the same time as did a precipitous drop in the birth rate, improvements in urban sanitation, and a more active lifestyle adopted by women at the turn of the century. Corsets were loosened. It was no longer chic to be frail. Women rode bicycles and cars, danced to big bands, and went to movies and beaches. The incidence of rickets, tuberculosis, and uterine prolapse declined (Fisher 1909). As is true so often today, the 'authorities' and the public gave medical 'science' credit for improved perinatal outcomes that were more likely to have been due to social improvements. Doctors generally accepted credit. Sir William Osler said at this time:

> 'If a poor lass, paralyzed apparently, helpless, bedridden for years, comes to me, having worn out in mind and body, and estate, a devoted family; if she in a few weeks or less, by faith in me, and faith alone, takes up her bed and walks, the saints of old could not have done more' (Cushing 1940).

So, with the popular health movement isolated, fragmented, and lacking newsworthy breakthroughs, with women and infants more obviously ill than before 1850, and with 'scientific' medicine attracting the support of civic leaders, the stage was set for the final important element in the eclipse of support for the Popular Health Movement in America. This was the recruitment of women themselves into the service of medicine, as charitable workers, ancillary medical professionals, and as doctors.

The nursing profession, for example, began in 1872, when a group of women calling themselves 'the best class of our citizens', formed a committee to monitor the conduct of New York hospitals and almshouses, conducting what would now be called a 'raid'. They found rats, patients in beds of 'indescribable filth', and nurses sleeping on the floors in the bathrooms. Physicians resisted the ladies' recommendations to upgrade the training and social status of nurses, who until then had been servants and 'deserving' poor girls. So the ladies went over the heads of the doctors to the hospitals' boards of directors, who were composed of their social equals. By 1873 Philadelphia, New York, Boston, and New Haven had schools for nurses and by 1910 there were over 1100 nursing schools in America, all modelled after Florence Nightingale's military nurses' school in England (Starr 1982). One of the first nursing textbooks cautioned:

> 'Loyalty to the physician is one of the duties demanded of every nurse, not solely because the physician is her superior officer, but chiefly because the confidence of the patient in his physician is one of the important elements in the management of his illness' (Aikens 1916).

Social workers and nurses were soon joined by laboratory technicians and growing legions of mostly female staff in the support of medicine.

These support personnel and volunteers were welcomed by 'regular' doctors, but midwives and women physicians were not (Abrams 1986). (see Chapter 9). Curiously, midwives and women doctors met different fates from 1850 to 1920. Although it is clear that 'regular' doctors opposed midwives, they campaigned against women doctors just as vociferously from 1840 onwards, with much less success. While midwifery declined (Litoff 1986), the drive for female physicians was remarkably successful. The extreme modesty so often linked with Victorian women did not lead them to seek out the services of midwives rather than doctors (except among immigrants and in the rural south). American women apparently agreed with Emmons and Huntington (1912), who wrote that midwives were:

> '. . . not a product of America . . . as soon as the immigrant is assimilated, and becomes part of our civilization, then the midwife is no longer a factor in his home'.

Many of the first female doctors were trained in schools opened by the popular health movement. Most practised what would now be called 'holistic' medicine (Abrams 1986; Stockham 1886). But, like the popular health movement itself, women doctors were divided and isolated in their loyalties and efforts—partly because they were ostracized by male physicians (Abrams 1986). Some opened clinics for women and children, but most practised in their own and their patients' homes. Many ardently pursued social reforms such as child labour restrictions, improved workplace health, and urban public health.

Not only were women, doctors and health advisors divided, but some seemed to hold themselves above other women. There is more than a trace of chauvinism in the quoted statements of some women doctors, and even those of some feminists from this period, towards less capable or less lucky women. Alice B. Stockham, a Hygienic 'irregular', wrote in 1886:

> 'We find in women of superior education and marked intelligence an exaggerated development of the emotional nature, and a corresponding deterioration of physical powers. Weakness, debility, and suffering is the common lot of most of them. Not one in a hundred has health and strength to pursue any chosen study, or to follow any lucrative occupation, and what is vastly worse, most are unfitted for the duties and perils of maternity'.

In the 1870s Elizabeth Cady Stanton, a feminist and mother of seven, forecast the teachings of some holistic childbirth educators a century later:

> 'If you suffer, it is not because you are cursed of God, but because you violate his laws . . . We know that among Indians the squaws do not suffer in childbirth . . .' (Saur 1891).

In conclusion, the first patients' movement lost popular support during a half-century in which startling medical discoveries won people's allegiance. Having begun among lay people as a reaction against the excesses of 'heroic' medicine, the popular remedies became competing systems. Their practitioners crowded under the wing of medicine where they lost identity and failed to develop powerful allies. Reproductive health was actually poorer between 1850 and 1900 than previously, as reflected in maternal and infant mortality statistics; women began to view their illnesses as warranting the 'best' that medicine could offer. Finally, doctors and hospitals began to attract women in large numbers as volunteers and ancillary health professionals, positions from which women became elite competitors and advocates, rather than critical users, of perinatal care.

3 Women as partners in obstetrics: 1900–1939

From 1900 until World War II, the role of educated women was one of partnership with obstetrics. In the settlement houses and immigrant slums, poor women were urged by doctors, and elite women community health workers, literally to *contribute their bodies* to obstetric advancement. Austin Flint, M.D., of Cornell Medical College said in 1898:

'... the homeless, friendless, degraded and possibly criminal sick poor in the wards of a charity hospital receiving aid and comfort in their extremity and contributing each one his modest share to the advancement of medical science ...'

Well-off women were also expected to agree to new obstetric procedures, but mostly they were appealed to for donations to 'improve' obstetrics. This approach had a long precedent in American medicine. Between 1902 and 1928 the Rockefeller Institute for Medical Research gave $65 million to medical schools, many times the amount of government funding. In 1908 the American Medical Association asked the Carnegie Foundation for a study which would raise the standards of medical schools. The Carnegie Foundation's Flexner Report (1910) (in concert with economic woes of small medical schools) accomplished the closing of most sectarian medical schools within five years (Starr 1982).

From 1912 to the mid-1920s, Johns Hopkins professor, J. Whitridge Williams wrote and lectured obstetricians and women's groups about the need to abolish midwives and to have all births occur in hospitals. He pleaded that safety was assured only if fewer medical schools could have better facilities to train fewer, but better, obstetricians. As newspapers and ladies' magazines carried Williams' message about the safety of hospitals, an outpouring of business and individual philanthropy resulted in the building of quiet, homelike maternity wings in most of the nation's major hospitals during the 1920s (Wertz and Wertz 1979). Midwife-attended births declined from 40 per cent in 1915 to 10.7 per cent in 1935; by the latter year 4.5 per cent of Caucasian babies and 54 per cent of black babies were delivered by midwives, nearly all of them in the rural south (Jacobson 1956).

Each obstetric 'advance' was announced in the popular press. The first 'method' of childbirth was the Twilight Sleep Method, publicized from 1914 through the 1920s by feminists (Tracy and Boyd 1915; Rion 1915) and by elite women and doctors. Mrs John Jacob Astor, member of the Twilight Sleep Association, announced, in the *New York Times*, plans to open an office, publish pamphlets answering women's questions, and establish a teaching hospital where German doctors who developed the method could teach it to American physicians (Wertz and Wertz 1979).

Both Williams and the other major obstetric leader of that time, Joseph B DeLee, spoke and wrote about the dangers of birth. DeLee said he was 'convinced the minority of births were normal' (DeLee 1920). In the first issue of the *American Journal of Obstetrics and Gynecology* DeLee expanded his thesis with his famous proposal that all women have prophylactic episiotomy and forceps assistance for birth:

'If a woman falls on a pitchfork, and drives the handle through her perineum, we call that pathologic—abnormal, but if a large baby is driven through the pelvic floor, we say that is natural ... If a baby were to have its head caught in a door ... enough to cause a cerebral haemorrhage, we would say that is decidedly pathologic, but when a baby's head is crushed against a tight pelvic floor and a haemorrhage in the brain kills it, we call this normal ...' (DeLee 1920).

Despite the warning of more conservative professors such as Williams, prophylactic episiotomy and forceps did become fairly routine; in 1932 a White House Conference survey of 233 hospitals, 37 per cent reported from 20 to 81 per cent of all deliveries as forceps assisted. From 1918 to 1925 infant deaths from birth injuries rose 44 per cent in a survey of 11 states (Frankel 1927). Plass and Alvis (1936) studied 129 500 births in Iowa in 1934, concluding that, 'the significant increase in the stillbirth rate in urban hospitals over that of other groups is probably related to the increased incidence of operative delivery'.

DeLee, Williams, and many other obstetricians during the 1920s became alarmed at the number of doctors performing invasive obstetric procedures for which they had been ill-trained. This spurred the development of the American Board of Obstetrics and Gynecology in 1930, which mailed standards for the training of the obstetrician–gynaecologist to all hospital maternity units (Danreuther 1931). However, DeLee blamed women and their bodies as much as poorly trained doctors for bad outcomes in childbirth:

'... I have often wondered whether Nature did not deliberately intend women to be used up in the process of reproduction, in a manner analogous to that of the salmon, which dies after spawning' (DeLee 1920).

Despite the initial alarm of obstetricians, 'twilight sleep' also became routine. In 1938 all Boston hospitals used twilight sleep (Boston Lying-in Hospital 1938), and the rate of anaesthesia accidents and asphyxiated newborns was enough to prompt Rudolph Holmes, the obstetrician who introduced scopolamine in the United States, to say in an interview with *Time Magazine* in 1936, 'I wish to God I hadn't done it' (Holmes 1936).

In the 1930s, even women community leaders had stopped campaigns for obstetric changes, apparently willing to be semiconscious partners on the obstetric 'team'. Debates over perinatal procedures were carried on between obstetricians; the interventionist camp won decisively. Asepsis was more stringently attempted, and obstetricians controlled the requirements for practitioners and hospital facilities more tightly through their voluntary examining board, the American Board of Obstetrics and Gynecology, which was set up in 1930. To the public, and to many doctors, the wisdom of this course seemed confirmed when maternal and infant mortality rates began to decline after 1936, even though other factors, such as the drop in the United States birth rate and the discovery of antibiotics, could have accounted for this improvement.

There is no record to suggest that childbearing women were aware of any obstetric data, such as the maternal and infant mortality statistics which worried the New York Academy of Medicine (1933), the forceps injuries studied by Frankel (1927), and the 1922 controlled trial which failed to show that routine perineal shaving made a difference in the bacteria present (Johnson and Siddall 1922).

4 The second maternity patients' movement

4.1 The rise of the second maternity patients' movement: 1939–1975

The seeds of the present patients' movement were sown in 1939 with a story in *The Atlantic Monthly* from a woman who had gone to Switzerland in order to have an unmedicated birth (Freidreich 1939). American women were not ready for this message; Freidreich's account of her ecstatic experience brought jeering letters to the editor. In that same year the anthropologist, Margaret Mead *was* able to arrange an unmedicated birth at Yale, thus inspiring the first United States hospital program in 'natural childbirth'.

After World War II the Maternity Center Association hosted a lecture tour by Grantly Dick-Read, author of *The Principles and Practice of Natural Childbirth* (1944). In 1948 Thoms began a pilot programme in natural childbirth at Yale. But what evolved during the 1950s was a sad vestige of what Dick-Read had described. Neither the support of midwife and doctor during labour, nor the woman-controlled environment of a home birth was possible in American hospitals. Fathers were strictly kept out of labour rooms until the end of the 1950s. Dick-Read had reported that only about ten per cent of mothers asked for pain relief, but at Yale about 50 per cent somehow 'required' pain medication (Thoms and Wyatt 1951). Dick-Read had wanted to avoid delivering sleepy babies who could not be put to breast immediately. But in American hospitals 'rooming-in' began (when it was available at all) only after babies were 'observed' in the nursery for 12 to 24 hours after birth. Breastfeeding was limited to three minutes on each breast every four hours during the daytime. Margaret Mead later wrote:

> 'It should be pointed out that natural childbirth, the very inappropriate name for forms of delivery in which women undergo extensive training so that they can cooperate consciously with the delivery of their children, is a male invention meant to counteract practices of complete anesthesia, which were also male inventions' (Mead and Newton 1967).

In any case, natural childbirth appealed to only a few women (Rich 1976) in the post-war period of America's highest recorded birth rate. The vast majority of parents-to-be assumed that medical procedures were safe and effective. In the 1950s women accepted diethylstilboestrol (DES) which continued to be widely prescribed by many doctors in the United States to prevent miscarriage, even after six controlled trials had failed to show the hormone to be effective (Robinson and Shettles 1952; Dieckmann *et al.* 1953; Ferguson 1953; Crowder *et al.* 1950; Randall *et al.* 1955; Reid 1955) (see Chapter 38). Women also continued to agree to prenatal and intrapartum X-rays despite wide publicity about the long term effects of ionizing radiation. Towards the end of the 1950s most women welcomed the 'advance' of spinal, and, later, caudal anaesthesia, which were generally used for delivery after a labour conducted with heavy sedation in combination with the amnesiac, scopolamine (Shaw 1974).

In 1958 natural childbirth, which had been conducted entirely under the auspices of obstetrics, became a somewhat more popular health movement. That year the *Ladies' Home Journal* carried an article by a nurse who described inhumane treatment of women during labour and delivery. This was the beginning of the nurse as patient advocate. For nearly a century nurses had been trained to equate professionalism with loyalty to doctor and hospital. This nurse's story evoked over 500 letters to the editor from women, many of whom told of callous, even brutal treatment during birth:

> 'When my baby was ready the delivery room wasn't. I was strapped to the table, my legs tied together, so I would "wait" until a more convenient and "safer" time to deliver. In the meantime my baby's heartbeat started faltering. At this point I was incapable of rational thought and cannot report fairly the following hour. When I regained consciousness I was told my baby would probably not live' (Anon., *Ladies' Home Journal* 1958).

When the husband's role was described in *Thank You Dr Lamaze* (Karmel 1959), some people concluded that the husband should be in the labour room if only to assure that his wife would obtain humane treatment. In fact, in the early 1960s there were newspaper reports of husbands who had handcuffed themselves to their wife's rolling bed or delivery table so that they could be removed only by police action (*Los Angeles Times* 1961).

In 1960 the need to popularize natural childbirth, and Karmel's description of 'painless childbirth', gave impetus to the starting of the International Childbirth Education Association (ICEA) and the American Society for Psychoprophylaxis in Obstetrics (ASPO). Both natural childbirth and psychoprophylaxis were quickly adapted to create a new ancillary profession: the childbirth educator. The classes were offered to both parents and the programmes were renamed 'prepared

pared childbirth' (Miller 1962) and the 'Lamaze Method'. Although most were community-based, nearly all the instructors in ASPO, and many of those in ICEA, were nurses or physiotherapists. The question of whether parents should be advised to co-operate with their caregivers or taught to question and to assert their own choices was settled in favour of co-operation (Miller 1962; Bing *et al.* 1961), even by those who rose later to champion 'true' natural childbirth (Bradley 1965) and 'painless childbirth' (Hommell 1969).

Surprisingly little attention was paid to adapting the two 'methods' to what American parents said they wanted. The first teaching manual for psychoprophylaxis cautioned:

'The questions of rooming-in and breast-feeding are always likely to arise in the classes. Although there is no reason not to discuss them, it is probably a mistake to make them part of the course. Many women have a great emotional involvement in these questions, perfectly justifiably' (Bing *et al.* 1961).

Most of the early childbirth educators were also careful to modulate any fixed ideas of parents about going through labour without medication:

'You must assure women that today most good obstetricians use fewer and better drugs than in the past and only those that they consider important to insure the best possible delivery with the best results to the health of mother and child' (Bing *et al.* 1961).

Yet even these attenuated approaches to natural childbirth and psychoprophylaxis elicited anger and ridicule from some women and doctors. In a woman's magazine the spectre of being thought masculine or neurotic was raised for women who insisted on medication-free birth:

'Thus it is a fairly aggressive, masculine-oriented, non-conservative woman who is most apt to elect "Natural Childbirth". She looks forward not so much to motherhood as to the potency she has always lacked. She is determined to miss not one moment, not one detail of the intensely awaited event, which she fantasies will establish her own psychic virility' (Gittleson 1961).

And women were warned that, even if they succeeded in their obstetrician's eyes, natural childbirth could still make them crazy:

'Mrs. A, four days after delivery, stated that the contractions had been "much worse" than anything she had expected. After some gas anesthesia, she had awakened and heard the baby cry, but "didn't give a damn about the baby". She regretted the experience and did not think she could ever go through it again. The doctor's opinion was that Mrs. A was a "successful" Natural Childbirth patient. The psychologist's conclusion: "This patient is apt to end up with great emotional problems"' (Fielding and Benjamin 1962).

Thus it is not surprising that most women who ventured into a 'prepared' childbirth were unusually compliant. Husbands demonstrated that they could behave properly so they would gain admittance to labour rooms. There they usually proved their value in giving labour support, which doctors and nurses had never been trained to provide (Bradley 1965; Chabon 1966). Doctors and hospital administrators began to realize that 'prepared' couples were nearly always grateful for whatever doctors could convince them that they needed (Shearer 1983). And they paid their bills.

In fact, by the end of the 1960s, it had become necessary to woo such paying obstetric patients as hospitals began to compete to be included in new regional perinatal systems. Pilot regional programmes had been operating since 1966; by 1970 it was clear within the obstetric profession that in order to equip and staff a fetal and neonatal intensive care unit a hospital would need a minimum of 1500 births each year, with enough paying patients, government 're-imbursements', and charitable contributions to support expansion and operation of such units (Quilligan 1972; Butterfield 1972). Doctors' specialty organizations even suggested that hospitals without perinatal intensive care capability should close their obstetric facilities or merge with nearby hospitals (Ryan *et al.* 1977). Yet, fewer than one in forty United States hospitals had 1500 births annually (American Hospital Association 1969) and, to complicate matters, the birth rate began to fall in 1965 and reached the lowest level ever recorded in the United States in 1974.

Thus, in the last half of the 1960s childbirth educators' views—and those of their clients—began to be solicited by obstetricians who were anxious to have their maternity units survive or expand to include 'perinatal intensive care' (Shearer 1977, 1980). More 'prepared' parents succeeded in having the shave and enema modified or omitted, vaginal instead of rectal examinations during labour, and smaller doses of sedative, hypnotic, and narcotic medication. Spinal anaesthesia gave way to pudendal and paracervical block among willing doctors (or for insistent patients); continuous caudal and, later, epidural anaesthesia, was introduced. Some mothers were propped up to see their babies born and some were given their baby to hold before their episiotomies were repaired. Some hospitals launched charity drives with newspaper articles and brochures about this new 'family centred' maternity care.

But the same decade in which childbirth education was thus incorporated by obstetrics was also a decade of disillusionment with authority in general, and medicine in particular, as evidenced by public disenchantment with atmospheric testing of atomic weapons, Rachel Carson's prediction of ecological cataclysm in *Silent Spring* (1962), and the widely publicized thalidomide disaster (Silverman 1985). Civil rights marches and mounting demands for better access to medical care for the poor confronted the Kennedy and Johnson administrations.

Government response to the mid-1960s unrest had profound effects on obstetrics: it paved the way for non-physicians to gain firsthand experience caring for expectant and labouring women—most with no supervision by physicians. Nurse practitioners, nurse midwives, and physicians' assistants, who had been trained in federally funded community health programmes for the 'medically underserved', provided perinatal care with an unheard of degree of independence from doctors, largely because they practised where few doctors would go: among the urban and rural poor. These 'physician extenders' also attracted a devoted following among patients. Virtually every evaluation of nurse practitioners and nurse midwives showed their outcomes to be as good or better than those of doctors (Montgomery 1969; Spitzer 1984). Increasingly, nurses at many levels found themselves competing with doctors. In 1973 the International Council of Nurses Code omitted any reference to 'loyal obedience to physicians', stating instead:

> 'The nurse's primary responsibility is to those who require nursing care' (Winslow 1984).

The obstetricians' monopoly was further challenged by family practitioners whose training programmes had been expanded to redress the 'health manpower shortage' that was thought to exist in the 1960s (Starr 1982).

Lay feminists also gained firsthand experience in delivering obstetric and gynaecologic care. By 1968 feminists had begun their own abortion and women's health clinics (Ruzek 1978) even though abortion was not legalized in the United States until 1973. Feminists attacked obstetrician gynaecologists for what they saw as inaccurate and degrading attitudes about women, especially their sexual lives. In a survey of the contents of 27 gynaecology textbooks, Scully and Bart (1973) concluded:

> 'In addition, they (gynecology textbooks) said most women were "frigid" and that the vaginal orgasm was the "mature" response. Gynecologists, our society's official experts on women, think of themselves as the woman's friend. With friends like that who needs enemies?'

Feminists protested about the seeming manipulation of women by doctors and the medicalization of puberty, marriage, sex, childbearing, menopause, and ageing; the doctors' pushing of pills, making moral judgements, and discounting real illnesses as behaviour disorders (Boston Women's Health Book Collective 1973; Rich 1976; Ehrenreich and English 1979).

These lay and professional birth practitioners were joined after 1968 by returning Peace Corps members who had acquired experience with birth in Third World countries and among the American poor. They were also joined by a growing number of dissatisfied 'prepared' parents who planned 'do-it-yourself' births the next time (Hazell 1969), and by childbirth educators who suspected that they and their teaching had been trivialized and transformed by obstetrics, to serve the needs of hospitals and doctors (Souza 1976).

By the end of the 1960s, the public began to pay attention to the feminist message regarding medicine. Oestrogen replacement therapy, touted as 'the pills to keep women young' (Walsh 1965) and birth control pills were causing widely publicized alarm (Seaman and Seaman 1977). By 1977 some intrauterine devices had been associated with pelvic inflammatory disease, sterility, and deaths (Dowie and Johnson 1977). Diethylstilboestrol, given to prevent miscarriage, became linked to genital abnormalities and cancers in offspring. There was said to be an 'epidemic' of unnecessary hysterectomies, breast biopsies, and mastectomies (Corea 1979; Mendelsohn 1979). Caesarean section rates were increasing at an average of 1 per cent per year (National Institutes of Health 1980).

By 1970 popular discontent with obstetrics had spread to medicine in general. There were nation-wide accusations of incompetence and greed. The January 1970 *Business Week* lead story, 'The $60 billion crisis', called American medicine inferior to national health services in European countries (Burns 1970). The January 1970 issue of *Fortune* lead article, 'It's time to operate', said in part:

> 'Much of United States medical care, particularly the every-day business of preventing and treating routine illnesses, is inferior in quality, wastefully dispensed, and inequitably financed. Medical manpower and facilities are so maldistributed that large segments of the population, especially the urban poor and those in rural areas, get virtually no care at all—even though their illnesses are more numerous and, in a medical sense, often easy to cure.'

It was in this climate that the underground home birth movement became public. Since the mid-1960s home births had flourished, with the help and growing authority of lay and professional home birth practitioners. Although at first identified with the counter culture, home births were increasingly being sought by middle and upper class people (Hazell 1975). The case for home over hospital birth was publicized by Hazell in 1969.

Home birth was also praised by Lang (1972) in photographs and accounts from parents, children, and birth attendants. In 1972 Hazell showed films of four home births to a large ICEA convention in Minneapolis. One woman hung on a makeshift 'squat bar' during her delivery, and her pelvis seemed to open in all dimensions to give birth to a very large baby, with no hands-on assistance, no apparent maternal tissue damage, and no fuss.

At the same conference Klaus described studies of mother–infant attachment in the first hours after birth (Klaus *et al.* 1972a, b). It was suggested that fathers (Rodholm and Larsson 1979) and others who are present and become involved immediately with the new baby also develop a special attachment, and that this might be a way humans have always had to ensure caretaking even in the absence of the mother. It seemed as if home birth and extended family–infant attachment offered the potential for birth to exceed the narrow obstetric definition of 'normal'.

As home birth thus surfaced, hospital obstetrics underwent even more heavy criticism. Haire's monograph, *The Cultural Warping of Childbirth* (1972), contrasted American hospital obstetrics and newborn care with those of other developed countries, showing that much more medication, surgery, unnecessary routines, and separation of families is part of American births.

But the case against birth as conducted by obstetricians was made most strongly by Nancy Shaw in *Forced Labor* (1974) and Suzanne Arms in *Immaculate Deception* (1975a). Both delivered searing indictments of obstetricians for being unprepared to conduct normal childbirth and, worse, for actually preventing normal birth from taking place. Shaw observed prenatal and intrapartum care at several United States hospitals and also at the Frontier Nursing Service (a nurse midwifery service for Appalachian people) during 1968 and 1969. The obstetric system for both clinic and private patients in all the hospitals Shaw observed contrasted starkly with births at the midwifery service. Obstetricians used routine interventions to speed labour, heavy sedation, spinal anaesthesia for delivery, episiotomy, and forceps.

> 'Drugs make the nurse's work much easier. She is called on less for physical and emotional support. The rate of changing bed pads, johnnies (gowns), and linen is reduced . . . Totally controlled patients can be examined . . . as often as the nurse wishes, without either asking permission or bothering to completely close the woman from view. When they are "ready" according to clinical signs, they are all delivered by spinal, low forceps, and episiotomy.
>
> . . . the residents, who for the most part are firmly opposed to the full use of prepared childbirth . . . sometimes seem eager for the patient to give up' (Shaw 1974).
>
> Arms (1975a) quoted an Irish midwife who worked as a labour and delivery nurse in a large American hospital: 'When a woman doesn't have any medication she'll deliver at her own pace. But an undrugged birth is a frantic event in a hospital. The doctors get very nervous. They are not in control and never quite prepared. "Get this!" "Get that!" "Oh! Move this here!" "Quick, it's coming!" Nothing is ready. But usually, when there's anesthesia, the doctor is prepared. He slits the perineum just so, and he casually looks around to see: Yes, his bulb syringe is right there, and his this and that are there' (Arms 1975a).

Childbirth educators joined the criticism. Elisabeth Bing (1974) wrote of the 'Catch-22' situation in which hospitals announced that fathers could attend delivery (if they had gone to childbirth education classes) while the hospital rules actually made fathers' attendance impossible. A nurse explained:

1. She can wait for her doctor to come and deliver her baby, and then her husband can be in the room.
2. If she does not wait the resident will deliver the baby, but the father cannot be in the room then.
3. She can have a spinal to slow her labor so she can wait for her own doctor, but then the father cannot be in the room because she has had medication (Bing 1974).

From 1972 to the end of the 1970s books appeared describing the benefits of home birth that were thought to be impossible in hospitals (Souza 1976; Gilgoff 1978; Gaskin 1978). At least seven national home birth organizations were formed, including the National Association of Parents and Professionals for Safe Alternatives in Childbirth (NAPSAC), the American College of Home Obstetrics (ACHO), Informed Home Birth, the Association for Childbirth At Home International (ACHI), Home Oriented Maternity Experience (HOME), Birth Day, and the Midwives' Alliance of North America (MANA). In 1975 the most active of these organizations was NAPSAC, whose published conference proceedings won the American Nurses' Association Award in 1977. The leaders of NAPSAC invited professionals and scientists to speak at their meetings, and were blunt in their debates:

> 'If we would have to wait for scientific studies on how we got pregnant and how a baby develops inside before we did it, the human race would be extinct'
>
> 'Hospitals have never been proven to be the safest place to give birth' (Stewart and Stewart 1976).

Medical response was often strident; an official of the American College of Obstetricians and Gynecologists wrote:

> 'Home birth is maternal trauma! Home birth is child abuse!' (Pearse 1977).

Nurses were divided. Some defended hospital obstetrics while others supported the lay challenge. Like other Americans, nurses also felt the 'stunning loss of confidence in medicine' so widely publicized (Starr 1982). Although some nurse practitioners and nurse midwives were competing with obstetricians in delivering perinatal care, other nurses were losing jobs to electronic monitors. In fact, reducing the need for bedside nursing and nurses' record keeping was one of the selling points for electronic monitors (Quilligan 1972). Some nurses responded to job changes by joining unions and some joined nursing agencies instead of hospital staffs, so they could better control their duties and hours. Some nurses found themselves agreeing with feminists, chafing in their roles as 'handmaidens' and at being obliged to carry out perinatal care with which they disagreed. 'It was hardly surprising, therefore, that leaders of the patients' rights movement turned to nurses in the search for "patient advocates"' (Winslow 1984). In 1974 George Annas, a scholar in health law, pointed out that, since nurses are held to legal account for care they provide, they should accept the role of patient advocate.

Nurses agreed with Annas; within a decade over fifty nursing books and articles dealt with the nurse as patient advocate (Winslow 1984).

Nurses also became independent midwives, nurse midwives, and nurse practitioners. In those states where lay midwifery laws allowed it, training programmes were set up for independent midwives (Seattle Midwifery School). Nurse midwifery programmes, which had expanded in the late 1960s, further expanded to train independent (lay) midwives. In the mid-1970s a statistically apparent shift towards midwife-attended birth occurred; while only 0.5 per cent of births were attended by midwives in 1970, by 1982 the figure had risen to 2.1 per cent (Litoff 1986).

Nurse midwives also organized home-like centres in which to care for normal childbearing women, at lower cost than hospitals and obstetricians charged. In the early 1970s the Maternity Center Association began planning for the nation's first freestanding birth centre, in a townhouse in New York City (Lubic 1980) and by the end of the 1970s there were over 150 freestanding birth centres throughout the United States (National Association of Childbearing Centers 1983). By 1980 many major cities in the United States had women's health centres providing low cost, 'women-centred' obstetric and gynaecologic care (Cassidy-Brinn *et al.* 1984).

Midwives were not the only primary caregivers with increasing roles in obstetrics. The United States government, alarmed at the escalating cost of specialist-dominated, hospital-based health care, increased the support of the training of family practitioners. The numbers of family doctors more than doubled in the early 1970s. Until malpractice insurance became difficult for family practitioners to afford, increasing numbers practised obstetrics each year after 1975 (United States Department of Health and Human Services 1981b).

The most unprecedented action of the patients' movement was to join clinicians and epidemiologists in evaluating research evidence about the effects of obstetric procedures instead of accepting, as in the past, obstetricians' clinical judgement.

As electronic fetal monitors were bought by hospitals, and staff were taught to use them, the first article to question the safety and efficacy of electronic fetal monitoring was published by a childbirth educator, in the first issue of the journal she began as a forum for lay and professional perinatal debate: a journal now called *Birth* (Shearer 1974). Researchers, parents, and spokesmen with contrary opinions have since then contributed to this journal; its conferences feature eminent speakers who debate home and hospital birth, circumcision, infant formulae, regionalization of obstetric care, parent–newborn attachment, maternal position in labour and delivery, episiotomy, siblings at birth, weight gain in pregnancy, the safety and efficacy of ultrasound imaging, rising caesarean section rates, and many other controversial issues.

Patients began to be represented nationally as well. As an outgrowth of government mandated citizen involvement in community health centres in the late 1960s, the Health Planning Law of 1974 required 'consumer' members on local boards which were to set priorities for the development of obstetric and neonatal facilities. In the late 1970s the National Institutes of Health (NIH) convened 'consensus development conferences' composed of invited panels of experts and a 'consumer' member. Three of these panels considered the scientific evidence on efficacy, safety, and indications of antepartum monitoring, caesarean section, and ultrasound imaging. Consensus reports were then disseminated widely among perinatal professionals and health service users. Also in the late 1970s, the Food and Drug Administration began to include 'consumer' representatives on panels considering maternal and infant drugs and devices. The Women's Health Network was formed as a national umbrella organization for consumer advocacy, from which many of the 'consumer' members for official panels were appointed. In 1979 Doris Haire, convinced that oxytocin was sometimes used for the convenience of doctors rather than the benefit of women, representing the Women's Health Network and the International Childbirth Education Association, led a move that resulted in having oxytocin disapproved by the FDA for elective induction of labour (i.e. induction without clear medical indication).

Compared to changes made by the Popular Health Movement a century earlier, these changes in obstetric care were modest. Yet, the monopoly of obstetricians had been challenged, if not altered, by the expansion of midwifery, family practice, and birth centres. Hospitals' share of obstetric cases did rise in proportion with the total number of births (American Hospital Association 1982), but there were new options for women, which still exist. The style of care for some patients, especially paying ones, changed to take account of their wishes. One lasting gain made by the patients' movement was to forge alliances and foster debate, through personal contacts, publications and conferences, between consumer groups and those branches of medicine that are concerned with evaluation of neonatal and obstetric procedures and public policy.

4.2 The fate of the second maternity patients' movement

The diverse branches of the patients' movement, each with their own agendas, were united on several points in 1975. They agreed that obstetric interventions were often unnecessary, dangerous, and poorly investigated prior to widespread use. They also agreed that parents should have the right to select the place of birth and should be free to choose among different types of care and caregivers; that parents should be offered full disclosure of the unknowns, and the risks, benefits, and alternatives to any perinatal care proposal; and that they should have the right to refuse a procedure altogether.

But by 1980 the second patients' movement was losing popularity. Many of the reasons for this loss bear uncanny similarity to those behind the decline of the Popular Health Movement after the Civil War. First, and most pervasively, during the 1970s the national mood shifted from populist anti-authoritarianism toward the political and social conservatism characteristic of the Victorian and Reagan periods.

Second, the vanguard of the patients' movements in both eras fragmented. Like the Eclectics of the 1840s, many leaders of the patients' movement of the 1970s became professionals themselves, competing with one another, working in parallel with obstetricians, or actually in their service. These included childbirth educators, midwives, lactation counsellors, and scores of even more narrowly focused 'new professionals' (Table 7.1, p. 126). At the same time, some former leaders of the patients' movement took up ever more radical or isolated positions from which they were less able to push effectively for the changes they wanted in perinatal care. These included separatist feminists and people active in single issues such as circumcision prevention, fetal stimulation and education, and birth under water. Many leaders of the home birth movement scattered under legal assaults, some fighting criminal charges of practising medicine without a licence, others seeking licensure or more covert ways to practise home birth, or leaving the field altogether (Arms 1975a).

Another reason for the loss of popularity of the patients' movement was that obstetricians and hospitals adopted the form, if not the substance, of the movements' most attractive initiatives. This accounted for people's perception (both within and outside medicine) that obstetrics had, in fact, incorporated the most important ideas of the patients' movement. Hospitals and their staffs publicized hospital birth rooms, where little medication and technological intervention would be used during birth, and where families could stay together (Abdellah *et al.* 1973; Bean 1975; *American Journal of Nursing* 1975; Sumner 1976). By 1982, over 150 out of 3780 hospitals with maternity services (American Hospital Association 1982) had opened alternative birth centres, also known as ABCs (Klein and Westreich 1983). In many other units women were allowed to deliver in labour rooms rather than being moved to delivery rooms. These changes, along with early discharge from hospital (3–48 hours), kept separation of family members to a minimum. Some hospitals hired nurse midwives to staff their alternative birth facilities. Most also began to sell a burgeoning array of educational programs to parents, nearly all of which had begun as patients' initiatives in the community. (See Table 7.1, p. 126)

Among maternity nurses, loss of support for the patients' movement began when the American College of Obstetricians and Gynecologists (ACOG) formed the Nurses' Association of the American College of Obstetricians and Gynecologists (NAACOG). By 1975 it had become clear to nurses that NAACOG offered elite status to members who would learn to operate the new electronic equipment and supervise subordinates. Many nurses took pride in their monitoring roles, while others questioned these and other interventions or preferred to give bedside support. This division subverted maternity nurses' unity and power (Boston Women's Health Book Collective 1984).

The nurse patient-advocate became an impossible rôle without the unified support of nursing. This was illustrated most poignantly by the story of Christine Spahn Smith (1980) who called public attention to the high postpartum infection rates and lower than expected Apgar scores at one hospital and was then ostracized by her department and quit before she could be fired. Winslow (1984) writes:

> 'Unfortunately, this is typical of most published nurse as advocate stories. They usually describe a nurse's attempt to defend a patient or a group of patients against mistreatment. Most often the endeavour fails because the system overpowers the nurse. The patient suffers or dies. The nurse get fired or resigns in outrage'.

'Consumer' advocacy was also subverted in government health agencies by what appeared to be the 'divide and conquer' tactics of organized medicine. For example, when the National Institutes of Health Consensus Development Panel on Ultrasound was looking for a consumer representative, an unknown group called The Women's and Health Roundtable was contacted instead of the Women's Health Network which has strong consumer advocates (Shearer 1984). A woman lawyer with no contacts in women's health groups was picked as the 'consumer' representative for the panel. In another example, the American Hospital Association, in 1985, sponsored a new profession to represent 'consumers', the National Society of Patient Representatives, whose duties include reducing the incidence of lawsuits by soothing disgruntled patients, even offering to cancel their hospital bills (National Society of Patients' Representatives 1985).

Probably the most important reason for the decline in popularity of the maternity patients' movement after 1975 was that the public became interested in well publicized obstetric discoveries at about the time that certain reproductive problems also became news. The problems were complications of the sexual revolution of the 1960s, of birth control methods, and of delayed childbearing. The discoveries included microsurgery to reverse vasectomies and tubal ligations, a very wide range of new screening tests for genetic and high risk maternal conditions, and treatments for infertility that included in vitro fertilization and embryo transfer.

The middle and upper class clientele of the maternity patients' movement gradually changed goals as the 1970s closed. They were less interested in ways to reduce unnecessary, perhaps harmful medical intrusions into pregnancy and birth. They seemed much less mistrustful of medical authority than were expectant parents a decade earlier. They wanted to know whether they had high risk conditions, and what obstetrics had to offer to make childbearing as painless and risk free as possible. Evidence of this was the change in subjects of books written for expectant parents, starting about 1978. After that year there were no new books on home birth and few on reducing medical interventions. The books were on 'miracle babies', birth after age 30, caesarean birth, neonatal intensive care, tests and procedures in pregnancy, prepregnancy preparation, nutrition and exercise, and other ways to cope with the exigencies of reproduction (Moen 1979, 1986).

For all these reasons the maternity patients' movement became fragmented. It lost the characteristics of a movement; neither parents nor caregivers are united under any identifiable flag. Remnants of the old movement remain, along with their legacy of wider choices in caregivers and place of birth, while new interests are forming among perinatal caregivers and patients with goals of preventing and treating problems of infertility and high risk pregnancy.

5 Effects of the maternity patients' movement

One undisputable effect of the patients' movement was to bring fathers into labour and delivery. It is easy to forget the opposition mounted by doctors, hospitals, and health departments, on the grounds of preventing infection, spoiling a man's sexual desire for his spouse, and even having no room for him in the delivery suite. These and other arguments persisted throughout the 1960s and early 1970s as state health laws, one by one, changed to allow fathers, and then other family members, to be with the woman in labour and then delivery. Most parents report they were glad to be together. Few ill effects have been reported; stories of infection or men fainting, for example, have never been adequately documented.

What about the effects of the father's presence on obstetrics? His presence probably curbed the excessive use of mind altering drugs given the mother. The couple had to be considered. Obvious unkindness or dishonesty, as in this published incident, could no longer be hidden:

> 'When the patient is ready for delivery and her doctor isn't there, she's given some anesthesia that puts her out and she is delivered by a different obstetrician. Then her own doctor comes roaring in with his white coat on, takes some blood . . . and smears it all over him and acts as if he's just finished the delivery. He walks out to greet the father and says, "It's a boy!"' (Sweeney 1973).

But a subtler, more important effect of men's presence at birth has been their vulnerability to feelings of undue responsibility for helping with labour, especially if the couple attended prenatal classes where fathers were encouraged to be 'coaches' and given little skill in getting support for themselves. Fathers often feel helpless and guilty during labour, especially as uterine contractions become hard to manage or if even minor problems occur. Under these stresses the 'support' fathers often get is to be asked to agree to some sort of 'help' for their partners, like an epidural, a caesarean section, or a shot of pethidine:

> 'Ed, I know you and Jean are planning to have a natural childbirth, but there's no reason for her to be a martyr . . . some women have easier labors than others . . . There's no reason on God's earth for her to suffer like that . . .' (Sweeney 1973).

Childbirth educators have often noticed that after the baby is born men are generally the most enthusiastic supporters of whatever medical interventions were taken. Women in postpartum classes, even if they are still coming to terms with the birth or the way they were treated, often seem to develop a loyalty to the 'story' they remember, perhaps filled in with details from the father and medical staff. Men, on the other hand, often align themselves with those making the monitoring and 'management' decisions in labour and delivery.

Critics of the maternity patients' movement have said that the views of men and women have not been systematically gathered. Charges heard in the 1970s that childbirth educators were socializing parents to accept obstetric interventions (Arms 1975a) are mixed with charges like this one from a father writing a syndicated newspaper column in 1984:

'The movement sells attitudes as much as controlled breathing . . . It promotes the completely natural birth as the ideal, the standard against which we are to judge our own experience. Little support is given to the idea that completely natural childbirth might not be right for everybody. In a sense, the tyranny of the obstetrician has been replaced by the tyranny of Lamaze. . . . The word "medication" was once synonymous with twilight sleep of a woman in labor. Not anymore. In modern obstetrics, medicine is used primarily to ease her pain. She is still very much awake, she just doesn't hurt so much. Why this is so terrible is beyond me, but our teacher made it implicitly clear that terrible it most certainly is' (Nocera 1984).

What *do* patients want? Maternity patients' expectations were systematically gathered in Washington, Colorado, and Maryland by Korte and Scaer (1984). The 2067 women who had one child agreed on five general, rather pragmatic wishes:

'They want their husbands present for the labor, delivery, and recovery, and to have unrestricted visiting rights.

They want co-operation and assistance from the hospital staff—doctors and nurses—in using prepared childbirth techniques.

Women who breastfeed want effective help from nurses and doctors.

They want a lot of contact with their babies, immediately after birth and throughout their entire hospital stay.

They want their other children to visit them and to see and hold the new baby' (Korte and Scaer 1984).

Critics also charge that the treatments and advice dispensed by the perinatal movement and 'alternative' caregivers have been evaluated as little as have other perinatal interventions. Examples are films and testimonials that seek to assure that the birth of a baby under warm water, and continued submersion of the newborn for up to 14 minutes, is without harm and offers benefits ranging from less traumatic birth to less warlike individuals (Daniels 1986).

It is in the realm of such 'prophylaxis' that 'alternative' birth advice givers may be criticized most broadly. Whether a recommended prophylaxis is 'positive thinking' and the hoped for result is 'birthing normally' (Peterson and Mehl 1982) or 'childbirth with insight' (Noble 1983), 'healing' (Star 1986), or 'transformation through birth' (Panuthos 1983), the prophylaxis is nearly always a vague sort of 'trying harder'. It dooms many of its patients to some degree of failure because thinking cannot always be positive; insight, transformation, or normalcy cannot be absolute. Women who wonder have only themselves to blame if their experience failed to be 'spiritual' (Gaskin 1978), painless (Vellay 1959), or relaxed (Jacobson E 1959).

More modest therapies of the user movement have been criticized for the same reasons: poorly defined treatment and outcomes, with little or no attempt at evaluation (Chalmers 1986). In some cases risks have been suggested, as in prenatal and postpartum stretching, strengthening, and 'toning' exercises (Shearer 1981; Shrock *et al.* 1981), and prepregnancy classes (Lumley 1986). Jogging, aerobics, multivitamins, and consumption of 125 grams of protein daily (Brewer and Brewer 1986) have also been recommended to promote the 'perfect birth', 'wellness', or 'better babies'.

Assertive approaches by parents to caregivers have been recommended (McKay 1983; Herzfeld 1985), and their effects have not been evaluated. The recommendations range from negotiating a list of wishes during the first prenatal visit to sending a four-page typed, single-spaced letter outlining every detail of the parents' preferred management, from walking to the labour room instead of being pushed in a wheelchair, to having the vernix left on the baby. Copies of the letter are to be sent to the hospital administrator, chiefs of obstetrics, anaesthesia, neonatology, and nursing, to one's personal obstetrician and paediatrician, to one's labour assistant, and mate (Herzfeld 1985). The hope is that the patient's preferences will be respected, and also perhaps that if enough such letters are received hospital policies and practices will change in the preferred direction. There is no data on hospital staff reactions to such letters, how often women are forced to change doctors, or whether the new doctor is any better than the first one. There is some evidence, however, that women who precede their arrival in hospital with such letters actually get mistreated (Harrison 1982).

Few in the patients' movement who make such recommendations agree that they are actually *interventions* which should be subject to the same trials of efficacy and safety that are expected for drug, surgical, and technologic interventions. They, and most holistic advice givers and former members of the patients' movement who are now practitioners of 'improved pregnancy outcomes', have faith that their advice entails little loss and great potential for gain, as in Thomas Chalmers' (1986) quote of this advice of Pascal:

'Go to church every Sunday. If there is no God you will have wasted an hour a week. If there is a God you will have avoided an eternity in hell.'

Of course, some perinatal therapies and prophylactic measures have been subjected to evaluation: whether there is a sensitive period for family–infant attachment in the hours and days after birth; effects of breastfeeding versus bottle-feeding on mothers and infants; and the indications, benefits, and risks of screening tests and medications, of caesarean section and electronic fetal monitoring, and many other interventions. The maternity patients' movement has been just as guilty as have those in medicine and nursing of selective reading and uncritical adoption of recommendations published in the medical literature.

A prime example has been 'bonding research', the work led by Klaus and Kennell (1972a) on the importance of the first postpartum hours and days on family-infant attachment. Videotapes of mothers who were left alone with their naked infants in the first hours after birth showed a pattern of mutual interaction which unfolded at quite individual rates, over hours, and ceased when other people entered the room. Up to two years later mothers who had been thus treated showed distinctive alertness to their babies' cues, were less peremptory in dealing with the child, and sought more clarification from the child than did mothers who were separated from their babies in the first few hours after birth (Klaus *et al.* 1972a and b; Ringler *et al.* 1975).

In retrospect, it is surprising that mothers and their newborn babies were kept apart after birth. The effort at infection control by isolating babies in a central nursery was an anachronism, a holdover from a time when nosocomial infection and the protective, immunostimulative effects of mothers' skin, breath, and milk were poorly understood. In any case, members of the patients' movement said about family–infant separation what they said about most other aspects of 'care': the burden of proof should be on those who wish to intervene. For the patients' movement, keeping the newborn infant with the mother and family became a *cause célèbre*, second only to keeping the father with them. About ten years after the first published 'bonding' study hospitals all over the United States were assuring parents that if the baby and mother were well they could stay together, at least for a few minutes after birth in order to 'bond'. DeVries (1984) has written that 'bonding research' has had the greatest impact on obstetric care of all the patients' initiatives.

Yet 'bonding research' was over-sold, primarily by members of the patients' movement, at the same time that it was trivialized in practice, and even turned against women on occasion. Some hospital birth centres, and virtually all freestanding birth centres, do provide parents and newborns several hours alone after birth. However, in most United States hospitals 'bonding' after delivery is a 10-minute 'charade' (Klaus and Kennell 1982) which bears no relation to conditions described in the many studies. Nearly all newborns are routinely wiped, weighed, footprinted, wrapped, given prophylaxis against ophthalmic gonorrhea, and then handed to the mother to 'bond' for a few minutes. The baby is generally taken to the nursery at this point, for 'observation'. One-quarter of United States births are caesarean sections as of 1986 (Rosen 1987); another 25 per cent of neonates in the United States need intensive care due to 'prematurity' (7 per cent), 'postmaturity' (10 per cent), suspected infection (5 per cent), low Apgar score (5 per cent), or have another reason to be monitored. Thus, 'bonding' research has actually made almost no difference in the routine care of at least half of all birthing parents and newborns.

However, the effect on parents whose 'attachment behaviours' are being scrutinized may be great. Some researchers have looked for clues to future child abuse in mothers' initial responses to their babies (Gray *et al.* 1979). Mothers may undergo a 'bonding' inspection with their baby regardless of the way they feel in the moments after delivery.

How important are those first minutes and hours after birth for parent–infant bonding? Even critics of the attachment studies (Lamb 1982) have now joined the investigators (Anisfeld *et al.* 1983) in concluding that being alone with the new baby probably affects short term parent–infant attachment (Lamb 1983) and that separation may undermine attachment in a subgroup of parents who are vulnerable to parenting difficulties, including future child abuse (see Chapter 78). Yet it is those parents who are most vulnerable whose babies are most likely to be whisked away at birth (Klaus and Kennell 1982).

Klaus and Kennell concluded that most human parents are adaptable to separation from their infant at birth, and that a variety of mechanisms exist for promoting parent–infant attachment. But many mothers worry about how they will feel toward their baby (or how the baby will feel toward them). For some, early extended time alone with the new baby became a sort of blessing on the parent–child relationship, while being separated assumed the proportions of a hex.

This curse was thought by some leaders of the patients' movement to be compounded by obstetric medications. From the 1940s they had argued that too much medication was used during labour (Dick-Read 1944). In the following decades, as 'twilight sleep' was replaced by regional anaesthetics and smaller doses of systemic pain medications, some in the patients' movement maintained that all medications cross the placenta and affect the fetus and newborn, and that none had been approved by the Food and Drug Administration for obstetric use nor been 'shown' to be safe (Haire 1981, 1984). Others observed that pain medications are often used in hospitals as substitutes for bedside support during labour (Hazell 1969; Arms 1975b). During the 1960s and 1970s expectant parents who attended childbirth education classes were likely to be warned to some extent against obstetric medications.

In regard to the use of medication, childbirth education classes were apparently effective; several investigators found that women who attended them had significantly reduced intrapartum medications (Thoms and Wyatt 1951; Timm 1979; Enkin 1982) (see Chapter 20), although whether this was an effect of childbirth education itself or simply of obstetric staff co-operation with the wishes of patients is unclear. Surprisingly, no systematic studies were done on how parents felt about using or foregoing pain medication during childbirth. Nor were the effects of supportive labour companion on the use of medications ever studied, although a recent study in Guatemala (Sosa *et al.* 1980) found significantly reduced intrapartum complications when labouring women had a supportive female companion. The early monitrice organizations (Hommell 1969; Sumner 1976) have disbanded but there is recent interest among some in the patients' movement in training labour companions, who would be hired by women to be with them during labour (Shearer CA *et al.* 1987; Peddicord *et al.* 1984).

Data on the neonatal effects of obstetric drugs filtered in over a twenty-year period after the warnings of childbirth educators began. The indictment of drugs were inconclusive (Brazelton 1971; Bowes *et al.* 1970; Scanlon 1976), as were the reassuring studies (Abboud 1985; Horowitz *et al.* 1977).

Although many in the debate called for further studies, as with the 'bonding' literature, leaders of both the patients' movement and perinatal caregivers engaged in selective reading and uncritical acceptance of favoured ideas. Some saw these studies as confirmation of at least short term effects of obstetric medications on the neonate (Haire 1981, 1984), while some doctors said that if there were effects, they were not of obvious significance for the mother or baby or their relationship (Abboud 1985; Horowitz *et al.* 1977).

The breastfeeding and anticircumcision efforts of the patients' movement had somewhat less equivocal effects than did the antimedication and 'bonding' campaigns. From the mid-1960s both parents and professionals worked to promote breastfeeding; significantly more women now breastfeed upon hospital discharge (Martinez and Dodd 1983). However, some forms of 'education' and encouragement to breastfeed amount to high pressure tactics for some women and generate needless guilt when they decide to wean (Blachman 1981). Patients' groups, the American Academy of Pediatrics, and the American College of Obstetricians and Gynecologists called attention to the lack of medical indication for routine neonatal circumcision in the 1970s. By 1985 the rate of circumcisions in the United States had dropped from 95 per cent overall to 49 per cent in the west; 56 per cent in the south; 65 per cent in the north-east; and 70 per cent in the midwest (Milos 1986). Yet the four anticircumcision films shown to parents (Shearer CA *et al.* 1987) are interventions that have not been investigated for possible negative effects on parents.

In contrast, the maternity patients' movement has had little effect on the rising rate of caesarean sections, despite published support from the American College of Obstetricians and Gynecologists for a trial of labour instead of routine repeat caesarean section if the indication for the prior surgery does not repeat itself (Gleischer 1984) (see Chapters 70 and 71). Nor has the use of electronic fetal monitoring been deterred by criticism from the patients' movement or by the seven randomized controlled trials that failed to show the expected benefit of electronic fetal monitoring (Simkin 1986) (see Chapter 28). Neither patients' resistance (Shearer 1984) nor equivocal results of randomized controlled trials of routine ultrasound scanning (Eik-Nes *et al.* 1984; Bakketeig *et al.* 1984), have slowed the rate at which ultrasound scanning is used in pregnancy. Disturbing reports of sequelae of amniocentesis (Tabor *et al.* 1986) have not curbed its use either.

Simkin (1986) suggested that electronic fetal monitoring continues to be used routinely for reasons entirely apart from its clinical efficacy: increased job satisfaction due to the challenge, and the time saving conferred by electronic fetal monitoring; financial profits to medical equipment industries; belief in the efficacy of electronic fetal monitoring—that it *does* predict and prevent mental handicap and that the randomized controlled trials were flawed; and protection from blame in a malpractice lawsuit.

Many of these considerations underlie the expanding use of other interventions that have been criticized by the maternity patients' movement and its professional allies. But another important reason underlying the increased use of electronic fetal monitoring and other interventions is that women increasingly accept, and even demand them.

6 The future of the maternity patients' movement

Most of the people and organizations that remain today from the maternity patients' movement have narrowed their focus to one of the 'new professions' listed in Table 1. They are engaged in training practitioners, providing professional services, and expanding opportunities to practise, rather than in calling for evaluation and regulation of innovations in perinatal care. Indeed, they may actively discourage such trials, and suggest that they would be unethical. Such trials might fail to show that their own interventions were beneficial, or might even find unintended harmful effects.

Those few members of the 1970s patients' movement who are still active in calling for evaluation and regulation of perinatal interventions have taken aim at procedures they consider riskier than those promulgated by the 'alternative' childbirth movement of the 1970s: perinatal and neonatal screening, diagnostic routines and tests, monitoring regimes, and drug and surgical interventions. Some have taken a public education approach. The recently passed Massachusetts bill

Table 7.1 The fragmentation and professionalization of patients' movement initiatives

Read Natural Childbirth
Lamaze (Psychoprophylaxis)
The Bradley Method
Leboyer (Gentle Birth)
Holistic Childbirth Preparation
Assertive Childbirth (Birth plans)
The Kitzinger Method
Prepregnancy Classes
Early Pregnancy Classes
Fathers' Classes
Sibling Classes
Caesarean Education
Adoption Classes
Lactation Counselling
Infertility Counselling and Support
Exercise in Pregnancy Programmes
Yoga or Dance in Pregnancy and Postpartum
Fetal Awareness Classes
Prevention of Preterm Birth Classes
Infant Stimulation
Bereavement Counselling
Nurse Midwifery Practice
Hospital Alternative Birth Centres
Home Birth
Women's Health Clinics
Anti-vaccination Publicity
Freestanding Birth Centres
Parents Roles in the Ethics of Neonatal Intensive Care
Circumcision Prevention
Monitrice and Doula Programmes
Birth Under Water
Vaginal Birth After Caesarean (VBAC) Classes
Caesarean Prevention
Midwifery Licensure
Evaluation of Perinatal Procedures, Drugs, and Devices
Allocation of Perinatal Care Resources
Malpractice and Insurance Issues
Hospital and Physician Truthful Reporting and Accountability
Women's Occupational Health
Workplace Adaptation for New and Lactating Mothers

requiring hospitals to provide all registering expectant parents with their current annual rates of major interventions and outcomes is an example (Shearer EC 1986). Others lobby on a national level for evaluation and regulation of perinatal drugs and devices (Haire 1984). Some collaborate with epidemiologists and perinatal caregivers in reviewing existing data on interventions, designing trials, and publishing them (Young 1983; Shearer and Estes 1985).

One of the problems for these remaining members of the patients' movement is that the longer and more effectively they work, the more isolated they may become. These 'lay–professional' critics of perinatal care will have to ally themselves more effectively with existing consumer health advocacy organizations, and with people in perinatal care and public policy who are interested in evaluation and regulation of perinatal interventions. They will also need to use existing forums more efficiently for public education regarding the potential for harm in unevaluated procedures.

Public education in these areas has become more difficult since the 1970s. Among childbearing parents today there is more resistance to regulation of perinatal interventions because it reduces the choices available. This is of special concern to women with fertility problems who want unrestricted access to the newest technologies and to women with high risk conditions who want everything done to ensure a healthy outcome of pregnancy. These women do not see themselves as passive victims of poorly evaluated perinatal interventions but rather as responsible choosers of the best care. Nothing is more antithetical to such women than to be *randomized* to receive or to not receive an intervention; this removes all choice and generally makes them feel like human guinea pigs.

One of the most pressing challenges to the patients' movement is to make clear to both the parents and caregivers that women can avoid being 'human guinea pigs', in the worse sense of the term, if they take steps to avoid becoming involved in poorly controlled experiments. Such involvement results from seeking or acquiescing in the offers of inadequately evaluated forms of care provided outside the context of well-designed and risk-limiting controlled trials. If an inadequately evaluated intervention is only applied to a randomly selected *half* of the patients who might want or need it, this will certainly help to reveal any merits or dangers it may have; but, just as importantly, this cautious strategy will ensure that, if there are harmful effects, just *half* of these patients, and *no* future patients, will have suffered harm, not *all* of them (Chalmers 1986).

A final challenge to the patients' movement is to remain optimistic but not unrealistic in their expectations of childbearing parents as critics of perinatal care. While they do form the most numerous, identifiable contingent of patients, their patient status is quite temporary and it most often comes at a time in life when people are inexperienced with medical care, as well as with sophisticated arguments for and against most of what is recommended. While as many women resist any limitation on free choice in perinatal care, others say they would actually pay money *not* to know their test results (Berwick and Weinstein 1985); presumably many patients would rather not know the potential for harm in unevaluated perinatal interventions.

References

Abboud TK (1985). Comparison of the effects of general and regional anesthesia for cesarean section on neonatal neurologic and adaptive capacity scores. Anesth Anal, 64: 996–1001

Abdellah F (1973). New Directions in Patient-centered Nursing: Guidelines for systems of service education and research. New York: Macmillan.

Abrams R J (1986). Pioneering Women Doctors of the Past. New York: Norton.

Aikens CA (1916). Studies in Ethics for Nurses. Philadelphia: W B Saunders. p 44.

American Hospital Association (1969). Guide to the Health Care Field. Chicago: American Hospital Association.

American Hospital Association (1982). Guide to the Health Care Field. Chicago: American Hospital Association.

America Journal of Nursing (1975). Developing maternity services women will trust (editorial). Am J Nurs, 75: 10.

Anisfeld E, Curry NA, Hales DJ, Kennell JH, Klaus NH, Lipper E, O'Connor S, Siegel E, Sosa R (1983). Maternal–infant bonding: A joint rebuttal. Pediatrics, 72: 569–572.

Annas GJ (1974). The patient's rights advocate: can nurses effectively fill the role? Supervisor Nurse, 5: 21–25.

(Anonymous) (1958). Somewhere in Georgia. Ladies' Home Journal, May.

Arms S (1975a). Immaculate Deception. Houghton Mifflin: Boston.

Arms S (1975b). How hospitals complicate childbirth. Ms Magazine, May: 53.

Ashford JL (1986). A history of accouchement force: 1550–1986 Birth, 13: 241–249.

Bakketeig LS, Jacobsen G, Brodtkort CJ, Erikson BC, Eik-Nes SH, Ulstein MK, Balstad P, Jorgensen NP (1984). Randomised controlled trial of ultrasonographic screening in pregnancy. Lancet, ii: 207–211.

Barker-Benfield GJ (1976). The Horrors of the Half-known Life: Male Attitudes toward Women and Sexuality in Nineteenth Century. New York: Harper and Row.

Bean C (1977). Labor and Delivery: An Observer's Diary. New York: Doubleday.

Bean MA (1975). Birth is a family affair. Am J Nurs, 75: 10.

Berwick DM, Weinstein MC (1985). What do patients value? Willingness to pay for ultrasound in normal pregnancy. Med Care, 23: 881–893.

Bing ED (1974). Catch-22 in labor and delivery. Birth Family J, 1: 103.

Bing ED, Karmel M, Tanz A (1961). A practical training course for the psychoprophylactic method of childbirth. New York.

Blachman L (1981). Dancing in the dark. Part I and II. Birth Family J, 8: 271–286.

Bolduen C, Winerl L (1935). Infant mortality in New York City one hundred years ago. J Pediatr, 7:55–59.

Boston Lying-in Hospital (1938). Annual Report for 1934.

Boston Women's Health Book Collective (1973). Our Bodies Ourselves. New York: Simon & Schuster.

Boston Women's Health Book Collective (1976). Our Bodies Ourselves (2nd ed). New York: Simon & Schuster.

Boston Women's Health Book Collective (1984). The New Our Bodies Ourselves. New York: Simon & Schuster.

Bowes WA, Brackbill Y, Conway E, Steinschneider A (1970). The effects of medication on fetus and infant. Chicago: Monogr Soc Res Child Dev, 35: Serial 137.

Bradley R (1965). Husband-coached Childbirth. New York: Harper & Row.

Brazelton TB (1971). What childbirth drugs can do to your child. Redbook, February: p 65.

Brewer G, Brewer T (1986). What Every Pregnant Woman Should Know: The Truth about Diet and Drugs in Pregnancy. New York: Viking.

Burns D (1970). The $60 billion crisis (Lead article): Business Week, January.

Burns D (ed) (1972). The Greatest Health Discovery: Natural Hygiene and Its Evolution Past Present and Future. Chicago: Natural Hygiene Press.

Butterfield LJ (1972). Regional newborn care. Rocky Mountain Med J, 69: 53–60.

Carson R (1962). Silent Spring. Boston: Houghton Mifflin.

Cassidy-Brinn G, Hornstein F, Downer C (1984). Woman-centered Pregnancy and Birth. San Francisco: Cleis Press.

Chabon IR (1966). Awake and Aware. New York: Delacorte Press.

Chalmers I (1986). Minimizing harm and maximizing benefit during innovation in health care: controlled or uncontrolled experimentation? Birth, 14: 155–164.

Chalmers T (1986). Should smoking be banned on airplanes? McNeil-Lehrer Report. KQED, Sept 18 (interview-transcript available from KQED, 680–8th St, San Francisco, CA 94103).

Cohen NW, Estner J (1983). Silent Knife. Cesarean prevention and vaginal birth after cesarean. Massachusetts: Bergin & Garvey.

Corea G (1979). The Hidden Malpractice: how American medicine mistreats women. New York: Harper & Row.

Crowder RE, Bills ES, Broadbent JS (1950). The management of threatened abortion: a study of 100 cases. Am J Obstet Gynecol, 60: 896–899.

Cushing HW (1940). The Life of Sir William Osler, Vol 1. Oxford: Oxford University Press, p 222.

Daniels K (1986). Water Baby (Film). Point of View Productions, 2477 Folsom St, San Francisco, CA 94110.

Danreuther WT (1931). The American Board of Obstetrics and Gynecology: its organization function and objectives. JAMA, 96: 797–798.

Davis NS (1855). History of the American Medical Association from its origin up to 1855. Philadelphia: Lippincott.

DeLee JB (1920). The prophylactic forceps operation. Am J Obstet Gynecol, 1: 34–44.

Devitt N (1977). The transition from home to hospital birth: 1930–1960. Birth Family J, 4: 47–58.

DeVries R (1984). Humanizing childbirth: the discovery and implementation of bonding theory. Int J Health Services Res, 14: 89–104.

Dick-Read G (1944). The Principles and Practice of Natural Childbirth. New York: Harper & Row.

Dieckman WJ, Davis ME, Rynkiewicz LM, Pottinger RE (1953). Does the administration of diethylstilbestrol during pregnancy have therapeutic value? Am J Obstet Gynecol, 66: 1062–1081.

Dowie M, Johnston T (1977). A case of corporate malpractice In: Seizing Our Bodies: The Politics of Women's Health. Driefus C (ed). New York: Random House.

Editorial (1986). Lancet, I: 777–778

Ehrenreich B, English D (1979). For Her Own Good: 150 Years of the Experts' Advice to Women. New York: Anchor Books.

Eik-Nes SH, Okland O, Aure JC, Ulstein M (1984). Ultrasound screening in pregnancy—a randomised controlled trial. Lancet, i: 1347.

Emmons AB, Huntington JL (1912). The midwife: her future in the United States. Am J Obstet Dis Women Children, 65: 393, cited in Kobrin FE (1966) The American midwife controversy: a crisis of professionalization. Bull Med Hist, 40: 363.

Engelmann GJ (1883). Labour among Primitive Peoples. St Louis: J H Chambers.

Enkin MW (1982). Antenatal classes. In: Effectiveness and Satisfaction in Antenatal Care. Enkin MW, Chalmers I (eds). London: Heinemann.

Fenloń A, Dorchak L, Oakes E (1979). Getting Ready for Childbirth A Guide for Expectant Parents. Boston: Little Brown.

Ferguson JH (1953). Effect of diethylstilbestrol on pregnancy compared to the effect of a placebo. Am J Obstet Gynecol, 65: 592–601.

Fielding WL, Benjamin L (1962). The Childbirth Challenge: Commonsense versus 'Natural' Methods. New York: Viking.

Fisher (1909). Report on national vitality: its wastes and conservation. Bull No. 30. Committee of One Hundred on National Health. Washington DC: US Government Printing Office.

Flexner A (1910). Medical Education in the United States and Canada. New York: IV Carnegie Foundation.

Flint A (1898). The use and abuse of medical charities in medical education. Proceedings of the National Conference on Charities and Corrections, New York, p 331.

Fortune (1970). It's time to operate. Lead article: January.

Frankel LK (1927). The present status of maternal and infant hygiene in the United States. Am J Public Health, 17: 1909–1939.

Freidreich LP (1939). I had a baby. The Atlantic Monthly, 163: 461.

Gaskin IM (1978). Spiritual Midwifery. The Farm, Summertown, Tennessee: Book Publishing Co.

Gilgoff A (1978). Home Birth. New York: G P Putnam.

Gilman CP (1973). The Living of Charlotte Perkins Gilman: An Autobiography. New York: Harper Colophon Books.

Gittleson N (1961). The case against natural childbirth. Harper's Bazaar, Feb., p 33.

Gleischer N (1984). Cesarean section rates in the United States: the short-term failure of the National Consensus Development Conference in 1980. JAMA, 252: 3273–3278.

Gray J, Cutler C, Dean J, Kempe CH (1979). Prediction and prevention of child abuse and neglect. J Social Issues, 35: 127–139.

Haire D (1972). The cultural warping of childbirth. Milwaukee: International Childbirth Education Association.

Haire D (1981). Effects of prescription drugs during pregnancy. Hearing of US Senate Health Subcommittee on Investigations and Oversight of the Committee on Science and Technology. Senator Albert Gore, Chairman. Washington DC: US Government Printing Office.

Haire D (1984). How the FDA determines the Safety of Drugs: Just how safe is safe? Washington DC: National Women's Health Network.

Harrison H (1986). Neonatal intensive care: parents' role in ethical decision-making. Birth, 13: 165–174.

Harrison M (1982). A Woman in Residence. New York: Penguin Books.

Hazell L (1969). Commonsense Childbirth. New York: G P Putnam.

Hazell L (1975). A study of 300 elective home births. Birth Family J, 2: 11–16.

Herzfeld J (1985). Sense and Sensibility in Childbirth: A Guide to Negotiating Supportive Obstetrical Care. New York: Norton.

Holmes R (1936). Childbirth: nature versus drugs. Time Magazine, 27: 36.

Hommell F (1969). Natural childbirth nurses in private practice as monitrices. Am J Nurs, 69: 1446–50.

Horowitz FD, Ashton J, Culp R, Gaddis E, Levin S, Reichmann B, (1977). The effects of obstetrical medication on the behavior of Israeli newborn infants and some comparisons with Uruguayan and American infants. Child Dev, 48: 1607–1623.

Howell M (1979). Helping Ourselves. Boston: Beacon Press.

Irving FC (1942). Safe deliverance. Boston: Houghton Miflin.

Jacobi MP (1972). On female invalidism. In: Roots of Bitterness: Documents of the Social History of American Women. Cott NF (ed). New York: E P Dutton.

Jacobson E (1959). How to Relax and Have Your Baby. New York: McGraw-Hill.

Jacobson PH (1956). Hospital care and the vanishing midwife. Millbank MemFund Qtrly, 34: 253–61.

Johnson R, Siddall RS (1922). Is the usual method of preparing patients for delivery beneficial or necessary? Am J Obstet Gynecol, 4: 645–650.

Jordan B (1978). Birth in Four Cultures. St Albans, Vermont: Eden Press.

Karmel M (1959). Thank You Dr Lamaze. Philadelphia: Lippincott.

Kay MA (1982). Anthropology of Human Birth. Philadelphia: F A Davis.

Kestermann G (1980). Assessment of individual differences among healthy newborns on the Brazelton Scale. Early Hum Dev, 5: 15–27.

Klaus MH, Jerauld R, Kreger NC, McAlpine W, Steffa M, Kennell JH (1972a). Maternal attachment: importance of the first post-partum days. New Engl J Med, 286: 460–463.

Klaus MH, Jerauld R, Kreger N et al (1972b). Maternal behavior at first contact with her young. Pediatrics, 46: 187–192.

Klaus MH, Kennell JH (1982). Parent-infant Bonding. St Louis: C V Mosby, p 56.

Klein M, Westreich R (1983). Birth room transfer and procedure rates—what do they tell about the setting? Birth, 10: 93–99.

Korte D, Scaer R (1984). A Good Birth; A Safe Birth. New York: Bantam.

Lamb M (1982). Early contact and maternal-infant bonding; One decade later. Pediatrics, 70: 763–768.

Lamb M (1983). Letter, in Pediatrics, 72: 750.

Lang R (1972). The Birth Book. Santa Cruz: Genesis Press.

Leijon I, Finnstrom O (1982). Correlation between neurological examination and behavioural assessment of the newborn infant. Early Hum Dev, 7: 119–130.

Levy BS, Marine WM (1971). Reducing neonatal mortality with nurse-midwives. Am J Obstet Gynecol, 109: 50–58.

Litoff JB (1986). The American Midwife Debate. New York: Greenwood Press.

Los Angeles Times (1961). Father cited after delivery room scuffle. Jan 31, p 4.

Lubic RW (1980). Evaluation of an out-of-hospital maternity center for low risk patients. In: Health Policy and Nursing Practice. Aiken L (ed). New York: McGraw-Hill.

Lumley J (1986). A randomized controlled trial of pre-pregancy counseling. Paper presented at Birth conference, Feb. 27, San Francisco.

McKay S (1983). Assertive Childbirth: future parents' guide to a positive pregnancy. New York: Prentice-Hall.

Marieskind H (1979). An Evaluation of Caesarean Section in the United States. Washington DC: Department of Health Education and Welfare.

Martinez GA, Dodd DA (1983). 1981 milk feeding patterns in the United States during the first 12 months of life. Pediatrics, 71: 166–170.

Mead M, Newton N (1967). Pregnancy childbirth and outcome: a review of patterns of culture and future research needs. In: Childbearing: Its social and psychological aspects. Richardson SA, Guttmacher AF (eds). Baltimore, Maryland: Williams & Wilkins.

Mendelsohn RS (1979). Confessions of a Medical Heretic. Chicago: Contemporary Books.

Miller JS (1962). Child Birth: A manual for pregnancy and delivery. New York: Atheneum.

Milos M (1986). Newsletter of National Organization of Circumcision Information Resource Centers (NOCIRC), 1:3 Fall.

Moen L (1979). Bookmarks 19: Summer, ICEA. Seattle: Bookstore.

Moen L (1986). Imprints 20: Fall. Seattle: Birth and Life Bookstore.

Montgomery T (1969). The case for nurse-midwives. Am J Obstet Gynecol, 105: 309–313.

National Association of Childbearing Centers (1983). NACC News. RD 1, Box 1, Perkiomenville, PA 18074.

National Institutes of Health (1980). Caesarean Childbirth. Bethesda, Maryland: Department of Health and Welfare Publication No. 77–1079.

National Society of Patients' Representatives (1985). Patient representation in contemporary health care. American Hospital Association, PO Box 99376, Chicago IL 60693.

Nevins A, Thomas MH (eds) (1952). The Diary of George Templeton Strong: the turbulent fifties 1850–1859. New York: Macmillan, p 92.

New York Academy of Medicine (1933). Maternal Mortality in New York City: A Study of All Puerperal Deaths 1930–1932, pp 32–186.

Noble E (1983). Childbirth with Insight. Boston: Houghton Mifflin.

Nocera J (1984). A father-to-be learns how to hate Lamaze. San Francisco Chronicle, August 9: 17.

Panuthos C (1983). Transformation through Birth. Massachusetts: Bergin & Garvey.

Pearse W (1977). The home birth crisis. (July) Bulletin of the American College of Obstetricians and Gynecologists—Executive Director's Column. Chicago: ACOG.

Peddicord K, Curran P, Monshower C (1984). An independent labor support nursing service. J Obstet Gynecol Neonatal Nurs, 13: 312–316.

Peterson G, Mehl L (1982). Birthing Normally. Berkeley: Mindbody Press.

Plass ED, Alvis HJ (1936). A statistical study of 129 539 births in Iowa. Am J Obstet Gynecol, 28: 293–305.

Quilligan E J (1972). The obstetric intensive care unit. Hospital Practice, 7: 161–163.

Quint R (1975). In: Immaculate Deception. Arms S. Boston: Houghton Mifflin, p 52.

Randall CL, Baetz RW, Hall DW, Birtch PK (1955). Pregnancies observed in the likely-to-abort patient with or without hormone therapy before or after conception. Am J Obstet Gynecol, 69: 643—656.

Reid DD (1955). (Report to the medical research council by their conference on diabetes and pregnancy). The use of hormones in the management of pregnancy in diabetics. Lancet, 2: 833–836.

Rich A (1976). Of Woman Born: Motherhood as experience and institution. New York: Norton.

Ringler NM, Kennell JH, Jarvella R, Navojosky BJ, Klaus MH (1975). Mother-to-child speech at two years—effect of early postnatal contact. J Pediatr. 86: 141–8.

Rion H (1915). The Truth about Twilight Sleep. New York.

Robinson D, Shettles LB (1952). The use of diethylstilbestrol in threatened abortion. Am J Obstet Gynecol, 63: 1330–1333.

Rodholm M, Larsson K (1979). Father—infant interaction at the first contact after delivery, Early Hum Dev, 3: 21–27.

Rosen MG (1987). The cesarean crisis: physician and patient. Address given in San Francisco, February 20.

Ruzek SB (1978). The Women's Health Movement: Feminist alternatives to medical control. New York: Praeger.

Ryan GM, Gardiner SH, James LS, Quello RN, Russell KJ (1977). Toward Improving the Outcome of Pregnancy. White Plains, New York: March of Dimes Birth Defects Foundation.

Saur L (1891). Quoted in Rossi AS (ed) (1973). In: The Feminist Papers: From Adams to DeBeauvoir. New York: Columbia University Press.

Scanlon JW (1976). Effects of local anesthetic administration to parturient women on the neurological and behavioral performance of newborn children. Bull NY Acad Med, 52: 231–240.

Scully D, Bart P (1973). A funny thing happened on the way to the orofice. Am J Soc, 78: 1045–1050.

Seaman B, Seaman G (1977). Women and the Crisis in Sex Hormones New York: Bantam.

Seattle Midwifery School 2524 S 16th Seattle WA 98144.

Shaw NS (1974). Forced Labor. New York: Pergamon Press.

Shearer EC (1986). Hospital disclosure now Massachusetts law. C/SEC News, Winter: 1986.

Shearer CA, Kaufmann AS, Shearer MH, Shrock P (1987). Directory of Instructional Materials in Perinatal Education. Oxford: Blackwell Scientific Publications.

Shearer MH (1974). Electronic fetal monitoring: do the benefits outweigh the drawbacks? Birth Family J, 1: 12–18.

Shearer MH (1977). The effects of regionalization of perinatal care on hospital services for normal childbirth. Birth Family J, 4: 139–151.

Shearer MH (1980). The economics of intensive care for the full-term newborn. Birth Family J, 7: 234–241.

Shearer MH (1981). Teaching prenatal exercise: Part I Posture. Birth Family J, 8: 105–108.

Shearer MH (1983). The difficulty of measuring satisfaction with perinatal care. Birth, 10: 77.

Shearer MH (1984). Revelations: A summary and analysis of the NIH Consensus Development Conference on Ultrasound Imaging in Pregnancy. Birth, 11: 23–28.

Shearer MH, Estes M (1985). A critical review of the recent literature on post-term pregnancy and a look at women's experiences. Birth, 12: 95–109.

Shrock P, Simkin P, Shearer MH (1981). Teaching prenatal exercise Part II exercises to think twice about. Birth Family J, 8: 167–173.

Shrylock RH (1966). Medical licensing in America 1650–1965. Baltimore: Johns Hopkins Press.

Siddall AC (1980). Bloodletting in American obstetric practice 1800–1945. Bull Hist Med, 54: 101–110.

Silverman WA (1985). Human Experimentation: A guided step into the unknown. Oxford: Oxford University Press.

Simkin P, Whalley J, Keppler A (1984). Pregnancy Childbirth and the Newborn. New York: Simon & Schuster.

Simkin P (1986). Is anyone listening? Lack of clinical impact of randomized controlled trials of electronic fetal monitoring. Birth, 13: 219–222.

Smith CS (1980). Outrageous or outraged: a nurse advocate story. Nursing Outlook, 28: 624–626.

Sosa R, Kennell JH, Klaus MH, Robertson S, Urrutia J (1980). The effect of a supportive companion on perinatal problems length of labor and mother–infant interaction. New Engl J Med, 303: 597–600.

Souza M (1976). Childbirth at Home. New York: Prentice-Hall.

Spitzer WO (1984). The nurse practitioner revisited: slow death of a good idea. New Engl J Med, 310: 1049–1052.

Star RB (1986). The Healing Power of Birth. Austin, Texas: Star Publishing.

Starr P (1982). The Social Transformation of American Medicine. New York: Basic Books.

Stewart D, Stewart L (1976). Safe Alternatives in Childbirth. Chapel Hill, NC: National Association of Parents and Professionals for Safe Alternatives in Childbirth.

Stinson P, Stinson R (1979). On the death of a baby. The Atlantic Monthly, July, 64–72.

Stockham AB (1886). Tokology: a book for every woman. Chicago: Alice B Stockham & Co.

Sumner PE (1976). The home-like labor-delivery room. Connecticut Medicine, 39: 190–196.

Sweeney WJ III (1973). Woman's Doctor. New York: Morrow.

Tabor A, Philip J, Madsen J, Bang J, Obel EG, Norgaard-Pedersen B (1986). Randomised controlled trial of genetic amniocentesis in 4606 low-risk women. Lancet i: 1287–1293.

Thoms H, Wyatt R (1951). One thousand consecutive deliveries under a training for childbirth program. Am J Obstet Gynecol, 91: 205–209.

Thomson S (1825). New Guide to Health. Boston: Thomson.

Timm MM (1979). Prenatal education evaluation. Nursing Res, 28: 338–41.

Tracy M, Boyd M (1915). Painless Childbirth. New York: Frederick A Stokes.

US Department of Health and Human Services (1981a). Cesarean Childbirth. Bethesda Maryland: National Institutes of Health Publication No. 82-2067.

US Department of Health and Human Services (1981b). Graduate Medical Education National Advisory Committee. Report to the Secretary. Washington DC: Government Printing Office.

Vellay P (1959). Childbirth Without Pain. New York: E P Dutton.

Walsh A (1965). ERT (Estrogen Replacement Therapy): The Pills to Keep Women Young. New York: Bantam.

Wertz RW, Wertz DC (1979). Lying-in: A History of Childbirth in America. New York: Schocken Books.

White House Conference on Child Health and Protection (1932) Fetal newborn and maternal mortality and morbidity. New York: Century, pp 215–217.

Winslow GR (1984). From loyalty to advocacy: a new metaphor for nursing. Hastings Center Report June: 32–40.

Wright CD (1889). The Working Girls of Boston. Boston: Wright & Potter Printing.

Young D (1983). Obstetrical Intervention and Technology in the 1980s. New York: Haworth Press.

8 Women's views of care during pregnancy and childbirth

Margaret Reid and Jo Garcia

1 Introduction

This chapter reviews studies of the maternity services that have sought women's views of care. As will become apparent, the majority of these studies have used so-called 'soft' data—women's words and women's feelings—as the primary data to assess women's views. This focus upon the client's perspective forces recognition of the fact that these data can be studied in just as useful and systematic a manner as can more easily quantifiable data about pregnancy and birth. Our review covers four main areas of concern to researchers in the field of pregnancy and birth; early pregnancy, antenatal care, screening, and labour and delivery. Although there are gaps and methodological differences between studies (which will be briefly discussed) these studies have many common themes and concerns. The aim of our review is to draw out these central themes and to show that research and evaluation can no longer neglect the woman's perspective, or relegate women's views to a secondary consideration.

2 Limitations of the research

Studies that focus on the perspective of women or more rarely, their partners (Richman 1982; Brown 1982; Lewis and O'Brien 1987; Barbour, in preparation) and other relatives (Trause 1978; Anderson 1979; Lumley 1983; Maloney *et al.* 1983) are a relatively recent phenomenon. They are distinguished from previous social science research that described service users in sociodemographic, psychometric, or psychological terms. The majority of these studies have used questionnaires or interviews as the main form of data collection. In some the researcher has also used direct observation, sitting in, for example, on doctor–mother consultations at an antenatal clinic. Giving birth is often a highly charged emotional subject, about which some women may be hesitant to give their personal views. In these circumstances interviews, and to a lesser extent questionnaires, allow women to choose their own words and to put their interpretation of the events to the researcher.

Many of the studies quoted below have been carried out with relatively small numbers of women, because each interview demands a trained researcher and considerable time. Perhaps because interviews are time consuming, most studies have asked only the mother about her experience. Both the small sample sizes, and the limited inquiry into the broader social impact of the pregnancy on the whole family affect the extent to which one can generalize the findings. For example, we have very little systematically collected information about how pregnancy and birth affect the family and its routines, how older children view the experience, or indeed, because of the first-child bias of many of the studies, the consequences of becoming pregnant with second and subsequent children.

Small scale studies have other drawbacks, among them the representativeness of the subjects sampled. The studies have tended to concentrate on specific groups, delineated, for example, by social class or ethnicity. Other problems with the available research result from the lack of control groups for comparison.

Studies from different countries have tended to examine different aspects of the care in pregnancy and childbirth; in part this reflects differences in the organization of maternity care among countries. Thus, very few American studies have covered women's views of overall care in pregnancy in any depth, possibly because of the rather more individual approach to the organization of prenatal care. On the other hand, North American researchers have produced a considerable amount of work on the psychological and sociological factors associated with prenatal screening.

Unlike much medical research, where measurement often appears more reliable, psychological and sociological research has revealed that attitudes are more elusive; and it may be difficult to arrive at 'definitive' answers. As will be discussed at greater length in the section on labour and birth, women's responses about their experience of their delivery have been shown to vary, depending, among other factors, on the person asking the questions, the place of the interview and the time interval since the birth.

Finally, it must be noted that the research discussed has almost all been reported in the English language. Not all of these studies have been formally published; some have remained in the form of reports or occasional papers. A number of such unpublished studies have no doubt been missed because they did not come to our attention.

3 Early pregnancy

Both American and British studies have considered it important to include women's early views on being pregnant, although the American literature on early pregnancy is dominated by psychological or psychoanalytic approaches (reviewed by Breen 1975; Chalmers 1982). One American study reported that the majority of respondents said that they were excited and happy about their pregnancy; the first time mothers, in particular, were 'in awe at being able to conceive' (Grossman *et al.* 1980). British studies produced more cautious responses; the various projects, in which the same question was asked about first reaction to pregnancy, all found that over 50 per cent of the women were pleased (Graham and McKee 1979; Macintyre 1981; Oakley 1979).

Researchers attempted to find if the 'cool' reaction was due to an unwanted pregnancy. Gallagher (1978) found a correlation between family size and social class, noting that ideas about family life, and family and personal aspirations, obviously affected the response, a view supported by Graham and McKee (1979). Another important reason given was the awareness of what lay ahead. British researchers indicated that pregnancy, (particularly first pregnancy) heralded a change in 'self' and in lifestyle for these women, and it was this adjustment that took time.

Indeed, what lay ahead was, by some accounts, not always very pleasurable. In early pregnancy, women faced an array of minor complaints and general health problems, such as nausea and vomiting. Later in pregnancy the list of complaints changed, and sleep problems and tiredness affected a woman's social life. Some women disliked the changed body image, and what they saw as the ungainliness of the pregnant woman. Relationships with the husband changed; some drew closer, others became distant.

In several studies women were asked about advice and advice seeking during the antenatal period. While advice from professionals will be dealt with in the following section, what emerged during the early months of pregnancy was the wide availability (and the influence) in Britain of a small booklet given out at antenatal clinics and doctors' surgeries. Women expecting their first babies and women in the higher social classes were most likely to read additional material, although television programmes on the topic appeared to reach a wider audience (Graham and McKee 1979). More recent evidence about health education material in pregnancy comes from Dickinson (1985), who studied the Health Education Council's change of approach in issuing a new book *The Pregnancy Book* (1984). Dickinson reports that women generally preferred it to other leaflets they had seen, and intended to keep it. They liked the fact that it contained detailed information about pregnancy and birth.

When the literature that pregnant women receive is analysed, one message comes across clearly; the theory and the reality of the situation of pregnant women are often discrepant (Graham 1977; Graham and McKee 1979; Macintyre 1981). The literature offers a more romantic image of pregnancy and of women's circumstances than does the reality. Graham (1977) underlined the ambiguity with which pregnancy is considered in antenatal publications, the image fluctuating between pregnancy as a medical condition and pregnancy as a 'natural' or healthy state.

4 Care during pregnancy

The style and content of pregnancy care varies considerably both among and within countries. Much of the English language research into women's views is from Britain, where women receive at least part of their care in hospital antenatal clinics. North American antenatal care is rather more diverse in its organization and women's views of the kind of care they received has attracted little attention.

Concern about late attendance or missed visits is widespread, and studies from many countries have described the characteristics of women who first attended late in pregnancy or who missed some or all of the antenatal care offered (McKinlay 1970; Taffel 1978; Blondel *et al.* 1980). British survey data suggest that less than 1 per cent of pregnant women receive no formal antenatal care (O'Brien and Smith 1981; Simms and Smith 1986). While it is relatively unusual to seek the opinions of such women, some studies (Perfrement 1982; Parsons and Perkins 1980; Simms and Smith 1986) have asked women for their reasons for first attending late in pregnancy or missing their antenatal care. The largest category was frightened young women, some of whom did not admit, even to themselves, that they were pregnant. Another group identified by Parsons and Perkins (1980) consisted of women who had already had successful pregnancies, and who felt little need for professional help.

In some settings the cost of care is a further disincentive to attend. This is most apparent in the United States, where there is evidence that the proportion of women with late or no prenatal care has increased as public funding for such care is declining (Evans *et al.* 1985; Himmelstein and Woolhandler 1984; Moore *et al.* 1986) (see Chapter 14). Even where care is free, as in Britain or France, costs may be incurred by some women through lost pay or travel expenses.

Some researchers have studied the reasons that women *do* attend for antenatal care, and their expectations about care. The women interviewed by Macintyre (1981) generally felt that attending for care, and attending early, was correct, even though they were often vague about why they should do so. In another British study (Graham and McKee 1979), first and second time mothers were asked if antenatal check-ups were important. Ninety per cent said that check-ups were important, and gave medical and personal reasons for their answers. Many said that they received reassurance from their care, but a few (17 per cent) reported that they had learned nothing either about their pregnancy or about the baby. Only 31 per cent of these women said that they had enjoyed the check-up.

Women expect personal care during pregnancy, an expectation that often remains unfulfilled by institutionalized antenatal care. This may be more apparent in countries where care is state-financed and administered through hospitals rather than through the smaller and more personal setting of individual practitioner care. Research has shown that women feel undervalued as individuals in hospitals. For example, the way in which care is organized in Britain means that most women are likely to meet a large number of caregivers in the course of their maternity care. Waiting times are long, and clinics uncomfortable and lacking in facilities. Each woman's time with the doctor is often extremely short, and women often see a different doctor each time (Garcia 1982; Reid 1986).

Research from many parts of the world has reported women's need for information, and the difficulties they face in asking questions and receiving satisfactory answers. Women want to know more than they are often told about the procedures carried out during pregnancy (Cartwright 1979; Reid and McIlwaine 1980; Macintyre 1982; Dickinson 1985; Oakley 1979). While the official ideology has been one of openness and free exchange of information, with caregivers providing the answers to consumers' questions (Kirke 1980), the reality has been rather different. One researcher reported that during the course of an interview study many requests for information about pregnancy and birth were made by respondents to the interviewers; altogether the 60 mothers in the study made 664 such requests (Oakley 1979), which strongly suggests that the caregivers were not adequately responding to women's perceived needs.

One problem that has arisen particularly for women receiving clinic rather than individual practitioner care is the impression of 'busyness' that makes questioning difficult. Women are aware of the queue that is building up behind them, and gain the impression that the clinic is not a place for relaxed discussion. When women do succeed in asking questions, the answers are sometimes in the form of bland reassurance rather than the provision of information. (Oakley 1980; Macintyre 1982).

As Riley (1977) has pointed out, different women want different kinds of experiences and different kinds of information about their pregnancies and birth. It can be difficult for caregivers to provide information in a way that fits with a woman's individual wishes as well as with her particular knowledge of medical terms (Perfrement 1982). Macintyre (1982) has pointed out that euphemisms can be misleading, and that caregivers tend to use them more when talking to working class women than to middle class women.

The issue of medical records is related to that of information giving. The usual procedure, in which women leave their records in the hands of the caregivers after consultations, often results in them being asked the same questions by several different caregivers (Macintyre 1981), as well as leaving them frustrated by their own lack of information. Giving the woman a summarized 'co-operation card' does not really solve the problem. Women have difficulty in reading the abbreviated notes on their summarized record. Two experimental comparisons of programmes in which women held their own obstetric records with the conventional systems (Elbourne *et al.* 1987; Lovell *et al.* 1987) showed that women who held their own record felt in control of their antenatal care (Table 8.1), more able to communicate effectively with their caregivers (Table 8.2), and would want to hold their maternity record in another pregnancy (Table 8.3). The authors also estimate that fewer records were lost or unavailable

Table 8.1 Effect of women carrying their own case-notes while receiving antenatal care on not feeling 'in control' during pregnancy

Study	EXPT		CTRL		Odds ratio	Graph of odds ratios and confidence intervals
	n	(%)	*n*	(%)	(95% CI)	0.01 0.1 0.5 1 2 10 100
Elbourne DR *et al.* (1987)	66/132	(50.00)	79/120	(65.83)	0.52 (0.32–0.86)	
Lovell A *et al.* (1986)	76/97	(78.35)	91/102	(89.22)	0.45 (0.21–0.95)	
Typical odds ratio (95% confidence interval)					0.50 (0.33–0.76)	

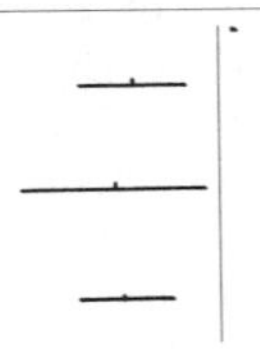

Table 8.2 Effect of women carrying their own case-notes while receiving antenatal care on poor communication with staff

Study	EXPT		CTRL		Odds ratio	Graph of odds ratios and confidence intervals
	n	(%)	*n*	(%)	(95% CI)	0.01 0.1 0.5 1 2 10 100
Elbourne DR *et al.* (1987)	84/132	(63.64)	95/120	(79.17)	0.47 (0.27–0.81)	
Lovell A *et al.* (1986)	85/97	(87.63)	93/102	(91.18)	0.69 (0.28–1.70)	
Typical odds ratio (95% confidence interval)					0.52 (0.33–0.83)	

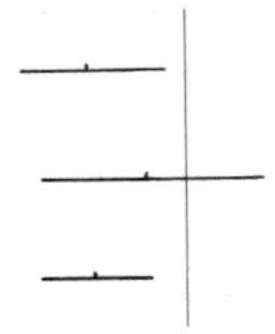

Table 8.3 Effect of women carrying their own case-notes whilst receiving antenatal care on 'preference for different care in future'

Study	EXPT		CTRL		Odds ratio	Graph of odds ratios and confidence intervals
	n	(%)	*n*	(%)	(95% CI)	0.01 0.1 0.5 1 2 10 100
Elbourne DR *et al.* (1987)	11/123	(8.94)	44/106	(41.51)	0.17 (0.09–0.31)	
Lovell A *et al.* (1986)	19/95	(20.00)	66/101	(63.35)	0.16 (0.09–0.28)	
Typical odds ratio (95% confidence interval)					0.16 (0.11–0.25)	

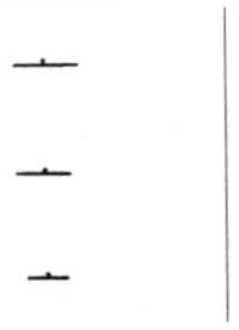

when required in the experimental (women-held) groups.

A common finding of many of the studies of women's views of care throughout the childbearing period has been the lack of respect shown by the caregivers, both to the women themselves, and to their family commitments and responsibilities. Graham (1984), for example, has drawn attention to women's attempts to follow medical advice about smoking or paid work, while at the same time fulfilling their responsibilities to the other family members (see Chapter 16). Researchers have also drawn attention to the need to take women's worries about the so-called minor complaints of pregnancy seriously (Oakley 1980) (see Chapter 32), and have reported on the discomfort engendered by the more subtle verbal and non-verbal signals that caregivers sometimes send in a busy clinic setting (Perfrement 1982; Oakley 1980).

For women who may be seen as in some way deviant, staff attitudes become even more crucial. One small study by Coyne on pre-16-year-old pregnant girls, revealed a mixture of experiences, some finding the staff supportive, while others reported hurtful and disapproving attitudes (Coyne (no date)). Women who are black or from other minorities may have special needs in maternity care (Homans and Satow 1982) and may experience difficulty in obtaining adequate and supportive care (Larbie 1985; Cornwell and Gordon 1984; Save the Children Fund 1983). If maternity care providers are concerned at the poor uptake of antenatal care in particular subgroups of the population, they should first consider the barriers to attendance. They can also take encouragement from some of the practical examples of ways that care can be made less threatening and more respectful of women's needs and circumstances. Dowling (1983) provides a general review;

Cornwell and Gordon (1984) and Winkler (1983) look at advocacy schemes for women from ethnic minorities; and Evans and Parker (1985) and Nunnerly (1985) describe clinics and classes set up for teenage women.

5 Pregnancy and screening

In the last decade there has been a growing interest in the social consequences of antenatal screening tests on the woman and her family, as will be seen in the remainder of this section. This may be related to the fact that the number of possible antenatal screening tests has increased rapidly in recent years (Rubin *et al.* 1983) (see Chapters 3 and 23).

In this section we shall divide screening into two sections, first concentrating upon diagnostic tests routinely undertaken during pregnancy, and later considering those tests used less routinely.

5.1 Routine screening

Routine pregnancy tests are so embedded in the pattern of antenatal care that women are scarcely aware of them (Macintyre 1981; Boyd and Sellars 1982). Virtually all women who attend either their general practitioner or a hospital antenatal clinic (or both) undergo a range of minor tests such as blood pressure, urinalysis and haemoglobin testing. Researchers have tended to be rather dismissive of these minor tests. The majority of studies reported in this chapter relate to British antenatal care, but this in no way suggests that such tests are confined to British practice. A recent survey of antenatal screening tests in European Community countries indicates that many more tests are routine in some European Community countries than in Britain (Heringa and Huisjes, 1988).

An important finding of many studies was that women wished to have more information than was normally given. There was a tendency for doctors to give women general reassurance about the test, rather than a proper explanation. If routine tests were used in non-routine situations, however, there was more likelihood of an explanation (Draper *et al.* 1984; Perfrement 1982). Macintyre (1981), asked fifty first time mothers about blood and urine sampling. She reported 'None refused to give, or queried the need for, samples of blood or urine, although most disliked providing samples and did not know their purpose' (Macintyre 1981, p. 135). Another British researcher asked women if they could name the antenatal checks they underwent during antenatal care and explain their purpose. She found that women's understanding of their tests rose as the pregnancy progressed (Perfrement 1982). Studying fetal kick charts, Draper and her colleagues (1984) found that while 98 per cent of the women complied, only 53 per cent were reassured. Nearly one quarter of the women surveyed worried about filling in the chart, in part because they did not fully understand the rationale for the task. The studies, thus, point to a high degree of compliance among pregnant women, but also a considerable lack of comprehension about the reasons for what they were asked to do.

Perfrement (1982) also asked women about their knowledge of the reason for vaginal examinations. She found that over half of the women could either give only one reason for the internal examination, or did not know why it was carried out at all. Women with more education could give more reasons. From the available literature (in a country where internal examinations are relatively infrequent) it seems that women dislike undergoing internal examinations. The women interviewed by Oakley (1979) reported their feelings of embarrassment at some length. Other researchers have also noted the discomfort with which women face such an examination (for a recent study and review of the literature on vaginal examinations, see Areskog-Wijma 1987). Women also want to be told about the risks of the test involved. For example, a number of women were alarmed at having a vaginal examination early in pregnancy (Macintyre 1981; Perfrement 1982).

One implication of the finding that women wished to know more about the often simple tests that they undergo at the clinic is that there is a lack of congruence between the amount of information that they desire and the amount that they are given. In an Australian study, Shapiro and her colleagues (1983) found that 84 per cent of the women they interviewed wanted to know about fetal deformities, while only 21 per cent of doctors correctly identified the women's desire for such information. Although most women have access to booklets and written information about pregnancy, clinics are often organized on the basis of 'only those who ask are told' (Reid *et al.* 1982). Shapiro and her colleagues explicitly note the class bias in this process: 'The lower the class of patient the less likely was the respondent to obtain the information she wanted' (Shapiro *et al.* 1983). A similar point is made by Cartwright (1979).

Finally, women are seldom told the results of their routine tests. It is assumed that they will understand that all is well unless they are told otherwise. While experienced mothers may understand this hidden rule (like the other rules that operate in antenatal care) ignorance of it may cause an unknowing mother to be unnecessarily concerned.

5.2 Non-routine testing

The availability and use of non-routine testing varies considerably both among and within countries. Availability is influenced partly by incidence of the particular disease, which has been shown to vary geographically; for example, Schnittger and Kjessler (1984) in Sweden, and Adams *et al.* (1981) and others in the United States have noted regional variations in screening for neural tube defects. However, attendance for testing has also been shown to depend upon a variety of other factors including physician and patient knowledge and patient age and class. (Lippman-Hand and Cohen 1980; Thomassen-Brepols *et al.* 1982; Schnittger and Kjessler 1984).

Non-routine tests, by their nature, cause women more concern than routine ones. If a woman is asked to undergo a non-routine test, such as amniocentesis, this may raise the fear that all is not well with the pregnancy. Women may be anxious about many aspects of the test, including possible injury to the baby caused by the test, possible miscarriage, pain, uncertainty about the test procedure, and the possibility of having to make a decision about terminating the pregnancy (Davies and Doran 1982; Finley *et al.* 1977; Golbus *et al.* 1974; Young and Young 1980). Families who had already experienced a previous fetal deformity reported an even higher level of anxiety (Robinson *et al.* 1975).

These studies show that, on average, the more information women receive, the less anxious they become. Support, as well as information, can be helpful when a women undergoes amniocentesis. Social support from friends and family has been shown to help, especially when the woman had friends or met other women who had the test (Robinson *et al.* 1984; Marion *et al.* 1980). Counselling from the clinic has also been shown to help (Finley *et al.* 1977; Nielson 1981; Robinson *et al.* 1975; Verjaal *et al.* 1982), although women have reported that genetic counselling, while technically good, did not lessen the psychological and emotional aftermath of the test (Davies and Doran 1982).

Supportive social interactions are important throughout the woman's contact with clinic staff. Having a partner with one at the time can help to reduce the anxiety (Milne and Rich 1981). Women value good social interactions in relation to many test procedures, including vaginal examinations (Oakley 1979), ultrasound (Hyde 1986; Jorgensen *et al.* 1985) or amniocentesis (Rothman 1986). Anxiety can be raised or reduced by the approach adopted by the technician or doctor administering the test (Campbell *et al.* 1982). Simple explanation and time spent on reassurance is well repaid: women report greater satisfaction with the whole procedure (Boyd and Sellars 1982; Nielson 1981).

Since most non-routine tests are more complicated than the usual routine screening measures, women report more anxiety about the procedure itself. Women like to know what is involved in the test procedure, and become anxious if they do not know (Milne and Rich 1981; Nielson 1981; Silvestre and Fresco 1980). Not all procedures turn out to be unpleasant; women have told researchers that being able to see and 'hear' the baby with ultrasound was very satisfying (Draper *et al.* 1984; Milne and Rich 1981; Perfrement 1982; Verjaal *et al.* 1982). Tests such as amniocentesis, however, which involve the removal of amniotic fluid raise fears in women about possible pain or harm to the fetus (Beeson and Golbus 1979; Davies and Doran 1982; Finley *et al.* 1977; Young and Young 1980). Rothman (1986) emphasizes the difficulties faced by the mothers who, through the combined use of ultrasound with amniocentesis are given the opportunity to see the fetus they may have to abort. She argues that the result can be a 'tentative pregnancy' until the results are confirmed.

Far more importance is attached to the results of non-routine than to those of routine tests and several authors have dealt with the results and aftermath of special tests (mostly amniocentesis). To summarize these findings, women wished to receive the report of results as quickly, and as personally as possible. They appreciate letters or telephone calls more than being left to assume that if not informed, all is well, but most of all prefer to be told in person (Fearn *et al.* 1982). Results, if normal, reduce the anxiety of both parents; if abnormal, they herald a new series of anxieties and decisions that must be made about the future of the pregnancy and the baby (Lippman-Hand and Fraser 1979; Blumberg *et al.* 1975). Few researchers have studied the effects of false positive (or false negative) results. One study by Burton and her colleagues (1985) shows that measured anxiety following a false positive alphafetoprotein (AFP) test was high and that the anxiety persisted until normal results were reached by further testing.

New developments in antenatal screening, such as chorion villus sampling for the early diagnosis of Down's Syndrome and other chromosomal abnormalities, may result in the need for some women to begin antenatal care considerably earlier than is presently the case. To have chorion villus sampling at eight weeks of pregnancy a woman must recognize her pregnancy within the first few weeks, and make contact with the maternity services almost immediately. In countries where referral from primary to specialist obstetric care is the usual pattern, both women and primary care-givers must be aware of the existence of early pregnancy diagnostic and screening tests. A lack of awareness of the facilities and their purpose may hinder good usage (Duncan 1978). There is at present considerable uncertainty about the degree of risk involved with the procedure. Lippman *et al.* (1985) reported that the women in their study liked the idea of early information about the fetus obtained by chorion villus sampling, provided that the risk of the procedure was not greater than that associated with amniocentesis. Small increases in the risk to their pregnancies would, however, change their preference.

6 Care around the time of birth

There is extensive research literature about women's

views of care during labour and childbirth. Three aspects in particular are addressed by this research: the place of birth, the style of care and the question of choice and power relations. There are a number of methodological difficulties in research in this field, an important one being the difficulty of determining women's immediate experiences of labour and delivery at the time that they occur. Women's views of the experience change over time (Erb *et al.* 1983; Bennett 1985). In addition, the type of answers received depend upon the place of asking and on the form of the questions (Lumley 1985; Oakley 1985; Shaw 1985). Researchers have also discussed the methodological difficulties which arise when women's views of specific techniques or interventions are studied (Garel and Kaminski, 1986; Shearer, 1983; Garcia *et al*, 1985; Lumley, 1985; Garel and Crost, 1982; Orleans 1985).

Another important dilemma for researchers concerns the interpretation of reported satisfaction with care (Lumley 1985). Service users may not find it easy to envisage alternatives to the care with which they are familiar and so may 'prefer' familiar styles of care (Porter and Macintyre 1984). Expectations and priorities influence women's reactions to care (McIntosh 1989). Studies can yield findings that later provoke some surprise. For example, a hospital-based interview study carried out in the United States in the mid-1970s reported, among other findings, that 72 per cent of respondents were satisfied with being strapped down during delivery (Light *et al.* 1976).

A telephone survey commissioned by the Canadian Medical Association (1986) was carried out on 2013 Canadian women who had a live birth in the previous 24 months. The survey reported that 96 per cent of the respondents were 'very satisfied' or 'somewhat satisfied' with their practitioner; over 90 per cent were satisfied with labour and delivery care, regardless of whether or not their prenatal practitioner had been present. Ninety-one per cent were satisfied with labour and delivery regardless of whether their expectations had been met. As acknowledged in the survey report, 'In interpreting these results it should be recognized that these women had up to two years to reflect on their experience of childbirth and obstetrical care. Certain issues may have been of more immediate and critical concern to them at the time of birth; others may have attained greater importance on reflection and in comparison with the experience of other women'.

6.1 Place of birth

Research about the place of delivery involves either asking women about their present choice of place of delivery (for example, home, hospital, or birth centre), or asking their preference for a future birth. In Britain, where less than 1 per cent of women have a planned home birth, women's preferences were very much affected by their experiences. In a study of 65 women who had expected a hospital birth, but who had their babies at home because of a hospital strike, 80 per cent of respondents said that they would like to have their next baby at home, in spite of some initial disappointment when they heard that they could not go to hospital (Goldthorp and Richman 1974). Cartwright (1979) found that of the small minority of women for whom the survey birth had been at home, 91 per cent would choose home for a subsequent birth. Of those who gave birth in hospital, 83 per cent would choose hospital the next time. The findings indicate some interest in home birth among those who had not experienced it. Those mothers who had the survey baby at home reported higher levels of satisfaction with several aspects of their care (O'Brien 1978). For example, they were more likely to be satisfied with their pain relief, less likely to be left alone by the caregiver(s), more likely to find the caregiver helpful about their worries during labour, and more likely to say that the caregivers were very helpful generally.

In the North American context the main alternatives to conventional hospital birth are home birth or birth in some kind of birthing room, either within or outside an obstetric hospital. These alternatives reflect a growing interest in a less technological and more flexible approach to birth and also reflect the high cost of hospital care to the individual (Romalis 1985). Studies asking women about their preferences or choices produce the unsurprising finding that families choose alternative birth settings either because of their dissatisfaction with the technological and social features of conventional hospital obstetrics or, more positively, because of a desire for natural childbirth or care from a midwife (Field 1985; McClain 1983). A representative sample survey of women delivering in a Canadian health district in 1978 (Hancock 1980) found that just over half the respondents would consider an alternative birth setting although they preferred an in-hospital birth centre as opposed to a separate birth centre or a home birth. A later study of a more selected Canadian sample (Hilditch *et al.* 1986) showed a stronger preference for alternatives to conventional care, but in-hospital birth centres were again preferred. In another Canadian study of eighty women choosing hospital birth and eighty choosing a home birth (Hodnett 1983, 1986), women in the home birth group were more likely to achieve their preferences for analgesia and anaesthesia, were less likely to say that they felt ashamed of their behaviour during labour and were more likely to report that they were treated as individuals during labour and birth.

6.2 Style of care

The growth of maternity pressure groups (see Chapter 7) and the increasing debate about the place of birth have both had an impact on the style of care in conventional hospital settings. In another chapter in this book (see Chapter 50) evidence is presented about the wide variation in hospital policies. While the move towards what is called 'family centred care' (Hanvey and Post 1986) can be observed in maternity, neonatal and children's wards, studies that have commented upon the father's role at birth (Brown 1982; Cartwright 1979; Danziger 1979b; Macintyre 1982; Richman 1982) have reported on some of the problems that arise when new policies are too rigidly applied. Authors have pointed out the mixed messages that fathers receive at birth; on the one hand their attendance is expected, while on the other, they are often made to feel awkward or marginal.

Attitudes of parents in relation to some of the other aspects of access to and contact between parents and the newborn have also been studied. Studies of maternity hospital length of stay (Burnell *et al.* 1982; Blondel *et al.* 1983) (see Chapter 78) show that women had widely varying preferences for, and satisfaction with, the length of their postnatal stay. These studies suggest that a move away from fixed lengths of stay to a flexible approach based on a woman's preference and circumstances would be beneficial. Williams (1985) who interviewed eighty women in two British hospitals about their postnatal stay in hospital noted that the length of stay was of less concern to these women than was the quality of postnatal care that they received.

6.3 Choice and power relations

In addition to their concern about family centred care, consumer groups have emphasized the themes of choice and power relations in childbirth. Their interest in these themes sometimes arose from the experiences of some members who have been subjected to obstetrical procedures to which they did not consent. Interview and observational studies of labour care have revealed examples where procedures such as amniotomy or episiotomy were carried out without informing the woman (Henderson 1984; Perfrement 1982; Oakley 1979) (see Chapter 51), and in some cases against her expressed wishes (Perfrement 1982). More generally, however, researchers have focused on women's perceptions of the degree of choice that they had; on their comments about the information that was available to them or that they felt they needed in order to make choices.

A picture of polarization between the medical model and the women's view of childbirth has been presented by several authors, including Nash and Nash (1979) and Graham and Oakley (1981), (see Chapters 6 and 7). Their argument is that while members of the medical profession see pregnancy as a kind of illness, and labour and delivery as a process that should be controlled by professionals, women themselves wish to see pregnancy as a natural condition, and birth as a natural process in which little interference from professionals should occur. Other researchers, however, have suggested that the professional/client split is more complex. Nelson (1983), for example, looked in detail at social class and women's preferences about aspects of labour care. In her study of 322 middle and working class North American women, she found that over 90 per cent of the whole sample had considered what they wanted in respect to a companion during labour and their first contact with the baby, although they had given less thought to some of the medical aspects of their care. Working class women were less likely to have thought about these procedures. In the event, all women had high levels of intervention. Working class women were more likely to have the kind of labour they wished for, that is, with considerable monitoring, including electronic fetal monitoring. Middle class women suffered a greater discrepancy between what they wished (little intervention) and their subsequent experience, although they were more likely than working class women to have their wishes respected concerning enemas, medication, and the presence of a companion.

In a Scottish study (McIntosh 1989) working class, first time mothers were interviewed once in late pregnancy and on several occasions after the birth. Their attitudes do not conform to a model of childbirth as natural and fulfilling. More than three-quarters had negative expectations of childbirth (62 of 88). Fear of pain was a major component of this expectation. Sixty per cent wanted pain relief and some of those who did not were afraid of the pain relief itself, or of its consequences for the baby. After the birth women were asked what they would wish for in future birth. Only six out of 80 expressed a desire for an 'intervention-free' birth. In another Scottish study (Reid *et al.* 1982) many working class women interviewed as part of a study of a community antenatal clinic, expressed an interest in epidural analgesia because of their concern to avoid pain in labour if at all possible.

In a large British study (Cartwright 1979) women were asked to assess retrospectively the adequacy of their knowledge about events around the time of birth. This study showed that while working class women were less likely than middle class women to report that they had discussed aspects of labour care with a caregiver antenatally, they also mentioned a larger number of items concerning labour about which they would have liked more information. Similar results were obtained in a smaller North American study (Shapiro *et al.* 1983). Cartwright (1979) also highlights the extra desire for information among those for whom all had not gone well, either during labour or when a baby had been admitted for special care.

A few studies have observed decision-making and information exchange during labour (Danziger 1979a; Kirkham 1983; Garforth and Garcia 1987; Oakley

1979; Barbour, in preparation; Henderson 1984). These studies are small, but provide examples of the ways that parents and caregivers interact. They reveal dilemmas for both parties. Parents found that staff fell into standard responses to questions about their progress and prospects, and developed devices for cutting short difficult discussions (Kirkham 1983). Caregivers sometimes intended to offer choice, but did it in a way that made it hard for the parents to exercise real choice.

The caregivers, however, may well find themselves faced with parents whom they do not know, and who are already under some strain. The extent of the parents' knowledge about labour and labour care may vary considerably, and they may go through changes of mind as they encounter different stages of labour (Flint 1986). People differ and change in the extent to which they wish to be consulted by caregivers about aspects of care (Cartwright 1979; Henderson 1984) (see Chapter 9).

7 Conclusions

The diversity of opinion reflected in the various studies should not be overlooked. The views of some women are not necessarily shared by all women. The opinions of service users are increasingly likely to be assessed when new techniques and services are evaluated. The views of parents are now more often than before included alongside the medical, administrative, and economic evaluation of care during pregnancy and childbirth. It is to be hoped that this trend will continue, and that the research agenda will increasingly reflect the priorities of childbearing families.

References

Adams M, Finley S, Hansen H, Jahiel R, Oakley G, Sanger W, Wells G, Wertelecki W (1981). Utilization of prenatal genetic diagnosis in women of 35 years of age and older in the United States 1977–1978. Am J Obstet Gynecol, 139: 673–677.

Anderson SVD (1979). Siblings at birth: A survey and a study. Birth Family J, 6: 80–87.

Areskog-Wijma B (1987). The gynaecological examination: women's experiences and preferences and the role of the gynaecologist. J Psychosom Obstet Gynecol, 6: 59–69.

Barbour R (in preparation). Fathers: The emergence of a new consumer group. In: The Politics of Maternity Care. Garcia J, Kilpatrick R, Richards M (eds). Oxford: Oxford University Press.

Beeson D, Golbus M (1979). Anxiety engendered by amniocentesis. Birth Defects, 15: 191–197.

Bennett A (1985). The birth of a first child: Do women's reports change over time? Birth, 12: 153–158.

Blondel B, Kaminski M, Breart G (1980). Antenatal care and maternal demographic and social characteristics: evolution in France between 1972 and 1976. J Epidemiol Community Health, 34: 157–163.

Blondel B, Garel M, Breart G, Sureau C (1983). La sortie précoce des femmes après l'accouchement. J Gynecol Obstet Biol Reprod, 12: 457–460.

Blumberg B, Golbus MS, Hanson KH (1975). The psychological sequelae of abortion performed for a genetic indication. Am J Obstet Gynecol, 122: 799–808.

Boyd C, Sellars L (1982). That's Life Survey of the British Way of Birth. London: Pan.

Breen D (1975). The Birth of the First Child: Towards an Understanding of Femininity. London: Tavistock.

Brown A (1982). Fathers in the labour ward: medical and lay accounts. In: The Father Figure. McKee L, O'Brien M (eds). London: Tavistock.

Burnell I, Elbourne D, McCarthy M, Chamberlain G, Hawkins D (1982). Patient preference and postnatal hospital stay. J Obstet Gynaecol, 3: 43–7.

Burton BK, Dillard RG, Clark EN (1985). The psychological impact of false positive elevations of maternal serum alpha-feto protein. Am J Obstet Gynecol, 151: 77–82.

Campbell S, Reading AE, Cox DN, Sledmere CM, Mooney R, Chudleigh P, Beedle J, Ruddick H (1982). Ultrasound scanning in pregnancy: the short term psychological effects of early real time scans. J Psychosom Obstet Gynecol, 1: 57–61.

Canadian Medical Association (1986). Obstetrics '87: a report of the Canadian Medical Association on obstetrical care in Canada. Can Med Assoc J, Mar 15: 136 (suppl).

Cartwright A (1979). The Dignity of Labour? London: Tavistock.

Chalmers B (1982). Psychological aspects of pregnancy: some thoughts for the eighties. Soc Sci Med, 16: 323–331.

Cornwell J, Gordon P (1984). An Experiment in Advocacy: The Hackney Multi-Ethnic Women's Project. London: Kings Fund Centre.

Coyne A-M (no date). Schoolgirl Mothers. London: Health Education Council, Research Report No. 2.

Danziger SK (1979a). On doctor watching—field work in medical settings. Urban Life, 7: 513–532.

Danziger SK (1979b). Treatment of women in childbirth: implications for family beginnings. Am J Public Health, 69: 895–901.

Davies B, Doran TA (1982). Factors in women's decision to undergo genetic amniocentesis for advanced maternal age. Nursing Res, 31: 56–59.

Dickinson R (1985). Publicising Pregnancy Care: An evaluation of the Pregnancy Book campaign. Leicester: Centre for Mass Communication Research, University of Leicester.

Dowling S (1983). Health for a Change: the provision of preventive health care in pregnancy and early childhood. London: Child Poverty Action Group.

Draper J, Field S, Thomas H (1984). An evaluation of a community antenatal clinic. Hughes Hall, Cambridge (unpublished report).

Duncan SLB (1978). Problems of a prenatal screening programme for Down's syndrome in older women. J Biosoc Sci, 10: 141–146.

Elbourne D, Richardson M, Chalmers I, Waterhouse I, Holt

E (1987). The Newbury Maternity Care Study: a randomised controlled trial to evaluate a policy of women holding their own obstetric records. Br J Obstet Gynaecol, 94: 612–19.

Erb L, Hill G, Houston D (1983). A survey of parents' attitudes towards their cesarean births in Manitoba hospitals. Birth, 10: 85–91.

Evans F, Hess C, Guyer B, Rosen SL (1985). Infant Health Status in Massachusetts. Mass J Community Health, Spring/Summer: 3–13.

Evans G, Parker P (1985). Preparing teenagers for parenthood. Midwives' Chron, 98: 239–240.

Fearn J, Hibbard BM, Robinson JO (1982). Screening for neural-tube defects and maternal anxiety. Br J Obstet Gynaecol, 89: 218–221.

Field PA (1985). Parents' reactions to maternity care. Midwifery, 1: 37–46.

Finley S, Varner P, Vinson P, Finley W (1977). Participants' reactions to amniocentesis and prenatal genetic studies. JAMA, 238: 2377–2379.

Flint C (1986). Sensitive Midwifery. London: Heinemann.

Garcia J (1982). Women's views of antenatal care. In: Effectiveness and Satisfaction in Antenatal Care. Enkin M, Chalmers I (eds). London: Spastics International Medical Publications, Heinemann Medical Books.

Garcia J, Corry M, MacDonald D, Elbourne D, Grant A (1985). Mothers' views of continuous electronic fetal heart monitoring and intermittent auscultation in a randomized controlled trial. Birth, 12: 79–85.

Gallagher E (1978). Infants, Mothers and Doctors. Lexington, Massachusetts: Lexington Books.

Garel M, Crost M (1982). L'analgésie péridural: Le point de vue des femmes. J Gynecol Obstet Biol Reprod, 11: 523–533.

Garel M, Kaminski M (1986). Psycho-social outcomes of caesarean childbirth. In: Perinatal Care Delivery Systems: Description and evaluation in European Community Countries. Kaminski M, Breart G, Buekens P, Huisjes H, McIlwaine G, Selbmann HK (eds). Oxford: Oxford University Press.

Garforth S, Garcia J (1987). Admitting—a weakness or a strength? Routine admission of a woman in labour. Midwifery, 3: 10–24.

Golbus MS, Conte F, Schneider EL, Epstein CJ (1974). Interuterine diagnosis of genetic defects: results, problems and follow-up of one hundred cases in a prenatal genetic detection centre. Am J Obstet Gynecol, 18: 897–905.

Goldthorp WO, Richman J (1974). Maternal attitudes to unintended home confinement. A case study of the effects of the hospital strike upon domiciliary confinements. Practitioner, 212: 845–853.

Graham H (1977). Images of pregnancy in antenatal literature. In: Health Care and Health Knowledge. Dingwall R, Heath C, Reid M, Stacey M (eds). London: Croom Helm.

Graham H, McKee L (1979). The first months of motherhood. Report of a Health Education Council Project concerned with women's experiences of pregnancy, childbirth and first months of life. York: University of York (unpublished).

Graham H (1984). Women, Health and the Family. Brighton: Harvester Press.

Graham H, Oakley A (1981). Competing ideologies of reproduction: Medical and maternal perspectives on pregnancy. In: Women, Health and Reproduction. Roberts H (ed). London: Routledge & Kegan Paul.

Grossman FK, Eichler LS, Winickoff SA (1980). Pregnancy, Birth and Parenthood. London: Jossey-Bass.

Hancock T (1980). A Matter of Balance: alternative approaches in maternity care and childbirth. Toronto: A Report for the Peel District Health Council.

Hanvey L, Post S (1986). Changing patterns in maternity care. Canadian Nurse, Sept., 28–32.

Health Education Council (1984). The Pregnancy Book. London, Health Education Council.

Henderson C (1984). Some facets of social interaction surrounding the midwife's decision to rupture the membranes. MA dissertation, University of Warwick.

Heringa M, Huisjes H J (1988). Prenatal screening: current policy in European Community Countries. In: Antenatal Screening: Current Policies in the European Community and evaluation. Huisjes HJ, Buekens P, Reid M (eds). Eur J Obstet Gynecol Reprod Biol (suppl).

Hilditch J, Hodnett E, Norton P (1986). Birth Centre Evaluation Fomulation Proposal. Final report. Ontario Ministry of Health.

Himmelstein DU, Woolhandler S (1984). Pitfalls of private medicine: Health care in the USA. Lancet, Aug. 18, 391–394.

Hodnett E (1983). The effects of person-environment interactions on selected childbirth outcomes of women having home and hospital births. Ph.D thesis, University of Toronto.

Hodnett ED; Abel SM (1986). Person-environment interaction as a determinant of labor length variables. Health Care for Women International, 7: 341–356.

Homans H, Satow A (1982). Can you hear me? Cultural variations in communication. J Community Nursing, Jan: 16–18.

Hyde B (1986). An interview study of pregnant women's attitudes to ultrasound scanning. Soc Sci Med, 22: 589–592.

Jorgensen C, Uddenberg N, Ursing I (1985). Ultrasound diagnosis of fetal malformation in the second trimester: The psychological reactions of the women. J Psychosom Obstet Gynaecol, 4: 31–40.

Kirke PN (1980). Mothers' views of obstetric care. Br J Obstet Gynaecol, 87: 1029–1033.

Kirkham M (1983). Labouring in the dark: Limitations on the giving of information to enable patients to orient themselves to the likely events and timescale of labour. In: Nursing Research—Ten studies in patient care. Wilson-Barnett J (ed). Chichester: John Wiley.

Larbie J (1985). Black Women and the Maternity Services. London: Training in Health and Race.

Lewis C, O'Brien M (eds) (1987). Reassessing Fatherhood. London: Sage.

Light HK, Solheim JS, Hunter GW (1976). Satisfaction with medical care during pregnancy and delivery. Am J Obstet Gynecol, 125: 827–831.

Lippman-Hand A, Fraser F (1979). Genetic Counselling—the post counselling period 1. Parents' perceptions of uncertainty. Am J Med Genetics, 4: 51–71.

Lippman-Hand A, Cohen D (1980). Influence of obstetricians attitudes on their use of prenatal diagnosis for the detection of Down's Syndrome. Can Med J, 122: 1381–1386.

Lippman A, Perry TB, Mandel S, Cartier S (1985). Chorionic Villi sampling: women's attitudes. Am J Med Genetics, 22: 395–401.

Lovell A, Zander LI, James CE, Foot S, Swan AV, Reynolds A (1987). The St Thomas's Maternity Case Notes Study: A randomized controlled trial to assess the effects of giving expectant mothers their own maternity case notes. Paedtr Perinat Epidemiol, 1: 57–66.

Lumley L (1983). Preschool siblings at birth: short term effects. Birth, 10: 11–16.

Lumley J (1985). Assessing satisfaction with childbirth. Birth, 12: 141–145.

McClain CS (1983). Perceived risk and choice of childbirth service. Soc Sci Med, 17: 1857–1865.

McIntosh J (1989). Models of childbirth and social class: a study of 80 working class primigravidae. In: Midwives, Research and Childbirth. Robinson S, Thomson A (eds). London: Chapman and Hall.

McKinlay JB (1970). The new late comers for antenatal care. Br J Prev Soc Med, 24: 52–57.

Macintyre S (1981). Expectations and experiences of first pregnancy. Occasional Paper No. 5. Aberdeen: MRC Medical Sociology Unit.

Macintyre S (1982). Communications between pregnant women and their medical and midwifery attendants. Midwives' Chron, November, 387–394.

Maloney MJ, Ballard JL, Hollister L, Shank M (1983). A prospective controlled study of scheduled sibling visits to a newborn intensive care unit. J Am Acad Child Psychiatry, 22: 565–570.

Marion JP, Kassam G, Fernhoff PM, Brantley KE, Carroll L, Zacharias J, Klein L, Priest LH, Elsas LT (1980). Acceptance of amniocentesis by low income patients in an urban hospital. Am J Obstet Gynecol, 138: 11–15.

Milne LS, Rich OJ (1981). Cognitive and affective aspects of the responses of pregnant women to sonography. Maternal–Child Nursing J, 10: 15–39.

Moore TR, Origel W, Key TC, Resnik R (1986). The perinatal and economic impact of prenatal care in a low-socioeconomic population. Am J Obstet Gynecol, 154: 29–33.

Nash A, Nash JE, (1979). Conflicting interpretations of childbirth: the medical and the natural perspectives. Urban Life, 7: 493–512.

Nelson M (1983). Working class women, middle class women and models of childbirth. Social Problems, 30: 284–297.

Nielson CL (1981). An encounter with modern medical technology: women's experiences with amniocentesis. Women and Health, 16: 109–124.

Nunnerley R (1985). Teenage dilemma. Midwives' Chron, 98: 244–248.

Oakley A (1979). Becoming a Mother. Oxford: Martin Robertson.

Oakley A (1980). Women Confined: Towards a Sociology of Childbirth. Oxford: Martin Robertson.

Oakley A (1985). Doctors, maternity patients and social scientists. Birth, 12: 161–166.

O'Brien M (1978). Home and hospital: a comparison of the experiences of mothers having home and hospital confinements. J R Coll Gen Pract, 28: 460–466.

O'Brien M, Smith C (1981). Women's views and experiences of antenatal care. Practitioner, 225: 123–125.

Orleans M (1985). Lessons from the Dublin study of electronic fetal monitoring. Birth, 12: 86.

Parsons W, Perkins ER (1980). Why don't women attend for antenatal care? Nottingham: Leverhulme Health Education Project, Occasional Paper No. 23.

Perfrement S (1982). Women's Information on Pregnancy, Childbirth and Babycare. Sussex: Centre for Medical Research, University of Sussex.

Porter M, Macintyre S (1984). What is, must be best: a research note on conservative or deferential responses to antenatal care provision. Soc Sci Med, 19: 1197–1200.

Reid M (1986). Non-medical aspects in the evaluation of prenatal care for women at low risk. In: Perinatal Care Delivery Systems: Description and Evaluation in European Community Countries. Kaminski H, Breart G, Buekens P, Huisjes H, McIlwaine G, Selbmann HK (eds). Oxford: Oxford University Press.

Reid ME, McIlwaine GM (1980). Consumer opinion of a hospital antenatal clinic. Soc Sci Med, 14A: 363–368.

Reid ME, Gutteridge S, McIlwaine GM (1982). A comparison of the delivery of antenatal care between a hospital and a peripheral clinic. University of Glasgow.

Richman J (1982). Men's experiences of pregnancy and childbirth. In: The Father Figure. McKee L, O'Brien M (eds). London: Tavistock.

Riley EMD (1977). What do women want? The question of choice in the conduct of labour. In: Benefits and Hazards of the New Obstetrics. Clinics in Developmental Medicine No. 64. Chard T, Richards M (eds). London: Spastics International Medical Publications/Heinemann Medical Books.

Robinson J, Tennes K, Robinson J (1975). Amniocentesis: its impact on mothers and infants; a 1-year follow-up. Clin Genet, 8: 97–106.

Robinson JO, Hibbard BM, Laurence KM (1984). Anxiety during a crisis: emotional effects of screening for neural tube defects. J Psychosom Res, 28: 163–169.

Romalis S (1985). Struggle between providers and recipients: the case of birth practices. In: Women, Health and Healing. Lewin E, Oleson V (eds). London: Tavistock.

Rothman BK (1986). The Tentative Pregnancy. Prenatal Diagnosis and Future of Motherhood. New York: Viking Penguin Books.

Rubin SP, Malin J, Maidman J (1983). Genetic counselling before diagnosis for advanced maternal age: an important medical safeguard. Obstet Gynecol, 62: 155–159.

Save the Children (1983). The Health of Traveller Mothers and Children in East Anglia. London: Save the Children.

Schnittger A, Kjessler B (1984). Alpha-feto protein screening in obstetric practice. Acta Obstet Gynaecol Scand (Supplement), 119: 25–31.

Shapiro MC, Najman JM, Chang A, Keeping JD, Morrison J, Western JS (1983). Information control and the exercise of power in the obstetrical encounter. Soc Sci Med, 17: 139–146.

Shaw I (1985). Reactions to transfer out of hospital birth centre: a pilot study. Birth, 12: 147–150.

Shearer M (1983). How do parents really feel after caesarean birth? Birth, 10: 91–92.

Silvestre D, Fresco N (1980). Reactions to prenatal diagnosis: an analysis of 87 interviews. Am J Orthopsychiat, 50: 610–617.

Simms M, Smith C (1986). Teenage mothers and their partners. Department of Health and Social Security Research Report No. 15. London: Her Majesty's Stationery Office.

Taffel S (1978). Prenatal Care in the United States, 1969–1975. Hyattsville, Maryland: National Centre for Health Statistics (DHEW publication No. (PHS) 78–1911).

Thomassen-Brepols LJ, Jahoda MGJ, Drogendijk AC, Galjaard H (1982). De lage opkomst in Nederland van oudere aanstaande Moeders voor prenatale diagnostick. Ned Tijdschr Geneeskd, 126: 2262–2266.

Trause MA (1978). Birth in the hospital—the effect on the sibling. Birth Family J, 6: 80–87.

Verjaal M, Leschot NJ, Treffers PE (1982). Women's experience with second trimester prenatal diagnosis. Prenatal Diagnosis, 2: 195–209.

Young D, Young RS (1980). Antenatal diagnosis. A patient study. J South Carolina Med Assoc, 76: 391–393.

Williams L (1985). Parents' views of maternity discharge policies. Dissertation, Middlesex Polytechnic (unpublished).

Winkler F (1983). Advocacy in health: racial minorities and maternity services. Radical Community Medicine, No. 16: 51–54.

9 Caregivers in pregnancy and childbirth

Raymond G. DeVries

1 Introduction

From a physiological point of view, human birth is quite similar to birth among other of earth's creatures. From a social point of view, human birth is unique. Because humans use symbols and create culture (Cassirer 1944) the context of human birth is unlike other creatures. Caregivers are an important part of that context. A few other species co-operate in nest building and in the care of the very young, but none separate a class of individuals to give care in pregnancy and childbirth and none have the highly systematized patterns of care found in human culture (Trevathan 1987). Patterns of care, however, vary considerably across cultures (see Chapter 6). The diversity is so great that care in one culture might not be recognized as care by members of another culture. When members of one culture confront the practices of another, they may be left scratching their heads, wondering how women survive childbirth.

This observation underscores the need to recognize the importance of culture in the provision of care at birth. Culture specifies the care available, but it also socializes and educates, creating the desire for a particular style of care. A woman from the Yucatan would be extremely ill at ease in a high technology hospital and would likely have a difficult birth there. Similarly, a housewife from Omaha or Glasgow would have great difficulty giving birth on a hammock or dirt floor.

Most caregivers regard themselves as members of a special sort of occupational group known as a profession. Professionals are distinguished by their prolonged and specialized training, by their submission to an ethical code developed and policed by the profession, and by their attitude of public service. Professions develop in characteristic ways; and although social scientists disagree about the motivators and outcomes of professionalization, they agree that this process is accompanied by increased authority of the professional, more effective organization of the occupation, and increased distance between those who give and those who receive care (Freidson 1986).

In this chapter, I examine the role of caregivers in pregnancy and childbirth, describing different types and identifying the forces that shape their availability, attitudes and performance. I begin by looking at the evolution of caregiving. Next I consider individual caregivers, including midwives, general and family practitioners, obstetricians, and a handful of emerging occupations, examining their motivation, socialization, and practice. Because it allows a close look at the professionalization of caregivers at birth, I provide a detailed comparison of nurse midwives and lay midwives as seen in the United States. This comparison provides a model for understanding the way caregiving at birth is shaped by professionalization and other social forces. To conclude I explore the power of caregivers to shape society's views of birth and the ways in which caregivers are constrained by social structure.

2 The evolution of care in pregnancy and childbirth

The history of caregiving in pregnancy and childbirth cannot be separated from political and social history. Styles of care are influenced by such things as patterns of immigration (Declerq and Lacroix 1985), social notions of the desirability of children (DeVries 1987), social movements (Ruzek 1978), and technological developments. Changes in the care of pregnant and childbearing women mirror changes in other parts of society, evolving in characteristic ways: from indigenous, folksy forms of care to sophisticated, professional care; from care given by generalists to care given by a variety of specialists; from non-technological to technological care. The modernization of caregiving in pregnancy and childbirth shifted the responsibility for care from family members and friends, to experienced midwives, and then to physicians, and finally on to obstetrical specialists.

In the brief history that follows, it is possible to identify three phases in caregiving: passive, active, and the most recent phase, 'controlled' caregiving. The passive phase was marked by a wait and see attitude. Little was done apart from support, encouragement, and the use of folk wisdom. With the advent of scientific medicine, care moved into a modern and active phase characterized by a readiness to intervene and by reliance on technology. Caregiving is, at least in the United States, currently moving into a third, controlled phase, marked by an 'active passivity'. Controlled care believes in non-intervention, and yet it is intrusive in its use of monitoring technology to anticipate and control intervention.

The turn towards restraining intervention is consistent with developments in society. Several observers note a widespread dissatisfaction with the over-use of technology and a general rejection of bureaucratic organization, and see this as evidence that society is moving into a 'postmodern' period (Cox 1984; Gablik 1984). Postmodernism questions science-based technology, endorses decentralized organization and acknowledges the validity of the experiential and spiritual dimensions of life, all of which are emphasized in new models of controlled and monitored care such as alternative birth rooms and centres.

The evolution of caregiving can be understood as a change in the relationship of caregiving to nature. Caregiving moved from a fatalistic view where nature overwhelmed care, to an exertion of power over nature. The active model offers caregivers power over nature and has proved effective in treating once untreatable complications of pregnancy. Controlled care seeks to work with nature and requires giving up some of that power. Controlled care recognizes that the experiential and spiritual dimensions of birth cannot be manipulated by the caregiver. The following history of caregiving shows no model to be absolute. There is overlap between models, and in practice, any one caregiver might draw on elements of all three.

It is not my intention to provide a definitive history of caregivers in pregnancy and childbirth. Several such histories, each with a different perspective, are available. The obstetric profession's history of itself is provided by Cianfrani (1960). Feminist revisions of this history are offered by Kobrin (1966), Ehrenreich and English (1973), Oakley (1976), Donegan (1978), and Wertz (1983). Shorter (1982) provides a revision of this revisionist history, suggesting that obstetric science saved women from ignorant midwives. Less polemic histories are offered by Wertz and Wertz (1977), Donnison (1977), Litoff (1978, 1986), Arney (1982), Oakley (1984), Scholten (1985), Leavitt (1986), and Towler and Bramall (1986). DeVries (1985) provides a history of the regulations governing midwives. Sorel (1984) gives a collection of personal and historical narratives on childbirth and Figes (1987) offers an interesting piece of historical fiction on English midwifery.

2.1 The rise of caregiving: from passive to active midwifery

The earliest distinct, non-family caregivers at birth were midwives. One of the oldest stories concerning midwives comes from the Jewish captivity in Egypt. The character of midwifery at that time is revealed by an account of the refusal of a group of midwives to obey an order by the Pharaoh to kill all male children born to the Hebrews. When the Pharaoh demanded an explanation for this disobedience, a spokeswoman for the group replied, 'The Hebrew women are not as the Egyptian women; for they are lively and are delivered ere the midwives come in unto them' (Exodus 1: 19). The Pharaoh's acceptance of this rather lame excuse is enlightening, for as Samuel Gregory noted in 1848, 'Even this tyrant dared not invade their sacred office to make special inquisition' (Gregory 1974: 7).

The Western midwife's autonomy was first challenged in the sixteenth century with the appearance of regulatory measures. The church was the primary agent of midwife regulation in medieval Europe; by the eighteenth century, municipal and state regulation predominated. Unlike modern legislation, which requires mastery of a specific body of knowledge, church regulation was more concerned with the social and religious aspects of midwifery; it required character witnesses, not technical examinations (Forbes 1966: 127; Oakley 1976: 23–30). The midwife's independence was further undermined by male involvement in birth, which began in a systematic way in the sixteenth and seventeenth centuries. Although culture still dictated that assistance at birth be provided by females, males proved useful in emergencies. Typically, barber-surgeons, who by virtue of guild membership had exclusive right to the wielding of surgical instruments, were called to assist in the most complicated cases. These ministrations were often disastrous for the mother and child as well as for the reputation of the male attendant. The gradual encroachment of an all-female domain by doctors and other males met some resistance, but the public was fascinated with and had increasing faith in the technology monopolized by males. The stage was set for a more active caregiver.

The invention of the forceps is generally acknowledged as the crucial factor in the rise of men to dominance as caregivers at birth (Rousch 1979; Litoff 1978: 7; Donnison 1977: 21–22). Midwives did not adopt the forceps and were reluctant to identify themselves with techniques and instruments characteristic of an activist male midwifery.

In America, the midwife played an important role at birth until the early twentieth century. At that point activist obstetrics and regulation combined to nearly eliminate her practice. Physicians generated a flood of articles and addresses on 'the midwife problem', spawning a rash of legislation restricting and regulating midwifery (Kobrin 1966). The number of midwives practising in New York City dropped from 1700 in 1919 to 170 in 1939, and finally to just 2 in 1957 (Kobrin 1966; Speert 1968). Professional belief and a sense of rivalry prompted the negative evaluation of midwives by physicians. Physicians believed in the benefits of the active approach and wanted to end the more passive approach of midwives. Commenting on the choice of titles for the many critical articles—most were variations of the 'Midwife Problem' rather than the 'Infant and Maternal Mortality Problem', Devitt (1979) believes that they reflect the desire of physicians for the expansion of their profession and the elimination of midwifery.

American physicians rejected the European idea of upgrading midwifery through education because it promulgated a double standard of obstetrics. The passive and the active models of care could not coexist. Two American physicians commented on the passage of the 1902 midwifery licensing law in England: 'The Midwife Bill . . . has given England a fairly well trained cleanly midwife, in place of the dirty midwife and the careless practitioner, but it has not instituted a new system, and in the light of modern medicine, it is of questionable advantage to the community, for it provides a double system in obstetrics, the midwife but scantily trained, depending upon the physician who is not certain to respond to her call. Some 30 000 women have taken enough practice away from physicians to obtain a livelihood. Unquestionably the field of physicians has been invaded and the community is the loser' (Emmons and Huntington 1911).

As physicians replaced midwives as the pre-eminent caregivers at birth, the place of birth shifted from home to hospital. Doctors preferred hospital birth for several reasons: it was convenient, eliminating the need to travel from home to home; it allowed access to equipment; the presence in hospitals of nursing staff and social workers eliminated the need for physicians to offer social support; and it provided a steady supply of patients for physicians in training (Wertz and Wertz 1977: 144–145).

The evidence suggests that styles of care influence public attitudes and that public attitudes and cultural themes influence styles of caregiving. Modernism supported the trends in caregiving during the first half of this century: the rise in popularity of hospital birth, the demise of home birth, the decline of the midwife, the proliferation of new techniques for intervening in and controlling childbirth and a sharp increase in the number of surgical deliveries. The modern mind is characterized by faith in science and technology and belief in the efficiency of bureaucratic rationalism (Cox 1984). Thus 'modern' women suffragists in America proclaimed the benefits of hospital birth and demanded access to the anesthetic technique of 'twilight sleep' (Wertz and Wertz 1977: 132–177) and in the 1950's women insisted that they be given diethylstilboestrol to prevent 'accidents of pregnancy' (Apfel and Fisher 1984).

Three significant changes characterize the shift from passive, premodern care to modern, active care at birth. First, care was rationalized. Styles of care moved from the realm of art to the realm of science. The science of birth was built on the canons of the empirical method and replaced a pot-pourri of legends and folk wisdom. Second, care moved from non-bureaucratic to bureaucratic settings, from the unstructured environment of the home to the organization of the hospital. Third, caregivers lost a measure of integration with the community because, coming from external professional education systems, they no longer served in the communities where they were raised. The catalyst for all these changes was clearly scientific and technological development. Scientific training became the sine qua non of caregiving, making personal familiarity between client and caregiver irrelevant.

Two aspects of this invasion of caregiving by science need further exploration: first, how scientific is 'science'?; and second, why was the public willing to accept a new 'scientific' approach to caregiving? Science has always been somewhat Janus-faced. The benefits won by a scientific method that formulates hypotheses and verifies (or falsifies) them by experimental test generate strong public faith in science. But this well earned prestige is easily abused. Unscrupulous medical merchants refer to their techniques and paraphernalia as 'scientific'. Even the scrupulous allow the mantle of science to justify techniques not subject to scientific scrutiny. True science becomes a 'science' that is useful to its practitioners. The transformation of birth by science did require complicity on the part of the public—a complicity that was achieved by the promise of medicine to control and reduce, perhaps eliminate, the risks of birth.

2.2 The demise of modernism and the rise of controlled care

Whereas modernism favoured the growing obstetric specialty, over the last two decades physicians and medical organizations have had to come to terms with the challenge of a postmodern culture that questions the 'benefits' of modernism. Consumers are influenced by a postmodern context that includes the feminist movement, a questioning of technology, renewed emphasis on naturalness and on the spiritual dimension of life, and serious concern about the rising cost of medical care. The generation giving birth over the last fifteen years lived through an era marked by civil disobedience, race riots, public protests over the war in Vietnam, and the call 'back to nature'. The resulting sensitivity to the abuse of power by institutions, sexism in medicine, and the benefits of naturalness led to questions concerning interventionist medical routines for birth (see Chapter 7). Active caregiving, which consumers had demanded a few decades previously, was now regarded as sexist, costly, overly technological, dangerous, and ignorant of the social, psychological, and spiritual needs of patients. There was a call for 'alternative', 'humanized' birth and for caregiving that did not separate birth from the rest of life.

The 'humanizing' of birth reflects a shift in focus from the product to the experience of birth. Among earlier generations, the primary concern in birth was with the health of mother and child. This attitude allowed activist obstetrics to flourish because it was a product oriented approach, promising better techniques for healthier babies. As birth became less dangerous and yielded better results, and as the nature of parents changed, concern shifted to the experiential elements of birth. Birth became not just a way to produce an heir, but a key experience for personal growth (Levesque-Lopman 1983). Obstetric routines that hindered that experience were challenged. A new model was needed, one in which caregiving was more controlled, one that used careful monitoring and practised restrained intervention.

Focus on experience places caregivers in a bind. It is difficult for focus on experience to coexist with focus on a healthy product: one or the other must take precedence. Writing in the *Journal of the American Medical Association*, two physicians note: 'We believe that certain priorities in the birthing process must be maintained if rational decisions regarding birth environments are to be made. The first priority is a live and healthy mother; the second, a live and healthy baby; and *third*, a psychologically rewarding experience for the parents and the baby' (Adamson and Gare 1980, emphasis added).

When the demands of consumers conflict with the tenets of medicine, caregivers find it difficult to give in. One reaction to this situation is an attempt by 'modern' caregivers to transform the desires of 'postmodern' parents into the terms of medicine. Parents come to medicine wanting to enhance the experience of birth, demanding less use of technology, more contact with their infant, and more emphasis on the relational aspects of birth. Medicine responds by scientizing experience, treating experience as any other variable that influences the outcome of birth. Experiences become quantifiable variables which can be incorporated as outcomes in randomized trials (Chalmers 1986). Arney and Bergen (1984) regard medicine's newly found interest in experience as a logical consequence of the evolution of medical technique. As the utility of looking into the body to solve health problems diminished, attempts to more fully understand and promote health adopted an ecological approach. The medical gaze was shifted from the body to the environment, to experience.

2.3 Controlled care: medicalized or demedicalized birth?

Controlled caregiving seeks to maximize experience without sacrificing product. This requires extending the bailiwick of medicine beyond physical ailments to the monitoring of personal habits, significant life transitions, and even private morality. The expansion of medical jurisdiction is a cause of concern to some who see it as medicalization, the extension of medical control of life (Zola 1972; Illich 1976).

Medicalization of birth was inherent in the activist model of caregiving. 'Modern' caregivers believed birth to be a dangerous event in need of medical supervision, a belief that also influenced public views. Kobrin (1966) observes that American obstetricians early in this century 'argued again and again that normal pregnancy and parturition are exceptions and that to consider them normal physiologic conditions was a fallacy'. An instructional book for expectant mothers published in 1935 warns: 'To consider childbirth as normal and natural is in a sense misleading, as every woman in childbirth is potentially a major surgical case. The risk of an emergency is always present whether with the first baby or the fifth. Therefore, in every maternity case selection of the doctor is as vital as it would be in a case of pneumonia or appendicitis' (Heaton 1935: 209).

Once birth was accepted as a risky and abnormal event, the task was to grade the level of risk in order to better plan its management. The gradation of risk allows for the controlled caregiving of the postmodern era. Levels of risk make it possible to divide tasks among medical personnel and to selectively use technology. High risk births are attended by highly trained experts; low risk births are handled by midwives and other lesser trained personnel and can be accomplished in birth rooms and other less technological settings. The most highly trained personnel monitor the situation by setting the parameters of risk, giving them the ability to control the flow of clients (Riessman and Nathanson 1986).

It is possible to regard recent concern with parent–infant bonding and alternative birth centres as marketing strategies of caregivers. Faced with a bevy of criticism and a small but worrisome trend toward home birth (Yankauer 1983), medicine needed an acceptable avenue of response. Study of attachment and bonding (see Chapter 78) provided that avenue (DeVries 1984). Attachment was easily subjected to scientific study and led researchers to the conclusion that there were important reasons to focus on the experiential aspects of birth (Klaus and Kennell 1976, 1981; Klaus *et al.* 1972; Kennell *et al.* 1974). This evidence gave key medical organizations acceptable grounds for restructuring hospital birth. In their 'Statement on parent and newborn interaction', the American Medical Association (1977) said: '. . . increasing evidence has accumulated to support the concept of an "attachment and bonding" process in the human race. It is timely to review all hospital procedures and professional practices for their appropriateness and thereby encourage the hospitals to reassess their policy in support of the bonding principle.' The sentiments of the American Medical Association were mirrored in a 1978 report, 'The development of family centered maternity/newborn care in hospitals', prepared by an Interprofessional Task Force composed of obstetricians, pediatricians, hospital representatives, and nurses (American College of Obstetricians and Gynecologists 1978). Thus was born the alternative birth centre. These centres promise enhanced parental control over birth, but ironically they can function to increase caregiver control of the experience.

Birth in alternative birth centres follows the model of controlled care; low risk patients are carefully monitored and protocols that define risk subject patients to medical authority (DeVries 1980 and 1983). Physicians and midwives also control the experiential dimension, 'helping mothers to love their babies' (*British Medical Journal* 1977; Ounsted *et al.* 1982; Jenkins and Westhus 1981; Rising 1974). Thus controlled care is something of an irony. It uses technology to reduce technology; the technology of monitoring and risk management allows some women to have less technological, less medical births.

3 The choice to give care in pregnancy and childbirth and the caregiving career

As society changes and as our knowledge of pregnancy and birth evolves, the requirements of compassion are altered. Those seeking to provide compassionate care to women in 1990 will approach their task differently from those who had the same desire in 1940. The desire to be compassionate is constant, but the operationalization of that desire is changed. The most obvious changes are those in the technical side of care, but there have also been important changes in the way the caregiving task is conceived by society.

It was once common to refer to one's life work as a vocation or a calling. Regarding one's occupation as a calling implies a moral dimension, because response to a call implies responsibility to a higher authority (Gustafson 1982). 'Premodern' caregivers saw their job as a vocation, a task they were called to do. By way of contrast, modern practitioners are professionals. Although some professionals might feel 'called', the defining criterion of caregiving is no longer motivation, but mastery of a technical body of knowledge. The word professional is rooted in the moral realm (as in a 'profession' of faith), but in current usage its connotations include a sense of the crass, one who performs a task simply for monetary reward as opposed to an amateur, who is involved for love and desire (Freidson 1986). Gustafson (1982) points out that a call is no substitute for the knowledge required to be a professional, but he adds that without a calling professionalization is empty, amoral, and unfulfilling.

A variety of factors causes an individual to choose a career in caregiving. These motivational factors determine the type of training that is sought and the style with which that training is applied. For example, the style of care offered by a woman who chose to become a midwife after an unpleasant hospital birth will differ from the style of care given by an obstetrician who chose his specialty as a fourth-year medical student after concluding that his first choice, surgery, was too bloody and too depressing. Although by definition motivations are personal, it is possible to observe characteristic motivations for different types of caregivers.

Motivation spills over into socialization. The motivations of the midwife and the obstetrician referred to above lead them to different educational programmes; in turn, these programmes direct and reinforce motivation. Socialization includes both technical training and informal, almost invisible, education in proper role behaviour. Novice caregivers learn techniques and appropriate ways of acting, and acquire proper attitudes about the clients they serve. The processes of education for different caregivers differ sharply and play a crucial role in defining the care offered.

Caregiving is also influenced by the type of clients seen by each practitioner. Consumers sort themselves according to their knowledge and desires, hence different types of caregivers see different types of clients. The type of client seen and the typical demands of that type of client influence patterns of care. As competition for clients becomes keener, caregivers may position themselves in the medical marketplace, with different caregivers having different strategies for marketing.

3.1 Midwives

3.1.1 A split in the ranks

Midwifery is unique among the caregiving occupations that are discussed, because, at least in the United States, there are two distinct categories of midwives: those with training in both nursing and midwifery, and those trained solely in midwifery. This is not the case everywhere. In The Netherlands, midwifery schools bear no relationship to nursing schools. Not only do they provide an entirely different type of training, gaining admission to one of the three midwifery schools in the country may be hampered by a prior training in nursing. In the United Kingdom, midwives trained in direct-entry (i.e. non-nursing) programmes work alongside midwives schooled in nursing. In the United States, however, certified nurse midwives rarely work with midwives who have not had a nursing training (variously referred to as lay or empirical midwives). This split in the ranks is unfortunate for the health care system, but fortuitous for the sociologist. It allows comparative analysis of the influence of motivation, socialization, and clientele on the profession. Given this advantage I will explore midwifery in the United States in depth, extending the analysis to midwives in other locations and then on to other occupations.

A certified nurse midwife in the United States is a registered nurse who has completed an additional course of training in obstetrics lasting between one and two years. In 1984 there were an estimated 2300 nurse midwives in the United States who could practise legally in 49 of the 50 states. In that year 26 schools offered training in nurse midwifery and together they produced about 250 graduates every year (Rooks and Haas 1986). Lay midwives have a more practical orientation toward birth and are often regarded as not being legitimate practitioners. While a few schools do exist for lay midwives (Baldwin 1979), their training is less formal and it usually consists of some combination of apprenticeship and self-education. Because lay midwives often practise without a licence, even in locations where licences are issued, there is no official record of their numbers.

The regulations which control midwifery reflect the differences between the two categories of midwives. Thanks to the efforts of their professional association, the American College of Nurse Midwives, the laws governing nurse midwives are fairly uniform across states. On the other hand, lay midwives, with no effective national organization, are regulated by a different set of statutes in each state. The legal status of lay midwifery varies radically from state to state and is constantly changing. According to a recent report, 21 states permit lay midwives to practise (Stickles 1986; Sallomi *et al.* 1981; Evenson 1982; Throne and Hansen 1981). Some of those states have formal licensing programmes which require schooling and involve state sponsored entry examinations; others simply require would-be midwives to register with the county or state.

In order to isolate the influence of the social context on the care offered by nurse and lay midwives, I will compare these two types of caregivers in four general areas: the nature of the practitioner; the nature of the client; the characteristics of the midwife-client relationship; and the structuring of the birth experience. Although the categories are presented distinctly, they overlap and interact.

3.1.2 The nature of the practitioner

The motivations and education of these two types of caregivers differ significantly. Lay midwives often come to the profession after giving birth at home or after witnessing home births. Training is usually acquired through a combination of self-education and apprenticeship. This training nurtures and sustains a naturalistic, non-interventionist view of birth assistance. Although health professionals are sometimes relied upon for training in seminars and workshops, the lay midwife's sceptical attitude toward organized medicine insulates her from the subtle propagandizing found in formal educational programmes. Training by apprenticeship supports a less fragmented approach to birth because the subject is not segmented into areas of study such as physiology, pharmacology, or anatomy. Lay midwives do not reject the knowledge made available by obstetric science, but they (and others) resist a view of birth that ignores its spiritual dimension or suggests that birth can be treated in a routine manner. In her book, *Spiritual Midwifery*, Gaskin (1978: 11) presents a view of birth that illustrates this orientation: 'The knowledge that each and every childbirth is a spiritual experience has been forgotten by too many people in the world today, especially in countries with high levels of technology . . . it is our basic belief that the sacrament of birth belongs to the people and that it should not be usurped by a profit-oriented hospital system'. This view of birth is reflected in attitudes toward training (Merz 1977): 'No matter how it is that a person acquired midwiving techniques, there is an element to being a midwife that cannot be taught. It is a gift, and one that must be shared to truly come to life'. The patterns of recruitment and training used by lay midwives are supportive of a view that maintains that the body is capable of giving birth with little or no outside intervention. In cases where intervention is required, it is most often a natural intervention; for example, to help ease the baby's head out of the birth canal, these midwives will use hot oil massages instead of episiotomies; to stimulate labour, they give their clients raspberry or cohosh tea rather than oxytocin (Peterson 1983).

The educational programmes mandated by licensing laws affect the type of person who chooses to become a midwife as well as her perception of the birth process. In contrast with lay midwives, to become a nurse midwife, an individual must first be a registered nurse and then complete a nationally approved educational programme in midwifery. By the time a nurse midwife is ready to practise, she has had a minimum of 6 years of specialized training: 4 years in an accredited school of nursing, 1 year or more job experience, and at least 1 year or more of midwifery education (Brennan and Heilman 1977: 16–17). Such educational requirements restrict entry into the profession and begin a socialization process that supports a more 'scientific' view of birth.

Only those with the resources necessary to survive a lengthy period of training can hope to achieve the status of certified nurse midwife. A recent study of applicants to nurse midwifery educational programmes made the interesting observation that nearly 70 per cent had no children (Warpinski and Adams 1979). This indicates that, in contrast to lay midwives, the majority of nurse midwives acquire their knowledge of childbirth in a medical setting rather than from personal experience. Arms (1977: 198–99) comments on the consequences: 'Nursing school, like medical school, teaches that pathology, not the normal is expected. In her education as a nurse, the nurse midwife is taught to expect anything and everything to go awry in birth, and she has a lusty respect for modern forms of interference which will protect a woman from her own working body . . . She is no longer the guardian of normal birth and watchful servant of mothers. She is a registered nurse with a postgraduate degree in a specialty called midwifery . . . She believes that the physician, not the birthing mother, knows best and holds the power to heal. By training, she sees life as a physician does, full of problems, abnormalities and complications'. In describing her experience with similarly trained British midwives, Comaroff (1977) confirms the observations of Arms. She notes that midwives view pregnancy as a 'condition akin to physical illness, suitably treated in terms of medical intervention'. Rothman (1982: 245–48 and 1983) also hints at the medical nature of the certified nurse midwife when she observes that home births 'radicalize' nurse midwives. She points out that nurse midwives who enter home delivery practice must relearn what constitutes a normal birth.

In examining the changing role of the midwife in Great Britain, Walker (1972) identifies other important changes that accompany licensure. She regards the British midwife's loss of independence as a threat to 'the continuation of midwifery as such, as distinct from obstetrics' (Walker 1972). In particular, she sees midwives as 'limited practitioners' (Wardwell 1972), who have been strongly affected by two factors: the concentration on the hospital for maternity care and the trend toward team-work in health care. Her perspective on British midwifery has direct application to American midwifery. Walker (1972) notes that as the use of domiciliary care declined, midwives became involved with several people other than their clients. In earlier days the midwife dealt primarily with her client; there was little interaction with doctors, supervisors, or other midwives. The modern midwife must interact with these people. This holds true both for the hospital-based and the few remaining domiciliary midwives.

Walker's analysis applies equally well to the licensed nurse midwives in America. Even the relatively autonomous nurse midwife who works in a birth centre is limited by hospital and medical staff policies, and it is evident that the midwife's intra-staff relationships often impinge upon the client–practitioner relationship. The nurse midwife is not free to provide her services to all who desire them. Written protocols prevent clients with high risk pregnancies from admission to the programme. Other policies also influence the midwife–client contract. A nurse midwife, interviewed as part of a study of alternative birth centres, expressed displeasure that her boss (the head of maternal and fetal medicine in her hospital) would not allow her to accept patients enrolled in a prepaid health service at another hospital. She was anxious to offer an alternative to these individuals, but had no choice but to obey her superior (DeVries 1980).

Protocols also set parameters on the care that a midwife may offer. Many of the policies contained in alternative birth centre protocols were inspired by licensing laws for midwives. For instance, the law governing California's nurse midwives, the California Business and Professional Code, states that the practice of midwifery '. . . does not include the use of any instrument at any childbirth, except such instrument as is necessary in severing the umbilical cord, nor does it include the assisting of childbirth by any artificial, forcible, or mechanical means, nor the performance of any version nor the removal of adherent placenta, nor the administering, prescribing, advising or employing, either before or after childbirth, of any drug, other than disinfectant or cathartic.' The code states that the certificate to practise midwifery may be revoked for failure to refer to, or summon, a physician for specified conditions during pregnancy, labour, or the lying-in period.

Unlicenced, lay midwives face fewer complexities. They accept the need to limit their practice to low risk pregnancies, but because of their independent position and extra-legal status, definitions of risk are more negotiable for them than for licenced midwives. One lay midwife notes (Merz 1977: 550): 'We have no agreement about what constitutes a pregnancy at risk, and therefore not viable for home birth. Each situation is handled individually as a negotiation between parents and midwife. Ultimately the decision is theirs. The midwife must then establish for herself whether or not she can take the responsibility for supporting them'. In their study of home birth, Mehl *et al.* (1977) point out that, unlike definitions of risk found in hospital settings, 'previous obstetric complications (with the exception of caesarean section) were not used as screening criteria because it was felt that they were iatrogenic to some extent'.

Unlicensed midwives typically require clients to see a doctor for some antenatal care, and to provide back-up care in the event of an emergency. The doctor and midwife thus enter into a relationship, but with no bureaucratic structure they have equal status with regard to the client. Only when it is necessary for the midwife and her client to enter the hospital does the hierarchical ordering between the doctor and the midwife become evident.

The relationships among unlicensed midwives serve some important functions. Because they feel a need to learn from each other, and because they share a distinctive and somewhat radical ideology with regard to birth, unlicensed midwives typically work in groups. In some areas these groups maintain contacts with other midwives in larger, informal networks to pass on referrals and to share knowledge. Sensitivity to their collective reputation also leads groups of unlicensed midwives to discipline those whose work they regard as sloppy or dangerous. They have set up self-certification programmes and will use peer pressure to discourage errant practice. The effectiveness of such informal control is difficult to assess. Licensed midwives lack these informal control networks. Because the authority for training and discipline belongs to state agencies, these midwives do not feel as strong a need to learn from each other or to patrol their ranks.

Nurse and lay midwives have different relationships with organized medicine. Nurse midwives have well-established relationships with obstetricians and physicians. Some licensed lay midwives have established working relationships with medical institutions, although it can be difficult to find supportive physicians. These relationships are often fragmentary because of the threat of professional sanction (loss of hospital privileges, for example) facing the doctors who collaborate. The formal ties between doctor and midwife necessitated by licensure lead midwives to resort more frequently to assistance from physicians. Donnison (1977: 185) reports that, in Britain, 'ever since the 1902 Act had come into operation, the proportion of cases in which midwives had sent for the doctor had been rising steadily'. In American cities where licensure was used earlier in this century, 'Midwives, more secure in their licensed status, were calling doctors earlier and oftener' (Kobrin 1966). The establishment of well-defined relationships with physicians alters the midwife's style of practice. Oakley (1977) comments: 'In a home confinement, where (a midwife) must summon a doctor for the repair of an episiotomy, she may be motivated to deliver the baby's head more slowly in order to stretch the perineum gradually and thus avoid the need for an incision.' In the case of lay midwives where physician back-up is not always well established, and where there is a disinclination to use hospitals, the motivations cited by Oakley result in a style of practice geared to avoid medical assistance.

When midwifery is legitimated by licensure, a different sort of individual is drawn to the profession. Licensed midwifery recruits individuals with motivations different from those of unlicensed midwives. Those who practise midwifery in states where it is not licensed, and perhaps prohibited, have a strong commitment to their occupation. If midwifery were to be licensed in those states, it would become a legitimate career opportunity, a job chosen by an individual because it appears an interesting way to make a living.

There may be other motivations, but for most nurse midwives, their occupation is their means of making a living. Being salaried, they are concerned with the efficient use of time, and client-practitioner interaction becomes part of business. Unlicensed lay midwives wish to be paid, but they have no desire to make midwifery especially lucrative. Midwifery is not seen as a commercial service, but as a 'calling for dedicated, spiritual women working in concert with like-minded patients' (Ruzek 1978: 138; Arms 1977: 195, 251–252). In her 'instructions to midwives' Gaskin (1978: 285) says: 'The spiritual midwife tries to find a way that she can practice without charging money, as this makes it easier to keep birthings spiritual. Her husband and/or community may assume her support. If she is helping ladies for free, she has a better moral position if she needs to talk to a lady about her attitude'. Because they are not interested in making a living, lay midwives typically have fewer cases and are freer to spend more time with their patients during both pregnancy and childbirth (Mills 1977).

3.1.3 The nature of the client

One characteristic common to clients of both nurse midwives and lay midwives is self-selection. The present structure of maternity care in the United States channels expectant parents toward a standard hospital delivery. It takes an active effort by parents to obtain a midwife-assisted delivery. This search for an alternative is often rooted in strong feelings of where the responsibility for birth should lie.

Parental desire to assume this responsibility varies widely. Interviews with parents reveal a range of feelings extending from total reliance upon medical personnel, as in hospital births where parents choose to allow a physician to direct and control care, to a desire for complete responsibility, as in home births where the father catches the baby (DeVries 1985; Milinaire 1974; Nash and Nash 1979). Hazell (1974: 24) concluded that the home birth couple usually feels that the primary responsibility for birth lies with parents, not with the doctor or the hospital. Those with such convictions often seek out the lay midwife because '. . . her function is to assist, not to take over responsibility' (Hazell 1974: 37). Lay midwives respect this feeling. One midwife notes that her clients are 'people who are taking control of their lives . . . and they're willing to take responsibility off me. That is what the doctors have done traditionally. They pat the lady on the hand and say, "Don't worry, dear, I'll take care of everything." But that is not the traditional role of the midwife' (Anderson 1978: 1).

Those who employ lay midwives to assist in home births are often inclined to accept the consequences of their decision as part of some larger plan. In case of mishap, these individuals tend to fall back on fateful explanations rather than faulting themselves for not choosing a hospital birth. A father whose child died five days after a home birth concludes: 'We believe that it was the hand of the Lord and we have accepted that. Nobody wanted that baby more than we did. We feel grieved about it, but we are at peace in this' (quoted in King and Saltus 1978).

When midwives are licensed, part of the parents' responsibility for childbirth is transferred to the state. The client often assumes that a licensed midwife is competent because she is certified. On the other hand, when midwives are not licensed, the client must assess the qualifications of the practitioner herself. Licensure actually encourages the client to forego any personal evaluation of the practitioners, even though most clients are not familiar with certification requirements. In Texas, before passage of a more restrictive law, many midwives took advantage of the registration requirement by advertising themselves as registered midwives. In turn, many of their clients confused registration with certification. Several clients noted that their midwife was registered, and though admitting that they did not know exactly what this implied, most assumed (incorrectly) that it involved some type of training and monitoring.

Inclusion of the state as a third party in the relationship between the midwife and her client undoubtedly alters feelings of where responsibility for birth lies. When licensure moves midwife assisted birth into the hospital, as it has for the nurse midwife, responsibility for the birth is shared not only with the state but with physicians. The nurse midwife's client is often more involved in the birth experience than the woman in a standard hospital delivery, but this is still very different from the total responsibility assumed by the mother delivering at home with an unlicensed midwife. In a birth centre, the client of the nurse midwife places the ultimate liability for her birth on medical professionals; responsibility for the birth is hers only as long as these medical experts define the situation as safe (i.e. low risk). Should a 'regular' hospital delivery be necessary, medical personnel take charge and the parents become bystanders. A proponent of natural birth comments: 'The mother who goes to the hospital to have her baby is in an impossible situation, really. If a doctor says he's doing something for the safety of her baby, there is nothing she can say. Once she is told a procedure is for her baby, she can offer no argument' (quoted in Arms 1977: 123).

Yet, there are subtle distinctions between those who choose to give birth at home and those who use a birth centre (DeVries 1979). Clients of a nurse midwife receive only minimal training in the physiology of birth; instead there is a heavy emphasis on psychoprophylaxis, breathing techniques employed during delivery as a substitute for analgesia. Those having births at home must learn more about the birth process. Most frequently this knowledge is gained through reading, but occasionally lay midwives organize a class for expectant parents. The classes stress 'getting in touch with your body' and encourage self-examinations which allow the mother to determine the progress of labour.

3.1.4 The practitioner-client relationship

Midwives establish close and personal relationships with their clients. In a study of nurse midwives in a hospital setting, Record and Cohen (1972) cite evidence of the client's personal satisfaction with the midwife: 'She thinks of all the little things the doctors don't have time to talk about. There are hundreds of things you don't want to bother your doctor with . . . I admit that I asked questions of (her) that I was shy to ask my doctor, or questions that I thought were too silly to take his time for since he is so busy.' The investigators conclude that 'such remarks suggest that either because of individual characteristics, or perhaps because she is a female, or perhaps because . . . she is less removed from (her clients) by professional mystique, the certified nurse midwife may not only be substituting for the doctor . . . but providing a service that the doctor cannot provide' (Record and Cohen 1972).

For many of the same reasons, the lay midwife also creates a personal relationship with her clients. But social context influences the nature of the relationship between midwife and client. Lay midwives often provide care in their own home or the client's home. These settings, coupled with the less demanding case-load of lay midwives, create relationships that go beyond concern with the ongoing pregnancy. Nurse midwives typically meet clients in more traditional medical environments. In this context the mother becomes little more than a 'maternity patient'. Although most nurse midwives are very approachable, the effects of the clinical setting are unmistakable. The contingencies of appointment schedules and staff responsibilities leave little time for discussion not directly related to the pregnancy. Furthermore, the large case-load of the nurse midwife often results in fragmented care because she is unable to attend to the needs of all her clients.

Client control of the caregiver also varies between lay and nurse midwives. The nurse midwife is in a bind because she is responsible both to her patient and to her supervisors. A woman entering a birth centre finds herself at the lower end of a chain of command since the licensing law stipulates that the midwife's treatment of her is regulated by physician supervisors. If a woman's request is not in accord with hospital and/or physician policy, it is often denied. The sole responsibility and ultimate accountability of the unlicensed lay midwife, on the other hand, is to her client, leaving much more room for negotiation on matters of treatment.

Location also helps to determine who controls the pregnancy. The client who enters a hospital is a guest of the practitioner and is less able to direct her care. 'A crucial means of control in the hospital is the strangeness of the setting to the client and the dependence of the client on hospital personnel for orientation to the setting, techniques and routines of the hospital' (Shaw, 1974: 125; see Chapters 50, and 51, 000, 000). On the other hand, if care is given in the client's home, the caregiver becomes the guest of her client and must respect her wishes. Most of those who choose to give birth at home are aware of this (Longbrake and Longbrake 1976; Ruzek 1978: 132).

3.1.5 The birth experience

The experience of birth is influenced by the degree to which it is standardized. The experience, the training, and the hospital location of the nurse midwife lead her to streamline her procedures. The alternative birth centre supplies written protocols to define normal progression through pregnancy and birth. Although these are negotiable to a certain extent, the definitions present an idealized frame of reference. Because any variation is regarded as abnormal, this routine view of birth anticipates intervention (Nash and Nash 1979). Approximately 25–30 per cent of those who begin labour in an alternative birth centre are in fact removed because of some complication (DeVries 1980). This compares to a 17 per cent hospitalization rate for lay midwives studied by Mehl *et al.* (1977).

Licensure encourages standardization of birth. A licensed lay midwife in Arizona, for instance, is prohibited from attending a woman over thirty-five years of age, with no allowance made for factors such as the health of the mother, number of previous pregnancies, or obstetric history. Furthermore, the training requirements and medical supervision that accompany licensing laws push midwives toward routinized birth. Altered recruitment patterns provide midwife trainees who are more likely to accept medical definitions of birth. In addition, the expanded practice that accompanies legitimation fosters standardization as an expeditious method of dealing with a large number of clients. When midwifery is practised in a hospital, midwife and client submit to the needs and regulations of the institution. Organizational demands often require the pacing of deliveries. A fixed amount of available space coupled with an unpredictable number of patients can create the need to speed up or slow down births. Such constraints are not found in the home. Ruzek (1978) points out that lay midwives operate on a different time frame than the professional: 'Rather than viewing midwifery as a full-time occupation, a job, or a task to be completed as quickly as possible, lay midwives look forward to births as meaningful, spiritual life-events to experience and enjoy. The long hours spent with labouring women are rewarding and satisfying because of the "birth energy": they are not draining, as are long hours worked in a frenetic hospital delivery service' (Ruzek 1978: 138).

The contrast between lay and nurse midwives demonstrates the influence of motivation, socialization, work setting, and clientele on caregiving. Although the same type of intra-professional comparison is not possible for the other caregivers I consider, the same influences are evident.

3.2 General/family practitioners: the dilemmas of general practice obstetrics

Reports from Australia (Chang *et al.* 1980) and from the United Kingdom (Marsh *et al.* 1985a, b) document the trend: general practitioners are assisting at fewer births. General practitioners disagree about the wisdom of this trend (see Chapter 11). Some believe birth is 'risky business' best left to obstetric specialists (McCormally 1984); others see caregiving at birth as central to family practice (Phillips and Stevens 1985; see also Matthies 1984; Taylor 1982). Debate over the advisability of general practice obstetrics is further confounded by the fact that general practitioners can assume a variety of caregiving roles during pregnancy and birth. Brundell (1983) outlines three: general practitioners can simply refer pregnant women to a specialist; they may assume full responsibility for care, providing ante-, intra-, and postnatal care; or they may provide antenatal care and refer to a specialist for intra- and postpartum care. The question is not simply *should* general practitioners be involved in birth?; but *how* should they be involved in birth?

In a world of specialization the general practitioner is

an anachronism, but the specialist in family practice survives. The family practice specialty has found a place in the medical market because of its emphasis on postmodern cultural themes, specifically 'wholeness' and 'holistic care'. Family practice physicians who believe in non-specialist obstetrics see this holistic approach as their contribution to care. In family practice obstetrics, the word holistic is typically replaced by the phrase 'continuity of care' (Shear *et al.* 1983). Supporters of family practice obstetrics also acknowledge that it is a valuable means of building and maintaining a practice, a point also noticed by sociologists (Wertz 1983).

Who chooses to become a family practitioner ? Sociological evidence suggests a good percentage (25 per cent) of those entering medical school intend a career in family practice (Oates and Feldman 1979). The image of a family practitioner corresponds closely to the ideals of freshman medical students, but ideals are altered by the experience of medical school and by the senior year many opt for more limited specialties (Oates and Feldman 1979). In their study of specialty selection in the United States, Sorlie and Essex-Sorlie (1985) found that those who choose to stay with family practice are likely to have chosen this field before medical school, to come from rural backgrounds, to believe that physicians must treat the emotional and social needs of clients and to have lower grades in medical school than those choosing other specialties. Family practice also draws more than its share of women (Berquist *et al.* 1985; Davidson 1979). Although there are no data on the special characteristics of family practitioners who choose to assist at birth, these general data suggest that those who choose to become family practitioners have a sense of calling to this career, have a less segmented view of life, and have a desire to provide holistic care. Given these characteristics, birth is likely to be viewed as a natural and normal event and birth assistance is likely to be regarded as a part of continuous care.

The training family practitioners receive, however, will undoubtedly influence these views. Like nurse midwives, family practitioners acquire a view of birth that anticipates intervention. The family practitioner's knowledge of birth is knowledge developed and presented by obstetric specialists. A recent edition of *Primary Care*, a journal intended for family practitioners, dedicated to 'Obstetrics in Family Practice', demonstrates the specialist perspective. The editor notes that family physicians play an important role in delivering care to 'obstetrical patients'. He goes on to point out that 'movement toward a more natural approach to the birthing process and the need for patients and their families to have a greater sense of control over their destiny and the destiny of the unborn infant have increased the number of patients seeking personalized and individualized care' (Avant 1983). But the chapters that follow seem to be based more on the obstetric specialist's obstetrics than on general practitioner obstetrics. A chapter on the induction and augmentation of labour notes that the hospital labour and delivery area might adversely affect labour, but rather than suggesting a non-interventionist strategy of modifying the environment, the suggestion is to 'familiarize the patient with the labor and delivery equipment' (Neese 1983). The chapter on obstetric anaesthesia and analgesia begins with this observation: 'Interest in "natural childbirth" as manifest by the various psychoprophylactic approaches, birthing rooms, and home deliveries is probably as strong now as it ever has been. Despite this, most women, and especially those having their first baby, do require some degree of anesthesia or analgesia for their delivery.' (Perry 1983).

In spite of the inclination of this training, family practitioners have set themselves apart from standard obstetric care. Clients are at least part of the reason for this. In a general sense, family practitioners have found their niche as caregivers at birth by providing an alternative and by emphasizing the differences in their approach to caregiving (see Chapter 11). More specifically, those who seek the assistance of a family physician, like those who choose midwives, are often avoiding specialist care and expect their doctor to be more flexible and less 'medical'. Even those who have no choice because of government or private insurance regulations will likely have different expectations for a general practitioner.

Family practitioners who give care at birth face the tension of balancing the expectations of clients and colleagues. They are expected to be less medical by their clients, but they need to demonstrate their knowledge and prove their effectiveness in terms recognized by their specialist colleagues. Research on continuity of care indicates that it is beneficial (Flynn 1985; Shear *et al.* 1983; Zander 1982) and several studies indicate that, at least in some respects, family practitioners can achieve equivalent, if not better outcomes than specialists (Klein *et al.* 1983a, b; see also Chapter 11). The tension between client and colleague expectations also emerges in the rates of referral to specialist care. While good comparative data are not available, it appears that rates of referral are higher for family practitioners situated in medical environments than for midwives assisting at home births (Nuovo 1985; Craig et al. 1985). Some of this difference is likely to be attributable to differences in the clients seen by these caregivers, but there is a large enough difference in referral rates to suggest that other factors, such as both socialization and the use of risk screening systems to anticipate the need for referral, account for some of the decisions to call in a specialist.

Another dilemma that family practitioners face, is the need to strike a balance between participation in enough births to maintain their skills, while preserving a small enough practice to provide a personal, non-bureaucratic approach to caregiving. In an era of increased concern with medical costs, care by family practitioners at birth is more attractive to policy makers. The State of California recently completed a study of alternative birth methods, that suggested that less technological birth would be more effective and less costly. Adams and Zuckerman (1984), discussing the high rate of malpractice suits against obstetricians, demonstrated a strong negative relationship between patient contact and the likelihood of malpractice actions. Increased patient contact and trusting relationships are the essence of care given by a family practitioner.

The care offered by general practitioners is shaped by motivation (the specialty is typically chosen before medical school), the nature of the specialty (emphasizing continuous, holistic care), training (guided by obstetric knowledge) and the expectations of clients (for non-specialist care). In addition, the viability of this model of care is assured by 'postmodern' cultural themes and by government policies that seek less costly ways to provide care at birth.

3.3 Obstetricians: the guardians of 'scientific' care

Obstetric medicine is something of a mixed blessing. Advances in obstetrics allow mothers and infants to be rescued from death, but those successes make the discipline heady. Heroic techniques are applied to women and babies who do not need to be rescued. Although many women feel uneasy about these techniques, they submit because of their genuine trust in the ability of obstetrics.

The more the specialized knowledge of the caregiver increases and becomes evident in interaction, the more the power of the client decreases. Among all the caregivers at birth, obstetricians have the most specialized knowledge and this knowledge is made evident both in their conversations with clients and visually, in the impressive technological tools they use. Shapiro *et al.* (1983) demonstrate how the control of information enhances the power of obstetricians. They note that in spite of the fact that few women get all the information they desire from their specialist, most are *highly satisfied* with their care. They conclude that obstetricians, because of their presumed knowledge, are able to control interaction, leading information-seeking patients to believe 'that if information is not provided, the information may not be needed or that it should be obtained from some other source'. This finding is important because it offers direct evidence of the ability of caregivers to mold the desires of their clients.

Unlike family practitioners, those who choose the obstetric specialty typically do so while in medical school (Oates and Feldman 1979; Scully 1980). After studying residents in obstetrics and gynaecology at two hospitals, Scully (1980) suggested factors responsible for their choice of this specialty. Scully believes that the specialty is chosen because of some combination of the following four reasons: obstetrics is a 'happy specialty' where outcomes are generally positive; it is an 'ego trip' because the doctor appears responsible for the large number of good outcomes; the specialty emphasizes life and avoids death, as the typical client is young and pleasant; and it allows control over women. Scully supports this last point by recounting the residents' preference for middle class women who are 'happy, obedient, respectful and thankful patients' (see also Inch 1985). These motivations are very different from those of midwives and family practitioners and they affect orientation toward clients and other aspects of caregiving.

As with the other caregivers, the motivations of those being trained in obstetrics are altered and refined by the educational process. Obstetricians in training develop their attitudes toward birth and their patients from a variety of sources, including texts, teachers, and the settings where they learn and work. An analysis of gynaecology textbooks suggests that they impart a view of women that is very traditional, emphasizing submission and motherhood (Scully and Bart 1973). 'Women are consistently described as anatomically destined to reproduce, nurture, and keep their husbands happy' (Scully and Bart 1973). The texts describe the feminine personality as masochistic and passive; they suggest that women need to be governed by the male sex drive. Physicians are regarded as the rightful arbiters of sexual problems: 'kindness and concern for his patient may provide her with a glimpse of God's image' (Scott 1968: 25, quoted in Scully and Bart 1973). Scully (1980) notes that the clinical settings in which obstetric residents are trained encourage depersonalization and teach students not to care. Women are often regarded as teaching material to be used to gain knowledge, judgement, and technique. Sociological studies of the obstetrician-supervised births witnessed by students often reveal decisions being made for the convenience of the caregiver, not the woman in labour (Rosengren and DeVault 1963; Shaw 1974; Danziger 1986). Savage (quoted in Inch 1985) points out that the majority of patients want pain relief, nursing care, relief from responsibility for their condition, and a cure for their illness: demands that cause medical students to become authoritarian, didactic, and all-knowing. She goes on to note that it is difficult for obstetric residents to shift gears and deal with pregnant women who seek information and autonomy and who want to share responsibility.

Patterns learned in medical school and in medical residencies are very important. Those who go on to become teachers perpetuate preferences and styles they have learned. For example, Healy and Laufe (1985) surveyed 105 obstetric training programmes and found that the type of forceps preferred was related to habit and the inclinations of the instructors, not to questions of design or function. Continuing education programmes do little to alter ingrained habits; studies of continuing education show that it results in only minor technical changes in practice (Mohide and Maudsley 1985).

Recent criticism suggests that the science of obstetrics taught in medical school might not be so scientific. Over the last decade, medical science has been criticized for being a science in name but not in deed (Richards 1975; Chalmers 1976; Chalmers and Richards 1977). Mendelsohn and his colleagues (1985) believe that the practice of medicine is shaped by habit, financial need, politics, and personal stubbornness, not by rigorous scientific technique. Much of the claim that modern medicine is scientific, rests on incidental features of similarity between scientific research and present-day medical practice. The use of technical gadgetry is a case in point. It is also common to find clinicians arguing that techniques are useful simply because they are of recent origin.

Richards (1975) finds it curious that such irrational practice could be regarded as scientific. But it is not so curious when the role of the client is considered. When obstetricians choose to look and act scientific, they are responding to the desires of clients for the best in birth. Convinced by a culture that finds efficacy in technical gadgetry, these clients feel reassured by the technology of obstetrics. Obstetrics is 'hoist with its own activist petard' forced to give the appearance of an activist science in situations that might require passivity and little outward display of science. For instance, carefully controlled studies might demonstrate that it is better not to intervene, but to stand idly during a long labour certainly does not look scientific.

Clients also push obstetricians toward change. Models of controlled caregiving are largely the result of agitation on the part of consumers. As competition becomes a more salient force, consumers have a greater voice. Obstetricians are beginning to tell each other that they need to meet the demands of their clients (Inch 1985; Haverkamp 1982). Pointing to the examples of unneeded separation of families at birth, poor nutritional advice, unnecessary sedation, and the use of dangerous drugs, Haverkamp (1982) credits dissatisfied clients with highlighting the lack of science in the science of obstetrics. He suggests that the activist caregiving of the past must be subject to true scientific scrutiny in an effort to weed out unnecessary intervention.

3.4 Emerging caregivers

The midwife, general practitioner, and obstetrician are the traditional caregivers at birth, but over the last few decades new professions have evolved and have influenced caregiving at birth. In the United States, these include childbirth educators, lactation consultants, mother's helpers, and exercise specialists. These new occupations follow a natural history of innovation, where the motivational contexts and training of the caregivers slowly change. In each of them it is possible to observe a move from the pioneers, who create the occupation with high ideals and a sacrificial spirit, to the professionals, whose concern with the image of the occupation leads them to create restrictive entry requirements and to formalize training and practice. Like other caregivers at birth, the impact of new caregivers is mixed: they have the potential to change common views of birth, but they can also diminish the development of parental competence.

Childbirth educators have the longest history as adjunct caregivers at birth. In reviewing that history, three themes emerge: the dependence of this profession on obstetric knowledge; the rise of professional attitudes; and the problem of parentism.

Childbirth education began as instruction in the various techniques of natural childbirth. As such, it had a distinctive body of knowledge, separate from the medical knowledge of birth. But the power of obstetric knowledge soon overwhelmed the field of childbirth education. The texts used by childbirth educators, which routinely include chapters on caesarean section and the pharmacology of birth, indicate that obstetric knowledge now sets the agenda (Hassid 1984). Childbirth education is also following the lead of medicine in another area: specialization. Shearer and Bunnin (1983) comment that childbirth educators are responding to the increasing complexity of obstetrics by specializing themselves, limiting their teaching to specialty areas like exercise, sibling preparation, caesarean birth, vaginal birth after caesarean section, or breastfeeding. Rather than pushing its own agenda, childbirth education responds to obstetrics. This is typical of adjunct occupations; often autonomy and special knowledge are abandoned to achieve the legitimacy and status that comes with recognition by an established occupation. Childbirth educators are now often hired by institutions (i.e. hospitals) and are beholden to their needs and desires.

Following that natural history, childbirth educators are moving from pioneers to professionals. Those who have been in the field for several years are calling for objective standards and mandatory programmes of certification (Shearer and Bunnin 1983; Sasmor and Grossman 1981). Veteran childbirth educators note that they are not as close to their clients as they were earlier in their careers, observing that as they have become more professional, they have become less involved with their clients (Birth 1984). Here the irony of professionalization emerges once again; professionals have the advantage of systematized knowledge and better organization, but they often lose empathy.

Childbirth educators can also suffer from parentism, deciding what is best for their clients. Early childbirth educators were often reverse dogmatists, who resisted the dogmatism of medicine with their own dogmatism of non-intervention. Although many childbirth educators now eschew the older dogmatic approach, they none the less help to define 'acceptable birth'. Cogan and Winer (1982) discovered that the clients of childbirth educators who had been trained in communication skills were more willing to discuss the pain of birth than clients whose childbirth educator had no such training. They conclude that childbirth educators might make it difficult for clients to admit to pain and fear, two elements that childbirth education is supposed to diminish. Similarly, Resnick *et al.* (1978) conclude that husbands are often not allowed to express fear and anxiety in childbirth classes, but are encouraged to be strong.

The field of childbirth education has also spawned a new specialty: the lactation consultant (Lauwers *et al.* 1985). The lactation consultant, also referred to as a breastfeeding consultant, breastfeeding co-ordinator etc., is available to guide the mother and her infant through their months of breastfeeding. This new profession has resulted from a desire for support and information on the part of an increasing number of breastfeeding women. The return to breastfeeding found physician specialists unprepared with little knowledge about the techniques and dynamics of breastfeeding, thus creating the need for a specialty adjunct like the lactation consultant.

Lactation consulting is still in a pioneering phase, but the pioneers are working to become more professional. A career in lactation consulting often begins as a lay breastfeeding counsellor. Lactation consultants are drawn from the ranks of childbirth educators, nurses, and 'La Leche League' leaders. As the occupation matures and seeks legitimacy, there is a move to recognize only those with certificates from approved training programmes. Currently, there is a push for state recognition of these certificates.

Certification is useful in enhancing status and allowing a wider audience to be reached, but, as shown with midwifery, state certification is not a neutral force. It begins a process that inevitably changes an occupation. Certification brings a new type of person to the occupation, one with an entirely different set of motivations. Certification brings an occupation into the medical fold, allowing it to influence established practices, but also inducing subtle changes.

Lactation consultants can play a role in changing social views of breastfeeding. They can provide a shield against a culture that discourages breastfeeding, and they can go beyond this shielding ability to change society. Their vested interest in breastfeeding—the more breastfeeding is accepted, the larger the pool of clients—will encourage them to change attitudes so that women no longer suffer the indignity of being leered at in public while breastfeeding, or feel compelled to nurse their children in lavatory cubicles. Separate studies in the United Kingdom (Jones and West 1985) and the United States (Auerbach 1985) show that lactation consultants extend the duration of breastfeeding. As these changes are aggregated, social attitudes will gradually begin to change.

4 The joys and pains of caregiving

Given the varied approaches represented by the variety of caregivers in pregnancy and childbirth, it is important to consider means of promoting co-operation among caregivers. All caregivers share a common goal of maximizing the health and well-being of the infant and its parents, but differing motivations, education, and clientele give various caregivers different ways of seeing birth and lead to different strategies for achieving the common goal.

Several co-operative models have been suggested. Feinbloom (1986) offers a model where midwives work with family practitioners. Robinson (1985a, 1985b) suggests a similar model for the United Kingdom. Schorfheide (1982) discusses a setting where nurse midwives work jointly with obstetricians. Keirse (1982) outlines a model of co-operation between midwives and physicians that works successfully in The Netherlands. Still others focus on the difficulties that attend co-operative efforts among caregivers, difficulties that most often begin with a lack of trust between caregivers in different categories (Massachusetts Nurse 1985; Sullivan and Weitz 1984; Hyde 1984; Rooks 1983). This lack of trust is sad, but not surprising given the divergent motivations and education of caregivers.

Cronenwett and Brickman (1983) present four models of helping and coping in childbirth that reflect the different approaches of various caregivers. The models vary in the degree of responsibility clients bear for 'problems and solutions'. The 'moral model' compels people to take action on their own behalf, because they are responsible for their situation and for finding appropriate solutions. Those who participate in home birth often subscribe to this model. The client is fully responsible for her birth; the caregiver is merely an assistant. The 'compensatory model' does not blame people for their problems, but holds them responsible for solving them. People are forced to compensate for structural obstacles and caregivers become resources toward that end. The caregiver presents a range of options and it is the responsibility of the client to choose the one that best fits her needs. Perhaps most familiar is the 'medical model' where people are not held responsible for either the origin or the solution to their problems. The caregiver is given ultimate authority and the client is expected to co-operate with caregiver's decisions. The 'enlightenment model' finds people responsible for their problems but sees solutions residing in caregiver provided enlightenment. Parts of the natural childbirth movement use this model, regarding women as weak and subject to the temptation of a medicated delivery and hence in need of caregiver direction.

Each model has its own pathology. The moral model puts a heavy burden on those with poor outcomes ('it was their own fault'). The compensatory model leads people to a bitter view of a health care system that presents a variety of obstacles in the way of an optimum birth. The medical model promotes dependency. The enlightenment model induces anxiety and guilt in those who cannot live up to the expectations of the caregiver.

Which model is preferable? It might be said that any model is acceptable as long as caregiver and client agree. But there is a danger here, a danger that emanates from the cultural authority of caregivers. Because of this authority, caregivers easily become tyrants giving clients the illusion of choice when, in fact, that choice is shaped by the motivation and training of the caregiver. It is here that the spectre of 'parentism' raises its head. When is it acceptable for caregivers to make decisions for, or exert influence over clients?

The issue of parentism is really an issue of power. Guggenbuhl-Craig (1982) explores this theme. He believes that many healers chose their profession 'out of a deep inner need' and concludes that those who choose to give care are often those who are uncomfortable with disease and illness. They feel powerless when confronted with the possibility of their own sickness and death. As a result, 'the power exercised by the physician makes ... a cheap and shabby impression. It is the result of a partial psychological and moral failure by both doctor and patient. The doctor is no longer able to see his own wounds, his own potential for illness; he sees sickness only in the other. He objectifies illness, distances himself from his own weakness, elevates himself and degrades the patient. He becomes powerful through psychological failure rather than through strength.' (Guggenbuhl-Craig 1982: 94–95). This power is most visible in the unwillingness to allow clients to make their own choices. Some caregivers eliminate choice by deciding what is best for the client based on their disinterested, professional knowledge. Other caregivers handicap their clients' choice by not giving complete information. Information is not withheld maliciously, but in the parents' 'best interest'. Bogdan *et al.* (1982) observed this in their study of communication in neonatal intensive care units. In that setting, caregivers commonly used euphemisms ('developmental delay' for retardation) and evasions ('you can never tell about these babies') in their interactions with parents. It is significant that caregivers often address labouring women in a style commonly used when talking to children, including tones of condescension and the use of dishonesty to 'protect' (Richards 1982).

Caregiving of any sort inevitably limits the client's choice to a certain extent. To receive care, the client must accept the caregiver's definition of the 'problem', a definition that will structure the choices available. This is the problem Richards (1982) alludes to when he discusses the trouble with choice in childbirth: '... pushing for alternatives in maternity care is not only too limited a tactic, but may be counterproductive because it fails to come to grips with the central issues of who is in control and the kind of process birth should be. An opposition exists between the physiological or engineering approach of obstetrics and the parents' social and psychological standpoint. In the guise of a concern for "safety"—in itself a dubious concept—birth has been redefined and parents made more or less completely powerless, to a point where it becomes irrelevant to discuss choice. Little can change without altering the fundamental relationship of mother and birth attendants.' (Richards 1982). It is not necessary to believe that people are the 'unwitting agents of professional puppeteers', as Chalmers (1986) puts it, in order to recognize that images and desires are shaped by caregivers. The primary sources of information about pregnancy and childbirth are caregivers and books authored by caregivers. As the marketing of childbirth care becomes more aggressive, caregivers (including hospital administrators) gain a new medium for influencing public attitudes about birth.

Caregivers should recognize both the source, in motivation, education and experience, and power of their attitudes toward pregnancy and birth. In some cases it seems clear that caregivers need to assume the parental role, as in situations where women are hurting themselves and their infant by excessive use of dangerous drugs. But what about situations where clients value their experience or religion more highly than their health or the health of the fetus? Kaunitz *et al.* (1984) studied such a situation. Their work revealed that the avoidance of care in pregnancy and childbirth among members of the Faith Assembly in Indiana resulted in drastically higher rates of perinatal and maternal mortality. It is instructive that Kaunitz and his colleagues close their article with this statement: 'These findings suggest that when women, even in the United States, avoid obstetric care, they greatly increase the risks of perinatal and maternal death.' Their response to the problem is to exert power ('you must have obstetric care!') But this exertion of power belies the psychological powerlessness noted by Guggenbuhl-Craig (1982): 'Don't these women recognize what they are doing? ...

Don't they know they will die unless they get good obstetric care? ... Don't they know they need me?' Kaunitz *et al.* (1984) do not explore less parentistic responses which might include strategies for working with members of the Faith Assembly, learning from them how caregiving threatens their faith and then working within those limitations.

It is often painful for caregivers to come to terms with the limits imposed on their practices. Caregivers are limited not only by the needs of clients, but by culture, by their individual histories, and by organizations. Culture specifies their knowledge of birth and their approach to caregiving. Their unique set of motivations and their educational experience shapes their methodology. Organizations, including hospitals, schools, professional associations, and insurance companies often limit the content of their care. Effective caregivers are those who recognize the limits within which they work and the limits that they impose on the women they serve.

The goal of effective care is to allow clients to flourish, not to alienate them from themselves. The skill of the caregiver can prevent the alienating experience of a bad outcome; but caregivers who look for a solution to their own powerlessness in the domination of clients or the domination of natural processes, can make good outcomes alienating experiences for their clients. They are less prepared to help clients when bad outcomes are unavoidable. Effective caregivers recognize their own powerlessness and work with clients. Effective caregivers are aware of the influence of culture and assess the care they give, not in terms of their own needs or the needs of a profession or a medical organization, but in terms of those who have entrusted them with their care.

References

Adams E, Zuckerman S (1984). Variation in the growth and incidence of medical malpractice claims. J Health Politics, Policy and Law, 9: 475–488.

Adamson G, Gare D (1980). Home or hospital births? J Am Med Assoc, 243: 1732–1736.

American College of Obstetricians and Gynecologists (1978). The Development of Family Centered Maternity/Newborn Care in Hospitals. Chicago: American College Obstetricians and Gynecologists.

American Medical Association (1977). Statement on Parent-newborn Interaction. Chicago: American Medical Association.

Anderson J (1978). Midwife. The Sacramento Bee, February 26: Scene 1,5.

Apfel R, Fisher S (1984). To Do No Harm: DES and the Dilemmas of Modern Medicine. New Haven: Yale University Press.

Arms S (1977). Immaculate Deception. New York: Bantam.

Arney WR (1982). Power and the Profession of Obstetrics. Chicago: University of Chicago Press.

Arney WR, Bergen B (1984). Medicine and the Management of Living. Chicago: University of Chicago Press.

Auerbach K (1985). The influence of lactation consultant contact on breastfeeding duration in a low-income population. Nebraska Med J, 70: 341–346.

Avant R (1983). Foreword. Primary Care, 10: 143–144.

Baldwin R (1979). An update on midwifery training. Mothering, 12: 51–54.

Berquist S, Duchac B, Schalin V, Zastrow J, Barr V, Borowiecki T (1985). Perceptions of freshman medical students of gender differences in medical specialty choice. J Med Education, 60: 379–383.

Birth (1984). Quantity, quality and money: still more on veteran childbirth educators. Birth, 11: 173–178.

Bogdan R, Brown M, Foster S (1982). Be honest but not cruel: staff/parent communication on a neonatal unit. Human Organization, 41: 6–16.

Brennan B, Heilman J (1977). The Complete Book of Midwifery. New York: E P Dutton.

British Medical Journal (1977). Helping mothers to love their babies (editorial). Br Med J, 2: 595.

Brundell J (1983). Future of general practitioner obstetrics: a discussion paper. J R Soc Med, 76: 197–199.

Burst H (1983). The influence of consumers on the birthing movement. Topics Clin Nursing, 5: 42–54.

Cassirer E (1944). An Essay on Man. New Haven: Yale University Press.

Chalmers I (1976). British debate on obstetric practice. Pediatrics, 58: 308–312.

Chalmers I (1986). Minimizing harm and maximizing benefit during innovation in health care: controlled or uncontrolled experimentation? Birth, 13: 155–164.

Chalmers I, Richards M (1977). Intervention and causal inference in obstetric practice. In: Benefits and Hazards of the New Obstetrics. Clinics in Developmental Medicine 64. Chard T, Richards M (eds). London: Spastics International Medical Publications. pp 34–61.

Chang A, Andersen M, Munro J, Morrison J (1980). Obstetric practice amongst Queensland general practitioners: a survey of needs and attitudes. Australian Family Physician, 9: 471–475.

Cianfrani T (1960). A Short History of Obstetrics and Gynecology. Springfield: Charles C Thomas.

Cogan R, Winer J (1982). Effect of childbirth educator communication skills training on postpartum reports of parents. Birth, 9: 241–244.

Comaroff J (1977). Conflicting paradigms of pregnancy: meaning ambiguity in antenatal encounters. In: Medical Encounters. Davis A, Horobin G (eds). New York: St. Martin's Press. pp 115–134.

Cox H (1984). Religion in the Secular City Toward a Postmodern Theology. New York: Simon & Schuster.

Craig A, Berg A, Kirkwood C (1985). Obstetric consultations during labor and delivery in a university-based family practice. J Family Practice, 20: 481–485.

Cronenwett L, Brickman P (1983). Models of helping and coping in childbirth. Nursing Res, 32: 84–88.

Danziger S (1986). Male doctor—female patient. In: The American Way of Birth. Eakins P (ed). Philadelphia: Temple University Press, pp 119–141.

Davidson L (1979). Choice by constraint. J Health Politics Policy and Law, 4: 200–220.

Declerq E, Lacroix R (1985). The immigrant midwives of Lawrence: The conflict between law and culture in twentieth century Massachusetts. Bull Hist Med, 59: 232–246.

Devitt N (1979). How doctors conspired to eliminate the midwife even though the scientific data support midwifery. In: Compulsory Hospitalization: Freedom of Choice in Childbirth? Stewart D, Stewart L (eds). Marble Hill: National Association of Parents and Professionals for Safe Alternatives in Childbirth.

DeVries R (1979). Responding to consumer demand: a study of alternative birth centers. Hospital Progress, 60: 48–51; 68.

DeVries R (1980). The alternative birth center: option or cooptation? Women and Health, 5: 47–60.

DeVries R (1983). Image and reality: an evaluation of hospital alternative birth centers. J Nurse Midwifery, 28: 3–10.

DeVries R (1984). 'Humanizing' childbirth: the discovery and implementation of bonding theory. Int J Health Services Res, 14: 89–104.

DeVries R (1985). Regulating Birth: Midwives, Medicine, and the Law. Philadelphia: Temple University Press.

DeVries R (1988). Normal parents: institutions and the transition to parenthood. Marriage and Family Review, 12: 287–312.

Donegan J (1978). Women and Men Midwives: Medicine, Morality and Misogyny in Early America. Westport, Connecticut: Greenwood Press.

Donnison J (1977). Midwives and Medical Men. London: Heinemann.

Ehrenreich B, English D (1973). Witches, Midwives and Nurses: A History of Women Healers. Oyster Bay, NY: Glass Mountain Pamphlets.

Emmons A, Huntington J (1911). A review of the midwife situation. Boston Med Surgical J, 164: 251–262.

Evenson D (1982). Midwives: survival of an ancient profession. Women's Rights Law Reporter, 7: 313–330.

Feinbloom R (1986). A proposed alliance of midwives and family practitioners in the care of low-risk pregnant women. Birth, 13: 109–113.

Figes E (1987). The Seven Ages. New York: Pantheon.

Flynn S (1985). Continuity of care during pregnancy: the effect of provider continuity on outcome. J Family Practice, 5: 375–380.

Forbes T (1966). The Midwife and the Witch. New Haven: Yale University Press.

Freidson E (1986). Professional Powers. Chicago: University of Chicago Press.

Gablik S (1984). Has Modernism Failed? New York: Thames & Hudson.

Gaskin I (1978). Spiritual Midwifery. Summertown, Tennessee: The Book Publishing Company.

Gregory S (1974 «1848»). Man Midwifery Exposed and Corrected. In: The Male Midwife and the Female Doctor. Rosenberg C, Smith-Rosenberg C (eds). New York: Arno Press.

Guggenbuhl-Craig A (1982). Power in the Helping Professions. Dallas: Spring Publications.

Gustafson J (1982). Professions as 'callings'. Social Service Review, 56: 501–515.

Hassid P (1984). Textbook for Childbirth Educators. Philadelphia: Lippincott.

Haverkamp A (1982). Restoring confidence in obstetric care. Perinatology/Neonatology, 6: 75–77.

Hazell L (1974). Birth Goes Home. Seattle: Catalyst.

Healy D, Laufe L (1985). Survey of obstetric forceps training in North America in 1981. Am J Obstet Gynecol, 151: 54–58.

Heaton CE (1935). Modern Motherhood. New York: Farrar & Rinehart.

Hyde E (1984). Territorial imperatives in health care. Nursing Outlook, 32: 136–138.

Illich I (1976). The Medical Nemesis. New York: Pantheon.

Inch S (1985). Attitudes of obstetricians and midwives: a neglected area of study. J R Soc Med, 78: 683–686.

Jenkins R, Westhus N (1981). The nurse role in parent-infant bonding. J Obstet Gynecol Neonatal Nurs, 5: 114–118.

Jones D, West R (1985). Lactation nurse increases duration of breast feeding. Arch Dis Childhood, 60: 772–774.

Kaunitz A, Spence C, Danielson T, Rochat R, Grimes D (1984). Perinatal and maternal mortality in a religious group avoiding obstetric care. Am J Obstet Gynecol, 150: 826–831.

Keirse MJNC (1982). Interaction between primary and secondary antenatal care, with particular reference to The Netherlands. In: Effectiveness and Satisfaction in Antenatal Care. Enkin M, Chalmers I (eds). London: Heinemann. pp 222–233.

Kennell J, Wolfe H, Jerauld R, Chesler D, Kreger N, McAlpine W, Steffa M, Klaus M (1974). Maternal behavior one year after early and extended post-partum contact. Dev Med Child Neurol, 16: 172–179.

King P, Saltus R (1978). Midwife faces murder charge in home-birth tragedy. San Francisco Sunday Examiner and Chronicle, June 9: 4.

Klaus M, Kennell J (1976). Maternal-Infant Bonding. St. Louis: Mosby.

Klaus M, Kennell J (1981). Parent-Infant Bonding. St Louis: Mosby.

Klaus M, Jerauld R, Kreger N, McAlpine W, Steffa M, Kennell J (1972). The importance of the first post-partum days. New Engl J Med, 286: 460–463.

Klein M, Lloyd I, Redman C, Turnbull A (1983a). A comparison of low-risk pregnant women booked for delivery in two systems of care. I: Obstetrical procedures and neonatal outcome. Br J Obstet Gynaecol, 90: 118–122.

Klein M, Lloyd I, Redman C, Turnbull A (1983b). A comparison of low-risk women booked for delivery in two systems of care. II: Labour and delivery management and neonatal outcome. Br J Obstet Gynaecol, 90: 123–128.

Kobrin F (1966). The American midwife controversy: a crisis of professionalization. Bull Hist Med, 40: 350–63.

Lauwers J, Woessner C, Bernard B (1985). The lactation consultant: a new health professional. Rental Roundup, 2: 5–7.

Leavitt J (1986). Brought to Bed: Childbearing in America, 1750–1950. New York: Oxford University Press.

Levesque-Lopman L (1983). Decision and experience: a phenomenological analysis of pregnancy and childbirth. Human Studies, 6: 247–277.

Linck K (1973). Legalizing a woman's right to choose. In:

Proceedings of the First International Childbirth Conference. Stamford, Connecticut. p 26.

Litoff J (1978). American Midwives—1860 to the Present. Westport, Connecticut: Greenwood Press.

Litoff J (1986). The American Midwife Debate. Westport, Connecticut: Greenwood Press.

Longbrake M, Longbrake W (1976). Control is the key. In: Safe Alternatives in Childbirth. Stewart D, Stewart L (eds). Chapel Hill, NC: NAPSAC, pp 154–160.

Marsh G, Cashman HA, Russell IT (1985a). General practitioner obstetrics in the northern region in 1983. Br Med J, 290: 901–903.

Marsh G, Cashman HA, Russell IT (1985b). General practitioner participation in intranatal care in the northern region in 1983. Br Med J, 290: 971–973.

The Massachusetts Nurse (1985). The lay midwifery controversy. The Massachusetts Nurse, 54: 4–5.

Matthies R (1984). Obstetric care: a family physician's affair. Postgrad Med, 75: 30–32.

McCormally T (1984). Doing obstetrics: risky business. Family Practice News, April 1–14, 12.

Mehl L, Peterson G, Whitt M, Hawes W (1977). Outcomes of elective home births: a series of 1,146 cases. J Reprod Med, 19: 281–290.

Mendelsohn R, ed. (1985). Dissent in Medicine. Chicago: Contemporary Books.

Merz T (1977). A working lay midwife home birth center, Madison, Wisconsin. In: 21st Century Obstetrics Now! Stewart D, Stewart L (eds). Chapel Hill, NC, *et al.* NAPSAC, pp 545–52.

Mills N (1977). A midwife's story. In: The Home Birth Book. Ward C, Ward F (eds). Garden City, NY: Doubleday, pp 47–52.

Milinaire C (1974). Birth. New York: Harmony Books.

Mohide P, Maudsley R (1985). Practice patterns and attitudes toward education among Canadian obstetricians and gynecologists. Am J Obstet Gynecol, 152: 989–994.

Nash A, Nash J (1979). Conflicting interpretations of childbirth: the medical and natural perspectives. Urban Life, 7: 493–511.

Neese R (1983). Normal labor and the induction and augmentation of labor. Primary Care, 10: 253–268.

Nelson M (1986). Birth and social class. In: The American Way of Birth. Eakins PS (ed). Philadelphia: Temple University Press.

Nuovo J (1985). Clinical application of a high risk scoring system on a family practice obstetric service. J Family Practice, 20: 139–144.

Oakley A (1976). Wise woman and medicine man: changes in the management of childbirth. In: The Rights and Wrongs of Women. Mitchell J, Oakley A (eds). Harmondsworth: Penguin.

Oakley A (1977). Cross-cultural practices. In: Benefits and Hazards of the New Obstetrics. Chard T, Richards M (eds). Philadelphia: Lippincott, pp 18–33.

Oakley A (1979). A case of maternity: paradigms of women as maternity cases. Signs, 4: 607–31.

Oakley A (1984). The Captured Womb: A History of the Care of Pregnant Women. Oxford: Basil Blackwell.

Oates R, Feldman H (1979). Longitudinal study of career choices of a SUNY-Upstate cohort of medical students. J Community Health, 5: 131–139.

Ounsted C, Roberts J, Gordon M, Milligan B (1982). Fourth goal of perinatal medicine. Br Med J, 284: 879–882.

Palkovitz R (1985). Fathers' birth attendance, early contact, and extended contact with their newborns: a critical review. Child Dev, 56: 392–406.

Perry L (1983). Current concepts of obstetric anesthesia and analgesia. Primary Care, 10: 269–284.

Peterson K (1983). Technology as the last resort in home birth: the work of lay midwives. Social Problems, 30: 272–83.

Phillips W, Stevens G (1985). Obstetrics in family practice: competence, continuity, and caring. J Family Practice, 20: 595–596.

Record J, Cohen H (1972). The introduction of midwifery in a prepaid group practice. Am J Public Health, 62: 354–60.

Resnick J, Resnick M, Packer A, Wilson J (1978). Fathering classes: a psycho-educational model. Counseling Psychology, 7: 56.

Richards M (1975). Innovation in medical practice: obstetricians and the induction of labour in Britain. Social Sci Med, 9: 595–602.

Richards M (1982). The Trouble with 'Choice' in Childbirth. Birth, 9: 253–260.

Riessman K, Nathanson C (1986). The management of reproduction: social construction of risk and responsibility. In: Applications of Social Science to Clinical Medicine and Health Policy. Aiken L. Mechanic D (eds). New Brunswick, New Jersey: Rutgers University Press. pp 251–281.

Rising S (1974). The fourth stage of labor: family integration. Am J Nurs, 74: 870–874.

Robinson S (1985a). Normal maternity care: whose responsibility? Br J Obstet Gynaecol, 92: 1–3.

Robinson S (1985b). Maternity care: a duplication of resources. J R Coll Gen Pract, 35: 346–347.

Rooks J (1983). The context of nurse-midwifery in the 1980's. J Nurse Midwifery, 28: 3–8.

Rooks J, Haas E (1986). Nurse-Midwifery in America. Washington DC: American College of Nurse-Midwives.

Rosengren W, DeVault S (1963). The sociology of time and space in an obstetric hospital. In: The Hospital in Modern Society. Freidson E (ed). New York: Free Press. pp 266–292.

Rothman B (1982). In Labor Women and Power in the Birthplace. New York: Norton.

Rothman B (1983). Midwives in transition: the structure of a clinical revolution. Social Problems, 30: 262–71.

Rousch R (1979). The development of midwifery—male and female, yesterday and today. J Nurse Midwifery, 24: 27–37.

Ruzek S (1978). The Women's Health Movement: Feminist Alternatives to Medical Control. New York: Praeger.

Sallomi P, Pallow A, O'Mara McMahon P (1981). Midwifery and the Law. Albuquerque: Mothering Publications.

Sasmor J, Grossman E (1981). Childbirth education in 1980. J Obstet Gynecol Neonatal Nurs, 10: 155–160.

Scholten C (1985). Childbearing in American Society, 1650–1850. New York: New York University Press.

Schorfheide A (1982). Nurse-midwives and obstetricians: a team approach in private practice revisited. J Nurse Midwifery, 27: 12–15.

Scott C (1968). The World of a Gynecologist. London: Oliver & Boyd.

Scully D (1980). Men Who Control Women's Health. Boston: Houghton Mifflin.

Scully D, Bart P (1973). A funny thing happened on the way to the orifice; women in gynecology textbooks. Am J Sociol, 78: 1045–1050.

Shapiro M, Najman J, Chang A, Keeping K, Morrison J, Western J (1983). Information control and the exercise of power in the obstetrical encounter. Soc Sci Med, 17: 139–146.

Shaw N (1974). Forced Labor: Maternity Care in the United States. New York: Pergamon Press.

Shear C, Gipe B, Mattheis J, Levy M (1983). Provider continuity and the quality of medical care. Medical Care, 21: 1204–1210.

Shearer M, Bunnin N (1983). Childbirth educators in the 1980's: a survey of 25 veterans. Birth, 10: 251–256.

Shorter E (1982). A History of Womens Bodies. New York: Basic Books.

Sorel N (1984). Ever Since Eve: Personal reflections on childbirth. New York: Oxford University Press.

Sorlie W, Essex-Sorlie D (1985). Specialty selection: relation of cognitive and noncognitive factors of prematriculation and undergraduate medical education. Evaluation and the Health Professions, 8: 267–298.

Speert H (1968). Midwifery in retrospect. In: Report of a Macy Conference: The Midwife in the United States. New York: Josiah Macy Jr. Foundation, pp 163–177.

Stickles P (1986). Lay-Midwifery regulation—1986. New Mexico: Maternal and Child Health Bureau. (Unpublished report).

Sullivan D, Weitz R (1984). Obstacles to the practice of licensed lay midwifery. Soc Sci Med, 11: 1189–1196.

Taylor G (1982). The general practitioner obstetrician. Practitioner, 226: 513–518.

Throne L, Hansen L (1981). Midwifery laws in the United States. Women and Health, 6: 7–26.

Towler J, Bramall J (1986). Midwives in History and Society. Wolfeboro, New Hampshire: Croom Helm.

Trevathan W (1987). Human Birth: An evolutionary perspective. New York: Aldine de Gruyter.

Walker J (1972). The changing role of the midwife. Int J Nursing Studies, 9: 85–94.

Wardwell W (1972). Limited, marginal and quasi-practitioners. In: Handbook of Medical Sociology. Freeman H, Levine S, Reeder L (eds). Englewood Cliffs, N.J: Prentice-Hall, pp 250–272.

Warpinski D, Adams C (1979). Characteristics of applicants to nurse-Midwifery educational programs. J Nurse Midwifery, 24: 5–9.

Wertz D (1983). What birth has done for doctors: A historical view. Women and Health, 8: 7–24.

Wertz R, Wertz D (1977). Lying-in: A History of Childbirth in America. New York: Free Press.

Yankauer A (1983). The valley of the shadow of birth. Am J Public Health, 73: 635–638.

Zander L (1982). The challenge of antenatal care: a perspective from general practice. In: Effectiveness and Satisfaction in Antenatal Care. Enkin M, Chalmers I (eds). London: Heinemann, pp 247–253.

Zola I (1972). Medicine as an institution of social control. Sociol Rev, 20: 487–504.

10 The role of the midwife: opportunities and constraints

Sarah Robinson

1 Introduction

The midwife has a central place in the provision of care in pregnancy and childbirth, as it is in her role in particular that the main elements of maternity care—clinical assessment and monitoring and the provision of advice and support—are combined. These elements are the focus of internationally accepted definitions of the role of the midwife (e.g. World Health Organization 1966; International Congress of Midwives/International Federation of Gynaecology and Obstetrics 1973). They recognize her as qualified to provide care throughout pregnancy, labour, and the puerperium, to recognize those signs of abnormality that require referral to medical staff, and to provide advice, information, and emotional support to women from the early stages of pregnancy to the end of the postnatal period.

An integrated and holistic approach to care in pregnancy and childbirth is facilitated when midwives are able to practise in accordance with these definitions. While the midwife is assessing fetal development at an antenatal examination, for example, she can at the same time provide the woman with advice on health care and preparation for breastfeeding. Similarly she can offer emotional support to a woman and her partner while monitoring the course of her labour and helping her to deliver. While assessing the clinical condition of the woman postnatally or helping her to establish infant feeding, the midwife has the opportunity to discuss infant care and the maintenance of the woman's own health, as well as facilitating the development of early mother-child relationships.

In practice, however, the range of midwives' responsibilities and the degree of clinical judgement they are able to exercise show considerable variation from one country to another and from one period of history to another. The role of the midwife in the maternity services has been the subject of much debate in recent years, particularly in Europe and North America. Differing views on childbirth and changing patterns and expectations of maternity care have led to considerable disagreement about the appropriate roles to be fulfilled by the various professionals involved in care during pregnancy and childbirth (see Chapter 9).

This chapter examines the factors which constrain the contribution of midwives to the maternity services, the benefits of midwifery care, the developments in the midwifery profession in the last few years, and the opportunities which exist for midwives to develop their role. It focuses primarily on the role of the midwife in the United Kingdom, with only brief reference to other countries. Apart from the author's familiarity with the British scene and the fact that midwifery in the United States is discussed elsewhere (see Chapter 9), there are two main reasons for this. First, international variations in midwifery education and practice are too wide for comprehensive review in this chapter. Second, the recent history of midwifery in Britain is a particularly good demonstration of the central issues in the debate about the midwife's place in maternity care. Issues raised by the British data are therefore relevant to countries in which midwives are seeking to restore their role in maternity care and to countries planning to introduce or reintroduce trained midwifery personnel in areas where they have long since declined.

2 Midwifery training and practice: some international variations

The variation in the training of midwifery personnel and the roles that they can potentially fulfil have been summarized by Hall and Meijia (1978). As shown in Table 10.1, they identify three levels of midwife: the professional midwife or nurse midwife; the intermediate auxiliary midwife or auxiliary nurse midwife, and the non-professional aide or traditional birth attendant. In many of the countries of Northern Europe, midwives are trained to practise in accordance with Hall and Meijia's first category, that of professional midwife. Considerable variation exists, however, in their employment status, their professional responsibilities, and whether or not they are likely to have qualified as nurses before commencing midwifery training. In the United Kingdom, for example, midwives are legally recognized as practitioners in their own right and may provide care for women throughout pregnancy, labour, and the puerperium on their own responsibility. Nearly all of them are employed by the National Health Service and work as members of teams alongside obstetricians,

Table 10.1 Classification and functions of midwifery personnel (Hall and Meijia, 1978, p.214)

Level/ classification	Titles used	Education/training required	Functions performed and independent judgement required
Professional			
Midwife	Midwife Feldsher-midwife	Secondary education plus minimum of 3 years' midwifery education.	Provides care and health education during pregnancy, labour and post-natal period. Manages apparently normal labour without supervision. Cares for newborn infant.
Nurse-midwife	Nurse-midwife	Secondary education, recognised nursing education plus 6–12 months' midwifery education; post-basic training in maternal and child health, advanced midwifery, community health nursing neonatal nursing.	Identifies and refers abnormal conditions and clients at risk. Carries out gynaecological and family planning activities. The above activities can be exercised in the areas of teaching, administration (including supervision), and research.
Intermediate			
Auxiliary or assistant midwife	Auxiliary midwife Assistant midwife Practical midwife Rural midwife Enrolled midwife	6–8 years' general education plus 1–2 years' midwifery training.	Provides care and health education and manages apparently normal labour, usually under direct professional supervision. May supervise lower-level aides. May be trained to work independently where manpower is in short supply e.g., in rural areas.
Auxiliary or assistant nurse-midwife	Auxiliary nurse-midwife Assistant nurse-midwife	6–8 years' general education and 1–2 years' training as an auxiliary nurse, plus 1–2 years' midwifery training or 2–3 years' integrated nursing and midwifery training at auxiliary level.	May qualify to train for professional-level positions through acquiring the requisite level of general education to enter professional education programmes, special curricula, etc, befitting requirements specified by the country.
Non-professional			
Aide	Maternal and child health aide Midwifery aide Trained traditional birth attendant	0–6 years' general education plus on-the-job training in midwifery. On-the-job training in midwifery	Carries out clearly specified tasks in the care of maternity patients and newborn infants, under direct supervision.
Traditional birth attendant	Numerous titles, varying from country to country	Training acquired through working with another traditional birth attendant in apprenticeship fashion.	Normally operates outside organised health system; assists mothers in deliveries; performs bulk of deliveries in rural areas of many countries, owing to inaccessibility of formally training health man-power and community acceptance of traditional practitioners.

general practitioners, health visitors, and other health service personnel. In France, a much larger proportion of midwives is in independent practice, and this is the case for the majority of the midwives in The Netherlands.

There is also considerable diversity in Europe in the way in which responsibilities for antenatal and intranatal care are shared by midwives and obstetricians and, in some countries, by general practitioners as well. A comparison of data from 13 European countries by Blondel *et al.* (1985) demonstrates a range from countries such as The Netherlands, where midwives are responsible for all the care of a substantial proportion of the women who have no complications, to countries like Switzerland where obstetricians supervise the care of most women. Variation also exists in the procedures which midwives are expected to perform. In France, for example, some midwives undertake breech deliveries and manual removal of the placenta, whereas in the United Kingdom these procedures would always be carried out by medical staff, except in an emergency (Bent 1982a).

The situation in North America is somewhat different. The virtual disappearance of the independent community midwife in America by the 1930s has been documented by a number of authors (DeVries 1982; Litoff 1978), and attributed to the medicalization of childbirth, the move from home to hospital delivery, and the hostility of many medical practitioners to midwifery. Nevertheless, midwifery is making a comeback in the United States as evidenced by an increase in the number of certified nurse midwives in practice and by the emergence of lay midwives (see Chapter 9). Recent data show that nurse midwives now work in a variety of settings (hospitals, private practice with physicians, private nurse midwifery practice, public health agencies, and maternity services operated predominantly by nurse midwives), and that there is an increasing trend to work administratively independently of physicians (Office of Technology Assessment 1986). Informally trained lay midwives, often known as 'grannies', had always provided care for women in poorer communities, learning their skills through apprenticeship; but a new generation of lay midwives has emerged to meet the needs of women who want to deliver at home (see Chapter 9). Their legal status varies from state to state, and many still work illegally.

In Canada too, independent community midwives gradually went out of practice, except in isolated rural areas (Barrington 1985). Small numbers of both lay midwives and nurse midwives practise in Canada, although neither are legally recognized at the time of writing. In a number of provinces, however, steps are being taken to recognize the profession of midwifery (see, for example, report by College of Nurses of Ontario 1986).

In any discussion about the role of the midwife it is important to remember that in developing countries 60 to 70 per cent of women give birth without the help of any formally trained personnel (Maglacas and Simons 1986), although they may have the help of traditional birth attendants (Table 10.1). In many countries training programmes for traditional birth attendants have been introduced as a means of increasing the quality of care available for women and children (World Health Organization 1982) and evaluation studies to assess their effectiveness have been undertaken (World Health Organization 1982; Pratinidhi *et al.* 1985; Maglacas and Simons 1986). The complex issues raised by the present and future role of the traditional birth attendant in developing maternal and child health services are not addressed here, however.

In a review of studies on the midwife's role in developed countries, Barclay (1985) has drawn attention to the consistent finding that midwifery skills are frequently under-utilized, mainly as a consequence of medical involvement in an increasing proportion of maternity care. This has meant that although training has created professional midwives or nurse midwives (Table 10.1), the actual practice of these trained professionals approximates more closely to that of auxiliary or assistant midwives. A report recently published by the World Health Organization on perinatal services in its European region also drew attention to this issue (World Health Organization 1985). Respondents in many of the 23 countries participating in the World Health Organization survey said that it was not known precisely what midwives did, but that their role was being diminished by a combination of such factors as 'the increasing role of obstetricians in the routine care of uncomplicated cases and the replacement of midwives by nurses and the moving of midwives into hospitals'.

3 Restriction of the midwife's contribution to maternity care

Three recently published reports of large scale surveys in the United Kingdom have demonstrated the ways in which the midwife's role is restricted. The first was a national survey which focused on the interrelationship of the midwife's role with that of other health professionals involved in maternity care (Robinson *et al.* 1983); the second was a study of the work and deployment of hospital midwives (Department of Health and Social Security 1984); the third was a national survey of policies within midwifery practice (Garcia *et al.* 1985).

The study undertaken by the present author and colleagues (Robinson *et al.* 1983) was commissioned by the Department of Health and Social Security in response to growing concerns in the 1970s about the role of the midwife. The history of the midwife in Britain had been one of a gradual change in role from an independent practitioner providing comprehensive care throughout pregnancy, labour, delivery, and the puerperium, to that of a member of a team of health professionals in which each midwife is likely to be involved in only part of this care (Cowell and Wainwright 1981; Robinson 1983; Towler and Brammall 1986). The view had been expressed that the midwife's skills were not fully utilized within this team, particularly in the provision of care during pregnancy. The Royal College of Midwives, for example, stated in its evidence to the Royal Commission on the National Health Service: 'the midwife is trained and capable of giving prenatal care on her own responsibility, but in practice the medical staff do not fully utilize this valuable resource'. It went on to suggest that 'clarification of the role of each member of the maternity services team is essential' (Royal College of Midwives 1977). Brain (1979) considered that the role of the midwife had contracted in the 1970s and that 'in some clinics midwives are only used as receptionists or chaperons, and to test urine and weigh women' (Brain 1979). Commenting on developments in the 1970s, Barnett (1979) felt that although midwives regarded doctors as their partners, the reverse was not always true.

Our survey (Robinson *et al.* 1983), undertaken in 1979, focused on the division of responsibility between midwives and other health professionals, but also looked at other factors, such as staff shortages, that could restrict the midwife's role. Sixty health districts were randomly selected from the regional health authorities of England and from Wales. Questionnaires were then sent to all midwives and medical staff in obstetrics in each district, and to a sample of the health visitors and general practitioners. The data cited here are drawn from information obtained from the midwives, 78 per cent of whom returned the questionnaire. Many of the findings have been substantiated by the two subsequent studies (Department of Health and Social Security 1984; Garcia *et al.* 1985).

3.1 Restrictions imposed by medical involvement

3.1.1 Antenatal care

Despite the fact that midwives are qualified to assess the health of the woman and the fetus, and to recognize those signs of abnormality that necessitate referral to medical practitioners, they were found to play only a minor role in antenatal care in 1979 (Robinson *et al.* 1983). The majority of both hospital and community midwives, who took part in the survey, did say that they performed most of the tasks that constitute normal antenatal care: interviewing the mother; recording her history; urine testing; weighing; taking blood pressures and performing abdominal examinations. However, nearly all the hospital midwives and two-thirds of the community midwives worked in clinics in which they were not required to take responsibility for the overall assessment of pregnancy.

As shown in Table 10.2, this was because the abdominal examination was performed by a doctor, even if it had already been carried out by a midwife. It is when this examination is performed and when the results of the other routine investigations are available that the overall assessment of pregnancy is made.

It can be argued that women attending hospital antenatal clinics were usually examined by a doctor because, since the advent of shared antenatal care between hospital and general practitioner, the primary purpose of the visits to the hospital clinic is assessment by an obstetrician. The data in Table 10.2 show, however, that at the community antenatal clinics women are also likely to be assessed by medical staff. In general, the main role for midwives in antenatal care in England and Wales at that time was shown to be one of ensuring that the medical staff had all the relevant information to make the assessment, and not one of interpreting the findings for themselves. Midwives do have the opportunity to make antenatal assessments on their own responsibility at midwives' clinics or when visiting women at home. The survey data showed, however, that there were few such clinics and that antenatal assessment at home visits was rare.

Similar conclusions were reached by the Central Management Services team after its survey of 18 hospitals (Department of Health and Social Security 1984). These hospitals, a random stratified sample of those in

Table 10.2 Hospital and community midwives responsibilities for abdominal examination during pregnancy (after Robinson *et al.* 1983)

Abdominal examination	Midwives in consultant units		Community midwives	
	No.	%	No.	%
Usually carried out by midwife only	27	4.3	161	13.9
Usually carried out by doctor only	212	33.4	193	16.7
Carried out by midwife but usually repeated by doctor	363	57.3	564	48.7
Carried out by midwife at one visit and by doctor at next	—	—	79	6.8
Situation varies from one clinic to another	—	—	100	8.6
No answer	32	5.0	62	5.3
Total	634	100.0	1159	100.0

England, represented a mix of general practitioner and consultant units. The data showed that medical staff undertook most of the examinations and diagnostic work and were assisted by midwives who undertook the various routine tasks and co-ordinated the running of the clinics (Department of Health and Social Security 1984).

3.1.2 Care during labour and delivery

The erosion of the midwife's role in the management of labour and delivery is more complex than that demonstrated for antenatal care. Although there was an increase in the 1970s in the proportion of operative and instrumental deliveries, the majority of deliveries in the United Kingdom, as in previous decades, continued to be undertaken or supervised by a midwife (Chamberlain *et al.* 1978; Cartwright 1979; Department of Health and Social Security 1984). Changes were, however, taking place in the extent to which the midwife was responsible for determining the pattern of care during labour and delivery. This was due both to an increase in the involvement of medical staff in the assessment of women in the labour ward, and to the introduction of policies specifying the procedures to be followed in the management of labour and delivery, such as the frequency of vaginal examinations, the length of time allowed for the second stage of labour, and whether or not to use routine continuous fetal heart rate monitoring. These policies were formulated by the senior medical staff, either alone or in conjunction with senior midwives. In either case they restricted the freedom of the individual midwife to exercise her clinical judgement in the care of individual women.

The studies by Robinson *et al.* (1983) and Garcia *et al.* (1985) demonstrated the extent to which midwives' responsibilities had been restricted in this way. As shown in Table 10.3, the majority of midwives who took part in the earlier study said that women in normal labour were cared for by a midwife and not examined by a doctor unless this was requested by the midwife. This proportion varied according to the type of unit in which the midwife worked, from slightly over 70 per

Table 10.3 Responsibilities of hospital midwives in the management of normal labour (data from Robinson *et al.* 1983)

Midwives' answers	No.	%
Patients in normal labour are cared for by a midwife and not examined by a doctor unless the midwife asks him/her to do so	1760	82.4
All patients are examined by a doctor on admission and then normal labours are managed entirely by a midwife unless a problem arises	224	10.5
All patients are examined by a doctor on admission, visited at regular intervals throughout labour and the decisions on management of labour are made by a doctor	83	3.9
No answer	69	3.2
Total	2136	100.0

Table 10.4 Responsibilities of hospital midwives in decision-making during normal labour and delivery by type of hospital and/or unit (after Robinson *et al.* 1983)

	Per cent of midwives working in				
	Consultant units within		General practitioner units/hospitals		
Decision making	Teaching hospitals (*n*=372)	Non-teaching hospitals (*n*=1062)	Within a consultant unit (*n*=85)	Separate from a consultant unit (*n*=225)	All types of units (*n*=1984)
1. *When to carry out vaginal examinations in normal labour*					
Decision usually made by midwife	30.4	53.2	72.9	93.3	56.3
Decision usually made by a member of medical staff	—	0.5	—	—	0.3
Unit policy which specifies the usual procedure	65.3	44.0	23.5	5.3	40.9
No answer	4.3	2.4	3.5	1.3	2.6
Total	100.–	100.–	100.–	100.–	100.–
2. *When to rupture membranes during normal labour*					
Decision usually made by midwife	43.–	61.–	60.–	82.7	59.7
Decision usually made by a member of medical staff	8.9	10.5	17.6	10.7	12.–
Unit policy which specifies the usual procedure	43.8	25.–	17.6	4.9	24.6
No answer	4.3	3.4	4.7	1.8	3.7
Total	100.–	100.–	100.–	100.–	100.–

cent in teaching hospitals, to 95 per cent in general practitioner units separate from a consultant unit.

The division of responsibility between midwives and medical staff in consultant units was explored in more detail by Garcia *et al.* (1985). They found that in only 15 per cent of units could a midwife send a woman home if she was admitted with intact membranes but was judged not to be in labour. They also found that in 1984 20 per cent of consultant units had a policy that women in normal labour should be seen by a doctor at regular intervals, whereas five years earlier, Robinson *et al.* had found this to be the case for less than 5 per cent of midwives working in consultant units.

Both the Robinson *et al.* (1983) and Garcia *et al.* (1985) studies looked at the effect of unit policies on the midwife's responsibilities. Robinson and her colleagues showed that a substantial proportion of those midwives who said that women in normal labour were only examined by a doctor when requested by a midwife, none the less worked in units in which decisions that are basic to the care during normal labour were determined by unit policy. This is shown in Table 10.4 for decisions about the frequency with which vaginal examinations should be carried out and about rupturing membranes during labour. These decisions were much more likely to be determined by unit policy in consultant units, particularly in teaching hospitals, than in separate general practitioner units. Garcia's study (1985) produced similar findings in that midwives in 70 per cent of consultant units followed a unit policy with regard to the timing of vaginal examinations. The study also explored unit policies and midwives' responsibilities for decision-making over a wide range of aspects of care in labour and delivery (see Chapters 14 and 51).

3.1.3 Postpartum care

The studies by Robinson *et al.* (1983) and Garcia *et al.* (1985) both demonstrated a duplication of roles in the clinical assessment of normal women after delivery similar to the duplication seen in antenatal care. Midwives are qualified to assess the condition of the mother postpartum and make daily examinations to do so. The majority of those who participated in the 1979 study, however, worked in consultant units in which medical staff also examined normal puerperal women, either once or twice during their stay (55 per cent) or daily (26 per cent). Only 17 per cent said that medical staff examined normal puerperal women only if asked to do so by a midwife (Robinson et al. 1983). Garcia's study, undertaken five years later, showed a similar situation: medical staff examined puerperal women routinely once or twice in two-thirds of consultant units, daily in a fifth of these units, and only if referred by a midwife in less than a fifth.

Data from both these studies and the Department of Health and Social Security study showed that it was usual practice for medical staff to make decisions as to whether mothers and babies were fit to be discharged. This is a decision which midwives are qualified to make on their own responsibility. Many of the respondents in the study of Robinson *et al.* (1983) felt that it was more appropriate for this decision to be made by the midwifery team than by the medical team, since they provided continuous care after delivery and were thus in a better position than the medical team to assess accurately whether women were emotionally and physically ready for discharge.

The study by Robinson *et al.* (1983) also showed that the midwife's degree of responsibility was likely to vary by the type of unit in which she worked. Thirty-five per cent of those working in teaching hospitals said that in the postpartum period normal women were examined daily by a doctor, whereas this proportion fell to 22 per cent in non-teaching hospitals, 14 per cent in general practitioner wards or units within consultant units, and 6 per cent in separate general practitioner hospitals.

3.2 Effects of restricting the midwife's role by medical involvement

Restrictions of the midwife's responsibilities for normal maternity care, as documented by these studies, have implications for the use of resources, for the self-confidence of midwives, for developing appropriate curricula for midwifery training and, most importantly, for the type of care available to women.

Under-using the midwife's skills wastes resources. Midwives are trained at some considerable cost, but the parts of their training that concern decision-making, particularly in the assessment of pregnancy, tend to be wasted. Resources are duplicated if medical staff repeat procedures that have already been carried out by midwives, who are qualified to do this on their own responsibility. Community antenatal care is a particular case in point. Midwives are specifically qualified to provide care for women with low risk pregnancies, and yet many general practitioners are also paid to provide care for the same group of women.

If decisions about the management of normal pregnancy, labour, and the puerperium are usually made by medical staff, opportunities for student midwives to develop confidence in their skills and in their ability to take responsibility for decisions will be limited. Opportunities for qualified midwives to develop and maintain their confidence in deciding about various aspects of care will also be restricted.

Similarly, stringent unit policies, whether they are formulated solely by the medical staff or by the medical staff in consultation with senior midwives, have a restricting effect on the development of clinical judgement. This can lead to problems when policies change, if the necessary skills have been lost with the retirement of experienced midwives and have not been developed in more recently trained practitioners. For instance, one of the senior midwives who took part in Robinson *et al.*'s 1979 survey said: 'Unit policy states that all primips must have an episiotomy. In some primips they are totally unnecessary, but students qualify without having delivered a primip with an intact perineum and never develop any judgement of their own.' Romney and White (1984), when considering the indications for setting up a controlled trial of the Brandt–Andrews technique for managing the third stage of labour, commented: 'It is important to conduct such research as soon as possible before the best exponents of non-active management have retired from the service'.

Obviously, some general guidelines about the management of labour are desirable, especially for newly qualified midwives and students. The expertise of senior midwives in conjunction with flexible application of these general guidelines, however, is likely to result in care that is at least as effective as that which results from rigidly interpreted policies but is not individualized. Of no lesser concern is the observation that many unit policies insist on practices of unproven benefit (see Chapters 50 and 51). The wide variation in the degree of responsibility that midwives are permitted to exercise once qualified creates difficulties in the development of appropriate curricula for midwifery training. If training is designed to enable midwives to take a particular level of responsibility, then many are likely to experience the frustration and lack of job satisfaction that results from unfulfilled expectations.

Failure to make full use of the clinical skills and judgement of the midwife also affects the kind of support they are able to provide for women. When medical staff assess normal pregnancy, care tends to be fragmented into a number of tasks undertaken by different personnel: not only doctors and midwives, but in some clinics, nursing and auxiliary staff as well. This fragmentation means that each woman has only brief contacts with each person involved in her care. In this situation midwives have neither the time nor the opportunity to develop the kind of supportive and continuous relationship within which women feel encouraged to discuss their pregnancy and any problems or concerns that they may have.

The fact that most women have to be seen by a doctor contributes to long waiting times. The medical staff in turn has less time available to spend with the women who have medical and obstetric problems that require their specialist expertise (see Chapter 78). Complaints about long waiting periods and lack of opportunities to discuss and voice concerns feature prominently in many of the reports of consumers' views of antenatal care (National Childbirth Trust 1981; Garcia 1982; see Chapter 8), and were certainly of concern to many of the midwives who participated in the 1979 survey (Robinson *et al.* 1983). One of the staff midwives said: 'More time is needed with patients to prepare them for the birth. The clinics are far too big and impersonal and midwives are too busy dashing from one patient to another with impatient mothers who are tired of waiting.' Another commented: 'We need more complete care of individual patients, rather than taking blood pressures, directing pregnant bodies on and off couches so that there is always one "prepared" and the doctor doesn't lose precious seconds as he rushes from one to the next.'

If a midwife is not entrusted with the care of normal pregnant women, a role for which she is qualified, she may cease to have confidence in her own ability and become less likely to be able to increase the self-confidence of the pregnant women who look to her for support. Cartwright (1979) reported that many women felt they were given insufficient information in the course of labour and a further study by Kirkham (1982) concluded that one of the reasons that midwives fail to provide women with information during labour, is that they are unhappy themselves with the policies they are required to implement in providing care.

3.3 Other factors restricting the midwife's role

Factors other than the increased involvement of medical staff in normal maternity care have also restricted the utilization of midwifery skills. Lack of opportunity to provide continuity of care and a shortage of midwives on duty also prevent the midwife from making her full contribution to the care of childbearing women.

The midwife is ideally qualified to provide continuity of care, as she is the only health professional whose training relates specifically to both the clinical and the advisory aspects of pregnancy, labour, and the puerperium. Historical accounts show that midwives working in the community and in hospital were able to follow women through from early pregnancy to the end of the postnatal period (Cowell and Wainwright 1981; Robinson 1983; Towler and Brammall 1986), but opportunities to give this continuity of care have gradually diminished.

Some of the reasons for this change include the move from home to hospital confinement, centralized delivery suites rather than combined wards, and the development of a staffing pattern in which hospital midwives tend to be based either in the antenatal clinic, on the labour ward, or on the postnatal ward, rather than to provide all these components of care. Data provided for the Peel Committee, for example, indicated that in 1968 approximately one-quarter of hospital midwives in Britain were working solely on one aspect of maternity care (Department of Health and Social Security 1970). By 1979 this proportion had risen to two-thirds (Robinson *et al.* 1983). The World Health Organization survey of perinatal services noted that this trend to fragment care was found in most European countries, with pregnancy, birth, and the puerperium being regarded as 'three separate clinical situations requiring different clinical expertise, different medical personnel and different clinical settings' (World Health Organization 1985). Lack of continuity of care within the antenatal, intranatal, and postnatal periods can, as discussed above, also be due to fragmentation of care between a number of health service personnel.

Shortage of midwifery staff is a longstanding problem. Since World War II, professional and statutory bodies for midwifery in the United Kingdom as well as a number of government working parties, have maintained that there are insufficient midwives in the service to provide adequate care (Robinson 1986a). A survey carried out by the International Confederation of Midwives and the International Federation of Gynaecology and Obstetrics (1976) showed that this was a problem in many other European countries as well (ICM/FIGO 1976). Data obtained by Robinson *et al.* (1983) showed staff shortages to be of major concern. Just over half of the midwives working in consultant units on day duty said that there were not usually enough midwives on duty to cope with the work. This feeling was expressed by almost three-quarters of those working on night duty. Midwives on postnatal wards were the most likely to express this view. Inadequate standards of care, lack of time to provide advice and support, lack of time to teach student midwives, and adverse effects on midwives' job satisfaction and working conditions were all cited as consequences of inadequate staffing levels in hospital (Robinson *et al.* 1983). Staffing levels were also a problem for community midwives, almost half of whom said that there were not enough midwives to cope with the work; some members of this group were making up to 15 postnatal visits a day. Evidence submitted to the Pay Review Body by the Royal College of Midwives indicates that the situation had not been improved in hospital or in the community in the United Kingdom since that study was undertaken (Royal College of Midwives 1984 and 1985).

4 The effects of midwifery care

The midwife's role has been constrained by medical involvement in normal maternity care, by fragmentation of care and by a shortage of staff; but does it matter? How essential is it in terms of perinatal outcome and experience of childbirth that midwifery skills, knowledge, and support are available and fully utilized? A number of studies have attempted to answer these questions. Some of these have focused on support and advice provided by midwives, others have looked at the outcome of pregnancy for women cared for primarily by midwives. Studies in the latter group fall into two categories: those that studied the effect of introducing midwifery personnel into situations where women previously had no access to such care; and those that compared systems of care based on midwives as the prime caregivers with systems where the medical staff was primarily responsible for care.

At least three randomized controlled trials have been conducted comparing the outcome of midwifery care with that of medical care. Two of these studies, Runnerstrom (1969) and Slome *et al.* (1976), sought to evaluate the effectiveness of care provided by certified nurse midwives in hospital settings in North America. In the former study, women who satisfied criteria for inclusion in the trial were randomly allocated to either an experimental group of women who were cared for solely by nurse midwives with medical referral when necessary, or to a control group who were cared for solely by the resident medical staff (Runnerstrom 1969). Similarly, in the study conducted by Slome and colleagues (1976) women were randomly allocated to care by nurse midwives or to care by resident medical practitioners. The third study (Flint and Poulengeris 1987), was undertaken in the United Kingdom in response to concerns about the lack of continuity of care in the maternity services and the resulting lack of opportunity for women to develop relationships of support and trust with their caregivers. Under the scheme, women were randomly allocated either to the care of a team of four midwives who provided them with all the care from early pregnancy to the end of the postnatal period, or to receive normal hospital care from a variety of different doctors and midwives.

The findings from these three studies are shown in Tables 10.5; 10.6; 10.7; 10.8, and 10.9. It should be noted, however, that there was some selection bias both at and after entry to the trial in all three of these studies. This applied in particular to the North American data, as is readily apparent from the differences between the number of women included in the midwifery care group and in the medical care group. It should be noted as well that the type of care provided by nurse midwives in the United States some twenty (Runnerstrom 1969) and ten (Slome *et al.* 1976) years ago, may not be exactly comparable to that provided by British midwives in the 1980s. This argument, however, is also likely to apply to the care received by the women included in the control groups of these studies.

There was no difference noted in these trials on the overall use of pharmacological analgesia by the women cared for by midwives and those cared for by medical practitioners. There was, however, a statistically significant decrease in the use of epidural analgesia by the woman cared for by midwives. Differences in the use of other pharmacological measures for pain relief did not reach statistical significance. (Table 10.6).

The data of Flint and Poulengeris (1987) showed that women cared for by the midwife team were more likely

Table 10.5 Effect of midwife vs. medical/shared care on Induction of labour

Study	EXPT		CTRL		Odds ratio	Graph of odds ratios and confidence intervals
	n	(%)	*n*	(%)	(95% CI)	0.01 0.1 0.5 1 2 10 100
Flint C and Poulengeris (1987)	51/465	(10.97)	60/458	(13.10)	0.82 (0.55–1.22)	
Typical odds ratio (95% confidence interval)					0.82 (0.55–1.22)	

Effect of midwife vs. medical/shared care on acceleration of labour

Study	EXPT		CTRL		Odds ratio	Graph of odds ratios and confidence intervals
Flint C and Poulengeris (1987)	80/465	(17.20)	114/458	(24.89)	0.63 (0.46–0.86)	
Typical odds ratio (95% confidence interval)					0.63 (0.46–0.86)	

Table 10.6 Effect of midwife vs. medical/shared care on use of pharmacological analgesia

Study	EXPT		CTRL		Odds ratio	Graph of odds ratios and confidence intervals
	n	(%)	*n*	(%)	(95% CI)	0.01 0.1 0.5 1 2 10 100
Flint C and Poulengeris (1987)	233/479	(48.64)	293/473	(61.95)	0.58 (0.45–0.75)	
Runnerstrom L (1969)	660/768	(85.94)	784/1005	(78.01)	1.69 (1.33–2.15)	
Typical odds ratio (95% confidence interval)					1.02 (0.86–1.22)	

Effect of midwife vs. medical/shared care on regional anaesthesia/analgesia

Study	EXPT		CTRL		Odds ratio	Graph of odds ratios and confidence intervals
Flint C and Poulengeris (1987)	88/479	(18.37)	143/473	(30.23)	0.52 (0.39–0.71)	
Runnerstrom L (1969)	7/768	(0.91)	48/1005	(4.78)	0.28 (0.16–0.48)	
Typical odds ratio (95% confidence interval)					0.45 (0.35–0.59)	

Table 10.7 Effect of midwife vs. medical/shared care on episiotomy

Study	EXPT		CTRL		Odds ratio	Graph of odds ratios and confidence intervals
	n	(%)	*n*	(%)	(95% CI)	0.01 0.1 0.5 1 2 10 100
Flint C and Poulengeris (1987)	152/443	(34.31)	185/438	(42.24)	0.72 (0.55–0.94)	
Runnerstrom L (1969)	515/768	(67.06)	754/1005	(75.02)	0.68 (0.55–0.83)	
Typical odds ratio (95% confidence interval)					0.69 (0.59–0.81)	

Table 10.7 *(continued)* Effect of midwife vs. medical/shared care on operative vaginal delivery

Study	EXPT *n*	EXPT (%)	CTRL *n*	CTRL (%)	Odds ratio (95% CI)	Graph of odds ratios and confidence intervals (0.01 0.1 0.5 1 2 10 100)
Flint C and Poulengeris (1987)	56/479	(11.69)	66/473	(13.95)	0.82 (0.56–1.19)	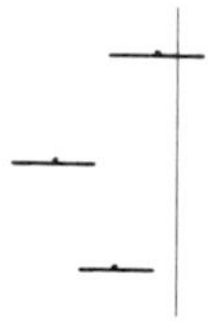
Slome C *et al*. (1976)	39/298	(13.09)	47/140	(33.57)	0.27 (0.17–0.45)	
Typical odds ratio (95% confidence interval)					0.55 (0.41–0.75)	

Effect of midwife vs. medical/shared care on caesarean section

Study	EXPT *n*	EXPT (%)	CTRL *n*	CTRL (%)	Odds ratio (95% CI)	Graph
Flint C and Poulengeris (1987)	37/479	(7.72)	35/473	(7.40)	1.05 (0.65–1.69)	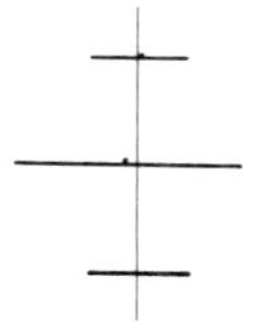
Slome C *et al*. (1976)	11/298	(3.69)	6/140	(4.29)	0.85 (0.30–2.41)	
Typical odds ratio (95% confidence interval)					1.01 (0.65–1.56)	

Table 10.8 Effect of midwife vs. medical/shared care on birthweight <2500g

Study	EXPT *n*	EXPT (%)	CTRL *n*	CTRL (%)	Odds ratio (95% CI)	Graph of odds ratios and confidence intervals (0.01 0.1 0.5 1 2 10 100)
Flint C and Poulengeris (1987)	31/478	(6.49)	38/471	(8.07)	0.79 (0.48–1.29)	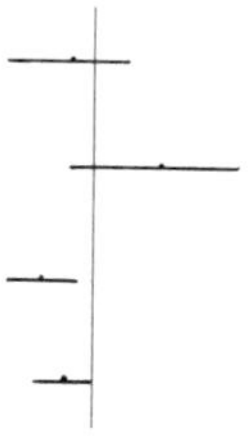
Slome C *et al*. (1976)	27/298	(9.06)	7/140	(5.00)	1.76 (0.83–3.73)	
Runnerstrom L (1969)	61/768	(7.94)	121/1005	(12.04)	0.64 (0.47–0.87)	
Typical odds ratio (95% confidence interval)					0.75 (0.59–0.97)	

Effect of midwife vs. medical/shared care on apgar score <8 at 1 minute

Study	EXPT *n*	EXPT (%)	CTRL *n*	CTRL (%)	Odds ratio (95% CI)	Graph
Flint C and Poulengeris (1987)	90/471	(19.11)	91/467	(19.49)	0.98 (0.71–1.35)	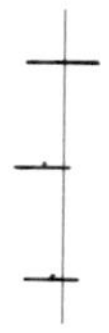
Runnerstrom L (1969)	100/768	(13.02)	149/1005	(14.83)	0.86 (0.66–1.13)	
Typical odds ratio (95% confidence interval)					0.91 (0.74–1.12)	

Effect of midwife vs. medical/shared care on neonatal resuscitation

Study	EXPT *n*	EXPT (%)	CTRL *n*	CTRL (%)	Odds ratio (95% CI)	Graph
Flint C and Poulengeris (1987)	97/474	(20.46)	128/465	(27.53)	0.68 (0.50–0.92)	
Typical odds ratio (95% confidence interval)					0.68 (0.50–0.92)	

Table 10.8 *(continued)* Effect of midwife vs. medical/shared care on stillbirth or neonatal death

Study	EXPT *n*	EXPT (%)	CTRL *n*	CTRL (%)	Odds ratio (95% CI)	Graph of odds ratios and confidence intervals (0.01 0.1 0.5 1 2 10 100)
Flint C and Poulengeris (1987)	8/470	(1.70)	4/467	(0.86)	1.95 (0.62–6.09)	
Slome C *et al.* (1976)	4/298	(1.34)	2/140	(1.43)	0.94 (0.17–5.27)	
Runnerstrom L (1969)	2/768	(0.26)	1/1005	(0.10)	2.59 (0.26–25.46)	
Typical odds ratio (95% confidence interval)					1.68 (0.70–4.05)	

Effect of midwife vs. medical/shared care on admission to special care nursery

Study	EXPT *n*	EXPT (%)	CTRL *n*	CTRL (%)	Odds ratio (95% CI)	Graph
Flint C and Poulengeris (1987)	23/475	(4.84)	21/470	(4.47)	1.09 (0.59–1.99)	
Runnerstrom L (1969)	90/768	(11.72)	162/1005	(16.12)	0.70 (0.53–0.91)	
Typical odds ratio (95% confidence interval)					0.75 (0.59–0.96)	

Table 10.9 Effect of midwife vs. medical/shared care on clinic waiting time 15 minutes or more

Study	EXPT *n*	EXPT (%)	CTRL *n*	CTRL (%)	Odds ratio (95% CI)	Graph of odds ratios and confidence intervals (0.01 0.1 0.5 1 2 10 100)
Flint C and Poulengeris (1987)	106/275	(38.55)	249/267	(93.26)	0.09 (0.06–0.13)	
Typical odds ratio (95% confidence interval)					0.09 (0.06–0.13)	

Effect of midwife vs. medical/shared care on poor ability to discuss anxieties

Study	EXPT *n*	EXPT (%)	CTRL *n*	CTRL (%)	Odds ratio (95% CI)	Graph
Flint C and Poulengeris (1987)	29/272	(10.66)	61/261	(23.37)	0.40 (0.26–0.64)	
Typical odds ratio (95% confidence interval)					0.40 (0.26–0.64)	

Effect of midwife vs. medical/shared care on poor ability to discuss post partum

Study	EXPT *n*	EXPT (%)	CTRL *n*	CTRL (%)	Odds ratio (95% CI)	Graph
Flint C and Poulengeris (1987)	89/246	(36.18)	108/220	(49.09)	0.59 (0.41–0.85)	
Typical odds ratio (95% confidence interval)					0.59 (0.41–0.85)	

Effect of midwife vs. medical/shared care on feeling ill-prepared for labour

Study	EXPT *n*	EXPT (%)	CTRL *n*	CTRL (%)	Odds ratio (95% CI)	Graph
Flint C and Poulengeris (1987)	131/275	(47.64)	152/254	(59.84)	0.61 (0.44–0.86)	
Typical odds ratio (95% confidence interval)					0.61 (0.44–0.86)	

Table 10.9 *(continued)* Effect of midwife vs. medical/shared care on dissatisfaction with pain relief

Study	EXPT n	EXPT (%)	CTRL n	CTRL (%)	Odds ratio (95% CI)	Graph of odds ratios and confidence intervals (0.01 0.1 0.5 1 2 10 100)
Flint C and Poulengeris (1987)	88/209	(42.11)	101/205	(49.27)	0.75 (0.51–1.10)	
Typical odds ratio (95% confidence interval)					0.75 (0.51–1.10)	

Effect of midwife vs. medical/shared care on lack of enjoyment of labour

Study	EXPT n	EXPT (%)	CTRL n	CTRL (%)	Odds ratio (95% CI)	Graph
Flint C and Poulengeris (1987)	142/246	(57.72)	151/223	(67.71)	0.65 (0.45–0.95)	
Typical odds ratio (95% confidence interval)					0.65 (0.45–0.95)	

Effect of midwife vs. medical/shared care on not feeling in control during labour

Study	EXPT n	EXPT (%)	CTRL n	CTRL (%)	Odds ratio (95% CI)	Graph
Flint C and Poulengeris (1987)	143/246	(58.13)	171/225	(76.00)	0.45 (0.31–0.66)	
Typical odds ratio (95% confidence interval)					0.45 (0.31–0.66)	

Effect of midwife vs. medical/shared care on feeling ill-prepared for child care

Study	EXPT n	EXPT (%)	CTRL n	CTRL (%)	Odds ratio (95% CI)	Graph
Flint C and Poulengeris (1987)	138/242	(57.02)	158/222	(71.17)	0.54 (0.37–0.79)	
Typical odds ratio (95% confidence interval)					0.54 (0.37–0.79)	

to have a spontaneous labour throughout, in that both the rates of induction and of acceleration of labour were higher in the group cared for by doctors (Table 10.5). Two of the studies provided data on the rate of instrumental vaginal delivery. Although a statistically significant decrease in the frequency of instrumental vaginal delivery was noted in the groups of women cared for by midwives, and the direction of the effect was consistent in both studies (Table 10.7), it should be noted that the pooled odds ratio is greatly influenced by the study of Slome *et al.* (1976), which was relatively weak in its experimental design. No differences in caesarean section rates emerged between women receiving care from midwives and those receiving medical care (Table 10.7). Women cared for by midwives were less likely to have an episiotomy than those cared for by medical practitioners (Table 10.7); a further sub-analysis of the British study (not shown) indicated that primiparae in particular were less likely to have an episiotomy when cared for by midwives.

Overall, midwifery care appeared to have a beneficial effect on the incidence of low birthweight (Table 10.8).

Data on stillbirth and neonatal death rates showed no disadvantage or advantage for midwifery care as compared to medical care, but the numbers of these adverse outcomes were too small to allow any confident conclusion (Table 10.8). The available data on resuscitation of the newborn and admission to special care nurseries seem to be in favour of midwifery care, although there were no differences in the incidence of low Apgar score at 1 min (Table 10.8).

Flint and Poulengeris (1987) also examined various aspects of maternal satisfaction, some of which are listed in Table 10.9. In general, maternal satisfaction was found to be greatly enhanced by the provision of midwife care; the possibility of assessment bias (see Chapter 50), however, needs to be taken into account before generalizations can be drawn from such data.

Overall, the randomized studies, while not of impeccable methodological quality indicate that there may be several advantages to the provision of midwife care. These relate mainly to less frequent interventions (such as epidural analgesia, drug-induced stimulation of uterine contractions, and episiotomy) on the one hand and to enhanced maternal satisfaction on the other.

Retrospective studies from areas where midwifery services were (re)introduced, especially the United States, as well as comparisons between midwifery and medical care, tend to give a more positive view on the effectiveness of midwifery care. These studies need to be interpreted with caution, however, given the inherent problems in their design.

A number of retrospective studies have drawn attention to the good results achieved by nurse midwives in the United States. The nurse midwifery service introduced in rural Kentucky in 1926 was followed by a reduction in maternal and neonatal mortality and stillbirth, leading the Metropolitan Life Insurance Company to conclude that the 'nurse midwives' care had effected a revolution in maternal and child health statistics' (quoted in Raisler 1985). Opportunities for nurse midwives to practise, though, have been restricted, as until recently few states have allowed them to do so. The effect which they may have on mortality rates has been shown, for example, in Madera County, California, when a shortage of medical manpower led to special legislation allowing them to practise for a three-year period in the early 1960s (Levy *et al.* 1971). Prior to the introduction of the nurse-midwifery programme, the rate of 'premature' births was 11 per cent and the neonatal mortality rate 23.9 per thousand. In the three years of the programme, these rates dropped to 6.6 per cent and 10.3 per 1000 respectively; there was a large increase in both the proportion of expectant mothers attending for antenatal care and in the average number of visits made by each woman.

Despite these improvements the programme was discontinued, as the California Medical Association refused to support a permanent change in the law which would allow nurse midwives to continue practising, and all care was again provided by inadequate numbers of medical staff. A retrospective analysis of the records showed that in the period over which medical care was restored (1960–1966) there was a significant rise in the incidence of 'premature' birth (from 6.6 to 9.8 per cent) and in the neonatal mortality rate (from 10.3 to 32.1 per 1000) and a decrease in the amount of antenatal care provided. Levy *et al.* (1971) examined a number of variables which might have accounted for these changes, but concluded that lower quantity and probably lower quality of care were the main causes.

In a retrospective comparison of records of women cared for by nurse midwives at Roosevelt Hospital in New York with a group of private patients cared for by obstetricians, Dillon *et al.* (1978) found no statistically significant difference in fetal outcome for the two groups. The authors concluded from the study that a low risk group of women suitable for midwifery care can be identified. Reviews of other studies which have evaluated the effectiveness of American nurse-midwifery programmes are provided by Thompson 1986 and Office of Technology Assessment 1986.

The success of nurse-midwifery teams, such as those employed at the North Central Bronx Hospital in New York, for example, has been attributed partly to a high degree of accountability among the midwives, through weekly outcome reviews—'someone must be responsible for the care of the patient. When that responsibility is diluted among many people, the outcome suffers. Nurse midwives here become keenly aware of the results of their practice . . .' (Dondeiro quoted in Raisler 1985). Commenting on the success of nurse-midwifery programmes, Raisler (1985) concluded that their good outcomes result from the 'provision of early, vigilant and personal maternity care that integrates the principles of continuity, participation and patient education'.

A number of studies have shown that many women consider the provision of support and information to be an important aspect of care. Kirkham's (1982) study, for example, showed that women felt they would be able to cope better with labour if they were kept regularly informed about its progress (see Chapter 49). Lack of support and advice was found by Filshie *et al.* (1981) to be a cause of complaints in the postnatal period (see Chapter 79), and a number of studies have revealed a similar situation in relation to the antenatal period (e.g. Graham and McKee 1980; Oakley 1980).

A number of authors have documented appreciation of the support and information that can be provided by midwives during the course of pregnancy, labour, and the puerperium. The majority of women who took part in a survey of the care received from community midwives, for example, commented favourably on many aspects of that care (Humphrey 1985). Continuity of care from one or two midwives, continuous help and support during labour, and adequate time to have questions answered (especially those 'the doctor might find silly') were all identified as being of particular importance. In a survey of attitudes to obstetric care, Morgan *et al.* (1984) found that 61 per cent of their sample of 1000 mothers agreed with the statement: 'Having a sympathetic midwife to help mothers through labour is more important than all treatment for pain relief.' Women interviewed by Williams *et al.* (1985) about epidural analgesia for pain relief in labour often commented on the importance of a supportive midwife; the authors suggested that perhaps 'midwives in this technological age have underestimated the importance of this aspect of their role'.

It has been proposed (Field 1984; Newson 1985) that support by midwives during pregnancy might have a beneficial effect on perinatal outcome, particularly for women at risk, and Davies and Evans (1987) have recently reported on the progress of such a scheme in an inner city area in the United Kingdom. Randomized controlled trials of social support by midwives, aimed at raising birthweight by an average of 150 g in women with a history of low birthweight delivery, are also currently in progress in a number of places (see Chapter 15).

5 Midwifery developments in the 1980s

5.1 Initiatives to develop and restore the midwife's role

In 1979 many of the midwives who took part in the study by Robinson *et al.* (1983) said that they wanted to take more responsibility for decision-making, particularly in the antenatal period. Since then midwives in Britain have been involved in developing schemes in which their skills are more appropriately deployed to meet womens' needs. Midwives' clinics have been established in a number of areas (e.g. Morrin 1982; Flint 1982; Stuart and Judge 1984). Also schemes in which consultant obstetricians visit community based clinics to give care in conjunction with the community staff have begun to restore the midwife's role in giving care during pregnancy (McKee 1984; Taylor 1984). Community based antenatal schemes do not necessarily make full use of the midwife's skills, however. When these clinics were first instigated in some of the districts included in the study by Robinson *et al.* (1983), antenatal assessments were made either by the consultant or by the general practitioner, but not by the midwife. Only after the issue was taken up by midwifery managers did obstetricians agree that at each clinic a group of women could be allocated to a midwife.

In some consultant units, delivery suites have now been established in which intrapartum care for low risk women is provided totally by midwives (Towler 1981; Rider 1983). Schemes in which midwives help special groups of women have also been developed: these include antenatal day wards for women who for one reason or another were not able to stay in hospital (Penny 1986) and support schemes for parents of preterm babies (Goodley 1986; Hughes 1986) and for those who experienced a perinatal or neonatal loss (Gilligan 1980; Mulkerrins and Gunn 1985; Collins 1986). As noted earlier, experimental schemes to assess the effects of midwifery support in pregnancy for women at risk of low birthweight delivery are now in progress (see Chapter 15).

Earlier in this chapter it was shown that women do not, as a rule, have direct access to midwives, and that they are likely to experience discontinuities in the care they receive. Both issues have been addressed by midwives in proposals put forward for reorganizing maternity care (Flint 1979; Thomson 1980; Cameron 1985; Walker 1985; Association of Radical Midwives 1986; Royal College of Midwives 1987) and in new schemes already implemented in some areas (Curran 1986; Flint and Poulengeris 1987). It is believed that women are more likely to develop confidence in themselves and will have more opportunity to discuss their concerns if they get to know a small number of midwives well, than if they are confronted with new faces at each antenatal visit and again during labour and the puerperium. In addition, it has been suggested that midwives are not only more likely to detect abnormalities and problems when they get to know a woman well over a period of time, but that their own job satisfaction is likely to be enhanced when their skills are fully used.

Recognizing that it is no longer practicable to return to a system in which one midwife provides sole care for a woman throughout pregnancy, labour, and the puerperium, these schemes have advocated that midwives work in small teams, each team providing total care for a group of women. Some of the proposals have advocated teams of midwives working in the community (Walker 1985); others have suggested separate teams with some based in the community and others in hospital (Association of Radical Midwives 1986); still others favour integrated teams of hospital and community midwives (Curran 1986; Royal College of Midwives 1987). Some of these schemes have now been implemented (e.g. Flint and Poulengeris 1987; Curran 1986) and one of these has been evaluated by means of one of the randomized controlled trials discussed earlier (Flint and Poulengeris 1987).

Midwives in some districts have also introduced individualized plans of care, often incorporating the woman's own birth plans (see, for example, Adams *et al.* 1981; Whitfield 1983; Kesby and Grant 1985; Bryar 1987). This approach to midwifery provides a more complete picture of a woman's emotional, social, and physical needs and preferences, which is then available to all those involved in her care. As with the move to team midwifery, organizational difficulties have been encountered in the introduction of these midwifery care plans (see Chapter 79), but once resolved it appears that the satisfaction of both the women and their caregivers increases.

Another significant development in midwifery in recent years has been the evaluation by midwives of the procedures they employ and the quality of care that they provide. The view is steadily gaining ground that midwifery practice should be based on research and should be constantly evaluated rather than being based on custom and tradition or being dictated by other health professionals. Midwives have, sometimes in collaboration with other professionals, undertaken randomized trials on the effects of midwife care (Flint and Poulengeris 1987) and on the effects of practices such as perineal shaving (Romney 1980), enemas in labour (Romney and Gordon 1981; Drayton and Rees 1984), and episiotomy (Sleep 1984). Other components of care that have been researched by midwives include postnatal support for mothers (Ball 1983), supportive care in labour (Kirkham 1982), the antenatal booking interview (Methven 1983), and the management of the third stage of labour (Moore and Levy 1983). A commitment to disseminate research findings to midwives in clinical practice, in education and in management became apparent in conferences (Thomson and Robinson 1985), information networks, and new professional journals (Flint 1985).

5.2 Continuing concerns

Despite the many positive developments in midwifery, the under-use of the midwife's skills continues to be a cause for concern. In Britain this has been evidenced in a number of recent reports on maternity care and in statements made by individual midwives and by the professional and statutory bodies for midwifery. The report of the House of Commons Social Services Committee (1980) on Perinatal and Neonatal Mortality stated that 'steps should be taken to make better use of the skills of the midwife in maternity care—particularly in the antenatal clinic . . . where they should be given greater responsibility for the antenatal care of women with uncomplicated pregnancies'. Reports from the multidisciplinary Maternity Services Advisory Committee, set up to develop guidelines for good practice in antepartum, intrapartum, and postpartum care, stressed the importance of the midwife's role, drawing particular attention to the under-use of her skills in the care of women during pregnancy (Maternity Services Advisory Committee 1982, 1984 and 1985).

Some members of the midwifery profession, however, felt that the recommendations in the Maternity Services Advisory Committee's second and third reports still restricted the exercise of independent clinical judgement by midwives. Flint (1984), for example, in commenting on the Committee's recommendations that to 'ensure a consistent standard of care and to avoid any confusion of practice each unit should have written operational policies', said: 'guidelines are acceptable but policies written in minute detail are for unthinking automatons, not for practitioners who are trying to give individualized care to a unique woman experiencing a unique labour'. The Committee recommended that policies should be drawn up by senior medical and midwifery staff, but in the experience of some senior midwives this was not the case. Kilvington (1985), for example, said that in her experience policies in many units were 'decreed by the consultant obstetricians . . . and instead of the broad policies that were present before, so that all staff taught the same thing to each student, we now have directions exactly when to do everything to the mother'. Henderson (1985) and Rider (1985) pointed out that the recommendations for postnatal care still left responsibility for the discharge of normal women and babies with medical staff, despite the fact that this activity falls within the midwife's sphere of practice.

Concern about the lack of recognition of the role of the midwife by the public and by other health professionals, particularly medical staff, led the profession's statutory bodies to issue a booklet in 1983 outlining the range of practice and level of responsibility for which the midwife is qualified (Central Midwives' Board for Scotland *et al.* 1983).

6 Role interrelationships

Boundaries between the roles of midwife, obstetrician, and general practitioner are not clearly defined in the United Kingdom and there is a considerable degree of overlap in their respective responsibilities. It is beyond dispute that the obstetrician should have overall responsibility for women with medical or obstetric complications; but there is a lack of clarity as to how much responsibility the obstetrician should have for the care of women who experience a normal pregnancy, labour, and puerperium, and how much of that care should be undertaken by midwives acting on their own responsibility. With regard to midwives and general practitioners, there is an inherent duplication of resources in the system of maternity care in Britain. We train a body of professionals, midwives, to provide normal childbearing women with clinical care, advice, and support, and yet at the same time, assign much of this care to general practitioners.

There is an increasing trend to see maternity care in terms of the relative roles of the consultant obstetrician on the one hand and the general practitioner on the other. Under the system of shared antenatal care which is now commonplace, the care of high risk women is assigned to the obstetrician and that of low risk women to the general practitioner with intermittent assessment by the obstetrician. Both may decide to delegate responsibility for low risk women to the midwife or they may decide to undertake all the assessments themselves. Shared care divides the responsibility for the assessment of women with normal pregnancies between two groups of medical staff, and yet not they but the midwife is specifically trained to provide that care.

A working party of obstetricians and general practitioners in the United Kingdom suggested that there should be an increase in the proportion of general practitioners trained to provide full care and that 'an expansion of general practitioner beds within or adjacent to specialist units in all districts would allow a substantial number of women to be cared for in labour by general practitioners with specialist assistance readily available' (Royal College of Obstetricians and Gynaecologists and Royal College of General Practitioners 1981). If such schemes are implemented intrapartum care will be subject to the same gross duplication of professional skills and resources that already exists in antenatal care.

Another important aspect of the interrelationship between the roles of midwives and medical staff is that of women's access to a midwife. Prior to the introduction of the National Health Service, the community midwife was the first point of contact with the maternity services for the majority of women. Once the new service had been introduced in 1948, an increasing number of general practitioners became involved in maternity care. At the same time the fact that women could book a general practitioner for delivery without payment of a fee led to a trend whereby women went to a general practitioner rather than to a midwife for confirmation of pregnancy (Bent 1982b). Increasingly, the general practitioner and not the midwife became the first point of contact with the maternity services.

In recent years a number of reports have questioned a system which 'makes the general practitioner the gatekeeper to all other health care services' (Clark 1984). In the context of maternity care, concern has been expressed for the women who are not registered with a general practitioner or who are reluctant to report their pregnancy in the first instance to a doctor. According to the Acheson report on primary health care in inner London, up to 30 per cent of people in some areas are not registered with a general practitioner (London Health Care Planning Consortium 1981). The report of the Social Services Committee on perinatal and neonatal mortality, remarked that it is often the women who are in greatest need of early antenatal care, the socially disadvantaged and the homeless in particular, who have no general practitioner or for whom the present system of reporting pregnancy to a doctor may act as a disincentive to receive early care (Social Services Committee 1980).

7 Conclusions

This chapter has demonstrated that there is a major role for midwives in achieving good perinatal outcomes and in providing women with a satisfying experience of pregnancy and childbirth. Concurrently, it has drawn attention to the constraints that were imposed on the midwife's role by the increased involvement of medical staff in normal maternity care, by the lack of opportunity to provide continuity of care and by understaffing. From recent developments in midwifery it may be concluded that, while erosion of the midwife's role is still a matter of concern, many midwives have none the less sought to restore their professional status by developing schemes in which the needs of women are met by their particular skills and knowledge. Most of the studies discussed have been undertaken in the United Kingdom. But the pattern of the midwife's central role in maternity care followed by an erosion of that role, and now some measure of restoration has been the history of midwifery in many countries.

There is no evidence to support a view that medical staff rather than midwives should be the providers of primary maternity care. The evidence in fact points in the opposite direction. Midwives should be the primary providers of care for the majority of women, with medical practitioners involved perhaps for interim assessment and certainly to take clinical responsibility for those women with obstetric or medical complications. The argument that childbirth is only 'normal in retrospect' should not be used to deprive midwives of their role in maternity care nor to deprive women of the particular benefits of midwifery care. Medical staff are needed to provide treatment and advice in the case of deviations from the normal, but it does not require a doctor to detect such deviations. Midwives are qualified to do this and can then refer to medical colleagues as and when appropriate (see Chapter 13). It is also far more cost-effective to base care for normal women on services provided by midwives and to keep obstetric expertise for high risk women, an argument not lost on those countries now seeking to reintroduce midwifery (College of Nurses of Ontario 1986; Kinch 1986).

General practitioners may argue that they should be responsible for providing care for women during pregnancy, and perhaps childbirth, on the grounds that this is an integral aspect of the long term relationship they develop with women and their families (see Chapter 11). The fact that a woman has a good relationship with her general practitioner does not mean, however, that she cannot also benefit from the support and care provided by a midwife, particularly since midwives are qualified to provide this care while this may not be the case for her particular general practitioner. There is no reason why the long term relationship between general practitioners and families should be weakened by the involvement of midwives in womens' maternity care, especially if the general practitioners also have some part in that care. In the present system, however, women can only gain access to midwives through general practitioners, and as already noted this poses problems for a small minority of women who do not have a general practitioner and for those who may prefer to receive care from a midwife rather than a doctor during pregnancy.

General practitioners may well have an important contribution to make to maternity care (see Chapter 11), but this need not mean that the maternity services at the primary level should focus on general practitioners in a manner that duplicates resources for some women and at the same time fails to reach others.

If the evidence and arguments presented here are accepted, those responsible for the maternity services should ensure, first, an organization of care that gives women access to midwives who can provide them with continuity of care on their own responsibility, and, second, that there are sufficient numbers of well-trained and confident midwives available to provide that care. Local antenatal clinics staffed by midwives and health visitors for women to attend without necessarily seeing a general practitioner first should be established, as recommended by the Social Services Committee (1980), by the Maternity Services Advisory Committee (1982) and by the Health Visitors' Association and the Royal College of Midwives (1982). Brain (1979) has questioned the policy of attaching midwives to general practices and indicated that it does not necessarily encourage early antenatal care. If instead the midwives were to relate to a specific geographic area, as indeed they used to do, they would get to know and be known by the women in the area. This in turn would facilitate the early provision of antenatal care by the midwife at local clinics or in womens' own homes. As documented in this chapter, a number of schemes have been implemented which fully use the midwife's skills in the antenatal period and during labour and the puerperium as well; many more such schemes should now be introduced and evaluated.

The tide is beginning to turn in favour of midwifery. Midwives must, however, feel confident and be willing to be accountable for their actions if they are to be the primary providers of maternity care. The increase in the length of training in Britain has led to an increase in the proportion of midwives who feel adequately prepared to practise (Robinson 1986b). But once qualified, they need support if they are to remain confident. As Flint (1986) has argued, they must care for and support each other if they are to be able to care for and support women and their families. Midwives can provide the kind of care which most women want and need: clinical assessment and monitoring, advice and emotional support. The midwife therefore should have a central role in the maternity services if women are to be provided with effective care in pregnancy and childbirth.

References

Adams M, Armstrong-Esther C, Bryar R, Duberly J, Strong G, Ward E (1981). Trial run—investigating the nursing process. Nursing Mirror, 7 October, 32–35

Association of Radical Midwives (1986). The Vision: Draft proposal for the future of the maternity services. Association of Radical Midwives.

Ball J (1983). Moving forward in postnatal care—some aspects of a research project. Midwives' Chron & Nursing Notes, 96: Supplement 14–16.

Barclay L (1985). Australian midwifery training and practice. Midwifery, 1: 86–96.

Barnett Z (1979). The changing pattern of maternity care and the future role of the midwife. Midwives' Chron & Nursing Notes, 92: 381–384.

Barrington E (1985). Midwifery in Canada. Toronto: New Canada Publications.

Bent EA (1982a). The Growth and Development of Midwifery. In: Nursing, Midwifery and Health Visiting since 1900. Allan P, Jolley M (eds). London: Faber & Faber.

Bent EA (1982b). The Midwives' Directives. J Adv Nursing, 7: 384–386.

Blondel B, Pusch D, Schmidt E (1985). Some characteristics of antenatal care in 13 European Countries. Br J Obstet Gynaecol, 92: 565–568.

Brain M (1979). Observations by a midwife. In: Report of a Day Conference on the Reduction of Perinatal Mortality and Morbidity. Children's Committee and Department of Health and Social Security. London: Her Majesty's Stationery Office.

Bryar R (1987). Implementing the midwifery process. In: Research and the Midwife Conference Proceedings for 1986. Robinson S and Thomson A (eds). King's College, London University.

Cameron J (1985). Midwifery in the real world. Nursing Mirror, 161: 42–44.

Cartwright A (1979). The Dignity of Labour. London: Tavistock.

Central Midwives' Board (1983). Final Report on the Work of the Board. Suffolk: Hymns Ancient and Modern Ltd.

Central Midwives' Board for Scotland, Northern Ireland Council for Nurses and Midwives, An Bord Altranais, Central Midwives' Board (1983). The Role of the Midwife. Suffolk: Hymns Ancient and Modern Ltd.

Chamberlain G, Philipp E, Howlett B, Master K (1978). British Births 1970. Vol 2, Obstetric Care. London: Heinemann Medical Books.

Clark J (1984). Opportunity knocks for primary health care nursing at long last. Nursing Standard, No. 354, 5.

College of Nurses of Ontario (1986). Midwifery: A CNO policy background paper. College of Nurses of Ontario 9002–03/86. Ontario, Canada.

Collins M (1986). Care for families following still-birth and first week deaths. Midwives' Chron & Nursing Notes, 99: Supplement xiii–xv.

Cowell B, Wainwright D (1981). Behind the blue door. The history of the Royal College of Midwives 1881–1981. London: Baillière Tindall.

Curran V (1986). Taking midwifery off the conveyor belt. Nursing Times, 20 August 1980, 42–43.

Davies J, Evans F (1987). Evaluating an inner city midwifery project. In: Research and the Midwife Conference Proceedings for 1986. Robinson S, Thomson A (eds). Nursing Research Unit, King's College, London University.

Department of Health and Social Security (1970). Report of the Sub-committee on Domiciliary and Maternity Bed Needs. London: Her Majesty's Stationery Office.

Department of Health and Social Security (1984). Study of Hospital Based Midwives—A report by Central Management Services. London: Department of Health and Social Security.

DeVries RG (1982). Midwifery and the problem of licensure. Research in the Sociology of Health Care, 2: 77–120.

Dillon T, Brennan B, Dwyer J, Risk A, Sear A, Dawson L, Wiele R (1978). Midwifery 1977. Am J Obstet Gynecol, 130: 971–926.

Drayton S, Rees C (1984). 'They know what they're doing';

the midwife and enemas. In: Research and the Midwife Conference Proceedings for 1983. Department of Nursing, University of Manchester.

Field P (1984). Management and nursing care in high risk pregnancy. In: Perinatal Nursing. P A Field (ed). London: Churchill Livingstone.

Filshie S, Williams J, Edith O, Osbourn M, Symonds EM, Backett ME. (1981). Postnatal care in hospital. J R Soc Health, 1O1: 70–73.

Flint C (1979). A continuing labour of love. Nursing Mirror, 15 November: 16–18.

Flint C (1982). Antenatal clinics. Nursing Mirror, 24 November; 1, 8, 15, and 22 December; and 5, 12, 19, and 28 January; Vol. 155 Nos 20–24, Vol. 156 Nos 1–4.

Flint C (1984). A mother's birthright. Nursing Times, 22 February: 18–19.

Flint C (1985). Three steps forward. Nursing Times, 11 September: 23.

Flint C (1986). Sensitive Midwifery. London: Heinemann.

Flint C, Poulengeris P (1987). The Know Your Midwife Report. London: C Flint, 49 Peckarman's Wood, London SE 26.

Garcia J (1982). Women's views of antenatal care. In: Effectiveness and Satisfaction in Antenatal Care. Enkin M, Chalmers I (eds). London: Spastics International Medical Publications. Heinemann Medical Books. pp 81–91.

Garcia J, Garforth S, Ayers S (1985). Midwives confined? In: Labour Ward Policies and Routines. Thomson A, Robinson S (eds). Research and the Midwife Conference Proceedings 1985. King's College, University of London.

Gilligan M (1980). The midwife's contribution to counselling parents who have suffered a perinatal death. Research and the Midwife Conference Proceedings 1979, 1980. Chelsea College, London University.

Goodley S (1986). Family care and the pre-term baby. Midwives' Chron & Nursing Notes, 99: Supplement, viii–x.

Graham M, McKee L (1980). The first months of motherhood—summary report of a survey of women's experiences of pregnancy, childbirth and the first six months after birth. London: Health Education Council Monograph No 3 HEC.

Hall TL, Meijia A (1978). Health Manpower Planning. Geneva: World Health Organization.

Health Visitors' Association and Royal College of Midwives (1982). Joint statement on antenatal preparation.

Henderson C (1985). Response to the third Maternity Services Advisory Committee Report. Midwives' Chron & Nursing Notes, 98: 162.

Hughes P (1986). Neonatal community liaison visiting. Midwives' Chron & Nursing Notes, 99: Supplement, xi–xii.

Humphrey C (1985). The community midwife in maternity care. Midwife, Health Visitor and Community Nurse, 21: 349–355.

International Congress of Midwives/International Federation of Gynaecology and Obstetrics (1973). Definition of the midwife. International Confederation of Midwives' Notices 1973.

International Federation of Gynaecology and Obstetrics and the International Confederation of Midwives (1976). Maternity Care in the World (2nd edn). FIGO/ICM.

Kesby O, Grant M (1985). Changing the system. Nursing Mirror, 160: 28–31.

Kilvington J (1985). Response to the Third Maternity Services Advisory Committee Report. Midwives' Chron & Nursing Notes, 98: 162.

Kinch R (1986). Midwifery and home births. Can Med Assoc J, 135: 280–281.

Kirkham M (1982). Information-giving by midwives during labour. In: Research and the Midwife Conference Proceedings for 1981. Thomson A (ed). Manchester University.

Levy B, Wilkinson R, Marine W (1971). Reducing neonatal mortality rate with nurse-midwives. Am J Obstet Gynecol, 109: 50–58.

Litoff J (1978). American Midwives: 1800 to the present. Westport, Connecticut: Greenwood Press.

London Health Care Planning Consortium (1981). Primary Health Care in Inner London (The Acheson Report). London Health Care Planning Consortium.

Maglacas A, Simons J, eds (1986). The potential of the traditional birth attendant. WHO Offset publications No. 95. Geneva: World Health Organization.

Maternity Services Advisory Committee (1982). Maternity Care in Action, Part I—Antenatal Care. London: Her Majesty's Stationery Office.

Maternity Services Advisory Committee (1984). Maternity Care in Action, Part II—Care during Childbirth. London: Her Majesty's Stationery Office.

Maternity Services Advisory Committee (1985). Maternity Care in Action, Part III—Care of the Mother and Baby. London: Her Majesty's Stationery Office.

McKee IH (1984). Community antenatal care: the Sighthill Community antenatal scheme. In: Pregnancy Care for the 1980's. Zander L and Chamberlain G (eds). London: Royal Society of Medicine and Macmillan Press Ltd.

Methven R (1983). The antenatal booking interview: recording an obstetric history or relating with a mother to be. In: Research and the Midwife Conference Proceedings for 1982. Thomson A, Robinson S (eds). Manchester University.

Moore J, Levy V (1983). Further research into the management of the third stage of labour and the incidence of postpartum haemorrhage. In: Research and the Midwife Conference Proceedings 1982, Thomson A, Robinson S (eds). Manchester University.

Morgan BM, Bulpitt CJ, Clifton P, Lewis PJ (1984). The Consumer attitude to obstetric care. Br J Obstet Gynaecol, 90: 624–628.

Morrin M (1982). Are we in danger of extinction? Midwives' Chron & Nursing Notes, 95: 17.

Mulkerrins M, Gunn P (1985). The visiting midwives participation in a confidential enquiry into perinatal death conducted by the North West Thames Regional Health Authority. Research and the Midwife Conference Proceedings for 1984. Thomson A, Robinson S (eds). Nursing Research Unit, King's College, London University.

National Childbirth Trust (1981). Change in Antenatal Care. Report from a working party set up for the National Childbirth Trust by Sheila Kitzinger.

Newson K (1985). The NHS could be fantastic. Interview in Nursing Mirror, 161: 16–17.

Oakley A (1980). Women Confined—Towards a sociology of childbirth. Oxford: Martin Robertson.

Office of Technology Assessment (1986). Nurse Practitioners, Physician Assistants and Certified Nurse Midwives: A policy analysis. Health Technology Case Study 37. Washington: Congress of the United States.

Penny Y (1986). Modern prenatal management—patterns of care for the future. Midwives' Chron & Nursing Notes, 99: Supplement, ii–iii.

Pratinidhi A, Shrotri A, Shah O, Chavan H (1985). Birth attendants and perinatal mortality. World Health Forum, 6: 115–117.

Raisler J (1985). Improving pregnancy outcome with nurse-midwifery care. J Nurse Midwifery, 30: 189–191.

Rider A (1983). Report on Dettol Sword Award. Midwives' Chron & Nursing Notes, 96: 165.

Rider A (1985). Midwifery after birth. Nursing Times, 7/8, 27–28.

Robinson S (1983). From independent practitioner to team member; some aspects of the history of the midwifery profession. In: Understanding Politics—An historical perspective. White R (ed). London: King's Fund Centre.

Robinson S, Golden J, Bradley S (1983). A study of the role and responsibilities of the midwife. NERU Report No. 1, Chelsea College, London University.

Robinson S (1986a). Career intentions of newly qualified midwives. Midwifery, 2: 25–36.

Robinson S (1986b). Midwifery Training: The views of newly qualified midwives. Nurse Education Today, 6: 49–59.

Romney M (198O). Predelivery shaving: an unjustified assault? J Obstet Gynaecol, 1: 33–35.

Romney M, Gordon J (1981). Is your enema really necessary? Br Med J, 282: 1269.

Romney ML, White VGL (1984). Current Practices in Labour. In: Perinatal Nursing. P A Field (ed). London: Churchill Livingstone.

Royal College of Midwives (1977). Evidence to the Royal Commission on the National Health Service. London: Royal College of Midwives.

Royal College of Midwives (1984 and 1985). Evidence to the Pay Review Body. Midwives' Chron & Nursing Notes, 97: 555 and 98: 165.

Royal College of Midwives (1987). The Role and Education of the Future Midwife in the United Kingdom. London: Royal College of Midwives.

Royal College of Obstetricians and Gynaecologists and Royal College of General Practitioners (1981). Report on Training for Obstetrics and Gynaecology for General Practitioners. Joint Working Party of the RCOG and RCGP, London.

Runnerstrom L (1969). The effectiveness of nurse-midwifery in a supervised hospital environment. Bull Am Coll Nurse-Midwives, 14: 40–52.

Sleep J (1984). The West Berkshire Episiotomy trial. In: Research and the Midwife Conference Proceedings for 1983. Department of Nursing, University of Manchester.

Slome C, Wetherbee H, Daly M, Christensen K, Meglen M and Thiede H (1976). Effectiveness of certified nurse-midwives : A prospective evaluation study. Am J Obstet Gynecol, 124: 177–182.

Social Services Committee—House of Commons (1980). Report on Perinatal and Neonatal Mortality. London: Her Majesty's Stationery Office.

Stuart B, Judge E (1984). The return of the midwife? Midwives' Chron & Nursing Notes, 97: 8–9.

Taylor RW (1984). Community-based specialist obstetric services. In: Pregnancy Care for the 1980's. Zander L. and Chamberlain G (eds). London: Royal Society of Medicine and Macmillan Press Ltd.

Thompson JB (1986). Safety and Effectiveness of Nurse Midwifery Care: Research Review in Nurse-Midwifery in America. Rooks HP, Haas JE (eds). A Report of the American College of Nurse-Midwives Foundation, Washington.

Thomson A (1980). Planned or unplanned? Are midwives ready for the 1980's? Midwives' Chron & Nursing Notes, 93: 68–72.

Thomson A, Robinson S (1985). Dissemination of midwifery research, how this has been facilitated in the UK. Midwifery, 1: 52–53.

Towler J (1981). Out of the ordinary. Park Hospital Maternity Unit. Nursing Mirror, 152: 32–33.

Towler J, Brammall J (1986). The midwife in history and society. Kent: Croom Helm.

Walker J (1985). Meeting Midwives Midway. Nursing Times, 23 October, 48–50.

Whitfield S (1983). The midwifery process in practice. Midwives' Chron & Nursing Notes, 90: 186–189.

Williams S, Hepburn M, McIlwaine G (1985). Consumer view of epidural analgesia. Midwifery, 1: 32–36.

World Health Organization (1966). The Midwife in Maternity Care. Technical Report Series No. 331, Chapter 3. Geneva: World Health Organization.

World Health Organization (1982). Traditional Birth Attendants: An annotated bibliography on their training, utilization and evaluation. Geneva: World Health Organization.

World Health Organization (1985). Having a baby in Europe. Public Health in Europe 26. Copenhagen: World Health Organization Regional Office for Europe.

11 The role of the family practitioner in maternity care

Michael Klein and Luke Zander

1 Introduction

Family doctors or general practitioners (we use both terms interchangeably in this chapter) are different from all other providers of health care, in that they alone are responsible for providing long term personal, comprehensive, and continuing health care to individuals and their families. The relationship of the specialist obstetrician and the midwife with the pregnant woman and her family is usually confined to the relatively short time period in and around pregnancy and childbirth. For the family doctor on the other hand, the care of a woman during pregnancy forms part of a continuum of care, care which often long predates conception, and extends onwards beyond birth and the postnatal period into the stages of motherhood, parenting, and child care that follow. In this way, care by the family doctor reflects the nature of pregnancy itself, which is not an encapsulated event to be considered in isolation, but an integral part of the life experience of both the mother and of those closest to her.

2 The decline of family doctor involvement in maternity care

In spite of these important features, throughout the Western world the family doctor's involvement in care for pregnancy and childbirth has declined markedly over the past 30 to 40 years and their continuing role in the delivery of obstetric care has become an important and contentious issue in many countries. The reasons for this change are many and varied. They relate to an era of increasing specialization that is uncomfortable with, and not infrequently hostile to, the generalist; to the changing pattern of maternity care; to a medical education that has tended to overemphasize the risks and hazards rather than the normal psychophysiological aspects of pregnancy; and to changes in the manner in which general practice itself is now being conducted in many countries.

There has been a tendency to assume that what constitutes good maternity care inevitably means the approach that has been adopted and propounded by the specialty of obstetrics. Obstetrics has taken over much of the control and decision making in the management of pregnancy. Increasingly it has been obstetricians who have set the objectives of and standards for care, and who to a very large extent, dictate and control the way that care is to be practised. This is the case even in systems where care is shared between general practitioner and specialist obstetrician. In the United Kingdom, for example, after an initial booking appointment to the hospital, many women see their own general practitioner throughout pregnancy, with intermittent attendances at the hospital, but it is almost always the specialist obstetrician who decides the nature and structure of that collaboration and care.

The shift in the place of birth from home to hospital and the subsequent dramatic increase in childbirth technology have been central influences in the decline of general practitioner involvement in pregnancy and childbirth. Few family doctors now have the expertise to employ many of these sophisticated techniques, or to interpret the results of many current monitoring and diagnostic modalities. This increasing use of technology during childbirth has played a major part in encouraging the attitude among many family doctors, as well as among many of their specialist colleagues, that the management of childbirth is something 'best left to the experts'.

The organization of general practice and the way in which it fits into the overall structure of health care, varies both from country to country and within each country. In urban areas in particular, the general practitioner now rarely functions alone in providing care. At the time of the inception of the National Health Service in Britain in 1948, over two-thirds of general practitioners worked in single-handed practices; by 1974 over 80 per cent of them were working in partnerships or group practices, often housed in purpose-built premises or health centres. A direct result of these trends has been the development of primary health care teams which, in addition to general practitioners, include various other health professionals such as midwives, district nurses, health visitors, and social workers and may even extend to include dieticians, physiotherapists, counsellors, and others. This may mean that, when considering the role of the family doctor in maternity care, one must think in terms of a closely integrated group of professionals with differing and complementary expertise and experience rather than in terms of a solo practitioner. The rationale for such health care teams is based on the belief that the care provided by a group of professionals with differing training and perspectives working together and in co-operation is superior to the care that can be provided by any of them working independently or alone. However, these teams of many individuals may not embody the personal, continuing, and total health care for individuals and their families that formerly was—and in some places still is—characteristic of family practice.

When the National Health Service was introduced in Britain in 1948, family doctors were responsible for approximately 50 per cent of all births—either at home or in a maternity unit. Thirty years later, in 1978, general practitioners' claims for payment for care during confinement had dropped to only 16 per cent of the total births in England and Wales. This does not, however, fully represent the general practitioners contribution to the provision of care for pregnancy and childbirth. On the one hand, the system of shared care in the United Kingdom ensures that general practitioners are responsible for a portion of the antenatal care of women whose pregnancies are supervised by specialist obstetricians, while on the other, a substantial proportion of the care provided for women delivering in general practitioner units or at home is in actuality given by community midwives. These data do document, however, the steady decline of the role of the general practitioner in the provision of care for pregnancy and childbirth in the United Kingdom.

In Canada, the attendance of family doctors at birth varies greatly among the provinces, ranging from approximately 80 per cent in Nova Scotia and Saskatchewan, to approximately 40 per cent in Quebec and 33 per cent in Ontario (Klein *et al.* 1984c). The family doctor's role is undergoing a steady erosion, especially in eastern Canada. This erosion has been so rapid that one of us was prompted to refer to the family doctor who carries out obstetrical care as an endangered species (Klein *et al.* 1984a). Yet even in Ontario, where family doctors attend less than a third of deliveries, approximately two-thirds of general practitioners still have privileges in obstetrics (Owen 1982). In 1979 over a quarter of Canadian family doctors were practising in small communities with a population of less than 25 000. Obstetrics is still a major and essential part of rural general practice in this country, where legalized midwifery is (at the time of writing) non-existent. In contrast, almost 80 per cent of Canadian obstetrical specialists practice in the 16 cities in which the medical schools are located, and only 6.4 per cent practise in communities with less than 25 000 people (Klein *et al.* 1984c; Klein 1986).

In the United States, although antenatal and postnatal care was the sixth most common ambulatory diagnostic entity, and childbirth was among the ten most common hospital diagnoses for family doctors (Black *et al.* 1980), they carried out only 20 per cent of deliveries in 1978 (Graduate Medical Education National Advisory Committee 1981).

Similar trends have taken place in Australia. Between 1981–1982 and 1984–1985 the proportion of all births attended by general practitioners fell from 24 per cent to 15 per cent (Hassett 1986). In 1985, 25 per cent of general practitioners in Australia were doing some obstetrics, but many of them attended fewer than five deliveries per year. As in North America, the activity level was highest in the rural areas, with 53 per cent of births in these areas being attended by general practitioners according to Medicare data (J Dickenson and R Alexander, personal communication).

Although the shift in the place of birth from the home to hospital is held responsible for much of the decline in general practitioner involvement, the role of the general practitioner in maternity care has been declining even in The Netherlands, where 35 per cent of deliveries are still conducted at home. In the home setting, where the birth attendants are furthest removed from the influences of specialist- and technology-dominated institutional care, it is the midwife, not the general practitioner who is the central professional attendant. The Dutch compulsory health insurance system will only remunerate general practitioners for care in pregnancy and childbirth in those districts where there are no practising midwives (Keirse 1982).

3 Range of maternity care provided by family doctors

Most studies on the effect of general practitioner care in pregnancy and childbirth have been descriptive rather than comparative. Data derived from such studies are useful to obtain insight into the practices concerned and may offer ideas as to how such practices are organized, but they are of little, if any, value for a generalizable overall assessment of the potential benefits and hazards of general practice maternity care.

Attempts to compare general practice obstetrics among different countries are made difficult by differences in terminology and in the organization of care. In England and Wales, so-called 'isolated' general practitioner maternity units are rarely truly isolated, but are usually located within an hour's drive of a specialist obstetric facility. In Northern Canada and in rural parts of the United States, on the other hand, the nearest referral unit may be 100 km or more distant, and family doctors often work with general surgeons who provide emergency services for caesarean section. In contrast to North America, where the general practitioner tends to attend the delivery personally, in Britain much of the so-called general practitioner care in pregnancy and childbirth is in fact provided by midwives working with general practitioners. Studies on general practitioner obstetrics in the United Kingdom, therefore, reflect not simply the effects of activities of general practitioners, many of whom have only a limited commitment to obstetrics, but the effects of a team in which the midwife plays the central role. (Needless to say, there are exceptions to this rule.)

Within any one country large differences will also exist between areas, so that descriptive studies of one team of general practitioners or of one general practice maternity unit will not necessarily reflect what goes on in the country as a whole. Discussions on the appropriate role of the family doctor in maternity care thus needs to take account of the geographical, social, cultural, and staffing characteristics of each locality. Roseveare and Bull (1982), for instance, described two types of general practitioner care in two different settings in the United Kingdom between 1976 and 1980; that of the closely integrated but still separate general practitioner maternity unit in Oxford and maternity care in Dulwich where two general practitioners work independently within the hospital specialist unit, referring very few women to specialist care. During the study period, only 65 per cent of women in the Oxford unit were ultimately delivered in the general practitioner unit, as compared with 98 per cent being cared for by the general practitioners in Dulwich. Intervention rates, including caesarean section and forceps delivery, were similar in the two units, as were the crude perinatal mortality rates. In Dulwich, the two experienced general practitioner–obstetricians appeared to be confident in dealing with most departures from the normal, while in Oxford, when problems were identified either in pregnancy or in labour, the matter tended to be resolved by transfer to specialist care.

In many of the rural areas of North America in particular, maternity care by family doctors is the only type of maternity care that is available. Black and Gick (1979), for instance, reported on the performance of a 40-bed hospital on the north-east coast of Newfoundland, staffed by six family doctors for whom the nearest specialist facility was two hours away by road, often under difficult weather conditions. In such settings, family doctors have no choice but to continue to provide most of the maternity care; there are neither specialist facilities nor practising midwives within reach.

4 Evaluation of maternity care provided by family doctors

A number of comparative studies, summarized in Table 11.1, have looked at the practice of family practitioner maternity care and compared it with that provided by specialist obstetricians. None of the studies listed in the Table have used random or quasi-random allocation of subjects. All except one (Klein *et al.* 1985) are retrospective and all but three (Taylor *et al.* 1980; Klein *et al.* 1983a, 1983b, 1985) suffer from the major methodological drawback of being delivery-based instead of booking-based. Delivery-based studies can introduce major bias because they do not account for the transfer of difficult and complicated cases from general practitioner to specialist care. The booking-based study of Taylor *et al.* (1980) showed that 66 per cent of women booked for general practitioner care were transferred to specialist care at some point in pregnancy, labour, or postpartum (Table 11.2). The first study by Klein *et al.* (1983a, 1983b, 1984a) showed a transfer rate of 34 per cent from the general practice unit to the consultant unit overall, and in the second prospective study Klein *et al.* (1985) reported a similar transfer rate of 36 per cent (Table 11.2).

In the delivery-based studies, women cared for by specialist obstetricians may be at considerably higher risk than those cared for by family doctors. Another way to address such a bias (neglecting for the moment the attitudinal and social factors that may lead women into one system or another) would be to introduce some kind of statistical weighting in an attempt to ensure that all study patients cared for by family doctors or by specialist obstetricians were at comparable initial risk. This, however, was not done in any of the comparative studies from the United States that are included in Table 11.1.

The British studies, while purporting to be studies of general practice, always involve midwives. Some of these midwives are working closely with family doctors only; others work with both family doctors and obstetric consultants; still others work exclusively with

Table 11.1 Comparative studies of maternity care given by family doctors and by specialist obstetricians*

Author Year Country	Numbers*	Rural Urban	Methods of comparison	Problems with the comparisons	Maternal outcomes	Newborn outcomes	Comments
Caetano 1975 USA	all live births in one county ($n=6612$)	rural + urban	delivery-based; census data using birth certificates (doctor who signed certificate)	FP more rural OB more urban more emergency care by FP	FP pregnancy complications ↑ delivery outcomes similar	birth injuries for FP ↑	dissimiliar samples & diagnostic criteria no information on asphhxia
Ely *et al.* 1976 USA	FP 111 OB 1197 FP 1972–75 OB 1972	urban (univ.)	retrospective; all patients in certain time period, but different time period for FP & OB; delivery-based	different time periods OB socioeconom. risk ↑	OB anaesthesia ↑ forceps rate ↑ FP postpartum haem. ↑ endometritis ↑ premat. rupt. membr. ↑	similar	comparable quality care by FP and OB given limitations of the study
Reeves and Anderson 1977 USA	22,857	one county hospital 1956–75	all deliveries from 1956 to 1975, while accoucheurs changed from FP + surgeons to OB specialists	not a true comparat. study study of births over time	increasing caesarian section rates over time	similar perinatal mortality	personnel changed; procedures increased; no change in perinatal mortality rates
Phillips *et al.* 1978 USA	FP 50 FPR 50 OB 50	urban (univ., inner city)	retrospective; delivery-based; 50 of 88 FP 50 of 79 FPR 50 of 413 OB deliveries	FM medical risk ↑ OB socioeconom. risk ↑	FP analgesia more than FPR and OB OB anaesthesia ↑ augmentation ↑ induction of labour ↑ artif. rupt. membr. ↑	similar	comparable quality care by FP, FPR and OB given limitations of study
Wanderer and Suyehira 1980 USA	FP 211 FPR 199 OB 193	urban	retrospective; delivery-based; all FPR births + all FP births + random sample of 4990 OB charts	FPR medical + socioeconom. risk ↑	OB epidural analgesia ↑ narcotic use ↑ FP & FPR oxytocin ↑	similar	comparable equality care by FP, FPR, and OB given limitations of study
Taylor *et al.* 1980 UK	GP-unit 1678 vs. OB-unit 1255	mixed urban + rural	retrospective; booking-based	GP and consultant units geographically separated; groups socioeconomically different	OB anaesthesia ↑ analgesia ↑ FP episiotomy ↑ forceps ↑ mat. complications ↑	similar	First booking-based study no apparent differences in outcome between GP and OB care
Meyer 1980 USA	FP 50 OB 50	rural	retrospective; hospital based; random sample of 73 pts. receiving care from FP + 131 pts. admitted by OB.	booking-based for FP, but delivery-based for OB; FP patients social risks ↑	OB analgesia ↑ other outcomes similar	similar	no difference OB vs. FP, but biased due to different selection methods
Black 1980 UK	all Oxfordshire births 1970–80	mixed rural + urban	epidemiological study of FP care vs. consultant OB care	—		similar perinatal mortality rates	when risk adjusted and birthweight adjusted, newborn outcomes similar

Richards and Richards 1982 USA	742 urban 435 rural urban = OB rural = FP	mixed rural + urban	delivery-based; maternal + infant records from 3 urban (OB) and 11 rural (FP) hospitals; focus on caesarean morbidity 1977–79	FP higher parity OB more post-term women	caesarean section rates: urban (OB) 9.3%; rural (FP) 7.9% rural (FP) more infection when based on culture + use of antibiotics	U low Apgar R RDS ↑ transfer for tachypnoea newborn ↑	no essential differences rural (FP) vs. urban (OB) Total admissions to neontal intens. Care similar
Shear *et al.* 1983 USA	FP 59 OB 101	urban county hosp. with FP & OB residents	delivery-based; retrospective; for each FP birth, 2 OB deliveries closest in time of day and date	FP socioeconom. risk FP more ante-natal visits	OB episiotomy	mean Apgars similar OB more admissions to neonatal intens. care	average number of doctors seen by pts. for FP 1.7 & OB 4.3 FP continuity care ↑ mat. satisfact. ↑
Klein *et al.* 1983 (a&b) UK	OB 1188 GPU 248 from total 5005 births in 1978	urban + rural	booking-based; retrospective; restrictive selection criteria	very low risk pregnancies only	almost all procedures lower in general practitioner unit than in OB consultant unit	similar, but birth asphyxia ↑ in primiparae with OB care	outcomes for FP and OB patients very similar
Klein *et al.* 1985	OB 85 GPU 86	urban + rural	prospective + booking-based; total FP care vs. shared OB/FP care enrollment in FP office; no selection bias		similar	similar	FP mat. satisfaction ↑ breastfeeding ↑ ambulation in labour ↑ early contact with infant ↑
Rosenblatt *et al.* 1985 New Zealand	206,054 births; 1388 fetal + 1084 1st. wk deaths 1978–81	rural + urban	all births in New Zealand divided: 5 level III hosp. 19 level II hosp. 89 level I hosp. preinat. mortality attributed to hosp. where birth occurred	not based on maternal residence; based on hospital where delivery took place			level I hospitals had lowest birthweight specific mortality rates in all but the lowest birthweight groups

* Abbreviations: FP = family doctors; FPR = family practice residents; GP-unit = general practitioner maternity unit; OB = obstetricians; R = rural; U = urban.

Table 11.2 Transfer rates from family doctor to specialist care in booking-based studies of maternity care by family doctors

Authors	Per cent transfer to specialist care			
	before labour	during labour	post partum	total
Taylor *et al.* 1980	35.2	20.3	11.5	65.9
Klein *et al.* 1983, 1984	13.2	20.7		33.9
Klein *et al.* 1985	10.4	13.0	4.7	36.0

obstetrical consultants. The largest study (Rosenblatt *et al.* 1985), while not strictly a comparison between general practitioner and specialist care, is included here because it reported on the perinatal mortality in all public maternity hospitals in New Zealand over the years 1978–1981, including the level I maternity units which were mostly rural and staffed by general practitioners and midwives. The second largest study, that of Reeves and Anderson (1977), again is not strictly a comparative study, but a study of all deliveries between 1956 and 1975 in one county hospital during the time that the principal birth attendants gradually changed from a system of family doctors working with general surgeons to a system in which labour and birth were managed almost entirely by obstetricians.

The data in Table 11.1 therefore give a general picture of, but not an evaluation of, the effects of general practitioner care as compared with specialist care. An unbiased comparison would need randomized trials in which an appropriate (and, of necessity, large) number of women were allocated to maternity care provided either by general practitioners or by specialist obstetricians. The minimum requirement for such a comparison would be a prospective cohort study of women, matched for identifiable risk factors, who attend for general practice or specialist care, with the results analysed by allocation at the time of booking. Such trials would be extremely difficult to mount, and their results would have limited generalizability in view of the large differences that exist both in family practice and in the organization of maternity care from one part of the world to another. It is doubtful whether such studies will ever be conducted, and indeed, it is questionable whether anyone should even attempt to mount them.

The only study in Table 11.1 that suggests that adverse perinatal outcomes may be attributable to family practice maternity care is that of Caetano (1975). The author reported an increase in the number of birth injuries in the population cared for by family practitioners as compared to that cared for by specialist obstetricians. Not only is it the oldest study in the series, it is also retrospective, based on census and birth certificate data, and the data are delivery-based, with the rural areas being over-represented in the family doctor group and the urban areas in the specialist care group. All other studies seem to indicate that the perinatal outcomes of general practitioner and of specialist care are similar, although it should be noted that several of the studies are too small to show any potential gain or loss for the rare outcomes such as mortality or severe morbidity. Moreover, it should be emphasized that crude perinatal mortality rates are poor indicators of the quality of perinatal care (Chalmers 1979). The retrospective study of Klein *et al.* (1983a, 1983b), that was booking-based and compared a subset of 'low risk' pregnancies cared for either in the consultant unit or in the general practice unit at the John Radcliffe Hospital in Oxford in 1978, found low Apgar scores (17 per cent versus 2 per cent) and intubation of the neonate (11 per cent versus 0 per cent) to be more frequent with consultant care (Klein *et al.* 1983b). In a subsequent study, conducted prospectively on a smaller number of pregnancies at the same institution, these differences in infant outcomes were no longer noted (Klein *et al.* 1985), overall outcomes having improved.

On the whole, the rates of various interventions tended to be higher with specialist care, although this was not a uniform finding across all of the studies reported in the Table. Consistent with this trend was that the length of labour tended to be somewhat longer in women cared for by family doctors than in those cared for by specialist obstetricians. This was reported in five of the studies listed in Table 11.1 (Ely *et al.* 1976; Wanderer and Suyehira 1980; Shear *et al.* 1983; Klein *et al.* 1983; Klein *et al.* 1985). One small study (Meyer 1981), however, reported the third stage of labour to be shorter in the family doctor than in the specialist care group. The few studies which took maternal satisfaction into account (Shear *et al.* 1983; Klein *et al.* 1985) suggested that this was enhanced by family doctor care.

On the whole and in spite of their limitations, these studies along with others from within and outside family practice, suggest that family doctors, midwives, and obstetricians working in settings which are specifically organized for the purpose of assisting women with apparently normal pregnancies can all obtain excellent outcomes. In fact, the professional membership of the birth attendant is of less consequence for the outcome of 'low risk' pregnancies than are the attitudinal or environmental factors which determine the attendant's actions.

Comparative studies of family practice obstetrics (Table 11.1) (Rosenberg and Klein 1987), population-based epidemiological studies (Black N 1982), descriptive studies and audits of family practice obstetrics (Owen 1981; Bull 1980; Koning 1984; Fleming 1983; Marsh 1977), hospital-based studies (Reynolds and

Yudkin 1987a,b), studies of rural practice (almost always involving family practitioners) (Black and Fyfe 1984; Casson and Sennett 1984), and studies of home births (Mehl *et al.* 1977; Mehl 1978; Tew 1985), birth rooms (Klein *et al.* 1984c), or alternative birthing facilities (which may or may not involve family practitioners) (Baruffi *et al.* 1984a,b; Ballard *et al.* 1985; Goodlin 1980), all appear to convey the same message. What seems to matter most in determining the outcomes of pregnancy for women and babies who are at relatively low prior risk, is not the extent to which care relies on technological advances, interventionist approaches, or specialist skills, but the establishment of a personal and continuing relationship between a mother and her principal caregiver, and the encouragement and facilitation of the normal physiological processes of pregnancy and childbirth. The general concept of preserving 'high touch/low tech care' for appropriately selected women by providers who are principally oriented to this type of care—whether they be general practitioners, midwives, or obstetricians—appears to be effective in terms of medical outcomes, cost, and satisfaction for both caregivers and care receivers.

It is in this context that we see the major advantages of family practice maternity care.

5 Family doctors and other providers of maternity care

In this age of specialization, many question whether there is still a role left for the true generalist. Those outside family practices often perceive the family doctor as occupying a midway position between the midwife on the one hand and the specialist obstetrician on the other. Some general practitioners themselves see their principal role as the provision of somewhat less complex obstetrical care than that provided by specialists, but still within the same model. They feel themselves to be less than adequate unless they are fully comfortable with most obstetrical approaches and procedures short of caesarean section. The other school of thought sees the general practitioner's principal role as facilitative to the midwife and supportive to the mother. These practitioners are in essence happy to leave the actual hands-on-management and the technological interventions to the specialist, whether it be the specialist in primary obstetric care—the midwife—or the specialist in secondary obstetric care—the obstetrician.

5.1 Family doctor and specialist obstetrician

Care by family doctors has often been considered within the same context as specialist obstetric care, albeit at a lower level of sophistication, with little consideration being given to the essential differences between these two types of care. Obstetricians with their everyday diet of obstetric problems, commonly perceive a pregnancy as a disaster waiting to happen, and consider that low risk can only be determined in retrospect. It is inevitable that high risk approaches, which are indispensable in the care of women at high risk, spill over to that of the vast majority of women who are of low risk, and tend to become the standard of care against which all performance is judged.

In this context, family practitioners do not provide the technological solutions that their specialist colleagues and frequently also the public, seem to feel are the essence of 'modern obstetrics'. There is a widespread (but not often explicitly stated) belief among obstetricians that care for pregnancy and childbirth should be left to the specialist. This attitude, which militates against general practitioners involvement, was clearly expressed by Sir Stanley Clayton, President of the Royal College of Obstetricians and Gynaecologists 1973–75, who said: 'If general practitioners want to practise obstetrics, they must practise modern obstetrics'.

Obviously, competence and technical expertise is not the sole province of the specialist. There are many family doctors, especially in rural areas, who practise a full range of obstetrical procedures up to and sometimes even including caesarean section, but this has become the exception rather than the rule. One can also find examples of maternity care given by family doctors that are just as meddlesome and interventionist as those found in some 'high tech' tertiary care centres. In our opinion, however, these stray far beyond the very essence of family doctor maternity care.

On the whole, the characteristics of family doctor maternity care can be contrasted with that of specialist care as shown in Table 11.3. These differences, which are most applicable in the United Kingdom, need some qualification when applied to North America, where obstetricians may often provide a greater degree of continuity of care for their patients, and frequently also

Table 11.3 Characteristics of family doctors and specialist obstetricians providing maternity care

General practitioner/family doctor	Specialist/consultant obstetrician
Responsible for total care	Responsible only for obstetrical care
Provides continuity of care	No continuity outside pregnancy
Usually cares for other family members	Does not care for other family members
Expertise centred on maternity care rather than on technical obstetrics	Expertise more in technical aspects of obstetrics than in maternity care

function as primary care physicians for obstetrical care and gynaecological complaints.

As a result of these differences, it is inevitable that the attitudes and orientation of the family doctor will be different from, though by no means less valid than those of the specialist. The specialist obstetrician's principal concern is to prevent, identify, and manage the abnormal. The general practitioner–obstetrician, on the other hand, is principally concerned with the care and nurturing of the normal and with identifying those deviations from the norm which indicate the necessity to seek specialist advice and help.

The family doctors' expertise in the care for pregnancy and childbirth is derived from their experience of providing comprehensive and continuing care, and from their responsibility for caring for the physical, psychological and social needs of the woman before, during, and after her pregnancy. This enables them to acquire an extensive and intimate knowledge about many aspects of their patients' lives and an awareness of how they respond to and cope with different forms of stress and challenge. The already established and ongoing relationship between a woman and her doctor is an important factor in encouraging communication, which in turn will assist the doctor to identify the woman's needs, and to provide appropriate care, advice and support.

Not only the content of care, but also its context, differs between the family doctor and the specialist obstetrician. Antenatal care provided in an office-based family practice is undertaken in familiar, usually easily accessible surroundings by a small number of individuals often limited to the woman's own doctor with whom she has an already established relationship. This is in sharp contrast with the circumstances in which much of specialist obstetric care in Britain tends to be provided, with overcrowded clinics, little time for communication between mother and health care professionals, and little possibility for the mother to establish a personal relationship with those providing care, due to the large number and frequently changing medical and nursing staff (see Chapter 8).

Such differences inevitably affect content, acceptability and accessibility of care. In fact, a British government document highlighted the poor attendance at hospital antenatal clinics and stressed that it was the women who are particularly 'at risk'—the very young, those of low social class, and those of high parity—that are particularly likely to receive a less than adequate form of care (see Chapter 14). A British national survey of women receiving antenatal care (O'Brien and Smith 1981) also showed that women attending hospital clinics were less likely to be satisfied with the care received than those attending their general practitioner.

The family doctor's knowledge of the social and psychological needs of his or her patients (Klein 1983c), enables him or her to modify and individualize programmes of care in order to make the best use of the available resources. Good and close working relationships between family doctors and their specialist colleagues, are of benefit to all concerned (Zander *et al.* 1978). Women at higher than average risk who need specialist expertise are able to receive both that expertise and the extra supportive psychological care from a doctor who knows them and their family well. With such collegial relationships, family doctors are able to increase their knowledge and expertise in obstetric care, and obstetric specialists can fulfil their proper role as consultants.

5.2 Family doctor and midwife

Both family doctors and midwives claim to provide continuity of care and a so-called 'holistic' approach to pregnancy care (see Chapter 10). Both are uncomfortable with excessive use of technology and its presumed dehumanizing effect. There are, however, some important differences between them.

General practitioners come from the same educational system as specialists, and are firmly rooted in the medical professional structure. Many midwives see the general practitioner as a representative of the medical model providing a type of care that is similar, albeit somewhat less complex, than that provided by the specialist obstetrician. Thus in the view of many midwives, general practitioners are inappropriate as providers of true primary maternity care. The Association of Radical Midwives in the United Kingdom, for example, have proposed that 'midwives will be the recognized point of entry into the care for all pregnant women' and that 'midwives will be seen as the professionals to consult in all matters relating to childbirth' (Association of Radical Midwives 1986). While such policy statements establish midwives as professionals in their own right, they also affirm that midwives are specialists rather than generalists. They are incompatible with the expressed aim of encouraging the 'holistic' care to which these professionals subscribe (see Chapter 10).

Many family physicians as well as many midwives combine clinical, advisory, and supportive skills in the care of childbearing women. While both midwives and family doctors can provide continuity of care, during the childbearing year, that of the general practitioner extends over a much longer period of time. The importance of this long term continuity should not be minimized.

Reid and McIlwaine (1981) studying consumer opinion about various aspects of antenatal care found that when women were asked whom they would consult if they had worries about their pregnancy, the most commonly mentioned person was their general practitioner; husbands and mothers came second and third and the hospital obstetricians, fourth on the list of 'confidantes'. Only a small proportion of women mentioned midwives.

Overall, the similarities between general practitioners and midwives far outweigh their differences. We hope that in time a truly collaborative relationship will develop between these two professions. General practitioners must come to look on midwives as colleagues rather than as auxiliary helpers or handmaidens and midwives be less concerned with regaining or retaining professional territory, and recognize the importance of the family doctor to the welfare of the childbearing woman. Both should acknowledge the contribution that each can make to effective care in pregnancy and childbirth.

5.3 The lack of choice in rural family practice

As mentioned earlier, the characteristics of family practice differ greatly both among and within countries. Discussions on the appropriate role, if any, of the family doctor in maternity care thus require careful assessment of the geographical, social, cultural, and staffing characteristics of each locality.

Moving all women away from their homes to centralized facilities to give birth would disrupt the life of the woman and her family. Moving those women with any degree of increased risk would so deplete the experience of the local family doctors that they would soon become unable to handle obstetrical crises when they do arise. Continuing educational activities for family doctors will achieve more than a general centralization of services.

The issue of centralization or decentralization must be firmly addressed by family practitioners and society as a whole, in order to avoid further depleting isolated and rural areas of competent family practitioners. Small units have been shown to have excellent perinatal outcomes provided that they approach their task in a highly organized fashion and have clear guidelines for maternal and infant consultation and transfer. New Zealand was considering closing half of its small units on the assumption that those doing less than 100 deliveries were unsafe. A survey (Rosenblatt *et al.* 1985) found that the level I maternity units, which were mostly rural and staffed by family doctors and midwives mostly without specialist coverage, had lower birthweight specific perinatal mortality rates than the better equipped level II and III hospitals to which they referred in all but the lowest low birthweight categories.

Family doctors who either of necessity or by choice desire to practise a wide range of maternity care will need to be appropriately trained for this task. In addition, general practitioner units, regardless of their size, should undertake regular quality assessments and have clear lines of authority and responsibility.

6 Conclusions

The family doctor has an important role to play in care during pregnancy and childbirth. This role is not to assume the right or responsibility to give that care in its entirety, but to assist the woman and her partner to obtain the care they need. The family doctor's ongoing relationship with the family makes her or him uniquely capable of fulfilling that role.

How the role of the family doctor will be most effectively played, will vary with the circumstances. In some settings, particularly isolated rural settings, family doctors will likely best serve by giving virtually total care. It would not be in the woman's interest to have her far from family and friends at the time of birth and more specialized personnel are not likely to be available in isolated settings. In other settings a genuine commitment to the needs of childbearing women and their families would suggest a close co-operation with community midwives.

Above all, the role of the family doctor should be to promote personalized maternity care in any setting (Klein *et al.* 1986). While this is a responsibility of all who give maternity care, the family doctor above all should identify with the pregnant woman and her family rather than with the institution and its rules.

References

Association of Radical Midwives (1986). Position Paper, July 15, 1986.

Ballard RA, Ferris C, Clyman RI, Read C, Sellars R, Berman F, Leonard C, Irvin D, Henning D, Roth R, Sniderman S (1985). The hospital alternative birth center: is it safe? Experience in 1000 cases from 1976 to 1980. J Perinatol, 5: 61–64.

Baruffi, G, Dellinger WS, Stobino DM, Rudolph A, Timmins RY, Ross A (1984a). A study of pregnancy outcomes in a maternity center and a tertiary care hospital. Am J Public Health, 74: 970–978.

Baruffi G, Stobino DM, Dellinger WS, Rudolph A, Timmons RY, Ross A. (1984b). The patterns of obstetric procedure use in maternity care. Obstet Gynecol, 64: 493–498.

Black DP, Gick S (1979). Management of obstetric complications at a small rural hospital. Can Med Assoc J, 12: 31–37.

Black DP, Fyfe IM (1984). The safety of obstetric services in small communities in northern Ontario. Can Med Assoc J, 130: 571–576.

Black N (1982). Do general practitioner deliveries constitute a perinatal mortality risk? Br Med J, 284: 488–490.

Black R, Schmittling G, Stern TL (1980). Characteristics and practice patterns of family practice residency graduates in the United States. J Family Practice, 11: 767–778.

Bull MJV (1980). Ten years' experience in a general practice unit. J R Coll Gen Pract, 30: 208–251.

Caetano DF (1975). The relationship of medical specialization (obstetricians and general practitioners) to complications in pregnancy and delivery, birth injury, and malformation. Am J Obstet Gynecol, 123: 221–227.

Casson RI, Sennett ES (1984). Prenatal risk assessment and obstetric care in a small rural hospital: comparison with guidelines. Can Med Assoc J, 130: 1311–1315.

Chalmers I (1979). Perinatal health: the search for indices. Lancet, ii: 1063–1065.

Ely JW, Ueland K, Gordon MJ (1976). An audit of obstetric care in a university family medicine department and an obstetrics-gynecology department. J Family Practice, 3: 397–401.

Fleming MF (1983). A family physician's approach to obstetrical practice. Family Med Rev, 2: 25.

Franks P, Eisinger S (1987). Adverse perinatal outcomes: Is physician specialty a risk factor. J Family Practice, 24: 152–156.

Graduate Medical Education National Advisory Committee (1981). US Department of Health and Human Services: Report of the Graduate Medical Education National Advisory Committee to the Secretary. Washington DC: US Government Printing Office.

Goodlin, RC (1980). Low-risk obstetrics for low-risk mothers. Lancet, 1: 1017–1019.

Hassett BR (1986). Newsletter: Victoria Faculty of the Royal College of General Practice, Aug: 12.

Keirse MJNC (1982). Interaction between primary and secondary antenatal care, with particular reference to The Netherlands. In: Effectiveness and Satisfaction in Antenatal Care. Enkin M, Chalmers I (eds). London: Heinemann, pp 222–233.

Klein M (1983). Contracting for trust in family practice obstetrics. Can Family Physician, 29: 2225–2227.

Klein M (1986). The Canadian Family Practice Accoucheur. Can Family Physician, 32: 533–540.

Klein M, Lloyd I, Redman C, Bull M, Turnbull AC (1983a). A comparison of low risk women booked for delivery in two different systems of care. Part I. Obstetrical procedures and neonatal outcomes. Br J Obstet Gynaecol, 90: 118–122.

Klein M, Lloyd I, Redman C, Bull M, Turnbull AC (1983b). A comparison of low risk women booked for delivery in two different systems of care. Part II. Labour and delivery management and neonatal outcome. Br J Obstet Gynaecol, 90: 123–128.

Klein M, Lloyd I, Redman C, Bull M, Turnbull AC (1984a). A comparison of general practitioner and specialist delivery service. In: Pregnancy Care for the 1980s. Zander L, Chamberlain G (eds). London: Royal Society of Medicine and Macmillan Press Ltd., pp 180–195.

Klein M, Papageorgiou A, Westreich R, Spector-Dunsky L, Elins V, Kramer MS Gelfand (1984b). Care in a birth room versus a conventional setting: a controlled trial. Can Med Assoc J, 131: 1461–1466.

Klein M, Reynolds JL, Boucher F, Malus M, Rosenberg E (1984c). Obstetrical practice and training in Canadian family medicine: conserving an endangered species. Can Family Physician, 30: 2093–2099.

Klein M, Elbourne D, Lloyd I (1985). Booking for maternity care: a comparison of two systems. Occasional Paper No. 31. London: The Royal College of General Practitioners.

Koning JH (1984). The obstetrical experience of 20 years in one family practice. J Family Practice, 14: 163–171.

Marsh GN (1977). Obstetric audit in general practice. Br Med J, 2: 1004–1006.

Mehl EL (1978). The outcome of home delivery research in the United States. In: The place of birth. Kitzinger SK, Davis JA (eds). Oxford: Oxford University Press, pp 93–117.

Mehl EL, Peterson G, Whitt M, Hawes W (1977). Outcomes of elective home births: a series of 1146 cases. J Reprod Med, 19: 281–290.

Meyer BA (1981). Audit of obstetrical care: comparison between family practitioners and obstetricians. Family Practice Res J, 1: 20–27.

O'Brien M, Smith C (1981). Women's views and experiences of antenatal care. Practitioner, 225: 123–125.

Owen G (1982). The occupational content of family medicine in Ontario. Toronto: College of Family Physicians of Canada, p 75.

Owen JD (1981). A review of general practitioner obstetric service in Colchester 1970–1979. J R Coll Gen Pract, 31: 92–96.

Phillips WR, Rice GA, Layton RH (1978). Audit of obstetrical care and outcome in family medicine, obstetrics and general practice. J Family Practice, 6: 1209–1216.

Reeves BD, Anderson ER (1977). Perinatal mortality rate at a community hospital, 1956–1975. Am J Obstet Gynecol, 128: 677–683.

Reid ME, McIlwaine GM (1981). Consumer opinion of hospital antenatal clinics. Soc Sci Med, 14A: 363–368.

Reynolds JL, Yudkin PL (1987a). Changes in the management of labour. 1: Length and management of the second stage. Can Med Assoc J, 136: 1042–1045.

Reynolds JL, Yudkin PL (1987b). Changes in the management of labour. 2: Perineal management. Can Med Assoc J, 136: 1045–1049.

Richards TA, Richards JL (1982). A comparison of cesarean section morbidity in urban and rural hospitals: a three-year retrospective review of 1177 charts. Am J Obstet Gynecol, 144: 270–275.

Rosenberg E, Klein M (1987). Is maternity care different in family practice? A pilot matched-pair study. J Family Practice, 25: 237–242.

Rosenblatt RA, Cherkin DC, Schneeweis R, Hart LG, Greenwald H, Kirkwood CR, Perkoff GT (1982). The structure and content of family practice: current status, future trends. J Family Practice, 15: 681–722.

Rosenblatt RA, Reinken J, Schoemach P (1985). Is obstetrics safe in small hospitals? Evidence from New Zealand's regionalized perinatal system. Lancet, 1: 429–432.

Roseveare MP, Bull MJV (1982). General-practitioner obstetrics: two styles of care. Br Med J, 284: 958–960.

Shear CL, Gipe TG, Mattheis JK, Levy MR (1983). Provider continuity and quality of medical care: a retrospective analysis of prenatal and perinatal outcome. Medical Care, 21: 1204–1210.

Taylor GW, Edgar W, Taylor A, Neal DG (1980). How safe is general practitioners' obstetrics? Lancet, 2: 1287–1289.

Tew M (1985). Place of birth and perinatal mortality. J R Coll Gen Pract, 35: 390–394.

Wanderer MJ, Suyehira JG (1980). Obstetrical care in a

prepaid co-operative: a comparison between family practice residents, family physicians, and obstetricians. J Family Practice, 4: 601–606.

Weiss BD (1986). The effect of malpractice insurance costs on family physicians' hospital practices. J Family Practice, 23: 55–58.

Zander LI (1981). The place of confinement—a question of statistics or ethics? J Med Ethics, 7: 125–127.

Zander LI (1984). Deciding on the home as the place of birth. Update, April 1: 821–827.

Zander LI, Watson M, Taylor RW, Morrell DC (1978). Integration of general practitioner and specialist antenatal care. J R Coll Gen Pract, 28: 455–458.

12 The role of the obstetric specialist

John Parboosingh, Marc J. N. C. Keirse, and Murray Enkin

1 Introduction

In recent decades, the obstetric specialist has played an increasingly large role in the provision of obstetrical care throughout most of the industrialized world. That same period of time has seen a dramatic fall in perinatal mortality, a growing increase in the use of sophisticated technology during pregnancy and childbirth, a major shift towards centralization of obstetrical services, and an exponential rise in the cost of maternity care despite a decrease in the number of births.

Although these trends are almost universal throughout the industrialized world, there are great differences in the way in which various countries provide patterns of specialist care. These depend on many factors including population density, social organization, health expenditure per capita, and the way in which health services are organized and funded (see Chapters 14 and 87).

This chapter will not attempt to address these important differences, as this would provide a perspective that is limited by local circumstances. Instead the chapter will try to provide a framework of general principles that would be universally applicable in spite of these differences.

2 Importance of the specialist

Concurrent with the increase in specialist involvement in obstetrical care there has been a dramatic drop in the risk of maternal death and a steady decline in perinatal mortality that is only beginning to level off at the present time (Macfarlane and Mugford, in preparation). While it is true that the major reasons for this decrease may have been general improvements in health, socioeconomic conditions, and changes in reproductive behaviour (Alberman 1980; Chalmers and Macfarlane 1980; Keirse 1984; Chalmers 1985), the contribution of the specialty of obstetrics has also been immensely important.

Control of infection and bleeding have contributed to the safety of childbirth for the mother in particular. Postpartum haemorrhage, once a major cause of maternal death, is now rarely life-threatening, because effective methods of prophylaxis and treatment have been developed (see Chapter 67). As far as the baby is concerned, conditions such as haemolytic disease of the fetus and newborn (see Chapter 35) have been virtually eliminated. Improved care of diabetic women has given them a prognosis that is now little different from that of non-diabetic women (see Chapter 36). Better methods of fetal surveillance have allowed more appropriate timing of delivery and a major decrease in antepartum and especially intrapartum deaths. The latter, which in the 1958 British Perinatal Mortality Survey accounted for 35 per cent of the total perinatal mortality (Butler and Bonham 1963), are now rarely observed. Early prenatal diagnosis now allows the detection of fetal abnormalities in time to give the woman the option of termination of pregnancy if she so chooses.

Many other examples could be cited to illustrate the important contribution of the obstetric specialty to maternal and perinatal health. Although the development of these elements of care has been a major achievement of the specialty, however, not all of them still need to be actually carried out by specialists. Many have now been incorporated into the care given by primary caregivers.

On the other hand, many of the practices and procedures of modern obstetrical care do require the skills and expertise that can only be attained by special training and practice. Sophisticated diagnostic technology, such as ultrasound, amniocentesis, cardiotocography, and fetal scalp blood sampling are beyond the usual range of expertise of primary caregivers. Similarly, many therapeutic interventions such as intrauterine transfusion (see Chapter 35), instrumental delivery (see Chapter 71), and caesarean section (see Chapter 72) require the skills of the obstetric specialist for their full potential to be realized.

In addition to the myriad of obstetric problems and disorders intrinsic to pregnancy that can occur, women with pre-existing disease can become pregnant, and pregnant women can become diseased. Effective care for these women requires thorough knowledge of reproductive physiology and pathophysiology and the technical know-how that can only be obtained by prolonged and focused study and be maintained by ongoing practice.

For some of these women the expertise of specialists in other fields will be necessary. These specialists, like general practitioners, often do not have the depth of understanding of the way in which physiological changes of pregnancy can modify concurrent disease processes. For this reason the obstetrician must take full responsibility for overseeing the care of these women, and for ensuring that the contribution which these other specialists have to offer is optimally used.

3 The nature of specialist care

There are three essential requirements for effective modern specialist care: knowledge, skills, and equipment.

Compared with the primary caregivers—midwives (see Chapter 10) and general practitioners (see Chapter 11)—obstetricians can be assumed to have superior technical competence and knowledge of obstetric disorders. While this is true for the majority of specialist obstetricians, it does not necessarily apply to the junior resident or to the practitioner whose interests and commitments are mainly with gynaecology. The special knowledge and skills required can only be achieved by focused study and concentrated training. Although the bulk of this education will be devoted to the pathophysiology and disorders of pregnancy and childbirth, consideration of the psychosocial needs of the woman and the way in which they are influenced by pregnancy and childbirth is an integral component of that education. Social skills must be as thoroughly mastered as technical skills.

In addition to learning how to carry out the many diagnostic and therapeutic procedures that may be required, the specialist in training must learn when and when not to use them. When they are required, it is equally important that the specialist know how to communicate this need to the woman in a way that she can understand, so that she will be left with the option of choice and the recognition that she remains in control. Results of a survey conducted among Canadian women revealed that the issues that had the most effect on dissatisfaction with the care they received during pregnancy and childbirth were the extent of communication between the doctor and woman, continuity of care, having explanations for interventions, and honouring choices made by women before labour (Canadian Medical Association 1987) (see Chapter 8).

Optimal utilization of the skills and knowledge of the specialist requires the use of sophisticated equipment. Specialist care, therefore, can only be carried out where such equipment is available, and often only in hospital. An inevitable consequence of this is that women will be subject to the rules and regulations that are necessary accompaniments of an institutional environment (see Chapter 50). A high level of technical care is often seen as being depersonalized or dehumanized, but this is by no means inevitable. The caregiver who is aware of this potential drawback should be able to prevent it. The woman who is most in need of a high level of technical care will often be most in need of a high level of personal care. Inadequate attention to either of these components is unlikely to result in effective care.

Efficient use of the knowledge, skills, and equipment of the specialist requires that they be directed to either consultation services for primary caregivers (Parboosingh and Kerr 1982) or to the care of women with pregnancy disorders or intercurrent disease.

4 Regionalization of care

Regionalization of perinatal care has become a major issue in many countries. The need to avoid excessive duplication of the costly equipment, high level technology, and specialized skills required for the care of tiny preterm and severely ill newborns makes centralization necessary. The need for this centralization is generally recognized. Such centralization of ill newborn care would be self-defeating if it were not matched by an equally high level of skill and judgement being applied before and at birth. There is ample evidence that the condition of the baby at birth is a major determinant of subsequent well-being and ultimate prognosis. The mortality and morbidity of conditions such as respiratory distress syndrome and haemolytic disease of the newborn are greatly determined by the condition of the baby at the time when responsibility shifts from the obstetrician to the neonatologist. Moreover, the transport of these tiny or ill babies can be a hazardous and harmful process (Shenai *et al.* 1981; Fetter *et al.* 1986), apart from the burden for the transport teams (Marshall and Kasman 1980) and the stress and expenses incurred by the parents (Smith and Baum 1983; Verloove-Vanhorick and Verwey 1987).

In recognition of the difference in neonatal outcomes, many neonatology departments publish separate statistics for babies born in their own institutions and for those transferred from outside units. However well transport from the latter is organized, the superior outcome of inborn infants is clear in all studies that present outcomes on a regional basis (Eksmyr *et al.* 1986; Hein and Lathrop 1986; Tenovuo *et al.* 1986; Verloove-Vanhorick and Verwey 1987; Northern Regional Health Authority Co-ordinating Group 1984).

Although the contribution of the neonatal intensive care unit to regionalized care is more readily apparent, obstetric intensive care including timing and mode of delivery, intrapartum surveillance, and the availability of skilled attention for the newborn at the immediate moment of birth, is equally important.

Regionalization does not necessarily mean that all women and babies perceived to be at increased risk must be brought to the regional centre. It can also mean that specialized care is brought to a woman in her own community in the form of consultation by telephone or by the perinatologist in person (Parboosingh and Kerr 1982).

Adverse effects of regionalization should not be underestimated, however. The very need to concentrate skills and facilities so that they can be most efficiently used to benefit as large a number of mothers and babies as possible, implies that these will often not be available within the near vicinity of those that need them. For most women, giving birth far away from one's home and family is distressful under any circumstances. The additional worries and concerns about the baby's survival and future well-being may make the burden virtually intolerable. Partners and other members of the family may have to travel long distances to visit the mother and baby and to help alleviate her feelings of alienation. This becomes particularly relevant when one considers that women are not infrequently transferred to, and give birth in, regional centres when in retrospect it is clear that they could have safely given birth in their own communities.

In the current climate of economic restraint, pressure on these scarce resources is such that at times mothers and babies must be separated. Regrettably, instances of multiple pregnancy in which the siblings have to be cared for in different cities are not rare.

When all mothers and babies who require special skills at the moment of birth are moved to regional centres, obstetricians and others working at the remaining centres will obviously lose the opportunity to maintain the skills and judgement necessary to deal effectively with a mother and baby who unexpectedly develop the need for such skills. There is a fine line between overcentralization and undercentralization.

5 Subspecialization

Throughout most of the world, obstetrics and gynaecology are one and the same specialty. Because of the increasing complexity of modern care, the disciplines of obstetrics and gynaecology have diverged. It is doubtful whether it is still possible for the specialist in training to learn all the skills that would be required to encompass both these fields with the level of competence that could be obtained in a more restricted field. It is equally difficult for the specialist in practice to be at the forefront of knowledge in the increasingly diverse elements that comprise obstetrics and gynaecology, and to develop and maintain the new technical skills that are necessary to apply that knowledge to clinical care.

In many countries these difficulties have led to the development of a number of subspecialties, one of them being obstetric perinatology, or feto-maternal medicine. In some countries such subspecialties have been or are on the point of being formally recognized as distinct branches of specialization. Such specialists then have tasks and responsibilities that are distinct and to some extent separate from those who practise the full specialty of obstetrics and gynaecology. The advantages of this are obvious in that the subspecialist, being freed from responsibilities in the wider sphere, will have the time and opportunity to concentrate in depth on a more limited area and to deal with the complexities of care and research that relate to it.

In many ways the relation between the subspecialist in obstetric perinatology and the general obstetrician–gynaecologist is similar to that between the latter and the general practitioner or midwife. There is sometimes resentment on the part of those who practise in the wider field about what they perceive as a take-over of tasks and responsibilities for which they (rightly or wrongly) feel competent. Sometimes the more specialized practitioner is irritated by what he or she perceives (rightly or wrongly) to be an inadequate application of current skills and knowledge working to the detriment of mother and baby. Some of these resentments on both sides are unquestionably justified; some are not.

The dividing line between the areas of competence and responsibility is often not clear-cut. The large grey area with its blurred boundaries demands flexibility by all parties concerned. Such flexibility should be possible to achieve when it is genuinely realized that the interests of the mother and baby, rather than those of the professional disciplines, are at stake.

It should be obvious that only a small proportion of pregnancies will require the direct attention of such subspecialists. Conditions such as clinically significant Rhesus isoimmunization, severe preeclampsia, diabetes, endocrine disorders, and cardiopathies that require a high level of specialized care, are not frequently encountered. Similarly, pregnancies that end with the birth of a liveborn baby at less than 32 weeks' gestation may account for as few as 0.6 per cent of deliveries and liveborn infants of less than 1500 g account for no more than 0.7 per cent of births (Verloove-Vanhorick et al. 1986).

The subspecialist's role is not confined to the direct provision of care, but includes the dissemination of the achievements in this narrow field to the wider body of practitioners. In this way the boundaries of the subspecialty will change continuously as former innovations become part of regular care while new horizons are reached.

6 Constraints on the specialty

So much has been achieved in making pregnancy and childbirth safe and in conquering previously devastating conditions, that expectations have risen to an unparalleled degree. Women who in former years could not dare to contemplate pregnancy without putting their lives at risk would at present achieve pregnancy outcomes that are hardly different from those of the population at large. Conditions that formerly could be faced with little but a philosophical acceptance of what fate would bring can now be brought to a safe and happy conclusion. Miracles are expected, and often occur.

While the results of specialization and modern technology are often taken for granted, the means to achieve them are often resented. Some feel that mothers, first time mothers in particular, 'will invariably be persuaded to agree to interventions, and many of those interventions are carried out routinely with little thought for the needs of individual mothers and babies' (Beech 1987). On the other hand, research conducted in the United States revealed that American women would be prepared to pay over 200 dollars for the information obtained by ultrasonography in an uncomplicated pregnancy (Berwick and Weinstein 1985). Arguments that modern obstetrical care is mechanized and dehumanized are heard, and there are many who genuinely believe, and publicize their opinion that technological advances and depersonalization go hand in hand (Arms 1975; Mendelsohn 1981).

The rise of alternative birth movements is a manifestation of this rejection of technology, but it is also a protest against what are perceived to be the excesses of the 'obstetrical establishment' (see Chapter 9). Such feelings of protest are not a recent phenomenon. In 1976, the International Childbirth Education Association accused organized obstetrics of: (1) ignoring the fact that the individual, not the professional, is responsible for her own health and for her choice of care; (2) contravening the individual's right to define health or illness in terms different from those of the professional; (3) operating a health care system that was not trustworthy and that often produced unnecessary physical and/or psychological trauma and interference; (4) disregarding the value systems of consumers and failing to give them a voice in the planning and operation of programs; (5) failing to acknowledge that childbirth is actually a normal physiological process, not a pathological one; and (6) taking full credit for improvement in maternal mortality and morbidity statistics when much of this may have been due to many other factors, 'such as improved living standards, hygiene, nutrition, antibiotics, and educational level of the populace' (International Childbirth Education Association 1976).

Obstetricians are caught in the middle, exposed to cross-fire from both sides. They cannot work miracles. Although they are expected to (and can) do more of value than ever before, the environment of antagonism and suspicion within which they must often function can result in insecurity and defensive behaviour.

In some countries the threat of malpractice litigation whenever a less than perfect outcome occurs is a constant preoccupation. The frustration and anger that a family must feel when faced with an unhappy outcome was formerly directed at a cruel amorphous destiny. It is now often directed at the obstetrician, and may be accompanied by legal action. Law suits, whether or not they are justified or successful, have a long lasting and devastating effect on the personal and professional lives of the obstetricians concerned (Lavery 1988). The threat of malpractice litigation undermines the obstetrician's self-confidence. Its effects extend far beyond the costs of malpractice insurance or the actuality of being sued. It can transform the potential for effective practice into the reality of defensive practice (Chalmers and Macfarlane 1979).

Obstetricians face other sources of anxiety. In addition to the serious consequences of many of the decisions that they must make, they are also faced with ethical dilemmas. Ultrasound, for example, can detect fetal abnormalities that have unpredictable but grave prognoses. The solutions that the obstetrician may have to offer are constrained by what society is ready to accept. Obstetricians who act in accordance with what they and the parents believe to be the best course of action, may still face societal consequences.

Unlike midwives and general practitioners, obstetricians cannot work alone. They are dependent on an ever increasing number of other health care professionals: midwives, general practitioners, neonatologists, anaesthesists, technicians, nurses, as well as specialists in other disciplines. Disagreements among such professionals with different perspectives about either the goals of care or the means to achieve them, may add to the strain of the obstetrician (Savage 1986), who must assume the ultimate responsibility for the well-being of mother and fetus.

Despite these constraints, developments in obstetrics are not at a standstill. The potential contribution to perinatal health is still enormous. If this potential is to be fully realized, the content and organization of care will require imaginative approaches in the future as it has in the past.

7 Conclusions

The specialist obstetrician plays a major role in the totality of care provided for pregnant women and their babies. That role should be limited in terms of the total volume of care, but it is indispensable for the total quality of that care.

References

Alberman E (1980). Prospects for better perinatal health. Lancet, i: 189–192.

Arms S (1975). Immaculate Deception. San Francisco: Houghton Mifflin.

Beech BL (1987). Who's Having your Baby? A health right's handbook for maternity care. London: Camden Press, p 10.

Berwick DM, Weinstein MC (1985). What do patients value? Willingness to pay for ultrasound in normal pregnancy. Medical Care 23: 881–893.

Butler NR, Bonham DG (1963). Perinatal mortality. The first report of the 1958 British Perinatal Mortality Survey. Edinburgh and London: Churchill Livingstone, p 194.

Canadian Medical Association (1987). Canadian Medical Association Policy Summary: obstetrical care. Can Med Assoc J, 136: 1312–1312B.

Chalmers I (1985). Short, Black, Baird, Himsworth and social class differences in fetal and neonatal mortality rates. Br Med J, 291: 231–3.

Chalmers I, Macfarlane A (1980). Interpretation of perinatal statistics. In: Topics in Perinatal Medicine. Wharton B (ed). London: Pitman Medical, pp 1–11.

Chalmers I, Macfarlane JA (1979). Towards defensive obstetrics (letter). Lancet 1: 53.

Eksmyr R, Larssen KE, Bakketeig LS, Bergsjo P, Finne P, Laurini R, Wasen G, Knoff H (1986). Perinatal mortality in a Swedish country 1973–1978. Time trends revealed by perinatal audit. Acta Paediatr Scand, 75: 17–23.

Fetter WPF, Baerts W, Borst LE (1986). Late morbiditeit bij kinderen met een geboortegewicht van minder dan 1500 gram, geboren in de periode 1979–1983. Ned Tijdschr Geneeskd 130: 1143–1146.

Hein HA, Lathrop SS (1986). The changing pattern of neonatal mortality in a regionalized system of perinatal care. Am J Dis Child, 140: 989–993.

International Childbirth Education Association (1976). International Childbirth Education Association replies to American College of Obstetricians and Gynecologists. ICEA News, 15: 1-?

Keirse MJNC (1984). Perinatal mortality rates do not contain what they purport to contain. Lancet, i: 1166–1169.

Lavery JP (1988). The physician's reaction to a malpractice suit. Obstet Gynecol, 71: 138–141.

Macfarlane AJ, Mugford M (in preparation). International trends in perinatal and infant mortality.

Marshall RE, Kasman C (1980). Burnout in the neonatal intensive care unit. Pediatrics, 65: 1161–1165.

Mendelsohn R (1981). Mal(e)Practice. Chicago: Contemporary.

Northern Regional Health Authority Co-ordinating Group (1984). Perinatal mortality: a continuing collaborative regional survey. Br Med J, 288: 1717–1720.

Parboosingh J, Kerr M (1982). Innovations in the role of obstetric hospitals in prenatal care. In: Effectiveness and Satisfaction in Antenatal Care. Enkin M, Chalmers I (eds). London: Heinemann, pp 254–265.

Savage W (1986). A savage enquiry: who controls childbirth? London: Virago.

Shenai JP, Johnson GE, Varney RV (1981). Mechanical vibration in neonatal transport. Pediatrics, 68: 55–57.

Smith MA, Baum JD (1983). Costs of visiting babies in special care baby units. Arch Dis Child, 58: 56–59.

Tenovuo A, Kero P, Piekkala, Sillanpaa, Erkkola R (1986). Advances in perinatal care and declining regional neonatal mortality in Finland, 1968–82. Acta Pediatr Scand, 75: 362–369.

Verloove-Vanhorick SP, Verwey RA (1987). Place of birth and transport. In: Project on Preterm and Small for Gestational Age Infants in The Netherlands 1983: A collaborative survey. MD thesis, Leiden University, pp 147–159.

Verloove-Vanhorick SP, Verwey RA, Brand R, Bennebroek Gravenhorst J, Keirse MJNC, Ruys JH (1986). Neonatal mortality risk in relation to gestational age and birthweight. Lancet, 1: 55–57.

13 Interaction between primary and secondary care during pregnancy and childbirth

Marc J. N. C. Keirse

1 Introduction

The second half of this century has seen enormous changes and improvements in not only the outcome of, but also the care given for, pregnancy and childbirth. Many of these improvements relate to general improvements in health care and public health systems that have made that care available to those who need it.

These improvements have by no means reached all segments of society. Large numbers of immigrants, with different socioeconomic and cultural backgrounds, now make up a large part of the childbearing population in many countries. From several countries there is ample evidence that these individuals are at a considerable disadvantage, both in terms of pregnancy outcome (Doornbos and Nordbeck 1985; Office of Population Censuses and Surveys 1986; Faur and Court 1987), and in terms of accessibility to and utilization of maternity care (see Chapter 14). Many of these countries, now in economic recession, are ill-prepared to take on the challenge that they invited in times of economic expansion. This may well become one of the most important barriers to effective maternity care in the next few years. It would be a grave error to assume that the major achievements in improving pregnancy outcome seen in recent years will continue and be realized forever.

The increasing heterogeneity of the childbearing population, with the different cultural and socioeconomic backgrounds represented among childbearing women, will in the future require a greater flexibility on the part of care providers than they have hitherto shown. Many of them place too much emphasis on the perceived achievements of their discipline and too little emphasis on the equally important question of whether the care that they offer is available and acceptable to, and utilized by, those who need it.

Patterns of care in pregnancy and childbirth have changed rapidly in two major ways. Birth has moved from the home or semi-domestic maternity unit to more technically equipped and specialist-staffed hospitals and has drawn all of maternity care in its wake. Many technical advances and procedures have evolved beyond the field of expertise and competence of those who formerly provided the bulk of care.

In many, if not most, countries these changes have led to rivalry, resentment, and territorial protection among different professional groups rather than to the co-operation that is so urgently needed. Vague terms such as 'holistic care', 'continuity of care' and 'superior knowledge' are used more often to defend professional prerogatives than to improve care. The use of these vague terms often expresses, implicitly or explicitly, the belief that one profession has a quality that is lacking in the others, and that this quality is more important than that which the others have to offer. The fact that the range of these qualities is far greater among the individuals within each of the caring professions than among the professions as a whole is often conveniently forgotten.

The thesis of this chapter is simple: adequate primary care can only exist where good secondary care is available; and adequate secondary care can only exist by virtue of good primary care. Neither can function properly without the other and their coexistence requires co-operation rather than competition.

2 Difference between primary and secondary care

While discussions abound on the merits and hazards of primary and secondary care, the content of these two types of care has not been clearly delineated. Primary care is usually defined as that provided by first-line health workers. In some countries (for example Canada where there is as yet no legal recognition of midwives), this means that care is given by general practitioners; in other countries (for example the United Kingdom) it refers mostly to general practitioners working with community midwives; in still others (for example The Netherlands) it refers to general practitioners as well as professional midwives, both of whom are fully qualified and licensed to provide independent care during normal pregnancy and childbirth. In contrast, secondary care is considered to be care given by specialists certified in obstetrics and gynaecology.

This distinction between primary and secondary care is arbitrary, artificial, and unrealistic for two reasons. First, throughout the world, true primary antenatal care is provided by the pregnant woman herself and it is essential that this is duly recognized in any evaluation of the quality of care. Second, it ignores the fact that the care provided by a specialist gynaecologist, whose main interest may be oncology or urodynamics for instance, is not likely to be better, even in purely technical terms, than that given by a first-line health worker whose main interests centre on care for pregnancy and childbirth. Differences in the quality of secondary care provided are now so well recognized that they have led to the introduction of the term 'tertiary care' to indicate yet another, still more specialized level of care.

A substantial part of the perceived distinctions between primary and secondary care, therefore, is an ill-conceived attempt to hide the really important issue of which individuals are properly qualified and/or experienced to provide care of adequate quality. Nevertheless, the terms primary and secondary care will be retained throughout this chapter in order to make the necessary distinction between care for women who do not require specialized care, and care for those women who do require that care. In theory, three patterns of care are possible: primary care only, for all women; secondary care only, for all women; and a balanced mixture of primary and secondary care.

The first of these, primary care only for all women, with no access to specialist services, is still unfortunately the predominant pattern in most of the developing world. In circumstances in which specialist care is not available, it is the best that can be offered. It is rarely, if ever, a pattern that would be preferred by choice, and it will not be further discussed. The two remaining patterns remain to be considered in detail.

3 Secondary care for all

The hazards inherent in any pregnancy are considered sufficient reason for specialized care. Hern (1975) graphically portrayed the concept of pregnancy as an illness. He outlined in exquisite detail the illness parameters of pregnancy: its known aetiology, its pathogenesis as a host–parasite relationship, and its multiphasic pathophysiology (including displacement of the abdominal contents, hypercoagulability of the blood and other derangements of body structures and function). He continued the simile by referring to the subclinical phase of the disease (before pregnancy is diagnosed), and the characteristic symptoms, signs, and laboratory findings which establish the diagnosis. He listed 25 acute and subacute complications which may occur, discussed the differential diagnosis and considered treatment under headings of medical management, early and late surgical intervention, and supportive therapy. The prognosis, he maintained, includes a characteristic duration that varies within certain limits; recovery that may be spontaneous or induced; and a risk of temporary or permanent sequelae. He noted that the condition 'carries a case fatality rate which varies according to the patient's general health status' and ended by observing that 'its recurrence is episodic in survivors' (Hern 1975).

The serious consequences of pregnancy to which Hern referred are rare today. Nevertheless, maternal deaths due to complications and disorders of pregnancy still occur, and, while in almost ninety-nine per cent of births the baby lives and is well, the minority who die or do not do well still represent a serious problem. To some these residual problems can loom so large that they occupy virtually their entire field of vision. For instance, the Canadian Medical Association (1987), in opposing the endeavours of some Canadian jurisdictions to license midwives as a separate health care profession, recently argued 'that without close medical supervision, problems beyond the scope of midwives' training could go unrecognized or that unexpected medical emergencies, which may develop during labour and delivery, would not receive appropriate attention.' (Canadian Medical Association 1987). Strangely enough, while denying a place for midwives, it also 'recognizes the major contributions of obstetrical nurses, and believes nurses could be trained to assume more obstetrical care responsibilities under the direction of physicians' (Canadian Medical Association 1987).

It is understandable that both caregivers and women giving birth feel that they should do everything possible to prevent even the rarest occurrence of disaster. Common sense tells us that it is far better to prevent a problem than to cure it. However, more careful consideration shows that even greater hazards would be incurred with a policy of secondary care for all pregnancies. Specialist care, no matter how competent, does not alter the basic fact that the majority of pregnancies are perfectly normal. This leaves the providers of secondary care with only two options: either to spend most of their time supervising purely physiological processes, or to neglect these normal pregnancies in order to concentrate their care on those with pathology. Both these options contain greater threats to the overall quality of care and to the care received by each individual woman than would a sensible division of responsibilities and collaboration between primary and secondary caregivers.

If the first option is chosen—that of concentrating on abnormal pregnancies—normal pregnant women would lose out in a number of ways. They would receive less (and probably later) care than they would have received from a primary attendant. The likelihood that a deviation from normal would be detected early would decrease, because infrequent attention, however sophisticated, cannot replace careful and regular surveillance. For instance, the detection of pregnancy-induced hypertension, one of the most frequent and most dangerous complications of pregnancy (see Chapter 24), demands little expertise or equipment. It does, however, require regular screening, particularly as symptoms are usually absent until the late stage of the condition.

This option, of drastically reducing the time spent with the woman who is (un)fortunate enough to have a normal pregnancy, would also decrease her opportunity to voice her fears and anxieties, or discuss her minor ailments. While this may have little influence on the physical outcome of the pregnancy, it would certainly affect her well-being. There would also be less opportunity for the education and counselling which could provide her, as the true primary provider of her own care, with the information that will enable her to make informed choices between alternatives. The ultimate effect of this option, then, is that a system of regular and careful attention would be replaced by the provision of only intermittent attention, albeit possibly with the attendant sense of false security engendered by occasional exposure to sophisticated techniques.

The second option—that of providing secondary level care for all during normal pregnancy—would require a considerable investment of time. If the required manpower were available, and one were to assume eight visits of 15 minutes each during the pregnancy as being a reasonable minimal time to spend with each woman, and no more than four hours for provision of all care during labour, delivery and the puerperium, this would amount to 6 hours of care per pregnancy. Thus a specialist working 60 hours per week, 50 weeks a year, at 100 per cent efficiency, would be able to have two weeks holiday and to care for exactly 500 pregnancies per year, provided that he or she has no gynaecological or other commitments.

Based on the known incidence of various pathological conditions, the yearly experience of the specialist would be 25 preterm births, 15 breech presentations, 6 twin pregnancies, four pregnancies complicated by essential hypertension, and less than three cases each of fetal death, placenta praevia, and accidental haemorrhage. He or she would not be able to devote more than 6 hours to each of these pathological pregnancies without working for more than 60 hours a week. Postgraduate education, undergraduate teaching, or professional reading to keep up with current developments would also be precluded. Dealing with fewer pregnancies would, of course, reduce the work load or increase the amount of time available for each pregnancy, but would also reduce the average number of pregnancy-related problems seen every year.

By choosing this second option, then, all pregnancies would receive care by trained and fully qualified specialists, but those women with pathological pregnancies, who desperately need such specialized care, would suffer significantly. They would now receive care from specialists who had neither the necessary time to devote to them, nor sufficient opportunity to develop or maintain the skills and experience necessary to deal with the various types of problems that may arise during pregnancy. Since these skills must also include the ability to carry out the necessary technical interventions during pregnancy, it would not be surprising if there were a tendency to maintain an appropriate level of expertise by carrying out these interventions in women who do not require them. To some this would seem better than to perform them clumsily due to a lack of experience when they are critically needed. This may well have contributed to the high rates of induction of labour, caesarean section, and other interventions observed in some countries which have tended to suggest the desirability of specialist care for all pregnancies (see Chapter 69).

Thus, a policy of secondary care for all women is not feasible even where manpower resources are available. If it could be realized, it would be inherently counter-productive.

Attempts are made in some countries or centres, to avoid the adverse consequences of total secondary care by entrusting care for pregnancy and childbirth to a team consisting of an experienced specialist in charge of less experienced junior staff. The specialist can then deal with the true secondary care problems, and the less experienced staff are left to cope with less complicated or routine cases. It is difficult to see how pregnant women can benefit more from a type of primary care provided by people aspiring to deal with pathology as soon as possible, rather than by caregivers more interested in and committed to the care of women who enjoy a normal pregnancy.

There can be little doubt that women will receive a better quality of care from persons who are experienced in and committed to the principle of primary care, with a true understanding of what pregnancy signifies to the pregnant woman and her family (see Chapters 10 and 11).

4 Limits of secondary and primary care

High risk and complicated pregnancies require specialized and technical care, which to be effective, requires a high level of expertise in, and experience with, the particular pathology. Neither of these qualities can be acquired by osmosis. They represent a major investment of time and effort over a long period of time. A complicated pregnancy will also constitute a time of worry and distress for the pregnant woman and her family. They are confronted not only with the pathology and its possible consequences for mother and baby, but also with an unfamiliar environment and a variety of unfamiliar interventions and their possible consequences. To the caregiver, all of these may be routine. This is rarely the case for the woman and her family. Care that concentrates on the physical aspects, and neglects the pregnant woman as a person, can only be described as inadequate care even when, in medical terms, her pregnancy is superbly managed against the worst odds. While at times intensive somatic medical care is the first priority, it is never in itself enough.

Individuals providing secondary care, therefore, have no choice but to limit their practice to those women who specifically need such care. This is necessary in order for them to maintain both adequate experience and expertise, and to afford them sufficient time to deal not only with pregnancy and its medical problems but with the pregnant woman and her family as well.

This leaves a majority of pregnant women who cannot, need not, and should not be dealt with by the sophisticated approaches required for women with high risk pregnancies. These women can more safely be cared for by primary caregivers who need not and should not attempt to give total care for the occasional complication that they will inevitably encounter. They can draw on, or refer to the expertise of the providers of true secondary care. Primary caregivers do not provide a lower level of care. They can more usefully be considered specialists in primary care providing a type of care which should be most suitable for the large majority of pregnant women.

In order to provide an appropriate level of care, those who provide care must know and work within the limits of their capabilities. This applies to both primary and secondary caregivers alike. Primary caregivers who stretch the boundaries of the care they give to, or beyond, the limits of their own capabilities, lose their margin of safety. By doing so, they create threats to the quality of care that are no less serious than would be created by a system of secondary care for all pregnant women. The women they care for will not have critical assessment and ready access to needed interventions when required, possibly with disastrous consequences. In the same way, providers of secondary care with limited information about the family and social circumstances of the woman may make recommendations that would clearly be unfeasible for her.

5 Co-operation between primary and secondary care

Competition between primary and secondary caregivers does harm to both of them, but most harm to the women over whose bodies the battle is fought. Territorial preoccupations and defensive attitudes are formidable barriers to effective care. They do not necessarily arise from an unwillingness of individuals at both ends of the spectrum to work together toward the common goal of effective care, but may have their origin in the regulations that govern obstetrical practice in most countries. These regulations differ widely from country to country. In The Netherlands, for example (though not in other Benelux countries), specialist care during pregnancy is remunerated only if medical reasons or obstetrical pathology warrant such care. Some European countries, such as the United Kingdom, have actively pursued policies of confining childbirth to large obstetrical units. Others (for example The Netherlands) have actively pursued policies to protect primary care and to favour midwifery, while still others (for example Canada) have not legalized midwives. Belgium and France have attached financial premium systems to childbirth and have tried to manipulate this tool to determine a minimum type of care that would be required. These variations in official policy have a major effect on the nature of the interaction between primary and secondary care (Keirse 1982; Blondel *et al.* 1985).

The appropriate dividing line between primary and secondary care is simple and straightforward. Secondary caregivers can only provide the type of care that is expected and required of them by abstaining from most, if not all, direct involvement in primary care. Primary caregivers will be able to provide adequate primary care only if they do not pretend to possess what is necessary to give adequate secondary care.

While the dividing line between these two types of care may be straightforward, it is not always clear whether an individual woman will require primary or secondary care for some, most or all of her pregnancy. Pathology, such as fetal growth retardation, pregnancy-induced hypertension or preterm labour, may arise, continue, or disappear. Adequate care for these women demands co-operation and close collaboration between primary and secondary caregivers.

There is no need and no place for rivalry between those whose expertise is in the supervision of health and the detection of disease and those whose specialty is the management of disease and, where possible, the restoration of health. The responsibility for achieving the co-operative interaction that is so necessary depends on an understanding and acceptance of this by all those concerned.

References

Blondel B, Pusch D, Schmidt E (1985). Some characteristics of antenatal care in 13 European countries. Br J Obstet Gynaecol, 92: 565–568.

Canadian Medical Association (1987). CMA policy summary: obstetrical care. Can Med Assoc J, 136: 1312–1312B.

Doornbos JPR, Nordbeck HJ (1985). Perinatal Mortality: Obstetric risk factors in a community of mixed ethnic origin in Amsterdam. MD thesis, University of Amsterdam.

Faur B, Court Y (1987). La situation démographique en 1985. Paris: Collections INSERM, serie D.

Hern W (1975). The illness parameters of pregnancy. Soc Sci Med, 9: 365–372.

Keirse MJNC (1982). Interaction between primary and secondary antenatal care, with particular reference to The Netherlands. In: Effectiveness and Satisfaction in Antenatal Care. Enkin M, Chalmers I (eds). London: Spastics International Medical Publications, Heinemann Medical Books.

Office of Population Censuses and Surveys (1986). Mortality statistics, perinatal and infant: social and biological factors. Series DH3, No. 17. London: Her Majesty's Stationery Office.

Part III

General care during pregnancy

14 The needs of childbearing families: social policies and the organization of health care

Jo Garcia, Béatrice Blondel, and Marie-Josèphe Saurel-Cubizolles

'What's the point in going to clinics if they repeat the same thing each pregnancy without giving you any way of putting it into practice?'

Debionne and Larcher (1982).

1 Introduction

1.1 The social context of maternity care

A woman's health, her response to, and utilization of, health care, and her ability to follow the advice that she is offered, are affected both by her social circumstances and by wider social, financial, and health care policies. Many caregivers take these factors into account when they offer advice or make clinical decisions. An obstetrician may, for example, weigh the advantages of asking a woman to make repeated visits to a specialist centre against the distance that she will have to travel in order to comply with this advice. Caregivers and medical policy makers may, however, lack relevant social information about the women for whom they care.

Concern about the way that social circumstances impinge on pregnancy and childbirth exists in all societies (see Chapter 6). A book first published in 1915 (Llewelyn Davies 1978) about the childbearing experience of members of the Co-operative Women's Guild, is a moving demonstration of women's concern about the conflict between their responsibility for their older children and other relatives, and their own pregnancies and health. One woman wrote: 'I myself had some very hard times as I had to go out to work in the mill. I was a weaver and we had a lot of lifting to do. My first baby was born before its time from me lifting my piece off the loom on to my shoulder . . . and when I had my second baby I had to work all through again, as my husband was short of work and ill at the time . . . I had to go out to work again at the month end and put the baby out to nurse. I had to get up by four in the morning and get my baby out of bed, wash and dress it, and then leave home by five' (p 107).

Another commented: '. . . and what a terrible time it is, to be sure, especially during the last two months—only just enough to live on and another coming. The mental strain in addition to bodily labour must surely affect the child . . . I did fairly well for a working man's wife, but the recollection is anything but pleasant. Fancy bending over a washing-tub doing the family washing perhaps an hour or two before baby is born' (p 53).

Working conditions for women in industrialized countries have improved considerably since the early part of this century, and maternity rights have become established in Europe (see Table 14.1). In spite of a

Table 14.1 Maternity rights in Europe

Country	Service requirement	Period of leave	Entitlement to pay	Additional points
Belgium	120 days of actual or credited work	14 weeks	Minimum 80%	
Denmark	At least 6 months' work in preceding year.	28 weeks	90% for 18 weeks (manuals); 50% for 5 months (non-manuals)	Last 10 weeks' leave taken by either parent.
France	200 hours' work in preceding 3 months	16 weeks	90% earnings	Greater period of leave if third or subsequent child. Also for multiple births.
Greece	200 days' work in preceding 2 years	12 weeks (4 months for public sector workers)	100%	Leave after can be extended to 14 weeks.
Ireland	26 weeks' employment	14 weeks	70%	
Italy	Must be employed at time of pregnancy.	5 months plus 6 months optional	80% and 30% during optional leave period	
Luxembourg	Social insurance coverage for 6 months in preceding year.	16 weeks	100%	Plus 4 weeks if premature/multiple births or feeding.
The Netherlands	Paid employment for 6 months	12 weeks	100%	
Portugal	Social insurance cover for 6 months	13 weeks (90 days)	100%	Period of leave may be extended in case of illness.
Spain	Registration with social security for minimum of 9 months and 180 days' contributions.	28 weeks	75%	Period of leave may be extended in case of illness.
Sweden	6 months or 12 in previous 2 years	6 weeks before birth. 18 months after	Not all paid	Partner can also claim 90% pay for up to 9 months.
West Germany	Must have worked 9 months (7 for premature births) in previous 12 or claimed unemployment benefit.	14 weeks	100%	Plus 4 weeks for premature births.
UK	2 years in same job (5 if working less than 16 hours)	40 weeks	6 weeks at 90% and 13 weeks at flat rate £32.85	If less than 2 years' service (but more than 26 weeks') 18 weeks' pay at lower rate.

Source: Labour Research Department (1987), 'Time off for childcare'. London: Labour Research Department

growing body of research about employment in pregnancy (Saurel-Cubizolles 1982; Chamberlain 1984; Romito 1986; Saurel-Cubizolles *et al.* 1986) there are still many uncertainties about the risks and benefits associated with particular aspects of employment. Caregivers will be able to give better care if they inform themselves about research in this field and become familiar with local employment patterns and employees' rights. In this way they can offer specific advice where the evidence exists to support it, and help women to make full use of special facilities or benefits to which they may be entitled, such as rest breaks, changes of job within a place of work, and maternity leave.

Public and private concerns meet in many aspects of maternity care. Antenatal advice about rest or admission to hospital during pregnancy, for example, too often does not take into account a woman's circumstances. She has to weigh up the financial and social benefits of employment against the possible risks. Soundly based dietary advice may be ineffective because women are unable to follow it. A British report (Durward 1984) showed that a mother receiving 'supplementary' benefit would be unable to afford a recommended basic diet in pregnancy. In one British study of unemployed families (Maternity Alliance 1985) a woman respondent said 'The doctor told me to eat fish, meat, vegetables . . . when I try to explain it's impossible, they get defensive.' Other small-scale studies of families on low incomes (Burghes 1980; Evason 1980) show that women often skip meals in order to feed their children adequately, and this may present them with a particular dilemma when they are pregnant. Current dietary advice may also be unsuitable for women in ethnic minorities because it fails to take into account the constraints of dietary exclusions and family customs about meals. These two examples—employment and diet—show how social factors can influence a woman's ability to comply with professional recommendations, her own health, and that of her child.

1.2 Inequalities in health

Although the association between health and prosperity both within a particular country and between countries is well documented (Whitehead 1987; Macfarlane and Mugford 1984; Mahler 1987), it is difficult to assess the extent to which social policies affect health. Policies are rarely introduced in an experimental way. The very extensive literature on the influence of unemployment on health reveals some of the methodological difficulties involved in attempting to do so (Smith 1987; Macfarlane and Cole 1985). We cannot attempt in this chapter to cover in detail the debate about the relative importance of health services, poverty, and individual behaviour in the shaping of health and disease (see, for example, Chalmers 1985; Reid 1986; Macintyre 1986; Blaxter 1983), but it is worth emphasizing that measurable health benefits are not the only ones that count when making social policies. Even if there was no evidence that unemployment could increase the risk of death or depression, most people would regard it as undesirable in itself. It is unlikely that paid time off work for fathers to enable them to be available for help around the time of birth would save lives, but there is demand for this, and men sometimes lose their jobs because they decide to look after their families at the time when a baby is born (Bell *et al.* 1983).

Even though, in world terms, standards of health are high in the countries with which we are concerned in this chapter, there are some important differences in the manifestations of health and disease between people categorized by occupation, wealth, race or other social variables. Inequalities in health are sometimes considered by looking at the full spectrum of a particular social variable such as income, and sometimes by focusing on those at the margin, the poor or poorest (Blaxter 1983; Boddy 1985). Different countries have tended to use different variables in presenting their national statistics. Income, for example, is rarely used in British data, while the social class classification, which has been widely used in the analysis of British data, seems inappropriate in the United States.

Occupational categories are commonly used for classification purposes in France and Britain. Striking differences in adult mortality are observed at all ages between those in professional and in manual occupations (Leclerc *et al.* 1984) Perinatal and neonatal mortality also differ by occupational grouping (Table 14.2) In France in 1970–1972, neonatal mortality varied from 8.7 per 1000, for children whose fathers were categorized as professionals or managers to 16.5 per 1000 for those in the unskilled manual group (Blondel *et al.* 1985a). More recent French survey data (1981) show that the proportion of preterm deliveries and low birthweight babies was higher in lower occupational groups (Kaminski and Blondel 1984) (recent national mortality data by occupation are not available). In England and Wales in 1984 (Office of Population Censuses and Surveys 1986) the perinatal mortality rate for legitimate births to women in Class I, the highest social class category (by virtue of their husband's occupation) was 7.1 per 1000 compared to 14.1 per 1000 for those in Class V. The use of occupational classifications is currently under discussion because rising levels of unemployment have made the categories less meaningful (Macfarlane and Mugford 1984). In addition, the use of husband's occupation to classify women by social class, which is problematic in itself (Irvine *et al.* 1979; Macfarlane 1980), is becoming more unsatisfactory as the proportion of births outside marriage increases (Office of Population Censuses and Surveys 1986).

Table 14.2 Perinatal and neonatal mortality by occupational classification: cross-national comparison

(a) Perinatal mortality rate (PNMR) by father's social class: legitimate births in England and Wales, 1984

Social class	PNMR
I	7.1
II	7.9
III N	8.2
III M	9.8
IV	11.6
V	14.1
All legitimate	9.5

Source: OPCS (1986)

(b) Neonatal mortality (NNMR) by father's occupational category: legitimate births in France, 1970–72

Category	NNMR
Agricultural, self-employed	11.4
Agricultural, employee	14.0
Other self-employed	11.2
Professional and intermediate	8.7
Clerical + shop workers	10.4
Foremen + skilled manual workers	11.4
Semi-skilled manual workers	13.2
Unskilled manual workers	16.5
All legitimate	11.4

Source: Blondel (1985a)

Although occupational classifications are not used in the United States, data on mortality by social variables like income or education are available. A detailed study of infant mortality in Massachusetts (Evans *et al.* 1985), however, showed that in that state, women with less than 12 years of education had a higher proportion of low birthweight babies (8.3 per cent) in 1983 than did those with more than twelve years of education (4.7 per cent). Their babies' neonatal mortality was also higher (7.6 per 1000 compared to 4.7 per 1000).

Race emerges as a very important variable in all the statistics from the United States. National data for 1977–79 show a black infant mortality rate of 22.8 per 1000 compared to a white rate of 11.9 per 1000 (McCormick 1985). In Massachusetts in 1983, neonatal mortality and low birthweight rates were both more than twice as high in the black population as in the white (Evans *et al.* 1985). Recent analyses have shown that race remains associated with low birthweight even after statistical adjustment for differences in obvious socioeconomic variables (Shiono *et al.* 1986).

No data about race are collected in France and Britain, but statistics are available about the country of birth of new parents. In 1984 in England and Wales the perinatal mortality rate was 9.7 per 1000 for mothers born in the United Kingdom compared to 13.7 per 1000 for mothers born in the 'New Commonwealth and Pakistan' (Office of Population Censuses and Surveys 1986). In France the stillbirth rate in 1985 was about twice as high for mothers of North African nationalities when compared with French mothers (Faur and Court 1987) but there was no statistically significant difference in the proportion of low weight or preterm births to mothers born inside or outside France in 1981 (Blondel *et al.* 1985a).

Young age and single marital status are also associated with poor perinatal outcome (Blondel *et al.* 1987; McCormick *et al.* 1984). Because these variables are associated with each other, and are linked to social class and education, there is considerable debate about their independent association with outcome, and in the case of young age, on the relative contributions made by biological and social factors (Blondel and Zuber 1988; Golding *et al.* 1986; McCormick *et al.* 1984).

1.3 Inequalities in the use of health services

In addition to differences in mortality and morbidity related to social inequalities, there are inequalities in the use of health care in the industrialized countries. The fact that poorer people receive *less* of particular kinds of care is not always a sign that they receive *worse* care. Some care may be ineffective or given to those who do not need it, and sometimes more 'advanced' forms of care may be associated with more risks than benefits. Given this proviso, the evidence of unequal access to care linked to social disadvantage is still important to those who plan national systems for providing and regulating health care.

As the main determinant of medical consumption should be the existence and seriousness of health problems (see Chapter 70), it is important to compare groups with the same needs when examining the social inequalities in the use of health care. Studies focusing on inequalities in antenatal care have tried to avoid the problem of obtaining equivalent groups by using as an indicator what they consider to represent minimal (or, in other cases, optimal) care in the absence of complications.

The most commonly chosen forms of this indicator are the stage of gestation at the first antenatal visit (McKinlay 1970; Taffel 1978; Wollast and Vandenbussche 1983; Cooney 1985; Ingram *et al.* 1986), or of a visit for screening for a congenital anomaly (Simpson and Walker 1980). Other studies have looked at the number of antenatal visits and at the place of care or person giving care (McKinlay and McKinlay 1972,1979; Kessner *et al.* 1973; Selbmann *et al.* 1980; Blondel *et al.* 1980,1982a,b,1985b; Robine *et al.* 1985; Task Force on Prevention of Low Birthweight and Infant Mortality 1985; Wollast *et al.* 1986).

The adequacy of care as measured by these indices varies according to the woman's sociodemographic characteristics (age, parity, social class, educational level, country of birth, race, place of residence, financial and family circumstances). In general, women in disadvantaged sociodemographic circumstances have less adequate antenatal care (McKinlay 1970; McKinlay and McKinlay 1972,1979; Kessner *et al.* 1973; Taffel 1978; Blondel et al. 1980, 1982a,b; Simpson and Walker 1980; Selbmann *et al.* 1980; Robine *et al.* 1985; Cooney 1985; Task Force on Prevention of Low Birthweight and Infant Mortality 1985; Ingram *et al.* 1986; Wollast and Vandenbussche 1983; Wollast *et al.* 1986).

In the countries that we have reviewed, which have widely different systems of care, late attendance for antenatal care is more common in women of lower social class (Blondel *et al.* 1980; Cooney 1985; Ingram *et al.* 1986). The same disparity between social classes exists for the number of antenatal visits; in France women married to or living with agricultural workers, unskilled manual workers and unemployed men, are more likely to make four or less antenatal visits, the minimum number recommended by the Ministry of Health (Table 14.3). In England and Wales, the proportion of women missing an antenatal visit rises somewhat, from 10 per cent in social class I, to 16 per cent in social class IV and V (Table 14.4).

Only a few studies have looked at social inequalities in care during delivery and the postnatal period. In France in 1981 the proportion of women having electronic fetal monitoring in labour and the proportion of caesarean sections and instrumental vaginal deliveries did not vary with social class. Induced labours were, however, less common for women married to or living with unskilled manual workers (Table 14.5) (Hubert *et al.* 1987) and this was also seen in England and Wales in 1975 (Cartwright 1979). In France, episiotomies are more likely among women of higher social class (Table 14.5). The type of health insurance also has an

Table 14.3 Antenatal care according to social class of the child's father in France in 1981

Social class	Number of visits	Place of care		
	≤4	Maternity unit or obstetrician only	GP only	Other[1]
	%	%	%	%
Professional, managerial	7.7 (440)	69.0	1.4	29.6 (429)
Intermediate	11.0 (686)	59.7	3.9	36.4 (637)
Clerical workers, shop assistants	14.1 (552)	49.5	4.1	46.4 (537)
Farmers	27.8 (212)	30.7	16.1	53.2 (205)
Other self-employed[2]	19.1 (267)	49.2	10.0	40.8 (260)
Skilled manual workers	19.5 (1085)	46.1	8.4	45.5 (1065)
Unskilled manual workers	28.6 (1205)	37.4	13.5	49.1 (1180)
Other	10.8 (204)	60.0	3.0	37.0 (200)
Unemployed	23.5 (264)	48.3	8.9	42.8 (259)
	$p<0.001$		$p<0.001$	

[1] Mainly maternity unit (or obstetrician) + GP
[2] Manual workers, shop keepers
Source: INSERM

Table 14.4 Antenatal care according to social class of the child's father[1] in England and Wales in 1975

Social class	First visit after 19 weeks of gestation	At least one visit missing	Place of care		
			Hospital only	GP only	Other[2]
	%	%	%	%	%
I	4.1 (194)	9.6 (198)	10.9	32.3	56.8 (192)
II	9.1 (384)	8.7 (392)	16.9	27.3	55.7 (384)
III N	5.9 (239)	12.2 (245)	16.2	24.6	59.2 (240)
III M	11.1 (854)	15.2 (875)	16.6	26.6	56.8 (866)
IV–V	11.7 (394)	16.2 (407)	18.8	22.7	58.5 (405)
	$p<0.01$	$p<0.01$		NS	

[1] National sample of legitimate live births
[2] Mainly hospital + GP
Source: Study of Childbearing and Induction (Cartwright)

Table 14.5 Obstetric intervention rates by social class of the child's father in France in 1981

	Caesarean section %	Induction[1] %	Episiotomy[2] %
Professional, managerial	10.1 (444)	14.7 (415)	51.0 (394)
Intermediate	10.1 (663)	15.1 (628)	45.4 (593)
Clerical workers, shop assistants	18.1 (561)	11.1 (523)	38.8 (484)
Farmers	9.9 (212)	11.4 (201)	33.7 (190)
Other self-employed[3]	12.5 (272)	14.7 (252)	34.0 (238)
Skilled manual workers	11.9 (1097)	10.5 (523)	39.2 (960)
Unskilled manual workers	9.9 (1238)	7.7 (1018)	31.7 (1107)
Other	7.8 (206)	11.6 (1172)	38.9 (190)
Unemployed	7.4 (207)	12.6 (262)	39.3 (247)
	NS	$p<0.001$	$p<0.001$

[1]Caesarean sections before onset of labour are excluded
[2]Caesarean sections are excluded
[3]Manual workers and shop keepers
Source: INSERM

influence during delivery: for US women the proportion of caesarean sections is lower for women without insurance or with public insurance and higher for women cared for by private physicians (Placek *et al.* 1983; Hurst and Summey 1984; Haynes *et al.*, 1986) (see Chapter 70).

Thus, we see that there is an association between a woman's social situation and both her health and her utilization of health services. In this chapter we will describe policies of social and financial support for childbearing women which may influence health (and which sometimes have improved health as one of their stated aims), and policies that are particularly aimed at reducing inequalities in health or in health care use. The two countries (Britain and France) that we use as our main examples have somewhat different overall approaches to welfare and the redistribution of resources. While differing in the details of their schemes (and, in particular, in their approach to health services) both have systems that are intended to provide universal, or almost universal national insurance and health care provision (Stacey 1985; Garcia and Saurel-Cubizolles 1986). Their systems are funded by a mixture of employment related contributions and taxation. In Britain, coverage of the population is more extensive in regard to health care, pensions and other income support, while in France benefits, where they apply, are more adequate in terms of income maintenance. Families with children generally receive larger benefits and tax concessions in France. (Saurel-Cubizolles and Garcia 1983; Ameline 1980).

2 Formal social and financial support for childbearing families

There are three main motives for government legislative and fiscal policies towards childbearing families. The first is a concern for the health and welfare of those sectors of the population that are seen to be particularly important or deserving; the second, seen particularly in employment protection legislation, is a commitment to equal opportunities for women; the third is pronatalism, manifested in countries that consider their population size or age structure to be unsatisfactory.

Countries vary enormously in the scope and content of the legislation that affects families. In this section we will give examples, rather than undertake a detailed comparison of the countries discussed. In order to evaluate the effects of a particular policy or piece of legislation, or to make proposals for change, it is not enough to know the text of the law; it is equally important to examine the practical consequences of policies and legislation, whether those consequences are intended or unintended. In complex societies, fiscal, economic, social and other policies interact.

2.1 Direct financial aid to childbearing families

Direct financial aid to childbearing families exists in most European countries (Table 14.1). This aid is generally available to all new parents, although a few women (for example, some very young women or women whose nationality status is uncertain) may be excluded. The amount of money paid to a woman around the time of birth varies dramatically among countries, and a direct comparison is made more difficult by the need to take into account the tax and insurance status of the family and the overlaps between general maternity benefits and employment-related maternity pay (Saurel-Cubizolles and Garcia 1983; Garcia and Saurel-Cubizolles 1986).

One aim of universal maternity benefits is to provide parents with resources at a time when costs are high. In recent years such benefits have been higher in France than in Britain. All women who attend specified antenatal and child health visits in France are eligible for a grant of nearly 800 francs (equals approx. US\$150) a month, paid monthly from the fourth month of pregnancy until the child is 3 months old. In Britain a new set of maternity benefits was introduced in early 1987. The small universal Maternity Grant was replaced by means-tested benefit for low income mothers. Mothers who fulfil certain employment and national insurance contribution criteria are eligible for either Statutory Maternity Pay or Maternity Allowance, and will receive a series of weekly payments totalling about £500 (equals approx. US\$300) with an additional amount of earnings-related pay for those who qualify for Statutory Maternity Pay. For many British women, especially those who do not qualify for the employment-related benefits (for example, many of those in households dependent on unemployment benefit or supplementary benefit), the extra costs of a pregnancy and a new baby are difficult to meet (Burghes 1980; Maternity Alliance 1985).

In addition to maternity benefits, there are other aspects of the welfare and taxation system to be considered. Family allowances in Britain are paid to all families with children, and, in France, to families with a second or subsequent child. Tax allowances may reduce the tax paid by families with children, and housing and other benefits take children into account. In France such policies benefit larger families because of a desire to increase the birth rate. Comparisons among countries are difficult, however, because of the different costs of various major cost of living items, such as food or housing.

2.2 Provision of preschool and out of school childcare

Although responsibility for the provision of schooling is accepted by most nations, preschool and out of school childcare is less likely to be seen as a priority. Policies vary from country to country. In France, children of 3 years and over can go to state or private infant schools but the availability of places at age 3 varies across the country. State infant schools are free of charge. Most schools provide lunch and some child care outside normal school hours, for which families pay according to their resources and which are subsidized by local councils. Attendance at school becomes compulsory at age 6. Of children who were under 4 in 1981, 25 per cent had places in crèches, infants' schools, and with registered child minders (Johanet 1982). In Britain schooling is compulsory and free of cost from 5 years of age onwards, but preschool provision is not seen as a responsibility of the state except for children thought to be in particular need because of poor home circumstances. In practice, very few nursery places are available free, although a few workplaces have them for employees. In a British study of women and employment carried out in 1980 (Martin and Roberts 1984), women with a preschool child who were in paid work (full or part-time) used relatives as their main source of childcare. Forty-seven per cent used their husband and 34 per cent the child's grandmother. Less than 3 per cent of women reported using either private nurseries or those provided by employers or local authorities. The main source of care outside the family was provided by childminders (who care for children in their own homes). They were used by 16 per cent of women in paid work.

2.3 Housing policies

Housing policies can have an important impact on the quality of life of families with young children, and there is some evidence of the adverse effect of poor housing on health (McCarthy *et al.* 1985; Elton and Packer 1986). In Britain, the recent increase in the number of families with children who are homeless, together with a statutory duty for local authorities to provide some accommodation for these families, has resulted in the phenomenon of families spending extended periods of time in private 'hotels'. This accommodation, which is paid for by local government, is often grossly inadequate. Various lay and professional groups have expressed concern about the influence of these poor conditions on the health of families, and on the families' ability to obtain health care (Durward 1988). Bad housing is often remote from shops and clinics and poorly served by public transport; women may have to negotiate steep stairs; lifts often do not work; accommodation may be noisy, crowded, and difficult to clean. It seems quite probable that poor housing conditions and pregnant women's domestic workload are among the factors mediating between low social status and adverse perinatal outcomes, but there has been little (Saurel-Cubizolles *et al.* 1986) research conducted to investigate this possibility (Romito 1986).

2.4 Home help

One response to the extra needs of pregnant women and families with young children is to provide publicly funded help in the home with domestic work. This was recommended for new mothers by Douglas in his report on the 1946 national British births survey (Douglas 1948). British women do receive 'home helps' in exceptional circumstances, such as multiple birth, but the provision is being reduced because of national financial difficulties and the competing needs of elderly and disabled people.

In some parts of France, the council or local agency that manages family benefits can provide family workers who do housework and so allow a woman to stay at home rather than be admitted to hospital or have children taken into care. They can also give health education advice. After the birth, women can be provided with help at home in special situations such as a multiple birth. Services are very unevenly distributed and do not generally meet the existing need. An experimental evaluation of a similar family worker scheme has been conducted in a British city (Spencer 1986) (see Chapter 15). In The Netherlands, provision for maternity aides to help postpartum is an integral part of the maternity care system, and specially trained maternity aides provide support for up to seven days postpartum for over 70 per cent of women having babies (van Teijlingen and McCaffery 1987).

2.5 Provisions for employed parents

In addition to those benefits or services already described, there are also special legal, administrative and financial provisions for working parents. While legislation varies considerably among countries, most European countries have legislation intended to protect the fetus, newborn, and mother from the general and specific harmful effects of work, protect employment by enabling parents to keep jobs while caring for children, and provide income maintenance for parents during breaks in employment.

Many countries have laws (often dating from early in the century) that restrict the type of work that pregnant women can do. Contact with low temperatures, lead, ionizing radiation, and other hazards, for example, may be controlled by law (Saurel-Cubizolles and Garcia 1983; Hunt 1979). Women may be barred from night work, or long working hours. In some countries employers must not allow a woman to work in the period just before or just after delivery. There has been considerable debate about this type of legislation (Coyle 1980; Henefin and Bertin 1984; Hunt 1979) because, while it has laudable aims, it can restrict women's employment opportunities and result in them losing earnings during the childbearing period, and conflicts with equal opportunities legislation. One practical difficulty with legislation of this nature is that, in the absence of adequate unemployment benefits or alternative work in the same enterprise, it may lead some women to conceal their pregnancies and to avoid seeking care. One way to avoid this effect is to have laws that protect women from dismissal on the grounds of pregnancy, and that offer alternative work or compensation to women if their usual jobs are thought to be dangerous. This is the case in both Britain and France. In addition, British women are allowed paid time off to attend for antenatal care, and in some other European countries there are work breaks for breastfeeding.

The other main area of legislation concerns leave, reinstatement and income maintenance during maternity or parental leave. Most European countries allow all employed women to have paid leave around the time of birth (Table 14.1). In France, for first and second births, women have 6 weeks maternity leave before the date that the baby is due, and 10 weeks thereafter. Two extra weeks can be added before delivery in the case of pregnancy problems. Women having a third or subsequent child have longer leave, 8 weeks before and 18 after the birth. Two extra weeks are added for any multiple birth. Maternity pay is set at 80 per cent of the usual salary. Some large employers, such as the Civil Service, pay 100 per cent of normal salaries during maternity leave. In the United Kingdom a woman must have been working for the same employer for at least two years (or five years for part-time workers) to qualify for leave and reinstatement. If she does qualify, she receives six weeks statutory maternity pay at 90 per cent of her usual salary and then a further twelve weeks off at the basic sick pay rate. She may take a further 22 weeks unpaid leave after the baby is born.

In practice, because of the qualifying conditions, many women may not be eligible for leave. A 1979 survey showed that just over half of the women who had worked during pregnancy qualified for leave and pay (Daniel 1981a). The complexity of the regulations was baffling for many women (Rodmell and Smart 1982), and also for many employers (Daniel 1981b).

In some countries employers have agreements with employees that provide some benefits when there is no government provision or better benefits than those that exist nationally (Labour Research Department 1987). These can include leave for fathers, where that is not part of legislation.

The level of income replacement during leave must be adequate for maternity protection legislation to be effective in protecting parents and infants from stress and hardship. In some countries (for example France, and Denmark) the maternity allowance is the same as, or close to a woman's usual earnings. In others (for example, the United Kingdom and the Federal Republic of Germany) it is fixed at a lower rate. If benefits are very low, women will be more likely to work during their period of maternity leave.

There is no evidence at present on which to determine the optimum length of leave. Some types and aspects of work seem to be more likely than others to compromise health during pregnancy (Mamelle *et al.* 1984; Saurel-Cubizolles *et al.* 1986). There may be a need for more flexible leave arrangements to allow some pregnant women to take time off earlier in pregnancy. One French policy document (Inspection Générale des Affaires Sociales 1980) argued that the extent of sick leave being taken during pregnancy suggested the need for some extension of the maternity leave provisions.

Although health researchers have drawn attention to the consequences of unemployment (Smith 1987), less attention has been paid to adverse work conditions, which may also flourish when there is a high level of unemployment. In this circumstance, employment protection legislation may be weakened and negotiating good working conditions may become more difficult. In some cases jobs may open up for women in areas where traditional 'male' jobs are lost. In these circumstances the pattern of women's work may shift and more families may depend on a female breadwinner. These changes may have an impact on the needs of pregnant women for advice about the work that they do, and for clinics and classes at appropriate times and places.

In concluding this section on formal social provisions for childbearing families, two further points should be made. First, this chapter has not attempted to look at the informal networks on which childbearing families rely, and which cannot be fully replaced by formal social systems, however good the latter may be. Second, any assessment of the effectiveness of national and local policies in terms of their expressed goals (such as income maintenance and employment protection) requires adequate surveys of those supposed to benefit from them. Family policies are complex and interact with broader fiscal and other social policies. There is a tendency for some people to fall through the net of social protection, however small the mesh.

3 Providing equal access to maternity care

3.1 Minimizing financial barriers to seeking care

The cost of getting care can be a major impediment to access. This is particularly obvious in the United States, where there is a close association between the lack of public or private coverage for low-income people and low uptake of medical services (Blendon *et al.* 1986). Among women with the same educational qualifications, antenatal care is commenced earlier by women who have third party insurance than those whose costs are to be met by Medicaid (Cooney 1985).

In the United States the system of financing health care does not cover the whole of the population: 16 per cent of the population was not covered for some or all of the year 1977 by either private insurance or public assistance (Davis and Rowland 1983). This proportion has increased recently because of unemployment and reductions in public assistance. Financial difficulties can therefore be significant during pregnancy, childbirth and, if the baby is in intensive care, in the weeks which follow. Recent figures show that 14.6 million women aged 15–44 (26 per cent of the women in that age group) have no insurance cover for maternity care. At delivery 550 000 women still have no cover from either state or private insurance (Alan Guttmacher Institute 1987).

A special study of pregnant women in Massachusetts showed that an estimated 7.8 per cent of births were not covered by private or public health insurance and that the proportion of women not covered for antenatal care was considerably higher. Some women who were eligible for Medicaid did not receive it, and some women have problems in getting care because so few obstetricians in their area are enrolled as Medicaid providers (Task Force on Prevention of Low Birthweight and Infant Mortality 1985). Doctors may be reluctant to provide care under Medicaid because reimbursement is slow, unreliable, and may be at a level well below normal fees charged. The factors vary between states. (Alan Guttmacher Institute 1987). Recent cuts in Medicaid funding have led to a significant reduction in the proportion of people covered. There is anxiety about the possible consequences of this, particularly for pregnant women and young children (Mundinger 1985; Fisher *et al.* 1985). A study conducted in the early 1970s in Indiana, attempted to investigate the effects of a financial intervention which was applied in a partially experimental way to low income families. This intervention supplemented family income to different ceilings. The author's analysis of the birthweight data, using a form of multiple regression, suggests that income supplementation may have a positive influence on birthweight in selected women but the study as published is very difficult to interpret (Kehrer and Wolin 1979).

In Britain, visits to a general practitioner or specialist, tests, and in-patient care are free at the point of use under the National Health Service. (Only 1 per cent of births in 1980 took place outside the NHS (Macfarlane and Mugford 1984).) Furthermore, pregnant women do not have to pay the part of the cost of prescribed drugs, dental care, spectacles, and artificial limbs, that most other people have to pay.

In France, on the other hand, there are still some financial barriers to access, even though several adjustments have been made to reduce the costs of care for pregnant women. In most places where care is provided, women must pay for the care at the time that it is received. One antenatal visit is fully reimbursed by Social Security during the first trimester of pregnancy, but until the sixth month, other care is reimbursed in the usual way—that is, to 70 or 80 per cent of the cost. After the sixth month of pregnancy all care is reimbursed by Social Security at 100 per cent, and this complete coverage lasts through to the end of pregnancy. It includes the birth and the first 12 postpartum days, or the first 30 days if the baby is still in hospital. (In 1980, 99 per cent of the French population were covered by Social Security, and 69 per cent had additional private insurance cover (Devouassoux and Morel 1984.) Women use their extra private insurance cover to reclaim some or all the costs of care that were not met by Social Security.)

In most countries where the cost of care represents a barrier to use, some measures have been taken to reduce these financial obstacles, either in a general way for the population as a whole, or specifically for pregnant women. In France, people who are not covered by Social Security can get medical assistance (*l'aide médicale gratuite*) to cover all or part of the costs. There are, however, some women, such as illegal immigrants, second or third wives of immigrant workers and a small number of other marginal ('Fourth World') women (Collin 1984; Comité Médico-Social 1985) who are either not eligible for Social Security or medical assistance, or who do not attempt to claim them because of the administrative hurdles. These women rarely receive antenatal care and they either deliver at home or else leave hospital very soon after the birth.

In addition, French hospitals designated as specializing in high risk maternity care, provide services that are entirely free. In 1976, only 6 per cent of pregnant women had made one or more visits to a hospital of this type and the women concerned were not socially more disadvantaged (Blondel 1979). In 1981, women with a higher level of education were more likely to deliver in a large hospital and were more likely to have their labour induced than other women (Hubert 1986; Hubert *et al.* 1987).

Other services are adjusted to the needs of the most disadvantaged. A specialized group of clinics in France are staffed by multidisciplinary teams made up of doctors, nurses, midwives, nursery nurses, and social workers. These clinics, which provide free care and carry out screening and vaccination, are located in disadvantaged neighbourhoods, which makes them more accessible to women who have difficulty approaching medical institutions. Some have adjusted their practice to the needs of the local population, especially in areas with a large proportion of immigrants (Comité Médico-Social 1985). Overall, however, antenatal care represents only a very small part of their activity (Service des Statistiques, des Etudes et des Systèmes d'Information 1984).

Programmes specifically aimed at disadvantaged women are supported by the federal government in some states in the United States. These programmes, which vary from state to state, can include routine antenatal care, special high risk care, social services, health education, nutrition, food supplements, free dental services and home visits. They are often provided by multidisciplinary teams (Sokol *et al.* 1980; Peoples *et al.* 1984; Kotelchuck *et al.* 1984). The Women, Infants and Children project in North Carolina, which included medical care, nutrition and social services, led to an improvement in the antenatal care provided to the most socially disadvantaged women between 1970 and 1977 (Peoples and Siegel 1983).

3.2 Incentives promoting minimum care for all pregnant women

Unlike most countries, which do not make provision of financial benefits to pregnant women dependent on their utilization of health care services, in France there is a system of incentives to promote at least minimum care for all pregnant women. The infant benefit (*allocation au jeune enfant*), which is a pronatalist measure not linked to the specific costs of medical care, provides monthly payments of 781 francs in 1987 (equals approx. US$140). It is paid to pregnant women on condition that they make at least three antenatal visits, one before the end of the third month of pregnancy, a second during the sixth month, and a third during the first half of the eighth month. In 1981, only 0.9 per cent of women had less than these three antenatal visits (Rumeau-Rouquette *et al.* 1984).

The French system of linking benefit payments to antenatal attendance was introduced in 1945, and was put forward in Britain in the 1970s as a way of encouraging early attendance for antenatal care. While the system had an important role in France at the time it was introduced, and still represents a safety net in areas of social disadvantage when the standards of care are low, in more 'medicalized' areas, the details of the regulations are little known and have little influence. Women receive antenatal care which is far more intensive than the legal minimum (Blondel *et al.* 1982b).

3.3 Patterns of perinatal care

Providing continuity of care for all pregnant women from the beginning of pregnancy to the postnatal period requires well-organized primary care, and co-ordination between the different services involved in giving care.

In Britain, access to hospital care and to specialists is only through a general practitioner (see Chapters 4, 11, 12, and 13). The system of shared care, in which pregnancy care is formally divided between a general practitioner and a hospital team, is the most common form of antenatal care (Chamberlain *et al.* 1978). In France, on the other hand, pregnant women can seek care in the local consulting rooms of a general practitioner, refer themselves directly to a specialist, or go to a maternity hospital out-patient clinic. In practice women are turning more and more to specialist care from the beginning of pregnancy, or to general practitioner care with a specialist taking over in the second or third trimester (Rumeau-Rouquette *et al.* 1984; Hubert *et al.* 1987). The general practitioner in France plays a relatively unimportant role in pregnancy and delivery care. Apart from care given by private or hospital doctors, primary care is also given by a public service specializing in preventive care for mothers and children (Protection Maternelle et Infantile). This service plays a very small part in antenatal care and often finds itself in competition with the private sector, where doctors' incomes relate directly to the number of medical tasks carried out.

The relation of socioeconomic status to the level of specialization of the caregiver varies greatly from country to country. In France, for example, care from a specialist is the usual pattern for middle and upper class women while care given exclusively by a general practitioner is more usual among women married to or living with self employed and unskilled manual workers (Table 14.3). In England and Wales, on the other hand, there is no association between social class, and the level of specialization of the caregiver (Chamberlain *et al.* 1978).

3.4 Accessibility of health services

The accessibility of health services depends on their location and the geographic pattern of facilities. Rural or urban place of residence has an influence (Blondel *et al.* 1982a; Robine *et al.* 1985). In two contrasting areas in the south-west of France, for example, rural residence was the most important factor associated with a relatively low number of antenatal visits and lack of specialist care: pregnancy complications, social class, and age showed a less significant association (Robine *et al.* 1985). This discrepancy arises, in part, from the uneven geographic spread of specialists. Problems associated with the location of hospitals are particularly acute in Britain where care is often centralized and women have to travel long distances for antenatal visits. In one national study the average time taken to travel to and attend hospital antenatal clinics was two and a half hours compared with one and a half hours for visits to a general practitioner (O'Brien and Smith 1981).

Community based clinics have been tried out in Britain (Zander and Chamberlain 1984; Draper *et al.* 1984; Dowling 1983; Reid *et al.* 1983; Kalizer and Kidd 1981) in an attempt to avoid the problems of busy clinics, the difficulties in communicating with staff and the time taken up in travel and waiting. These clinics enable women to receive care at a local clinic throughout their pregnancies, by the same professional team, often of the same cultural background as themselves. A specialist usually visits regularly to carry out examinations and assessments at specified stages of pregnancy and to look after women with problems requiring specialist care.

Domiciliary midwives provide another kind of contact with pregnant women. Their role is to provide information and advice for parents and to provide a link between the family and the health services. In France, there is less than one domiciliary midwife for every 1000 births. There are no strict national guidelines for their work but in most areas, priority is given to women in poor social circumstances. In Britain, where community midwives visit all newly delivered mothers regularly at home in the ten days following the delivery, 53 per cent of recent mothers had also received a visit at home from a community midwife or a health visitor during pregnancy (Martin and Monk 1982).

Local initiatives are often taken by health professionals responding to the specific needs of women living in their area, aimed at people who find the services difficult to approach (Dowling 1983; Commeau 1985). Among the most successful schemes are places where women can meet to speak their own language, posters appropriate to women's language or cultural needs, antenatal clinics or groups for teenagers, and volunteer projects to provide support for isolated women. These innovations are set up to meet local needs but they are relatively few in number, not well known outside the local area, and lacking in contacts with other such experiments.

3.5 Inequalities in the utilization of care

In consideration of the unequal use of perinatal care associated with the mothers' social characteristics, there is often an underlying belief that women have not done as much as they could, given the available services, and that, at the extreme, they have behaved irresponsibly. This is rarely the case. The system of care itself plays a major role in the creation of inequalities as has been described in the preceding sections. In France, women at high risk because of demographic factors or social disadvantage most often find themselves receiving care from care givers who are less well qualified in obstetrics, and often actually receive less care than women without these risks (Blondel *et al.* 1982a). In Britain, late attendance for antenatal care has received considerable attention partly because it prevents screening for neural tube defects (Pearson 1982). The delay in a first hospital visit is often due to the time taken for the general practitioner's referral letter to result in an appointment (Garcia and Oakley 1982; Simpson and Walker 1980). In addition, the system of care based on access through a general practitioner can result in gaps in provision. Asian women, for example, are less likely to have a general practitioner who is on the obstetric list and so the beginning of their antenatal care may be delayed (Clark 1981).

The social needs of childbearing women do not seem to have played a large role in the development of perinatal care in the last 20 years. This period has been marked principally by the introduction of new screening and diagnostic tests and techniques for intervention, which have directed the focus of care towards the recognition and prompt treatment of pregnancy complications and abnormalities rather than toward the encouragement of health and primary prevention of problems. Although, in the last 15 years French researchers have given considerable attention to the social and employment circumstances of pregnant women, a French 5-year programme instituted in 1971 had its impact mainly on the technical standards of maternity hospitals (Rumeau-Rouquette and Blondel 1985). French policies of that period were concerned mainly with women at high risk of pathology rather than those living in difficult social circumstances. The improvement of care has not, therefore, primarily benefited the socially disadvantaged women who need it most (Rumeau-Rouquette and Blondel 1985). The complete reimbursement of costs of care from the sixth month of pregnancy, and the creation of some community midwifery posts, are recent measures which go in the direction of taking social needs into account. Their impact, however, is limited.

Clinics and maternity hospitals are not always welcoming to women with particular needs and problems. In one English Health District, teenagers were over-represented among the very small proportion of women having two visits or less (Parsons and Perkins 1980). They were more likely to conceal their pregnancy because of the fear of hostile reactions from those who knew them, and they were concerned about feeling ill at ease in conventional care settings. Some other socially marginal women may also delay seeking care because of the reactions of caregivers. To announce that one is pregnant when the last baby was very recent, or too soon or too late in a life which is already precarious, may lead to humiliating comments from health or social service professionals, and can set in train a succession of social interventions which will disrupt a woman's private life (Debionne and Larcher 1982). Women at the margins do not have any confidence in the services (Collin 1984). Added to this is the possibility of shame about their bodies or their clothes, their difficulty in communication with staff and the impossibility of following the advice they are given.

The decision to seek care also depends on the needs that women themselves perceive. If in the course of previous pregnancies a woman had no health problems, or if she received care which was not useful, she may decide that it would not be useful to go regularly for care during the next pregnancy (Parsons and Perkins 1980). Young first time mothers may have only vague notions about what is abnormal in pregnancy, and confronted with serious or lasting symptoms may think them normal and not go for care or discuss them during a visit (Hubert 1979).

Women from lower social classes are less likely to feel that they know enough about the progress of pregnancy and birth (Cartwright 1979) and express a desire for more information than do middle class women (Table 14.6). Often this is because of their difficulties in communicating with care givers (Macintyre 1982). This is accentuated by rapidly changing treatments, tests and medical opinions. The diffusion of new information starts with higher social classes; there is a lag between social classes in knowledge and in the adoption of new practices (Boltanski 1969). This has been observed in the development of a new hospital antenatal clinic in a French provincial town (Rumeau-Rouquette *et al.* 1977). Changing professional opinion can result in contrasting behaviour in different social classes, as, for example, in the choice between breast and bottle feeding (McIntosh 1985).

Differing values between people classified as belonging to different social classes can explain differences in behaviour with respect to prevention (Milio 1975). In giving priority to the reduction of risks of future problems, the system of antenatal care is more adapted to the behaviour of middle and upper class women. People from lower social classes may be less oriented towards the future (perhaps because they have few expectations of improvement in their circumstances) and so may attach less importance to preventive care.

More specifically, when resources of money, time and energy are limited, the possibility of making choices that promote health are also limited. People may behave in a way which seems irrational to an outsider but which is the best choice for them (Graham 1984). Even in less extreme situations, pregnant women may have other priorities besides care; for example, finding the time and money to provide for children already in the household.

Table 14.6 Desire for extra information and social class; national sample survey of legitimate births 1975, England and Wales

Social class	Average number of items about which women would have liked more information	Number of mothers (=100%)
I	3.3	195
II	3.9	369
III N	4.4	239
III M	4.7	856
IV	4.6	311
V	5.5	114
Unclassified	4.1	94
All mothers	4.4	2178

Source: Cartwright (1979)

4 Conclusions

4.1 Implications for current practice

The overall aim of this chapter has been to emphasize the importance of the social circumstances of child-bearing families, and to look at the various public policy responses that have been adopted in different countries. A key theme has been the extent to which social policies have health implications, and health policies have social consequences. Our aim has not been to downplay individual needs, but to put each person in a wider context where political, social and financial forces all have their effects. A pregnant woman does not leave her work, or community and family responsibilities behind when she steps into the clinic or doctor's office.

Rather than offering any specific recommendations for practice; we would like to suggest a list of questions for caregivers. These questions draw attention to the social needs of families in a practical way:

- What sort of work do employed women do in this neighbourhood? Who are the major employers?
- What are the provisions for women to change the work they do in pregnancy if their usual work is hard or dangerous?
- What about leave and benefits for pregnant women who work?
- Are there benefits for all pregnant women or at least for women in need?
- Where would you send a woman to enquire about services and benefits?
- Are home helps available? How could a woman get one?
- How do women and their families get to the places where care is provided?
- Are there neighbourhoods in this area with very bad transport?
- Are there neighbourhoods with housing problems?
- Where would you refer a family with serious social problems?
- Are there groups of women who have no access to maternity care because of cost or entitlement?
- Could care be sited in more convenient places or at more convenient times?
- Do members of the team give counselling on diet? If so, is the advice practical? Does it take into account the special needs and wishes of sectors of the population?
- Are there language barriers which exclude some women from good care? What is being done to overcome this problem?

- Could some care be given more appropriately in women's own homes?
- Are there local organisations which give support and advice to families with special problems—multiple births, babies with disabilities, babies who have died?

4.2 Implications for future research

Monitoring of perinatal care and perinatal outcomes by social and demographic circumstances of parents should continue or be established at local and at national level.

There should be evaluation of social and health service provision for childbearing families to see if policies correspond with needs. In practice there are frequent changes in both medical care and in the social environment (new patterns of family life; changes in the distribution of wealth) which necessitate regular checks to see if policies are adequate. Are there high risk groups not covered by social protection? Are new forms of screening accessible to women who need them most? Can women at work take advantage of maternity leave, given the employment situation and the financial situation of their families?

More general links between health policies and wider social policies should be explored by researchers. Housing, taxation, and employment policies all have consequences for the health of families.

Randomized controlled trials of innovations in health care organisation and social policy are at an early stage of development. Outcomes of such trials can include medical, social, and psychological assessments of the well-being of child and family. Topics which could be addressed using this methodology include: extra help for women at home; modifications of women's workplace conditions; alternative maternity leave arrangements; taking aspects of perinatal care into the community, or to women's homes; special perinatal care for groups with social needs (travellers, very young women, etc.).

References

Alan Guttmacher Institute (1987). Blessed Events and the Bottom Line: Financing Maternity Care in the United States. New York: Alan Guttmacher Institute.

Ameline C (1980). Les prestations sociales, les cotisations et l'impôt sur les salaires en Grande Bretagne et en France. Revue Française des Affaires Sociales, 2: 151–169.

Bell C, McKee L, Priestley K (1983). Fathers, Childbirth and Work. Manchester: Equal Opportunities Commission.

Blaxter M (1983). Health service as a defence against poverty in industrialised societies. Soc Sci Med, 17: 1139–1148.

Blendon R, Aiken L, Freeman H, Kirkman-Liff B, Murphy J (1986). Uncompensated care by hospitals or public insurance for the poor. Does it make a difference? New Engl J Med, 314: 1160–1163.

Blondel B (1979). Les limites d'une politique de prévention basée sur le haut risque. Application à la période périnatale. Thèse de 3ème cycle. Paris (document polycopié).

Blondel B, Zuber MC (1988). Marital status and cohabitation: relationship with social condition, antenatal care and pregnancy outcome. Pediatr Perinat Epidemiol, 2: 125–137.

Blondel B, Kaminski M, Bréart G (1980). Antenatal care and maternal demographic and social characteristics. Evolution in France between 1972 and 1976. J Epidemiol Community Health, 34: 157–163.

Blondel B, Saurel-Cubizolles MJ, Kaminski M (1982a). Impact of the French system of statutory visits on antenatal care. J Epidemiol Community Health, 36: 183–186.

Blondel B, Kaminski M, du Mazaubrun C, Rumeau-Rouquette C (1982b). Surveillance prénatale et filières médicales pendant la grossesse. Rev Epidem et Santé Publ, 30: 21–34.

Blondel B, Bréart G, Kaminski M (1985a). Indicateurs de l'état de santé pendant la période périnatale. In: Mises à jour en Gynécologie Obstetrique. Tournaire M (ed). Collège National des Gynécologues et Obstétriciens. Vigot: Paris.

Blondel B, Pusch D, Schmidt E (1985b). Some characteristics of antenatal care in 13 European countries. Br J Obstet Gynaecol, 92: 565–568.

Blondel B, Kaminski M, Saurel-Cubizolles MJ, Bréart G (1987). Pregnancy outcome and social condition of women under 20: evolution in France from 1972 to 1981. Int J Epidemiol, 16: 425–430.

Boddy A (1985). Poverty and health services. In: Recent advances in Community Medicine No. 3. Smith A (ed). Edinburgh: Churchill Livingstone.

Boltanski L (1969). Prime éducation et morale de classe. Cahiers du Centre de Sociologie Européenne. Paris: Mouton

Burghes L (1980). Living from Hand to Mouth: A Study of 65 Families on Supplementary Benefit. Poverty Pamphlet 50, Child Poverty Action Group and Family Service Units, London.

Cartwright A (1979). The Dignity of Labour? A Study of Childbearing and Induction. London: Tavistock.

Chalmers I (1985). Short, Baird, Himsworth and social class differences in fetal and neonatal mortality rates. Br Med J, 291: 231–233.

Chamberlain G (ed) (1984). Pregnant Women at Work. London: Macmillan.

Chamberlain G, Philipp E, Howlett B, Masters K (1978). British Births 1970, Vol. 2. London: Heinemann.

Clark M (1981). The quality and organisation of medical care provided to immigrants in pregnancy in Leicestershire. In: Obstetric Problems of the Asian Community in Britain. London: Royal College of Obstetricians and Gynaecologists.

Collin C (1984). Grossesse, risques et prévention en milieu urbain très défavorisé: le quart monde. Prévenir, 10: 59–68.

Comité Médico-Social pour la Santé des Migrants (1985).

Maternité chez les femmes noires en France. Migrations Santé, 44: 46–49.

Commeau A (1985). Notre experience de terrain d'une PMI. Migrations Santé, 44: 46–49.

Cooney JP (1985). What determines the start of prenatal care. Medical Care, 23: 986–997.

Coyle A (1980). The protection racket. Feminist Rev, 4: 1–12.

Daniel WW (1981a). Maternity Rights: The Experience of Women. In: Report No. 588. London: Policy Studies Institute.

Daniel WW (1981b). Maternity Rights: The Experience of Employers. Report No. 596. London: Policy Studies Institute. London.

Davis K, Rowland D (1983). Uninsured and undeserved: inequities in health care in the United States. Health and Society, 61: 149–175.

Debionne F-P and Larcher P (1982). Pour une politique de la maternité. Igloos Quart Monde: 22.

Devouassoux J, Morel B (1984). Les modes de protection sociale en cas de maladie. In: Institut National de la Statistique et des Etudes Economiques. Paris: Données Sociales.

Douglas WB (1948). Maternity in Great Britain. A survey of social and economic aspects of pregnancy and childbirth undertaken by a joint committee of the Royal College of Obstetricians and Gynaecologists and the Population Investigation Committee. Oxford: Oxford University Press.

Dowling S (1983). Health for a Change. The Provision of Preventive Health Care in Pregnancy and Early Childhood. London: Child Poverty Action Group.

Draper J, Field S, Thomas H (1984). The Early Parenthood Project. An Evaluation of a Community Antenatal Clinic. Hughes Hall, Cambridge (unpublished report).

Durward L (1984). Poverty in Pregnancy: The Cost of an Adequate Diet for Expectant Mothers. London: Maternity Alliance.

Durward L (1988). Report on Bed and Breakfast. London: Maternity Alliance, Shelter, London Housing Aid Centre, London Food Commission.

Elton PJ, Packer JM (1986). A prospective randomised controlled trial of the value of rehousing on the grounds of mental ill-health. J Chron Dis, 39: 221–227.

Evans F, Hess C, Guyer B, Rosen SL (1985). Infant health status in Massachusetts. Mass J Community Health, Spring/Summer: 3–13.

Evason E (1980). Just Me and the Kids: a Study of Single Parent Families in Northern Ireland. Belfast: Equal Opportunities Commission.

Faur B, Court Y (1987). La situation démographique en 1985. Paris: Collections d'INSERM, serie D.

Fisher E, Logerfo J, Daling J (1985). Prenatal care and pregnancy outcomes during the recession: the Washington State experience. Am J Public Health, 75: 866–869.

Garcia J, Oakley A (1982). Is early antenatal attendance so important? Br Med J, 284: 1474.

Garcia J, Saurel-Cubizolles MJ (1986). Legal measures for the promotion of maternal and child health and the protection of working women in Europe. In: Prevention of Preterm Birth. Papiernik E, Bréart G, Spira N (eds). Colloque INSERM, Vol 138.

Golding J, Henriques J, Thomas P (1986). Unmarried at delivery. II Perinatal morbidity and mortality. Early Hum Dev, 14: 217–227.

Graham H (1984). Women, Health and the Family. London: Harvester Press.

Haynes de Regt R, Minkoff H, Feldman J, Schwarz R (1986). Relation of private or clinic care to the cesarean birth rate. New Engl J Med, 315: 619–624.

Henefin MS, Bertin J (1984). Making healthy babies: it's not just women's work. Science for the People, March/April: 18–22.

Hubert B (1986). Spécialisation de la surveillance prénatale: effets sur les soins pendant la grossesse et sur les conditions de l'accouchement. Mémoire de DEA de Statistique et Santé. Université de Paris sud.

Hubert B, Blondel B, Kaminski M (1987). Contribution of specialists to antenatal care in France: Impact of the level of care during pregnancy and delivery. J Epidemiol Community Health, 41: 321–328.

Hubert J (1979). Belief and reality: social factors in pregnancy and childbirth. In: The Integration of a Child into a Social World. Richards M (ed). Cambridge: Cambridge University Press, pp 37–51.

Hunt V (1979). Work and the Health of Women. Florida: CRC Press.

Hurst M, Summey P (1984). Child birth and social class: the case of cesarean delivery. Soc Sci Med, 18: 621–631.

Ingram D, Makuc D, Kleinman J (1986). National and state trends in use of prenatal care 1970–83. Am J Public Health, 76: 415–423.

Inspection Générale des Affaires Sociales (1980). Protection Sociale et Limitations Socio-économique. Paris: Rapport Annuel.

Irvine J, Miles I, Evans J (eds) (1979). Demystifying Social Statistics. London: Pluto.

Johanet G (1982). La nouvelle politique familiale. Droit Social, 6: 503–507.

Kalizer M, Kidd M (1981). Some factors affecting attendance to antenatal clinics. Soc Sci Med, 15D: 421–424.

Kaminski M, Blondel B (1984). Mortalité et morbidité des nouveau-nés et des jeunes enfants. Prévenir, 10: 49–58.

Kehrer BH, Wolin CM (1979). Impact of income maintenance on low birthweight: evidence from the Gary experiment. J Human Resources, 24: 434–462.

Kessner D, Singer J, Kalk C, Schlesinger E (1973). Infant Death: An Analysis by Maternal Risk and Health Care. Institute of Medicine. Washington DC: National Academy of Sciences.

Kotelchuck M, Schwartz JB, Anderka MT, Finison KS (1984). WIC participation and pregnancy outcomes: Massachusetts statewide evaluation project. Am J Public Health, 74: 1086–1092.

Labour Research Department (1987). Time Off for Childcare. London: Labour Research Department.

Leclerc A, Lert F, Goldberg M (1984). Les inegalités sociales devant la mort en Grande-Bretagne et en France. Soc Sci Med, 19: 479–487.

Llewelyn Davies H (ed) (1978). Maternity: Letters from Working Women. London: Virago.

Macfarlane A, Mugford M (1984). Birth Counts. Statistics of Pregnancy and Childbirth. London: Her Majesty's Stationery Office.

Macfarlane A, Cole T (1985). From depression to recession: evidence about the effects of unemployment on mothers' and babies' health 1930s-1980s. In: Maternity Alliance. Born Unequal: Perspectives on Pregnancy and Child Rearing in Unemployed Families. London: Maternity Alliance.

Macfarlane A (1980). Official statistics and women's health and illness. Equal Opportunities Commission Res Bull, 4: 43–47.

Macintyre S (1982). Communications between pregnant women and their medical and midwifery attendants. Midwives' Chron, Nov: 387–394.

Macintyre S (1986). The patterning of health by social position in contemporary Britain: Directions for sociological research. Soc Sci Med, 23: 393–415.

Mahler H (1987). The safe motherhood initiative: a call to action. Lancet, 1: 668–670.

Mamelle N, Laumon B, Lazar P (1984). Prematurity and occupational activity during pregnancy. Am J Epidemiol, 119: 309–322.

Martin J, Monk J (1982). Infant Feeding 1980. London: Office of Population Censuses and Surveys.

Martin R, Roberts C (1984). Women and Employment: A Lifetime Perspective. London: Department of Employment, Office of Population Censuses and Surveys, Her Majesty's Stationery Office.

Maternity Alliance (1985). Born Unequal: Perspectives on Pregnancy and Child Rearing in Unemployed Families. London: Maternity Alliance.

McCarthy P, Byrne D, Harrison S, Keithley J (1985). Respiratory conditions: effect of housing and other factors. J Epidemiol Community Health, 39: 15–19.

McCormick M (1985). The contribution of low birth weight to infant mortality and childbirth morbidity. New Engl J Med, 312: 82–90.

McCormick M, Shapiro S, Starfield B (1984). High risk young mothers: Infant mortality and morbidity in 4 areas in the United States 1973–78. Am J Public Health, 74: 18–23.

McIntosh J (1985). Barriers to breastfeeding: Choice of feeding method in a sample of working class primiparae. Midwifery, 1: 213–224.

McKinlay JB (1970). The new late comers for antenatal care. Br J Prev Soc Med, 24: 52–57.

McKinlay JB and McKinlay SM (1972). Some social characteristics of lower working class utilizers and under utilizers of maternity health care services. J Health Soc Behav, 13: 369–381.

McKinlay JB and McKinlay SM (1979). The influence of premarital conception and various obstetric complications on subsequent prenatal health behaviour. J Epidemiol Community Health, 33: 84–90.

Milio N (1975). Values, social class and community health services. In: A Sociology of Medical Practice. Cox and Mead (eds). London: Collier Macmillan, 49–61.

Mundinger M (1985). Health service funding cuts and the declining health of the poor. New Engl J Med, 313: 44–47.

O'Brien M, Smith C (1981). Women's views and experiences of antenatal care. The Practitioner, 225: 123–125.

Office of Population Censuses and Surveys (1986). Mortality Statistics, Perinatal and Infant: Social and Biological Factors Series DH3, No 17. London: Her Majesty's Stationery Office.

Parsons WD, Perkins ER (1980). Why Don't Women Attend for Antenatal Care? Occasional Paper No. 23. Nottingham: Leverhulme Health Education Project.

Pearson JF (1982). Is early antenatal attendance so important. Br Med J, 284: 1064–5.

Peoples M, Siegel E (1983). Measuring the impact of programs for mothers and infants on prenatal care and low birthweight: the value of refined analyses. Medical Care, 21: 586–608.

Peoples MD, Grimson RC, Daughtry GL (1984). Evaluation of the effects of the North Carolina Improved Pregnancy Outcome project: implications for state-level decision-making. Am J Public Health, 74: 549–554.

Placek P, Taffel S, Moien M (1983). Cesarean section delivery rates: United States 1981. Am J Public Health, 73: 861–862.

Reid M (1986). The persistence of social inequalities in perinatal statistics. In: Prevention of Preterm Birth. Papiernik E, Bréart G, Spira N (eds). Colloque INSERM, Vol 138.

Reid M, Gutteridge S, McIlwaine G (1983). A Comparison of the Delivery of Antenatal Care between a Hospital and a Peripheral Clinic. Glasgow: Social Paediatric and Obstetric Research Unit.

Robine JM, Maguin P, Nicaud V, Hatton F (1985). Facteurs déterminants des pratiques de santé. Exemple de la surveillance de la grossesse en milieu rural et urbain. Rev Epidem et Santé Publ, 33: 203–211.

Rodmell S, Smart L (1982). Pregnant at Work: The Experiences of women. Milton Keynes: The Open University.

Romito, P (1986). La place du travail non payé des femmes dans les recherches sur la santé. Paper presented at a meeting 'Housework and Household Production', 4 March 1986, Paris: Centre National de la Recherche Scientifique and Institut National de la Statistique et des Etudes Economiques.

Rumeau-Rouquette C, Blondel B (1985). The French perinatal programme. In: Health Policy, Social Policy and Mortality Prospects. Vallin J, Lopez A (eds). Liège: Ordina, pp 299–314.

Rumeau-Rouquette C, Kramar A, Sandrock R, *et al.* (1977). Evolution de la surveillance prénatale en relation avec les catégories socio-culturelles à la maternité d'Haguenau. Rev Franç Gynec, 72: 699–709.

Rumeau-Rouquette C, du Mazaubrun C, Rabarison Y (1984). Naître en France. Dix ans d'évolution. Paris: INSERM-Doin, 57–73.

Saurel-Cubizolles MJ (1982). Activité professionelle des femmes enceintes, comportement médical et issue de la grossesse. Thèse, Université de Paris I.

Saurel-Cubizolles MJ, Garcia J (1983). Activité professionelle pendant la grossesse en France et en Grande Bretagne. Rev. Française des Affaires Sociales, Sept: 177–187.

Saurel-Cubizolles MJ, Kaminski M, Garcia J (1986). Conditions de travail des femmes enceintes et prematurité. In: Prevention of Preterm Birth. Papiernik E, Bréart G, Spira N (eds). Colloque INSERM, Vol 138.

Selbmann HK, Brach M, Elser H, Holzmann K, Johannigmannn J, Riegel K, Münchner (1980). Perinatal-Studie 1975–1977. Deutscher Arzte-Verlag, Köln-Lövenich, 1.

Services des Statistiques, des Etudes et des Systèmes d'Information (1984). Annuaire des statistiques sanitaires et sociales. Paris: Ministère des Affaires Sociales et de la Solidarité Nationale.

Shiono PH, Klebanoff MA, Graubard BI, Berendes HW, Rhoads GG (1986). Birthweight among women of different ethnic groups. JAMA, 255: 48–52.

Simpson H, Walker G (1980). When do pregnant women attend for antenatal care? Br Med J, 2: 104–107.

Smith R (1987). Unemployment and Health: A Disaster and a Challenge. Oxford: Oxford University Press.

Sokol RJ, Woolf RB, Rosen MG, Weingarten K (1980). Risk, antepartum care, and outcome: impact of a maternity and infant care project. Obstet Gynecol, 56: 150–156.

Spencer B (1986). The family worker project: social support in pregnancy. In: Prevention of Preterm Birth. Papiernik E, Bréart G, Spira N (eds). Colloque INSERM, Vol 138.

Stacey M (1985). Women and health: the United States and the United Kingdom compared. In: Women, Health and Healing. Lewin and Olsen (eds). London: Tavistock.

Taffel S (1978). Prenatal care in the United States 1969–1975. Hyattsville, Maryland: National Centre for Health Statistics (DHEW publication No. (PHS) 78–1911).

Task Force on Prevention of Low Birthweight and Infant Mortality (1985). Closing the gaps: Strategies for improving the health of Massachusetts infants. Report to the Massachusetts Department of Public Health.

van Teijlingen E, McCaffery P (1987). The profession of midwife in The Netherlands. Midwifery, 3: 178–186.

Whitehead M (1987). The Health Divide: Inequalities in Health in the 1980's. London: Health Education Council.

Wollast E, Vandenbussche P (1983). Evaluation de la surveillance prénatale dans la région francophone de Belgique. ULB, Bruxelles, document polycopié.

Wollast E, Vandenbussche P, Buekens P (1986). Evaluation de la surveillance prénatale en Belgique et comparaison entre les secteurs médicaux publics et privés. Rev Epidem et Santé Publ, 34: 52–58.

Zander L, Chamberlain G (eds) (1984). Pregnancy Care for the 1980s. London: Royal Society of Medicine and Macmillan Press.

15 Social and psychological support during pregnancy

Diana Elbourne, Ann Oakley, and Iain Chalmers

1 Introduction

'I'm not saying that they've got time—that they should go into the social side of it. But if they knew a bit more about your state of mind, perhaps it would help them.'

Pregnant woman, cited in Oakley (1979).

Women in some parts of the world are more than 200 times more likely to die during pregnancy and childbirth than women in most industrialized countries (Mahler 1987). It was this appalling world-wide variation in maternal mortality rates that prompted Rosenfield and Maine to ask, in 1985, what had happened to the 'M' in 'MCH'. They charged professionals with having forgotten about the interests of mothers while pursuing their attempts to further the interests of children.

Similar charges of omission have been made in relation to the 'care' component of antenatal care. The development of the maternity services over the last thirty years or so has increasingly led to an emphasis on clinical surveillance of fetal well-being (Oakley 1984). There has been a tendency to lose sight of the idea of 'caring' for mother and child in a more comprehensive sense—a philosophy that inevitably demands that attention be given to the mother's social and psychological needs and resources (Lewis 1980; Oakley 1984).

It is thus not only in developing countries that the interests of mothers are sometimes forgotten by those who profess an interest in promoting maternal and child health. A tendency also exists among professionals working in industrialized societies to focus on the care of the fetus and the newborn child, and to downplay or ignore the mother's interests. It sometimes seems as if pregnant women are perceived as little more than containers for the 'real patients'—their unborn children (Oakley 1984).

This tendency manifests itself in a number of ways. There are demands, for example, that, from the moment conception is contemplated, women should alter various aspects of their way of life in the supposed interests of the fetus (see Chapter 16). Rather than provide opportunities to discuss and resolve the often very tangible problems and concerns that women experience during pregnancy (see Chapter 8), professionals expect women to tolerate arrangements for antenatal care that revolve around the application of largely unvalidated attempts to unearth relatively intangible problems ('intrauterine growth retardation' and 'reduced placental function', for example) in the fetus (see Chapters 22–31). In spite of the lack of any good evidence to justify the view (Campbell and Macfarlane 1987), some professionals suggest that the minority of women who wish to give birth in the familiar surroundings of their own homes are selfishly engaging in the earliest form of child abuse (Jeffcoate 1976). At its most extreme, the tendency of health professionals to attempt to provide care for fetuses in ways which ignore the problems being experienced by their mothers is manifested in women being charged with criminal offences against their unborn children (Oppenheimer 1986). The low priority given to problems experienced by women during pregnancy and childbirth is also manifested in the rarity with which clinical researchers seeks their views about alternative forms of care (see Chapter 8), and they way in which maternal morbidity has received such little attention from researchers (see, for example, Chapters 32, 79 and 86).

The tendency among some health professionals to ignore the problems perceived by pregnant women is (to say the very least) regrettable. Professional discounting of women's own perspectives and experiences can be harmful and upsetting enough in itself. The ways in which these attitudes can prejudice effective care during pregnancy and childbirth have been reiterated repeatedly both by those working in the services (Morris 1960; Atlee 1963; Kerr 1975) and by others (Chalmers *et al.* 1980). Because the social, psychological, and physical problems experienced by pregnant women are often substantial (Oakley 1979; McIntosh, in press), care during pregnancy and childbirth cannot be as effective as it might be if those providing it are insufficiently aware of the particular problems experienced by individual pregnant women and uninformed about the wider social circumstances in which these are occurring (see Chapter 14).

Earlier chapters in this book have discussed the relative strengths and weaknesses of different kinds of caregivers in providing effective care in these respects (see chapters in Section II of this volume). Subsequent chapters will deal with a variety of physical and other problems experienced by women during pregnancy. In this chapter we wish to focus on the importance of offering general social and psychological support to women during pregnancy. In some senses it is sad that a chapter with this focus should be considered a necessary component of a review of strategies for effective care during pregnancy and childbirth: it should be taken for granted by caregivers that social and psychological support are integral elements of any and all of the care they provide for pregnant women. But, as we have noted above, these elements of good care often seem to be missing from much of the care currently on offer. Indeed, it is because of this reality that it has been possible to mount controlled trials in which some pregnant women received forms of care which were explicitly intended to increase above average the amount of general social and emotional support usually available to women in their contacts with the maternity services.

2 Controlled trials of enhanced social and psychological support in pregnancy

The characteristics of the 14 trials which provide the basis for our assessment of the effects of providing enhanced social and psychological support during pregnancy are described in Table 15.1. The final column of this table gives examples of the form of words which helped us to decide that they should be included in this review. The provision of social and psychological support was the primary aim in six studies (Carpenter *et al.* 1968; Dance 1987, unpublished; Heins and Nance 1986 and Heins *et al.*, unpublished; Oakley *et al.*, unpublished; Olds *et al.* 1986a, b, and in press; Spencer and Morris 1986; Spencer *et al.* in press). In the remaining eight trials, the provision of social and psychological support was an explicit objective, but was not the main focus of the study. In two trials the main focus was information feedback and information sharing (Elbourne 1987; Elbourne *et al.* 1987; Lovell *et al.* 1986, 1987; Lovell and Elbourne 1987); in four others it was the organization of care (Blondel *et al.*, unpublished; Reid *et al.* 1983; Yanover *et al.* 1976; Yauger 1972). The remaining two trials focused on preparation for pregnancy, childbirth and parenthood (Shereshefsky and Lockman 1973; Spence Cagle 1984). No quantitative information was provided in the published reports of two of the trials selected (Yauger 1972; Spence Cagle 1984) and our attempts to obtain this information from the authors was unsuccessful. The results of some of the trials presented here have not yet been published (Blondel *et al.*; Dance; Heins *et al.*; Oakley *et al.*; Spencer *et al.*) and so must be considered still provisional. We are indebted to the investigators for making the data available to us.

3 Psychological and behavioural effects

The available evidence from these controlled trials suggests that enhanced social and psychological support during pregnancy has a number of beneficial psychological and behavioural effects. During pregnancy, women who received enhanced social and psychological support were less likely than controls to feel unhappy, nervous, and worried during pregnancy, and less likely to have negative feelings about the forthcoming birth (Table 15.2). These findings were also reflected in the results of the trial conducted by Shereshefsky and Lockman (1973) (who reported their results as proportions with no raw data): pregnant women in the supported group in their trial were more confident than controls that they would be able to adjust to motherhood. The available data from the totality of the studies suggest that supported mothers were more likely than controls to report having had no difficulties in communicating with staff, to feel 'in control' during their pregnancies, to attend antenatal classes and to have been satisfied with the antenatal care they had received (Table 15.3).

Women who had received enhanced social and psychological support during pregnancy were also more likely than controls to have had a companion with them during labour, to be satisfied with their care, and to report that they had enjoyed a worry-free labour (Table 15.4), findings which are supported by the results of the

Table 15.1 Characteristics of trials of explicit social and psychological support in pregnancy

Study (papers and dates)	Type(s) of interventions	Entry criteria	Allocation to interventions	Numbers	Outcomes	Inclusion criteria (for overview)
Blondel *et al.* (unpublished)	*Organization of care*	Women attending hospital out-patient clinics or hospitalized with threatened preterm labour; 26–36 weeks' gestation.	Random (sealed enveloped)		Costs; women's views including satisfaction with care; birthweight; gestational age.	Social support.
	Usual care + 1–2 home visits a week by midwives.			79		
	Usual care for women with threatened preterm labour.			73		
Carpenter *et al.* (1968)	*Emotional support*	Women registered in a hospital prenatal clinic.	Time of prenatal visits		Nervousness and use of medication before, during and after labour; length of labour.	'provision of emotional support' (p 109)
	Interviews at intervals throughout pregnancy, labour and the puerperium with 1st year medical students.			52		
	Usual care.			50		
Dance (unpublished)	*Social support*	Immigrant Pakistani women from rural villages in Azad Kashmir and Rawlpindi, with history of one or more low birthweight babies, not associated with elective caesarean, gross malformation or multiple birth.	Alternate		Birthweight, maternal physical and psychosocial health, intrapartum care, neonatal health, knowledge of health.	'Social intervention . . . to give information/education on health needs, facilities and services available to pregnant women . . . to advise/counsel, befriend and support' (p 3).
	Usual care + 'link-workers' (minimum 3 home visits and 2 telephone calls).			25		
	Usual care.			25		
Elbourne *et al.* (1987) Elbourne (1987)	*Information feedback/sharing*	Women <34 weeks' gestation booked for antenatal care with one obstetrician in a peripheral antenatal clinic.	Random (consecutively numbered, sealed opaque envelopes)		Women's feelings of satisfaction, being informed, anxious, confident, in control; father's involvement; depression; health-related behaviour; analgesia/anaesthesia; mode of delivery; length of labour; birthweight; gestational age; administrative effects.	Hypothesized that [women holding their own obstetric notes] would feel 'less anxious, more confident, more in control . . . and would find it easier to communicate with staff' (Elbourne *et al.* (1987), p 613).
	Women held sole obstetric record from booking until 10 days postpartum.			147		
	Women held usual co-operation cards.			143		
Heins and Nance (1986); Heins *et al.* (unpublished)	*Social support*	<30 weeks' gestation; previous low birthweight baby; ≥10 cm Creasy risk scoring system; free of medical or obstetric complications, e.g. hypertension, renal disease, diabetes, or multiple pregnancy.	Random (computer-generated random numbers in sealed opaque envelopes at co-ordinating centre, opened in response to telephone call from one of 5 tertiary centres)		Birthweight; gestation at delivery; maternal weight-gain.	'social support and stress reduction'
	Intensive antenatal care from nurse/midwife in 5 regional low birthweight clinics; social support and stress reduction; increased number of visits; assessment of cervix; education re signs of preterm labour and on health-related behaviour; emphasis on weight gain; continuity of care.			684		
	Usual antenatal care in high-risk clinic.			687		

Table 15.1—*continued*

Study (papers and dates)	Type(s) of interventions	Entry criteria	Allocation to interventions	Numbers	Outcomes	Inclusion criteria (for overview)
Lovell *et al.* (1986) Lovell *et al.* (1987) Lovell and Elbourne (1987)	*Information feedback/ sharing* Women held sole obstetric record from booking to delivery. Women held usual co-operation cards.	Women attending hospital antenatal clinic of one obstetrician.	Randomly (consecutive numbered sealed envelopes)	 115 120	Women's feelings of satisfaction; sense of control; communications with staff; father's involvement; health-related behaviour; clinical outcomes such as birthweight, gestation, intrapartum anaesthesia, length of labour, mode of delivery; administrative effects.	'communication . . . women's choices' (p 1) 'encourage information sharing and increased participation in decision making'
Oakley *et al.* (unpublished)	*Social support* Social support including home visiting by midwives, and telephone calls to women and 24-hour 'hot-line' to midwives. Usual antenatal care.	Previous low birthweight baby (without major malformation, multiple pregnancy or elective delivery). Fluent English-speakers.	Random by central telephone allocation	 251 253	Birthweight; gestational age at delivery; maternal and infant morbidity; maternal psychological condition postpartum, and satisfaction with care.	Social support to 'influence mother's physical and mental health (antenatally and postnatally), affect process of labour and delivery . . . and increase women's self-confidence about mothering'.
Olds *et al.* (1986a,b)	*Social support* A Control (no services provided through research project). B Free transportation and regular prenatal and well child care. C As (B) plus nurse–home visitor during pregnancy. D As (C) plus nurse–visitor until child aged 2.	Primiparous women either < 19 years or single parent or low socioeconomic status; ≤25 weeks' gestation.	Stratified by marital status, race, geographical regions. Assigned at random. Women drew assignment from deck of cards. Decks reconstituted periodically to over-represent treatment with smaller number of subjects. (As Efron's biased coin design.)	 90 94 100 116	Obstetrical, labour and neonatal details; use of health services; health habits including diet and smoking; gestational age at delivery; birthweight.	'Appreciation for the full set of stressful family and community influences on women's health habits and behaviours' (p 16). 'home visitation by nurses should be an effective means of . . . responding flexibly to the stressful life circumstances with which socially disadvantaged women must contend' (p 17) 'parent education, enhancement of the women's informal support systems . . . to emphasize the strengths of the women and their families' (p 17)
Reid *et al.* (1983)	*Organization of care* Community antenatal clinic.	Women referred by GP from Easterhouse area for delivery at Glasgow Royal Maternity Hospital.	Random with stratification	100	Obstetric morbidity and mortality; birthweight; intrapartum anaesthesia and analgesia; instrumental/operative	To deal with 'failure of communication and lack of continuity of care' (p 3).

	Routine hospital service.			100	delivery rate; pattern of usage of clinics; financial effects; communication; women's perceptions of pregnancy and childbirth and reported management of first 3 months of infant life.	
Shereshefsky and Lockman (1973)	*Preparation for pregnancy/childbirth/parenthood*	'Normal' women and their husbands during first pregnancy.	Random		Emotional disturbance in pregnancy; physical complications in pregnancy and childbirth; relationship between husband and wife in the pregnancy.	'counselling service' (p 151)
	Social work; counselling service.			?		'directed to emotional needs of pregnant women and their families' (p 152)
	Control			?		
Spence Cagle (1984)	*Preparation for pregnancy*	Couples participating in Lamaze classes.	Random		Caring relation-inventory; fundamental interpersonal relations, orientation behaviour.	'aimed at couple interpersonal needs for control, affection and inclusion' (p 56)
	In-class homework aimed at couple. Interpersonal needs for control, affection and inclusion during pregnancy.			?		
	Usual Lamaze classes.			?		
Spencer and Morris (1986) Spencer *et al.* (unpublished)	*Social support*	Women at increased risk of having low birthweight baby booking in at 2 maternity units in south Manchester.	Random		Birthweight; outcome of pregnancy; gestational age; intrapartum analgesia and anaesthesia; length of labour; mode of delivery.	'social support service'
	Offer of family worker. Client-centred approach.			655		
	Usual care.			633		
Yanover *et al.* (1976)	*Organization of care*	Parity 0, 1; 19–35 years old; low risk medically; 12th grade education; parents living together; father prepared to attend antenatal classes.	Random		Length of labour; analgesia; anaesthesia; mode of delivery; length of hospital stay; complications in mother or baby.	'endeavour to respond to wishes of numerous families to enhance family participation . . . collaborative perinatal . . . continuity of care'
	Family-centred care mainly postpartum but including continuity of care from prenatal classes.			44		
	Traditional care.			44		
Yauger (1972)	*Organization of care*	Residents of specified areas; 3–8 months pregnant; at least one child $\leqslant 5$ years.	Random		Health knowledge; health behaviour; health status.	'family-centred care . . . identification of problem and needs of family and provision of appropriate service for every member' (p 320)
	Family-centred care; nursing service, identifying problems and needs of family and providing appropriate care. Minimum of 4 home visits.			30		
	Usual care.			31		

Table 15.2 Effect of general social support from caregivers during pregnancy on unhappiness in pregnancy

Study	EXPT *n*	EXPT (%)	CTRL *n*	CTRL (%)	Odds ratio (95% CI)	Graph of odds ratios and confidence intervals (0.01 0.1 0.5 1 2 10 100)
Oakley *et al.* (unpub)	31/230	(13.48)	40/226	(17.70)	0.73 (0.44–1.20)	
Elbourne *et al.* (1987)	2/132	(1.52)	5/120	(4.17)	0.38 (0.08–1.69)	
Dance (unpub)	4/25	(16.00)	15/25	(60.00)	0.16 (0.05–0.50)	
Typical odds ratio (95% confidence interval)					0.54 (0.35–0.85)	
Effect of general social support from caregivers during pregnancy on worry/nervousness in pregnancy						
Elbourne *et al.* (1987)	15/131	(11.45)	20/120	(16.67)	0.65 (0.32–1.32)	
Carpenter *et al.* (1968)	13/44	(29.55)	27/43	(62.79)	0.27 (0.12–0.62)	
Typical odds ratio (95% confidence interval)					0.45 (0.26–0.77)	
Effect of general social support from caregivers during pregnancy on negative feelings about forthcoming birth						
Elbourne *et al.* (1987)	29/127	(22.83)	38/113	(33.63)	0.59 (0.33–1.03)	
Lovell *et al.* (1986)	3/96	(3.13)	4/102	(3.92)	0.79 (0.18–3.57)	
Dance (unpub)	1/25	(4.00)	11/25	(44.00)	0.12 (0.03–0.42)	
Typical odds ratio (95% confidence interval)					0.48 (0.29–0.78)	

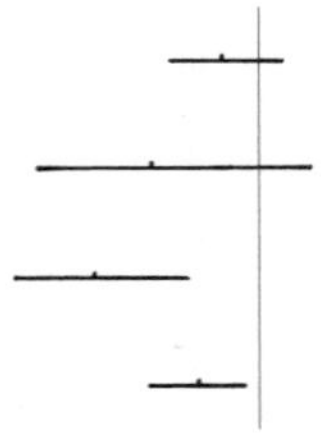

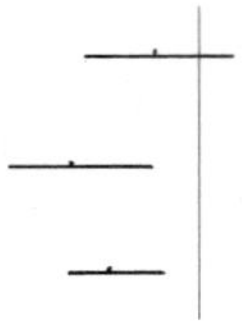

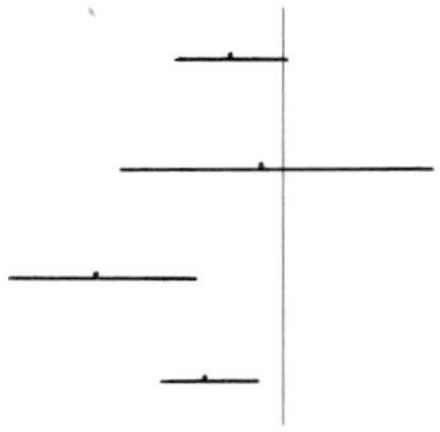

Table 15.3 Effect of general social support from caregivers during pregnancy on poor communication with staff

Study	EXPT *n*	EXPT (%)	CTRL *n*	CTRL (%)	Odds ratio (95% CI)	Graph of odds ratios and confidence intervals (0.01 0.1 0.5 1 2 10 100)
Elbourne *et al.* (1987)	84/132	(63.64)	95/120	(79.17)	0.47 (0.27–0.81)	
Lovell *et al.* (1986)	85/97	(87.63)	93/102	(91.18)	0.69 (0.28–1.70)	
Reid *et al.* (1983)	16/75	(21.33)	19/78	(24.36)	0.84 (0.40–1.79)	
Typical odds ratio (95% confidence interval)					0.60 (0.40–0.89)	
Effect of general social support from caregivers during pregnancy on not feeling 'in control' during pregnancy						
Elbourne *et al.* (1987)	66/132	(50.00)	79/120	(65.83)	0.52 (0.32–0.86)	
Lovell *et al.* (1986)	76/97	(78.35)	91/102	(89.22)	0.45 (0.21–0.95)	
Typical odds ratio (95% confidence interval)					0.50 (0.33–0.76)	

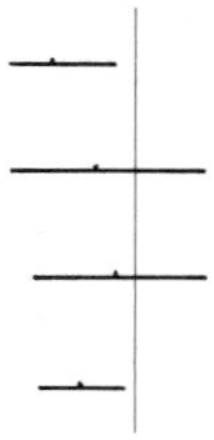

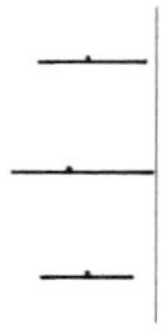

Table 15.3—*continued* Effect of general social support from caregivers during pregnancy on non-attendance at antenatal classes

Study	EXPT		CTRL		Odds ratio	Graph of odds ratios and confidence intervals
	n	(%)	*n*	(%)	(95% CI)	0.01 0.1 0.5 1 2 10 100
Elbourne *et al.* (1987)	55/133	(41.35)	59/123	(47.97)	0.77 (0.47–1.25)	
Olds *et al.* (1986a)	55/129	(42.64)	65/120	(54.17)	0.63 (0.38–1.04)	
Typical odds ratio (95% confidence interval)					0.70 (0.49–0.99)	

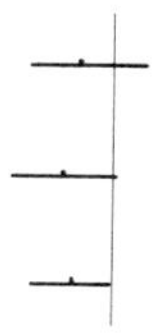

Effect of general social support from caregivers during pregnancy on dissatisfaction with antenatal care

Study	EXPT		CTRL		Odds ratio	Graph of odds ratios and confidence intervals
Blondel *et al.* (unpub)	17/79	(21.52)	41/73	(56.16)	0.23 (0.12–0.45)	
Elbourne *et al.* (1987)	7/133	(5.26)	1/120	(0.83)	4.22 (1.03–17.26)	
Lovell *et al.* (1986)	2/87	(2.30)	3/80	(3.75)	0.61 (0.10–3.59)	
Typical odds ratio (95% confidence interval)					0.41 (0.23–0.71)	

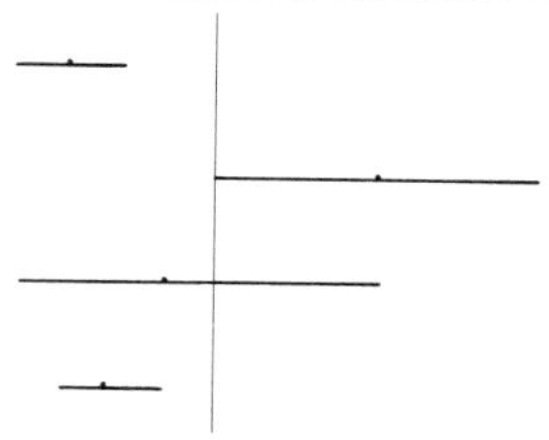

Table 15.4 Effect of general social support from caregivers during pregnancy on lack of companion in labour

Study	EXPT		CTRL		Odds ratio	Graph of odds ratios and confidence intervals
	n	(%)	*n*	(%)	(95% CI)	0.01 0.1 0.5 1 2 10 100
Oakley *et al.* (unpub)	51/228	(22.37)	53/224	(23.66)	0.93 (0.60–1.44)	
Lovell *et al.* (1986)	16/94	(17.02)	32/99	(32.32)	0.44 (0.23–0.85)	
Olds *et al.* (1986a)	7/142	(4.93)	17/127	(13.39)	0.35 (0.15–0.82)	
Dance (unpub)	12/25	(48.00)	21/25	(84.00)	0.21 (0.07–0.66)	
Typical odds ratio (95% confidence interval)					0.60 (0.44–0.83)	

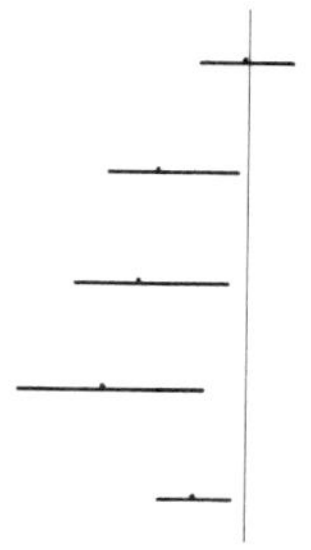

Effect of general social support from caregivers during pregnancy on dissatisfaction with intrapartum care

Study	EXPT		CTRL		Odds ratio	Graph of odds ratios and confidence intervals
Elbourne *et al.* (1987)	4/131	(3.05)	3/120	(2.50)	1.23 (0.27–5.50)	
Lovell *et al.* (1986)	8/88	(9.09)	20/89	(22.47)	0.37 (0.16–0.82)	
Shereshefsky *et al.* (1974)	22/29	(75.86)	26/28	(92.86)	0.28 (0.07–1.17)	
Typical odds ratio (95% confidence interval)					0.43 (0.23–0.82)	

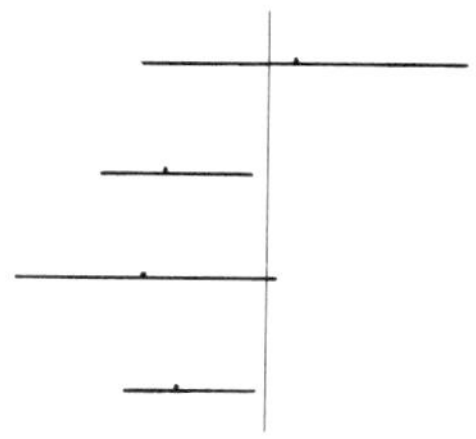

Table 15.4—*continued* Effect of general social support from caregivers during pregnancy on worry/non-enjoyment in labour/birth

Study	EXPT		CTRL		Odds ratio	Graph of odds ratios and confidence intervals
	n	(%)	*n*	(%)	(95% CI)	0.01 0.1 0.5 1 2 10 100
Oakley *et al.* (unpub)	79/230	(34.35)	96/226	(42.48)	0.71 (0.49–1.03)	
Carpenter *et al.* (1968)	15/44	(34.09)	25/43	(58.14)	0.38 (0.17–0.89)	
Typical odds ratio (95% confidence interval)					0.64 (0.45–0.90)	

Table 15.5 Effect of general social support from caregivers during pregnancy on unhappiness after childbirth

Study	EXPT		CTRL		Odds ratio	Graph of odds ratios and confidence intervals
	n	(%)	*n*	(%)	(95% CI)	0.01 0.1 0.5 1 2 10 100
Oakley *et al.* (unpub)	92/230	(40.00)	107/226	(47.35)	0.74 (0.51–1.07)	
Elbourne *et al.* (1987)	8/132	(6.06)	10/122	(8.20)	0.72 (0.28–1.89)	
Typical odds ratio (95% confidence interval)					0.74 (0.52–1.04)	
Effect of general social support from caregivers during pregnancy on father not being involved with baby						
Oakley *et al.* (unpub)	13/222	(5.86)	16/219	(7.31)	0.79 (0.37–1.68)	
Elbourne *et al.* (1987)	15/124	(12.10)	13/114	(11.40)	1.07 (0.49–2.35)	
Lovell *et al.* (1986)	3/94	(3.19)	13/102	(12.75)	0.28 (0.10–0.78)	
Typical odds ratio (95% confidence interval)					0.70 (0.44–1.14)	

Table 15.6 Effect of general social support from caregivers during pregnancy on not breastfeeding at hospital discharge

Study	EXPT		CTRL		Odds ratio	Graph of odds ratios and confidence intervals
	n	(%)	*n*	(%)	(95% CI)	0.01 0.1 0.5 1 2 10 100
Oakley *et al.* (unpub)	124/229	(54.15)	139/226	(61.50)	0.74 (0.51–1.07)	
Elbourne *et al.* (1987)	38/140	(27.14)	30/125	(24.00)	1.18 (0.68–2.04)	
Lovell *et al.* (1986)	20/96	(20.83)	23/102	(22.55)	0.90 (0.46–1.78)	
Dance (unpub)	5/25	(20.00)	17/25	(68.00)	0.15 (0.05–0.45)	
Typical odds ratio (95% confidence interval)					0.78 (0.59–1.02)	

Table 15.6—*continued* Effect of general social support from caregivers during pregnancy on not breastfeeding at 6 weeks

Study	EXPT *n*	(%)	CTRL *n*	(%)	Odds ratio (95% CI)	Graph of odds ratios and confidence intervals
Oakley *et al.* (unpub)	166/230	(72.17)	167/226	(73.89)	0.92 (0.61–1.39)	
Dance (unpub)	10/25	(40.00)	25/25	(100.0)	0.06 (0.02–0.20)	
Typical odds ratio (95% confidence interval)					0.69 (0.46–1.02)	

Effect of general social support from caregivers during pregnancy on introduction of solid food before 6 weeks

Study	EXPT *n*	(%)	CTRL *n*	(%)	Odds ratio (95% CI)	Graph of odds ratios and confidence intervals
Oakley *et al.* (unpub)	35/230	(15.22)	48/226	(21.24)	0.67 (0.42–1.07)	
Typical odds ratio (95% confidence interval)					0.67 (0.42–1.07)	

Effect of general social support from caregivers during pregnancy on lack of control postpartum

Study	EXPT *n*	(%)	CTRL *n*	(%)	Odds ratio (95% CI)	Graph of odds ratios and confidence intervals
Oakley *et al.* (unpub)	65/230	(28.26)	83/226	(36.73)	0.68 (0.46–1.01)	
Elbourne *et al.* (1987)	15/125	(12.00)	19/118	(16.10)	0.71 (0.35–1.47)	
Typical odds ratio (95% confidence interval)					0.69 (0.49–0.97)	

Graph scale: 0.01 0.1 0.5 1 2 10 100

Table 15.7 Effect of general social support from caregivers during pregnancy on admission to hospital during pregnancy

Study	EXPT *n*	(%)	CTRL *n*	(%)	Odds ratio (95% CI)	Graph of odds ratios and confidence intervals
Oakley *et al.* (unpub)	99/243	(40.74)	126/243	(51.85)	0.64 (0.45–0.91)	
Elbourne *et al.* (1987)	35/141	(24.82)	24/129	(18.60)	1.44 (0.81–2.56)	
Reid *et al.* (1983)	34/75	(45.33)	31/78	(39.74)	1.26 (0.66–2.38)	
Typical odds ratio (95% confidence interval)					0.87 (0.66–1.14)	

Effect of general social support from caregivers during pregnancy on mother feeling physically unwell at 6 weeks

Study	EXPT *n*	(%)	CTRL *n*	(%)	Odds ratio (95% CI)	Graph of odds ratios and confidence intervals
Oakley *et al.* (unpub)	49/230	(21.30)	61/165	(36.97)	0.46 (0.29–0.72)	
Elbourne *et al.* (1987)	5/133	(3.76)	1/23	(4.35)	0.85 (0.09–8.47)	
Typical odds ratio (95% confidence interval)					0.47 (0.30–0.73)	

Graph scale: 0.01 0.1 0.5 1 2 10 100

trial by Shereshefsky and Lockman (1973). After delivery they were less likely to be unhappy, and the father of the baby was more likely to be involved in its care (Table 15.5). Mothers who had received extra support during pregancy were more likely to be breastfeeding on discharge from hospital; at six weeks postpartum, they were still more likely than controls, to be feeling 'in control', to be breastfeeding and less likely to have introduced solid foods into their babies' diets (Table 15.6).

4 Other effects

In view of the intimate relationship between psychological and physical health it would be surprising if the beneficial psychological effects of social and psychological support during pregnancy were not reflected in some manifestation of improved physical health. Six weeks after delivery mothers who had received enhanced social and psychological support during pregnancy were less likely than controls to be feeling physically unwell (Table 15.7). Furthermore, their babies were less likely to have worrying health problems after discharge from hospital (Table 15.8).

5 Discussion

In none of the controlled trials that we have included in this review were any negative effects of enhanced social and psychological support during pregnancy reported. As the data we have presented above have shown, the beneficial effects in psychological and behavioural terms can be substantial. The available evidence also suggests that caregivers who provide this kind of support may reduce the frequency of some of the physical morbidity which so often dominates the various problems perceived by those providing professional care during pregnancy and childbirth.

The results of these experiments are consistent with some of the results of non-experimental studies in which the relationships between social class, stress and aspects of reproduction have been examined (Oakley *et al.* 1982; see Chapter 87). Other hypotheses derived from such studies have not yet been confirmed in controlled experiments. For example, the observed association between anxiety and complications of labour might lead one to expect that efforts to reduce stress during pregnancy would be reflected in a reduced use of pharmacological methods of pain relief and a reduced incidence of prolonged labour and operative delivery. None of these hypotheses are supported by the available data (Table 15.9).

Similarly, the observation of a social class gradient in the incidence of surrogate indicators of adverse outcome of pregnancy like preterm delivery and low birthweight, taken together with evidence suggesting a relationship between stressful life events and preterm delivery (Newton and Hunt 1984), suggest that one might expect enhanced social and pyschological care during pregnancy to reduce the frequency of these indicators (Oakley et al. 1982; Oakley 1985; Bryce *et al.* 1988). The data so far available, however, suggest that if such an effect exists then it is likely to be relatively modest (Table 15.10; Elbourne and Oakley, in press).

The failure of the experiments in this field to confirm these hypotheses does not detract from the substantial positive effects of enhanced social and psychological support during pregnancy. The 'bottom line' is that in

Table 15.8 Effect of general social support from caregivers during pregnancy on baby having health problems since discharge

Study	EXPT		CTRL		Odds ratio	Graph of odds ratios and confidence intervals
	n	(%)	*n*	(%)	(95% CI)	0.01 0.1 0.5 1 2 10 100
Oakley *et al.* (unpub)	56/214	(26.17)	73/215	(33.95)	0.69 (0.46–1.04)	
Dance (unpub)	1/25	(4.00)	2/25	(8.00)	0.50 (0.05–5.03)	
Typical odds ratio (95% confidence interval)					0.68 (0.46–1.03)	
Effect of general social support from caregivers during pregnancy on worry about baby postpartum						
Oakley *et al.* (unpub)	36/230	(15.65)	63/226	(27.88)	0.49 (0.31–0.76)	
Elbourne *et al.* (1987)	7/127	(5.51)	3/121	(2.48)	2.18 (0.62–7.72)	
Typical odds ratio (95% confidence interval)					0.58 (0.38–0.88)	

Table 15.9 Effect of general social support from caregivers during pregnancy on use of intrapartum regional block/general anaesthesia

Study	EXPT *n*	EXPT (%)	CTRL *n*	CTRL (%)	Odds ratio (95% CI)	Graph of odds ratios and confidence intervals (0.01 0.1 0.5 1 2 10 100)
Oakley *et al.* (unpub)	68/241	(28.22)	82/238	(34.45)	0.75 (0.51–1.10)	
Spencer and Morris (1986)	326/603	(54.06)	327/581	(56.28)	0.91 (0.73–1.15)	
Elbourne *et al.* (1987)	32/139	(23.02)	37/127	(29.13)	0.73 (0.42–1.26)	
Lovell *et al.* (1986)	44/95	(46.32)	33/102	(32.35)	1.79 (1.01–3.17)	
Reid *et al.* (1983)	38/75	(50.67)	29/78	(37.18)	1.72 (0.91–3.26)	
Yanover *et al.* (1976)	40/44	(90.91)	44/44	(100.0)	0.13 (0.02–0.93)	
Dance (unpub)	2/25	(8.00)	1/25	(4.00)	2.00 (0.20–20.20)	
Typical odds ratio (95% confidence interval)					0.95 (0.80–1.12)	

Effect of general social support from caregivers during pregnancy on use of intrapartum injected narcotic/oral analgesic

Study	EXPT *n*	EXPT (%)	CTRL *n*	CTRL (%)	Odds ratio (95% CI)	Graph
Oakley *et al.* (unpub)	125/241	(51.87)	106/238	(44.54)	1.34 (0.94–1.92)	
Spencer and Morris (1986)	226/603	(37.48)	225/581	(38.73)	0.95 (0.75–1.20)	
Elbourne *et al.* (1987)	45/139	(32.37)	41/127	(32.28)	1.00 (0.60–1.68)	
Reid *et al.* (1983)	22/75	(29.33)	29/78	(37.18)	0.70 (0.36–1.38)	
Dance (unpub)	2/25	(8.00)	17/25	(68.00)	0.08 (0.03–0.26)	
Carpenter *et al.* (1968)	19/44	(43.18)	27/43	(62.79)	0.46 (0.20–1.06)	
Typical odds ratio (95% confidence interval)					0.91 (0.76–1.07)	

Effect of general social support from caregivers during pregnancy on rate of prolonged labour (> 12 hours)

Study	EXPT *n*	EXPT (%)	CTRL *n*	CTRL (%)	Odds ratio (95% CI)	Graph
Oakley *et al.* (unpub)	17/202	(8.42)	14/189	(7.41)	1.15 (0.55–2.39)	
Spencer and Morris (1986)	326/603	(54.06)	327/581	(56.28)	0.91 (0.73–1.15)	
Elbourne *et al.* (1987)	12/132	(9.09)	8/118	(6.78)	1.37 (0.55–3.41)	
Lovell *et al.* (1986)	15/91	(16.48)	14/98	(14.29)	1.18 (0.54–2.61)	
Typical odds ratio (95% confidence interval)					0.97 (0.79–1.19)	

Table 15.9—*continued* Effect of general social support from caregivers during pregnancy on instrumental/operative delivery rate

Study	EXPT		CTRL		Odds ratio	Graph of odds ratios and confidence intervals
	n	(%)	*n*	(%)	(95% CI)	0.01 0.1 0.5 1 2 10 100
Oakley *et al.* (unpub)	46/243	(18.93)	61/243	(25.10)	0.70 (0.45–1.07)	
Spencer and Morris (1986)	226/603	(37.48)	225/581	(38.73)	0.95 (0.75–1.20)	
Elbourne *et al.* (1987)	32/138	(23.19)	29/127	(22.83)	1.02 (0.58–1.81)	
Reid *et al.* (1983)	25/75	(33.33)	22/78	(28.21)	1.27 (0.64–2.52)	
Lovell *et al.* (1986)	29/95	(30.53)	16/102	(15.69)	2.31 (1.19–4.49)	
Yanover *et al.* (1976)	14/53	(26.42)	22/44	(50.00)	0.37 (0.16–0.84)	
Dance (unpub)	4/25	(16.00)	5/25	(20.00)	0.77 (0.18–3.20)	
Carpenter *et al.* (1968)	19/44	(43.18)	27/43	(62.79)	0.46 (0.20–1.06)	
Typical odds ratio (95% confidence interval)					0.91 (0.77–1.08)	

Table 15.10 Effect of general social support from caregivers during pregnancy on preterm delivery rate (<37 weeks)

Study	EXPT		CTRL		Odds ratio	Graph of odds ratios and confidence intervals
	n	(%)	*n*	(%)	(95% CI)	0.01 0.1 0.5 1 2 10 100
Blondel *et al.* (unpub)	14/79	(17.72)	11/73	(15.07)	1.21 (0.51–2.85)	
Oakley *et al.* (unpub)	34/243	(13.99)	33/243	(13.58)	1.04 (0.62–1.73)	
Spencer and Morris (1986)	60/602	(9.97)	54/581	(9.29)	1.08 (0.73–1.59)	
Elbourne *et al.* (1987)	10/140	(7.14)	9/127	(7.09)	1.01 (0.40–2.56)	
Lovell *et al.* (1986)	5/95	(5.26)	4/102	(3.92)	1.36 (0.36–5.16)	
Olds *et al.* (1986a)	11/166	(6.63)	12/142	(8.45)	0.77 (0.33–1.80)	
Dance (unpub)	5/25	(20.00)	4/25	(16.00)	1.30 (0.31–5.44)	
Typical odds ratio (95% confidence interval)					1.06 (0.82–1.36)	

Table 15.10—*continued* Effect of general social support from caregivers during pregnancy on low birthweight rate (<2500g)

Study	EXPT *n*	(%)	CTRL *n*	(%)	Odds ratio (95% CI)
Blondel *et al.* (unpub)	9/79	(11.39)	6/73	(8.22)	1.43 (0.49–4.13)
Oakley *et al.* (unpub)	45/243	(18.52)	52/243	(21.40)	0.84 (0.54–1.30)
Heins *et al.* (unpub)	127/667	(19.04)	139/679	(20.47)	0.91 (0.70–1.19)
Spencer and Morris (1986)	54/602	(8.97)	50/581	(8.61)	1.05 (0.70–1.56)
Elbourne *et al.* (1987)	11/143	(7.69)	12/130	(9.23)	0.82 (0.35–1.92)
Lovell *et al.* (1986)	5/95	(5.26)	11/102	(10.78)	0.48 (0.17–1.33)
Reid *et al.* (1983)	6/76	(7.89)	10/79	(12.66)	0.60 (0.21–1.68)
Olds *et al.* (1986)	10/166	(6.02)	4/142	(2.82)	2.09 (0.71–6.11)
Dance (unpub)	3/25	(12.00)	4/25	(16.00)	0.72 (0.15–3.51)
Typical odds ratio (95% confidence interval)					0.92 (0.77–1.10)

Graph of odds ratios and confidence intervals: 0.01 0.1 0.5 1 2 10 100

Table 15.11 Effect of general social support from caregivers during pregnancy on preference for different care in future

Study	EXPT *n*	(%)	CTRL *n*	(%)	Odds ratio (95% CI)
Blondel (unpub)	9/79	(11.39)	29/73	(39.73)	0.22 (0.11–0.46)
Elbourne *et al.* (1987)	11/123	(8.94)	44/106	(41.51)	0.17 (0.09–0.31)
Lovell *et al.* (1986)	19/95	(20.00)	66/101	(65.35)	0.16 (0.09–0.28)
Typical odds ratio (95% confidence interval)					0.18 (0.12–0.25)

Graph of odds ratios and confidence intervals: 0.01 0.1 0.5 1 2 10 100

all three of the experiments from which data on the matter are available, far smaller proportions of the women in the experimental groups than in the control groups receiving standard care would seek other forms of care in a future pregnancy (Table 15.11).

6 Conclusions

Social and psychological support of pregnant women should be an integral part of all forms of care given during pregnancy and childbirth. Unfortunately it is not. The available data from relevant controlled trials suggest that penalties of ignoring these aspects of care can be expected not only in terms of psychological morbidity, but also in less desirable health behaviour and avoidable physical morbidity in both women and their babies.

Serious investigation of this field has only begun very recently. A number of controlled trials in addition to those reviewed above have completed recruitment and at least five are still in progress (Table 15.12). As the results from these trials accumulate, we are likely to obtain more definitive answers to questions about the effects of social and pyschological support during pregnancy. No adverse effects of these forms of care have been reported, however, so they should be adopted forthwith so that more women and their babies begin to enjoy their beneficial effects.

Table 15.12 Uncompleted trials of social and psychological support in pregnancy

Principal investigator and place	Nature of the intervention	Sample	Allocation	Outcomes of intervention
A. Recruitment complete: Awaiting data analysis and report(s)				
S. Elliot T. Leverton London, England	Social support—education groups led by psychologist or health visitor	First and second time mothers ($n=200$)	Week of clinic booking	Incidence of psychiatric disorder, especially postnatal depression; psychological well-being; use of support networks; birthweight
C. Larson Montreal, Canada	Prenatal home visits by community health nurses	? ($n=1548$)	Random	Health and social status of mother and child to 3 years postpartum, childrearing attitudes and behaviour of mother
B. In progress				
S. Ng New York, USA	Intense prenatal care including weekly visit, pelvic examination; education on self-palpation; home uterine contraction monitor; social service referral	History of preterm delivery, stillbirth or spontaneous abortion $>20/52$; age <16, >35; registered for prenatal care before 26/52 ($n=450$)	Stratified randomization so that equal numbers assigned to each treatment at any point in time	Preterm delivery; stillbirths; spontaneous abortions in 2nd or 3rd trimester; birthweight
F. Stanley R. Bryce Perth, Australia	Social support via home visiting by midwives	Any of: previous preterm birth; perinatal death; spontaneous 2nd trimester abortion; $\geqslant 3$ first trimester abortions; APH; low birthweight ($n=2000$)	Computer-generated random numbers in blocks of 4	Preterm delivery; birthweight; cost; anxiety; social support; locus of control; conduct of labour
J. Villar E. Kestler Latin America (Argentina, Brazil, Cuba, Guatemala, Mexico)	Home visits by trained women (including nurses, social workers and lay workers) to provide personal and family support, health education and use of social and health services	Women attending specified antenatal clinic before 20/52, without important clinical problems, but having one or more risk factors: previous low birthweight birth; age $\leqslant 17$; malnutrition; low income; low maternal education, unsupported women ($n=2000$)	Random, stratified by centre	IUGR, LBW, preterm delivery; maternal weight gain; obstetric interventions, labour complications, breastfeeding, neonatal morbidity; use of health and social services; satisfaction; support; postpartum depression
C. Hobel R. Bemis Los Angeles, USA	Psychosocial support/social work to reduce stress	High-risk women in 5 experimental clinics	Random assignment of clinics to experimental or control status. Then random assignment of high-risk women within 5 experimental clinics to one of 5 interventions—one of which is support	Gestational age at delivery; birthweight
A. Stevens Birmingham, England	Relocation of antenatal care from hospital into community so convenient for mothers and appropriate to their needs; antenatal home visits; midwife care; intensive link-worker support	Women booking at 2 hospitals (unless need specialist care) ($n=1665$)	Computer-generated list of random numbers	Patient satisfaction; antenatal clinic attendance; antenatal complications; birthweight

References

Atlee HB (1963). The fall of the Queen of Heaven. Obstet Gynecol, 21: 514–519.

Blondel B, Bréart G, Llado J (unpublished). Prevention of preterm deliveries by home visiting midwives: results of a French randomised controlled trial.

Bryce RL, Stanley RJ, Enkin MW (1988). The role of social support in the prevention of preterm birth. Birth, 15: 19–23.

Campbell R, Macfarlane AJ (1987). Where To Be Born? The Debate and the Evidence. Oxford: National Perinatal Epidemiology Unit.

Carpenter J, Aldrich K, Boverman H (1968). The effectiveness of patient interviews. A controlled study of emotional support during pregnancy. Arch Gen Psychiatry, 19: 110–112.

Chalmers I, Oakley A, Macfarlane JA (1980). Perinatal health services: an immodest proposal. Br Med J, 1: 842–845.

Dance J (unpublished) (1987). A social intervention by link-workers to Pakistani women and pregnancy outcome.

Elbourne D, Richardson M, Chalmers I, Waterhouse I, Holt E (1987). The Newbury Maternity Care Study: a randomized controlled trial to assess a policy of women holding their own obstetric records. Br J Obstet Gynaecol, 94: 612–619.

Elbourne D (1987). Subjects' views about participation in a randomised controlled trial. J Reprod Infant Psychol, 5: 3–8.

Elbourne D, Oakley A (in press). An overview of trials of social support in pregnancy: effects on gestational age at delivery and birthweight. In: Advances in the Prevention of Low Birthweight. Berendes HW, Kessel W, Yaffe S (eds). New York: Perinatology Press.

Heins HC, Nance NW (1986). A statewide randomized clinical trial to reduce the incidence of low birthweight/very low birthweight infants in South Carolina. In: Prevention of Preterm Birth. Papiernik E, Breart G, Spira N (eds). Paris: INSERM, 138: 387–410.

Heins HC, Nance N, Efird C (unpublished). Multicenter randomized controlled clinical trial for the prevention of low birthweight in South Carolina.

Hobel C, Bemis RL (1986). West Area Los Angeles prematurity prevention demonstration project. In: Prevention of Preterm Birth. Papiernik E, Breart G, Spira N (eds). Paris: INSERM, pp 205–222.

Jeffcoate N (1976). Medicine versus nature. J R Coll of Surg Edinb 21: 263–277.

Kerr MG (1975). Problems and Perspectives in Reproductive Medicine. Inaugural Lecture No. 61. University of Edinburgh.

Lewis J (1980). The Politics of Motherhood. London: Croom Helm.

Lovell A, Elbourne D (1987). Holding the baby—and your notes. Health Service J, 19 March: 335.

Lovell A, Zander LI, James CE, Foot S, Swan AV, Reynolds A (1986). St. Thomas's Maternity Case Notes Study: why not give mothers their own case notes? In: Cicely Northcote Trust, London: United Medical and Dental School of St. Thomas's Hospital, pp 1–155.

Lovell A, Zander LI, James CE, Foot S, Swan AV, Reynolds A (1987). The St. Thomas's Hospital Maternity Case Notes Study: a randomised controlled trial to assess the effects of giving expectant mothers their own maternity case-notes. Pediatr Perinat Epidemiol, 1: 57–66.

McIntosh J (in press). Models of childbirth and social class: a study of 80 working class primigravidae. In: Research in Midwifery and Childbirth Care. Robinson S, Thomson A (eds). London: Croom Helm.

Mahler H (1987). The motherhood initiative: a call to action. Lancet, 1: 668–670.

Morris N (1960). Human relations in obstetric practice. Lancet 2: 913–915.

Newton RA, Hunt LP (1984). Psychosocial stress in pregnancy and its relation to low birthweight. Br Med J, 288: 1191–1193.

Oakley A (1979). Becoming a Mother. London: Martin Robertson.

Oakley A (1984). The Captured Womb: a History of the Medical Care of Pregnant Women. Oxford: Blackwell.

Oakley A (1985). Social support: the 'soft' way to improve birthweight? Soc Sci Med, 21: 1259–1268.

Oakley A, Macfarlane JA, Chalmers I (1982). Social class, stress and reproduction. In: Disease and the Environment. Rees AR, Purcell H (eds). Chichester: John Wiley, pp 11–50.

Oakley A, Rajan L, Grant A (unpublished). Social support during pregnancy.

Olds DL, Henderson CR, Tatelbaum R, Chamberlin R (1986a). Improving the delivery of prenatal care and outcomes of pregnancy: a randomized trial of nurse home visitation. Pediatrics, 77: 16–28.

Olds DL, Henderson CR, Chamberlin R, Tatelbaum R (1986b). Preventing child abuse and neglect: a randomized trial of home nurse visitation. Pediatrics, 78: 65–78.

Olds DL, Henderson CR, Tatelbaum R, Chamberlin R (in press). Improving the life course development of socially disadvantaged mothers: a randomized trial of home nurse visitation. Am J Public Health.

Oppenheimer I (1986). The civil liberties of the unborn. New York Times, October 23.

Reid ME, Gutteridge S, McIlwaine GM (1983). A comparison of the delivery of antenatal care between a hospital and a peripheral clinic. Report to Health Services Research Committee, Scottish Home and Health Department.

Rosenfield A, Maine D (1985). Maternal mortality—a neglected tragedy. Where is the M in MCH? Lancet, 2: 83–85.

Shereshefsky PM, Lockman RF (1973). Comparison of counselled and non-counselled groups and within-group differences. In: Psychological Aspects of a First Pregnancy and Early Postnatal Adaptation. Shereshefsky PM, Yarrow LJ (eds). New York: Raven Press, pp 151–163.

Spence Cagle C (1984). Changed interpersonal needs of the pregnant couple: nursing roles. J Obstet Gynecol Neonatal Nurs, 13: 56.

Spencer B, Morris J (1986). The family worker project: social support in pregnancy. In: Prevention of Preterm Birth. Papiernik E, Breart G, Spira N (eds). Paris: INSERM, 138: 363–382.

Spencer B, Thomas H, Morris J (in press). The family worker project: a randomised controlled trial of the provision of social support service during pregnancy. Br J Obstet Gynaecol.

Stanley FJ, Bryce RL (1986). The pregnancy home visiting program. In: Prevention of Preterm Birth. Papiernik E, Breart G, Spira N (eds). Paris: INSERM, 138: 309–328.

Yauger RA (1972). Does family-centred care make a difference? Nursing Outlook, 20: 320–323.

Yanover MJ, Jones D, Miller MD (1976). Perinatal care of low-risk mothers and infants. New Engl J Med, 94: 702–705.

16 Advice for pregnancy

Judith Lumley and Jill Astbury

All who drink of this remedy recover in a short time, except those whom it does not help, who all die.

Silverman (1980).

1 Introduction

William Silverman quotes this aphorism, ascribed to Galen, in his book *Retrolental Fibroplasia: A Modern Parable*, in order to illustrate the well-established tendency in perinatal medicine to explain away failures of treatment. The idea of inevitable effect has widespread popularity in medicine, and is especially evident in medical thinking about appropriate maternal behaviour in pregnancy. Here, a welter of prescriptions and proscriptions is justified on the grounds that they ensure reproductive perfection and/or avoid reproductive disaster.

The content of any advice or remedy used to bring about recovery 'in a short time' is its least important feature. The ingredients used can vary so greatly that one may sample dozens of remedies related to the goal of a perfect pregnancy, labour and delivery without finding the same ingredient used twice. What is important and invariant is the assumption that all the salient factors relating to that goal are both known and controlled for. Knowledge and control, or the belief that one has them, supply the basis for making predictions about future outcome with the confident certainty associated with infallible remedies. The idea of certainty, coupled with the ability and desire to act quickly, is an almost irresistible combination in any situation in which it is believed that suffering, death, or permanent disability will follow unless 'something is done'.

Considerable psychological gains stem from feeling certain about something, particularly when that something is viewed as a means of saving lives. Certainty reduces apprehension, ambivalence, and anxiety in both doctor and patient. It can act like a misguided Ockham's razor, cutting down alternative courses of action, including no action at all, to one pristine 'solution'. At a subconscious level, some clinicians may even prefer to take a course of action which is ineffective or worse, rather than be seen to do nothing at all.

The most common form of remedy offered to pregnant women comes in the guise of 'advice'. However, this is no ordinary advice, there being no option of refusal. Those believed to be authorities on reproduction, like obstetricians and childbirth educators, can give advice which appeals powerfully to the pregnant woman's desire for a physically and emotionally satisfying birth experience for herself and her infant. The self-evident desirability of these ends imbues the means suggested for their attainment with a strong prescriptive force. The Association for Preconceptual (*sic*) Care (Foresight, no date) states that pregnancy advice makes a major contribution to raising 'a generation of children virtually free from the disadvantage of malformation, allergic illness, and compromised development', not to mention 'an easy pregnancy and birth, abundant lactation and sturdy, healthy children'. Who could dissent from such aims?

The 'remedies' related to childbearing can take two forms. One is directed to 'curing' current ills, the other to preventing future ills. Encouragement to take the preventive remedies may be expressed positively—take it now and enjoy the benefits later, or negatively—don't take it now and experience the hazards later on. If a woman fails to accept a remedy offered in the positive form, she may find herself presented with the negative version in an atmosphere of 'shroud-waving' (Cartwright 1979).

In the following pages we intend to examine some of

the most potent 'remedies' available to pregnant women, namely advice about sexual activity, cigarettes and alcohol, work and exercise, and maternal anxiety.

2 Advice before pregnancy

Although prepregnancy advice has been a possibility ever since effective contraception permitted the planning of pregnancy, the terms prepregnancy counselling and prepregnancy care have come into use only in the last eight or nine years. (Alternative names include preconceptional, preconceptual, and interpregnancy care.) Whatever the term used, the basic idea of providing advice *before* pregnancy to improve pregnancy outcome has become increasingly popular with diverse groups. The Institute of Medicine in the United States devoted a chapter to prepregnancy counselling in its major review of low birthweight and its prevention (Committee to Study the Prevention of Low Birth Weight 1985). In Britain, both the Royal College of Obstetricians and Gynaecologists and a consumer coalition, Maternity Alliance, have called for the establishment of prepregnancy clinics.

The appeal of prepregnancy advice is easy to see. Care during pregnancy has yet to have a significant impact on rates of preterm delivery. It has even less to offer for the other major cause of perinatal death and disability, congenital malformations, since almost all birth defects are already determined by the time of the earliest antenatal visit. As in other cases of therapeutic impotence the response has been to redouble the efforts, i.e. extend care and advice backwards into the period before conception.

Two controversies have lent impetus to prepregnancy advice. The first is the possibility that alcohol use around the time of conception might be harmful to the fetus, with the corollary that women need to be warned to give up alcohol as soon as they stop using contraception. The second is the debate about the prevention of neural tube defects, among women with a previous affected infant, by supplementation with micronutrients before and just after conception. Despite the many scientific uncertainties in both cases they have somehow legitimized the provision of prepregnancy advice, not just in the two areas mentioned but well beyond them into the occupations and hobbies of both parents and their whole way of life (Lehrmann 1988).

Territorial rivalries have also played a part in the development of the prepregnancy industry. For advice-givers who do not currently have a major role in antenatal and birth care (childbirth educators, community health nurses, some midwives, some self-help and support organizations), the prepregnancy period offers an opportunity to intervene in an area which is not yet fully medicalized. It is also one in which the emphasis can be seen as health-related rather than illness-related.

The range of activities covered by the general heading 'advice before pregnancy' is very great. The difference between the provision of information requested by the woman or the couple in order for decisions to be made about the next pregnancy, the provision of advice as to how to achieve a good outcome of pregnancy and the provision of counselling in order to deal with previous poor outcomes are not always clear even to those running prepregnancy services. The information and counselling aspects mostly apply to parents who are, or believe themselves to be, in a high-risk category for pregnancy or those requiring regular medical care outside pregnancy (Chamberlain and Lumley 1986). Some of those seeking or being offered advice will be in the same categories but many will be the 'worried well', those with strong beliefs about nutrition, exercise, or wellness, and increasingly those who see 'preconceptual care' as the right and proper way to go about becoming a parent.

The fundamental problem with advice before pregnancy is the threadbare state of our knowledge about how to avoid preterm delivery, birth defects, stillbirths, or fetal growth retardation. Apart from ensuring that the woman has been immunized against rubella and will not be taking any drugs, including over the counter preparations and natural remedies, except those for which a careful risk–benefit analysis has been made, what sensible advice can be given? Smokers, as discussed later, need practical assistance for quitting rather than advice. Suggestions to adopt the prudent diet (less fat, less sugar, less salt, more fruit, vegetables, and complex carbohydrates) although probably beneficial as general dietary guidelines, are not warranted in terms of preventing malformations or low birthweight (Rush 1986). Supplementation with trace minerals and vitamins cannot be justified in the present state of knowledge (*Lancet*, leading article 1985). Evidence on the effects of physical activity, work, exercise and travel is still inconsistent and that on paternal exposures is extraordinarily rudimentary. The identification of uncertain gestation as a risk factor for a whole host of adverse outcomes (Hall and Carr-Hill 1985) may suggest a factor which could be modified by careful recording of menstrual data and early presentation for antenatal care but the underlying factors are likely to be more complex.

The possible unwanted side-effects of prepregnancy advice for clients are those of reduced self-confidence, reduced self-reliance and increased anxiety. For advice givers, the side-effects may be more dangerous; a reduced awareness of the social factors beyond individual health behaviours which are associated with recalcitrant obstetric disorders such as preterm birth, and a misguided though sincere belief that they have the answers.

In Britain the Association for Preconceptual Care is collecting information on the outcome of pregnancy after preconceptional advice, compared with the outcome of earlier pregnancies to the same couple (Foresight Newsletter 1986). The fallacies inherent in this form of evaluation have been well documented in relation to spontaneous abortion treated by diethylstilboestrol, and preterm delivery treated by cervical suture, (see Chapters 38 and 40) among many examples. One randomized trial of a prepregnancy package (information, advice, screening, support) is under way in Melbourne (Plovanic, Burrell, Lumley, in preparation). The population is a demographically high-risk one, and the primary outcome of interest in the trial is birthweight.

It would be premature to make any judgements about prepregnancy advice except to say that on present knowledge its beneficial effects are likely to be extremely modest and it cannot automatically be regarded as harmless.

3 Sexual activity

A patient attending the antenatal clinic in a London teaching hospital before the birth of her third child was accidentally discovered to have a cardiac disorder complicating a congenital heart defect. The consultant who went to tell her this, as tactfully as possible, was amazed to discover that she already knew about the defect, which had been diagnosed at the same hospital during adolescence. 'Didn't they tell you it would be dangerous for you to have children?' he asked. 'No. No one ever mentioned that. They did say I should never get married—so I never have.'

Although one could tell this story as a joke, it is also an awful warning about the ways in which advice is often given: inexact, inexplicit, euphemistic, misleading, allowing no opportunity for clarification and discussion of alternatives—not to mention being downright dangerous in terms of unintended side-effects.

As recently as the mid-1960s, sex during pregnancy was a relatively straightforward issue. If one can generalize from a single survey carried out among Australian public hospital patients at that time, almost all women worried that sexual activity might harm the fetus (though fewer multiparae worried). However, very few indeed (less than 5 per cent) mentioned this fear to a doctor, and no doctor raised the topic with any of the women (Blankfield and Wood 1971).

Fifteen years later the following conversation in the antenatal clinic at the same hospital demonstrates how radically attitudes have changed.

Doctor (talking to a woman who went into preterm labour in her last pregnancy and who is to have a cervical suture inserted): 'By the way, once you've had the stitch put in you can't have sex until after the birth.'
Woman (angrily): 'Well, what are we supposed to do?'
Doctor: 'Your husband can always go to a massage parlour.'

Although this exchange may not be typical, it does exemplify some important contemporary elements: the willingness of both parties to mention the topic of sex; the belief that sexual activity may cause preterm labour; the woman's view of sexual activity as something to which she and her partner have a right; and the doctor's view that abstaining from sex is a 'problem' for men but not for women.

There are at present two conflicting attitudes to sexual activity in pregnancy, and two corresponding sorts of advice. The first is illustrated by Dr Pierre Vellay in his preface to *Making Love During Pregnancy* (Bing and Coleman 1977):

> Until recently sex during pregnancy was a taboo subject. Traditional obstetrics observed the law of silence on this matter. Conditioned by tradition and alienated by convention, both the pregnant woman and her husband did not dare to discuss making love during pregnancy, although both thought about it . . . Through detailed studies of couples facing pregnancy (the authors) demonstrate that sex during pregnancy can be fulfilling for both husband and wife. They show, too, how the husband can be entirely involved in his wife's pregnancy from the moment of conception to the birth of the child. Through a continued, shared experience of sex during these nine months, a couple begins to define in a context of mutual trust and love their individual responsibilities towards the child they will have together.

The emphasis here is on personal and mutual pleasure and fulfilment, with pregnancy and birth seen as conjugal processes of delight. The tone goes well beyond encouragement and reassurance to extreme enthusiasm. There is no hint in Vellay's preface of the now well-established fact that all forms of sexual activity decline progressively through pregnancy (Falicov 1973; Solberg *et al.* 1973; Morris 1975; Tolor and Di Grazia 1976; Lumley 1978; Grudzinskas *et al.* 1979; Mills *et al.* 1981) and that for a variety of reasons, enjoyment of sexual activity is highly problematic for many men and women during pregnancy (Falicov 1973; Tolor and Di Grazia 1976; Lumley 1978).

The second attitude is typified by the following newspaper extract headlined 'Sex Harmful':

> *New York*: Sexual intercourse for a pregnant woman is more dangerous to the foetus than the combined effects of the use of alcohol and cigarettes . . . Dr Richard Naeye of the Pennsylvania State University told a medical meeting in Providence, Rhode Island. (*The Age*, Melbourne, 15 June 1981).

The belief that sexual intercourse is harmful to the fetus unites the views attributed to Dr Naeye with those of figures as diverse as Seneca, St. Ambrose, and Avicenna (Noonan 1965). *The Ladies' Guide to Health and Disease* (Kellogg 1902) warns of dangers to the mother as well: 'sexual indulgence during pregnancy may be suspended with decided benefit to both mother and child'. The good sense of this course of action was supported by the authority of 'the most ancient medical writers (who) call attention to the fact that by the practice of continence during gestation, the pains of childbirth are greatly mitigated'. If women rejected this line of reasoning, Kellogg had another to which they surely felt vulnerable. He warned that 'the injurious influences upon the child of the gratification of the passions during the period when its character is being formed, are undoubtedly much greater than is generally supposed'.

Obstetric textbooks of this era (reviewed by Enkin 1980) mentioned different but equally compelling risks, notably of abortions, preterm labour, and puerperal infection. The last of these was dropped from editions after the 1930s when the general acceptance of aseptic and antiseptic procedures after nearly a century of struggle, finally controlled puerperal infection and, in addition, drugs became available to treat it. Concern over abortion lessened too as the overt demand for illegal (and later legal) abortion provided proof that abortion could not be a common side-effect of sexual intercourse and it was discovered that most early spontaneous abortions are of embryos with major defects or chromosomal abnormalities. Only women with recurrent abortion (another obstetric mystery) are now counselled about sexual activity in early pregnancy. 'Sexual abstinence has been an important part in the therapeutic regimen for habitual abortion' said Javert in 1957. The specific injunction such women are still commonly given—to avoid intercourse when the next three menstrual periods would have been due—is less straightforward than it sounds; try calculating the forbidden days in the first trimester, given a menstrual cycle of even low variability, such as 29 days +2.

Figure 16.1 summarizes the scope of the possible hazards of sex during pregnancy. The best-documented of these is maternal death from air embolism (Aronson and Nelson 1967). By a tragic irony, these deaths may have been the result of an injunction 'not to have sex' in the last six weeks of pregnancy. The substitution of blowing air into the vagina for genital intercourse proved fatal—an example of the way in which inexplicit advice may have unintended side-effects.

The second hazard focuses on female orgasm, which may produce painful and prolonged uterine contractions in pregnancy (Masters and Johnson 1966) with concurrent or subsequent fetal bradycardia (Goodlin *et al.* 1972). Note that these are not invariable consequences of genital intercourse. In the study of Solberg and colleagues (1973), 86 per cent of the women had coitus during pregnancy; 50 per cent mostly or always had an orgasm, but only 25 per cent had cramps or contractions after coitus.

In the book *Sex and the Unborn Child*, Limner (1969) has suggested that these episodes of fetal bradycardia damage the brain and result in mental retardation. He adduces as supportive evidence the comment of Javert (1957) that his patients who abstained from sexual activity throughout pregnancy had highly intelligent offspring. This extraordinary claim seems not even to deserve the compliment of rational opposition or refutation except for its potential to increase the grief and guilt of parents with a mentally retarded child.

As an extension of the studies on fetal bradycardia, Grudzinskas *et al.* (1979) have reported an association of borderline statistical significance between coitus in

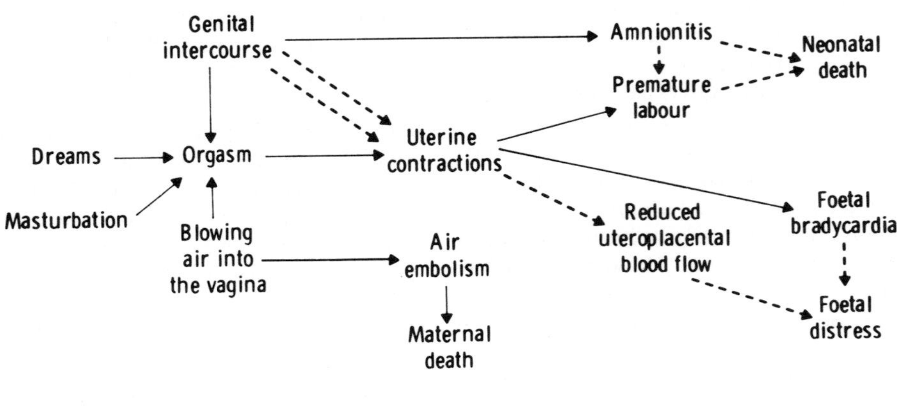

Fig. 16.1 Scope of possible hazards of sex during pregnancy.

the last four weeks of pregnancy and fetal distress during labour (or, rather two 'soft signs' of fetal distress). The mechanism they propose is possible compromise of the fetal circulation associated with the contractions of orgasm, but in fact they provide no information at all about orgasm, their figure referring to 'sexual activity' and their table to 'coitus', as if all three were interchangeable. This is no pedantic quibble. If it is orgasm that is harmful, then women must be advised that masturbation is more dangerous than genital intercourse, because Masters and Johnson have shown that the former produces more powerful uterine contractions (1966). It is difficult to imagine what reasonable advice could be given to the 5 or 10 per cent (Goodlin *et al.* 1971) whose orgasms result from dreams.

The major proposed hazard of orgasm is preterm labour (Goodlin *et al.* 1971, 1972)). Although Goodlin and others have found an association between orgasm and preterm labour, other studies have failed to find an association with either coitus or orgasm (Pugh and Fernandez 1953; Solberg *et al.* 1973; Perkins 1979; Rayburn and Wilson 1980; Mills *et al.* 1981). In comparing pre-labour sexual activity of women delivering preterm and women delivering at term, Goodlin and colleagues introduce a systematic bias, as the normative studies quoted earlier all show a progressive decline in sexual activity as pregnancy progresses to term.

The power of the theory that sexual activity is an important factor in preterm labour can be demonstrated by the extent to which the data have been rearranged in the attempt to find some association. The large Seattle study (Solberg *et al.* 1973) included 19 women who gave birth to infants of low birthweight. This group was a mixed bag of preterm birth or retarded fetal growth, or both. No association with labour itself could be found, but it was proposed that frequent or very intense or multiple orgasm, especially in the first trimester, might be a factor in the ultimate poorer outcome (Wagner *et al.* 1976). Neither Perkins (1979) nor Rayburn and Wilson (1980) could confirm this possibility, but the latter found yet another association: the 18 women whose preterm labour had no known predisposing factor reported coitus more often than controls (1.67 times per week compared with 0.85 times per week). Although this difference is statistically significant, its practical significance remains elusive.

Most recent discussion about the hazards of sexual activity in pregnancy has been related to genital intercourse as the primary danger, with orgasm demoted to a secondary role. The suggested mechanism is that coitus promotes infection and amnionitis, leading to premature rupture of the membranes and preterm delivery. One analysis showed an increased frequency of amnionitis, by histologic rather than by clinical criteria, when women reported coitus once a month or more in the month before delivery (15.6 per cent compared with 11.7 per cent), and an increased death rate among infected infants (1.7 per 1000 compared with 0.3 per 1000) (Naeye 1979a). Interpreting Naeye's findings is made more difficult by the fact that the pregnancies studied occurred from 1959 to 1966, a period when preterm labour, the main associated feature of amnionitis, resulted in a much greater perinatal mortality than it does today. In addition, information on coital activity collected on admission to hospital differed dramatically from that collected in the antenatal clinic, which casts doubt on the reliability of the information which was the basis of the analysis. The differences in infection rates were statistically significant only before 33 weeks and after 38 weeks, and at most coitus explained only 25 per cent of infections. Finally, the crucial question of the extent to which neutrophilic infiltration of the membranes constitutes firm evidence of amniotic fluid infection remains unresolved.

Subsequent publications have pointed to possible interactions between poor hygiene and impaired host resistance, possibly nutritional, and the presumptive introduction of infection. Semen itself is said to play a part, enhancing bacterial growth and providing additional prostaglandins (Naeye and Ross 1982). Pressure of the penis on the cervix in late pregnancy might also release prostaglandins as vaginal examination has been shown to do (Mitchell *et al.* 1977). The final element in the theory is that orgasm may also have an effect by increasing the chances that the damaged membranes will rupture under the extra force exerted by uterine contractions.

Attempts to replicate Naeye's findings in another large data set with methodologically superior data on sexual activity were unsuccessful (Mills *et al.* 1981).

An editorial in the *New England Journal of Medicine*, commenting on Naeye's work, quoted two papers which do claim to show harmful effects of sexual activity (Goodlin *et al.* 1971; Grudzinskas *et al.* 1979) but failed to mention any of the papers which found no ill effects. It went on to ask the rhetorical question 'Where does all this leave the gravid patient?' and added 'in view of the fragmentary evidence, patients receive a wide range of advice' (Herbst 1979).

The research on sexual activity and pregnancy has been presented in very great detail to make it clear that on the basis of available evidence, any prohibition (except to avoid blowing air into the vagina) is wholly inappropriate.

Those who give advice, counselling or reassurance should bear in mind what Marie Stopes wrote in 1918:

> 'Much has been written, and may be found in the innumerable books on the sex problem, as to whether a man and a woman should or should not have relations while the wife is bearing an unborn child. In this matter experience is very various, so that it is

difficult or impossible to give definite advice without knowing the full circumstances of each case. I have heard from a number of women that they desire union urgently at this time; while to others the thought is incredible . . .

The accumulating evidence which I have acquired through direct personal confidences about this subject points in absolutely conflicting directions, and there is little doubt that in this particular, even more so than in many others, the health, needs and mental conditions of women who are bearing children vary profoundly.'

4 Smoking

If prohibition of various forms of sexual activity in pregnancy illustrates one category of inappropriate advice—that based on inadequate evidence—prohibition of cigarette smoking and the consumption of alcohol illustrate another problem altogether. The evidence that these behaviours may have harmful effects on the fetus in some circumstances is compelling. However, most anti-smoking 'advice' and propaganda ignore the problem of physical and psychological addiction, the meaning of the behaviour for the women involved, and the guilt and anxiety felt by those who continue to smoke in the face of exhortations to give it up. Much health-promotional material for use in pregnancy is characterized by its particularly strident tone.

Between 1957 and 1986 over a hundred publications, based on studies of more than half a million births, reported that women who smoked during pregnancy had infants of lower birthweight than women who did not. The size of the difference (175–200 g) was remarkably constant across investigations and remained even after adjustment for social class, parity, maternal age, height and weight, level of education, previous low birthweight infant, and alcohol consumption (Butler and Alberman 1969; Fabia 1973; van den Berg 1977; Rush and Cassano 1983; Lumley *et al.* 1985). A similar birthweight difference has been demonstrated between the infants of smoking and non-smoking women doctors (Alberman *et al.* 1977). In one Australian state non-smokers of all social classes had infants with the same mean birthweight suggesting that here at least smoking accounts for much of the quite marked class difference in outcome (Lumley *et al.* 1985).

The strength of the association between maternal smoking and lower birthweight, the consistency of the findings, the existence of dosage effects, and the evidence on biological mechanisms outlined below, all add up to strong evidence that the association is causal. This inference has not gone unchallenged, the most detailed criticisms being those of Yerushalmy (1971, 1972), who viewed the birthweight differences as a manifestation of the smoker rather than of the cigarettes. It is true that smokers are more likely nowadays to be at risk on other grounds such as socioeconomic status, extremes of parity and low maternal age. Smoking is also associated with a low prepregnancy weight for height (Naeye and Tafari 1983). In addition, the effect of stressful life events on pregnancy outcome is partly mediated by increased smoking (Newton and Hunt 1984) and smoking rates are increased by unemployment of the pregnant woman or her partner (Najman *et al.* 1983). However, when these confounding factors are taken into account, as they were in the studies cited above, the birthweight difference remains.

The association between paternal smoking and lower birthweight reported by Yerushalmy (1971) is in part likely to be confounded by social class differences in smoking rates, but is also likely to be explained by passive exposure of the mother and fetus to paternal side stream smoke. The relative risk of delivering a term low birthweight infant in non-smoking women increased to 2.17 if they are thus exposed for at least two hours a day (Martin and Bracken 1986; Rubin *et al.* 1986)

Research into the pathophysiology of cigarette smoking has documented ways in which nicotine, carbon monoxide, or both adversely affect the fetus and placenta (Gennser *et al.* 1975; Longo 1977; D'Souza *et al.* 1978; Davies *et al.* 1979; Naeye 1979b). Two small randomized controlled trials have confirmed immediate effects of smoking a single cigarette in late pregnancy on fetal heart rate (Pijpers *et al.* 1984a) and on fetal heart rate patterns and fetal movements (Goodman *et al.* 1984).

Further support for the hypothesis that smoking causes the observed difference in birthweight comes from two of the randomized controlled trials discussed in more detail below (Sexton and Hebel 1984; MacArthur *et al.* 1987). Suggestions that fetal growth might be increased in smokers by increasing maternal food intake and weight gain have not been supported by analyses of weight gain in smokers and non-smokers (Meyer 1978; D'Souza et al. 1981), though the effects of heavy smoking on birthweight were partially reversed by both of the dietary supplements evaluated in the randomized controlled trial of nutritional supplementation in New York (Rush *et al.* 1980).

The association between smoking and average gestational duration at delivery is very weak, a matter of a few days only. But this small average difference masks a significant excess of deliveries between 24 and 34 weeks' gestation in smokers, which is even greater for those smoking 20 or more cigarettes a day (Meyer 1977). Three pregnancy complications: placenta praevia, abruptio placentae, and premature rupture of the membranes are more common in smoking mothers. All three are precursors of preterm birth.

Though the birthweight findings are consistent

between studies, those on perinatal mortality are not. The most likely explanation is that the birthweight effect is the major factor with perinatal mortality secondary to it. The effect on perinatal mortality risk appears to be much more marked in women whose babies are already at high risk on biological or social grounds. Such women have an unfavourable birthweight distribution which becomes even more unfavourable as a result of maternal (and to a lesser extent paternal) smoking (Fabia 1973; Goldstein 1977; Rush and Cassano 1983). In women at low prior risk there is no convincing evidence that, in addition to its effect on birthweight, smoking increases the risk of perinatal death.

The association between cigarette smoking and spontaneous abortions is also inconsistent, and is possibly secondary to an association of both of them with alcohol (Harlap and Shiono 1980; Kline *et al.* 1980). Any effect of smoking on congenital malformations is vanishingly small (Evans *et al.* 1979). Long term effects of antenatal exposure to maternal smoking on the growth and development of the child are markedly reduced once social class, family size, birth order, and maternal height are taken into account (Goldstein 1977). Observational studies have consistently shown an apparently protective effect of smoking against pregnancy induced hypertension (see, for example, Butler and Alberman 1969; Donovan 1977; Lumley *et al.* 1985) but no such effect was observed in the one randomized controlled trial that assessed complications of pregnancy (M Sexton, personal communication).

The recent finding that maternal smoking in pregnancy was associated with an increased risk of certain childhood cancers (Stjernfeldt *et al.* 1986) was not confirmed in three similar case-control studies elsewhere (McKinney and Stiller 1986; Buckley *et al.* 1986; Li 1986). The reported association lacks both strength and consistency and it would be inappropriate to invoke this as a reason for quitting smoking in pregnancy.

Major reviews of the evidence on smoking and reproduction, including paternal effects not discussed here, have been published since 1980 (Abel 1980; US Department of Health and Human Services 1980; Sexton 1986).

The assumption among health professionals is that smoking during pregnancy is due to ignorance or to selfishness. Women either do not know the facts about the dangers, or they do not care about the fetus. The official response to this analysis is a mixture of information giving and moral persuasion. Such advice and exhortation may go well beyond the evidence:

'Do you want a cigarette more than you want your baby?' (poster headline).

'Almost certainly (smoking 30 cigarettes a day) causes mental and physical retardation in later childhood' (Bourne 1975).

Pregnant women are seen as a very suitable target group for health education because they have regular contact with the health care system. They are thought to be highly motivated to do anything which will promote fetal welfare (that is, when they are not being ignorant or selfish). The fact that many women's altered perceptions of food and smells in the first trimester causes at least some of them to give up smoking spontaneously may contribute to the belief that anti-smoking advice is particularly effective at this time.

The view from the other side, the target group, is rather different. Knowledge of the official view on the dangers of smoking is almost universal (Baric and MacArthur 1977; Graham 1977; Ryan *et al.* 1980), but action on the official view is much less common. However, the official explanation for the lack of action (that such women do not care about fetal welfare) is very different from the self-perceptions of women about their smoking behaviour.

Some reject the official view as untrue, basing their belief on other evidence which they see as much more relevant: 'Smoking can't be dangerous because all the midwives smoke a lot', or 'Smoking is okay—if there was anything wrong with it they wouldn't be allowed to advertise cigarettes'. Hilary Graham (1977) discusses some of the reasons why women may prefer to assess the costs and benefits of smoking during pregnancy from information acquired outside the medical profession, from personal and lay networks of information and advice.

Some accept the official view as probably true in general but not applicable to them personally : 'Smoking didn't affect my baby so I think it's okay in moderation.' (Ryan *et al.* 1980); 'It's supposed to make them underweight but I've always smoked nearly 40 a day and mine were all around 11 lb—that's with the smoking.'; 'Well, I smoke and they say you shouldn't, but our Paul was 8½ lb and he's never backward' (Graham 1977). The speakers regard personal experience as being more reliable than other sources of information, a behaviour not restricted to pregnant women or even to women in general. In professional settings, a regard for sincere personal beliefs held in opposition to scientific or statistical evidence is called 'acting on my clinical experience'.

Some women accept the official view and regard it as relevant to themselves, but view giving up smoking as something that would harm other people for whom they are already responsible. That is, fetal welfare conflicts with the welfare of her existing children or partner: 'I've cut down and I'm on 10 a day. If I cut down any more, I take it out on the baby which isn't fair on him. So it's one bairn or the other.' 'I gave up smoking for a bit, and I was even more irritable . . . I reckon if I get much worse, Dave'll move out!' (Graham 1977).

For the remaining women, smoking was an essential element in structuring their day, often defining brief times of freedom from the total demands of children, making explicit the end of the working day and adult time. For some women, smoking was the only thing they did for themselves. Housewives without paid employment may particularly value such structuring, since being a housewife/mother lacks the built in structuring devices of morning breaks, lunchtime, evenings after work, weekends and holidays.

It is not easy to stop smoking, and a recent review of smoking cessation provides evidence that it may be more difficult for women to do so than for men (Gritz 1978). The review by Jacobson (1986) points out that the social factors positively correlated with becoming an ex-smoker in men do not have the same predictive power in women. She sees women as stressed by their multiple responsibilities, lacking practical and emotional support, and at the same time blocked by social pressure from some types of reaction to stress, so that they become more vulnerable to accessible reducers of tension such as cigarettes.

The campaign against smoking in pregnancy has not been free of unwanted side-effects—many smokers spend the whole of their pregnancy in a state of guilt and inadequacy: 'I smoked a lot and I was scared all the way through about the effect it would have.' (Ryan *et al.* 1980); 'It's the cigarettes really that made me worry. I knew if anything went wrong with her, I'd blame the cigarettes and I'd know I'd done it myself, and my husband would know I'd done it. Knowing that, afterwards, that's what frightened me.' (Graham 1977). We do not know what the effects of such chronic stress and anxiety might be on the course of pregnancy and labour, or on the ultimate relationship with the child. We do know that more than half of the smoking women worry about smoking during pregnancy and that 10 per cent of smokers actually smoke more heavily in pregnancy (Baric *et al.* 1976; Ryan *et al.* 1980).

The global nature of much anti-smoking exhortation means that any bad outcome of pregnancy (including malformations and mental retardation) may be blamed on smoking retrospectively, even when this could not have been the cause. One randomized trial of anti-smoking advice tried to avoid this particular side-effect by excluding from the trial all the women who had previously had a perinatal death (Donovan 1977), but sometimes health professionals unwittingly reinforce the self-blame. A senior midwife, reporting on individual interviews held with mothers after a perinatal death, made the following comment: 'Some of the mothers pledged that they would in no way jeopardise another pregnancy and, *regardless of the cause of death*, intended to stop smoking in the event of conceiving again' (emphasis added) (Gilligan 1980).

4.1 Interventions to stop smoking in pregnancy

Despite the validity of the comments quoted above and the victim-blaming inherent in much anti-smoking activity, the strength of the evidence as to the harmfulness of cigarettes in pregnancy and the prevalence of smoking among pregnant women (30 per cent or more in the US, UK, Canada, Australia, New Zealand, and Norway (Sexton 1986) makes this behaviour a primary target for intervention.

Over the past decade the reported proportion of smokers who quit by the time of their first antenatal visit has been around 18 per cent (Baric *et al.* 1976; Donovan 1977; Sexton and Hebel 1984), with a few recent papers suggesting that this proportion is increasing (King and Eiser 1981; Windsor *et al.* 1985). Women who give up smoking in this way go on to have infants of equivalent weights to those of non-smokers (Butler and Alberman 1969; Donovan 1977). Typically, such women usually smoke less, have been able to stop before, have stronger beliefs about the dangers of smoking and have more support and encouragement at home for giving up (Baric *et al.* 1976; Ryan *et al.* 1980).

By contrast, to judge from the experience of control groups in randomized trials, very few smokers (<6 per cent) give up later in pregnancy (Baric *et al.* 1976; Sexton and Hebel 1984; Windsor *et al.* 1985; Lilley and Forster 1986). The implication of these findings is that the routine advice that is offered during antenatal care is relatively ineffective. Are there more effective interventions which can change women's smoking behaviour during pregnancy?

Ten randomized trials have tried to answer this question. Five trials aimed to ensure that information about the hazards of smoking plus firm advice to quit was actually given to every pregnant smoker. This advice seems to have had some, albeit limited success (Baric *et al.* 1976; Donovan 1977; Lilley and Forster 1986; MacArthur *et al.* 1987; Burling *et al.* unpublished, but discussed in Windsor and Orleans 1986). One possible exception to this conclusion is Donovan's study (1977), which appeared to show significant reductions in mean cigarette consumption, but its documentation of the extreme unreliability of self-reported smoking behaviour, and the possibility that socially desirable answers were given makes it difficult to be confident that the reported reductions in mean number of cigarettes smoked actually did occur. No data were available on the numbers who said that they had stopped smoking in this trial. Data from the other four trials are presented in Table 16.1.

The two trials utilizing feedback have yielded conflicting results (Table 16.2). One could detect no effect at all (Bauman *et al.* 1983); the other found a very marked increase in the number of women who stopped smoking (Reading *et al.* 1984). Both were assessed

Table 16.1 Effect of anti-smoking advice in pregnancy on continued smoking during pregnancy

Study	EXPT		CTRL		Odds ratio	Graph of odds ratios and confidence intervals
	n	(%)	*n*	(%)	(95% CI)	0.01 0.1 0.5 1 2 10 100
Baric *et al.* (1976)	54/63	(85.71)	45/47	(95.74)	0.33 (0.09–1.16)	
Burling (unpub)	62/69	(89.86)	68/70	(97.14)	0.30 (0.08–1.16)	
MacArthur *et al.* (1987)	484/493	(98.17)	483/489	(98.77)	0.67 (0.24–1.86)	
Lilley and Forster (1986)	73/77	(94.81)	72/73	(98.63)	0.31 (0.05–1.82)	
Typical odds ratio (95% confidence interval)					0.42 (0.22–0.80)	

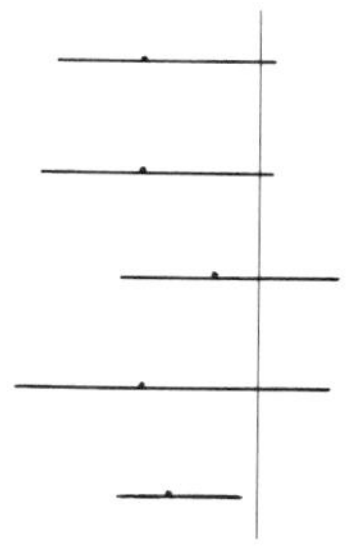

Table 16.2 Effect of feedback for smoking cessation in pregnancy on continued smoking during pregnancy

Study	EXPT		CTRL		Odds ratio	Graph of odds ratios and confidence intervals
	n	(%)	*n*	(%)	(95% CI)	0.01 0.1 0.5 1 2 10 100
Bauman *et al.* (1983)	36/36	(100.0)	43/43	(100.0)	1.00 (1.00–1.00)	
Reading *et al.* (1984)	20/39	(51.28)	20/26	(76.92)	0.34 (0.13–0.95)	
Typical odds ratio (95% confidence interval)					0.34 (0.13–0.95)	

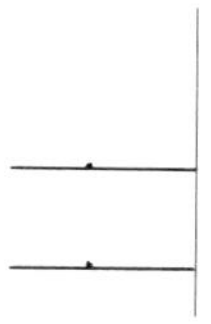

relatively soon after the feedback episode, so the longer term effects are uncertain. The 'ineffective' information was a demonstration of the carbon monoxide levels in the blood after smoking; the 'effective' information was an ultrasonogram of the fetus, discussed with and shown to the pregnant woman while it was being taken. Feedback may need to be related to the fetus to be perceived as relevant. This is borne out by the serendipitous finding, in a randomized controlled trial of the effect of cigarette smoking on fetal and maternal heart rate patterns, that 19 per cent of women stopped smoking after taking part in the study and that 37 per cent halved their smoking though all were heavy smokers who had continued to smoke through pregnancy (Kelly and O'Conor 1984).

Another trial (Loeb *et al.* unpublished observations, cited in Windsor and Orleans 1986) used individual and group counselling, but this intervention has not been tested properly since fewer than 10 per cent of participants received any of the counselling (Windsor and Orleans 1986). Lilley and Forster's trial (1986) refers to individual counselling in the title, but the detailed account of the intervention makes it clear that this was advice rather than counselling.

One quasi-experimental intervention was a mass media campaign about the risk of cigarettes, alcohol, and drugs in pregnancy. An unusual feature was the attempt to link the campaign with improved support, both family and social, for pregnant women, though no major change in facilities or resources was made available (Ryan *et al.* 1980). An evaluation of this relatively expensive project was unable to detect a significant increase in quitting among pregnant smokers within the city exposed to the campaign, but the post-intervention survey was too small to detect any likely effect (Chapman *et al.* 1982).

More successful interventions (Table 16.3) have emphasized *how* to give up smoking and have developed pregnancy-specific behavioural strategies (Sexton and Hebel 1984; Windsor *et al.* 1985). Sexton and Hebel supplemented written material with a home visit and intermittent telephone and mail contact (Nowicki *et al.* 1984) and so this intervention was relatively expensive though also more effective.

Only three trials have attempted to assess whether smoking cessation increases birthweight (Table 16.4). Although the trial by Donovan (1977) found no statistically significant difference in birthweight, that by Sexton and Hebel (1984) found a 92 g difference in favour of the intervention group, an effect compatible with the

Table 16.3 Effect of behavioural strategies for smoking cessation in pregnancy on continued smoking during pregnancy

Study	EXPT		CTRL		Odds ratio	Graph of odds ratios and confidence intervals
	n	(%)	*n*	(%)	(95% CI)	0.01 0.1 0.5 1 2 10 100
Windsor *et al.* (1985)	88/102	(86.27)	102/104	(98.08)	0.19 (0.07–0.54)	
Sexton and Hebel (1984)	221/326	(67.79)	316/328	(96.34)	0.14 (0.10–0.21)	
Typical odds ratio (95% confidence interval)					0.15 (0.10–0.22)	

Table 16.4. Birthweight effects in anti-smoking trials

Trial	Intervention gp		Control gp			
	Birthweight	(*n*)	Birthweight	(*n*)	D1	D2
Donovan (1977)	3172	263	3184	289	12	–
Sexton and Hebel (1984)	3278	326	3186	328	+90	–
MacArthur *et al.* (1987) all	3164	493	3130	489	+34	+28
para 0	3164	182	3068	196	+96	+68
para 1+	3163	311	3171	293	−8	−0.5

D1 Crude difference in birthweight
D2 Difference standardized for gestation, sex of child and height of mother

smoking cessation rates in the two groups. MacArthur *et al.* (1987) were able to show a small impact on the smoking behaviour of women having their first child and they detected a 68 g higher mean birthweight (standardized for gestational age at delivery, sex, and maternal height) in primiparae in the experimental group than in those in the control group, thus supporting the findings of Sexton and Hebel (1984).

The main problem with this most recent study is that the analysis by parity was not specified in the original design. Strictly speaking then, the conclusion that the intervention worked in primiparae but not in other women is a new hypothesis to be confirmed elsewhere. However, the differences in exposure to the intervention, in altered behaviour and in fetal size among women having their first child were consistent and coherent. The design of this study virtually rules out the possibility that the effect on fetal size was mediated by increased social support rather than a reduction in smoking. The former explanation had been proposed to explain why Sexton and Hebel (1984) showed an impact on fetal size while Donovan (1977) did not. The reason that Donovan's study findings are different probably has to do with the self-reporting problems discussed above.

Although MacArthur *et al.* (1987) also relied upon self-reports about smoking they tried to ensure the validity of the information and its comparability between the groups. The other great strength of their study was to test an inexpensive intervention, which could be incorporated into routine antenatal care, and to test it on a scale large enough to assess the effect on fetal size. An additional problem with this trial was the intervention itself: knowledge about the risks of smoking is already widespread, as discussed earlier and as the paper describes, the intervention was poorly implemented. Once again, the problem of staff compliance in a randomized trial is shown to be as important as patient compliance.

The policy implications of these findings are twofold. Since it is possible to alter smoking behaviour during pregnancy in a small minority of continuing smokers by a variety of strategies, one step is to repeat the trials with a stronger intervention such as the self-help manual already tested in the United States (Windsor *et al.* 1985) on a scale large enough to be able to detect an improvement in fetal size.

As with other interventions, it will be important to be aware of the possibility that adverse effects may occur in a subgroup of those exposed. In this regard it is encouraging that no trial has shown an increase in cigarette consumption in the intervention group compared with the controls. Recognition of the social and environmental context in which individuals take up or continue certain behaviours has led some people to condemn health education activities addressed to individuals as 'victim blaming'. (Perhaps fear of victim blaming was another factor in reducing staff compliance in the trial of MacArthur *et al.* 1987.) Interventions which focus on self-help and behavioural strategies are less likely to be perceived in this way and, in relation to quitting smoking can be soundly based on the current evidence that they seem to be more effective than advice.

At the same time, obstetricians and midwives should support the population strategies towards a progressive reduction in cigarette smoking in the whole of society: to increase cigarette excise taxes; to ban all forms of tobacco advertising; to challenge legally whether tobacco manufacturers are responsible for health outcomes; to enforce the laws which prohibit sales to children and adolescents; to make public areas non-smoking and to develop smoking policies for institutions and workplaces. The aim should be to make healthy choices easy choices.

5 Alcohol

The damaging effects of alcohol in pregnancy were described in the nineteenth century (Sullivan 1899) and rediscovered in France in the 1960s (Lemoine *et al.* 1968) and elsewhere in the 1970s. They comprise spontaneous abortion at relatively low levels of daily consumption (Harlap and Shiono 1980; Kline *et al.* 1980); fetal growth retardation (in which length is more affected than weight); mental retardation and a dysmorphic syndrome with variable features (all at much higher levels of consumption); and altered neonatal behaviour (see reviews by Streissguth 1978; Newman and Correy 1980). Only regular consumption of at least 28.5 ml alcohol per day was found to be associated with the developmental abnormalities, though one case has been reported following a single massive exposure to alcohol in the early weeks of pregnancy (Turner 1978, quoting a personal communication). Animal experiments confirm that alcohol administration to pregnant females causes severe fetal malformations, depressed growth and increased mortality in at least six species (see the reviews cited above and Newman 1986 for detailed references).

One slight puzzle in the evidence is that even women who are alcoholic may have an unaffected infant (Jones *et al.* 1974). There is also the undoubted fact that heavy alcohol use is highly correlated with heavy use of nicotine and caffeine, and often occurs with multiple nutritional deficiencies as well, raising the possibility that alcohol alone might not be a single causal factor. Unbiased, prospective ascertainment of maternal drinking status has been one of the major methodological problems in papers on the fetal alcohol syndrome (Neugut 1981). However, no other substance and no deficiency has been implicated in the specific pattern of abnormalities.

Ironically, many books on pregnancy, even those written in the 1970s, state that alcohol in moderation is harmless, and some even recommend a glass a day for relaxation (Wood and Reed 1973; Llewellyn-Jones 1978). As late as 1975 Baric and MacArthur (1977) found that 17 per cent of a sample of pregnant women in Bolton were drinking stout in the belief that it was particularly beneficial in pregnancy.

Campaigns to increase public awareness of the dangers of alcohol during pregnancy run the risk of arousing anxiety in some women already pregnant, partly because of the uncertainty about the safe lower limit for alcohol intake and also because of the possibility that the most dangerous time for dysmorphic effects may be the first trimester, even before the time when pregnancy is recognized. The very first weeks of pregnancy are often reported to be a period of high anxiety and depression (Ryan *et al.* 1980), which may increase drinking to relieve tension, even though alcohol often becomes unpalatable by six to eight week's gestation (Little *et al.* 1976). Some such reactions have been documented in reactions to a campaign in Seattle:

> 'An unexpected problem has been the considerable resistance and even anger that resulted . . . Complaints of sensationalism and scare tactics, as well as disbelief, have been heard . . . Also under attack was the program's recommendation of abstinence during pregnancy. Not all persons working in the field agree . . . (but) until a safe level of drinking is established, avoiding alcohol altogether is the safest course. Women who have been drinking infrequently are sometimes unduly alarmed by this recommendation . . .' (Little *et al.* 1980).

As the fetal alcohol syndrome includes those most feared outcomes, malformations, and mental retardation, it is no wonder that women are 'unduly alarmed' by the stated need for total abstinence prior to conception.

A large, population based study of prospectively recorded alcohol and pregnancy outcome in Australia was unable to detect any association with adverse outcomes below two standard drinks a day. The optimum birthweight was found among occasional social drinkers, who fared better than abstainers (Lumley *et al.* 1985).

The hard sell on maternal drinking—the Seattle paper states 'an interesting question still unanswered is whether drinking heavily during pregnancy constitutes child abuse *in utero*'—contrasts with the paucity of studies on those infants exposed to very high levels of alcohol (0.10 mg per cent) iatrogenically in the management of preterm labour in the 1960s.

Government action on alcohol and pregnancy has been to recommend, as the Food and Drug Administration did in the United States, that all alcoholic beverages contain a warning that ingestion by pregnant women can cause irrevocable fetal damage.

Policy development on alcohol and pregnancy requires, first of all, clarification as to the degree of risk around conception for low levels of regular alcohol consumption (fewer than two standard drinks a day), and for weekly or monthly 'binge' drinking. No formal trials of interventions to reduce high levels of consumption in pregnancy have been reported and it may be that in this regard the priority is better detection of heavy drinkers during antenatal care. A population policy is more difficult to define for alcohol than for tobacco, since there is no safe consumption level for the latter while for the former low levels of consumption may be not just harmless but actually beneficial. Policies in this area, other than ones to reduce total alcohol consumption and thus per capita consumption in order to reduce the numbers of people drinking at hazardous levels, are premature.

6 Working

When the *American College of Obstetrics and Gynecology* issued its guidelines on work in pregnancy (1977) the most striking exclusion from them was any mention of housework and child care as work, whether the discussion was about exposure to toxic chemicals (pesticides, household spray cleaners?) or lifting heavy weights (a toddler plus a folding push chair, a handicapped 7-year-old?). For example, although women who have previously given birth to two infants weighing less than 2 kg each are strongly advised not to work, no one suggested that such women be provided with free child care and daily household help throughout pregnancy. Equally, discussions of whether pregnant women should work usually pay scant attention to the implications for family health and welfare of the concomitant reduction in family income. In fact, the benefits of paid employment are rarely mentioned.

Research on the conflict between 'production' and 'reproduction', as well as ignoring women's unpaid work, has often failed to take into account parity, social class, maternal age, alcohol and tobacco use (Saurel-Cubizolles and Kaminski 1986). Healthy worker and infertile worker effects have also been excluded from consideration (Joffe 1985). The other methodological confusion has been to regard paid employment as a unitary category, lumping together women working with much less physical effort or stress than they would be exercising at home, with those whose work involves standing all day, or carrying heavy loads, or exposure to extremes of temperature or humidity. No wonder then that the results (reviewed recently by Garcia and Elbourne 1984; Joffe 1985; Saurel-Cubizolles and Kaminski 1986) of the 40 post-1945 studies are so confusing. The most consistent and clear-cut finding is the association between preterm delivery and an index of occupational fatigue which comprises measures of posture, machine work, physical effort, repetitive gestures, and environmental components of the workplace (Mamelle *et al.* 1984).

General advice on employment in pregnancy is clearly inappropriate. Where working conditions meet the criteria for occupational fatigue, women's requests for a change of work during pregnancy should be supported by those providing antenatal care. Apart from this situation it is extremely difficult to weigh up the net benefits and risks.

The research needs in this field have been summarized by Garcia and Elbourne (1984). It is difficult to generalize about the policy implications while nations differ so much in terms of maternity leave, income maintenance, paid leave to attend for antenatal care, availability of antenatal care outside usual working hours, subsidized or free home help and child care, taxation, child allowance, etc. (see Chapter 14). Most policy changes introduced with the aim of improving health and well-being are poorly evaluated: unintended consequences are likely when interventions are made in an already complex situation. Research on aspects of housework and child care which might lead to a comparable occupational fatigue index for unpaid employment is a priority.

7 Exercise

A letter to the *Lancet* implies that the attention paid to work has been misleading: we should have been worrying about the dangers of relaxation instead:

> '. . . it is often more important to prevent the annual holiday at the thirty-second week in a patient with a history of premature labour' (Smith 1981).

This recapitulates an old theme : in 1860 it was written that 'Pregnant women should stop running and dancing and avoid tiring journeys' (cited in Saurel-Cubizolles and Kaminski 1986). Travel remains a relatively unexplored research territory but running and dancing, not to mention aerobics, swimming, and cycling, currently generate a great deal of research and advice.

In 1980 9 per cent of Australian women aged 25–29 and 11 per cent of those from 30 to 34 engaged in vigorous exercise at least three times a week (National Heart Foundation 1982). Increasing emphasis on exercise in health promotion and illness prevention, plus the recognition of its subjectively rewarding nature, is leading some women—though still a minority and mostly advantaged—to wish to continue exercising through pregnancy. Unlike smoking, drinking, work and sex—all viewed as hazardous during pregnancy—exercise might possibly be beneficial. Elizabeth Cady Stanton, nineteenth-century feminist and mother of seven wrote:

> 'My girlhood was spent mostly in the open air . . . I would walk five miles before breakfast, or ride ten on horseback . . . so (in pregnancy) I dressed lightly, walked every day . . . The night before the birth I walked three miles. The child was born without a particle of pain' (Wertz and Wertz 1977).

Not all autobiographies of energetic and physically fit women bear out her assertions about the benefits of regular exercise, but it has been suggested intermittently for at least 200 years that complications of labour, especially failure to progress, may be prevented by maternal exercise before and during pregnancy.

Most studies have been small; most carried out on selected healthy women. More than half the women studied before 1983 were top class European or Russian athletes. The strongest evidence for any harmful effects of exercise is for a prepregnancy risk, that of infertility and menstrual dysfunction associated with strenuous endurance sports and the maintenance of a low bodyweight (Baker 1981). Maternal exercise in pregnancy was used as a stress test in the late 1960s and early 1970s. Adverse changes in fetal heart rate were detected in women with pregnancy complications. Most were very minor but occasional major ones have been described (Hon and Wohlgemuth 1962). Two recent observational studies have detected a lower birthweight (−500 g) among women exercising vigorously into the third trimester (Clapp and Dickstein 1984; Kulpa *et al.* 1987). Apart from these two findings there is insufficient evidence to support any recommendations on exercise in pregnancy. Beliefs about its dangers and beliefs about its benefits are equally unwarranted (reviewed by Lumley 1986).

Table 16.5 Randomized controlled trials of maternal exercise in pregnancy

Trial size	Intervention	Effects
Erkkola and Makela (1976) 21 + 23	Strenuous, 1 hr × 3/wk	Training effect heart volume ↑
Collings *et al.* (1983) 15	Strenuous, 50 min, regular 22–34 weeks	Training effect ↑ FHR
Pijpers *et al.* (1984b) 28	2 × 10 min semirecumbent cycling	MHR; MBP; FHR nc
Veille *et al.* (1985) 17	Running or cycling	MHR; MBP; FHR nc UA nc

FHR fetal heart rate
MHR maternal heart rate
MPB maternal blood pressure
UA uterine activity
nc no significant change
All trials were restricted to healthy women

Four randomized controlled trials of maternal exercise have been reported, all carried out in healthy women (Table 16.4). Two demonstrated training effects (Erkkola and Makela 1976; Collings *et al.* 1983)—the former on heart volume and the latter on fetal heart rate. Two other trials, using mild to moderate short term exercise, were unable to detect changes in fetal heart rate (Pijpers *et al.* 1984b) or uterine activity (Veille *et al.* 1985).

8 Relaxation

> 'There is nothing to fear but fear itself.'
> 'Don't be anxious, relax, there's nothing to worry about.'

Advice like this from doctor to pregnant patient is commonplace. Whether it is useful or easily acted upon is another matter. Since the 1940s, anxiety has been singled out as the most crucial negative emotion in childbearing. Read's description of the inevitable results of fear and pain in labour (1944) is a perfect example of the negative prescription remedy, or what a woman can expect if she does not do what she is told:

> 'This disrupting emotion of fear, and the concomitant pain, not only alters the course of labour but is directly or indirectly responsible for interference, haemorrhage, tissue injury, and the psychopathies in the mother as well as anoxemia, respiratory failure and exhaustion in the newborn infant. By these misfortunes not only the early progress of the child, but its physical and psychological development may be delayed or permanently damaged. Therefore the pain of labour, and its initiating cause, fear, extend their evil influence into the very roots of our social structure. They corrupt the minds and bodies of successive generations and bring distress and calamity where happiness and prosperity are the natural reward of a simple physiological performance'.

If a fraction of these dire predictions were true, only a brave or foolish woman would risk ignoring the role of fear in childbirth.

Certainly Read has no patience with women who refuse to believe in the possibility of painless childbirth. For Read, once information about childbirth replaced ignorance there remained no rational basis for fear of the reproductive process (1933, 1942). He was exasperated with women who did not agree with him:

> 'Their minds are irrational; they become abnormal. If a woman's mind is so constituted that it cannot admit a fact, her labour is as pathological as that of a woman whose pelvis is so constricted that it cannot admit a fetus'.

Read's intractable belief in his own theory prevents him from regarding those women whom he fails to convince as anything other than deluded in some way. Nothing can be done for women whose minds are constituted in this way; they are beyond help. Conveniently for Read, such an explanation of the method's failures precludes the need to question whether all fears can be attributed to ignorance or cured by knowledge.

These ideas have been echoed by others over the years and may have helped to prompt some of the empirical studies of maternal anxiety which have been conducted during the last 30 years or so. Much of this research has been directed by the belief that anxiety in pregnant women is a negative, destructive emotion, likely to lead to obstetrical complications. An unavoidable consequence of this dominant view of maternal anxiety has been a reduction in the scope of studies and a corresponding lack of recognition of other possible functions of anxiety and other significant variables that should be taken into account.

Anxiety in pregnant women is often seen as irrational. Women's fears that something will hurt their babies or themselves are thought to be unrealistic and unwarranted. In other words their anxiety is conceptualized as fundamentally neurotic. Obviously this view is inconsistent with an alternative formulation in which anxiety is seen as an adaptive response to real stress, with this response facilitating the development of coping behaviour.

There is evidence to suggest that both these views of anxiety may be relevant. For instance, several studies have reported that high levels of anxiety in pregnant women are correlated with obstetrical abnormalities in labour (Davids *et al.* 1961; McDonald *et al.* 1963; Crandon 1979); others have reported that moderate levels of anxiety in late pregnancy are associated with better postnatal adjustment (Pitt 1968; Breen 1975). Further studies have found that the level of anxiety in pregnancy is unrelated to complications in labour (Beck *et al.* 1980; Astbury 1980). Such seeming contradictory results demand closer scrutiny of the way in which anxiety has been conceptualised and assessed.

Apart from the distinction between 'neurotic' and 'objective' anxiety, much empirical research fails to distinguish between anxiety as a 'trait' and anxiety as a 'state'. 'Trait anxiety' refers to relatively stable individual differences between people in the tendency to perceive situations as threatening; 'state anxiety' refers to a transitory emotional state that varies in intensity and fluctuates over time (Spielberger *et al.* 1970). This distinction is important in determining the practical relevance of findings from studies on maternal anxiety. For example, those studies which have reported a significant correlation between high maternal anxiety late in pregnancy and obstetrical complications in labour have all measured anxiety as a 'trait' (Davids *et al.* 1961; McDonald *et al.* 1963; Crandon 1979). Thus the women classified as being highly anxious in these studies were anxious in the 'stable personality trait' sense of the term. They were anxious women who happened to be pregnant. Even if stable personality traits can be demonstrated to be counterproductive (and this is by no means conclusive), they are unlikely to be altered in a short period of time. Nevertheless, the finding that high levels of trait anxiety may be associated with obstetrical complications is used as the basis for advising a reduction of anxiety, usually through some form of childbirth preparation (see Chapter 20). Yet any progress aimed at reducing anxiety must have as a starting point an understanding of the source or sources of that anxiety. A high score on a measure of anxiety in late pregnancy does not mean in itself that a woman is highly anxious about pregnancy or the prospect of labour.

Studies since 1970 have indicated the importance of identifying the sources of stress and anxiety rather than assuming that they must necessarily be related to pregnancy. Gorsuch and Key (1974) investigated abnormalities of pregnancy and labour as a function of both anxiety and life stress. They measured 'state anxiety' and 'trait anxiety' at different stages during pregnancy. They found that whereas 'state anxiety' contributed significantly to difficulties in the first trimester of pregnancy, life stress was more significant in the second and third trimesters. Moreover, the greater the stress of live events in the second and third trimesters, the more likely it was for obstetrical complications to occur.

Although they were not specifically investigating anxiety, Nilsson and Almgren (1970) also found that a lower than average level of education was significantly correlated with the reporting of a higher number of psychological symptoms during pregnancy. Allied emotions such as depression (of which anxiety is a major component) have been reported to be significantly affected by social and environmental factors operating on young working class mothers (Brown and Harris 1978). Recognition that social and environmental factors may trigger stress and anxiety (see Newton and Hunt 1984) is very relevant if useful advice is to be given to anxious pregnant women. If, for example, anxiety stems largely from crowded housing conditions, unemployment, marital conflict, or inadequate income, it is unlikely that it will be alleviated by a course of childbirth preparation which stresses relaxation and breathing patterns in labour or by other forms of stress management. Social support might be more helpful.

Apart from social factors, the health of pregnant women needs to be considered in interpreting their psychological well-being. While early work in psychosomatic medicine during the 1940s considered that the body was as powerful a causative agent on the mind as the mind was on the body, this has not been a popular view in thinking about childbirth. A study by Erickson (1976a) suggests it is a view which deserves reconsideration. In a large study of 717 primiparae and multiparae, Erickson examined the link between psychological variables, health problems and later obstetrical complications. Though she found that there was a significant correlation between psychological variables in pregnancy and obstetrical problems in labour, after controlling statistically for the effect of health problems during pregnancy, no statistically significant relationship remained for primiparae. For multiparae, psychological variables continued to have predictive power even after health problems were taken into account (Erickson 1976b).

Finally, there is some evidence which challenges the long held view that anxiety is a central emotion in pregnancy and labour. Barclay and Barclay (1976) compared non-pregnant with pregnant women in order to assess knowledge and attitudes towards pregnancy and labour. Although pregnant women were more knowledgeable than non-pregnant women, this greater knowledge did not appear to contribute to reduced anxiety; in fact, there was no significant difference in anxiety between the two groups of women. Unexpectedly, non-pregnant women expressed more fear for the unborn fetus and expected they would feel a greater degree of depression in pregnancy than was actually experienced by the pregnant women. Another study comparing women who attended childbirth preparation classes with those who did not found that, while prepared women were significantly more knowledgeable about reproduction, they were not significantly less anxious (Astbury 1980).

A randomized controlled trial of counselling in 57 women having their first pregnancy was unable to detect any psychological benefits from the intervention. The authors commented that neither group showed more regression, introversion, or primitive affect than would be engendered by the stresses of other life periods (Shereshefsky and Lockman 1974).

These more recent studies suggest that, contrary to the claims of Dick Read and others, complications in childbirth arise from a variety of causes. Where anxiety is involved, it is clear that it can derive from the actual conditions of women's lives, not just from their ignorance about the reproductive process. Very little of the published research has managed to clarify the nature and function of maternal anxiety and there is urgent need for well-designed studies in which hypotheses can be rigorously tested. (See Chapter 15).

9 Conclusions

The images which underlie the advice industry are threefold: the perfect child, the perfect mother, and the perfect birth. The perfect child, attainable by following the right instructions, is of course a mirage. All children are less than perfect. In order to be a perfect mother and have the perfect birth, a pregnant woman is exhorted to lead a selfless, healthy life, uncontaminated by sex, cigarettes, alcohol, employment, or anxiety. As we have shown, the evidence for most of these exhortations is slight. Where the evidence is stronger, the flaw has been in the way that research and prescription fail to take into account the real lives and responsibilities of women.

References

Abel EL (1980). Smoking during pregnancy: a review of effects on growth and development of offspring. Hum Biol, 52: 593–625.

Alberman E, Pharaoh P, Chamberlain G (1977). Smoking and the fetus. Lancet, ii: 36–37.

American College of Obstetricians and Gynecologists (1977). Guidelines on pregnancy and work. Washington DC: US Department of Health, Education and Welfare, Contract No. 210–76–1059.

Aronson ME, Nelson PI (1967). Fatal air embolism in pregnancy resulting from an unusual sexual act. Obstet Gynecol, 30: 127–130.

Astbury J (1980). Labour pain: the role of childbirth education, information and expectation. In: Problems in Pain. Peck C, Wallace M (eds). Oxford: Pergamon Press.

Baker E (1981). Menstrual dysfunction and hormonal status in athletic women: a review. Fertil Steril, 36: 691–696.

Barclay RL, Barclay MD (1976). Aspects of the normal psychology of pregnancy: the mid trimester. Am J Obstet Gynecol, 125: 207–211.

Baric L, MacArthur C (1977). Health norms in pregnancy. Br J Prev Soc Med, 31: 30–38.

Baric L, MacArthur C, Sherwood M (1976). A study of health education aspects of smoking in pregnancy. Int J Health Educ, 19: Suppl.

Bauman KE, Bryan, ES, Dent, CW, Koch GG (1983). The influence of observing carbon monoxide levels on cigarette smoking by public prenatal patients. Am J Public Health, 73: 1089–1091.

Beck NC, Siegel LJ, Davidson NP, Kormeier S, Breitenstien A, Hall DG (1980). The prediction of pregnancy outcome:

maternal preparation, anxiety and attitudinal sets. J Psychsom Res, 24: 343–352.

Berg BJ van den (1977). Epidemiologic observations of prematurity: effects of tobacco, smoking and alcohol. In: The Epidemiology of Prematurity. Reed DM, Stanley FJ (eds). Baltimore: Urban & Schwarzenberg, pp 157–176.

Bing E, Coleman L (1977). Making Love During Pregnancy. New York: Bantam Books.

Blankfield A, Wood C (1971). A profile of the obstetric patient: a social psychology report on patients from a Melbourne public hospital. Med J Austral, 1: 1320–1325.

Bourne G (1975). Pregnancy. London: Pan Books.

Breen D (1975). The Birth of a First Child. London: Tavistock.

Brown GW, Harris T (1978). The Social Origins of Depression. London: Tavistock.

Buckley JD, Hobbie WL, Ruccione K, Sather HN, Woods WG, Hammond GD (1986). Maternal smoking during pregnancy and the risk of childhood cancer. Lancet, ii: 520.

Burling T, Bigelow G, Robinson C, Mead A (1983)—cited in Windsor and Orleans (1986).

Butler N, Alberman E (1969). Perinatal Problems. The Second Report of the British Perinatal Mortality Survey. Edinburgh: Churchill Livingstone.

Cartwright A (1979). The Dignity of Labour? A Study of Childbearing and Induction. London: Tavistock.

Chamberlain GVP, Lumley J (eds) (1986). Prepregnancy Care. Chichester: John Wiley.

Chapman A, Coates D, Dawbin D, McGregor C, Outram S, Roff C, Spencer S (1982). The pregnant pause campaign. An intervention programme to reduce drug use in pregnancy. Part B: Programme evaluation. New South Wales Department of Health, Division of Drug and Alcohol Services, DAS 82–021.

Clapp JF, Dickstein S (1984). Endurance exercise and pregnancy outcome. Med Sci Sports Exer, 16: 556–562.

Committee to Study the Prevention of Low Birth Weight, Division of Health Promotion and Disease Prevention, Institute of Medicine (1985). Preventing low birth weight. Washington DC: National Academy Press.

Collings CA, Curet LB, Mullin JP (1983). Maternal and fetal responses to a maternal aerobic exercise program. Am J Obstet Gynecol, 145: 702–707.

Crandon AJ (1979). Maternal anxiety and obstetric complications. J Psychosom Res, 23: 109–111.

Davids A, De Vault S, Talmadge M (1961). Anxiety, pregnancy and childbirth abnormalities. J Consult Psychol, 25: 76–77.

Davies JM, Latto IP, Jones JG, Veale A, Wardrop CAJ (1979). Effects of stopping smoking for 48 hours on oxygen availability from the blood: a study on pregnant women. Br Med J, 2: 355–356.

Donovan JW (1977). A randomized controlled trial of anti-smoking advice in pregnancy. Br J Prev Soc Med, 31: 355–356.

D'Souza SW, Black P, Richards B (1981). Smoking in pregnancy: Associations with skinfold thickness, maternal weight gain and fetal size at birth. Br Med J, 1: 1661–1663.

D'Souza SW, Williams N, Jennison RF (1978). Effect of smoking during pregnancy upon the haematological values of cord blood. Br J Obstet Gynaecol, 85: 495–499.

Enkin M (1980). What the health professional can do to influence life styles. Proceedings of the Second Symposium on the Prevention of Handicapping Conditions of Prenatal or Perinatal Origin, Calgary, Alberta, Alberta Social Services and Community Health.

Erickson MT (1976a). The influence of health factors on psychological variables predicting complications of pregnancy, labour and delivery. J Psychosom Res, 20: 21–24.

Erickson MT (1976b). The relationship between psychological variables and specific complications of pregnancy, labour and delivery. J Psychosom Res, 20: 207–210.

Erkkola R, Makela M (1976). Heart volume and physical fitness of parturients. Ann Clin Res, 8: 15–21.

Evans DR, Newcombe RB, Campell H (1979). Maternal smoking habits and congenital malformations: A population study. Br Med J, 2: 171–173.

Fabia J (1973). Cigarettes pendant la grossesse, poids de naissance et mortalite perinatale. Can Med Assoc J, 109: 1104–1109.

Falicov C (1973). Sexual adjustment during first pregnancy and post partum. Am J Obstet Gynecol, 117: 991–1000.

Foresight (no date). The Association for Preconceptual Care. Guidelines for future parents. Surrey: Foresight, pp 5–42.

Foresight Newsletter (1986). 1.

Garcia J, Elbourne D (1984). Future research on work in pregnancy. In: Pregnant Women at Work. Chamberlain G (ed). London: Royal Society of Medicine and Macmillan Press, pp 273–278.

Gennser G, Marsal K, Brantmark B (1975). Maternal smoking and fetal breathing movements. Am J Obstet Gynecol, 123: 861–867.

Gilligan M (1980). Perinatal mortality enquiries at district level. In: Perinatal Audit and Surveillance. Chalmers I, McIlwaine G (eds). London: Royal College of Obstetricians and Gynaecologists, pp 148–158.

Goldstein H (1977). Smoking in pregnancy: some notes on the statistical controversy. Br J Prev Soc Med, 31: 13–17.

Goodlin RC, Keller DW, Raffin M (1971). Orgasm during late pregnancy. Obstet Gynecol, 38: 916–920.

Goodlin RC, Schmidt W, Creevy DC (1972). Uterine tension and fetal heart-rate during maternal orgasm. Obstet Gynecol, 39: 125–127.

Goodman JDS, Visser FGA, Dawes GS (1984). Effects of maternal cigarette smoking on fetal trunk movements, fetal breathing movements and the fetal heart rate. Br J Obstet Gynaecol, 91: 657–661.

Gorsuch RL, Key MK (1974). Abnormalities of pregnancy as a function of anxiety and life stress. Psychosom Med, 36: 352–362.

Graham H (1977). Smoking in pregnancy: the attitudes of expectant mothers. Soc Sci Med, 10: 399–405.

Gritz ER (1978). Women and smoking: a realistic appraisal. In: Progress in Smoking Cessation. Schwartz JL (ed). New York: American Cancer Society, pp 119–141.

Grudzinskas JG, Watson C, Chard T (1979). Does sexual intercourse cause fetal distress? Lancet, ii: 692–693.

Hall MH, Carr-Hill RA (1985). The significance of uncertain gestation for obstetric outcome. Br J Obstet Gynaecol, 92: 452–460.

Harlap S, Shiono PH (1980). Alcohol, smoking and incidence

of spontaneous abortion in the first and second trimester. Lancet, ii: 173–176.

Herbst AL (1979). Coitus and the fetus (Editorial). New Engl J Med, 301: 1235–1236.

Hon EH, Wohlgemuth R (1962). The electronic evaluation of fetal heart rate. IV: The effect of maternal exercise. Am J Obstet Gynecol, 81: 361–372.

Jacobson B (1986). Beating the Ladykillers: Women and Smoking. London: Pluto Press.

Javert CT (1957). Spontaneous and Habitual Abortion. New York: McGraw-Hill.

Joffe M (1985). Biases in research on reproduction and women's work. Int J Epidemiol, 14: 118–123.

Jones KL, Smith DW, Streissguth AP, Myrianthopoulos NC (1974). Outcome in offspring of chronic alcoholic women. Lancet, i: 1076–1078.

Kellogg JH (1902). The Ladies' Guide in Health and Disease. Melbourne: Echo Publishing Co.

Kelly J, O'Conor M (1984). Smoking in pregnancy: effects on mother and fetus. Br J Obstet Gynaecol, 91: 111–117.

King J, Eiser JR (1981). A strategy for counselling pregnant smokers. Health Educ J, 40: 66–68.

Kline J, Shrout P, Stein Z, Susser M, Warburton D (1980). Drinking during pregnancy and spontaneous abortion. Lancet, ii: 176–180.

Kulpa PJ, White BM, Visscher R (1987). Aerobic exercise in pregnancy. Am J Obstet Gynecol, 156: 1395–1403.

Lancet (1985), Misconceptions about preconceptional care (Leading article). Lancet, ii: 1046–1047.

Lehrmann E (1988). Prepregnancy counselling. Birth (in press).

Lemoine P, Harrousseau H, Borteyni JP (1968). Les enfants des parents alcooliques. Anomalies observees. A propos de 127 cas. Ouest Médicale, 21: 476–482.

Li FP (1986). Maternal smoking during pregnancy and the risk of childhood cancer. Lancet, ii: 520.

Lilley J, Forster DP (1986). A randomized controlled trial of individual counselling of smokers in pregnancy. Public Health, 100: 309–315.

Limner RR (1969). Sex and the Unborn Child. New York: Julian Press.

Little RE, Schulz F, Mandell W (1976). Drinking during pregnancy. J Stud Alcohol, 37: 375–379.

Little RE, Streissguth AP, Guzinski GM (1980). Prevention of fetal alcohol syndrome: a model program. Alcoholism: (NY) Clinical and Experimental Research, 4: 185–189.

Llewellyn-Jones D (1978). Everywoman: A Gynaecological Guide for Life (2nd edn). London: Faber & Faber.

Loeb B, Bailey J, Waage G, Feldman V (1983)—cited in Windsor and Orleans (1986).

Longo LD (1977). The biological effects of carbon monoxide on the pregnant woman, fetus and newborn infant. Am J Obstet Gynecol, 129: 69–103.

Lumley J (1978). Sexual feelings in pregnancy and after childbirth. Austral J Obstet Gynaecol, 18: 114–117.

Lumley J (1986). Exercise and stress. In: Prepregnancy Care. Chamberlain GVP, Lumley J (eds). Chichester: John Wiley, pp 209–221.

Lumley J (1987). The epidemiology of prematurity. In: Prematurity. Yu V, Wood C (eds). London: Churchill Livingstone, pp 1–24.

Lumley J, Correy J, Newman N, Curran J (1985). Cigarette smoking, alcohol consumption and fetal outcome in Tasmania, 1981–2. Austral NZ J Obstet Gynaecol, 25 33–40.

MacArthur C, Newton JR, Knox EG (1987). Effect of anti-smoking health education on fetal size: A randomised controlled trial. Br J Obstet Gynaecol, 94: 295–300.

McDonald RL, Gynther MD, Christakos AC (1963). Relations between maternal anxiety and obstetric complications. Psychosom Med, 25: 357–363.

McKinney PA, Stiller CA (1986). Maternal smoking during pregnancy and the risk of childhood cancer. Lancet, ii: 519.

Mamelle N, Laumon B, Lazar P (1984). Prematurity and occupational activity during pregnancy. Am J Epidemiol, 119: 309–322.

Martin TR, Bracken MB (1986). Association of low birth weight with passive smoke exposure in pregnancy. Am J Epidemiol, 124: 633–642.

Masters WH, Johnson VE (1966). Pregnancy and sexual response I: Anatomy and physiology. In: Human Sexual Response. Masters WH, Johnson VE (eds). Boston: Little, Brown.

Meyer MB (1977). Effects of maternal smoking and altitude on birth weight and gestation. In: The Epidemiology of Prematurity. Reed BM, Stanley FJ (eds). Baltimore: Urban & Schwarzenberg, pp 81–101.

Meyer MB (1978). How does maternal smoking affect birth weight and maternal weight gain? Am J Obstet Gynecol, 131: 888–893.

Mills JL, Harlap S, Harley EE (1981). Should coitus late in pregnancy be discouraged? Lancet, ii: 136–138.

Mitchell MD, Flint APF, Bibby J, Brunt J, Arnold JM, Anderson ABM (1977). Rapid increases in plasma prostaglandin concentration after vaginal examinations and amniotomy. Br Med J, 2: 1183–1185.

Morris NM (1975). The frequency of sexual intercouse during pregnancy. Arch Sex Behav, 4: 510–507.

Naeye RL (1979a). Coitus and associated amniotic fluid infections. New Engl J Med, 301: 1198–2000.

Naeye RL (1979b). The duration of maternal smoking and fetal and placental disorders. Early Hum Dev, 3: 229–237.

Naeye RL, Ross S (1982). Coitus and chorioamnionitis: a prospective study. Early Hum Dev, 6: 91–97.

Naeye RL, Tafari N (1983). Risk Factors in Pregnancy and Diseases of the Newborn. Baltimore: Williams & Wilkins, pp 198–212.

Najman JM, Keeping JD, Chang A, Morrison J, Western JS (1983). Employment, unemployment and the health of pregnant women. New Doctor, 28: 9–12.

National Heart Foundation (1982). Risk Factor Prevalence Study. Canberra: National Heart Foundation.

Neugut RH (1981). Epidemiological appraisal of the literature on the fetal alcohol syndrome in humans. Early Hum Dev, 5: 411–429.

Newman N (1986). Alcohol. In: Prepregnancy Care. Chamberlain GVP, Lumley J (eds). Chichester: John Wiley and Sons, pp 183–208.

Newman N, Correy JF (1980). Effects of alcohol in pregnancy. Clinical Review. Med J Austral, 2: 5–10.

Newton RW, Hunt LP (1984). Psychosocial stress in pregnancy and its relation to low birth weight. Br Med J, 288: 1191–1194.

Nilsson A, Almgren PE (1970). Paranatal emotional adjustments: a prospective investigation of 165 women. Acta Psychiatr Scand (Suppl), 220.

Noonan JT (1965). Contraception. New York: Mentor-Omega; Cambridge, Massachusetts: Harvard University Press.

Nowicki P, Gintzig L, Hebel JR, Lathem R, Miller V, Sexton M (1984). Effective smoking intervention during pregnancy. Birth, 11: 217–224.

Perkins RP (1979). Sexual behavior and response in relation to complications of pregnancy. Am J Obstet Gynecol, 134: 498–505.

Pijpers L, Wladimiroff JW, McGhie JS, Bom N (1984a). Acute effects of maternal smoking on the maternal and fetal cardiovascular system. Early Hum Dev, 10: 95–101.

Pijpers L, Wladimiroff JW, McGhie JS, Bom N (1984b). Effect of short term maternal exercise on maternal and fetal cardiovascular dynamics. Br J Obstet Gynaecol, 91: 1081–1086.

Pitt B (1968). 'Atypical' depression following childbirth. Br J Psychiatry, 114: 1325–1335.

Plovanic P, Burrell R, Lumley J (in preparation).

Pugh WE, Fernandez FL (1953). Coitus in late pregnancy. Obstet Gynecol, 2: 636–642.

Rayburn WF, Wilson EA (1980). Coital activity and premature delivery. Am J Obstet Gynecol, 137: 972–974.

Read GD (1933). Natural Childbirth. London: Heinemann.

Read GD (1942). Revelation of Childbirth. London: Heinemann.

Read GD (1944). Childbirth without Fear. New York: Harper Bros.

Reading AE, Campbell S, Cox DN, Sledmere CM (1984). Health beliefs and health care behaviours in pregnancy. Psychol Med, 2: 379–383.

Rubin DH, Krasilnikoff PA, Leventhal JM, Werle B, Berget A (1986). Effect of passive smoking on birthweight. Lancet, ii: 415–417.

Rush D (1986). Nutrition in the preparation for pregnancy. In: Prepregnancy Care. Chamberlain GVP, Lumley J (eds). Chichester: John Wiley, pp 113–139.

Rush D, Cassano P (1983). Relationship of cigarette smoking and social class to birth weight and perinatal mortality among all births in Britain, 5–11 April 1970. J Epidemiol Community Health, 37: 249–255.

Rush D, Stein ZA, Susser M (1980). A randomised controlled trial of prenatal nutritional supplementation in New York City. Pediatrics, 65: 683–697.

Ryan P, Booth R, Coates D, Chapman A, Healy P (1980). Experiences of pregnancy. Pregnant Pause Campaign. Health Commission of New South Wales, Division of Drug and Alcohol Services.

Saurel-Cubizolles MJ, Kaminski M (1986). Work in pregnancy: its evolving relationship with perinatal outcome. A review. Soc Sci Med, 22: 431–442.

Sexton M (1986). Smoking. In: Prepregnancy care. Chamberlain GVP, Lumley J (eds), Chichester: John Wiley and Sons, pp 141–164.

Sexton M, Hebel JR (1984). A clinical trial of change in maternal smoking and its effect on birth weight. JAMA, 251: 911–915.

Shereshefsky PM, Lockman RF (1974). Comparison of counselled and non-counselled groups and within group differences. In: Psychological Aspects of a First Pregnancy and Early Postnatal adaptation. Shereshefsky PM, Yarrow LJ (eds). New York: Raven Press, pp 151–163.

Silverman W (1980). Retrolental fibroplasia: a modern parable. New York: Grune & Stratton.

Smith AW (1981). Bed rest in pregnancy. Lancet, i: 1319–1320.

Solberg DA, Butler J, Wagner NN (1973). Sexual behavior in pregnancy. New Engl J Med, 288: 1098–1103.

Spielberger CD, Gorsuch RL, Lushene RE (1970). Manual for the State-Trait Anxiety Inventory. Palo Alto, California: Consulting Psychologists Press.

Stjernfeldt M, Lindsten J, Berglund K, Ludvigsson J (1986). Maternal smoking during pregnancy and risk of childhood cancer. Lancet, i: 1350–1352.

Stopes M (1918). Married Love: A New Contribution to the Solution of Sex Difficulties. New York: Eugenics Publishing Co. (reissued 1930).

Streissguth AP (1978). Fetal alcohol syndrome: an epidemiological perspective. Am J Epidemiol, 107: 467–478.

Sullivan WC (1899). A note on the influence of maternal inebriety on the offspring. J Med Sci, 45: 489–503.

Tolor A, Di Grazia PV (1976). Sexual attitudes and behavior patterns during and following pregnancy. Arch Sex Behav, 5: 539–551.

Turner G (1978). The fetal alcohol syndrome (Editorial). Med J Austral, 1: 18–19.

US Department of Health and Human Services (1980). The health consequences of smoking for women. A report of the Surgeon-General. Washington DC: Department of Health and Human Services, Public Health Service, Office of the Assistant Secretary for Health, Office on Smoking and Health.

Veille JC, Hohiner AR, Burry K, Speroff L (1985). The effects of exercise on uterine activity in the last eight weeks of pregnancy. Am J Obstet Gynecol, 151: 727–730.

Wagner NN, Butler JC, Sanders JP (1976). Prematurity and orgasmic coitus during pregnancy; data on a small sample. Fertil Steril, 27: 911–915.

Wertz RW, Wertz DC (1977). Lying-in: A History of Childbirth in America. New York: Schocken Books.

Windsor RA, Orleans CT (1986). Guidelines and methodological standards for smoking cessation research among pregnant women: improving the science and art. Health Educ Qtrly, 13: 131–161.

Windsor RA, Cutter G, Morris J, Reese Y, Manzella B, Bartlett EE, Samuelson C, Spanos D (1985). The effectiveness of smoking cessation methods for smokers in public health maternity clinic: a randomized trial. Am J Public Health, 75: 1389–1392.

Wood C, Reed D (1973). ABZ of Pregnancy. Melbourne: Nelson.

Yerushalmy J (1971). The relationship of parents' cigarette smoking to the outcome of pregnancy—implications as to the problem of inferring causation from observed associations. Am J Epidemiol, 93: 443–456.

Yerushalmy J (1972). Infants with low birth weight born before their mothers started to smoke cigarettes. Am J Obstet Gynecol, 112: 277–284.

17 Effects of changes in protein and calorie intake during pregnancy on the growth of the human fetus

David Rush

1 Introduction

The relationship between the diet of the mother and the well-being of the fetus and infant continues to be a matter of great importance, uncertainty, and controversy. A great deal of information has become available since my previous review of the effects of changing protein and calorie intake during pregnancy (Rush 1982).

Observational studies, in which there has been no change from the diet the pregnant woman would otherwise have taken, have generated conflicting and uncertain results. Since only relatively small changes in birthweight are likely to occur, study of large populations is required. The precise techniques of nutritional balance studies cannot be applied on such a large scale, and we are left with a variety of field methods for determining nutritional status and diet, all of which are plagued by problems of precision or meaning.

Observational studies must also cope with the many other aspects of the pregnant woman's life that covary with diet and nutrition. Whenever there are limits to nutritional intake imposed by economic, educational, social or other constraints, there are likely to be accompanying stresses, such as exposure to infection, the need for physical labour, inadequate housing or frequent family disruption. Studies of groups with isolated nutritional deprivation, such as middle class women imposing the macrobiotic diet on themselves and their offspring (Grieve *et al.* 1979), remain of great interest and where possible should be pursued.

2 Studies of the effects of famine imposed on previously well-nourished populations

In most chronically deprived populations, average birthweights are lower than in more affluent populations. The amount that birthweight is depressed specifically by diet, however, will probably remain uncertain in the absence of well-designed feeding experiments. During acute famine, dietary restriction is accompanied by other insults, but the effects of severe food deprivation can probably be inferred when the deprivation has been abrupt and involves populations that have been previously well nourished. This chapter will address three studies of the effects of maternal famine: Antonov (1947) described the effects of the seige of Leningrad from 1941 to 1943; Stein *et al.* (1975), following the original report of Smith (1947), studied the acute starvation of the winter of 1944–45 in Holland; and Dean (1951) studied residents of Wuppertal in 1945–46 and reviewed the earlier literature. (Table 17.1)

Table 17.1 Studies of the effects of famine on previously well-nourished population

Authors	Population studied	Assignment method/ research design	Study group No.	Study group Treatment	Control group No.	Control group Treatment	Results	Comments
Antonov (1947)	Leningrad; famine during siege of 1941–43, especially winter of 1941–42	Comparison with pre- and post-famine births in one clinic	414	Born Jan.–June 1942 (height of famine)	11319	Born 1939–41, and July–Dec. 1942	Jan.–June 1942 / Other Stillbirth (%) 5.6 (23) / 2.6 (300) Premature live birth (%) 41.2 (161) / 6.5 (5)* Neonatal death (%) 21.2 (83) / 5.2 (1)* <2500 g (%) 49.2 (181) / ? Mean birthweight (g) 2789 (255) / 3338 (2828) * rate for July–Dec. 1942 only ( ) = *n*, numerator	Winter of 1941–42 was very severe, and fuel and other supplies were non-existent. Population under great physical strain. Fertility drastically reduced.
Stein *et al.* (1975) Smith (1947)	Holland; acute starvation 1944–45. For reproductive processes, data from 5 teaching hospitals	Retrospective cohort study; comparison with period before and after famine, and with areas not exposed	2411	Famine area	2439	Control areas	Birthweight (g) D.o.B. / Famine area, No. / Control areas: North, No., South, No. Pre-famine 8–11/1944: 3358, 453 / 3385, 209, 3324, 181 12/44–1/45: 3126, 222 / 3309, 123, 3357, 74 2/45–6/45: 3019, 519 / 3199, 350, 3302, 276 Total famine 12/44–6/45: 3051, 741 / 3228, 473, 3313, 350 Post-famine 7/45–3/46: 3320, 1214 / 3361, 608, 3367, 617 Excessive very early prematurity: ↑ infant mortality With exposure early in pregnancy: ↑ perinatal mortality ↑ CNS abnormality, ↑ later obesity With exposure late in pregnancy: ↓ later obesity No behavioural effects in young men exposed *in utero*	Differential fertility not an adequate explanation for results (i.e. results for those who conceived before famine, in general, not different from those who conceived during famine).
Dean (1951)	Wuppertal, Germany; period of extreme scarcity of food, 1945–46, particularly 1945	Comparison with pre-scarcity births in one clinic	1906 2438	1945: severe shortages 1946: official rations: 1052 cal/d (6/46) to 1550 cal/d	2434	1937–38	1945 / 1946 / 1937–38 Mean birthweight (%) Private patients 3325 / 3414 / 3495 Others 3103 / 3213 / 3330 Median birthweight 3250 / 3300 / 3400 % ⩽2400 g 8.2 / 6.7 / 4.3	Decrease in amount of breast milk during scarcity. 20% of births in study clinic in 1937–38, 70% in 1946.

In both Leningrad and The Netherlands, famine was associated with a marked decrease in fertility. Because of the sudden onset and cessation of the Dutch famine, however, the effects on fetal growth could be distinguished from those on fertility; the effects on birthweight were among infants conceived before the onset of famine.

Conditions in Leningrad were extremely severe. The famine was during a long and bitter winter, in which fuel was almost non-existent, and grinding physical labour was inescapable. Mean birthweight during the worst period in Leningrad was 2789 g, a depression of almost 550 g compared with birthweight during the period prior to 1941. During the Dutch famine, in which official rations fell to as low as 590 calories a day, mean birthweight fell by 300 g; there was little difference between those exposed to the famine during the third trimester alone or during both the second and third trimesters. There was no birthweight depression among infants who were conceived during the famine but whose mothers received adequate rations during the third trimester. This suggests that adequate nutrition during the third trimester can alleviate the effect on birthweight of earlier acute nutritional deprivation.

In Wuppertal, when food shortages were worst (official rations were down to 1052 calories a day) the mean birthweight was depressed by 170 g in babies born to women receiving private care, and by 227 g in those born to women receiving public care. Later, when rations varied between 1052 and 1550 calories per day, the depression was 81 g among babies of women receiving private care and 117 g among those of women receiving public care. It is not possible from published reports to distinguish between the effects of food deprivation on those who conceived before the onset of famine and the effects on those who were fertile during the famine. Thus, the relatively small fall in birthweight in Wuppertal might be due partly to the relative privilege of those who remained capable of conceiving.

Even though data collected under these devastating conditions have inherent limitations, some conclusions seem warranted. The Leningrad experience probably represents the outer limits of endurance of a population which was previously well-nourished, and a fall in mean birthweight of 550 g was observed. With very severe famine, the Dutch experienced a 300 g depression. In Wuppertal, shortage of food was great and there were long periods during which rations were down to half the usual intake, but birthweight was depressed at most by 227 g, and by considerably less among private patients, or when food shortage was intermediate, but with official rations still under 1500 calories per day.

3 Studies of iatrogenic dietary limitation

There are surprisingly few systematic studies of the formerly widespread medical practice of advising women to limit their diet and weight-gain during pregnancy. (Table 17.2)

Campbell and MacGillivray (1975) prescribed a 1200-calorie low carbohydrate diet for 51 primigravidae who had average weight gains over 570 g per week between the 20th and 30th weeks of gestation. Fifty-one matched controls received no intervention, and an additional 51 matched women received a diuretic (two tablets a day of cyclopenthiazide with potassium). The restricted diet was associated with lower maternal weight-gain, and the infants of the women who dieted and of those who received diuretics were lighter at birth than those of controls. When the children were examined between 4 and 6 years of age, over 40 per cent of the infants whose mothers had been put on restricted diet were at or below the 50th centile in weight, compared with only 17.6 per cent of infants whose mothers had been given diuretics and 18.2 per cent of controls (Blumenthal 1976).

This issue was later restudied by the same group, with somewhat different results (Campbell 1983). Ninety-one primigravidae over the 75th centile in weight for height at 28 weeks gestation were matched on height, weight gain from 20 to 30 weeks gestation, and smoking, with 91 controls, and placed on 1250-calorie reducing diets from 30 weeks gestation to term. Towards the end of pregnancy the women on restricted diets reported eating 1479 calories a day, almost 500 calories less than controls. Although mean birthweights were similar in the two groups, 25 per cent of the women who had been prescribed restricted diets had infants with birthweights under the 25th centile of weight for gestational age, as opposed to 18 per cent of controls. Twice as many of these women had durations of gestation of over 40 weeks (32 per cent versus 15 per cent). Whether this difference in duration of gestation was a treatment effect is uncertain, but it would certainly influence birthweight. Fetal growth thus probably was impaired by dieting.

Grieve *et al.* (1979) studied primigravidae in a consultant obstetrician's practice in Motherwell, Scotland. For thirty years he had counselled a diet high in animal protein and low in carbohydrates and calories. Both the weight-gains of the mothers and the birthweights of the babies in his practice were lower than those in a population of similar stature and social status in Aberdeen. Calculated from the data presented, the median weight-gain in the Motherwell women was 0.32 kg per week, compared with 0.46 kg per week in Aberdeen. Birthweights in Motherwell were more than 400 g lower than in Aberdeen, a remarkable difference.

Table 17.2 Studies of iatrogenic dietary limitation

Authors	Population studied	Assignment method/ research design	Study group No.	Study group Treatment	Control group No.	Control group Treatment	Results				Comments
Naeye *et al.* (1973)	1044 consecutive autopsies, perinatal deaths, Columbia-Presbyterian Medical Center, New York City, 1960–68, with exclusions 'which had any fetal or maternal disorder known to influence (a) fetal or placental growth (b) amniotic fluid volume (c) mother's extracellular fluid volume . . .'	Retrospective cohort study	123 (32 underweight*, 91 overweight) * Below WHO standards, wt for ht. Others above	1200–1500 cal diet prescribed	344 (181 underweight*, 163 overweight)	General dietary advice			Low cal diet	Others	Exclusions not enumerated, nor causes for exclusion identified. No information about whether dietary advice preceded or followed weight-gain, nor of duration of diet. Stillbirths not analysed separately from live births. Impossible to judge whether dichotomizing population provided sufficient control.
							Low weight-gain (%)				
							among underweight		34.3	59.7	
							among overweight		59.3	64.4	
							Birthweight, % normal value				
							Total		103	105	
							among underweight only		98	102	
							with low weight-gain		78	97	
							with high weight-gain		108	110	
							among overweight only		105	108	
							with low weight-gain		101	103	
							with high weight-gain		111	118	
Cambell and MacGillivray (1975) Blumenthal (1976)	Primigravidae, at 30 wks gestation, with ≥570 g/wk weight-gain between 20–30 wks	Subjects matched with controls on age, height, weight for height at 20 wks gestation, social class, cigarette and blood pressure in pregnancy	(A) 51	1200 cal, low CHO diet	(B) 51 (C) 51	Cyclopenthiazide 2 tabs/d No dietary intervention, no diuretics	Pre-eclampsia (%)	A	B	C	Matching categories not stated. Allocation of those at 50th growth centile confusing. No data on stature of parents or sibs.
							with proteinuria	11.8	15.7	17.7	
							without proteinuria	25.5	19.6	23.5	
							Other outcomes (normotensives only)				
							weight-gain/wk(kg), 30–38 wks	0.19	0.32	0.52	
							change, skinfold thickness (mm), 30–38 wks	−0.17	−0.18	2.98	
							Birthweight <25th centile (%)				
							Weight	43.2	17.6	18.2	
							Height	45.5	23.5	18.2	
							Head circumference	52.3	26.5	54.5	

Barsa Gregory and Rush (1987)	1137 term singleton births in the Natl. Collab. Perinatal Study, Columbia Univ. 1959–63 registered < 25 wks gest.	Births < 31st centile for birthweight, within strata of ethnic group and duration of gestation	255	⩾ 31st centile for birthweight matched with cases for ethnicity, gestation, smoking, parity and prepregnant weight	255			Low birthweight	Matched controls	Difference	No differences in results statistically significant. Late pregnancy weight-gain unrelated to diet, after controlling for prior weight-gain.
							Low calorie diet (%)	37.3	40.4	− 3.1	
							Adjusted for weight-gain				
							(a) in early pregnancy	–	–	− 1.7	
							(b) + midpregnancy	–	–	+ 1.7	
							(c) + late pregnancy	–	–	+ 2.2	
Campbell (1983)	Aberdeen Primigravidae > 75th centile weight for height, normal GTT at 28 wks gest.	Pair matched on height, weight-gain from 20 to 30 wks gest., and smoking	91	1250 kcal reducing diet from 30 wks to term (1479 kcal reported mean intake at 38 wks gest.)	91	Regular care (1957 kcal reported mean intake at 38 wks gest.)		Cases	Controls		Head circumference not reported.
							Change, from 30 to 38 wks gest.				
							Weight (kg)	2.92	4.21		
							Total body water (l)	2.88	3.81		
							Plasma (l)	0.20	0.32		
							Pre-eclampsia (%)	39.6	37.4		
							Perinatal death (*n*)	2	0		
							Birth > 40 wks gest. (%)	31.9	15.4		
							Birthweight (g)	3291	3285		
							Birthweight < 25th centile (%)	25.3	17.6		
							Length (cm)	49.8	49.8		
Grieve *et al.* (1979)	Motherwell Maternity Hospital, Scotland	Retrospective evaluation of diet used by clinician from 1938–1977 Comparable group from Aberdeen used as controls	295 251	(1965) (1975) High protein, low CHO and kcal diet prescribed. (Substudy, $n = 10$; 1465 cal, 84 g protein/d)	1829	(1968–70) Routine care (Substudy, $n = 489$; 2449 cal, 75 g protein/d)		Motherwell	Aberdeen		Report limited to effects on primigravidae.
							Median weight-gain/wk(kg)	0.32	0.46		
							Birthweight (g)				
							1965	3008			
							1975	2940			
							1968–70		3393		

While perinatal mortality in Motherwell was not reported, it has been said not to have been excessive. Compared with the three famine studies, the 400 g depression in mean birthweight is exceeded only by that experienced in Leningrad. Some of this difference almost certainly would have resulted from the liberal use of induction of labour that was practised in Motherwell, but it is also likely that the high protein content of the diet, along with the restriction of calories, contributed to this dramatic depression in birthweight (see Table 17.2).

Barsa Gregory and Rush (1987) studied the relationship of a low calorie diet to weight-gain and birthweight among women who participated in the National Collaborative Perinatal Project from 1959 to 1963. From the this data set, singleton term infants were identified who were below the 31st centile in birthweight; these 255 births were matched to higher weight infants for ethnicity, duration of gestation, smoking, parity, and prepregnant weight. Women who had given birth to low birthweight babies were somewhat *less* likely to have been advised to restrict their diet (37 per cent versus 40 per cent), but the difference was not statistically significant.

The relationship between prescription of a low calorie diet and the birthweight of the infant is confounded by weight-gain during pregnancy. A mother who gains more weight during pregnancy has a greater likelihood both of being prescribed a low calorie diet and of giving birth to a heavier infant. We therefore adjusted this outcome sequentially, first for weight gain in early pregnancy, then in midpregnancy and finally in late pregnancy. Again, no statistically significant differences were observed. Late pregnancy weight-gain was not statistically significantly related to whether or not a low calorie diet had been prescribed.

Since women who were asked to limit caloric intake continued to gain more weight than others, the discrepancy in the findings between this observational study and those of the intervention studies might be poor compliance with the prescribed dietary regimen.

4 Studies of dietary advice without emphasis on restriction

Two of the three reported trials of dietary advice without suggestions for dietary restriction (Cameron and Graham 1944; Berry and Wiehl 1952) showed a lower rate of both low birthweight and perinatal death in the counselled group than in the controls. (Table 17.3) Dietary intake was not presented, nor is it known whether diet was monitored. The rate of low birthweight among those supervised was 6 per cent compared with 10 per cent in controls.

The small study of Sweeney *et al.* (1985) is not easily interpreted. Twenty-two women were randomly assigned to counselling by the 'Higgins method' (see Rush 1982 for further evaluation of this method). Unfortunately, the authors did not present outcome by experimental group, and in their tables it appears that there were 25 subjects, rather than 22. The estimated experimental effect (calculated from their data) was 12 g heavier birthweight in the counselled group.

The results of Dr Thomas Brewer's programme at the prenatal clinic of the Contra Costa County Hospital, Richmond, California, were compared with those of the same clinic prior to his programme, and those of two other clinics in the same county, in which the programme was not used (Lundin and Stark 1980). Brewer gave lectures on nutrition in which he stressed the advisability of eating high-quality protein, vegetables, and fruits, whilst discouraging high-carbohydrate and high-fat 'junk' foods and beverages. Weight control was avoided, as was salt restriction. No statistically significant differences were detected in the mean birthweights, the proportion born under 2500 g birthweight, the proportion delivered preterm, and the neonatal death rates among the babies born to women attending the different clinics. The results were unchanged when subgroups deemed to be at particular nutritional risk (those under 19 years of age or those having their first pregnancies), or considered to have had the best exposure to the therapeutic regimen (those registering under 28 weeks gestation and seen for at least four visits over the least four weeks duration) were considered separately. (See also Chapter 18.)

5 Studies in which the decision to supplement (or the level of supplementation) were in part controlled by the participant

Although the study by Habicht *et al.* (1974) in Guatemala began as a controlled trial with random allocation of villages to two different programmes (Table 17.4) in analysis, the original design was abandoned, and women who chose to consume over 20,000 calories as supplementary food during pregnancy were compared with those who did not. No data on total dietary intake were presented. There was a 110 g difference in mean birthweight, favouring those babies whose mothers had eaten more supplement.

There are several problems in accepting the authors' conclusions that the increased birthweight observed was a result of the supplementation. Thirty-eight per cent of births were excluded from analysis because they were not weighed immediately after birth, and the relationship of supplementation to duration of gestation was not presented, a serious omission. There is a confounding bias in favour of those taking over 20,000

Table 17.3 Studies of dietary advice without emphasis on restriction

Authors	Population studied	Assignment method/ research design	Study group No.	Study group Treatment	Control group No.	Control group Treatment	Results				Comments
Cameron and Graham (1944)	Glasgow Royal Maternity Women's Hospital, 1942–43, in last 3 months of pregnancy	Alternate	400	Dietary advice; encouraged to apply for priority allowance of food	500	None		Supervised	Control		Numbers of drop-outs not given; monitoring of diet implied but not certain; observers probably not blind.
							Stillbirth (%)	4.2	7.2		
							Low birthweight (%)	6.2	10.0		
							Neonatal death (%)	1.6	2.0		
Berry and Wiehl (1952)	Prenatal clinic, Morrisania Hospital, New York City, 1948–50	Prospective intervention, of counselling; alternate assignment	116 (+21 with unknown outcome)	Instruction only	110 (+13 with unknown outcome)	None		Instructed	Control		
							Perinatal death (%)	5.2	6.4		
							(excluding early fetal death	3.7	3.7)		
							% <2500 g birthweight	6.2	9.9		
Lundin and Stark (1980)	Richmond, CA, public prenatal clinic, singleton live births (Brewer)	All patients registering in clinic, contrasted with (a) same clinic, prior to programme, and (b) 2 other clinics, same county and same hospital of delivery	584 (black) 638 (white)	'... nutrition lectures and prompting by the physician avoiding maternal weight control, salt restriction ... saluretic diuretics were not prescribed. The nutritional emphasis was on eating high-quality protein, vegetables and fruit and on discouraging high carbohydrate, high fat 'junk food' and beverages.'	155 Black 92 White*	Richmond, < 1964		Richmond Clinic 1965–70 (Brewer)	Richmond Clinic 1/61–6/63 (Before Brewer)	Other clinics 1965–70	The results were unaffected by restricting analysis to patients registering < 28 wks gestation, and seen for at least 4 visits, over at least 4 weeks, and under 19 years of age, or in first pregnancy.
					243 Black 1951 White*	Other clinics	Mean birthweight (g)				
					* Includes Spanish Americans		Black	3146	3163	3178	
							White	3321	3359	3301	
							% <2500 g birthweight				
							Black	9.4	8.4	7.8	
							White	6.3	5.4	7.1	
							% delivered <37 wks gestation				
							Black	16.5	N/A	17.3	
							White	8.1	N/A	8.8	
							% neonatal death (28 d)				
							Black	1.20	N/A	0.41	
							White	1.73	N/A	1.08	
Sweeney *et al.* (1985)	Tertiary care centre patients, Salt Lake City, registered < 20 wks gest.	Random assignment within strata; 'approx. equal' number of women with lowest weight-gain in each group	22	Counselling by 'Higgins method' (see Rush 1982) 2653 kcal/d and 92 g protein/d reported	21	Unspecified 2373 kcal/d and 81 g protein/d reported		Counselled	Control		Data on comparability of groups not presented; 'no significant differences between groups'. Numbers inadequate to test hypothesis. Outcome data not presented by experimental intervention and results therefore calculated from authors' data. No explanation why 25 subjects presented in table, while only 22 were said to be assigned for counselling.
							Birthweight (g): ( ) = *n*	3255 (25)	3243 (18)		

Table 17.4 Studies in which the decision to supplement was in part controlled by the participant

Author	Population studied	Assignment method/ research design	Study group		Control group		Results	Comments
			No.	Treatment	No.	Treatment		
Habicht *et al.* (1974) Lechtig *et al.* (1975)	4 rural villages in Guatemala; 2 supplied with protein-rich gruel, 2 with beverage containing carbohydrate only	Supplement taken *ad libitum*	178	⩾20,000 cal taken over entire pregnancy	240	< 20,000 cal taken over entire pregnancy	About 110 g difference in birthweight, favouring well supplemented. ↑ weight gain; ↑ placental weight; ↓ placental RNase; ↓ perinatal death (NS)	Intake of supplements observed. Neither inclusion of protein nor when in pregnancy consumed related to effect. 38% of births not weighed. No data presented on duration of gestation. Result confounded by gestation: i.e. with longer gestation, more likely to have had chance to take > 20,000 cal.

calories. Given longer duration of pregnancy, there is greater opportunity to pass this threshold, and an unspecified amount of the observed differences in birthweight could therefore be due to an artefactually longer gestation in the more highly supplemented group.

6 Studies in which the decision to supplement and the level of supplementation were not under the subjects' control

6.1 Studies in developed countries

The results of a number of studies of dietary supplementation are summarized in Table 17.5. These studies are of varied quality, and show conflicting results. Supplementation was associated with *increases* in mean birthweight in some studies (Dieckmann *et al.* 1944; Higgins 1976; Rush *et al.* 1980a,b, (balanced calorie/protein supplementation); Adams *et al.* 1978 (balanced calorie/protein supplementation); Elwood *et al.* 1981; Campbell Brown 1983), but with *decreases* in mean birthweight in others (Ebbs *et al.* 1941, 1942; Osofsky 1975; Rush *et al.* 1980a,b, (high protein supplementation); Adams *et al.* 1978 (high protein supplementation); Viegas *et al.* 1982a; Watney and Alton 1986). The differences in mean birthweights ranged from 32 to 114 g. Not enough data are given in the reports of the studies to permit a meta-analysis, but it is obvious from these trials that no dramatic effect on birthweight can be expected from dietary supplementation of women who are not significantly undernourished.

The incidence of low birthweight was lower in the supplemented groups in all studies that reported this outcome (Ebbs *et al.* 1941, 1942 (assuming that 'premature' meant <2500 g in 1942); Tompkins *et al.* 1955; Higgins 1976). The incidence of preterm births was also lower in the studies that reported this outcome (Dieckmann *et al.* 1944; Campbell Brown 1983).

There were small differences in stillbirth rates or perinatal mortality in favour of the supplemented groups reported in some studies (Balfour 1944; Ebbs *et al.* 1941, 1942), but not in others (Dieckmann *et al.* 1944). The extent of these differences are reported in Table 17.5.

We performed a randomized, partially double-blind, controlled trial of nutritional supplementation in a black, public clinic population in New York City (Rush *et al.* 1980a,b). The balanced protein/calorie 'complement' was associated with a 41 g increase in birthweight compared with controls (non-significant) and with slightly longer duration of gestation and lower proportion of births under 2500 g compared with the other two groups combined (both at the margins of statistical significance). The high protein 'supplement' was associated with 32 g *lower* birthweight than among the controls (not statistically significant), with statistically significantly depressed birthweight among those born preterm, and with *increased* very early preterm delivery and neonatal death, at the margins of statistical significance.

The small study of Adams *et al.* (1978) used the same supplements developed for our study and resulted in similar outcomes. The mean birthweight of the babies born to women in the group who received the balanced protein/calorie 'complement', was 92 g greater than among controls, while that of the babies born to women in the high protein 'supplement' groups was 45 g lower than that of the controls.

Elwood *et al.* (1981), in a randomized trial carried out in South Wales, offered their treatment group tokens which allowed the daily purchase of 20 ounces of whole milk at half price, beginning in midpregnancy and continuing until the children were 5 years old. Their report does not give birthweights for the 212 children in the trial who were not assessed at age 5. Among those for whom birthweights are reported, after correcting for the disproportionately high number of smokers in the study group, there was about a 55 g increase in birthweight associated with supplementation.

Viegas, *et al.* (1982a,b) performed two supplementation trials among women of Asian origin in Birmingham, England. In the first, women were randomly allocated to one of three treatment groups, 47 to a daily regimen of 26 g of protein and 273 kcal, 50 to a comparable level of caloric supplementation, but without protein, and 45 to an unsupplemented control group. All received iron and vitamin C. The results are confusingly presented, since it is unclear whether they are for the total treatment groups, or exclude women with vaginal bleeding, hypertension, or 'low compliance'. In this first trial, the control group had higher mean birthweight than those who receive energy supplementation alone (30 g) or those receiving protein and energy supplements (40 g). However, the control differed from the supplemented group in potentially important ways, and these differences were not adjusted for in analysis. For instance, there were a quarter as many Hindus among controls (5 per cent versus 20 per cent in the supplemented groups); controls were considerably less likely to have been vegetarians or to have had previous low birthweight infants or fetal or perinatal losses; their body weights were higher, as were their initial triceps skinfold thickness. Thus, the meaning of the results of the trial are obscure.

The meaning of the group's second trial (Viegas *et al.* 1982b) is even more questionable. A subsequent group of pregnant women of Asian origin living in Birmingham, England, were stratified by amount of change in triceps skinfold between 20 and 28 weeks of ges-

Table 17.5 Studies in which the decision to supplement (or the level of supplementation) were not under the subjects' control in developed countries

Authors	Population studied	Assignment method/ research design	Study group No.	Study group Treatment	Control group No.	Control group Treatment	Results	Comments
Osofsky (1975)	Philadelphia, Temple University Hospital prenatal clinic, 'low-income' women	Subjects recruited after completion of all control pregnancies	122	'Meritene', a high protein–mineral supplement. Amount prescribed not stated; contains 6.5 g protein in every 100 kcal. Total intake of 80.3 g protein/d reported.	118	Routine care. 92% black. Intake of 71.8 g protein/d reported	Subjects / Controls Birthweight (g) 3005 / 3119 $p<0.05$ Length (cm) 49.0 / 50.0 $p<0.05$ Head circ. (cm) 33.4 / 34.1 $0<0.05$ Apgar (5 min) 9.4 / 9.7 $p<0.05$	Subjects had significantly fewer years of school, lower occupational status and lower initial Hgb, but magnitude of differences not stated. Racial composition of subject group not presented. Results not controlled for these differences.
Higgins (1976) Rush (1981)	Public patients at Royal Victoria Hospital, Montreal; 1963–74	Patients referred to care of Montreal Diet Dispensary in non-systematic way, matched on 5 characteristics with other patients from same clinic in a retrospective cohort study	1213	Dietary evaluation, advice and for 75% of population, milk, eggs, and oranges	1213	Regular care	Treated / Controls % <2500 g birthweight 5.7 / 6.8 NS Birthweight (g) 3291 / 3251 $p<0.05$ No significant difference in mortality or gestation. Effect greater in women <140 lb at conception and women of lower parity	
Rush *et al.* (1980a,b)	Public clinic population, New York City, 1970–74; black; registered <30 wks gestation; <140 lb at conception; plus at least one other risk factor (low weight-gain, weight <110 lb at conception, past low birthweight and/or ingestion of <50 g protein in past 24 hours)	Randomized, partially double-blind prospective intervention; treatment from registration to term	263 272	Supplement (40 g protein/470 kcal/d) Complement (6 g protein/322 kcal/d). Participants reported taking 74% (326 kcal) of supplement, 20% (65 kcal) as replacement to regular diet. For complement, 72% (233 kcal) with 11% (26 kcal) as replacement.	272	Control (routine multivitamin/ mineral tablets)	Suppl. / Comp / Controls Birthweight (g) (based on 768 liveborn singletons) 2938 / 3011 / 2970 Increase in very early delivery and neonatal death at margins of significance in Supplement group. Significant depression of birthweight among prematures with Supplement. No residual toxicity at age 1 year. Significant difference in attentional measures with Supplement at age 1 year, interpretable as beneficial. Increased duration of gestation, and % >2500 g in Complement group, versus other two groups combined.	Effects of heavy smoking on weight-gain partially reversed, and on birthweight reversed by both dietary supplements.
Adams *et al.* (1978)	Kaiser-Permanente group. San Francisco, with chronic HBP, or past fetal loss, or heart disease, or smoking >1/2 pack per day or unmarried, or stature <5 ft 2 in. or	Assignment method unstated; prospective trial	36 23	(A) As Supplenent developed for Rush *et al.* (1980a,b) (B) As Complement developed for Rush *et al.* (1980a,b)	43	(C) Multivitamin/ mineral tablet	A / B / C Birthweight (g) 3227 / 3365 / 3272 (NS)	Distribution of risk characteristics among treatment groups unclear; only 45% completion rate, 3 infants <2500 g excluded from analysis (1 in A, 2 in C).

(1981)	South Wales, from 1972; treatment from booking for half of pregnancy (on average), and through to age 5 years		 234	smokers) (B) Females (30% smokers). Study group received 20 oz milk/day at half price. At 4½ years, supplemented children took 71 ml/d more milk than controls	 204	smokers) (D) Females (43% smokers)	A 3460 B 3320 C 3390 D 3240 A–C = 70 g† B–D = 80 g† † If smoking caused 200 g decrease in birthweight, controlling for smoking would lower A–C to 56 g and B–D to 54 g	Data on intake during pregnancy not given. Birthweight × treatment status of 212 children not followed to age 5 years not available but they weighed 70 g less at birth than those completing trial. Outcome not controlled for marked disparity in smoking.
Balfour (1944)	28 areas, South Wales and North of England, 1937–39; wives of unemployed or low-wage earners	Discretion of doctors; controls were others at clinic; parity lower in controls, social status higher	11,618	q2w: 1 lb dried milk, ½ lb 'Ovaltine', plus 'Marmite' or 8 oz 'Minadex'	8095 or 9912(?)	None; however, local authorities often reserved their milk for controls	(Fed / Controls) Perinatal deaths (%): 5.9 / 7.1 $x^2 = 12.48$ (Birthweight not reported)	Selective assignment; allocation of local authority milk-supplies only to controls in some areas.
Ebbs *et al.* (1941, 1942)	Toronto General Hospital; *c.* 1940; prior to 7th month; no major disease	Alternate among patients with poor diet; a third group with good diet also followed	90	(A) 45 g protein, 840 kcal, vitamins, minerals and advice given (original intake 56 g protein; 1690 kcal; later 94 g protein, 2424 kcal/d)	120 170	(B) Capsules of corn old (original intake 56 g protein, 1672 kcal; later 62 g protein, 1837 kcal/d) (C) Normal good diet: 81 g protein, 2206 kcal; later 92 g protein, 2521 kcal/d)	(A / B / C) Birthweight (g): 3377 / 3462 / 3392 'Prematurity' (%): 2.2 / 8.0 / 3.0 Miscarriage (%): 0.0 / 6.0 / 1.2 Stillbirth (%): 0.0 / 3.5 / 0.6 Infant death <6 m (%): 0.0 / 2.8 / 0.0	Prematurity not defined; some attempt to monitor compliance; supervising obstetrician blind; no information about drop-outs.
Dieckmann *et al.* (1944)	Chicago, *c.* 1942; low income	'Random'	179 102	(II) 100 g/d cereal (for mineral content) (IV) Cereal and vitamin A and D 100 g cereal given; average amount taken 'ranged from 30 to 50 g' daily	175 98	(I) None (III) Vitamin A and D	Groups (II and IV / I and III) Fetal death (%): 5.1 / 3.7 Delivery <36 wks (%): 2.2 / 4.4 Total wt-gain (kg): 11.0 / 10.1 Weight-gain/wk (g): 494 / 477 Duration preg. (wks): 40.3 / 40.2 Birthweight (g): 3397 / 3352	Unequal assignment to treatment conditions not explained; some monitoring of compliance—patients overstated intake; observer blindness unknown; no indication of drop-out rate.
Tompkins *et al.* (1955)	Philadelphia Lying-in Hospital, 1948–52; less than 15 weeks' gestation; married; no major complication, 74% white	'Seriatim'; prospective intervention	332 334	50 g protein, 1.5 g Ca/d given As above, plus vitamins (+instruction)	467 447	None Vitamins (+instruction)	(Protein (+vitamins) / No protein (+vitamins)) % <2500 g birthweight White: 3.8 / 5.0 Black: 8.7 / 13.2 Total: 5.2 / 7.0	Protein + vitamin group included fewer very poor. In prior pregnancy multiparae in protein group had more frequent low birthweight (10.5 vs. 5.0%), stillbirth (3.1 vs. 1.1%), and neonatal death (3.1 vs. 2.0%). Those initially assigned to protein supplements who did not use them were transferred to control group, hence differing cell sizes.
Viegas *et al.* (1982a)	Birmingham, England S. Asian pregnant women living in defined area, April–Oct. 1979	Random allocation. Treatment from 18 to 20 wks gest. to 38 wks gest.	47 (or 33?) 50 (or 28?)	273 kcal + 26 g prot./d + vit. C + Fe 273 kcal/d + vit. C + Fe (Smaller number of subjects excludes those with vaginal bleeding, hypertension, or 'low compliance')	45 (or 34?)	Fe, 3 mg/d vit. C, 30 mg/d	Treatment groups (Energy and protein / Energy / Controls) Wt gain/wks (g) —28 wks: 465 / 460 / 360 28–35 wks: 360 / 335 / 300 *n*: (47 or 33?) / (50 or 28?) / (45 or 34?) Duration gest. (wks)[1]: 38.9 / 39.0 / 39.0 Birthweight (g): 3010 / 3020 / 3050 *n*: 47 / 50 / 45 [1] From authors, not in publication	Data analysed both including and exclusing those with vaginal bleeding and hypertension (7, 10, and 2 respectively in the 3 treatment groups) or who were low compliers (7, 12, and 9 respectively in the 3 treatment groups). Not specified which results present in publications. Results not adjusted for initial disparities in population groups: Treatment groups (Protein + Energy / Energy / Controls) Hindus (%): 19 / 22 / 5 Vegetarians (%): 13 / 16 / 9 Past LBW, fetal or perinatal loss (%): 49 / 42 / 29 Weight (kg): 53.0 / 54.6 / 56.3 Triceps SF (mm): 16.9 / 17.1 / 18.4 (Not mentioned when weight measured) No mention of whether any women delivered preterm. Number of subjects too small to test hypothesis. No dietary assessment during treatment reported.

Table 17.5—*continued*

Authors	Population studied	Assignment method/ research design	Study group No.	Study group Treatment	Control group No.	Control group Treatment	Results	Comments
Viegas *et al.* (1982b)	Birmingham, England S. Asian pregnant women living in defined area, Nov. 79–June 80	Random allocation, stratified by change in triceps SF between 20 and 28 wks gest. Treatment from 28 to 38 wks gest.	 14 (or 12) 17 (or 15)	Small prior increment in triceps skinfold 425 kcal + 40 g prot./d (37% of energy as protein: text states 10%) 425 kcal/d	14 (or 12)	'Orovite 7'	Treatment groups: Energy and protein / Energy / Controls Wt gain/wks (g), prior gain in triceps SF Low: ~480 / ~300 / ~310 High: ~500 / ~320 / ~340 *n*: ? / ? / ?	Results stratified by change in prior triceps skinfolds, but data on comparability only presented for total (unstratified) groups; comparability therefore uncertain across treatment groups. Number too small to test hypotheses. Results inconsistent with authors' interpretations.
			   (30 (or 21) 26 (or 23)	Large prior increment in triceps skinfold Protein + cal (as above) Cal as above) (Smaller number of subjects excludes those with vaginal bleeding, hypertension, or 'low compliance'	27 (or 19)	'Orovite 7'	Birthweight (g) Low triceps gain No exclusions: 3340 (14) / 2950 (17) / 3010 (14) exclusions: 3350 (12) / 2900 (15) / 3020 (12) High triceps gain No exclusions: 2980 (30) / 3110 (26) / 3160 (27) exclusions: 2940 (21) / 3080 (23) / 3210 (19) ( ) = *n*	
Campbell Brown (1983)	Aberdeen 1975–80 Primigravidae 30 wks gest., in lowest quartile of at least 2 of the following: Height; Weight and wt./ht. at 20 wks gest.; wt. gain from 20 to 30 wks gest.	First member of matched pair assigned to supplementation. If delivery <37 wks, replaced by next matchable recruit	No. 90	Treatment / Cal as protein (%) 276 ml flavoured milk (293 kcal, 15 g prot.) or — 20.5 554 ml whole milk (387 kcal, 20 g prot.) or — 20.7 75 g cheese (319 kcal, 18 g prot.) or combinations — 23.8	90	Regular care	Cases / Controls / Diff. Gestation <37 wks (%): 7.2 / 8.2 / −1.0 Weight-gain/wks (kg): 0.40 / 0.36 / 0.04 ($p = 0.08$) During gest. (wks): 39.7 / 39.6 / 0.1 Birthweight (g): 3032 (+372) / 2995 (+395) / 37 Length (cm): 48.5 / 48.2 / 0.3 Head circ. (cm): 34.3 / 34.2 / 0.2	r, reported nitrogen intake and urine N excretion = 0.51 in cases, 0.58 in controls (both $p < 0.001$) Controls had sign. increase of N excretion in week of recruitment. r, energy from suppl. and diff. in birthweight from matched control = 0.24, $p = 0.03$. r, protein from suppl. and diff. in bthwt from matched control = 0.26, $p = 0.01$.
Watney and Alton (1986)	W. Bromwich, England Pregnant women with low 2nd trimester triceps skinfold gain (per criterion of Viegas *et al.* 1982b), half 'White' and half Asian.	Half assigned to supplementation, 3rd trimester	78	Milk based supplement 'comparable to the protein energy supplement' of Viegas *et al.* (1982b)	78	Unspecified	'The babies of supplemented women were lighter than those of unsupplemented women'.	

Mean daily intake (Campbell Brown (1983))

	Calories on-set	Calories during trial	Calories diff	Protein (g) on-set	Protein (g) during trial	Protein (g) diff
Cases	2035	2214	179	69	83	14
Controls	2089	2043	−46	71	70	−1

tation. Women within low and high change groups were then randomly allocated to either 425 kcal and 40 g of protein a day; 425 kcal a day; or to a control group. Presumably, all women received vitamin supplementation. Among those with low triceps gain, the treatment groups varied in size between 14 and 17 per treatment. The authors found one statistically significant difference: the 14 women who had low prior triceps skinfold gain and received the high protein energy supplement had infants with mean birthweight of 3340 g, compared to 2950 g in the energy alone group, and 3010 g for the control group. However, the birthweights in the high triceps gain groups were 2980, 3110, and 3160 g respectively. Thus, the 14 women with low triceps gain and with protein and energy supplementation had infants with mean birthweights that were 180 g greater than the infants of unsupplemented high triceps gain controls, and 130 g heavier than high triceps gain energy supplemented women, and 360 g heavier than the high triceps gain group who received protein energy supplementation. This pattern is not consistent with a coherent treatment effect. There is no rational reason to expect treatment among those at high risk to do any more than to bring them to parity with those at low risk. In fact, they did considerably better than those at presumably lower risk. Further, the presentation of the data makes it impossible to judge whether the supplemented and control women were comparable, since comparability was judged on the combined low and high triceps gain groups, while the treatment results were presented separately.

Watney and Alton (1986) replicated the design of Viegas *et al.* (1982b) and increased the study group to 78, with 78 randomly matched controls. The authors stated 'the babies of supplemented women were lighter than those of unsupplemented women', but gave no data to quantitate this statement.

Balfour (1944) reported the results of supplementing the diets of over 11,000 women in the poorer areas of England and Wales with dried milk, 'Ovaltine', and iron-rich food. Although relatively more deprived areas were probably chosen for supplementation, they experienced a lower perinatal death rate than the control areas (5.9 per cent vs. 7.1 per cent). Birthweights were not reported.

Ebbs *et al.* (1941), at a public antenatal clinic, identified by interview women judged to be having a poor diet. High protein and calorie supplements were given for at least one trimester to alternate pregnant women so identified. The mean birthweight of infants of supplemented mothers was 85 g *lower* than among the untreated alternate controls, although 'prematurity' rates (prematurity was not defined) and perinatal death rates were lower among the supplemented group.

Dieckmann *et al.* (1944), in Chicago, studied the effects of supplementation with 100 g of cereal daily. The reported daily intake of cereal ranged from 30 to 50 g. Mothers with cereal supplementation gained 0.9 kg more than controls. These women had infants that were, on average, 45 g heavier than the controls. They were slightly less likely to deliver preterm, but had slightly higher fetal death rates.

Tompkins *et al.* (1955) gave supplements of 50 g protein daily to women in Philadelphia. Rates of low birthweight were slightly lower with than without protein supplementation (5.2 per cent vs. 7.0 per cent), but women who did not co-operate with dietary supplementation were reallocated to the control group. Unfortunately, the original data of this study have been destroyed and cannot be reanalysed, so the results remain problematical. (Birthweights were not presented.)

Osofsky (1975), after studying 118 controls in the prenatal clinic at the Temple University Hospital, supplemented a further 122 women with 'Meritene', a dietary supplement containing 26 per cent of calories as protein. He found statistically significantly lower birthweight, infant length and head circumference, and lower Apgar score among those given dietary supplementation. However, these analyses did not control for differences in the composition of the supplemented and control groups.

The impact of the dietary programme of the Montreal Diet Dispensary, under the guidance and direction of Mrs Agnes Higgins, was evaluated in a retrospective matched pair cohort study (Rush 1981). This intensive programme of dietary education and (for three-quarters of the population) provision of milk, eggs, and oranges, was associated with a statistically significant increase in birthweight of 40 g. Differences in gestation and perinatal mortality were small and not statistically significant. Weight-gain patterns of the woman were consistent with the effect on birthweight, but were not statistically significant.

Campbell Brown (1983) matched primigravidae at 30 weeks gestation on height, weight, and height to weight ratio at 20 weeks gestation, as well as weight-gain from 20 to 30 weeks gestation. The first member of 90 matched pairs was assigned to dietary supplementation with dairy products which contained between 15 and 20 g of protein, and between 293 and 387 kcal per day. The supplemented women gained more weight (at the margins of statistical significance). The mean birthweight of infants of supplemented women was 37 g higher than that of controls, and the head circumference was 0.2 cm larger. (Neither of these differences were statistically significant.)

6.2 Studies in developing countries

Most studies of protein and calorie supplementation in developing countries showed increased mean birthweight with supplementation. This is not surprising

Table 17.6 Studies in which the decision to supplement and the level of supplementation were not under the subjects' control in developed countries

Author	Population studied	Assignment method/ research design	Study group No.	Study group Treatment	Control group No.	Control group Treatment	Results				Comments
								A	B	C	
Iyengar (1967)	Indian women, age 25–40 in manual labour; monthly income 'rarely exceeded' 125 rupees	How assigned to groups A and B not stated; controls recruited when presenting in labour		Hospitalized 4 weeks before EDC, plus	26	(C) Women arriving in labour	4 wks weight-gain (kg)	1.25	1.27	unknown	Not controlled for gestation; results therefore could be artefactual and a function of premature delivery among controls. Controls had not registered for services, therefore of doubtful comparability.
			12	(A) 2450 kcal, 95 g protein/d (55 g as animal protein)			Birthweight (kg)	3029	3029	2704	
			13	(B) 2450 kcal, 60 g protein/d (20 g as animal protein) ('about' 1400 kcal and 40 g protein/d at onset)			Cord plasma protein (g%)	6.09	6.11	5.34	
								A	B	C	
Qureshi *et al.* (1973)	Rural Indian multiparae, age 20–35, manual labourers	Alternate; from 20 weeks' gestation; method of selection of untreated controls unclear	39	(A) 500 kcal/d, 20 g protein plus iron and folate (Survey of other subjects suggested usual diet contained 1800 kcal and 42 g protein/d)	37	(B) Iron and folate	Weight-gain from 20th wk (kg)	3.9	2.9	unknown	Duration of gestation not reported; outcome not controlled for gestation, but infants premature by dates excluded from analysis. Selection method for untreated controls not stated, nor is it clear whether they were followed prospectively.
					50	(C) Untreated	Birthweight (g)	3320	2780	2510	
								+470	+270	+250	
Herriott *et al.* (1978) McDonald *et al.* (1981) (Bacon Chow study)	Taiwan, rural villages	Randomized, controlled, double-blind trial	81* 108†	(A) 40 g protein. 800 kcal/d given: 36.7 g protein. 1133 kcal taken from regular diet*. 539 kcal, 26.9 g protein taken from supplements†	88* 105†	(B) 80 kcal/d given: 37.7 g protein, 1202 kcal taken from regular diet*. 59 kcal taken from supplements†	Birthweight (g)				Supplementation began just after previous pregnancy. Analysis of Herriott *et al.* limited to those taking >50% prescribed supplements; Ingestion observed.
				* Heriott *et al.* † McDonald *et al.*			Herriott *et al.*	A	B	A–B	
							First (untreated) preg.	3064	3021		
							Second (treated) preg.	3188	3094		
							Difference, total group	124	73	51	
							Difference, males	196	117	79	
							Difference, females	50	16	34	
							McDonald *et al.*	A	B	C	
							First (untreated) preg.	3062	3033		
							Second (treated) preg.	3118	3073		
							Difference, total group	56	40	16	
							Difference, males	162	73	90	
							Difference, females	−59	2	−61	
							No difference in maternal weight-gain, infant length, or head circumference				
Mora *et al.* (1979) Waber *et al.* (1981)	Bogotá, Colombia; women with at least half their children under 5 years malnourished	Prospective intervention, random assignment. Postnatal feeding and stimulation, with crossover design	200	(A) 38.4 g protein/d and 856 kcal/d supplied. 55.4 g/d protein taken vs. 34.9 g initially; 1766 kcal taken vs. 1611 initially. Third trimester only	207	(B) Health care only no data on diet	Birthweight (g)				Birthweight difference not significant on 2-tailed test. On testing later in infancy, 'females were more sensitive to treatment than were males'.
								A	B	A–B	
							Total	2978	2927	51	
							Males	3040	2951	89	
							Females	2911	2905	6	
							% < 2500 g	11.0	8.7		
							Increased attention and accelerated visual habituation at 15 days. Cognitive 'effects of supplementation during pregnancy and first 6 months of life were short lived'.				

Merchant and Sheth (pers. comm., 1980)	Bombay, working class women registered for prenatal care	Random	 97 136 122 157	Protein, g/d — kcal/d A 45* — 450 B 30* — 300 C 7.5 — 450 D 5.0 — 300 * 25% as animal protein	501 134	E F (No supplements)	Group — Birthweight (g) — bw (vs. gsp E and F combined) A — 2669 ± 382 — −17 B — 2663 ± 408 — −23 C — 2769 ± 428 — +83 $p < 0.05$ D — 2722 ± 418 — +36 E — 2695 ± 398 F — 2650 ± 370 2868 ± 392	All received iron, folate, B_{12}, except group F. Half also received lysine and methionine, which were unrelated to outcome. Dose of supplements raised half-way through study (i.e. groups B and D preceded groups A and C).
Prentice *et al.* (1981, 1983a,b,c) Lamb *et al.* (1984) Lawrence *et al.* (1984)	All births in one Gambian village during 2 years of supplementation, compared to outcome during prior 4 years	Outcome during supplementation vs. prior experience Observed supplementation	51 42	'Wet season', 1100 kcal/d, 6 d/w 'Dry season', 950 kcal/d, 6 d/w Actual increments (24 hr weighing) kcal/d Wet season 430 Dry season 433 'On average women were attending by the 16th week of pregnancy'	95 86	Wet season Dry season Diet intake/d (kcal) Wet season 1464 Dry season 1468	— Supplemented — Control — Difference Wet season Mean birthweight (g)* — 3030 — 2844 — 186 % < 2500 g — 4.7 — 28.2 — −23.5 Dry season Mean birthweight (g)* — 2892 — 2889 — 3 % < 2500 g — 11.7 — 8.0 — 3.7 Combined seasons: Head circ. (mm) — ? — ? — 5 Duration of gest. (wks) Boys — ? — ? — −0.33 Girls — ? — ? — 0.65 * Adjusted for sex, parity, and month of birth	Magnitude of interaction with season uncertain because of small sample. Patterns of outcome do not conform to authors' interpretations.
Girija *et al.* (1984)	Low SES multip. women (< 100/m family income) in third trimester	Random assignment	10	30 g protein 417 kcal/d Intake shown by semiquantitative bargraphs; no apparent differences between supplemented and control groups	10	Not specified	— Supplemented — Controls 3rd trimester Wt-gain (kg) — 3.90 — 3.95 Hgb increase (g%)* — 1.97 — 0.17 Birthweight (g) — 2939 — 2676 Length (cm) — 47.7 — 45.9 * Not specified whether increase followed or preceded supplementation	Primary goal of research was to assess effect of supplementation on lactational performance and infant growth.
Ross *et al.* (1985)	Consecutive births among Zulus in clinic near Durban, South Africa, with expected original vaginal delivery, 1977	Randomized allocation Observed supplementation from 20 wks gestation	31 31 32	773 kcal/d, 'high bulk' 5 d/w 697 kcal/d, 'low bulk' 5 d/w 30 to 90 mg Zn gluconate/d 1403 to 1537 avg kcal/d prior to supplementation; no data on intake during supplementation	33	Placebo	— Low bulk — High bulk — Zn — Controls Wt-gain to 20 wks gest. (kg) — 8.1 — 8.3 — 7.2 — 8.8 Duration gest. (wks) — 38.6 — 29.2 — 39.4 — 38.9 Birthweight (g) — 3376* — 3082 — 3088 — 3171 (diff. from Controls) (g) — 205 — −89 — −83 — −)	Numbers of subjects too small to test hypothesis.

given that levels of nutrition were often very low. Birthweight effects, however, varied widely, and reported results were often internally inconsistent. Details of these trials (in chronologic order) are presented in Table 17.6.

Iyengar (1967) hospitalized two small groups of women, starting four weeks before their expected date of confinement.

They received different amounts of protein, but caloric intake was kept identical. There was virtually no difference in either the mothers' weight-gain or the mean birthweight of the babies associated with differing protein intake. The babies of the antenatally hospitalized mothers had a mean birthweight 325 g higher than that of 26 infants whose mothers were first seen when in labour, but the difference in birthweight between those hospitalized and supplemented and the women presenting in labour cannot be attributed to either nutritional intervention, or to hospitalization. Study mothers were excluded unless they went to full term, while women arriving in labour could have been at differing stages of gestation, including an unknown number who were delivering before term. Also, the women in the control group clearly differed from the supplemented women, as they had received no antenatal care, whether by choice or because of limited access.

Qureshi *et al.* (1973) alternately assigned women to either protein/calorie supplementation plus iron and folate, or to iron and folate alone. Supplementation began at 20 weeks gestation, and was associated with a 1 kg greater increase in maternal weight from the 20th week to delivery, and a 540 g difference in birthweight in favour of the protein/calorie supplemented group. The study appears to be well-designed and executed, but there are several problems. Preterm infants were excluded from the analysis, duration of gestation was not reported, and outcome was not otherwise controlled for gestation. Prior survey had indicated that the usual diet among pregnant women was about 1800 calories and 42 g of protein a day, and these are not levels associated with marked nutritional deprivation (see the studies of famine, above). The standard deviation of birthweight was much larger for the treated group than for the control group (470 g vs. 270 g): it is biologically implausible to have such differing variability in subgroups drawn from the same population. Finally, the differences in maternal weight-gain appear to be small, given the birthweight differences. This study stands out: the effect of supplementation on birthweight is five to ten times greater than in any other controlled trial.

The study of Chow in Taiwan, initially analysed by Herriott *et al.* (1978) and more recently by McDonald *et al.* (1981), was double-blinded and supplementation was observed. The analysis of Herriott *et al.* was limited to those taking over 50 per cent of the prescribed supplements, thus vitiating the utility of random allocation. Supplementation began at the end of the previous pregnancy, so feeding was initiated before conception. Taking into account birthweight differences from the previous pregnancy, the data of Herriott and colleagues suggested a 51 g difference in mean birthweight favouring the supplemented group (79 g for male and 34 g for female infants), while in the analysis of McDonald *et al.* there was a 16 g difference (90 g for males and a negative relationship of 61 g for females).

Mora *et al.* (1979) performed a well-designed randomized controlled trial of third trimester supplementation in Bogotà, Colombia. They found a 51 g greater mean birthweight with supplementation (not statistically significant on a two tailed test). The effect was apparently confined to males.

Merchant and Sheth (personal communication, 1980) carried out a large randomized trial in Bombay among a group of working class mothers registered for prenatal care. The study design evolved from that of Rush *et al.* (1980a,b) in New York. There were four levels of nutritional supplementation, two of different amounts of a supplement of low protein density, and two with different amounts of a high density protein supplement. Compared to controls, both of the groups receiving the low protein density supplement showed increments in birthweight (36 g and 83 g among those who received larger amounts of supplementation). In contrast, those who received the high density protein supplements experienced birthweight decrements of 17 g and 23 g. The only statistically significant difference was the 83 g increment with larger amounts of the low protein density supplement.

The studies in the Gambia conducted by Prentice and his colleagues (1981, 1983a,b,c) appear to have been seriously performed. Baseline birthweights were collected for four years among all births in one village, 95 during the wet season, and 96 during the dry season. Supplementation was then instituted in the subsequent two years (1100 kcal for six days a week for 51 births during the wet season, and 950 kcal a day for six days a week during the dry season for 42 births). Supplemented women had infants of higher birthweight compared to the prior control years, but only during the wet season. The investigators interpreted this result to mean that only with the additional stress of the wet season (greater field work, and lower food supply) could any effect of supplementation be detected.

The data they present are not consistent with this interpretation. During the control years, daily diet intake during the wet season was not lower than in the dry season (1464 vs. 1468 kcal per day); the incremental intake in the years of supplementation were also identical (430 kcal during the wet season and 433 kcal during the dry season). Their interpretation demands that, prior to supplementation, wet season birthweights should have been markedly lower than those in the dry season, but this was not the case. During the control period, dry season mean birthweight was 2889 g, and in the wet season, 2844 g. Further, their logic dictates that supplementation during the wet season would bring birthweights up to levels already extant during the dry season. In fact, what was observed was that wet season supplemented women had infants with birthweights considerably higher than any others. Control women during the wet or dry seasons, or supplemented women during the dry season, had infants nearly identical birthweights. This pattern of results is as consistent with a chance finding as with a treatment effect.

Girija *et al.* (1984) supplemented 10 low income pregnant women in the third trimester in Hyderabad, India, and studied 10 controls. The very large birthweight difference, 263 g, between the supplemented and control women was not statistically significant.

Ross *et al.* (1985) performed a study in which 127 pregnant women were randomly allocated at 20 weeks gestation to one of four treatments. The size of treatment groups ranged between 31 and 33. The group in which mothers received a high energy supplement of 'low bulk' had a higher mean birthweight than the other three groups. Those who received a high energy 'high bulk' supplement or a zinc supplement (30 to 90 ml of zinc gluconate a day) actually had slightly lower mean birthweight than controls. There was no dietary assessment during supplementation, so that differences in actual intake between the groups cannot be judged.

7 The effect of protein density

Table 17.7 shows the effect of protein density of dietary supplementation on birthweight difference between subjects and controls, with the controlled trials of dietary supplementation ranked in order of protein density. The effect of protein density is striking; higher protein densities are associated with a *lower* birthweight among the supplemented group, whereas lower protein density supplements (under 20 per cent of supplemented calories) are associated with a higher mean birthweight in the supplemented group.

Table 17.7 Controlled trials of dietary supplementation in pregnancy; protein density and birthweight difference between subjects and controls, in rank order by protein density of supplementation

Study	% of calories as protein	Birthweight diff. (g) Subjects minus controls	No. subjects/ controls
Merchant and Sheth (pers. comm., 1980)	40.0 (larger amt.)	−17	(97/635)
	40.0 (smaller amt.)	−23	(136/635)
Rush *et al.* (1980)	34.0	−32	(263/272)
Adams *et al.* (1978)	34.0	−45	(36/43)
Osofsky (1975)	26.0	−113	(122/118)
Ebbs *et al.* (1941, 1942)	21.4	−85	(90/120)
Elwood *et al.* (1981)	21.2	55*	(510/441)
Campbell Brown (1983)	20.5–23.8	37	(90/90)
Herriott *et al.* (1978)	20.0	51	(81/87)
McDonald *et al.* (1981)	20.0	16	(108/105)
Mora *et al.* (1979)	17.9	51	(200/207)
Qureshi *et al.* (1973)	16.0	540	(39/37)
Rush *et al.* (1980)	7.5	41	(263/272)
Adams *et al.* (1978)	7.5	92	(36/23)
Merchant and Sheth (pers. comm., 1980)	6.7 (larger amt.)	83	(122/635)
	6.7 (smaller amt.)	36	(157/635)

* Controlling (approximately) for disparity in frequency of smoking.

8 The Special Supplemental Food Programme for Women, Infants, and Children (WIC)

The Special Supplemental Food Programme for Women, Infants and Children (WIC) was begun in the United States in 1973, and is available to women with low income and with at least one other characteristic that might make her subject to nutritional risk. Currently the programme, which also supplements postpartum women and preschool children up to the age of five, serves 3,000,000 clients at any one time, and costs 1.6 billion dollars a year. Approximately one-third of American pregnant women meet the income eligibility criterion, and in 1980, we estimated that 40 per cent of income eligible women were actually enrolled in the programme. This proportion had probably risen to about 46 per cent in 1986. The supplements are substantial: approximately 800 kcal per day of dairy products, cereals, vitamin C rich juices, and several miscellaneous items, such as eggs, peanut butter, and lentils. The programme aims not only at an adequate diet, but at co-ordination and improvement of health care.

In 1978, when the US Congress reauthorized the WIC programme, it mandated that a thorough evaluation of the health effects of the programme be carried out. As part of the evaluation, we reviewed some 85 past

Table 17.8 Studies of effects of the United States WIC programme

Authors	Difference in birthweight (g)	Difference in % <2500 g birthweight	*n*, subjects	*n*, controls	Comments
MEDICAID OR POSTPARTUM WIC CONTROLS					
Edozien *et al.* (1976a,b, 1979)	102* or 136* NA	NA −2.0†	139 1651	41 4976	Two regression models for mean birthweight: 6+ months' WIC treatment in pregnancy vs. postnatal WIC recruits: relationship of duration of WIC benefits to mean birthweight confounded by duration of gestation. Postpartum WIC recruits were controls.
Fleshood *et al.* (1983)	NA	−5.9‡	12,533	7961	Tennessee, all 1982 prenatal WIC recipients, vs. postnatal WIC recruits.
Goldberg (1982)	368‡	−17.6	46	63	Prenatal vs. postnatal WIC recruits. Results confounded to the extent that low birthweight was the criterion for postnatal recruitment into WIC.
Heimendinger (1981)	60*	NA	476	1536	Three WIC sites in Boston; controls: postnatal WIC recruits (438) and children at neighbourhood clinics (1098). Difference controlled for whether low birthweight/premature, probably leading to underestimate of true difference.
Kennedy *et al.* (1982a,b)	122‡ or 67*	−2.8*	897	400	Lower figure for mean birthweight adjusted for social and biological differences between WIC and control groups. Comparability of WIC group and controls (e.g. race) not certain.
Langham *et al.* (1975, addendum 1981)	NA	−4.8‡	11,817	6214	Controls: postpartum WIC recruits; Louisiana WIC programme, 1979–81.
Schramm (1983, 1985)	6	−1.9*	1883	5745	Medicaid births, Missouri, 1980. Subpopulation of those studied by Stockbauer and Blount (1983).
Williams (1982)	NA	−5.1†	506	750	Prenatal vs. postnatal WIC recruits, Wyoming, 1978–80.
COMMUNITY OR OTHER CONTROLS					
Bailey *et al.* (1983)	−47	−5.0	35	46	WIC group from the Maternal and Infant Care (MIC) project. Controls from public clinic; controls reported greater calorie intake.
Brevard County, Florida (1977)	NA	−5.5	NA	NA	Total *n* = 1847; countywide data pre-WIC and post-WIC.
Centres for Disease Control (CDC) (1978)	NA NA	−3.6‡ −1.8*	1580	20,257	Louisiana WIC recipients vs. Charity Hospital, New Orleans. No data on comparability of WIC recipients and controls.
Collins *et al.* (1981)	0	2.6	342	178	Study among those receiving prenatal care in 6 Alabama Appalachian county health departments.

studies of effects of the WIC programme, both published and unpublished. Those relevant to this review are summarized in Table 17.8. These previous studies are aggregated into two groups: those that included Medicaid patients or women whose children were recruited postpartum into the WIC programme as controls and a second group of studies that used community or other controls. The first group of studies would tend to overestimate the effects of the programme, because Medicaid, the federal financing scheme for health care for the low income and indigent, has far more stringent economic criteria for programme receipt than the WIC programme. Presumably controls drawn from that roster would be, on average, worse off than WIC participants. The bias toward overestimating programme effects by using postpartum WIC recruits as controls is

Table 17.8—*continued*

Authors	Difference in birthweight (g)	Difference in % <2500 g birthweight	*n*, subjects	*n*, controls	Comments
Kotelchuck *et al.* (1981)	21	−1.9†	4126	4126	Massachusetts, 1978, WIC recipients matched with controls on several characteristics known from birth certificates. Probable undermatching and consequently low estimate of mean birthweight difference. Internal evidence of systematic exclusion of very premature deliveries from WIC group, with probable overestimate of effect on rates of very low birthweight and neonatal death.
Nutt *et al.* (1981)	72†	NA	104	104	WIC and 'matched' control group widely discrepant for race and welfare status. Results not controlled for infant sex; sex difference could account for about 12 g of difference between WIC recipients and controls.
Rye *et al.* (1978)	NA	−0.9	1976–77: 1360 1977–78	All births in Arizona 1977	All WIC recipients in 14 counties and 9 tribal WIC programme in Arizona vs. statewide rates.
Schelzel and Britton (1978)	NA	−5.3	64 (<6 months' benefits) 55 (>6 months' benefits)		Comparison with past reproductive history. Results confounded by regression to the mean, if adverse past outcome a criterion for programme eligibility.
Sharbaugh *et al.* (1977)	57*	NA	452	222	Maternal and Infant Care (MIC) project recipients, central Florida; 6 counties with WIC, 3 without, 1975–76.
	NA	−1.8*	2126	6944	MIC recipients, central Florida; comparison of rates before (<1974) and after (1975–76) the introduction of WIC.
Kotelchuck *et al.* (1982, 1984)	28	−1.7*	1309	1309	Subset of same study population, as in Kotelchuck *et al.* (1981), comparing differential increase in birthweight and rates of low birthweight across pregnancies. Probable systemic exclusion of very preterm deliveries from index pregnancies.
Metcoff *et al.* (1982, 1985)	Lowest tercile, predicted birthweight:				Published article (Metcoff *et al.* (1985) omits mention of marked imbalance in risk of low birthweight between WIC and control groups. No treatment effect after adjusting for group disparities in maternal weight. Birthweight presented in publication only with adjustment for duration of gestation, obscuring actual effects.
	−146	NA	63	37	
	Middle tercile, predicted birthweight:				
	−14	NA	83	101	
	Upper tercile, predicted birthweight:				
	111	NA	92	34	
Total	−4	1.8	238	172	
Silverman *et al.* (1982)	94‡	−3.3*	1047	1361	MIC recipients, Alleghany County, Pennsylvania; most controls prior to WIC programme (1974).
Stockbauer and Blount (1983); Stockbauer (1986)	16* (non-white: 48*	−0.9* −3.1*	6657 2200	71,931 NA)	All births, Missouri, 1980; results controlled for maternal weight at conception, smoking, education, and race.

* $p<0.05$ † $p<0.01$ ‡ $p<0.001$

even more severe, as one of the most frequent criteria used to enrol infants into the programme is that they were of low birthweight. On the other hand, there is probably a bias *against* the programme with controls selected from other sources, such as matching on the limited number of items available on the birth certificate. Thus, the choice of control group will influence the estimate of programme effects.

Probably the best of the studies described in Table 17.8 are the ones of all births in Missouri in 1980 (Stockbauer and Blount 1983; Stockbauer 1986) and the subset of the same births who were Medicaid recipients (Schramm 1983 and 1985). Stockbauer and Blount found a statistically significant higher mean birthweight of 16 g associated with WIC participation, almost entirely contributed by non-whites, for whom the difference was 48 grams. The comments in Table 17.8 may be helpful to those who are particularly interested in this array of studies. A more detailed presentation is available (Rush *et al.* 1988a). In summary, the array of results, showing supplementation to be associated with modest increases in birthweight and reductions in low birthweight is reasonably consistent with the studies presented in Tables 17.1 to 17.7 above.

Two of the four large studies executed between 1982 and 1984 and released by the US government (Rush *et al.* 1986) are relevant to this review. One was a retrospective study which related WIC benefits to perinatal outcome in 1322 counties in 19 states over the first decade of the programme's existence; the other was a prospective controlled study of over 7000 births to income eligible women, done in 58 randomly selected areas in the continental United States, performed at 174 randomly chosen WIC clinics and 55 public or hospital prenatal clinics without WIC programmes. Some of the results are presented in Tables 17.9 and 17.10.

It was our judgment that several research studies with different research strategies were necessary to seek convergent evidence in order to quantitatively estimate the impact of the programme. Any contemporary study would be biased towards underestimating the programme effect for two reasons. First, we cannot assume that women not formally participating in the programme, who might therefore serve as controls, would not be affected by the existence of the programme. The WIC programme employs more nutrition professionals than any other single programme nationwide, and it is likely that these people, as well as former participants, may have positively affected the dietary habits of women not formally enrolled in the programme. An improvement in the diet of non-participants would tend to lead to underestimation of the effect of participation in the programme. In addition, as this is an eligibility (as distinct from an entitlement) programme, the number of beneficiaries is limited. In general, clinic staff would tend to allocate precious places in the programme to those who appear to be at greatest need, and hence at greatest nutritional risk. Comparison of these women with the residuum of eligible non-enrolled women would thus also tend to underestimate programme effects.

One solution to this problem was to perform a study at the ecological level, relating the rate of receipt of WIC benefits within geographical areas (in this case, counties) with countywide changes in perinatal outcome, specified from linked birth and death certificates for a period going back before the program started. There were many technical and administrative problems in executing this study. First, only 19 states and the District of Columbia had all three necessary data sets in reasonably convenient and accessible form (the US census; fetal death and/or linked birth and infant death certificates; WIC service data). Second, even for these 19 states, which had a total of over 13,000,000 births between 1972 and 1981, the years of study, there were many incomplete data elements, which precluded the use of some entire states or sets of counties in any particular analysis. In fact, the largest number of counties used in complete time series analyses was just under 900.

A further limitation was that the birth certificates include few indices of social or physiological status. The social indices that were usually available were maternal race, years of education, and legitimacy of the birth. Legitimacy proved to be inconsistently recorded, and we therefore depended on stratification by race and education (see Table 17.9).

We were able to estimate the effect of one unit of WIC service, but it was not possible to say that the effects of WIC service were limited to those who were formally enrolled: the estimate was rather of how much community change occurred for service to one WIC beneficiary.

The limitations of this study design relate to possible confounding from unmeasured mediating variables. We are moderately assured that this did not occur in our analysis, since a coherent confounding variable is difficult to conceive of or specify, and it seems to us unlikely that there is some alternative explanation for the results.

While there are weaknesses to a geographically based study, and among them is a tendency to underestimate effects, there are special strengths. First, the estimates of effect apply to the total population, and are not confined to some limited subset of participants recruited into a trial. With other designs it takes a leap of faith to generalize results among trial participants to a larger population, since the participants cannot always be presumed to be representative of the population from which they were drawn. Second, trial results are achieved in the special circumstances of an expensive, small scale study and may not be achievable when a

Table 17.9 National evaluation of the special supplemental food programme for women, infants, and children (Rush *et al.* 1988b)

Historical study of pregnancy outcome

(A) Total population

Study design	Outcome measure	Mean	Change/yr	Change/yr	Difference associated with WIC participation	No. of counties
Relationship of perinatal outcome, from fetal death certificates and linked birth ($n=13{,}434{,}000$) and infant death certificates, to rate of WIC benefits to income eligible pregnant women, within 1322 counties, by year; 19 states from 1972 to 1981; analysis limited to counties with at least 100 births at midpoint of time series (1975) and with all data elements necessary to specific analysis	First trimester registration for prenatal care (%)	73.9	0.9‡	0.9‡	4.1‡	822
	Inadequate no. of prenatal visits (%)	6.3	−0.4‡	−0.4‡	−5.0‡	765
	Preterm delivery (<37 wks; %)	6.6	−0.1	−0.1	−0.7	1255§
	Duration of gestation (wks)	39.1	0.0	0.0	0.2*	1255§
	Birthweight <2500 (%)	6.8	−0.1	−0.1	−0.4	888
	Mean birthweight (g)	3335	6.7‡	6.7‡	23.9†	1321§
	Fetal deaths, 28+ wks gest./1000	6.2	−0.3‡	−0.3‡	−2.3†	1018§
	Neonatal death/1000	10.6	−0.7‡	−0.7‡	−1.5	1149§

(B) WIC effect, by maternal race and education

		Race: White, Education (yrs) <12	White 12+	Black <12	Black 12+
Comparison of time trends with WIC effects on duration of gestation, fetal and neonatal death rates, and birthweight strongly suggests nutritional effect rather than mediation by improved medical care (see text).	First trimester registration for prenatal care (%)	1.4 (475)	−0.8 (730)	6.7‡ (110)	5.0* (118)
	Inadequate no. of prenatal visits (%)	−2.5* (420)	−1.1 (674)	−1.1 (98)	0.5 (106)
	Preterm delivery (<37 wks; %)	−1.8‡	0.1	−2.0*	−1.3
	Duration of gestation (wks)	0.2†	0.0	0.0	0.1
	Birthweight <2500 (%)	−0.4	−0.4	−1.5*	−1.8
	Mean birthweight (g)	46.6‡	43.7‡	26.1*	33.6
	Fetal deaths, 28+ wks	−0.5 (437)	−2.8 (665)	−1.4 (105)	−2.7 (111)
	Neonatal death/1000	−2.3 (306)	−6.2* (445)	−4.7 (83)	0.6 (85)

( ) = n, counties
n's = to first row, unless specified

(C) Change in outcome/yr by maternal race and education

	Race: White, Education (yrs) <12	White 12+	Black <12	Black 12+
First trimester registration for prenatal care (%)	0.5‡	0.7‡	1.3‡	1.5‡
Inadequate no. of prenatal visits (%)	−0.4‡	−0.2‡	−0.9‡	−0.7‡
Preterm delivery (<37 wks; %)	−0.08*	−0.03	−0.08	−0.09
Duration of gestation (wks)	0.01	0.00	0.01	0.01
Birthweight <2500 (%)	−0.7‡	−0.08‡	−0.03	−0.15‡
Mean birthweight (g)	1.5*	7.4‡	1.0	6.0‡
Fetal deaths, 28+ wks	−0.4‡	−0.2‡	−0.8‡	−0.4†
Neonatal death/1000	−0.8‡	−0.5‡	−1.1‡	−0.6†

(n's = to (B), above)

* $p<0.05$ † $p<0.01$ ‡ $p<0.001$ §includes additional counties with incomplete years

Table 17.10 The special supplemental food programme for women, infants and children (WIC) Longitudinal study, Rush *et al.* (1988c,d)

Population studied	Assignment method/ research design	Study group No.	Study group Treatment	Control group No.	Control group Treatment	Results: Dietary advice and maternal anthropometry	WIC	WIC at follow-up[2]	Control	Control at follow-up	Comments
First time registrants for WIC, or prenatal care, first 2 trimesters, in 58 randomly selected areas in US, 1983	WIC patient from 174 of 185 randomly selected WIC sites, controls income eligible women from 55 of 80 prenatal clinics without WIC programmes and in areas of low WIC penetration	5205	Standard WIC benefits	1358	Routine prenatal care (25.1% enrolled in WIC by 8th month gestation)	Diet in 8th month					One-quarter of controls enrolled in programme by 36–38th week gestation. Control group had higher income, education, and social status.
						kcal	+111†	+142*		1905	
						Protein (g)	+ 5.2†	+ 6.5		75.5	
						Iron (mg)	+ 3.2‡	+ 4.5†		14.1	
						(n	2762	181		530)	
						Wt. (kg)					
						Registration[3]	− 0.7†	− 0.7		65.9	
						Follow-up	+ 0.1	− 0.3		72.1	
						(n	3576	214		598)	
						Triceps skinfold (mm)					
						Registration	− 0.5	− 0.4		20.7	
						Follow-up[4]	− 0.9‡	− 0.4		22.5	
						(n	3619	218		612)	
						Subscapular skinfold (mm)					
						Registration	− 0.3	+ 0.5		17.8	
						Follow-up[4]	− 0.8‡	− 0.2		20.9	
						Prenatal outcome					
							WIC		Control[5]		
						Duration gestation (d)	−0.1		276.0		
						<37 wks gest. (%)	−1.2		15.1		
						Mean birthweight (g)	−9		3258		
						<2500 g (%)	+0.5		7.4		
						Length (mm)	−0.2		50.3		
						Head circ. (cm)	+0.2†		33.8		
						Fetal mort. (/1000)	−5.5		15.1		
						(n	2536–3192		693–813		

[1] All results adjusted for race, age, income, education, welfare status, etc.
[2] Control women who had enrolled in WIC before late pregnancy evaluation.
[3] Wt. at registration adjusted for wt. at conception; therefore not interpretable as weight-gain.
[4] Follow-up skinfold adjusted for value at registration; follow-up values therefore interpretable as change in skinfold thickness.
[5] Includes those who enrolled in WIC after registration.

$^*p<0.05$ $^\dagger p<0.01$ $^\ddagger p<0.001$.

programme is fully implemented, with all the limitations associated with large programmes. Thus, while this type of study does not have the methodologic rigour of the randomized trial, the results are likely to be more readily generalizable.

We found statistically significant positive correlations between the intensity of WIC service and early registration for prenatal care, more frequent prenatal visits, duration of gestation, mean birthweight, and, possibly most importantly, a reduction in the late fetal death rate (Rush *et al.* 1988b). The magnitude of reduction in neonatal death rate was somewhat less than that of fetal death rate, and the result was not statistically significant. The pattern of results strongly suggests to us that this was an effect on maternal physiology, and not mediated primarily by better obstetrical care. First, there were major effects in our contemporary study on the woman's diet, weight gain, and skinfold thickness (see Table 17.10). Also, we found that there were marked changes over time in the entire population in some perinatal outcomes, particularly a fall in infant death rates. (Table 17.9). On the other hand, in the entire population, there was no change in duration of gestation over the decade under study. Thus, that WIC significantly affected duration of gestation, birthweight, and fetal death rate seems coherent with improved maternal physiologic status, rather than mediation by improved health care. Since these are all indices that reflect change prior to the onset of labour (other than for intrapartum fetal death), they cannot be related to improvements in intrapartum or neonatal care.

The relationship with lowered fetal death bears some special attention. In the past, work on the effect of nutritional supplementation during pregnancy has focused almost exclusively on birthweight. Studies of effects on mortality have not been undertaken because of the much larger numbers of subjects needed. This may thus be the first secure demonstration of a direct relationship between a feeding programme in pregnancy and lowered mortality rates in the offspring. Further, the results stratified by race and education suggest that WIC programme benefits were more pronounced among the subsets of women most likely to have been enrolled in the programme: blacks and those with less formal education.

While for those outcomes specified in the birth certificate, this retrospective ecological study probably gave a less biased estimate of programme effect (but likely an underestimate, given the relatively crude and imprecisely measured indices of numbers of WIC beneficiaries that were available to us), the outcome measures are limited. In order to study issues other than these included on birth certificates, we also executed an extensive prospective study on a large nationwide representative sample of low income pregnant women, some of the results of which are presented in Table 17.10 (Rush *et al.* 1988d). Diets were increased in energy and in nutrient density, weight-gain was accelerated, and late pregnancy fat deposition lowered. Further, while birthweight and duration of gestation were not different, after adjusting for a wide variety of social and physiological indices, the head circumferences of infants of mothers who participated in WIC were statistically significantly larger than those of controls (0.21 cm, $p < 0.01$). As with mortality, this has been an infrequently studied outcome, and the likelihood that this was a real, rather than a chance, finding is strengthened because we found a similar, although not statistically significant relationship, among preschool children whose mothers had been enrolled in the WIC programme during pregnancy (not present among children enrolled after birth). This association with accelerated head, and presumably brain, growth is potentially of great importance and requires follow up in early childhood to test its constancy over time, and whether it reflects changes in cognition and behaviour.

We found significant relationships between the quality of the individual WIC programme, as judged by the administrator responsible for all WIC programmes within a state, and rate of fetal growth. Further, we found no relationship between the response to WIC programme benefits on perinatal outcome with maternal skinfold thickness at the onset of programme participation. Prior skinfold thickness was not an index of responsiveness to programme.

9 Conclusions

9.1 Implications for current practice

We can draw two main conclusions from the studies reviewed. On the one hand, dietary restriction can cause markedly decreased birthweight. During famine, mean birthweight can be depressed by as much as 550 g. Iatrogenic dietary manipulation and restriction can have almost as serious an effect. Although the extent to which such decrements in birthweight are associated with perinatal mortality and morbidity is unknown, there can be no rational justification for either allowing pregnant women to go hungry or for imposing either dietary restriction or marked manipulation of the dietary constituents upon them.

On the other hand, attempts at nutritional supplementation, while well-intentioned, have not always had the desired effect. First, it is clear that high density protein supplements are consistently associated with depression, rather than increase, in mean birthweight. Second, although consistent increments (on average, about 30 to 50 g) in mean birthweight have been found in association with programmes of aggressive nutritional counselling and/or supplementation with preparations of lower protein density, the magnitude of these increments is nevertheless lower than had been hoped.

9.2 Implications for future research

Since the increase in mean birthweight associated with nutritional counselling and supplementation has been relatively small, further trials of these interventions must concentrate on the subsets of women in which a beneficial effect is most likely to be demonstrated. This notion is supported by the fact that in our New York study (Rush *et al.* 1980a,b), nutritional intervention matched our expectations only among those women who were heavy smokers. Women who are likely to benefit most from dietary supplementation might be identified in a number of ways. Reliance on dietary history alone has been unrewarding. Possibly biochemical assessment (Metcoff *et al.* 1973) or anthropometric measurements (Habicht *et al.* 1974) may prove more useful.

Further research is also urgently needed to determine whether the observed range of increments in birthweight are consistently associated with decreased perinatal morbidity and mortality, and with improved long term growth and development of the infant and child. New studies with new research designs are needed. Much larger populations are required to study effects on mortality and careful longitudinal research is essential to understand long term development. In addition, since there is some evidence that prenatal feeding may influence subsequent development independent of changes in birthweight (Rush 1984), the possibility of such effects must not be neglected.

While there is obvious need of further research into the best means of promoting optimal nutrition in pregnancy, hungry women cannot wait for the results of such studies. They must have access both to adequate amount of food and to informed, sympathetic care.

References

Adams SO, Barr GD, Huenemann RL (1978). Effects of nutritional supplementation in pregnancy I: Outcome of pregnancy. J Am Diet Assoc, 72: 144–147.

Antonov AN (1947). Children born during the seige of Leningrad in 1942. J Pediatr, 30: 250–259.

Bailey LB, O'Farrell-Ray B, Mahan CS, Dimperio D (1983). Vitamin B6, iron, and folacin status of pregnant women. Nutr Res, 3: 783–793.

Balfour MI (1944). Supplementary feeding in pregnancy. Lancet, l: 208–211.

Barsa Gregory P, Rush D (1987). Iatrogenic caloric restriction in pregnancy and birthweight. Am J Perinatol, 4: 365–371.

Berry K, Wiehl DG (1952). An experiment in education during pregnancy. Milbank Mem Fund Qtrly, 30: 119–151.

Blumenthal I (1976). Diet and diuretics in pregnancy and subsequent growth of offspring. Br Med J, 2: 733.

Brevard County, Florida (1977) Report of WIC data. Unpublished report. Florida: Rockledge.

Cameron CS, Graham S (1944). Antenatal diet and its influences on still births and prematurity. Glasgow Med J, 1420: 1–7.

Campbell DM (1983). Dietary restriction and its effect on neonatal outcome. In: Nutrition in Pregnancy. Campbell DM, Gillmer MDG (eds). Proceedings of the Tenth Study Group of the Royal College of Obstetricians and Gynaecologists, pp 243–250.

Campbell DM, MacGillivray I (1975). The effect of a low calorie diet or a thiazide diuretic on the incidence of pre-eclampsia and on birthweight. Br J Obstet Gynaecol, 82: 572–577.

Campbell Brown M (1983) Protein energy supplements in primigravid women at risk of low birthweight In: Nutrition in Pregnancy. Campbell DM, Gillmer MDG (eds). Proceedings of the Tenth Study Group of the Royal College of Obstetricians and Gynaecologists, pp 85–98

Centers for Disease Control, Nutrition Section (1978). CDC analysis of nutritional indices for selected WIC participants. Atlanta, Georgia: US Dept of Health and Human Services, Public Health Service, Centers for Disease Control.

Collins T, Leeper J, Northrup RS, Demeillier S (1981). Integration of WIC program with other infant mortality programs Final report, Appalachian Region Commission Report, University of Alabama, Tuscaloosa.

Dean RFA (1951). The size of the baby at birth and the yield of breast milk In: Studies of Under-nutrition. Wuppertal 1946–9. Medical Research Council Special Report Series, No. 275. London: Her Majesty's Stationery Office, pp 346–378.

Dieckmann WJ, Adair FL, Michael H, Kramer S, Dunkle F, Arthur B, Costin M, Campbell A, Wensley AC, Lorang E (1944). Calcium, phosphorus, iron and nitrogen balances in pregnant women Am J Obstet Gynecol, 47: 357–368.

Ebbs JH, Tisdall FF, Scott WA (1941). The influences of prenatal diet on the mother and child. J Nutr, 22: 515–526.

Ebbs JH, Brown A, Tisdall FF, Moyle WJ, Bell M (1942). The influence of improved nutrition upon the infant. Can Med Assoc J, 46: 6–8.

Edozien JC, Switzer BR, Bryan RB (1976a). Medical evaluation of the special supplemental food program for women, infants and children (WIC), 6 volumes. Chapel Hill, North Carolina: University of North Carolina, School of Public Health.

Edozien JC, Switzer BR, Bryan RB (1976b). Medical evaluation of the special supplemental food program for women, infants, and children. Select Committee on Nutrition and Human Needs, United States Senate. Washington DC: US Government Printing Office.

Edozien JC, Switzer BR, Ryan RB (1979). Medical evaluation of the special supplemental food program for women, infants and children. Am J Clin Nutr, 32: 677–692.

Elwood PC, Haley TJL, Hughes SJ, Sweetman PM, Gray OP, Davies DP (1981). Child growth (0–5 years) and the effect of entitlement to a milk supplement. Arch Dis Child, 56: 831–835.

Fleshood L, Buckner MH, Hatchett AF, Hayes JA, Seals J, Smith CM, Scanlon PA, Wallace JN (1983). Is WIC reducing the prevalence of low birthweight and infant mortality? Paper presented during the 160th American Public Health Association meeting, 1978.

Girija A, Geervani P, Nageswara Rao G (1984). Influence of dietary supplementation during pregnancy on lactation performance. J Trop Pediatr, 30: 79–83.

Goldberg HE (1982). An Evaluation of the Effectiveness of the WIC Program in Terms of Height, Birthweight, Weight, and Hematocrit. Unpublished report. New York: The Mount Sinai Medical Center.

Grieve JFK, Campbell Brown BM, Johnstone FD (1979). Dieting in pregnancy: a study of the effect of a high protein low carbohydrate diet on birthweight on an obstetric population. In: Carbohydrate Metabolism in Pregnancy and the Newborn 1978. Sutherland MW, Stowers JM (eds). Berlin: Springer Verlag, pp 518–533.

Habicht JP, Lechtig A, Yarbrough C, Klein RE (1974). Maternal nutrition, birthweight and infant mortality In: Size at Birth. Elliott K, Knight J (eds). Ciba Foundation Symposium 27 (New Series). Amsterdam: Elsevier, pp 353–377.

Heimendinger G (1981). I. The Effect of WIC on the Growth of Infants and Children. II. The Use of Growth Standards in Assessing WIC Impact on Infants and Children. Unpublished doctoral thesis. Boston: Harvard University.

Herriott RM, Hsueh AM, Aitchison R (1978). Influence of maternal diet on offspring: growth, behaviour, feed efficiency and susceptibility (human); a study in Suilin, Taiwan, initiated by Chow, BF. Final report on AID/CSD 2944, contract with the Johns Hopkins University.

Higgins AC (1976). Nutritional status and the outcome of pregnancy. J Can Diet Assoc, 37: 17–36.

Iyengar L (1967). Effects of dietary supplements late in pregnancy on the expectant mother and her newborn. Indian J Med Res, 55: 85–89.

Kennedy ET, Gershoff S (1982a). Effect of WIC supplemental feeding on hemoglobin and hematocrit of prenatal patients. J Am Diet Assoc, 80: 227–230.

Kennedy ET, Gershoff S, Reed R, Austin JE (1982b). Evaluation of the effect of WIC supplemental feeding on birth weight. J Am Dietetic Assoc, 80: 220–227.

Kotelchuck M, Schwartz JB, Anderka M, Finison K (1981). Massachusetts Special Supplemental Food Program for Women, Infants and Children (WIC) evaluation project: Final report Boston: Massachusetts Department of Public Health.

Kotelchuck M, Anderka M, Stern LJ, Hudson M, Graham-Mero L (1982). Massachusetts Special Supplemental Food Program for Women, Infants, and Children (WIC) follow-up study: Final Report Boston: Massachusetts Department of Public Health.

Kotelchuck M, Schwartz J, Anderka M, Finison K (1984). WIC participation and pregnancy outcomes: Massachusetts Statewide Evaluation Project. Am J Public Health, 74: 1086–1092.

Lamb WH, Lamb CMB, Foord FA, Whitehead, RG (1984). Changes in maternal and child mortality rates in three isolated Gambian villages over ten years. Lancet, 2: 912–914.

Langham RA, Dupree BW, Atkins EH, Schilling PE (1975). Impact of the WIC program in Louisiana. Unpublished report. New Orleans: Louisiana State Health Department. [Addendum (1981)]

Lawrence M, Lamb WH, Lawrence F, Whitehead RG (1984). Maintenance energy cost of pregnancy in rural Gambian women and influence of dietary status. Lancet, ii: 363–365.

Lechtig A, Habicht JP, Delgado H, Klein RE, Yarbrough C, Martorell R (1975). Effect of food supplementation during pregnancy on birthweight. Pediatrics, 56: 508–520.

Lundin FE, Stark CR (1980). A maternal nutrition education project-evaluation of effects of birthweight, gestational age, and infant mortality. Personal communication.

McDonald EC, Pollitt E, Mueller W, Hsueh AN, Sherwin R (1981). The Bacon Chow study: Maternal nutritional supplementation and birthweight of offspring. Am J Clin Nutr, 34: 2133–2144.

Merchant S, Sheth P (1980). Personal communication.

Metcoff J, Wikman-Coffelt J, Yoshida T, Bernal A, Roasado A, Yoshida P, Urristi J, Frenk S, Madraso R, Velasco L, Morales M (1973). Energy metabolism and protein synthesis in human leukocytes during pregnancy and in the placenta related to fetal growth. Pediatrics, 51: 866–867.

Metcoff J, Costiloe P, Crosby W, Sandstead H, Bodwell CE, Kennedy E (1982). Nutrition in pregnancy ('NIP') final report (USDA). Report to the Food and Nutrition Service, USDA. Oklahoma City: University of Oklahoma Health Sciences Center.

Metcoff J, Costiloe P, Crosby W, Dutta S, Sandstead H, Milne D, Bodwell CE, Majors S (1985). Effect of food supplementation (WIC) during pregnancy on birth weight. Am J Clin Nutr, 41: 933–947.

Mora JO, de Paredes B, Wagner M, de Navarro L, Suescun J, Christiansen N, Herrara MG (1979). Nutritional supplementation and the outcome of pregnancy I: birthweight. Am J Clin Nutr, 32: 455–462.

Naeye RL, Blanc W, Paul C (1973). Effects of maternal nutrition on the human fetus. Pediatrics, 52: 494–503.

Nutt PC, Wheeler M, Wheeler RA (1981). Social Program Evaluation Revisited: The WIC Program. The Ohio State University, American Institute of Decision Sciences.

Osofsky HJ (1975). Relationships between prenatal medical and nutritional measures, pregnancy outcome, and early infant development in an urban poverty setting I: the role of nutritional intake. Am J Obstet Gynecol, 123: 682–690.

Prentice AM, Whitehead RG, Roberts SB, Paul AA (1981). Long-term energy balance in child-bearing Gambian women. Am J Clin Nutr, 34: 2790–2799.

Prentice AM, Lunn PG, Watkinson M, Whitehead RG (1983a). Dietary supplementation of lactating Gambian women II: Effect on maternal health, nutritional status and biochemistry. Hum Nutr Clin Nutr, 37: 65–74.

Prentice AM, Watkinson M, Whitehead RG, Lamb, WH (1983b). Prenatal dietary supplementation of African women and birthweight. Lancet, 1: 489–491.

Prentice AM, Prentice A, Lamb WH, Lunn PG, Austin S (1983c). Metabolic consequences of fasting during Ramadan in pregnant and lactating women. Hum Nutr Clin Nutr, 37: 283–94.

Qureshi S, Rao NP, Madhavi V, Mathur YC, Reddi YR (1973). Effect of maternal nutrition supplementation on the birthweight of the newborn. Indian Pediatr, 10: 541–544.

Ross SM, Nel E, Naeye R (1985). Differing effects of low and high bulk maternal dietary supplements during pregnancy. Early Hum Dev, 10: 295–302.

Rush D (1981). Nutrition services during pregnancy and birthweight: a retrospective matched pair analysis. Can Med Assoc J, 125: 567–574.

Rush D (1982). Effects of changes and calorie intake during pregnancy on the growth of the human fetus In: Effectiveness and Satisfaction in Antenatal Care, Clinics in Developmental Medicine Series. Enkin M, Chalmers I (eds). London: Spastics International Medical Publications, pp 92–113.

Rush D (1984). The behavioural consequences of protein-energy deprivation and supplementation in early life: an epidemiological perspective. In: Nutrition and Behaviour, Vol 5 of Human Nutrition: A Comprehensive Treatise. Galler JR (ed). New York: Plenum Press, pp 119–157.

Rush D, Stein Z, Susser M (1980a). A randomized controlled trial of prenatal nutritional supplementation in New York City. Pediatrics, 65: 683–697.

Rush D, Stein Z, Susser M (1980b). A Randomized Controlled Trial of Prenatal Nutritional Supplements. March of Dimes Birth Defects Foundation, Vol XVI, 3, 200 pp + xvii. New York: Alan R Liss.

Rush D, Leighton J, Sloan NL, Alvir JM, Garbowski GC (1988a). The national WIC evaluation: Evaluation of the special supplemental food program for women, infants, and children. II Review of past studies of WIC. Am J Clin Nutr, 48: 394–411.

Rush D, Alvir JM, Kenny DA, Johnson SS, Horvitz DG (1988b). The national WIC evaluation: Evaluation of the special supplemental food program for women, infants, and children. III Historical study of pregnancy outcomes. Am J Clin Nutr, 48: 412–428.

Rush D, Horvitz DG, Seaver WB, Leighton J, Sloan NL, Johnson SS, Kulka RA, Devore JW, Holt M, Lynch JT, Virag TG, Woodside MB, Shanklin DS (1988c). The national WIC evaluation: Evaluation of the special supplemental food program for Women, Infants, and Children. IV Study methodology and sample characteristics in the longitudinal study of pregnant women, the study of children, and the food expenditures study. Am J Clin Nutr, 48: 429–438.

Rush D, Sloan NL, Leighton J, Alvir JM, Horvitz DG, Seaver WB, Garbowski GC, Johnson SS, Kulka RA, Holt M, Devore JW, Lynch JT, Woodside MB, Shanklin DS (1988d). The national WIC evaluation: Evaluation of the special supplemental food program for women, infants, and children. V Longitudinal study of pregnant women. Am J Clin Nutr, 48: 439–483.

Rye J, White M, Majchrzak M (1978). Intervention outcomes in Arizona's WIC program, July 1976 through March 1977. Unpublished report. Pima County, Tucson, Arizona.

Schelzel G, Britton MA (1978). An assessment of the WIC program in Pennsylvania. Unpublished report. Pennsylvania Health Department.

Schramm WF (1983). WIC Prenatal Participation and Its Relationship to Newborn Medicaid Costs in Missouri: A Cost/Benefit Analysis. Jefferson City, Missouri: Missouri Center for Health Statistics.

Schramm WF (1985). WIC prenatal participation and its relationship to newborn Medicaid costs in Missouri—a cost/benefit analysis. Am J Public Health, 75: 851–857.

Sharbaugh C, Morris C, Mahan C (1977). The North Central Florida WIC evaluation. Unpublished report. Gainesville, Florida: North Central Florida Maternity and Infant Care Project.

Silverman PR, Kuller LH, Kolodner DC (1982). The effect of a local prenatal nutrition supplementation program (WIC) on birth weight. Unpublished manuscript. Pittsburgh, Pennsylvania: Allegheny County Health Department.

Smith CA (1947). The effect of wartime starvation in Holland upon pregnancy and its product. Am J Obstet Gynecol, 53: 599–608.

Stein Z, Susser M, Saenger G, Marolla F (1975). Famine and Human Development: The Dutch Hunger Winter of 1944/45. New York: Oxford University Press.

Stockbauer JW (1986). Evaluation of the Missouri WIC Program: Prenatal Component. J Am Diet Assoc, 86: 61–67.

Stockbauer J, Blount CR (1983). Evaluation of the prenatal participation component of the Missouri WIC program. Jefferson City, Missouri: Missouri Department of Social Services Division of Health.

Sweeney C, Smith H, Foster JC, Place JC, Specht J, Kochenour NK, Prater BM (1985). Effects of a nutrition intervention program during pregnancy. J Nurs Midwifery, 3: 149–158.

Tompkins WT, Mitchell RM, Wiehl DG (1955). Maternal nutrition studies at Philadelphia Lying-in Hospital, 2 Prematurity and maternal nutrition. In: The Promotion of Maternal and Newborn Health. New York: Milbank Memorial Fund, pp 25–50.

Viegas OAC, Scott PH, Cole TJ, Mansfield HN, Wharton P, Wharton BA (1982a). Dietary protein energy supplementation of pregnant Asian mothers at Sorrento, Birmingham 1: Unselective during second and third trimesters. Br Med J, 285: 589–592.

Viegas OAC, Scott PH, Cole TJ, Needham PG, Wharton BA (1982b). Dietary protein energy supplementation of pregnant Asian mothers at Sorrento, Birmingham II: Selective during the third trimester only. Br Med J, 285: 592–595.

Waber DP, Vuori-Christiansen L, Ortiz N, Clement JR, Christiansen NE, Mora JO, Reed RB, Herrera MG (1981). Nutritional supplementation, maternal education, and cognitive development of infants at risk of malnutrition. Am J Clin Nutr, 34: 807–813.

Watney PJM, Alton C (1986). Dietary supplementation in pregnancy. Br Med J, 293: 1102.

Williams JT (1982). Wyoming WIC evaluation. Unpublished letter report to Food and Nutrition Service.

18 Diet and the prevention of pre-eclampsia

Jane Green

'(Pre-eclampsia) can almost always be avoided if the pregnant woman understands the importance of antenatal care, keeps her antenatal appointments religiously and carries out her doctor's instructions, especially those regarding diet . . . A total weight gain of 8–9 kg is all that should be allowed throughout pregnancy . . .'

Bourne (1984).

'. . . there is no evidence that control of the weight by calorie restriction reduces the incidence of preeclampsia'

Chesley (1978).

'. . . there is conclusive evidence why pregnant women get toxemia . . . there is an inexpensive way to prevent it in every pregnancy . . . No mother who is able to eat, digest, absorb and metabolize a diet adequate for pregnancy will develop MTLP (metabolic toxemia of late pregnancy) . . . the overall aim is for the mother to have 2600 calories and 100 g of protein each day, plus all the salt and other essential minerals and vitamins she needs. . . .'

Brewer and Brewer (1985).

'There is no scientific basis for believing that deficiency or excess of any essential nutrient predisposes to pre-eclampsia/eclampsia'

Davies (1971).

1 Introduction

Since the development of formal antenatal care there has been no shortage of advice for pregnant women and their medical attendants on the ideal diet or weight gain in pregnancy (and, more recently, in the preconceptional period as well). Much of this advice, in the developed world at least, has been restrictive in nature and characterized by extremes of dogmatism. 'If only women will eat as they are told', the story runs 'most of the complications of pregnancy and birth for mother and child can be avoided'.

The effects of changes in nutritional intake on various outcomes of pregnancy have been discussed in other chapters in this book (see Chapters 17 and 19). This chapter addresses the relation of these changes to the development or progression of pre-eclampsia.

Pre-eclampsia has been one of the focal points of dietary advice to pregnant women since the beginning of this century. While the current 'orthodox' medical view in Europe and the United States is that diet and control of weight gain play no significant role in the onset or course of pre-eclampsia, some of the previously widely held beliefs, in particular those concerning weight gain, continue to influence antenatal care. There are also a number of people who continue to believe that there is a direct link between diet and pre-eclampsia. The quotations above reflect these conflicting views.

Pre-eclampsia is a common and potentially serious complication of pregnancy (see Chapter 24). It would evidently be of immense importance were a relatively simple factor like maternal diet really to have a major influence on the development of pre-eclampsia. Equally if it is shown that there is no evidence for such a claim then it should be possible for both doctors and their critics to refrain from giving ill-founded and unnecessary advice about diet to women in pregnancy.

1.1 Sources and methods

In this chapter the association between maternal diet and pre-eclampsia will be examined using evidence from epidemiology, the study of populations under conditions of war and famine, dietary surveys of affected and unaffected women, and intervention studies that have attempted either by advice or by supplementation to alter the diets of pregnant women.

A major difficulty in assessing this evidence is the use of variable and often imprecise criteria for the diagnosis of 'pre-eclampsia' by different authors (see Chapter 24). In this chapter true 'pre-eclampsia' implies both hypertension (diastolic pressure of 90 mm Hg or more) and significant proteinuria (above 0.2 g/l) arising in the second half of pregnancy, with the obvious proviso that other causes of these signs (essential hypertension, renal disease, urinary tract infection) have been ruled out (MacGillivray 1983; Chesley 1985). The term 'toxaemia' is used only where the author's usage requires this. Variations in the definitions of 'pre-eclampsia' and 'toxaemia' make it virtually impossible to assess and compare fully a great many of even the most recent studies on diet and pre-eclampsia.

Other difficulties in assessment arise from the problems inherent in methods of dietary survey and assessment (Johnstone 1983).

2 Epidemiology

Comparisons of the incidence of pre-eclampsia in different population groups could at best provide only indirect evidence about a possible link with diet; in practice their usefulness has been even more limited by the difficulty of obtaining reliable comparative data from studies using widely ranging diagnostic criteria.

It has been argued that the substantially lower incidence of pre-eclampsia in second and subsequent pregnancies is difficult to reconcile with nutritional theories of its aetiology, particularly those involving dietary deficiencies. Indeed, it is assumed that the woman's diet will, if anything, get worse as family size increases (MacGillivray 1983). Little is known, however, about actual differences in diet between first and subsequent pregnancies.

If diet were an important factor in the development of pre-eclampsia, the incidence of pre-eclampsia might be expected to vary with social class (on the whole, poorer women have poorer diets, although as Brewer has pointed out (Brewer and Brewer 1985), it is quite possible for a wealthy woman to self-impose or have imposed upon her, a diet sufficiently restricted to cause relative malnutrition). Unfortunately, there is little reliable evidence on the true incidence of pre-eclampsia in different social groups in the developing countries where extremes of poverty and malnutrition might highlight any differences in incidence due to diet (Davies 1971; MacGillivray 1983). In the developed world, persistent claims that pre-eclampsia is more common among poorer women, particularly in the United States (Ross *et al.* 1938; Brewer and Brewer 1985) have not been substantiated (Chesley 1978).

The only good population study using an adequate definition of pre-eclampsia is that of Nelson in Aberdeen (Nelson 1955a; and updated by Liston, quoted in MacGillivray 1983). He found no clear relationship between social class and the incidence of 'severe pre-eclampsia' (late pregnancy hypertension with proteinuria). There is similarly no evidence for a significant difference in the incidence of pre-eclampsia in different social classes in the British Births Survey of 1970 (Chamberlain *et al.* 1978), although the criteria used to define pre-eclampsia and essential hypertension for this analysis do not allow a clear distinction to be made between true pre-eclampsia and other forms of hypertension in pregnancy. (It is interesting that both Nelson and the British Births Survey found a clear effect of social class on the *outcome* of pre-eclamptic pregnancy, with perinatal mortality and morbidity increasing with lower social class (Nelson 1955b; Chamberlain *et al.* 1978).)

Davies *et al.* (1970) found some evidence for an increased incidence of pre-eclampsia in poor women in their careful population study in West Jerusalem, where the incidence of pre-eclampsia among illiterate women (educational standard being used as a measure of social class) was higher than that in women of other educational groups; however, the definition of pre-eclampsia used in this study was unfortunately not ideal, being based on criteria which allowed the inclusion of women as 'pre-eclamptic' on the basis of hypertension or oedema alone.

There have been a number of attempts to use geographical and racial differences in the reported incidence of pre-eclampsia and eclampsia to support dietary theories. Specific components of the diet such as dietary fibre (Hipsley 1953), calcium (Belizan and Villar 1980), and essential fatty acids (Dyerberg and Bang 1985) have all been implicated on this basis, but the paucity of reliable comparative data on differences in incidence even of eclampsia, let alone pre-eclampsia, is such that it is virtually impossible to draw any conclusions that might serve as a useful basis for investigating dietary (or any other) aetiological factors (Davies 1971; Davies and Dunlop 1983; MacGillivray 1983).

In summary, the limited epidemiological data available do not suggest any important association between diet and pre-eclampsia.

3 War and famine

Severe food shortages in parts of Europe during the

World Wars I and II have been variously associated with reports of increased, unchanged, and decreased incidences of pre-eclampsia and eclampsia (for references, see MacGillivray 1983, p 34). These reports have been used to support conflicting views about the relationship between diet and pre-eclampsia. Unfortunately, many of these studies deal only with the incidence of eclampsia in hospital populations and do not take into account changes in the age and parity distribution of the childbearing population in wartime. There are, however, a few reports from World War II where changes in the incidence of pre-eclampsia are relatively well documented.

The best of these deal with the Dutch 'hunger winter' of 1944–45 (Smith 1947; Mastboom 1948; Ribeiro *et al.* 1982) (see Chapter 17) and show a fall in the incidence of hypertension, pre-eclampsia, and eclampsia in areas affected by the famine (during which the official rations fell as low as 600 calories a day) as compared with the periods immediately preceding and following the famine. While the rates of 'toxaemia', 'pre-eclampsia' and 'eclampsia', are based on recorded clinical diagnoses, and the criteria for the diagnoses are not always made explicit, it should be noted that the rates of all three diagnoses fell during the famine period. These studies do not, however, fully take into account differential fertility and known changes in the age and parity composition of the populations compared.

The deficiencies of the evidence from war studies are obvious and have been pointed out since the first reports appeared (Hauch and Lehmann 1934). It should be equally obvious that in any case an association between a change in the incidence of pre-eclampsia and a period of war or famine is far from proof that one is caused by the other, and even further from evidence relating pre-eclampsia to specific dietary factors. Yet it seems that an uncritical assumption of a causal relationship between famine and a reported fall in incidence of toxaemia was one of the influences that led to the introduction of widespread dietary restriction in pregnancy in the United States (Chesley 1978).

4 Weight and weight-gain

4.1 Body weight and pre-eclampsia

Attempts to evaluate the obstetric risks associated with maternal obesity began to appear in the literature in the 1930s and 1940s. In early studies 'toxaemia' was said to occur more frequently in obese women than in the general obstetric population (e.g. Matthews and der Brucke 1938; Odell and Mengert 1945) and this view has generally been reiterated in subsequent reports of controlled studies (Tompkins and Wiehl 1951, Tompkins *et al.* 1955; Woodhill *et al.* 1955; Kerr 1962; Williams 1957; Emerson 1962; Fields and Davis 1962; Stewart and Hewitt 1960; Peckham and Christianson 1971; Treharne *et al.* 1979; Efiong 1975; Roopnarinesingh and Pathak 1970; Edwards *et al.* 1978). Only a minority of authors have found no clear association between obesity and 'toxaemia' or pre-eclampsia (Lowe 1961; Gillmer 1983). Obesity is today widely regarded as a proven risk factor for the development of pre-eclampsia (MacGillivray 1983; Ruge and Andersen 1985).

Doubts have been raised about this interpretation of the evidence (Lowe 1961; Emerson 1962; Redman 1982a) and indeed many of the 'controlled' studies have such serious flaws in design (notably, failure to allow for differences in age and parity between obese and control groups, and imprecision in the diagnostic criteria used) that it is difficult to assess the validity of their results. It does appear, however, from the few relatively well designed studies (Efiong 1975, Roopnarinesingh and Pathak 1970; Edwards *et al.* 1978; Treharne *et al.* 1979) that there probably is a true association between obesity and pre-eclampsia. This is not surprising; obese women have a higher incidence of hypertension both before and during pregnancy. Essential hypertension is known to be associated with an increased incidence of superimposed pre-eclampsia (MacGillivray 1961; Butler and Bonham 1963), so an association between obesity and pre-eclampsia would be expected.

The situation is complicated by evidence that the overall increase in incidence of pre-eclampsia among obese women is accompanied by a *fall* in the incidence of *severe* pre-eclampsia (Thomson and Billewicz 1957; Treharne *et al.* 1979). To regard obesity as a 'risk factor' for pre-eclampsia would appear at the least to be an over-simplification, and not very helpful in practice. It should also be remembered that unless an appropriately sized cuff is used to measure the blood pressure, obese women are likely to show artificially high readings.

Underweight women have in this context received less attention than those considered overweight. Tompkins and Wiehl (1951) reported an increased incidence of 'toxaemia' (not defined) among women more than 20 per cent below standard weight for height (using reported prepregnancy weights) of the same order as that in obese women (more than 20 per cent above standard weight for height), but although this trend was still present in their later expanded series (Tompkins *et al.* 1955) it was no longer statistically significant. Lowe (1961) also found a high incidence of toxaemia among thinner women, but again this trend was of doubtful significance.

4.2 Weight-gain in pregnancy

It seems clear that a higher than average weight-gain in the second half of pregnancy is associated with the development of pre-eclampsia (Redman 1982a,b; MacGillivray 1983). This is particularly well illustrated in the excellent studies of Aberdeen primigravidae by Thomson and his colleagues (Thomson 1959b; Thomson and Billewicz 1957). The rate of weight-gain in the first half of pregnancy is probably also higher in women who later develop pre-eclampsia (Tompkins and Wiehl 1951; Tompkins et al. 1955; MacGillivray 1983). (It has been claimed that women with especially *low* rates of weight-gain in the second trimester also have an increased risk of pre-eclampsia (Tompkins *et al.* 1955) but this was not seen in Thomson and Billewicz's 1957 study.) Thomson and Billewicz found, however, that the weight-gains of the normotensive and pre-eclamptic populations overlapped to such an extent that it was impossible to predict the occurrence of pre-eclampsia for an individual woman from the rate of weight-gain in the second trimester, despite unsubstantiated claims to the contrary (Hamlin 1952).

The Aberdeen women studied by Thomson (1958; 1959a,b) were apparently free from medical pressures to control weight-gain in pregnancy; the same cannot be said of many women in Europe, Australia and the United States over the past 50 years. So widespread has been the advocacy of restriction of weight-gain that it has proved surprisingly difficult to obtain figures for a normal range of weight-gain (Hytten and Chamberlain 1980). Studies such as those in Aberdeen suggest that Western women eating normally will gain on average about 24–30 lb (12–14 kg) at an average rate in the 2nd trimester of about 1 lb (0.5 kg) a week, but it cannot be too strongly stressed that the *range* of normal weight gain is very wide indeed (Thomson and Billewicz 1957; Hytten and Chamberlain 1980). Many women in developing countries gain much less weight than this during an apparently normal pregnancy. Figures on the relationship between weight-gain and pre-eclampsia in these women would be of considerable interest.

The correlation of higher than average weight-gain (and to a lesser extent prepregnancy obesity) with pre-eclampsia has been one of the main reasons for attempts by the medical profession to prescribe dietary restriction of weight-gain in pregnancy. The restrictions advocated have been quite severe (a maximum total weight-gain in pregnancy of about 20 lb (9 kg); and a maximum rate of weight-gain in the 2nd trimester of 0.5-0.8 lb (0.3 kg) per week (e.g. Hamlin 1952, 1958; Kerr Grieve 1974; Bourne 1984), and the measures adopted to ensure compliance often extreme: hospital admission for dietary instruction and control (Hamlin 1952; Kerr Grieve 1974), the use of the police to chase up poor attenders at antenatal clinics (Hamlin 1952), and the prescription of amphetamines to control appetite (Stevenson 1958).

The illogicality of this restriction has been pointed out many times (Thomson and Billewicz 1957; Brewer 1966; Brewer and Brewer 1985). If the weakness of the theoretical basis for dietary restriction as a means of preventing pre-eclampsia did not influence most clinicians, neither, it appears, did the lack of any good evidence that restricting weight-gain had the desired effect.

Some of the most influential (although not authoritative) work in this respect was published by Hamlin and his followers from Australia and New Zealand in the 1950s (Hamlin 1952, 1958; Hughes 1956; Stevenson 1958; Dawson 1953) and it remains widely quoted in support of weight restriction today (e.g. Myles 1981; Dewhurst 1981). Hamlin observed a striking reduction in the rate of eclampsia (from 1 in 350 before 1948 to 1 in 7000 between 1948 and 1953) and 'albuminuric pre-eclampsia' (not defined) (10 per cent in 1946 to 1.8 per cent in 1957) in Sydney after the introduction of an intensive campaign of antenatal supervision including a strong emphasis on dietary advice and education and an attempt to control weight-gain to less than 8 lb between 20 and 30 weeks. He was convinced (though he produced no evidence to support his conviction) that a weight-gain higher than this would lead inexorably to pre-eclampsia, and attributed the reduction in eclampsia and pre-eclampsia almost entirely to weight control and a high protein, low carbohydrate diet (Hamlin 1952, 1958). (He also claimed (Hamlin 1958) that a low calorie (low carbohydrate and low salt) diet would reverse or slow down the progress of pre-eclampsia if it did develop.) Hamlin's was not a controlled study, and he provides no evidence to support his contention that it was the dietary component of his regimen, rather than some other aspect of the increased intensity of antenatal care that caused the observed effect.

In more recent years a number of controlled studies of weight restriction have been carried out in Aberdeen (Table 18.1). In a study based on the observation by Thomson and Billewicz (1957) that the 'optimal' rate of weight-gain between 20 and 30 weeks was about 1 lb a week (in terms of the incidences of pre-eclampsia and low birthweight), Baird *et al.* (1962) compared two large groups of women, one of which received normal antenatal care with no advice to restrict the diet, and the other of which was given advice to adjust high or low weight-gains towards the 'ideal'. They achieved some success in terms of adjusting weight-gain in the experimental group, but there was no difference in the incidence of pre-eclampsia between the two groups. Campbell and MacGillivray (1975) using matched groups, compared the effects of a low calorie (1200 cal/day) diet, a diuretic, and no intervention, in primigravidae with a high weight-gain (>1.25 lb/wk) between 20 and 30 weeks, but found no difference in the incidence of hypertension or pre-eclampsia between the three groups (although there was a significant reduction in weight-gain over the experimental period (30–38

Table 18.1 Controlled studies of dietary restriction

Authors	Population studied	Study design	Groups		Results			Comments
Baird *et al.* (1962)	Aberdeen Hospital antenatal clinic patients—primigravidae	Experimental group—attending one clinic. Controls 'selected at random' from women attending the ordinary antenatal clinics. Details of allocation to clinic not available. 'Mild pre-eclampsia' (hypertension) = Diastolic BP > 90 mmHg after 26 weeks Proteinuric pre-eclampsia = Diastolic BP > 90 mmHg + proteinuria > 0.25 g/l (Nelson 1955a)	Experimental ($n = 880$)	Dietary advice aimed at adjusting weight-gain to ~1 lb/week		Mild pre-eclampsia (%)	Proteinuric pre-eclampsia (%)	Full data on allocation not available.
			Control ($n = 880$)	No dietary advice	Experimental group	22.5	4.9	
					Control group	21.1	5.4	
Campbell and MacGillivray (1975)	Aberdeen Hospital antenatal clinic patients—primigravidae with high weight-gain (> 1.25 lb (570 g) per week) at 20–30 weeks	Patients matched in 3's for age, height, social class, smoking, weight-for-height at 20 weeks, BP in early pregnancy. Allocation to groups by record number of 1st of each 3 recruited. 'Mild pre-eclampsia' (hypertension) = Diastolic BP > 90 mmHg after 26 weeks Proteinuric pre-eclampsia = Diastolic BP > 90 mmHg + proteinuria > 0.25 g/l (Nelson 1955a)	Diet ($n = 51$)	Advised 1200 cal/day, low carbohydrate diet		Mild pre-eclampsia No. (%)	Proteinuric pre-eclampsia No. (%)	Gestation at onset of pre-eclampsia—same in all groups
			Diuretic ($n = 51$)	Cyclopenthiazide with potassium (Navidrex K), ii daily	Diet	13 (25.5)	6 (11.8)	
			Control ($n = 51$)	No treatment	Diuretic	10 (19.6)	8 (15.7)	
					Control	12 (23.5)	9 (17.7)	
Campbell Brown (1983)	Aberdeen Hospital antenatal clinic Obese primigravidae (> 75th percentile weight for height at booking) with normal glucose tolerance test at 28 weeks	Pairs matched for height, smoking, weight gained 20–30 weeks One of each pair to experimental group (basis of allocation not given). 'Mild pre-eclampsia' (hypertension) = Diastolic BP > 90 mmHg after 26 weeks Proteinuric pre-eclampsia = Diastolic BP > 90 mmHg + proteinuria > 0.25 g/l (Nelson 1955a)	Diet ($n = 91$)	1250 calorie reducing diet + dietary advice		Mild pre-eclampsia (%)	Proteinuric pre-eclampsia (%)	
			Control ($n = 91$)	No treatment	Diet	27.5	12.1	
					Control	30.8	6.6	

weeks) in the dieted group). A similar result was obtained by Campbell (1983) in a comparison of two matched groups of obese primigravidae, one of which was asked to restrict their diet to 1250 calories per day from 30 weeks. Thus none of the controlled studies supports the idea that limiting weight-gain (at least towards the end of pregnancy) affects the incidence of pre-eclampsia. (see Chapter 17).

In view of the lack of either a theoretical or an empirical basis for the prevention of pre-eclampsia by weight restriction, the idea shows an interesting persistence. It is true that in the last ten years there has been a relaxation in medical attitudes towards weight restriction in pregnancy, along with explicit recognition from official bodies of the lack of evidence that control of weight-gain prevents pre-eclampsia (Royal College of Obstetricians and Gynaecologists 1983; Suter and Ott 1984), and that this change of attitude is reflected in the reduced emphasis on weight restriction in recent editions of many obstetric textbooks (Walker *et al.* 1976; Garrey *et al.* 1980; Iffy and Kaminetsky 1981; Pritchard *et al.* 1985) and in several current popular books about pregnancy (Stoppard 1985; Reader's Digest Association 1986; Phillips 1983). It is difficult, however, to avoid the impression that clinical practice has not yet changed to the same extent. There are certainly those who continue to advocate dietary restriction as strongly as ever as a reliable means of preventing pre-eclampsia (Bourne 1984; Llewellyn-Jones 1986; Holme 1985; Ashcroft and Owens 1986), using in some cases the specific threat of the possible death of the baby from 'toxaemia' to reinforce their views (Holme 1985; Ashcroft and Owens 1986).

5 Dietary surveys and interventions

5.1 Overall dietary adequacy and energy intake

5.1.1 Surveys

In an early survey often quoted in support of a causal link between poverty, poor diets and pre-eclampsia, Burke *et al.* (1943) claimed a dramatic correlation between the overall adequacy of the diet and the incidence of pre-eclampsia in 216 'average middle-class American women' attending a Boston antenatal clinic (Burke *et al.* 1943). Diets were assessed by repeated dietary histories and graded from 'excellent' to 'very poor' on the basis of the then current recommended daily allowances for pregnancy. There were no cases of pre-eclampsia among 31 women with 'good' or 'excellent' diets, but 16 cases among the 36 women with 'poor' or 'very poor' diets. Unfortunately 'toxaemia' and 'pre-eclampsia' were not defined and insufficient information is given on other variables (such as parity, age, and previous hypertension) that might correlate either with diet or with pre-eclampsia. A similar survey carried out in Sydney (Woodhill *et al.* 1955) also suggested an association between poor diets and 'toxaemia', which in this case included some women with hypertension alone. The association was apparently confined to multiparae. Woodhill and her colleagues (1955) also refer to a survey (using dietary interviews) carried out by the National Health and Medical Research Council of Australia, in which a correlation between poor diets and toxaemia was found in multiparae but not in primiparae.

The results of surveys in which a direct comparison has been made between the diets of pre-eclamptic and non pre-eclamptic women do not support the idea that there are consistent differences in overall food intake between the two groups. The most convincing studies are those of Thomson in Aberdeen and Davies in Jerusalem (Thomson 1958, 1959a,b; Davies *et al.* 1970, 1976). In his careful prospective dietary survey of 500 Aberdeen primigravidae, using supervised 7-day weighed food records, Thomson found that both hypertensive and pre-eclamptic women reported slightly but significantly *higher* intakes (at seven months of pregnancy) of calories (2600 compared with 2400 calories daily), protein, carbohydrate and fats than women who remained normotensive. He suggested that a higher energy intake might be one factor related to the higher rate of weight-gain seen in pre-eclamptic women. In a survey of all pregnant women in West Jerusalem, Davies and his colleagues identified over 200 women with 'suspected toxaemia' (based on hypertension, proteinuria, oedema, or high weight-gain) during pregnancy; a dietary survey of these women and controls matched for age, parity, gestation, years of schooling, year of immigration, and country of origin was carried out using a questionnaire and dietary history at a single interview shortly after selection. The final analysis was based on the results for 180 women in whom the diagnosis of pre-eclampsia (using 1952 American Committee on Maternal Welfare criteria) had been confirmed after delivery. The pre-eclamptic women had slightly lower food intakes than controls, but on further analysis the difference was found to be confined to those pre-eclamptic women (about two-thirds of the sample) who reported a change in their diet during pregnancy. The author concluded that the differences were the *result* rather than the cause of pre-eclampsia. Certainly their results would be consistent with, though not confirmatory of this hypothesis.

Hunt and her colleagues, in preliminary surveys (using 24-hour dietary recall) for their study of zinc supplementation in 213 Hispanic women in Los Angeles (Hunt *et al.* 1983, 1984) also found evidence that pre-eclamptic women tended to change their diets during pregnancy. They found no difference in the reported diet during the first trimester between women who remained normotensive and those (numbering 16) who later developed pregnancy-induced hypertension, but these women reduced their intake of protein and carbohydrate towards the end of pregnancy, whereas the normotensive women increased theirs. It is not clear from the reports to what extent this difference may have been due to medical advice, but it emphasizes again the difficulty of drawing conclusions from dietary surveys without taking such factors into account.

Most of the remaining surveys, all of which are open to criticisms of design or execution, have found no significant differences in energy intake between pre-eclamptic and non-pre-eclamptic women (Hankin and Symonds 1962; Chaudhuri 1969, 1970; Mack *et al.* 1956; Williams *et al.* 1981; Williams and Fralin 1942). McGanity *et al.* (1954) found that toxaemic women enrolled in the Vanderbilt Cooperative Study of Maternal and Infant Nutrition reported a slightly lower intake of calories (and correspondingly of all the specific nutrients measured) compared with their total survey population, but they felt that this reflected the advice given to obese women (over-represented in the toxaemic group) to restrict weight-gain.

Thus only inconsistent and unimpressive differences in energy intake between pre-eclamptic and non pre-eclamptic women emerge from the most careful surveys. It should be noted that few, if any, of the women in these populations were overtly malnourished and the mean energy intake even among the most impoverished was well above the level (1500 calories a day) at which other evidence of impairment of reproductive performance has been seen (Rush 1982).

5.1.2 Interventions

Controlled trials of calorie restriction during pregnancy have already been discussed.

Most studies of dietary supplementation have concentrated on specific nutrients rather than on overall energy intake, and are discussed later (although it is obviously difficult to separate the effects of, for instance, additional protein from the additional energy which the protein supplement provides). In two studies, an attempt has been made to assess the effects of dietary *advice* aimed at ensuring an optimal diet (Table 18.2). Hankin and Symonds (1962) gave advice (based on the 1958 United States Food and Nutrition Board recommendations of 80 g of protein per day) to 96 women, and compared their reported diets and the incidence of pre-eclampsia with those of 40 women given no routine dietary advice. There was a small increase in the reported daily nutrient intake in the group given advice (protein 83 g vs. an already high 74 g) but no difference in the rates of pre-eclampsia. The remaining study is an unpublished report of the effects of nutritional counselling provided by Brewer in California in the late 1960s (Stark, Lundin, and Harley, personal communication), which will be discussed later.

5.2 Protein

The persistent idea that a lack of dietary protein might be responsible for pre-eclampsia seems to have arisen from observations of hypoproteinaemia in 'toxaemic' women, and from the subsequent reports of the apparently successful treatment (Strauss 1935; Dodge and Frost 1938) or prevention (Hamlin 1952, 1958) of pre-eclampsia by high protein diets. (Until the 1930s the fashion had been to *restrict* dietary protein in toxaemia, presumably to avoid metabolic 'toxins' (Theobald 1935).) Protein intake has in consequence been the focus of much of the work on dietary surveys, and protein supplementation one of the commonest forms of intervention. The protein deficiency hypothesis is, however, not supported by the experimental evidence.

5.2.1 Surveys

Dietary surveys (Thomson 1959b; Davies *et al.* 1970, 1976; Chaudhuri 1971; Williams and Fralin 1942; Williams *et al.* 1981) have shown no clear relationship between reported protein intake and pre-eclampsia. There is typically a wide range of reported protein intakes in these surveys, and in several studies further analysis has shown no obvious relationship between protein intakes (in the range less than 50 g to more than 90 g daily) and the incidence of pre-eclampsia (MacGillivray and Johnstone 1978; Hankin and Symonds 1962; Williams and Fralin 1942). Similar results have been obtained in recent studies using biochemical markers such as urinary nitrogen, urea, and creatinine in an attempt to obtain a more objective measure of protein intake (MacGillivray 1983; Ojengbede *et al.* in MacGillivray 1983; Zlatnik and Burmeister 1983).

5.2.2 Supplementation

Some of the early reports of the benefits of protein supplementation seem to have exerted an unwarranted influence on practice. Strauss (1935) treated 15 'toxaemic' women with a very high protein, low carbohydrate diet (260 g protein/day) and five others with a low protein (20 g/day) diet containing the same number of calories (about 2200). No attempt was made to ensure comparability of these groups. All of the women in the high protein group, and two on low protein diets, showed a loss of weight (attributed to loss of oedema fluid) and a general improvement in their condition (there was also a tendency for the arterial blood pressure to fall, but Strauss cautioned against attributing this to any more specific feature of the treatment than rest in hospital).

Table 18.2 Advice to improve diet

Authors	Population studied	Study design	Groups	Results: Treatment	Results: Group	Results	Comments
Hankin and Symonds (1962)	Adelaide Hospital antenatal clinic patients, first or second pregnancy, <20 weeks at booking Initial diastolic BP <80 mmHg	3 groups based on day of clinic attendance Dietary records for 4 days in 2nd and 3rd trimesters NB All patients with excessive weight gain advised to limit fat and carbohydrates Pre-eclamptic toxaemia: any 2 of 1. Diastolic BP >90 mmHg 2. Excessive weight-gain (not defined) or oedema 3. Proteinuria (catheter specimen)	n	Treatment		Pre-eclamptic toxaemia No. (%)	Unsatisfactory definition of pre-eclampsia. Groups not matched. Unknown number of women given advice to restrict diet.
			A and B (n=96)	Dietary advice and discussion with dietician after initial dietary record (USA Food and Nutrition Board 1958 recommended diet ~80 g protein/day).	A and B	17 (7.7)	
			C (n=40)	No routine dietary advice	C	8 (20.0)	
Stark, Lundin, and Harley (unpublished results)	California Antenatal clinic patients with singleton live births, <28 weeks at booking, seen at least 4 times over at least 4 weeks (Identified from total population delivered at Contra Costa County hospital 1965–70)	Retrospective cohort study comparing patients seen by Brewer with those seen by other doctors in same or other clinics. Data from clinics and hospital records up to 36 weeks' gestation.	Test (n=195)	Brewer— Dietary counselling (good diet, no junk foods, no calorie or salt restriction, no diuretics)		Change in diastolic BP up to 36 weeks No. (%) Fall / No change / Rise 1–14 mmHg / Rise >15 mmHg / Diastolic BP >90 mmHg at first visit	Data available up to 36 weeks' gestation only. Results apparently not related to differences between groups in age, parity, or timing of antenatal visits, but details not available. Figures for change in BP appear to refer to women with diastolic BP <90 mmHg at first visit, but this is not clearly stated.
			Usual (n=1246)	Other doctors— No dietary counselling 38% received at least one of diuretics, or salt, or calorie restriction.	Test	62 (32) / 49 (25) / 73 (38) / 9 (4.7) / 2	
					Usual	412 (33) / 243 (19.8) / 438 (35) / 139 (11.3) / 14	
						(x^2)=7.9 p<0.01)	

studies of protein and energy supplementation

Authors	Population studied	Study design	Groups		Results	Comments
Ross *et al.* (1938)	USA Inmates of antenatal hospital for young impoverished primigravidae in last weeks of pregnancy Included 6 with hypertension or 'nephritis' on admission	Alternate allocation to groups Written dietary records by all patients Toxaemia = some or all of BP > 140/90 mmHg, oedema, albuminuria, headache	Supplemented ($n = 27$) Control ($n = 26$)	Skimmed mild powder, bone meal, yeast, and iron (~60 g daily) No supplements to normal diet	Toxaemia No. Supplemented 9 Control 11	Small numbers; groups not matched Unsatisfactory definition of toxaemia
Ebbs *et al.* (1941, 1942)	Toronto Hostel antenatal clinic patients, < 6th month of pregnancy	Dietary assessment at 4–5 months and 34–36 weeks (7-day food record); diets assessed 'good' (~2400 cal, 75 g protein daily) or 'poor' (1700 cal, 55 g protein daily) Alternate 'poor diet' patients given food supplements to bring them to level of 'good diet' Pre-eclampsia/toxaemia not defined. (Comparison of results in 1941 and 1942 papers suggest 'toxaemia = eclampsia')	Supplemented ($n = 90$) Control ($n = 120$)	Given eggs, milk, oranges, cheeses, tomatoes, vit. D, and wheatgerm capsules, dietary advice Placebo (corn oil) capsules	Pre-eclampsia No. (%) Supplemented 5 (5.7) Control 6 (5.0) Toxaemia No. (%) Supplemented 3 (3.4) Control 9 (7.6)	Unexplained difference in size of groups— ? 'alternate' allocation Groups differ *re* advice as well as supplements No check on compliance Unsatisfactory def. of pre-eclampsia and toxaemia
Tompkins and Wiehl (1951, 1955)	Philadelphia Nutrition research clinic patients; married women, < 16 weeks at booking, excluding 'major complications' (TB, cardiovascular disease)	Seriatim assignment to study groups, 'taking into account' age, race. NB. Patients reassigned during study if failed to take supplements Criteria for 'toxaemia' unclear—based on American Committee Maternal Welfare 1952 'Borderline' toxaemia = high weight-gain/oedema or hypertension alone	Control ($n = 467$) Vitamin ($n = 447$) Protein ($n = 332$) Vit. + protein ($n = 334$)	No treatment Daily multivitamin capsules Protein concentrate (~50 g protein/day) Vitamins and protein supplements	Toxaemia No. (%) Severe/Moderate Control 10 (2.1) Vitamin 5 (1.1) Protein 3 (0.9) Mild Control 7 (1.5) Vitamin 1 (0.2) Protein 3 (0.9) Vit. + prot. 1 (0.3) Borderline Control 5 (1.1) Vitamin 4 (0.9) Protein 1 (0.3) Vit. + prot. 1 (0.3) Total Control 22 (4.7) Vitamin 10 (2.2) Protein 7 (2.2) Vit. + prot. 2 (0.6)	Groups differed in parity, income, outcome previous pregnancy Confusing and unsatisfactory definition of toxaemia Unsatisfactory study design—reallocation of large numbers during study
Campbell Brown (1983) Campbell and MacGillivray (1983)	Aberdeen Hospital antenatal clinic patients Primigravidae considered at risk of low birthweight infant on basis nutrition indices: maternal weight, weight for height at 20 weeks, weight-gain 20–30 weeks, maternal height	Admission to trial at ~29 weeks (range 25–32 weeks) Pairs matched by indices of selection and for smoking First of pair recruited allocated to group by case record number Cases ending with delivery < 37 weeks withdrawn and replaced by next recruited with same indices (applied to 9.7%) Pre-eclampsia: diastolic BP > 90 mmHg after 26 weeks, with proteinuria > 0.25 g/l	Supplemented ($n = 90$) Control ($n = 90$)	Given flavoured milk, cheese, or fresh milk to provide ~300 kcal and 15–20 g protein daily for 3rd trimester No treatment	Proteinuric pre-eclampsia (No.) Supplements 4 Control 6	Not designed to study pre-eclampsia; small numbers

Strauss himself restricted his conclusions to the comment that high protein diets did not appear to be harmful, and that the improvements seen 'may well have been due' to the high protein intake and the provision of vitamins. Others have not shown such restraint, however, and this paper has frequently been cited in support of the importance of high protein diets in preventing and treating pre-eclampsia (Hamlin 1952; Brewer and Brewer 1985). Other anecdotal reports of the apparent benefits of adding protein foods to the diets of impoverished toxaemic women (e.g. Dodge and Frost 1938; Primrose and Higgins 1971) have also been misrepresented in this way, as have the reports, already discussed, from Hamlin and his followers (e.g. Hamlin 1952, 1958). More recently, Kerr Grieve conducted an interesting but unfortunately uncontrolled experiment in Scotland (Kerr Grieve 1974) in which he prescribed a diet high in protein (with 1 lb of red meat a day), but low in carbohydrate and total calories, as the basis for the routine antenatal care of all women attending his maternity clinic (they represented about 70 per cent of all deliveries in the district). He used an indirect measure of 'diet success'; women with a high haemoglobin (> 12 g/dl) and a low weight-gain (< 250 g/week) were assumed to have a high protein intake, and he found such women to have a much lower incidence of 'gestosis' (equivalent to toxaemia) than those whose low haemoglobin and high weight-gain put them into the 'low diet success' category. Unfortunately, from the data presented it is impossible to say whether or not Grieve's dietary regimen had any effect on the incidence of pre-eclampsia, despite his claim that '. . . the overall rates of gestosis . . . speak to their own compelling conclusion'.

Controlled studies have also failed to reveal any convincing benefit of protein supplementation in the prevention of pre-eclampsia (Table 18.3). The small study by Ross *et al.* (1938) is of interest because Ross, again, has often been referred to in support of claims for the value of supplementation. In fact, in this study the addition of a protein–mineral supplement to the diets of alternate inmates of a hostel for young pregnant women made no difference to the rate of toxaemia.

Ebbs *et al.* (1941, 1942) assessed their patients' diets by interview and a 7-day food record at 4–5 months of pregnancy. Those with 'poor' diets at this stage (on average 1700 calories and 55 g protein a day) were divided into two groups, one of which received food and vitamin supplements and dietary advice designed to take their intake to about 2400 calories and 75 g protein per day. The remaining patients received only placebo 'vitamin' (corn oil) capsules. The rate of pre-eclampsia (not defined) was the same in both groups; the rate of 'toxaemia' was less in the supplemented group. This result means little in the light of the several serious flaws in the design of the study: most notably, the unexplained discrepancy between 'alternate' allocation and the different sizes of the two groups (90 and 120 women); and the inadequate definitions of pre-eclampsia and toxaemia.

There are also major flaws in the design of the only study that showed a positive association between protein supplementation and toxaemia (Tompkins and Wiehl 1951, 1955). These authors assigned patients serially to four groups, receiving vitamins, protein (as a concentrate providing about 50 g protein/day), both vitamins and protein, or no supplement. Compared with the control group, there was a small reduction in the rate of 'toxaemia' in the 'vitamin' and 'protein' groups, and a greater reduction in the group receiving both vitamins and protein. Results were analysed in terms of the women's reported intake, however, rather than by the group to which they had been allocated, thus vitiating the value of the serial allocation. Finally, MacGillivray has provided information on the rates of pre-eclampsia among women in a well designed study of protein-energy supplementation recently carried out in Aberdeen by Campbell Brown (1983). Ninety matched pairs of primigravidae considered to be at risk of producing low birthweight babies were allocated by case record number of first of the matched pair to be recruited) at 30 weeks to receive no treatment (controls) or a supplement of milk or cheese designed to add an extra 20 g protein and 300 calories per day to the normal diet containing 2050 calories and 70 g protein. No difference was found in the rates of pre-eclampsia in these two groups (macGillivray 1983).

These studies do illustrate the difficulties that confront the investigator who attempts to assess the effects of dietary manipulation on the development of pre-eclampsia. One of the most striking is the importance—and technical difficulty—of measuring dietary compliance; it cannot be assumed that the amount of supplement given, or advised, is that eaten, or eaten in addition to, rather than as a partial substitute for, the normal diet. Campbell Brown's study (1983) provides a particularly well documented example where dietary intake was closely monitored by 7-day weighed food records and urinary nitrogen analysis; she concluded that supplementary food was eaten as a partial substitute for the normal diet, and that the increase in protein and energy intake was only about 60 per cent of the food value of the additional food provided. It should also be noted that the women in many of these studies did not start out with a particularly low (reported) protein intake. Nor did supplementation apparently raise the protein intake by very much; for example, from 70 g to 83 g a day in Campbell Brown's study. Certainly, accurate measures of the actual protein intakes of supplement and non-supplement groups would be necessary before any effect could be attributed to protein supplementation rather than simply to advice, increased antenatal care, or indeed simply increased calorie intake. Any adequate study would also need to be on a much larger scale than those quoted in order to detect a change in the already low rate of proteinuric pre-eclampsia.

5.3 Vitamins and minerals

Although attempts to prevent pre-eclampsia by vitamin and mineral supplementation have a long, if sporadic history, they appear often to have been based more upon speculation and the desire to provide a generally 'good' diet than on any evidence linking pre-eclampsia to deficiencies of specific vitamins or minerals. There have been a number of unsubstantiated claims. In the 1930s, for instance, Theobald (1935) was convinced that toxaemia was the result of 'an absolute or relative insufficiency of some substance or substances in the diet, the most important of which is calcium'. He described dramatic improvements in the condition of 68 toxaemic women given a mixed diet and supplements of calcium, iron, sulphur, thyroid extract, and vitamins A, B, and D. He produced no evidence from controlled experiments, however, to substantiate his claims. Belizan and Villar have recently resurrected the idea that calcium deficiency may predispose towards pre-eclampsia (Belizan and Villar 1980). While current interest in the role of calcium in the control of blood pressure certainly provides a basis for their speculation, many of their arguments are unconvincing and they have yet to provide evidence in favour of their hypothesis.

5.3.1 Surveys

No consistent differences in vitamin or mineral content between the diets of pre-eclamptic and non-pre-eclamptic women have emerged from the more convincing dietary surveys. Thomson (1959b) in Aberdeen found that the diets of women with pre-eclampsia tended to contain less vitamin C than those of normotensive or hypertensive women, but rather more of other vitamins and calcium, as is consistent with their generally greater food intake. Hunt *et al.* (1983, 1984) found no difference in the first trimester intakes of vitamins and minerals, including zinc, between women who remained normotensive and those who later developed pregnancy-induced hypertension. Chaudhuri's dietary survey in Calcutta (oral questionnaire) of toxaemic and non-toxaemic women in the third trimester revealed some differences in mineral and vitamin intake, with the toxaemic women reporting lower intakes of calcium, iron and vitamins A, B, B_2, and C (Chaudhuri 1969, 1971). A number of other surveys of dubious merit have included figures on vitamin and mineral intakes but have not produced either consistent or convincing results (e.g. Mack *et al.* 1956; McGanity *et al.* 1954; Williams and Fralin 1942; Lu *et al.* 1981; Williams *et al.* 1981).

5.3.2 Supplementation

Controlled studies of vitamin and mineral supplementation have, however, produced some interesting findings (Table 18.4).

In their recent randomized double-blind study of zinc supplementation, Hunt *et al.* (1983, 1984) found a lower incidence of 'pregnancy-induced hypertension' in the supplemented group. Only two out of 87 women in the supplemented group developed pregnancy-induced hypertension, compared with 14 out of 90 in the control group. These were women whose reported dietary intake of zinc was low, and in whom Hunt *et al.* were primarily studying the effects of zinc supplementation on serum and hair zinc levels. The difference in pregnancy-induced hypertension between the groups was the 'only difference in sub-optimal outcomes of pregnancy between women in the control and zinc-supplemented groups'. The results must be viewed with some caution as far as pre-eclampsia is concerned; women with 'pregnancy-induced hypertension' did not necessarily all have true pre-eclampsia, and in any case the results may well have represented a chance finding. No prior hypothesis as to a possible effect on pre-eclampsia was stated, and we are not told how many outcomes were examined. A statistically significant difference would be expected 5 per cent of the time even if in truth there were no differences between the groups. It is also interesting that the incidence of pregnancy induced hypertension did not correlate with low serum zinc levels, despite its association with zinc supplementation. Indeed, zinc supplements did not significantly alter mean serum zinc levels in these women (Hunt 1983).

Two recent studies, on the other hand, have found significantly lower plasma zinc concentrations in women with severe pre-eclampsia than in non-pre-eclamptic controls (Jenkins and Soltan 1983; Kiiholma *et al.* 1984). The dangers of too hasty an interpretation of such results in turns of dietary deficiency have recently been pointed out (Hytten 1985). Whether or not this proves to be a fruitful line of enquiry into the prevention of pre-eclampsia remains to be seen.

None of the remaining studies dealing with specific vitamins or minerals has produced a positive result. A number of authors included toxaemia or pre-eclampsia in their investigation of the effects of routine folic acid supplementation in pregnancy (Fletcher *et al.* 1971; Willoughby 1967; Trigg *et al.* 1976; see also Hemminki and Starfield 1978, and Chapter 19 in this volume); none found any difference in the incidence of toxaemia between supplemented and control groups. A number of trials of B vitamin supplementation, none particularly well designed, found no difference in the incidence

Table 18.4 Vitamin and mineral supplementation

Authors	Population studied	Study design	Groups		Results	Comments
Hunt *et al.* (1983, 1984)	Los Angeles Low income women of Mexican descent, over 17 years and <27 weeks at booking Excluding diabetes, heart, renal, and thyroid disease	Randomized double-blind trial Compliers—in a study for at least 60 days, and collected more capsules after 60 days. 213 entered in trial. Results for 177 analysed (3 abortions, 2 twin pregnancies, 31 lost records). Pregnancy-induced hypertension (PIH) = (a) BP >140/90 mmHg *or* rise of 30 mmHg systolic *or* rise of 15 mmHg diastolic with (b) Proteinuria >0.3 g/l and/or (c) Persistent oedema	Supplemented ($n=87$) Control ($n=90$)	Daily vitamin–mineral capsules + 20 mg zinc/day Daily vitamin–mineral capsules without zinc	PIH: *n* / No. / (%) Supplemented All 87 / 2 / (2.3) Compliers 65 / 1 / (1.5) Non-compliers 22 / 1 / (4.5) Controls All 90 / 14 / (16) Compliers 81 / 10 / (12) Non-compliers 9 / 4 / (44)	'PIH' could include essential hypertension
Fletcher *et al.* (1971)	London Antenatal clinic patients	Random allocation at booking (14 weeks) Pre-eclampsia: not defined	Study ($n=321$) Control ($n=332$)	200 mg $FeSO_4$ + 5 mg folic acid daily 200 mg $FeSO_4$ daily	Pre-eclampsia: No. / (%) Iron + folate ($n=321$) 64 / (19.3) Iron 50 / (15.2)	No dietary assessment No measure of compliance No definition of pre-eclampsia
Trigg *et al.* (1976)	England Antenatal patients from General Practice clinics	Prospective Pairs of consecutive patients entered into trial by GPs at booking Allocation initially random, then in sequence Pre-eclampsia not defined	Study ($n=82$) Control ($n=76$)	Iron and folate tabs daily (minimum 50 mg $FeSO_4$ and 0.5 mg folic acid Iron tablets (minimum 50 mg $FeSO_4$)	No differences between groups in prevalence of pre-eclampsia	Inadequate data
Willoughby (1967)	Glasgow Hospital antenatal clinic patients	Random allocation at booking Patients withdrawn if Hb <10 Excluded from analysis if suspected non-compliant Toxaemia: not defined	I ($n=706$) II ($n=736$) III ($n=716$) IV ($n=715$) V ($n=726$)	Controls (no supplements) Supplemented 105 mg iron/day 105 mg iron + 100 μg folic acid/day 105 mg iron, 300 μg folic acid/day 105 mg iron, 450 μg folic acid/day	No differences between groups in rates of toxaemia	Inadequate data
Browne (1943)	London Hospital antenatal clinic patients, <20 weeks pregnant	Alternate allocation Of initial 200 in trial, 31 dropped out (miscarriage, moved, etc.) Toxaemia— Standard I —BP 130/70 mmHg Standard II—BP >140/90 mmHg *or* >130/70 mmHg with albuminuria	Study ($n=88$) Control ($n=81$)	3 mg vit. B1 daily No treatment	Toxaemia: No. / (%) Std I Supplemented 32 / (36.3) Control 20 / (24.6) Std II Supplemented 7 / (7.9) Control 4 / (4.9)	Unsatisfactory definition of toxaemia No dietary assessment or check of compliance Not placebo-controlled
Ferguson (1955)	New Orleans Hospital 'toxaemia' clinic patients	Four categories: (1) Hypertension at referral (2) Excessive weight-gain (3) Toxaemia in previous pregnancy (4) Other 'high risk', e.g. diabetes Seriatim allocation within these categories	Study ($n=130$) Control ($n=139$)	Caps. methionine + vit. B daily Placebo capsules	Pre-eclampsia: No. / (%) Study without chronic hypertension ($n=65$) 23 / (35) with chronic 21 / (32)	Unsatisfactory definition of toxaemia Insufficient data on selection and composition of groups

		albuminuria (catheter) after 24 weeks; or rise in BP of > 30 mmHg systolic or > 15 mmHg diastolic and/or albuminuria in women with chronic hypertension (BP > 90 diastolic before 24 weeks postpartum)			with chronic hypertension ($n=71$) 27 (38)	
Hillman *et al.* (1963)	New York Hospital antenatal clinic patients, all stages of gestation Consecutive	Randomized, double-blind trial 'Toxaemia' = diagnosis in hospital records	1 ($n=576$) 2 ($n=588$) 3 ($n=368$)	1 multivitamin–mineral capsule daily 1 multivitamin–mineral capsule with added pyridoxine 20 mg + 3 placebo lozenges daily 1 multivitamin–mineral capsule + 3 lozenges of pyridoxine (total 120 mg) daily	Toxaemia (%) 1 2.1 2 3.6 3 3.0	Insufficient data Unsatisfactory definition of toxaemia
Dieckman *et al.* (1944)	Chicago Hospital antenatal clinic Patients with 'low income'	Groups selected 'at random'. Details not given Toxaemia not defined	I ($n=175$) II ($n=179$) II ($n=98$) IV ($n=102$)	Controls—no treatment 100 mg cereal daily (for minerals) Vitamins A and D daily Cereal and vitamins A and D daily	Toxaemia No. (%) I 15 (8.6) II 11 (5.9) III 14 (14.5) IV 5 (4.9)	Insufficient data on allocations and exclusions Toxaemia not defined
People's League of Health (1942, 1946)	London Antenatal clinic patients at 10 hospitals, excluding those with disease or physical abnormality, or > 24 weeks at booking	Alternate allocation at each hospital. 5644 enrolled; 622 dropped out (494 war evacuees, 39 with twins, 89 miscarriages) Toxaemia— Initially— (a) BP > 140/90 mmHg and/or (b) albuminuria Later—albuminuria, oedema + (usually with) hypertension Pre-eclampsia— hypertension (> 140/90) with albuminuria, oedema, etc.	Supplemented ($n=2510$) Control ($n=251$)	Daily supplements of vitamins and minerals (iron, calcium, iodine, manganese, copper, vit. A, B, C, D) No supplements Primiparae Supplemented ($n=1530$) Control ($n=1513$) Multiparae Supplemented ($n=980$) Control ($n=999$)	Hypertension No. (%) / Pre-eclampsia (hypertension + albuminuria, oedema, etc.) No. (%) Primiparae Supplemented: 332 (21.7) / 69 (4.5) Primiparae Control: 368 (24.3) / 97 (6.4) ($x^2=5.31$, $p<0.05$) Multiparae Supplemented: 179 (8.3) / 31 (3.2) Multiparae Control: 166 (16.6) / 46 (4.6) ($x^2=2.37$: N.S.)	Not placebo-controlled No measurement of compliance
Robinson (1958)	Derby Hospital antenatal clinic patients	Alternate allocation at booking 58/2077 excluded from analysis (not pregnant, miscarried, moved) Toxaemia: BP > 140/90, and/or oedema and albuminuria	S ($n=1019$) S− ($n=1000$)	Advised to eat more salt Advised to eat less salt	'Toxaemia' (No.) / BP > 140/90 + albuminuria, + oedema (No.) Primiparae S ($n=144$) 16 / – S− ($n=146$) 38 / – ($x^2=8.09$, $p<0.01$) Multiparae S ($n=975$) 22 / – S− ($n=854$) 59 / – ($x^2=23.1$, $p<0.001$) Total S ($n=1019$) 38 / 20 S− ($n=1000$) 97 / 44 ($x^2=28$, $p<0.001$) ($x^2=8.9$, $p<0.01$)	No data on compliance
Chaudhuri (1969)	India Antenatal clinic patients booking before 24 weeks	Initial 'random selection' of 500 patients; those with gross anaemia or other nutritional disorders excluded and remainder allocated alternately Later exclusion of patients who were un-co-operative or developed nutritional deficiency 'Pre-eclampsia' = BP > 490/90 after 24 weeks, with oedema and/or proteinuria	Study ($n=164$) Control ($n=164$)	Routine antenatal care, dietary advice and multivitamin tablets Routine antenatal care and dietary advice	Toxaemia No. (%) Supplemented 8 (4.8) Control 26 (14.6)	Insufficient data on large numbers excluded No check on compliance. Study group asked to buy own tablets but no check that controls did not also do this No assessment of diet No comparability of groups (other than by parity) given

of toxaemia with supplementation (Browne 1943; Ferguson 1955; Hillman *et al.* 1963) (see Table 18.4).

The remaining studies are of multiple vitamin and mineral supplementation. Dieckmann *et al.* (1944) compared the incidence of toxaemia in a control group and three treatment groups given supplements of cereal (for its mineral content) and/or vitamins A and D. Differences between the groups in the incidence of toxaemia were not striking. Chaudhuri (1969) in India reported a clear advantage in the multivitamin–mineral supplemented group compared with the non-supplemented control group; the incidence of pre-eclampsia (defined reasonably well) was 4.8 per cent in the supplemented group and 14.6 per cent in the controls. Unfortunately a very large number of women were excluded from the study or from the analysis of the results after the initial 'random' allocation, and without more information than is available the comparability of the final groups must remain in doubt. The study was not placebo-controlled.

The third, and most interesting, of these studies is the large-scale controlled trial of vitamin–mineral supplementation given to alternate pregnant women attending hospitals in London in the late 1930s for the People's League of Health (People's League of Health 1942, 1946). This included over 5000 women, half of whom were given a multivitamin–mineral supplement throughout the second half of pregnancy. Fewer women in the supplemented group than in the control group developed pre-eclampsia (hypertension > 140/90 mm Hg, and albuminuria); the difference was statistically significant for primiparae, though not for multiparae (see Table 18.4).

A frequent, but invalid, criticism of this study is that there were large differences in the rates of 'toxaemia' between the 10 participating hospitals; however, since patients were allocated alternately to the supplemented and control groups at *each* hospital, differences between hospitals are not relevant to the comparison between treatment groups. More significant criticisms are that allocation to the groups was not formally randomized; that the trial was not placebo-controlled; and that no check was made of compliance. In practice, the alternate allocation of large numbers probably provides an acceptable substitute for randomization; certainly the groups were closely comparable in terms of age and parity. The lack of placebo controls may be of more importance; and it is not clear whether provision of the vitamins and mineral supplements was associated with a difference in the amount of attention or dietary advice given to the two groups. Failure to check on compliance means simply that it is not possible to say how closely the effect seen was associated with supplement actually taken, rather than provided. These are reasons for caution in assessing the results of the People's League of Health trial, but not for dismissing them out of hand. A clear difference in the incidence of proteinuric pre-eclampsia was seen between supplemented and unsupplemented primiparae. While this difference may not have been due directly to the vitamin–mineral supplement this remains one of the few good studies in the field to produce a positive result.

5.4 Salt

The use of low salt diets in treating oedema in both non-pregnant and pregnant patients in the early years of this century appears to be behind the idea of restricting salt intake to help prevent pre-eclampsia (De Snoo 1937; Chesley 1978). By the late 1940s it was considered daring to allow pregnant women, especially those with toxaemia, to eat a diet containing a normal amount of salt, though a few clinicians did begin to question the wisdom of salt restriction. Interest in dietary salt waned somewhat in the 1960s, possibly as attention was now focused instead on the recently introduced diuretic drugs. The recent resurgence of the debate about the role of salt in the aetiology of essential hypertension seems likely to raise the issue of salt in pregnancy once again.

Despite many enthusiastic clinical reports, no convincing evidence has ever been produced that salt restriction helps in the treatment of pre-eclampsia (see Chesley 1978; Redman 1982b). The widespread extension of salt restriction to attempts to *prevent* pre-eclampsia appears to have been almost entirely without either theoretical or empirical foundation. The only attempts to assess the use of salt-restricted diets in prevention or treatment in a controlled way were published in the 1950s as a more critical approach to the practice emerged. Of the three available controlled studies, two (Bower 1961; Mengert and Tacchi 1961) deal with the use of salt restriction in the hospital treatment of established pre-eclampsia. Neither found any differences in outcome between their 'high' (between 10–25 g salt daily) and 'low' (about 1–2 g salt daily) salt groups. Both studies can be criticized for aspects of their design, and in particular for lack of information about the general composition of the diets and about compliance. The third study (Robinson 1958) has aroused considerable interest as the only large-scale attempt to assess the effect of 'low' and 'high' salt diets in the prevention of pre-eclampsia. Robinson allocated over 2000 antenatal clinic patients alternately to groups receiving advice to eat a diet high in salt (salty meat, salt butter, added salt at table) or low in salt (avoiding salty foods, and no added salt at table). There were statistically significantly *fewer* cases of 'toxaemia' among both primiparae and multiparae in the '*high salt*' group (Table 18.4). Robinson's definition of toxaemia was very broad, but the difference remains statistically significant if only those women who developed both hypertension and albuminuria are considered.

Robinson's study has been criticized for the lack of information on compliance (Chesley 1978; MacGillivray 1983). While this criticism is valid, the difference in the incidence of pre-eclampsia between two groups given the contrasting advice about salt intake is still important. At the very least this report suggests that considerable caution should be exercised in applying current recommendations on reduction of salt intake (National Advisory Committee on Nutrition Education 1983) to pregnant women (see also Brown *et al.* 1984). It would be a pity if salt restriction in any form were to be reintroduced to antenatal care with, once again, no evidence as to the benefits or harm that it might cause.

5.5 Polyunsaturated fatty acids

It has recently been suggested that the dietary intake of polyunsaturated fatty acids, as precursors for the production of prostaglandins with a hypotensive effect, might be important in pre-eclampsia (McCarty 1982). A high ratio of polyunsaturated to saturated fat in the diet has been reported to reduce blood pressure in men and non-pregnant women (Iacono *et al.* 1982; Norris *et al.* 1986). Preliminary evidence from dietary surveys has not shown any association between dietary polyunsaturated fat and pre-eclampsia. Hunt *et al.* (1984) examined the ratio of polyunsaturated to saturated fat in the diets of women in their study and found no difference between those developing pregnancy-induced hypertension and the remainder. MacGillivray and his colleagues, in a small-scale study in Aberdeen, also found no difference in the amount or type of polyunsaturated fatty acids between the diets of women with hypertension or pre-eclampsia and those of normotensive controls (MacGillivray 1983, p 229).

6 'Metabolic toxemia of late pregnancy'

The most outspoken current advocate of a nutritional theory of the aetiology of pre-eclampsia is Thomas Brewer of California. Brewer is convinced that what he calls 'metabolic toxemia of late pregnancy' is a disease of maternal malnutrition, often caused or exacerbated by the 'iatrogenic starvation' of restrictions on weight-gain in pregnancy, and by the use of diuretic and appetite suppressant drugs (Brewer 1982; Brewer and Brewer 1985).

It is worth considering Brewer's work in detail. Although largely dismissed by the medical profession (Davies 1971; Redman 1982b; Chesley 1978; MacGillivray 1983), Brewer's theories form the basis of the advice given to women by self-help and information groups throughout the world, such as the Preeclamptic Toxaemia Society (PETS) in the United Kingdom, the Nutrition Action Group (NAG) in the United States, and the Arbeitsgemeinschaft Gestose-Frauen in West Germany. As reference and referral to these groups becomes more common (e.g. Phillips 1983; Boston Women's Health Book Collective 1984) the significance of Brewer's ideas as the only readily available 'alternative' advice to women about pre-eclampsia should not be underestimated.

Brewer's recommendations to pregnant women are straightforward and have not changed significantly since he first published his work in 1966 (Brewer 1966): women should avoid any attempt to reduce weight-gain; they should avoid all drugs, especially appetite suppressants and diuretics; and should eat a well-balanced diet of good foods with salt and water to taste. Brewer recommends about 2600–3000 calories and 100–120 g protein a day (Brewer and Brewer 1983; 1985), not as 'minimum' but as optimum amounts. He stresses the importance of eating mainly unprocessed food and he does not believe that vitamin or other supplements should be necessary. In his more recent publications he has began to warn women that they should not go without good food for more than a few hours; in 'The Brewer Medical Diet for Normal and High Risk Pregnancy' (Brewer and Brewer 1983) women are urged to eat snacks mid-morning, afternoon, and at least once during the night, as well as three main meals a day.

Brewer does not claim that his regimen will eliminate all of the symptoms of pre-eclampsia/toxaemia (such as oedema, hypertension, proteinuria, convulsions) but that if these occur in a well-nourished woman they must be due not to pre-eclampsia but to other conditions such as essential hypertension, renal disease, urinary tract infection, cerebral tumours, or epilepsy. He dismisses the claims of his critics who find pre-eclampsia in well-nourished women as due to their incompetence in differential diagnosis.

Brewer's theories about the nutritional basis of toxaemia are based on his clinical experience in California and the Southern United States in the 1950s and 1960s. He stands in a direct line of succession to clinicians such as Theobald (1935) and Hamlin (1952, 1958) who were equally convinced from their clinical practice of the importance of good nutrition in preventing toxaemia. Brewer was struck by the contrast between the poor diets of women attending a public clinic in New Orleans, where there was a high rate of toxaemia, and the well-nourished women he saw in private practice in Missouri where apparently there was virtually no toxaemia at all. Over the next few years he began to elaborate his theory of the metabolic nature of toxaemia, based on the work of Strauss (1935) and Dodge and Frost (1938) on hypoproteinaemia in pre-eclampsia. Brewer's hypothesis, that a lack of protein, calories, and vitamins in the diet leads to a failure of hepatic synthesis of plasma proteins, and to hypoproteinaemia and hypovolaemia as the central problem in toxaemia, is supported largely by a selective and speculative interpretation of some of the pathological findings in pre-eclampsia and eclampsia (see Chesley 1978 for a critique). Brewer finds further support for his theories in the work of, in particular, Ross, Theobald, and Hamlin. These studies have already been discussed; it seems clear that they do not, in fact, provide scientific proof of Brewer's nutritional thesis, as he claims.

The central part of Brewer's argument for the nutritional prevention of toxaemia is based, however, not on theory but on his observations of the effects of a nutritional counselling programme that he ran for several years in the 1960s and 1970s in an antenatal clinic in California.

Brewer was opposed to the 'interventionist' approach to antenatal care then at its peak in the United States, with the common, if not routine, advocacy of weight limitation and the use of appetite suppressants and diuretics (see Chapter 35). In his antenatal clinic there was no weight limitation, no use of drugs and (to use Brewer's own phrase) an 'aggressive programme of nutritional counselling throughout pregnancy'. He claims that he virtually eradicated pre-eclampsia (and completely eradicated eclampsia) among over 7000 women attending his clinics.

It is this antenatal programme that Stark, Lundin, and Harley attempted to evaluate in an unpublished study for the National Institutes of Health (Table 18.2). This is the only study in which an attempt has been made to assess Brewer's claims in a controlled way. They carried out a retrospective analysis, using hospital and clinic records, to assess the outcome for women at Brewer's clinic compared with women attending other clinics in the same area over the same 5-year period, and who subsequently gave birth at the same hospital. The 'control' group of women had received routine antenatal care; the extent to which weight limitation, salt restriction, and the use of diuretics were common practice is clear from the fact that 38 per cent of the 'control' women had undergone one or more of these interventions.

Among the outcomes assessed were blood pressure (specifically, the change in diastolic pressure during pregnancy), proteinuria, and oedema. The data on proteinuria and oedema available to the study are difficult to interpret usefully (there was no agreed method of measuring or recording oedema among the various clinicians and no information to distinguish infective from non-infective proteinuria). The authors did their best to eliminate the most obvious sources of bias in the assessment of blood pressure, for instance by using the change in recorded diastolic pressure rather than absolute values; the results (Table 18.2) showed that significantly fewer women in Brewer's group than in the control group experienced a rise in diastolic blood pressure of more than 15 mm Hg during pregnancy.

Although there are many problems with this study (most of them inevitable with a retrospective analysis), as a preliminary study the evaluation certainly suggested a possible advantage for Brewer's regimen. It would have been most useful if this observation could have been followed up by a properly designed prospective study. Brewer maintains that the Stark, Lundin, and Harley study provides support for his views on the prevention of pre-eclampsia and alleges that the results have been suppressed by an unsympathetic medical establishment (Brewer 1974, 1982).

There is no doubt that much of Brewer's advice over the past 20 years has represented a valuable counterbalance to the tendency towards excessive and unfounded intervention in the name of the prevention of pre-eclampsia. Women following Brewer's regimen probably did have healthier pregnancies than if they had been subject to the routine use of weight restriction, salt restriction, and diuretics. Brewer's concern for the nutritional needs of pregnant women and his recognition that it is not only 'poor' women who may have inadequate diets represent a valuable contribution. His criticisms of a widespread lack of interest in, and knowledge of the principles of nutrition in pregnancy are probably justified. His central thesis, however, that pre-eclampsia is a metabolic disease caused by maternal malnutrition, remains unproven.

7 Conclusions

Attempts to use dietary manipulation to prevent pre-eclampsia continue to influence antenatal care, despite the fact that the evidence and arguments on which they are based are almost all unconvincing.

With very few exceptions, the better designed studies have failed to show any effect on the incidence of pre-eclampsia of dietary restriction or supplementation, or any correlation of pre-eclampsia with dietary factors. In some areas (for example, vitamin and mineral supplementation) there are very few good studies at all. Supporters of dietary theories of the aetiology of pre-eclampsia have based their claims upon uncontrolled clinical reports and inadequate research investigations. The persistence of some of these claims, with an apparent disregard both for logic and for experimental evidence, is remarkable and attests to the powerful feelings which the question of food in pregnancy provokes. The subject is an emotive one, so it is perhaps particularly important that an attempt be made to distinguish fact from feeling so that women may make informed decisions about their diet in pregnancy.

It is clear that the present evidence provides no

justification for any form of dietary intervention with the aim of preventing pre-eclampsia. In particular, women should not be told to restrict their diet to reduce 'high' weight-gain; as already discussed, the still widespread idea that this helps to prevent pre-eclampsia was based on false arguments. Dietary restriction has been found to be ineffective in controlled trials and may have unwanted adverse effects such as reduction of birthweight (see Campbell Brown 1983). (Restriction of weight-gain in pregnancy has also been advised for other reasons, none of which stands up to scrutiny (Hytten 1979)). Equally, there is no evidence to support the alternative view that eating sufficient of a good diet will reliably protect against pre-eclampsia.

We know too little about the effects of high or low salt consumption on the development of pre-eclampsia to be able to offer well-informed advice. The intriguing but unconfirmed results of Robinson's study in which the incidence of pre-eclampsia was lower in women advised to eat more salt than those advised to eat less (Robinson 1958) do suggest that women should be very cautious about restricting salt intake during pregnancy.

Both the People's League of Health trial of vitamin and mineral supplementation (People's League of Health 1942, 1946) and Hunt's more recent study of zinc supplementation (Hunt *et al.* 1983, 1984) raise the possibility of some benefit from vitamin or mineral supplements in preventing pre-eclampsia. Both should be replicated before any decision on vitamin or mineral supplementation can be taken.

More than half a century of research on diet and pre-eclampsia has produced disappointingly little in the way of reliable, and therefore interesting, or useful, results. While pre-eclampsia remains an enigma attempts to relate it to dietary factors are likely to continue, even if, as in the past, often in an opportunistic and haphazard fashion. One of the most important lessons to be learnt is that confusing and unhelpful results will continue to emerge unless an effort is made to use only an agreed and precise definition of pre-eclampsia (MacGillivray 1983; Chesley 1985) for all future research; and unless interventions are introduced in the proper context of a controlled trial.

References

Ashcroft JJ, Owens RG (1986). Weight control in pregnancy. Wellingborough, NY: Thorsons.

Baird D, Thomson AM, Hytten F (1962). Weight gain in pre-eclampsia (Letter). Lancet, 1: 1297–1298.

Belizan JM, Villar J (1980). The relationship between calcium intake and edema-, proteinuria-, and hypertension-gestosis: an hypothesis. Am J Clin Nutr, 33: 2202–2210.

Boston Women's Health Book Collective (1984). The New Our Bodies Ourselves. New York: Simon & Schuster.

Bourne G (1984). Pregnancy (new and revised edition). London: Cassell.

Bower D (1961). The influence of dietary salt intake on pre-eclampsia. J Obstet Gynaecol Br Commnwlth, 81: 601–605.

Brewer GS, Brewer TH (1983). The Brewer Medical Diet for Normal and High Risk Pregnancy. New York: Simon & Schuster.

Brewer GS, Brewer TH (1985). What Every Pregnant Woman Should Know. The Truth about Diet and Drugs in Pregnancy (revised edition). New York: Penguin.

Brewer TH (1966). Metabolic Toxemia of Late Pregnancy: A Disease of Malnutrition. Springfield, Illinois: Charles C Thomas.

Brewer TH (1974). Metabolic toxemia of late pregnancy in a county prenatal nutrition education project: a preliminary report. J Reprod Med, 13: 175–176.

Brewer TH (1982). Metabolic Toxemia of Late pregnancy: A Disease of Malnutrition (2nd edn). New Canaan, Connecticut: Keats Publishing.

Brown JJ, Lever AF, Robertson JI, Semple PF, Bing RF, Heagerty AM, Swales JD, Thurston H, Ledingham JG, Laragh JH, Hansson L, Nicholls MG, Espiner EA (1984). Salt and hypertension (letter). Lancet, 2: 1333–1334.

Browne FJ (1943). On the value of vitamin B_1 in prevention of toxaemia of pregnancy. Br Med J, 1: 445–446.

Burkē BS, Beal VA, Kirkwood SB, Stuart HC (1943). Nutrition studies during pregnancy. Am J Obstet Gynecol, 46: 38–52.

Butler NR, Bonham DG (eds) (1963). Perinatal Mortality: The First Report of the 1958 British Perinatal Mortality Survey. Edinburgh: Churchill Livingstone, pp 86–100.

Campbell DM (1983). Dietary restriction in obesity and its effect on neonatal outcome. In: Nutrition in Pregnancy. Proceedings of the Tenth Study Group of the Royal College of Obstetricians and Gynaecologists, September 1982. Campbell DM, Gillmer MDG (eds). London: Royal College of Obstetricians and Gynaecologists, pp 243–250.

Campbell DM, MacGillivray I (1975). The effect of a low calorie diet or a thiazide diuretic on the incidence of pre-eclampsia and on birthweight. Br J Obstet Gynaecol, 82: 572–577.

Campbell Brown M (1983). Protein energy supplements in primigravid women at risk of low birthweight. In: Nutrition in Pregnancy. Proceedings of the Tenth Study Group of the Royal College of Obstetricians and Gynaecologists,

September 1982. Campbell DM, Gillmer MDG (eds). London: Royal College of Obstetricians and Gynaecologists, pp 85–98.

Chamberlain G, Philipp E, Howlett B, Masters K (1978). British Births 1970. Vol 2: Obstetric Care. London: Heinemann Medical Books.

Chaudhuri SK (1969). Effect of nutrient supplement on the incidence of toxemia of pregnancy. J Obstet Gynaecol India, 19: 156–161.

Chaudhuri SK (1970). Relationship of protein–calorie malnutrition with toxaemia of pregnancy. Am J Obstet Gynecol, 107: 33–37.

Chaudhuri SK (1971). Role of nutrition in the etiology of toxaemia of pregnancy. Am J Obstet Gynecol, 110: 46–48.

Chesley LC (1978). Hypertensive Disorders in Pregnancy. New York: Appleton-Century-Crofts.

Chesley LC (1985). Diagnosis of pre-eclampsia (Editorial). Obstet Gynecol, 65: 423–425.

Davies AM (1971). Geographical Epidemiology of the Toxemias of Pregnancy. Springfield, Illinois: Charles C Thomas.

Davies AM, Czaczkes W, Sadovsky E, Prywes R, Weiskopf P, Sterk VV (1970). Toxemia of pregnancy in Jerusalem. I: Epidemiological studies of a total community. Israel J Med Sci, 6: 253–266.

Davies AM, Dunlop W (1983). Hypertension in pregnancy. In: Obstetrical Epidemiology. Barron SL, Thomson AM (eds). London: Academic Press.

Davies AM, Poznansky R, Weiskopf P, Prywes R, Sadovsky E, Czaczkes W (1976). Toxemia of pregnancy in Jerusalem. II: The role of diet. Israel J Med Sci, 12: 508–518.

Dawson B (1953). The prevention of eclampsia. J Obstet Gynaecol Br Empire, 60: 80–84.

Dieckmann WJ, Adair FL, Michel H, Kramer S, Dunkle F, Arthur B, Costin M, Campbell A, Wensley AC, Lorang E (1944). Calcium, Phosphorus, iron and nitrogen balances in pregnant women. Am J Obstet Gynecol, 47: 357–368.

De Snoo K (1937). The prevention of eclampsia. Am J Obstet Gynecol, 34: 911–926.

Dewhurst J (1981). In: Integrated Obstetrics and Gynaecology for Postgraduates (3rd edn). Dewhurst J (ed), Oxford: Blackwell Scientific Publications, p 267.

Dodge EF, Frost TT (1938). Relation between blood plasma proteins and toxemias of pregnancy. JAMA, 111: 1898–1901.

Dyerberg J, Bang HO (1985). Pre-eclampsia and prostaglandins (Letter). Lancet, i: 1267.

Ebbs JH, Tisdall FF, Scott WA (1941). The influence of prenatal diet on mother and child. J Nutr, 22: 515–526.

Ebbs JH, Scott WA, Tisdall FF, Moyle WJ, Bell M (1942). Nutrition in pregnancy. Can Med Assoc J, 46: 1–6.

Edwards LE, Dickes WF, Acton IR, Hakanson EY (1978). Pregnancy in the massively obese: course, outcome and obesity prognosis in the infant. Am J Obstet Gynecol, 131: 479–483.

Efiong EI (1975). Pregnancy in the overweight Nigerian. Br J Obstet Gynaecol, 82: 903–906.

Emerson RG (1962). Obesity and its association with the complications of pregnancy. Br Med J, 2: 516–518.

Ferguson JH (1955). Methionine-vitamin B therapy: effect of a supplement of methionine and vitamin B on pregnancy and prematurity. Obstet Gynecol, 6: 221–227.

Fields H, Davis RE (1962). The overweight nullipara. Obstet Gynecol, 19: 423–427.

Fletcher J, Gurr A, Fellingham FR, Prankerd TAJ, Brant HA, Menzies DN (1971). The value of folic acid supplements in pregnancy J Obstet Gynaecol Br Commwlth, 78: 781–785.

Garrey MM, Govan ADT, Hodge C, Callander R (1980). Obstetrics Illustrated (3rd edn). Edinburgh: Churchill Livingstone.

Gillmer MDG (1983) Obesity in pregnancy—clinical and metabolic effects. In: Nutrition in Pregnancy. Proceedings of the Tenth Study Group of the Royal College of Obstetricians and Gynaecologists, September 1982. Campbell DM, Gillmer MDG (eds). London: Royal College of Obstetricians and Gynaecologists, pp 213–230.

Hamlin RHJ (1952). The prevention of eclampsia and pre-eclampsia. Lancet, 1: 64–68.

Hamlin RHJ (1958). Prophylaxis against toxaemia. Clin Obstet Gynecol, 1: 369–377.

Hankin ME, Symonds EM (1962). Body weight, diet and pre-eclamptic toxaemia of pregnancy. Austral NZ J Obstet Gynaecol, 4: 156–160.

Hauch E, Lehmann K (1934). Investigations into the occurrence of eclampsia in Denmark during the years 1918–1927. Acta Obstet Gynaecol Scand, 14: 425–475.

Hemminki E, Starfield B (1978). Routine administration of iron and vitamins during pregnancy: review of controlled clinical trials. Br J Obstet Gynaecol, 85: 404–410.

Hillman RW, Cabaud PG, Nilsson DE, Arpin PD, Tufano RJ (1963). Pyridoxine supplementation during pregnancy. Am J Clin Nutr, 12: 427–430.

Hipsley EH (1953). Dietary 'fibre' and pregnancy toxaemia. Br Med J, ii: 420–422.

Holme R (1985). Pregnancy and Diet. Harmondsworth: Penguin Books.

Hughes TD (1956). Antenatal care and the prevention of eclampsia and severe toxaemia. Med J Austral, 2: 48–50.

Hunt IF, Murphy NJ, Cleaver AE, Faraji B, Swendseid ME, Coulson AH, Clark VA, Laine N, Davis CA, Smith JC (1983). Zinc supplementation during pregnancy: zinc concentration of serum and hair from low-income women of Mexican descent. Am J Clin Nutr, 37: 572–582.

Hunt IF, Murphy NJ, Cleaver AE, Faraji B, Swendseid ME, Coulson AH, Clark VA, Browdy BL, Cabalum MT, Smith JC (1984). Zinc supplementation during pregnancy: effects on selected blood constituents and on progress and outcome of pregnancy in low-income women of Mexican descent. Am J Clin Nutr, 40: 508–521.

Hytten FE (1979). Restriction of weight gain in pregnancy: is it justified? J Hum Nutr, 33: 461–463.

Hytten FE (1985). Do pregnant women need zinc supplements? Br J Obstet Gynaecol, 92: 873–874.

Hytten F, Chamberlain G (1980). Clinical Physiology in Obstetrics. Part 2: Nutrition and Metabolism. Oxford: Blackwell Scientific Publications.

Iacono JM, Dougherty RM, Puska P (1982). Reduction of blood pressure associated with dietary polyunsaturated fat. Hypertension, 4: 34–42.

Iffy L, Kaminetzky H (eds) (1981). Principles and Practice of Obstetrics and Perinatology. New York: John Wiley.

Jenkins DM, Soltan MH (1983). Plasma zinc and copper in pregnancy. In: Nutrition in Pregnancy. Proceedings of the

Tenth Study Group of the Royal College of Obstetricians and Gynaecologists, September 1982. Campbell DM, Gillmer MDG (eds). London: Royal College of Obstetricians and Gynaecologists, pp 173–8.

Johnstone FD (1983). Assessment of dietary intake and dietary advice in pregnancy. In: Nutrition in Pregnancy. Proceedings of the Tenth Study Group of the Royal College of Obstetricians and Gynaecologists, September 1982. Campbell DM, Gillmer MDG (eds). London: Royal College of Obstetricians and Gynaecologists, pp 9–18.

Kerr MG (1962). The problem of the overweight patient in pregnancy. J Obstet Gynaecol Br Commwlth, 69: 988–995.

Kerr Grieve JF (1974). Prevention of gestational failure by high protein diet. J Reprod Med, 13: 170–174.

Kiiholma P, Paul R, Pakarinen P, Gronroos M (1984). Copper and zinc in pre-eclampsia. Acta Obstet Gynecol Scand. 63: 629–631.

Llewellyn-Jones D (1986). Fundamentals of Obstetrics and Gynaecology (4th edn). London: Faber and Faber.

Lowe CR (1961). Toxaemia and pre-pregnancy weight. J Obstet Gynaecol Br Empire, 68: 622–627.

Lu LY, Cook DL, Javia JB, Kirmani ZA, Liu CC, Makadia DN, Makadam TA, Omasayie OB, Patel DP, Reddy VJ, Walker BW, Williams CS, Chung RA (1981). Intakes of vitamins and minerals by pregnant women with selected clinical symptoms. J Am Diet Assoc, 78: 477–482.

MacGillivray I (1961). Hypertension in pregnancy and its consequences. J Obstet Gynaecol Br Commwlth, 68: 557–569.

MacGillivray I (1983). Pre-eclampsia: The Hypertensive Disease of Pregnancy. London: WB Saunders.

MacGillivray I, Johnstone FD (1978). Dietary protein and pre-eclampsia. In: Hypertensive Disorders of Pregnancy. Beller FK, MacGillivray I (eds). Stuttgart: Georg Thieme.

Mack HC, Kelly HJ, Macy IG (1956). Complications of pregnancy and nutritional status. I: Toxemias of pregnancy. Am J Obstet Gynecol, 71: 577–592.

Mastboom JL (1948). De frequentie van eclampsie in oorlogstijd. Ned Tijdschr Geneeskd, 92: 3604–3616.

Matthews HB, der Brucke MG (1938). Normal expectancy in the extremely obese pregnant woman. JAMA, 110: 554–558.

McCarty MF (1982). Nutritional prevention of pre-eclampsia—a special role for 1—series prostaglandin precursors? Med Hypotheses, 9: 283–291.

McGanity WJ, Cannon RO, Bridgforth EB, Martin MP, Densen PM, Newbill JA, McClellan GS, Christie A, Peterson JC, Darby WJ (1954). The Vanderbilt Cooperative Study of Maternal and Infant Nutrition. VI: Relationship of obstetric performance to nutrition. Am J Obstet Gynecol, 67: 501–527.

Mengert WF, Tacchi DA (1961). Pregnancy toxemia and sodium chloride. Am J Obstet Gynecol, 81: 601-605.

Myles MF (1981). Textbook for Midwives (9th edn). London: Churchill Livingstone.

National Advisory Committee on Nutrition Education (NACNE) (1983). A Discussion Paper on Proposals for Nutritional Guidelines for Health Education in Britain. London: The Health Education Council.

Nelson TR (1955a). A clinical study of pre-eclampsia. J Obstet Gynaecol Br Commwlth, 62: 48–57.

Nelson TR (1955b). A clinical study of pre-eclampsia. Part II. J Obstet Gynaecol Br Commwlth, 62: 58–66.

Norris PG, Jones CTH, Weston MJ (1986). Effect of dietary supplementation with fish oil on systolic blood pressure in mild essential hypertension. Br Med J, 293: 104–105.

Odell LD, Mengert WF (1945). The overweight obstetric patient. JAMA, 128: 87–89.

Peckham CH, Christianson RE (1971). The relationship between pre-pregnancy weight and certain obstetric factors. Am J Obstet Gynecol, 111: 1–7.

The People's League of Health (1942). Nutrition of expectant and nursing mothers. Lancet, ii: 10–12.

The People's League of Health (1946). The nutrition of expectant and nursing mothers in relation to maternal and infant mortality and morbidity. J Obstet Gynaecol Br Empire, 53: 498–509.

Phillips A (1983). Your Body, Your Baby, Your Life. London: Pandora Press.

Pritchard JA, MacDonald PC, Gant NF (eds) (1985). Williams Obstetrics (17th edn). Englewood Cliffs: Prentice-Hall International.

Primrose T, Higgins A (1971). A study in human antepartum nutrition. J Reprod Med, 7: 257–264.

Reader's Digest Association (1986). Reader's Digest Mother and Baby Book. London: Reader's Digest Association.

Redman C (1982a). Screening for pre-eclampsia. In: Effectiveness and Satisfaction in Antenatal Care. Enkin M, Chalmers I (eds). London: Spastics International Medical Publications, William Heinemann Books, pp 69–80.

Redman, C (1982b). Management of pre-eclampsia. In: Effectiveness and Satisfaction in Antenatal Care. Enkin M, Chalmers I (eds). London: Spastics International Medical Publications, William Heinemann Books, pp 182–197.

Ribeiro MD, Stein Z, Susser M, Cohen P, Neugut R (1982). Prenatal starvation and maternal blood pressure near delivery. Am J Clin Nutr, 35: 535–541.

Robinson M (1958). Salt in pregnancy. Lancet, i: 178–181.

Roopnarinesingh SS, Pathak UN (1970). Obesity in the Jamaican parturient. J Obstet Gynecol Br Commwlth, 77: 895–899.

Ross RA, Perlzweig W, Taylor H, McBryde A, Yates A, Kondritzer A (1938). A study of certain dietary factors of possible etiologic significance in toxemias of pregnancy. Am J Obstet Gynecol, 35: 426–440.

Royal College of Obstetricians and Gynaecologists (1983). Nutrition in Pregnancy. Proceedings of the Tenth Study Group of the Royal College of Obstetricians and Gynaecologists, September 1982. Campbell, DM and Gillmer MDG (eds). London: Royal College of Obstetricians and Gynaecologists.

Ruge S, Andersen T (1985). Obstetric risks in obesity. An analysis of the literature. Obstet Gynecol Surv, 40: 57–60.

Rush D (1982). Effects of changes in protein and calorie intake during pregnancy on the growth of the human fetus. In: Effectiveness and Satisfaction in Antenatal Care. Enkin M, Chalmers I (eds). London: Spastics International Medical Publications, William Heinemann Books, pp 92–113.

Smith CA (1947). The effect of wartime starvation in Holland upon pregnancy and its product. Am J Obstet Gynecol, 53: 599–606.

Stark CR, Lundin FE, Harley E. Effects of different prenatal regimens on pregnancy outcomes. (Unpublished.)

Stevenson RBC (1958). The prevention of eclampsia and severe pre-eclampsia. J Obstet Gynaecol Br Empire, 65: 982–987.

Stewart A, Hewitt D (1960). Toxaemia of pregnancy and obesity. J Obstet Gynaecol Br Empire, 67: 812–818.

Stoppard M (1985). The Pregnancy and Birth Book. London: Dorling Kindersley.

Strauss MB (1935). Observations on the etiology of the toxemias of pregnancy. The relationship of nutritional deficiency, hypoproteinemia, and elevated venous pressure to water retention in pregnancy. Am J Med Sci, 190: 811–824.

Suter CB, Ott DB (1984). Maternal and infant nutrition recommendations: a review. J Am Diet Assoc, 84: 572–573.

Theobald GW (1935). The dietetic deficiency hypothesis of the toxaemias of pregnancy. Proc R Soc Med, 28: 1388–1399.

Thomson AM (1958). Diet in pregnancy. 1: Dietary survey technique and the nutritive value of diets taken by primigravidae. Br J Nutr, 12: 446–461.

Thomson AM (1959a). Diet in pregnancy. 2: Assessment of the nutritive value of diets, especially in relation to differences between social classes. Br J Nutr, 13: 190–204.

Thomson AM (1959b). Diet in pregnancy. 3: Diet in relation to the course and outcome of pregnancy. Br J Nutr, 13: 509–525.

Thomson AM, Billewicz WZ (1957). Clinical significance of weight trends during pregnancy. Br Med J, i: 243–247.

Tompkins WT, Wiehl DG (1951). Nutritional deficiencies as a causal factor in toxemia and premature labor. Am J Obstet Gynecol, 62: 898–918.

Tompkins WT, Wiehl DG (1955). Maternal and newborn nutritional studies at Philadelphia Lying-In Hospital. Maternal studies III: toxemia and maternal nutrition. In: The Promotion of Maternal and Newborn Health. Tompkins WT, Wiehl DG (eds). New York: Milbank Memorial Fund, pp 62–90.

Tompkins WT, Wiehl DG, Mitchell RM (1955). The underweight patient as an increased obstetric hazard. Am J Obstet Gynecol, 69: 114–123.

Treharne IAL, Sutherland HW, Stowers JM, Samphier M (1979). Reproduction in obese women. In: Carbohydrate Metabolism in Pregnancy and the Newborn 1978. Sutherland HW, Stowers JM (eds). Berlin: Springer Verlag, pp 479–499.

Trigg KH, Rendall EJC, Johnson A, Fellingham FR, Prankerd TAJ (1976). Folate supplements during pregnancy. J R Coll Gen Pract, 26: 228–230.

Walker J, MacGillivray I, MacNaughton M (eds) (1976). Combined Textbook of Obstetrics and Gynaecology. Edinburgh: Churchill Livingstone.

Williams C, Highley W, Ma EH, Lewis J, Tolbert B, Woullard D, Kirmani S, Chung RA (1981). Protein, amino acid, and calorie intakes of selected pregnant women. J Am Diet Assoc, 78: 28–35.

Williams CD (1957). Weight in relation to pregnancy toxaemia. Br Med J, ii: 1338–1340.

Williams PF, Fralin FG (1942). Nutrition study in pregnancy. Am J Obstet Gynecol, 43: 1–20.

Willoughby MLN (1967). An investigation of folic acid requirements in pregnancy II. Br J Haematol, 13: 503–509.

Woodhill JM, Van den Berg AS, Burke BS, Stare FJ (1955). Nutrition studies of pregnant Australian women. Am J Obstet Gynecol, 70: 987–1003.

Zlatnik FJ, Burmeister FF (1983). Dietary protein and preeclampsia. Am J Obstet Gynecol, 147: 345–346.

19 Iron and folate supplementation in pregnancy

Kassam Mahomed and Frank Hytten

1 Introduction

About one hundred years ago there was a sudden change of view about pregnancy, from a belief that all pregnant women were 'plethoric' and would benefit from blood letting, to an equally firm belief that they were all anaemic and needed haematinics. The concept that healthy pregnant women might be neither plethoric nor anaemic is a recent and more rational concept, which has not had the same clinical appeal, possibly in part because it deprives the clinician of the opportunity to do something active.

The now discredited hypothesis that pregnant women were plethoric was well-supported by observation and the 'scientific' understanding of the day: pregnant women did not menstruate, they were often flushed and had dilated veins; they sometimes had fits which were 'known' to be caused by excessive blood in the body (Siddal 1980). Similarly, the anaemia hypothesis, still part of some clinical thinking, is supported by a great deal of laboratory evidence which shows changes in pregnancy similar to those characteristic of iron deficiency in the non-pregnant person: haemoglobin concentration and packed cell volume fall, there are fewer red cells per millilitre, serum iron falls, and iron binding capacity rises. When these and other generally accepted indices of iron deficiency were first demonstrated they undoubtedly provided a plausible basis for iron supplementation, just as the observations mentioned earlier provided a plausible basis for blood-letting. Now, however, an increasing understanding of the physiology of pregnancy has made it clear that those haematological changes do not represent iron deficiency, but are rather normal physiological adaptations that constitute an elaborate mimicry of iron deficiency anaemia, for which 'treatment' would clearly be inappropriate.

The understanding that pregnancy is not a deficiency disease is not new; it was discussed in detail more than 30 years ago (Hytten and Duncan 1956), and yet many obstetricians and even haematologists continue to insist that routine iron supplementation is necessary even in well-nourished populations.

The changes in pregnancy physiology which have led to the confusion were discussed in detail by Hytten and Leitch (1971) and are by now well-known. Briefly, the fall in haemoglobin concentration and red cell count is due to a greater dilution of the circulating red cell mass by what is often described as a 'disproportionate' rise in the plasma volume. The description is unfortunate, because the two components are controlled quite separately and bear no necessary relation to one another. The red cell mass is governed by the need to transport oxygen; it increases at high altitude and in athletic training, and falls as a result of prolonged confinement to bed. Plasma volume expands and contracts in relation to the need to fill the vascular bed and maintain blood pressure; for example, it rises during peripheral vasodilatation as may be seen in a hot climate or as a response to acclimatization to heat, and falls in the colder months of the year. Single indices that reflect the ratio of total red cell mass to plasma volume, such as haemoglobin concentration or red blood cell count, cannot be interpreted without a knowledge of the separate background changes in red cells and plasma. While the average healthy woman living at sea-level has a haemoglobin concentration of about 13–14 g/dl, that ratio is not sacred (Hytten 1985). In pregnancy, the changes in blood volume are greater, and the control mechanisms of plasma volume and total red cell mass are more obviously distinct and separate than at any other time in adult life.

Red cell mass rises by an average of some 18 per cent, more than is necessary for the somewhat smaller increase of about 16 per cent in oxygen uptake. Plasma volume increases by an average of about 50 per cent, largely to take account of vasodilatation and greatly increased circulation to areas where extra oxygen carriage is not needed: the skin and the kidneys. It is also related to the 'size' of the pregnancy so that bigger babies are associated with bigger increases in plasma volume than small babies, and multiple pregnancies with volume increases which are correspondingly bigger still.

While the falls in haemoglobin concentration and haematocrit, which result from the differential changes in red cell mass and plasma volume, provide the most common diagnostic pitfalls in pregnancy, there are a number of others. For example, in common with almost all water soluble nutrients, and for reasons which are not clear (Hytten 1980), serum levels of iron and folate fall. The concentration of transferrin (iron binding capacity) rises in response to increased oestrogen during pregnancy, as it does in iron deficiency states; and free protoporphyrin in the red cell, which is also increased in iron-deficiency anaemia, rises in normal pregnancy for reasons which have not been explained (Hytten and Duncan 1956).

In spite of all these arguments the notion persists that the fall in haemoglobin concentration may be, at least in part, due to iron deficiency if only because it can be reversed by treatment with iron. It suggests 'cure by replacement', the classic test of deficiency.

In this chapter we will consider the published evidence as to whether routine haematinic supplements confer any advantage on healthy pregnant women, and suggest criteria which will allow haematinics to be prescribed to those who need them.

Iron supplements have been given with two objects in view: one is to try to return the blood picture towards the normal non-pregnant state, a strange objective when millions of years of evolution have determined otherwise; the other is to improve the clinical outcome of the pregnancy and the future health of the mother. The first objective can certainly be accomplished; the key question is whether or not in achieving the 'normalized' blood picture we benefit or harm the woman and her baby. But genuine anaemia does occur in pregnancy, and we will consider it first.

2 Anaemia

Nothing has caused more confusion about the extent of 'anaemia' among pregnant women than attempts to define the condition. From the physiological point of view, anaemia can be crudely defined as a state in which insufficient haemoglobin is present in the blood to carry the oxygen required by an individual to perform normal activities. Thus for example, in terms of haemoglobin concentration, anaemia means different things in different circumstances; a person with a haemoglobin concentration of 13 g/dl who would not be anaemic at sea-level, would certainly be anaemic at an altitude of 25,000 feet.

While that functional definition may be the only certain way of establishing the presence of anaemia, it is not possible to apply it in practice without elaborate exercise tolerance testing. Perforce it has been necessary to decide on a definition which can be applied widely to populations of pregnant women and can be accommodated by a simple blood test; by tradition, haemoglobin concentration has been selected.

It was a poor choice. To dichotomize a continuous variable at some arbitrary point into normal and abnormal (a common device in medicine to decide such things as who is hypertensive or who has stunted growth) is philosophically dubious, and in the case of haemoglobin, biologically unsound. An individual's haemoglobin concentration, as we have discussed, depends on circumstances most of which have nothing to do with nutrient deficiency.

After struggling with this problem, the World Health Organization (1979) have adopted the general device of clinicians in setting a norm for pregnant women, in this case 11 g/dl, below which 'anaemia or deficiency should be considered to exist'. Other workers have chosen other arbitrary dividing lines: the most popular are 10.5 and 10.0 g/dl.

The advent of electronic blood counters has given an opportunity for more appropriate criteria to be applied for the diagnosis of anaemia. Mean cell volume may be the most useful; it is not closely related to haemoglobin concentration and declines quite rapidly in the presence of iron deficiency. It is not foolproof; microcytosis due to thalassaemia must be borne in mind.

And perhaps iron deficiency is the diagnosis we need to make since there is evidence that the blood picture changes only at a late stage when iron reserves are seriously depleted. The use of serum ferritin as a screening device may turn out to be more useful than haematology.

Megaloblastic anaemia, due almost always to folate

deficiency, also presents problems of definition. Measurement of folate levels in serum or red cells is the most common screening test, and again, the choice of arbitrary levels in pregnant women to decide who has a deficiency has caused confusion. Megaloblastic changes in peripheral blood, a rising mean red cell volume, can be equally confusing since it is clear that supplemental iron can cause an increase in red cell volume in pregnancy sufficient to mimic pathology (Taylor and Lind 1976). The definitive diagnosis requires the finding of megaloblastic changes in the bone marrow.

2.1 Prevalence

In the light of what we have said about the difficulty in defining anaemia it is hardly surprising that the true prevalence is nowhere known. There have been numerous published surveys which give the distribution of haemoglobin concentration among pregnant women, but none has distinguished between true anaemia and the effects of haemodilution; the techniques of blood sampling and of haemoglobin estimation have varied widely; and the way in which the women were selected is seldom stated. There would be little profit in attempting to list these studies, but some general observations are possible.

In a collection of data from developing countries representing some 68 million pregnant women, the World Health Organization (1979) found that about two-thirds had haemoglobin levels 'below those laid down by World Health Organization as being indicative of anaemia'. There was a range from 0 per cent (Panama) to 98 per cent (India and Pakistan) of pregnant women who fell below this arbitrary level of 11 g/dl.

As an example from a British population, Scott *et al.* (1975) showed that booking haemoglobins of less than 10 g/dl fell from 14 per cent in 1946–47 to under 1 per cent in 1968–72, due, it was thought to improved nutrition and supplementation. But over the same period the prevalence of diagnoses of megaloblastic anaemia in pregnancy rose from 1 per cent to over 12 per cent, apparently as a result of changing methods of diagnosis.

The studies of Garn and his colleagues have shown the effect of diagnostic criteria on the prevalence of 'anaemia' in a study of nearly 18,000 women (Garn *et al.* 1977). Black women had a haemoglobin level 1 g/dl below white women. This confirms their earlier findings of a constant 1 g difference between the mean haemoglobin concentrations of black and white individuals in a sample of 27,000 from infancy to old age (Garn *et al.* 1975) and the similar difference found by Kraemer *et al.* (1975) between black and white athletes in the University of Washington. As Garn *et al.* (1977) put it 'The net effect of race-specific haemoglobin and haematocrit norms would be to reduce the proportion of American blacks considered to be 'anaemic' or the proportion of black women needlessly given iron supplementation during pregnancy'.

That true anaemia occurs in the apparently healthy female population and that its prevalence increases during pregnancy is not disputed. But whether in any developed country there is a lot or a little of it is seldom possible to say. How the clinician might cope with this uncertainty is discussed below.

2.2 Association with adverse outcomes

Despite contention about the definition and the prevalence of anaemia in pregnancy, the underlying assumption which pervades the literature is that a low haemoglobin is causally associated with an adverse clinical outcome, and that the maintenance of a high or 'normal' haemoglobin is bound to be advantageous. The facts suggest otherwise, although it is remarkable how many trials have sought to raise the haemoglobin level or the iron stores, without apparently looking to see if any subjective, or clinical advantage followed.

Whether the 'improvement' in haematological indices associated with iron and/or folate supplementation leads to a better (or worse) clinical outcome is dealt with below in relation to controlled trials, but there is some compelling observational data, particularly relating haemoglobin levels to clinical outcome.

Both ends of the range of haemoglobin concentrations are associated with an impaired obstetric performance, but high haemoglobins are particularly sinister.

In late pregnancy the haemoglobin concentration will be high, that is to say, within or above the normal non-pregnant range, if the plasma has failed to rise to its normal high pregnancy volume, or if it has declined. Both phenomena occur. Koller (1982) pointed out the association between high haemoglobin and pre-eclampsia and Koller *et al.* (1980) showed that women whose infants were below the 10th centile of weight for gestation had relatively high haemoglobin levels: those whose infants died *in utero* had particularly high levels. Similar observations were made by Dunlop *et al.* (1978). Garn *et al.* (1981) in a study of nearly 60,000 pregnancies in the (United States) National Collaborative Perinatal Project, found that the highest rates of preterm labour, low birthweight, and fetal death were associated with haemoglobin levels which did not fall below 13–14 g/dl (Fig. 19.1).

In a study which included women with a history of reproductive failure, and where no iron supplements were given, Gibson (1973) found the expected positive relation between the increase in plasma volume and birthweight, and its obverse, a negative correlation between the lowest haemoglobin concentration reached by the women and the eventual birthweight of their babies (Fig 2). It is particularly noteworthy that two of the largest babies were associated with a haemoglobin

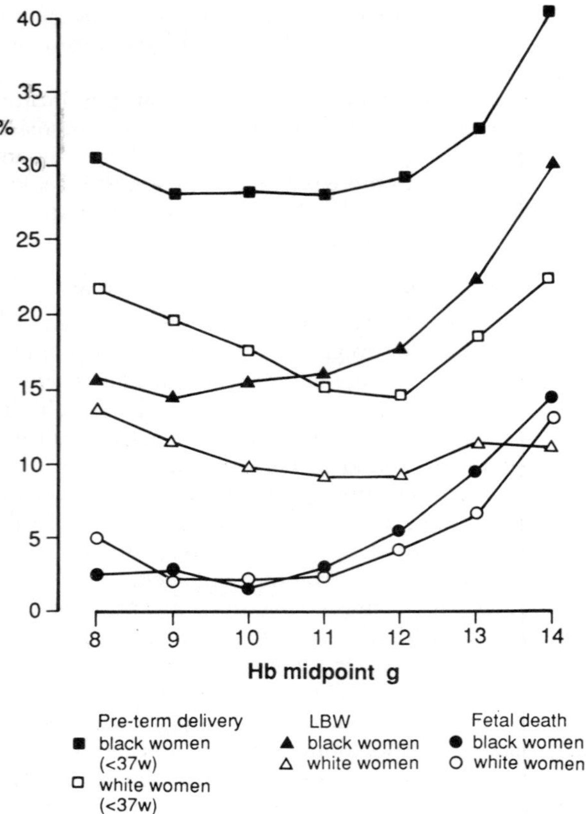

Fig. 19.1 Relation between lowest haemoglobin and pregnancy outcome (Garn *et al.* 1981)

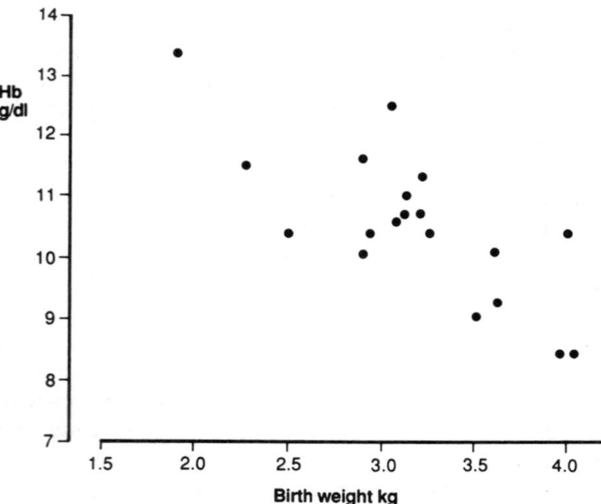

Fig. 19.2 Relation between lowest haemoglobin and birthweight (Gibson 1973)

level of 8.5 g/dl and yet these women had a normal red cell mass and no evidence of anaemia.

Particularly low haemoglobin levels in general may be associated with some excess fetal pathology (Garn *et al.* 1981), probably because the effects of genuine anaemia will be included. Note that the haemoglobin level associated with the optimum performance in that study (Fig. 19.1) was about 1 g lower in black women than white, confirming the ethnic difference in haemoglobin concentrations. A similar optimum level, which it will be noted fulfills the World Health Organization criterion of 'anaemia', was found by Murphy *et al.* (1986). The reason for the association between high haemoglobin concentration and obstetric pathology may be complex. For the women whose pregnancy, for whatever reason, is of poor quality, the fetus will grow poorly, the endocrine response will be impaired and the maternal adaptations which include the rise in plasma volume, will therefore be diminished. Thus the high haemoglobin is a consequence of, and not a reason for the poor obstetric performance. But if the plasma volume is normally expanded and then contracts as a result of some vasoconstrictive process, such as pre-eclampsia, then the rising haemoglobin will add an increasing viscosity to a diminishing uteroplacental circulation and will add directly to the fetal jeopardy.

These are examples of pathology. Whether raising the haemoglobin by the administration of iron has any direct effect in promoting poor fetal growth is not known, but there is little doubt that the red cells are enlarged as a result of supplemental iron (Taylor and Lind 1976) and may be less flexible, so that resistance to flow may be increased in the uteroplacental circulation.

2.3 Treatment

Generally in medicine, diagnosis of disease is made following complaints by patients: symptoms lead to investigation and diagnosis. But anaemia in pregnancy is seldom diagnosed that way; most women are screened routinely, and the diagnosis is made on the basis of some arbitrary laboratory measurements which may or may not be abnormal, and may or may not include some real pathology. For that reason it is difficult to discuss treatment and this section inevitably shades into the one which follows on routine supplementation.

Ideally, randomized controlled trials of treatment should be based on women whose anaemia has been diagnosed on sound criteria, but such trials do not seem to exist. Only two types of anaemia associated with pregnancy have received attention; in the case of iron deficiency anaemia it is usually the haemoglobin concentration which is being treated, only rarely are there examples of attempts to repair a proven iron deficiency. With megaloblastic anaemia the basis for treatment has been generally better founded, usually on the findings of a megaloblastic bone marrow. And since the treatment of iron deficiency anaemia with iron and megaloblastic anaemia with folate is almost universally successful, most trials have dealt with no more than comparisons of different forms and formulations of these compounds. The many papers which compared different types of oral iron were summarized by Hytten and Duncan (1956).

2.3.1 Iron deficiency anaemia

Treatment with iron in pregnancy is probably seldom necessary. It will be clear from what has been said earlier in this chapter that a 'low' haemoglobin without other evidence of iron deficiency requires no treatment; indeed, treatment may be harmful.

If there is genuine evidence of iron deficiency, iron treatment is obviously needed, and the usual approach is to give iron salts by mouth. There is a large literature reporting the effects of many preparations of iron, alone or in combination with other haematinics. All are effective, and there is no convincing evidence that the addition of copper, manganese, molybdenum or ascorbic acid improve the efficiency with which the iron is used, although some salts, and combined preparations are better tolerated than others. Ferrous sulphate causes more side-effects such as nausea and vomiting than most other preparations, but is better tolerated when given with molybdenum (Benstead and Theobald 1952); ferrous gluconate causes fewer gastrointestinal complications and the more complex iron chelates fewer still (Jennison 1958). In the very large doses given, particularly in the earlier studies where 1200 mg was not unusual, a high proportion of women had digestive disturbances. It could be that the lack of haematological response reported for some women in most studies may be due to their failure to take the iron because of its side-effects, rather than to their failure to absorb or use it.

A more certain method of introducing iron into the body is to give it parenterally, and several iron-carbohydrate complexes are available for intramuscular and intravenous use. It is generally agreed that the haematological response is no better, though possibly a little faster, than with oral iron (Allaire and Campagna 1961; Pritchard and Hunt 1958). Moreover, there can be serious side-effects with injected iron compounds: anaphylactic reactions, sometimes severe; thrombosis in the vein used for injections; even deaths have been reported. And although most haematologists believe that there is seldom a case for injected iron, there are enthusiasts such as Dawson *et al.* (1965) who said that 'In our opinion the most satisfactory method of treating iron deficiency anaemia in pregnancy in hospital is by the intravenous injection of large doses of 'imferon'.

Although a case could be made for the occasional use of injectable iron, particularly in areas of the world where iron deficiency is serious and compliance in pill-taking poor, there can be no case for the kind of heroics shown by Bare and Sullivan (1960). These authors had patients who were all taking iron supplements in pregnancy, but if their haemoglobin was below 10 g/dl at 30 weeks they were subjected to a trial of intravenous iron versus blood transfusion.

2.3.2 Megaloblastic anaemia

The cause of megaloblastic anaemia in pregnancy is almost always folate deficiency, and for practical purposes the possibility of a vitamin B_{12} deficiency can be ignored. As we have said, a megaloblastic picture in the peripheral blood occurs at a late stage of folate deficiency and is rare; the condition is more often diagnosed from the finding of megaloblastic changes in the bone marrow during the investigation of an anaemia not responding to iron. Chanarin (1985) suggests that iron deficiency may 'conceal evidence of a mild megaloblastic process' and that the rarity of recognizable megaloblastic anaemia is due to the 'dominant role played by iron deficiency in anaemia in pregnancy'.

In most patients the diagnosis is made in the final few weeks of pregnancy or in the puerperium. Presentation earlier in pregnancy is more likely if there is an associated condition causing an increased folate requirement, such as twin pregnancy or treatment with anticonvulsant drugs.

Once megaloblastic haemopoiesis is established, treatment of folic acid deficiency becomes more difficult (Letsky 1984) and there are some patients who fail to respond to parenteral folic acid treatment and only recover after delivery (Giles 1966). But in general treatment is straightforward: 5 mg of folic acid continued until after delivery, or for 4 weeks for those first diagnosed in the puerperium.

2.3.3 Other anaemias

Other anaemias not specifically related to pregnancy may occasionally occur, and are generally made worse by the pregnancy. They are included here for the sake of completeness, but it is neither possible, nor sensible to discuss their management: all require expert help from a haematologist.

Of the haemoglobinopathies, thalassaemia minor may present with a low haemoglobin concentration and microcytosis and be mistaken for a simple iron deficiency; oral iron and folic acid are recommended but parenteral iron should not be given. Women with the more serious thalassaemia major have generally had a lifetime of blood transfusions (few become pregnant) and suffer from iron overload; for them iron treatment is contraindicated and parenteral iron should never be given (Letsky 1984).

Sickle cell disease is associated with a particularly low haemoglobin concentration, which is usually reduced still further by pregnancy. These women are much more subject to most of the complications of pregnancy, and the complications of the haemoglobinopathy itself may pose serious problems for the pregnancy. They require meticulous care from a knowledgeable medical team (Charache and Niebyl 1985). Rarer and serious forms of anaemia which may develop in pregnancy are aplastic anemia, autoimmune haemolytic anaemia and anaemia associated with an exacerbation of systemic lupus erythematosus (Letsky 1984).

3 Routine supplementation

The evidence so far presented suggests that, excepting genuine anaemia, the best reproductive performance seems to be associated with levels of haemoglobin which are traditionally regarded as pathological. Further, there is little doubt that supplementation with iron, or in some circumstances folate, can change the blood picture towards its non-pregnant state. The key question is whether or not in achieving the 'normalized' blood picture we benefit or harm the woman and her baby.

The following analyses were based on the results of trials where supplements of iron or folate or both were given to pregnant women who were not anaemic on entry to the trial. Trials were excluded if supplementation began after 30 weeks of pregnancy, contained no adequate controls, or where insufficient data were presented for analysis. If data were missing, or presented in such a way that they could not be used, then an attempt was made to contact the authors, and in many cases more information was obtained.

3.1 Iron

Many aspects of the blood picture have been examined over the years, but the current almost universal use of the automatic blood counter, while improving the accuracy of results, has also narrowed the range of measurements available to the clinician. We will concentrate here on the two measurements which are generally available and most useful: haemoglobin concentration and mean red cell volume (MCV).

3.1.1 Haematological indices

3.1.1.1 Haemoglobin There is no doubt that supplemental iron prevents or greatly reduces the normal fall in haemoglobin concentration in pregnancy; this has been demonstrated in many controlled trials and comparisons of all kinds. Raising the mean haemoglobin concentration is, in itself, not important. What matters is that the lowest haemoglobin concentrations, where one might reasonably expect any true iron deficiency anaemias to lie, will become less frequent or be eliminated. That also is true. An analysis of well-conducted controlled trials demonstrates that considerably fewer women had a low haemoglobin (less than 10 or 10.5 g/dl) at 36–40 weeks if they had received supplemental iron compared with controls (Table 19.1).

3.1.1.2 Mean cell volume Mean cell volume, which characteristically falls when there is iron deficiency (microcytosis) does not usually change in normal pregnancy, but a slight increase in mean red cell volume

Table 19.1 Effect of routine iron administration in pregnancy on Hb <10–10.5 g/dl at 36–40 weeks

Study	EXPT		CTRL		Odds ratio	Graph of odds ratios and confidence intervals
	n	(%)	*n*	(%)	(95% CI)	0.01 0.1 0.5 1 2 10 100
Chisholm (1966)	6/72	(8.33)	37/72	(51.39)	0.13 (0.06–0.26)	
Batu *et al.* (1976)	0/30	(0.00)	7/25	(28.00)	0.08 (0.02–0.41)	
Fleming *et al.* (1974)	2/29	(6.90)	4/31	(12.90)	0.52 (0.10–2.77)	
Taylor *et al.* (1982)	0/22	(0.00)	7/24	(29.17)	0.11 (0.02–0.54)	
Holly (1955)	0/94	(0.00)	6/55	(10.91)	0.06 (0.01–0.33)	
Pritchard and Hunt (1958)	0/74	(0.00)	8/49	(16.33)	0.07 (0.02–0.30)	
Morgan (1961)	0/27	(0.00)	0/38	(0.00)	1.00 (1.00–1.00)	
Typical odds ratio (95% confidence interval)					0.12 (0.07–0.20)	

has been shown to occur in almost all women given haematinics compared to controls (Zittoun *et al.* 1983; Taylor *et al.* 1982; Dommisse *et al.* 1983; Edgar and Rice 1956; Fenton *et al.* 1977). Taylor and Lind (1976) showed that while normal pregnant women who are not given iron supplements maintain their mean red cell volume at around the average non-pregnant value of 85 fl, the distribution of mean red cell volume in those given iron showed a shift to the right of some 5 fl with a number displaying frank macrocytosis. Chanarin *et al.* (1977) interpreted similar findings differently, suggesting that the trend towards bigger red cells was normal, and that the unsupplemented group whose cells did not enlarge were, on the frail basis of a falling serum iron, iron deficient.

3.1.1.3 Serum iron There is universal agreement that the serum iron level falls in pregnant women who do not receive iron supplements, and even in some who do (Cantlie *et al.* 1971; Svanberg *et al.* 1975; Castren *et al.* 1968; Taylor *et al.* 1982; Buytaert *et al.* 1983; Wallenberg and Van Eijk 1984). Despite the widespread use of serum iron measurement as an index of iron status, interpretation of changes in serum iron is almost impossible. The level varies widely from time to time in the same individual and is poorly related to demonstrable iron stores (Hytten and Duncan 1956); as Bentley (1985) commented, it is 'a poor and frequently misleading indication of iron status'. The same could be said for measurements of the iron binding protein, transferrin (iron binding capacity) which rises, as it does characteristically in iron deficiency, in response to increased oestrogen levels in pregnancy. There is no merit in retaining serum iron, or iron binding capacity, as part of the investigation of iron deficiency in pregnancy.

3.1.1.4 Iron stores Stainable iron stores in the marrow were for many years regarded as the ultimate objective evidence of iron sufficiency, and it would indeed be difficult to argue that a falling haemoglobin concentration was due to iron deficiency when there was demonstrable iron in the marrow. But it is widely believed that menstruating women have very little storage iron, and a Scientific group of the World Health Organization (World Health Organization 1968) said that 'In estimating the dietary iron requirements of pregnant women reliance should not be placed on the iron stores since these have been found to be small or absent in most women'. There is no good epidemiological evidence to support that pessimistic assertion, and none is likely to be forthcoming since a study using marrow puncture in normal women would be ethically dubious, and the search for stainable iron is in any event inefficient and misleading. Even if information on iron status were available it is doubtful whether the entrenched opinions about iron deficiency in pregnancy would be modified. As an example of the illogicality it is possible to achieve, Hancock *et al.* (1968), who examined sternal marrow samples from 78 pregnant women, and who decided whether they were anaemic or not on conventional non-pregnant criteria, stated 'These results indicate that the presence of adequate iron in the bone marrow does not preclude the subsequent development of iron deficient anaemia in pregnancy . . .'

Nevertheless, Puolakka *et al.* (1980), who reported that some two-thirds of their women had stainable marrow iron in early pregnancy, were able to find none in most women at term if they had not had iron supplements.

3.1.1.5 Ferritin An apparently more reliable, and certainly more accessible criterion of iron status is the level of ferritin in serum and all investigations have shown it to fall in pregnancy (Fenton *et al.* 1977; Van Eijk *et al.* 1978; Taylor *et al.* 1982; Romslo et al. 1983). The pattern is of a rapid fall up to about 28 or 30 weeks followed by a plateau during the last trimester and a rapid rise after delivery. The fall occurs even if iron supplements are given, but is much more profound if they are not, with a majority of women falling to levels

Table 19.2 Effect of routine iron administration in pregnancy on serum ferritin <10 ug/l at 36–40 weeks

Study	EXPT		CTRL		Odds ratio	Graph of odds ratios and confidence intervals
	n	(%)	*n*	(%)	(95% CI)	0.01 0.1 0.5 1 2 10 100
Romslo *et al.* (1983)	1/22	(4.55)	19/23	(82.61)	0.05 (0.01–0.15)	
Taylor *et al.* (1982)	3/22	(13.64)	22/24	(91.67)	0.05 (0.01–0.15)	
Puolakka *et al.* (1980)	0/16	(0.00)	2/16	(12.50)	0.13 (0.01–2.12)	
Typical odds ratio (95% confidence interval)					0.05 (0.02–0.11)	

below 10 μg/l. The 3 randomized trials which have examined the effect show clearly that while many unsupplemented women will have serum ferritin concentrations below 10 μg/l in late pregnancy, very few who have taken supplements fall to that level (Table 19.2).

3.1.2 Outcome of pregnancy

If the effect of routine iron is to 'improve' the peripheral blood picture, it has not been shown to have any beneficial effects on the outcome of pregnancy. The women certainly do not feel any subjective benefit from having their haemoglobin concentration raised (Fisher and Biggs 1955; Paintin *et al.* 1966), and Magee and Milligan (1951) commented that in their large series 'the great bulk of women, whether taking iron or not, were perfectly healthy and had no complaints, which raises the question whether a haemoglobin level raised by iron therapy is in itself an advantage'. A possible advantage which has been claimed for a high level of haemoglobin in pregnancy is that the woman is in a stronger position to withstand haemorrhage, and even that she has less tendency to haemorrhage postpartum. There is no evidence to support the first part of that claim and it is difficult to see how it could be proven. Indeed, if a low haemoglobin in healthy pregnant women generally implies a large circulating blood volume then it is at least possible that women with a *low* haemoglobin might better withstand a given loss of blood. Wills *et al.* (1947) reported a greater incidence of haemorrhage in women who took no additional iron, but Lund (1951) and Willoughby (1967) found no difference in the prevalence of haemorrhage between treated and untreated women, and Benstead and Theobald (1952) said that 'the only disadvantage of maintaining the haemoglobin level at its normal value throughout pregnancy would appear to be a slightly increased risk of post partum haemorrhage'.

In the very few randomized trials where clinical outcome was examined, there was no influence of iron supplementation on the prevalence of proteinuric hypertension (Table 19.3), antepartum haemorrhage (Table 19.4), or maternal infection (Table 19.5). The only cause for concern is an agreement in two well-conducted trials of a clear though not entirely convincing increase in the prevalence of preterm delivery (Table 19.6) and low birth weight (Table 19.7). If that association is confirmed by further trials, a possible mechanism is not self-evident. Perhaps there is a primary effect on fetal growth due to the increased viscosity of maternal blood, which follows the iron-induced macrocytosis and increased haemoglobin concentration, impeding uteroplacental blood flow.

3.1.3 The situation in developing countries

What has been said so far refers almost entirely to relatively well-fed Western populations where the women are generally healthy; the situation is quite otherwise in most developing countries. It is difficult to know the extent of anaemia because of the general use

Table 19.3 Effect of routine iron in well-nourished women in pregnancy on proteinuric hypertension

Study	EXPT		CTRL		Odds ratio	Graph of odds ratios and confidence intervals
	n	(%)	*n*	(%)	(95% CI)	0.01 0.1 0.5 1 2 10 100
Paintin *et al.* (1966)	3/56	(5.36)	5/57	(8.77)	0.60 (0.14–2.50)	
Taylor *et al.* (1982)	1/24	(4.17)	0/24	(0.00)	7.39 (0.15–99.99)	
Typical odds ratio (95% confidence interval)					0.80 (0.21–3.08)	

Table 19.4 Effect of routine iron in well-nourished women in pregnancy on APH

Study	EXPT		CTRL		Odds ratio	Graph of odds ratios and confidence intervals
	n	(%)	*n*	(%)	(95% CI)	0.01 0.1 0.5 1 2 10 100
Paintin *et al.* (1966)	1/56	(1.79)	1/57	(1.75)	1.02 (0.06–16.48)	
Taylor *et al.* (1982)	0/24	(0.00)	0/24	(0.00)	1.00 (1.00–1.00)	
Typical odds ratio (95% confidence interval)					1.02 (0.06–16.48)	

Table 19.5 Effect of routine iron in well-nourished women in pregnancy on maternal infection

Study	EXPT		CTRL		Odds ratio	Graph of odds ratios and confidence intervals
	n	(%)	*n*	(%)	(95% CI)	0.01 0.1 0.5 1 2 10 100
Paintin *et al.* (1966)	0/56	(0.00)	3/57	(5.26)	0.13 (0.01–1.30)	
Taylor *et al.* (1982)	2/24	(8.33)	2/24	(8.33)	1.00 (0.13–7.58)	
Typical odds ratio (95% confidence interval)					0.41 (0.09–1.87)	

Table 19.6 Effect of routine iron in well-nourished women in pregnancy on short gestation

Study	EXPT		CTRL		Odds ratio	Graph of odds ratios and confidence intervals
	n	(%)	*n*	(%)	(95% CI)	0.01 0.1 0.5 1 2 10 100
Paintin *et al.* (1966)	1/56	(1.79)	0/57	(0.00)	7.52 (0.15–99.99)	
Fleming *et al.* (1974)	1/29	(3.45)	1/31	(3.23)	1.07 (0.07–17.55)	
Taylor *et al.* (1982)	3/24	(12.50)	0/24	(0.00)	8.08 (0.80–81.60)	
Typical odds ratio (95% confidence interval)					4.04 (0.80–20.48)	

Table 19.7 Effect of routine iron in well-nourished women in pregnancy on low birthweight

Study	EXPT		CTRL		Odds ratio	Graph of odds ratios and confidence intervals
	n	(%)	*n*	(%)	(95% CI)	0.01 0.1 0.5 1 2 10 100
Paintin *et al.* (1966)	3/56	(5.36)	2/57	(3.51)	1.54 (0.26–9.19)	
Taylor *et al.* (1982)	2/24	(8.33)	0/24	(0.00)	7.72 (0.47–99.99)	
Typical odds ratio (95% confidence interval)					2.46 (0.54–11.07)	

of the World Health Organization definition of less than 11g/dl, but it seems reasonable to assume that true, often gross anaemia is a major problem in most of the developing world. In the Indian subcontinent anaemia makes a large contribution to the high maternal death rate (World Health Organization 1979). Dietary inadequacies, aggravated in many countries by food taboos in pregnancy, are a common background, but it is obvious that in most areas, anaemia represents much more than that; it is associated with widespread disease, the most conspicuous of which are intestinal parasites and malaria.

Because of the local circumstances, generally with an illiterate population and a high rate of non-cooperation, and because of the complexity of the clinical background, few trials of treatment have been undertaken and all suffered subject losses which make interpretation difficult. In tropical Africa, the picture is dominated by haemolysis due to malaria, and a randomized blind trial in Northern Nigeria (Fleming *et al.* 1986), inevitably dogged by problems of non-compliance and dropouts, showed clearly that vigorous anti-malarial treatment together with iron and folic acid supplements gave the best clinical results and the best postpartum haematological status. Malaria prophylaxis was undoubtedly the most important of these elements, and folic acid the least important although there is some evidence that with very young girls characteristic of Muslim Northern Nigeria, folate supplements may be important to allow them to continue their own growth during pregnancy (Harrison *et al.* 1985).

Sood *et al.* (1975) who gave iron supplements to Indian pregnant women in a good randomized trial, showed that compared to a control group where 42 out of 70 women had low birthweight infants, only 33 out of 107 did so when supplemented, an odds ratio of 0.31 (95 per cent confidence limits 0.17—0.56).

3.2 Folate

3.2.1 Haematological indices

Almost all trials of folic acid supplementation have been made in women also receiving supplementary iron, so that the effect if any on haemoglobin concentration is inevitably submerged and the pooled overview (Table 19.8) shows no effect on the proportion of women having a low haemoglobin concentration in late pregnancy. Where folate alone is compared to iron alone there is a much higher proportion of low haemoglobin

Table 19.8 Effect of routine folate administration in pregnancy on Hb <10–10.5 g/dl at 36–40 weeks

Study	EXPT		CTRL		Odds ratio	Graph of odds ratios and confidence intervals
	n	(%)	*n*	(%)	(95% CI)	0.01 0.1 0.5 1 2 10 100
Chisholm (1966)	21/155	(13.55)	6/72	(8.33)	1.64 (0.69–3.88)	
Giles PF*et al.* (1971)	117/265	(44.15)	126/263	(47.91)	0.86 (0.61–1.21)	
Batu *et al.* (1976)	14/46	(30.43)	17/55	(30.91)	0.98 (0.42–2.28)	
Fleming *et al.* (1974)	2/57	(3.51)	2/29	(6.90)	0.47 (0.06–3.88)	
Iyengar and Apte (1970)	7/69	(10.14)	7/77	(9.09)	1.13 (0.38–3.39)	
Iyengar (1971)	5/27	(18.52)	2/80	(2.50)	13.40 (2.32–77.59)	
Giles C and Burton (1960)	37/758	(4.88)	54/721	(7.49)	0.64 (0.42–0.97)	
Menon and Rajan (1962)	17/95	(17.89)	33/88	(37.50)	0.37 (0.20–0.72)	
Iyengar and Rajalakshmi (1975)	14/110	(12.73)	13/114	(11.40)	1.13 (0.51–2.53)	
Typical odds ratio (95% confidence interval)					0.82 (0.66–1.01)	

Table 19.9 Effect of routine folate vs routine iron administration in pregnancy on Hb <10–10.5 g/dl at 36–40 weeks

Study	EXPT		CTRL		Odds ratio	Graph of odds ratios and confidence intervals
	n	(%)	*n*	(%)	(95% CI)	0.01 0.1 0.5 1 2 10 100
Chisholm (1966)	60/156	(38.46)	6/72	(8.33)	4.30 (2.33–7.95)	
Batu *et al.* (1976)	13/21	(61.90)	0/30	(0.00)	24.42 (6.88–86.70)	
Fleming *et al.* (1974)	5/29	(17.24)	2/29	(6.90)	2.61 (0.54–12.48)	
Menon and Rajan (1962)	54/90	(60.00)	33/88	(37.50)	2.45 (1.36–4.40)	
Typical odds ratio (95% confidence interval)					3.83 (2.59–5.66)	

Table 19.10 Effect of routine folate administration in pregnancy on serum folate <2.5–5 μg/ml at 36–40 weeks

Study	EXPT		CTRL		Odds ratio	Graph of odds ratios and confidence intervals
	n	(%)	*n*	(%)	(95% CI)	0.01 0.1 0.5 1 2 10 100
Batu *et al.* (1976)	0/44	(0.00)	29/52	(55.77)	0.07 (0.03–0.17)	
Fletcher J *et al.* (1971)	10/321	(3.12)	32/322	(9.94)	0.33 (0.18–0.61)	
Rolschau *et al.* (1979)	0/20	(0.00)	0/15	(0.00)	1.00 (1.00–1.00)	
Srisupandit *et al.* (1983)	0/107	(0.00)	39/92	(42.39)	0.07 (0.03–0.14)	
Typical odds ratio (95% confidence interval)					0.14 (0.09–0.21)	

Table 19.11 Effect of routine folate administration in pregnancy on low red cell folate at 36–40 weeks

Study	EXPT		CTRL		Odds ratio	Graph of odds ratios and confidence intervals
	n	(%)	*n*	(%)	(95% CI)	0.01 0.1 0.5 1 2 10 100
Batu *et al.* (1976)	0/43	(0.00)	13/52	(25.00)	0.12 (0.04–0.40)	
Weil and Maurascher (1977)	0/8	(0.00)	3/13	(23.08)	0.17 (0.01–1.94)	
Rolschau *et al.* (1979)	0/20	(0.00)	3/15	(20.00)	0.08 (0.01–0.89)	
Iyengar (1971)	2/32	(6.25)	15/26	(57.69)	0.09 (0.03–0.27)	
Typical odds ratio (95% confidence interval)					0.11 (0.05–0.22)	

Table 19.12 Effect of routine folate in well-nourished women in pregnancy on proteinuric hypertension

Study	EXPT		CTRL		Odds ratio	Graph of odds ratios and confidence intervals
	n	(%)	*n*	(%)	(95% CI)	0.01 0.1 0.5 1 2 10 100
Fletcher J *et al.* (1971)	62/321	(19.31)	49/322	(15.22)	1.33 (0.88–2.00)	
Typical odds ratio (95% confidence interval)					1.33 (0.88–2.00)	

values in the groups having no iron (Table 19.9), and where combined iron and folate supplements are compared to placebo there is also a considerable effect in reducing the number of women with a low haemoglobin in late pregnancy.

As would be expected, folate supplements almost eliminated low serum (Table 19.10) and red cell folate (Table 19.11) levels in late pregnancy.

3.2.2 Outcome of pregnancy

In generally well-nourished women the addition of folate to iron supplements had no evident effect on proteinuric hypertension (Table 19.12), antepartum haemorrhage (Table 19.13), preterm delivery (Table 19.14) and low birthweight (Table 19.15). In less well-nourished women from developing countries the addition of folate may be more important although the evidence is sketchy. For proteinuric hypertension there are only two randomized trials (Table 19.16) in which the pooled overview shows no convincing effect, and the better trial no effect at all. For antepartum haemorrhage (Table 19.17) and maternal infection (Table

Table 19.13 Effect of routine folate in well-nourished women in pregnancy on antepartum haemorrhage

Study	EXPT		CTRL		Odds ratio	Graph of odds ratios and confidence intervals
	n	(%)	*n*	(%)	(95% CI)	0.01 0.1 0.5 1 2 10 100
Fletcher *et al.* (1971)	19/321	(5.92)	14/322	(4.35)	1.38 (0.69–2.78)	
Hall (1972)	9/925	(0.97)	16/2024	(0.79)	1.24 (0.53–2.90)	
Willoughby (1967)	0/706	(0.00)	1/736	(0.14)	0.14 (0.00–7.11)	
Typical odds ratio (95% confidence interval)					1.27 (0.74–2.17)	

Table 19.14 Effect of routine folate in well-nourished women in pregnancy on short gestation

Study	EXPT		CTRL		Odds ratio	Graph of odds ratios and confidence intervals
	n	(%)	*n*	(%)	(95% CI)	0.01 0.1 0.5 1 2 10 100
Tchernia *et al.* (1982)	2/54	(3.70)	7/54	(12.96)	0.30 (0.08–1.17)	
Fleming *et al.* (1974)	2/57	(3.51)	1/29	(3.45)	1.02 (0.09–11.47)	
Fletcher *et al.* (1971)	28/321	(8.72)	28/322	(8.70)	1.00 (0.58–1.74)	
Rolschau *et al.* (1979)	1/20	(5.00)	1/16	(6.25)	0.79 (0.05–13.44)	
Typical odds ratio (95% confidence interval)					0.85 (0.52–1.39)	

Table 19.15 Effect of routine folate in well-nourished women in pregnancy on low birthweight

Study	EXPT		CTRL		Odds ratio	Graph of odds ratios and confidence intervals
	n	(%)	*n*	(%)	(95% CI)	0.01 0.1 0.5 1 2 10 100
Fletcher *et al.* (1971)	16/321	(4.98)	18/322	(5.59)	0.89 (0.44–1.77)	
Rolschau *et al.* (1979)	0/20	(0.00)	2/19	(10.53)	0.12 (0.01–2.02)	
Typical odds ratio (95% confidence interval)					0.79 (0.40–1.55)	

Table 19.16 Effect of routine folate in poorly nourished women in pregnancy on proteinuric hypertension

Study	EXPT		CTRL		Odds ratio	Graph of odds ratios and confidence intervals
	n	(%)	*n*	(%)	(95% CI)	0.01 0.1 0.5 1 2 10 100
Fleming *et al.* (1968)	2/28	(7.14)	2/26	(7.69)	0.92 (0.12–6.96)	
Iyengar and Rajalakshmi (1975)	1/117	(0.85)	2/122	(1.64)	0.53 (0.05–5.17)	
Typical odds ratio (95% confidence interval)					0.72 (0.16–3.28)	

Table 19.17 Effect of routine folate in poorly nourished women in pregnancy on antepartum haemorrhage

Study	EXPT		CTRL		Odds ratio	Graph of odds ratios and confidence intervals
	n	(%)	*n*	(%)	(95% CI)	0.01 0.1 0.5 1 2 10 100
Iyengar and Rajalakshmi (1975)	0/117	(0.00)	1/122	(0.82)	0.14 (0.00–7.11)	
Typical odds ratio (95% confidence interval)					0.14 (0.00–7.11)	

Table 19.18 Effect of routine folate in poorly nourished women in pregnancy on maternal infection

Study	EXPT		CTRL		Odds ratio	Graph of odds ratios and confidence intervals
	n	(%)	*n*	(%)	(95% CI)	0.01 0.1 0.5 1 2 10 100
Fleming *et al.* (1968)	2/28	(7.14)	2/26	(7.69)	0.92 (0.12–6.96)	
Iyengar and Rajalakshmi (1975)	4/117	(3.42)	4/122	(3.28)	1.04 (0.26–4.26)	
Typical odds ratio (95% confidence interval)					1.00 (0.32–3.18)	

Table 19.19 Effect of routine folate in poorly nourished women in pregnancy on short gestation

Study	EXPT		CTRL		Odds ratio	Graph of odds ratios and confidence intervals
	n	(%)	*n*	(%)	(95% CI)	0.01 0.1 0.5 1 2 10 100
Iyengar and Rajalakshmi (1975)	19/117	(16.24)	31/122	(25.41)	0.58 (0.31–1.07)	
Typical odds ratio (95% confidence interval)					0.58 (0.31–1.07)	

Table 19.20 Effect of routine folate in poorly-nourished women in pregnancy on low birthweight

Study	EXPT		CTRL		Odds ratio	Graph of odds ratios and confidence intervals
	n	(%)	*n*	(%)	(95% CI)	0.01 0.1 0.5 1 2 10 100
Baumslag *et al.* (1970)	4/65	(6.15)	19/63	(30.16)	0.20 (0.08–0.49)	
Iyengar and Apte (1970)	12/57	(21.05)	8/45	(17.78)	1.23 (0.46–3.27)	
Iyengar (1971)	5/23	(21.74)	12/26	(46.15)	0.35 (0.11–1.12)	
Iyengar and Rajalakshmi (1975)	18/98	(18.37)	31/91	(34.07)	0.44 (0.23–0.85)	
Typical odds ratio (95% confidence interval)					0.43 (0.28–0.67)	

Table 19.21 Effect of routine folate in poorly nourished women in pregnancy on stillbirths

Study	EXPT		CTRL		Odds ratio	Graph of odds ratios and confidence intervals
	n	(%)	*n*	(%)	(95% CI)	0.01 0.1 0.5 1 2 10 100
Fleming *et al.* (1968)	0/28	(0.00)	1/26	(3.85)	0.13 (0.00–6.33)	
Iyengar and Rajalakshmi (1975)	1/117	(0.85)	4/122	(3.28)	0.31 (0.05–1.80)	
Typical odds ratio (95% confidence interval)					0.26 (0.05–1.33)	

Table 19.22 Effect of routine folate in poorly nourished women in pregnancy on admission to neonatal unit

Study	EXPT		CTRL		Odds ratio	Graph of odds ratios and confidence intervals
	n	(%)	*n*	(%)	(95% CI)	0.01 0.1 0.5 1 2 10 100
Iyengar (1971)	3/60	(5.00)	5/57	(8.77)	0.56 (0.13–2.32)	
Iyengar and Rajalakshmi (1975)	8/117	(6.84)	15/122	(12.30)	0.54 (0.23–1.26)	
Typical odds ratio (95% confidence interval)					0.54 (0.26–1.13)	

Table 19.23 Effect of routine folate in poorly nourished women in pregnancy on neonatal deaths

Study	EXPT		CTRL		Odds ratio	Graph of odds ratios and confidence intervals
	n	(%)	*n*	(%)	(95% CI)	0.01 0.1 0.5 1 2 10 100
Iyengar (1971)	2/60	(3.33)	3/57	(5.26)	0.63 (0.11–3.73)	
Iyengar and Rajalakshmi (1975)	5/117	(4.27)	8/122	(6.56)	0.64 (0.21–1.96)	
Typical odds ratio (95% confidence interval)					0.64 (0.25–1.64)	

19.18) there is no obvious effect. For preterm delivery (Table 19.19) a single study suggests some beneficial influence, and a pooled overview of five randomized trials suggests that women given folate supplements have fewer low birthweight infants (Table 19.20). The result is somewhat unconvincing in that the largest study by Sood *et al.* (1975) showed the opposite effect, and three of the other four studies were from the same team of Iyengar *et al.* (1970,1971,1975) in India. There was a slight beneficial trend suggested for stillbirths (Tables 19.21) and for neonatal morbidity (Table 10.22) and mortality (Table 10.23), but there were few studies and almost all of these were from Iyengar's group.

In summary, folate itself seems to have little influence on clinical outcome, although there are persistent indications of possible benefit to fetal growth in ill-nourished communities, and perhaps some value in young pregnant teenagers when both fetal and maternal growth are competing.

4 Conclusions

4.1 Implications for current practice

In spite of persistent recommendations from haematologists that iron and folate supplementation is an important aspect of antenatal care, the evidence that it benefits the mother and her fetus is, to say the least, unconvincing.

There is no clinical benefit to be seen either in the pregnancy itself or in the infant, and the only beneficial results may be to build up the woman's iron stores. On the other hand there are hints that the reversal of the normal fall in haemoglobin concentration and the iron-induced macrocytosis may increase blood viscosity to a degree which could impair uteroplacental blood flow.

For the obstetrician caring for generally healthy well-nourished women in a developed country the indication is clear: anaemia, which is undoubtedly more common in pregnancy, should be looked for in all pregnant women and treated if found. But to treat all pregnant women as if they were iron deficient is both therapeutically misguided and possibly harmful.

In developing countries, where many, perhaps most women are nutritionally deficient and generally unhealthy, and where constant supervision in pregnancy is impracticable, there is an excellent case for universal supplementation, and for malaria prophylaxis if appropriate. In this situation any possible ill-effects of unnecessary iron supplementation are far outweighed by the life-saving benefits of eliminating serious anaemia. And where the pregnant women are particularly young, perhaps still growing themselves, folate supplements are likely to be beneficial.

Even where nutritional supplements are indicated we should heed the warning of Hemminki (1982) that there is '. . . the danger that pharmaceutically prepared supplements may divert attention from the need to improve the circumstances which lead to malnutrition in the first place'.

4.2 Implications for future research

While all the evidence indicates that iron supplementation tends to reverse the characteristic haematological changes of pregnancy, and adds to body iron store, it also suggests that no clinical benefit follows and there may even be some clinical disadvantage.

That general impression urgently needs to be clarified, not only because of the huge cost of supplementation, but because more and more supplements are being proposed as necessary for pregnant women and will tend to be carried along in the wake of iron and folate unless a more critical climate is promoted.

These questions deserve an answer: Is the iron added to body stores in pregnancy of any lasting benefit to the women? Does she have less chance of becoming anaemic in later life or in a later pregnancy and does she gain any advantage in terms of general health?

Does the child of the supplemented pregnancy have bigger iron stores which might confer some long term benefit?

Does a haemoglobin level in pregnancy, raised by iron treatment, confer any clinical benefit or disadvantage?

In developing countries, where anaemia is a major public health problem, there can be no argument about the need for supplementation, but the specific problem of the young pregnant girl growing herself deserves closer study. What are the long term benefits to her of allowing her to express her own growth potential during pregnancy, and does that harm the fetus? What supplements are needed to achieve the best results?

The time has come for large scale multicentre randomized trials to be mounted, preferably in several countries, to answer these questions. The studies will have to be very big and meticulously planned, but there are now sufficient obstetricians who doubt the wisdom of routine supplementation for that to be possible.

Whether it may also be possible to examine in more detail any detrimental effects of iron supplementation deserves exploration. If iron-induced macrocytosis coupled with the raised red cell concentration increases blood viscosity, then changes in uteroplacental blood flow may be visible by Doppler ultrasound techniques.

References

Allaire BI, Campagna FA (1961). Iron-deficiency anaemia in pregnancy. Evaluation of diagnosis and therapy by bone marrow hemosiderin. Obstet Gynecol, 17: 605–610.

Bare WW, Sullivan AA (1960). Comparison of intravenous saccharated iron oxide and whole blood in treatment of hypochromic anemia of pregnancy. Am J Obstet Gynecol, 79: 279–285.

Batu AT, Toe T, Pe H, Nyunt KK (1976). A prophylactic trial of iron and folic acid supplements in pregnant Burmese women. Israel J Med Sci 12: 1410–1417.

Baumslag N, Edelstein T, Metz J (1970). Reduction of incidence of prematurity by folic acid supplementation in pregnancy. Br Med J, 1: 16–17.

Benstead N, Theobald G W (1952). Iron and the 'physiological' anaemia of pregnancy. Br Med J, i: 407–410.

Bentley DP (1985). Iron metabolism and anaemia in pregnancy. In: Haematological Disorders in Pregnancy. Letsky E A (ed). Clin Haematol, 14: 613–628.

Buytaert G, Wallenburg HCS, Van Eijk HG, Buytaert P (1983). Iron supplementation during pregnancy. Eur J Obstet Gynecol Reprod Biol, 15: 11–16.

Cantlie GSD, De Leeuw NKM, Lowenstein L (1971). Iron and folate nutrition in a group of private obstetrical patients. Am J Clin Nutr, 24: 637–641.

Castren O, Levanto A, Rauramo L, Ruponen S (1968). Preventive iron and folic acid therapy in pregnancy. Ann Chir Gynaecol Fenn, 57: 382–386.

Chanarin I (1985). Folate and cobalamin. Clin Haematol, 14: 629–641.

Chanarin I, McFadyen IR, Kyle R (1977). The physiological macrocytosis of pregnancy. Br J Obstet Gynaecol, 84: 504–508.

Charache S and Niebyl JR (1985). Pregnancy in Sickle Cell disease. Clin Haematol 14: 729–746.

Chisholm M (1966). A controlled clinical trial of prophylactic folic acid and iron in pregnancy. J Obstet Gynaecol Br Commwlth, 73: 191–196.

Dawson DW, Goldthorp WO, Spencer D (1965). Parenteral iron therapy in pregnancy. J Obstet Gynaecol Br Cmmnwlth, 72: 89–93.

Dommisse J, Bell DJH, Du Toit ED, Midgley V, Cohen M, (1983). Iron-storage deficiency and iron supplementation in pregnancy. S Afr Med J, 64: 1047–1051.

Dunlop W, Furness C and Hill LM (1978). Maternal haemoglobin concentration, haematocrit and renal handling of urate in pregnancies ending in the births of small-for-dates-infants. Br J Obstet Gynaecol, 85: 938–944.

Edgar W, Rice HM (1956). Administration of iron in antenatal clinics. Lancet, 1: 599–602.

Fenton V, Cavill I, Fisher J (1977). Iron stores in pregnancy. Br J Haematol, 37: 145–149.

Fisher M, Biggs R. (1955). Iron deficiency in pregnancy. Br Med J, i: 385–386.

Fleming AF, Hendrickse JP de V, Allan NC (1968). The prevention of megaloblastic anaemia in pregnancy in Nigeria. J Obstet Gynaecol Br Commwlth, 75: 425–432.

Fleming AF, Martin JD, Hahnel R, Westlake AJ (1974). Effects of iron and folic acid antenatal supplements on maternal haematology and fetal wellbeing. Med J Austral, 2: 429–436.

Fleming AF, Ghatoura GBS, Harrison KA, Briggs OD and Dunn DT (1986). The prevention of anaemia in pregnancy in preimigravidae in the Guinea Savanna of Nigeria. Ann Trop Med Parasit, 80: 211–233.

Fletcher J, Gurr A, Fellingham FR, Prankerd TAJ, Brant HA, Menzies DN (1971). The value of folic acid supplements in pregnancy. J Obstet Gynaecol Br Empire, 78: 781–785.

Garn SM, Shaw HA, Guire KE and McCabe KD (1977). Apportioning black-white hemoglobin and hematocrit differences during pregnancy. Am J Clin Nutr, 30: 461–462.

Garn SM, Keating MT and Falkner F (1981). Haematological status and pregnancy outcomes. Am J Clin Nutr, 34: 115–117.

Garn SM, Smith NJ and Clark DC (1975). The magnitude and the implications of apparent race differences in hemoglobin values. Am J Clin Nutr, 28: 563–564.

Gibson HM (1973). Plasma volume and glomerular filtration rate in pregnancy and their relation to differences in fetal growth. J Obstet Gynaecol Br Commnwlth, 80: 1067–1074.

Giles C (1966). An account of 335 cases of megaloblastic anaemia of pregnancy and the puerperium. J Clin Pathol, 19: 1–11.

Giles C, Burton H (1960). Observations on prevention and diagnosis of anaemia in pregnancy. Br Med J, 2: 636–640.

Giles PF, Harcourt Ag, Whiteside MG (1971). The effect of prescribing folic acid during pregnancy on birthweight and duration of pregnancy. A double blind trial. Med J Austral, 2: 17–21.

Hall MH (1972). Folic acid deficiency and abruptio placentae. J Obstet Gynaecol Br Commwlth, 79: 222–225.

Hancock KW, Walker DA Harper TA (1968). Mobilization of iron in pregnancy. Lancet, ii: 1055–1058.

Harrison KA, Fleming AF, Briggs ND and Rossiter CE (1985). Growth during pregnancy in Nigeria teenage primigravidae. Br J Obstet Gynaecol, 92, Suppl 5: 32–39.

Hemminki E (1982). Effects of routine haematinic and vitamin administration in pregnancy. In: Effectiveness and Satisfaction in Antenatal Care. Enkin M and Chalmers I (eds). London: Heinemann, pp 114–121.

Holly RG (1955). Anemia in pregnancy. Obstet Gynecol, 5: 562–569.

Hytten FE (1985). Blood volume changes in normal pregnancy. Clin Haematol, 14: 601–612.

Hytten FE (1980). In: Clinical Physiology in Obstetrics. Hytten F and Chamberlain G. (eds). Oxford: Blackwell Scientific Publications.

Hytten FE and Duncan DL (1956). Iron deficiency anaemia in the pregnant woman and its relation to normal physiological changes. Nutrition abstracts and reviews, 26: 855–868.

Hytten FE and Leitch I (1971). Physiology of Human Pregnancy (2nd edn). Oxford: Blackwell Scientific Publications.

Iyengar L (1971). Folic acid requirements of Indian pregnant women. Am J Obstet Gynecol, 111: 13–16.

Iyengar L, Apte SV (1970). Prophylaxis of anemia in pregnancy. Am J Clin Nutr, 23: 725–730.

Iyengar L, Rajalakshmi K (1975). Effect of folic acid supplement on birth weights of infants. Am J Obstet Gynecol, 122: 332–336.

Jennison RF (1958). Trial of an iron chelate in the treatment of anaemia of pregnancy. Practitioner, 181: 731–735.

Koller O (1982). The clinical significance of hemodilution during pregnancy. Obstet Gynecol Surv, 37: 649–652.

Koller O, Sandvei R, Sagen N (1980). High hemoglobin levels during pregnancy and fetal risk. Int J Gynaecol Obstet, 18: 53–56.

Kraemer MJ, McFarland RM, Dillon TL and Smith NJ (1975). Reply to letter of Garn *et al.* Am J Clin Nutr, 28: 566.

Letsky E (1984). Blood Volume, Haematinics, Anaemia in Medical Disorders in Obstetric Practice. M de Sweit (ed). Oxford: Blackwell Scientific Publications.

Lund CJ (1951). Studies on the iron deficiency anaemia of pregnancy. Am J Obstet Gynecol, 62: 947–961.

Magee HE, Milligan EHM (1951). Haemoglobin levels before and after labour. Br Med J, ii: 1307–1310.

Menon MKK, Rajan L (1962). Prophylaxis of anaemia in pregnancy. J Obstet Gynaecol Br Commwlth, 12: 382–389.

Morgan EH (1961). Plasma-iron and haemoglobin levels in pregnancy. Lancet, 1: 9–12.

Murphy JF, O'Riordan J, Newcombe RG, Coles EC and Pearson JF (1986). Relation of haemoglobin levels in first and second trimester to outcome of pregnancy. Lancet, 1: 991–994.

Paintin DB, Thomson AM, Hytten FE (1966). Iron and haemoglobin level in pregnancy. J Obstet Gynaecol Br Commwlth, 73: 181–190.

Pritchard JA, Hunt CF (1958). A comparison of the hematologic responses following the routine prenatal administration of intramuscular and oral iron. Surg Gynecol Obstet, 106: 516–518.

Puolakka J, Janne O, Pakarinen A, Jarvinen PA, Vihko R (1980). Serum ferritin as a measure of iron stores during and after normal pregnancy with or without iron supplement. Acta Obstet Gynecol Scand, 95: 43–51.

Rolschau J, Date J, Kristoffersen K (1979). Folic acid supplement and intrauterine growth. Acta Obstet Gynecol Scand, 58: 343–346.

Romslo I, Haram K, Sagen N, Augensen K (1983). Iron requirements in normal pregnancy as assessed by serum ferritin, serum transferrin saturation and erythrocyte protoporphyrin determinations. Br J Obstet Gynaecol, 90: 101–107.

Scott JM, Goldie H and Hay SH (1975). Anaemia of pregnancy: the changing postwar pattern. Br Med J, i: 259–261.

Siddal AC (1980) Blood letting in America, 1800 to 1945. Bull Hist Med, 54: 101–110.

Sood SK, Ramachandran K, Mathur M, Gupta K, Ramalingaswami V, Swarnabai C, Ponniah J, Mathan VI, Baker SJ (1975). WHO sponsored collaborative studies on nutritional anaemia in India. I. The effects of supplemental oral iron administration to pregnant women. Qtrly J Med, 174: 241–258.

Srisupandit S, Poorakul P, Areekul S, Neungton S, Mokkaves J, Kiriwat O, Kanokpongsukdi S (1983). A prophylactic supplementation of iron and folate in pregnancy. Southeast Asian J Trop Med Public Health, 14: 317–323.

Svanberg B, Arvidsson B, Norrby A, Rybo G, Solvell L (1975). Absorption of supplemental iron during pregnancy—a longitudinal study with repeated bone marrow studies and absorption measurements. Acta Obstet Gynecol Scand, 48: 87–108.

Taylor DH and Lind T (1976). Haematological changes during normal pregnancy: iron induced macrocytosis. Br J Obstet Gynaecol, 83: 760-767.

Taylor DJ, Mallen C, McDougall N, Lind T (1982). Effect of iron supplementation on serum ferritin levels during and after pregnancy. Br J Obstet Gynaecol, 89: 1011–1017.

Tchernia G, Blot I, Rey A, Kaltwasser JP, Zittoun J, Papiernik E (1982). Maternal folate status, birthweight and gestational age. Dev Pharmacol Ther, 4: 58–65.

Van Eijk HG, Kroos MJ, Hoogendoorn GA, Wallenburg HCS (1978). Serum ferritin and iron stores during pregnancy. Clin Chim Acta, 83: 81–91.

Wallenburg HCS, Van Eijk HG (1984). Effect of oral iron supplementation during pregnancy on maternal and fetal iron status. J Perinat Med, 12: 7–12.

Weil A, Mauracher E (1977). Folic acid and pregnancy, a real problem? Schweiz Med Wochenschr, 107: 1943–1947.

Willoughby MLN (1967). An investigation of folic acid requirements in pregnancy. II. Br J Haematol, 13: 503–509.

Wills L, Hill G, Bingham K, Miall M, Wrigley J (1947). Haemoglobin levels in pregnancy. The effect of the rationing scheme and routine administration of iron. Br J Nutr, 1: 126–138.

World Health Organization (1968). Nutritional Anaemias. Technical Report Series No. 405. Geneva: WHO.

World Health Organization (1979). The prevalence of nutritional anaemia in women in developing countries. Geneva: WHO.

Zittoun J, Blot I, Hill C, Zittoun R, Papiernik E, Tchernia G (1983). Iron supplements versus placebo during pregnancy: its effects on iron and folate status on mothers and newborns. Ann Nutr Metab, 27: 320–327.

20 Antenatal classes

Penny Simkin and Murray Enkin

1 Introduction

A woman's education for childbirth is shaped by the cultural expectations of her society, her family values, her self-image, and the life experiences to which she has been exposed since her own birth. As the culture of her society changes, all the other influences shift to compensate for what was lost in the change, so that they still serve the function of guiding the woman in her role and behaviour during childbearing.

Western society has undergone massive shifts in attitudes toward childbearing since the early twentieth century. The development of medicine as a science, the creation of the medical specialty of obstetrics, and the shift from home to hospital as the usual place for parturition all contributed to an increasing medicalization of childbirth. Efforts to improve the safety of birth succeeded, but, many believed, at the expense of women's sense of dignity, fulfilment, and autonomy. Major societal changes such as the Industrial Revolution, and the increased mobility of the nuclear family with its resultant isolation deprived women of their traditionally strong, informal networks of support and education.

As maternity care became the province of scientific professionals, so did the dissemination of information. The accumulated experience shared among women, and passed from mother to daughter, no longer met women's needs in a society where birth had become so complex. Antenatal classes perhaps evolved at least in part as an attempt to substitute for these lost sources of vital information, and to respond to these new needs.

'Natural childbirth' and 'psychoprophylaxis' began as alternatives to the new, but firmly established, conventions of 'scientific obstetrics', with its liberal use of pain-relieving drugs and operative delivery. A variety of different programmes with a single common aim appeared at about the same time. Their professed goal was straighforward; the use of psychological or physical, non-pharmaceutical modalities for the prevention of pain in childbirth. Their multifocal origins and complex cross-fertilizations have been well described (Buxton 1962; Beck and Siegel 1980; Beck and Hall 1978; Lumley and Astbury 1980; and Katona 1981).

Grantly Dick Read (1933) described a vicious cycle of culturally induced fear leading to tension, which then led to pain and in turn to greater fear. He proposed to combat this cycle with education to dispel fear of the unknown, and muscular relaxation to relieve tension. In addition, he prescribed specific progressive breathing patterns for the woman to learn and practise during pregnancy and to use during labour, as well as physical exercises to improve her general health, muscle tone, and sense of well-being (Heardman 1948). The term, 'natural childbirth' was coined by Read (1956). Robert Bradley (1965), an obstetrician, and Margaret Gamper (1971), a nurse, began using the Read method in the United States in the late 1940s, and later introduced American modifications. Bradley brought in the concept of the father as a 'coach' for the labouring woman, helping her to carry out the prescribed breathing and relaxation routines.

The psychoprophylactic method, based on Pavlov's concepts of conditioned reflexes, originated in the Soviet Union about 1945 (Velvovsky *et al.* 1960) and was introduced to the West by Lamaze and Vellay (1952). This method has become so closely associated with Lamaze's name that in some quarters 'Lamaze' has become an eponym for all forms of antenatal education. His approach was popularized in North America by Marjorie Karmel (1959) and Elisabeth Bing and colleagues (Bing *et al.* 1962; Bing 1967).

Psychoprophylaxis was 'aimed very definitely at abolishing the so-called unavoidable pain associated with uterine contractions during labour' (Lamaze 1958, 1984). Conceptually, it recognized the potentially painful stimulus of the uterine contraction, but suggested that by the development of new conditioned reflexes, pain transmission, or perception could be inhibited or blocked. In practice, like 'natural childbirth', psychoprophylaxis includes lectures or discussions for imparting knowledge and attitudes, training in voluntary muscle relaxation, body building exercises, and a progression of specific breathing techniques. The emphasis is on the importance of a strong focus of attention to blot out unwanted sensations, and light massage (effleurage) is recommended as a counter stimulus to the uterine contraction.

Sheila Kitzinger (1962, 1980) emphasized greater awareness of the psychological, sexual, and sociological significance of childbearing, incorporating them into her 'psychosexual method'. She also promoted a model of acceptance of labour pain as opposed to the avoidance model, which characterizes the other major methods in the 1960s and 1970s.

Kitzinger helped women to perceive labour pain as a 'side-effect of a task willingly undertaken', (Kitzinger 1978) or 'pain with a purpose.'

There have been a number of variants of these methods. 'Respiratory Autogenic Training' (Schultz and Luthe 1959) essentially teaches a woman how to hypnotize herself into relaxation and tranquillity by concentrating on her bodily sensations. Among others, formal hypnosis (Gross and Posner 1963), autohypnosis (Ringrose 1966) and mental concentration (Earn 1962) all have had their proponents. While there are major differences in the conceptual frameworks underlying these differing approaches, there is a remarkable similarity in their practical applications. All share the approach of group sessions to establish a community of experience and include voluntary muscular relaxation, specific breathing patterns to serve as a focus of attention or distraction, verbal suggestion for both pain reduction and for appropriate behaviour, and the provision of accurate and reliable information about pregnancy, birth, and the experiences which women will undergo or encounter.

2 Content of antenatal classes

There is a great deal of difference in emphasis between different types of prenatal classes. Some, started early in pregnancy, are aimed primarily at teaching self-care and hygiene. Some, often held in the latter part of pregnancy, are primarily a physical preparation for labour, while others are fundamentally a preparation for parenthood and early child care. Still others are specialized, such as abbreviated refresher classes for multiparae, or classes for women who have had a previous caesarean section. Nevertheless, all have some common components, which may be grouped into three main areas: imparting information, skill, and attitudes.

Health professionals tend to overestimate the knowledge, and underestimate the desire for information by their clients. An understanding of the anatomy and physiology of the reproductive tract and the changes which take place in the body assumes a new importance during pregnancy. The information content of modern prenatal classes may include the relation of pregnancy symptoms to underlying mechanisms, and suggest ways of alleviating these symptoms. The emotional shifts of pregnancy may be explored, and issues of sexuality, relationship to spouse and other children discussed as well.

Antenatal classes allow an opportunity to review the mechanisms of labour and birth in adequate detail, and to explain medical and obstetrical terminology. Information need not come from the instructor alone. Discussion with other participants allows for the reassurance and sense of community that comes from sharing experience, and the imparting of a better understanding of what to expect during childbirth. This would include both the sensations of labour and birth and the procedures and practices the woman is likely to experience in her chosen place of birth.

Many classes today are directed not only to pregnant women, but to their partners, husbands, loved ones, and friends as well. The classes prepare the partners to help interpret the events of labour and respond appropriately with useful comfort measures and emotional support (see Chapters 49 and 56).

In addition to knowledge and information, most antenatal classes attempt to impart skills for coping with the stress of labour. These often include a variety of relaxation techniques, various forms of attention, focusing and distraction techniques, numerous comfort measures, and various types of controlled breathing patterns. Finally, the antenatal class is a vehicle for attitude modification, towards on the one hand increased self-reliance and questioning on the part of the woman or couple, or on the other to increased compliance with and adherence to prescribed medical regimens. All classes have as a goal to enhance each woman's sense of optimism and confidence as she approaches childbirth.

Recently, antenatal education has become more complex as it has expanded beyond its primary goal of two and three decades ago, the reduction of pain. The development of safer regional anaesthetics, the rise of feminism and patients' rights, the holistic health movement, the greatly increased popularity of antenatal classes among all social classes, the changing economics of health care, emphasis on reduction of maternal and neonatal morbidity, and the increasingly technological approach to perinatal care have exerted profound influences on expectant parents and their educators.

Whereas in the 1950s and 1960s the goal of non-pharmaceutical pain reduction was universal in antenatal education, this is no longer the case. Antenatal education no longer attracts only the highly motivated people who wish to avoid pain medication. A small minority of expectant parents for whom this is the primary goal still exists. Vocal and assertive, this small minority exerts a disproportionately large influence on maternity care practices. They carefully investigate and select antenatal classes, read extensively, exercise their right to choose their caregivers and places for birth (changing in midpregnancy if they feel unsatisfied), and expect full participation in the decisions concerning their own and their baby's care. They take responsibility for becoming informed and making choices.

But today vast numbers of people attend classes for other reasons as well: simply to learn what to expect in labour and afterwards; to learn about procedures, interventions, and hospital routines; to obtain advice and answers to questions; to reduce anxiety; to meet other expectant parents; and to learn baby care and feeding. Many parents know little or nothing about classes when they decide to attend; they come because they are told to, by their doctor, midwife, friend, or spouse. Therefore, antenatal classes today are not unified in the goal of pain reduction; they vary in ideology, objectives, quality, structure, methods, content, and qualifications of the instructors, reflecting the diversity of the clientele who attend.

Antenatal education is sometimes perceived as a vehicle for those outside the mainstream of medical thinking (both lay and professional) to influence or change the course of maternity care. Indeed, this was an integral component of the early programmes. Unconventional medical care providers, independent childbirth educators and parents have banded together for decades to assure the availability of the maternity care options they desire.

On the other hand, antenatal education is also utilized as a way to maintain control of maternity care by the providers of that care. Katona (1981) traces the history of antenatal education, showing how obstetricians and midwives dealt with the threat of 'natural childbirth' by offering their own classes to offer reassurance and relieve anxiety and to encourage compliance and acceptance of the existing models of care. Depending on the ideology, preferences, and biases of the teacher, antenatal education may either promote or discourage parent decision making, use of medications, acceptance of routine interventions or alternatives, formula or breast feeding, and anxiety or confidence in the caregiver and place of birth.

The polarization among maternity care providers over the appropriate use of obstetric technology also exists among childbirth educators and the public. Those providers and users who have faith in an aggressive medical and technological approach to child bearing tend to seek out childbirth educators who promote the value of this approach and who emphasize patient compliance more than decision-making by the woman. Those who have faith in a conservative, non-medical physiological approach tend to seek out educators who emphasize women's rights and responsibilities to participate in all aspects of their care, including pain-control measures and alternatives to medical interventions.

Regardless of orientation, however, most classes today attempt to accomplish other goals as well: good health habits, stress management, anxiety reduction, enhancement of family relationships, feelings of 'mastery' (Humenick 1981), enhanced self-esteem and satisfaction, successful infant feeding, smooth postpartum adjustment, and family planning.

With the broadened emphasis of today's antenatal classes, educators look outside the obstetrical literature to the biological and social sciences, to Eastern philosophies and meditation techniques, to athletics, to the disciplines of law, ethics, and history, to poetry, music, theatre, dance, and art for guidance and new applications in hopes of better preparing women to give birth with fulfilment and satisfaction.

3 Evaluation of antenatal classes

How effective are antenatal classes as a form of preparation for childbirth? Because of their complex, often disparate goals and ideologies, one cannot make general statements about the effects of antenatal classes as if they were a single intervention, like protein supplementation or the presence of a labour support person. Research on the effectiveness of antenatal classes over the years reflects their changing emphasis. The early studies focused on the effects of class attendance on labour pain, medication use, and other qualities of labour. Today the emphasis has shifted to study of the psychological effects, parenting behaviours, and the effectiveness of specific teaching, counselling, or labour-coping techniques.

Evaluation is further complicated by the difficulty in separating the questions of whether the skills taught in the classes *can* work if appropriately used, and whether or not women actually use (or even have the opportunity to use) the skills that they are taught. One study (Charles *et al.* 1978) reported that of 95 women (57 primigravidae) who had received Lamaze training, 72 per cent said they were able to use the techniques learned to reduce pain effectively throughout labour. Only 15 per cent of the comparison group of 154 women without training were able to use the techniques when taught by their nurses during labour. On the other hand, Copstick *et al.* (1985), using postpartum self reports from 60 primiparae regarding their use of breathing and postural techniques, found that while most used their coping techniques at the onset of contractions, as labour progressed they were less likely to do so. By the second stage of labour less than a third were using any coping techniques at all, many because they had received epidural analgesia. Even among those without epidural analgesia, however, less than half continued to use coping strategies, despite the fact that 'All midwives had routinely encouraged women to use any techniques they had learned'. The authors suggest that the coping strategies may become less effective as labour progresses, or that some mothers find it progressively more difficult to use their coping skills.

One can only speculate as to possible explanations for the failure to use the techniques taught. Were they ineffective, and abandoned when the parents discovered that they were not helping? Some authors (Geden *et al.* 1985; Stevens 1976) suggest that the most effective coping strategies have not yet been developed. Were the techniques taught poorly, so that the women and their partners were uncertain of what to do? Did the students not master the techniques, or were they not motivated to use them? Did the staff make it difficult for the parents to do as they had been taught?

The effectiveness of an individual teacher or class programme is unquestionably one factor in determining the effectiveness of antenatal classes in any particular setting. Because attendance at antenatal classes is voluntary, and there are no tests, 'grades', or other secondary incentives to attend or master the material, the burden falls on the teacher and the programme to provide inherently interesting and relevant content. Continued success of any programme largely depends on its usefulness as perceived by its graduates. Teachers vary in their ability to present information in an interesting manner, and to motivate students to attend classes, to master labour-coping techniques, and to use them in labour. To date, there are no studies of which teacher qualities or teaching methods are associated with the greatest compliance in applying classroom learning to labour. Variation in teaching effectiveness, however, may account for some of the variation found in evaluations of antenatal education.

Other influences, such as the quality of support provided by her partner and the attitudes and philosophy of the labour staff where the woman gives birth, may be major determinants of whether or not a woman uses the techniques she learns. If not encouraged by her partner and the experts around her to use her coping techniques, even a well-prepared and highly motivated woman may experience doubts and be unable to continue using the techniques throughout a stressful labour. On the other hand, if she is encouraged and is complimented on how well she is working, she is more likely to continue. Both effective teaching and consistent follow-up in labour, encouraging use of the learned strategies, is required to assure that women can indeed use what they have learned.

Four research teams (Brant 1962; Campbell and Worthington 1981; Henneborn and Cogan 1975; Copstick *et al.* 1986) investigated the importance of labour support in contributing to the effectiveness of prepared childbirth. Brant stated, 'Previous experience had shown that, during labour, patients frequently forget what they have been taught antenatally.' In his study all women received antenatal education. The treatment group of 123 primigravidae was randomly selected from among women booked for care at the hospital clinic. The control group consisted of 66 primigravidae who delivered within a prescribed period of time. The treatment group received four individual half-hour sessions with a trained assistant who accompanied each woman throughout labour. Preparation emphasized the sensations and emotional reactions to be expected at the various phases of labour. Relaxation and patterned breathing were also emphasized. The control group received lectures and exercise classes and some support in labour. Length of labour was similar in the two groups, although the second stages were shorter in the treatment group, as were incidences of low and mid forceps operations. The dosage of pethidine during first stage and the percentage and length of time trilene analgesia was used during second stage were all markedly lower in the treatment group. Apgar ratings were higher in the treatment group. The author concluded that realistic expectations of pain and emotional stress during labour combined with expert labour support brought superior results.

Henneborn and Cogan (1975) studied two groups of husband–wife Lamaze-prepared couples: in one group the husbands attended only the first stage of labour; in the other they attended both labour and birth. When husbands were present throughout, the women received less medication and reported more positive feelings about the birth. The study was limited by a low return of completed questionnaires (49 of 317 couples contacted completed all three questionnaires which comprised the study), and the self-selection factor which separated the two groups. The possibility exists, however, that the greater participation and satisfaction were related to the continuous labour support.

Campbell and Worthington (1981) compared two types of training for husbands to assist their wives with labour and delivery. One group engaged in unstructured discussion. The other received behaviourally explicit structured training, reviewing techniques from class and other techniques for handling discouragement, panic, and conflict. Results indicated that the men preferred the structured training, the women had more confidence in the men who had the structured training, and those men managed panic better than the men in the discussion group.

Copstick *et al.* (1986) found similar results in their study of the relationship between the type of labour support provided to women receiving and not receiving epidural blocks. The women who received epidurals, had been less likely to use the pain-control techniques they learned in class than those who had not received epidurals. Moreover, they had also received a different type of labour support. Their partners were more likely to have given 'general support' in the form of holding the mother's hand, and giving verbal encouragement and reassurance. In contrast, the partners of the woman who did not receive epidurals, gave more specific and directive support; timing contractions, giving abdominal and back massage, and actively encouraging the use of breathing, distraction, relaxation, and other pain control techniques.

Although both groups of women rated their pain as 'the worst pain imaginable', those who received epidural blocks were more likely to feel 'overwhelmed' and panicked by the pain, and exhausted by the labour. The quality of labour support may have influenced the meaning of the pain to the woman.

Thus, in these four studies the quality of labour support appears to have been an important variable in the women's abilities to utilize what they learn in antenatal classes. Specific content, teacher effectiveness, and quality of labour support are rarely considered as possible confounding variables in studies of effectiveness of antenatal classes. Nevertheless there are useful findings reported in the obstetrical, nursing, and social sciences literature.

Cogan (1983) has divided the goals of childbirth preparation into two broad categories: pain relief during childbirth; and 'diffuse mental hygiene,' through which the birth experience might be happier and more fulfilling. In the latter, labour without pain medications is not a desired effect. Such results as anxiety reduction, positive attitudes toward pregnancy, knowledge, labour support and emotional satisfaction are generally clustered together as constituting 'mental hygiene.'

4 Effectiveness in reducing use of pain medications in labour

4.1 Comparisons of prepared versus unprepared women

According to Beck and Hall (1978), the minimum essentials for an adequate trial of antenatal preparation for childbirth should be: random assignment of subjects, the raters' unawareness of the subject's group membership; and a three-group design to include no-treatment controls and attention-placebo controls, as well as the experimental subjects. Both the necessity for trials of this nature and the difficulties involved in mounting them are acknowledged. Only one such trial has been reported to date.

Timm (1979) studied a group of very low income women attending two urban hospital clinics in Pittsburgh. Medical records of all women attending the clinics were reviewed. The study excluded those who attended for pregnancy termination, had major complications, were scheduled for elective caesarean, or who planned to attend a prenatal class. Of those eligible, all who agreed to be in the study were stratified according to age, race and parity, and randomly assigned to one of three treatment groups: prenatal classes of a standard format; knitting classes, as an attention-placebo in which the woman was guided in knitting a shirt for the expected infant; and a group which did not attend classes but were encouraged to consult the physicians and nurses if they had any questions regarding any aspect of childbearing. In order to encourage continued participation, women were paid for their attendance at a series of six prenatal classes or knitting classes, or for serving as controls.

Of the 146 women who agreed to participate, 28 delivered before completing the study, leaving 40 who were assigned to the prenatal class, 31 to the knitting class, and 47 to the no class programme. At the time of entry into the hospital, study participants were not identified as such but were treated as all other women using the hospital facility. The women who had attended the prenatal class used significantly smaller amounts of medication than did those in the two control groups. This is an important finding because this low income population group is recognized to be at high perinatal risk. In reducing the medications used in labour, added risk to the infant may be minimized.

Huttel *et al.* (1972) took the opportunity of working in a cultural setting in which psychoprophylaxis was completely unknown. This precluded any preconditioning of either hospital staff or women. 132 primiparae due to give birth within an 8-week span were randomly allocated to an experimental or control group. All were invited to the hospital by similar letters; 95 women appeared. The 49 women who had been allocated to the control group were given the opportunity to meet the obstetrician and to visit the delivery room; the 46 women allocated to the experimental group were offered a five-session course of psychoprophylactic training. Women who did not complete the training, or who had a caesarean section, were excluded from the study.

The final sample contained 31 women in the experimental group and 41 in the control group. Medication was used significantly less often, and in smaller quantities, in the trained group than in the control group. Unfortunately, the validity of this study was marred by failure to report on the women who were excluded; this failure introduced the possibility of a serious selection bias into the samples.

Nichols (1987) conducted a randomized trial of prenatal classes on 49 single adolescents, but reported on only 16 in the class group and 10 in the control group who completed the study. No differences between the groups were found in the psychological tests of self-esteem, or evaluation of labour and delivery, conducted at 7 and 9 months of pregnancy and one month after childbirth.

Numerous studies comparing outcomes in prepared and unprepared women have appeared since the early 1950s. Early reports of antenatal preparation classes, as well as some more recent ones, are descriptive, anecdotal, and uncontrolled. Those reporting benefits from classes may have testified more to the enthusiasm of their proponents than to the effectiveness of the approaches. It is important, however, to bear in mind that at the time these studies were reported, massive narcosis and virtually universal general anaesthesia for delivery had become accepted as standard obstetric practice, in North America and elsewhere. In this setting, Thoms and Karlovsky's (1954) report of 2000 consecutive deliveries, 34 per cent of which were conducted without analgesia and 29 per cent without anaesthesia, was most impressive, despite the self-selection of the women who chose to attend their clinic and the possibly distorting effect of the enthusiasm of the investigators. Other investigators of that period reported similar findings (Roberts, *et al.* 1953; Castallo 1958).

Quite contrary findings were published a few years later by Davis and Morrone (1962). They compared 355 self-selected prepared women with 108 women who had not attended classes, and found no differences between the two groups in the use of analgesia or anaesthesia. In contrast to the findings of Thoms and Karlovsky (1954) in the same clinic eight years previously, only 8 per cent of their patients did not receive analgesia, and only 0.2 per cent escaped anaesthesia for the second stage of labour. These authors suggested that 'with the passage of time, the original evangelical zeal is gone'. Differences in class content and in follow-up support in labour may also have contributed to the vastly different outcomes in the two studies.

A major problem with the early studies was the lack of comparability between those women who chose to attend classes and those who did not. Davis and Morrone (1962) found that those who elected to attend classes were older, better educated, and of a higher socioeconomic group. Similar studies have addressed the specific question of the differences between those who chose to attend classes and those who did not (Leonard 1973; Cave 1978). As motivation to take classes may, in itself, be a significant determining factor in the results obtained, several later studies attempted to control for that variable.

A recent study (Patton *et al.* 1985) reported similar findings. A retrospective chart review of 64 primiparae who attended 'prepared childbirth classes' compared with 64 similar but unprepared primiparae failed to show any significant differences in use of analgesia or anaesthesia.

Patton's *et al.* (1985) groups were comparable in age, antenatal risk score, ethnic group, and socioeconomic group, but the retrospective nature of their study precluded them from learning how many classes were attended, the content of the class (which may very well have contained a bias toward the use of anaesthesia), or other important factors. In other words, class attendance or non-attendance, as indicated by a 'Yes' or 'No' in the chart, may not have represented a real difference between the groups.

Enkin *et al.* (1972) compared women who took psychoprophylactic preparation classes with two control groups: those who requested classes, but could not be accommodated because the classes were full; and a group of women drawn from the general hospital population. Having requested and applied for classes, it was presumed that the women in both the trained group and the first control group would have been similarly motivated, thus correcting for self-selection. For analysis, the three groups were matched into triads according to age, parity, and date of delivery. The trained group used significantly less analgesia and anaesthesia than either of the control groups. There was no statistically significant difference between the two control groups. This would indicate that in this setting the effects of the training outweighed those of motivation.

Doering and Entwisle (1975) chose their subjects by 'acquaintance networks' in order to provide a sample from a wide variety of doctors and hospitals, and thus a diversity of childbirth experiences. One hundred and sixteen doctors and 38 hospitals were represented in the final sample. Most of their trained women were contacted through childbirth preparation classes. They chose the subjects randomly from the lists of women who registered for classes and then contacted them after delivery. In this way they avoided the risk of contacting only 'success stories.' At the close of the interview, the interviewee was asked if she knew any other pregnant women. These women were contacted in turn. All of the untrained women, and a few trained ones, were located by referral from other women.

Of a total of 290 women invited, 269 (93 per cent) participated; 132 had had Lamaze training, 137 had not. The two groups did not differ significantly in age, parity, socioeconomic status or education. The outcome measures related to analgesia were based on the woman's report of the medication she had received. The women were classified into three groups: fully conscious (including no medication, pudendal block or local infiltration); semiconscious (including first stage sedatives or analgesics and major regional blocks, such as epidural or spinal); and unconscious (general anaesthesia). There was a strong association 'both in statistical and practical terms' between Lamaze training and reduced use of analgesia and anaesthesia. Other cohort studies (Zax *et al.* 1975; Scott and Rose 1976) have also suggested a reduced need for pharmacological analgesia in women who have had some formal training in childbirth preparation, thus lending some slight additional support to the conclusions of the few small randomized trials.

4.2 Comparison of different methods of antenatal preparation

There are few studies comparing pain-relieving effects of different methods of childbirth preparation. The two major methods, Read's natural childbirth and Lamaze's psychoprophylaxis, have never been compared systematically, using random assignment and a control group. Other comparisons have been made, however, between some less widely known methods of preparation and psychoprophylaxis.

One such study (Zimmermann-Tansella *et al.* 1979) compared the effects of traditional psychoprophylaxis with respiratory autogenic training. Relaxation and anxiety during the course as well as pain and behaviour during delivery were compared in two randomly assigned groups: 14 women with respiratory autogenic training and 20 with traditional psychoprophylaxis. Assessments were made by observers blind to the method of preparation. Outcomes showed some advantages to the respiratory autogenic training: less anxiety before labour, less reported pain during labour, and shorter expulsion periods. Other parameters—controlled behaviour during delivery, condition of the neonate, and positive attitudes toward childbirth showed no differences. Although it was a controlled trial, a high drop-out rate (only 34 of the original 90 enrolled completed the trial) diminishes its significance.

A comparison of a Lamaze prepared group and a Lamaze plus biofeedback group (all multiparas) showed far fewer women requesting pain medication during labour (45 per cent) in the group who received biofeedback training and used a biofeedback instrument to aid relaxation during labour (Gregg 1978). All (100 per cent) the women in the Lamaze only group received pain medication. This study suffered from potential bias, since it was conducted by the manufacturer of the biofeedback device. There was no control group of untrained women. Also surprising was the 100 per cent rate of medication use among the Lamaze only group, since in no other studies have there been 100 per cent medication rates.

Biofeedback in conjunction with 'conventional antenatal training' was evaluated in another study (St. James-Roberts *et al.* 1982). Primiparae were divided into 4 groups: 13 women receiving antenatal education plus autonomic relaxation training with skin-conductance biofeedback; 13 women with antenatal education only who were similar to the experimental group in age, social class and State-Trait Anxiety scores; 11 women receiving antenatal education plus voluntary-muscle relaxation training with electromyographic biofeedback training and 11 controls. Those with biofeedback training also used the biofeedback instruments during labour.

Results from this controlled trial indicated that the electromyographic biofeedback group was able to 'achieve a profound level of muscle relaxation,' while the skin-conductance biofeedback group was not able to lower skin conductance. There was no advantage from use of either biofeedback device on labour performance. There were no significant differences between the experimental and control groups in mean length of first stage, mean dosage of anaesthesia, or proportion of women using epidural anaesthesia (100 per cent in all groups), or mean 1 minute Apgar scores. Seventy per cent of the biofeedback group and 50 per cent of the class alone groups underwent an operative delivery.

Another attempt to compare different methods of childbirth preparation failed to detect significant differences, except in women's pain ratings (Beck *et al.* 1980). The authors randomly assigned women requesting Lamaze preparation either into Lamaze only ($n=37$) or Lamaze plus group systematic desensitization ($n=30$). These were compared to a non-treatment control group ($n=35$) who had not requested training. Although the two Lamaze groups rated their pain as lower than the control group, the difference may be due more to self-selection for training than the training itself. The type of training had no significant associations with labour length, patient 'manageability' during labour, incidence of complications, Apgar scores, or the use of analgesia or anaesthesia.

Freeman *et al.* (1986), in a randomized trial compared a group of 36 primigravidae who attended routine antenatal classes with a similar group of 29 women who attend the classes and also received training in self-hypnosis. Although there was no difference in the proportion of women receiving epidural analgesia or in their assessments of pain-relief derived from their preparation between the hypnosis and control groups, the hypnosis group reported a higher satisfaction with labour. Fifteen of the 29 women in the hypnosis group (52 per cent) rated their satisfaction with labour as 'very high' compared with 8 of the 36 women in the control group (22 per cent) ($p=0.08$)

Moore (1983) compared Lamaze prepared couples and hospital class prepared couples for differences in labour variables and in marital satisfaction attributable to type of training. She found no differences in marital satisfaction, but did find longer labours and less use of pain medication and pitocin among the Lamaze couples. She felt differences might have been more pronounced if the content of hospital classes had been less varied. Some were very similar to Lamaze classes while others were very different.

Thus far, then, studies comparing different types of preparation have failed to show significant differences in most of the outcomes measured, with the exception of possible slight advantages from Respiratory Autogenic Training over Traditional Psychoprophylaxis, and of Psychoprophylaxis over hospital classes.

5 Relationship between medication use and experience of pain

A reduction in the use of pain medications was found in the best designed trials which partially or fully controlled for possible inherent differences between women who took classes and those who did not (Timm 1979; Huttel *et al.* 1972; Enkin *et al.* 1972), as well as in a majority of cohort studies. These findings were reported in different countries, different cultures, and with different study designs. It cannot be assumed, however, that a reduction in use of pain medication is necessarily associated with reduced pain. The use of pain medications is related only in part to the pain experienced by the woman. Other factors such as availability (many hospitals do not have 24-hour anaesthesia services), quality of labour support, wish of the mother, or hospital customs, may be major determinants of whether she will receive medication, what kind and how much.

For these reasons many investigators (Melzack *et al.* 1981; Niven and Gijsbers 1984; Bonnel and Boureau 1985; Davenport-Slack and Boylan 1974; Cogan *et al.* 1976; Charles *et al.* 1978; Nettelbladt *et al.* 1976; Copstick *et al.* 1986) have attempted to evaluate the pain of labour using outcome variables other than medication use. Questionnaires such as the McGill Pain Questionnaire and other verbal descriptive scales, visual analogue scales such as pain thermometers, and observed behaviour are examples of methods used to assess labour pain. Each method has its avid supporters. Labour pain has been assessed both during labour, by observing or questioning women, and afterwards by asking them to recall their pain. Two findings have been consistently reported: first, that there is a wide variation in the pain experienced by women, with some reporting little or no pain while others report very severe pain; second, that the average level of pain experienced by women in labour is very high.

No recent systematic trials have reported consistently low levels of pain among prepared women. For many women, childbirth pain is willingly accepted, even if medications are freely available (Morgan 1984). The reasons given for this vary: fear of side-effects on mother or baby; a high motivation and adequate support to have a 'natural' childbirth; perception of the pain as manageable, normal, and non-threatening.

The problem of pain in labour was addressed directly in a study by Melzack *et al.* (1981). Using the McGill Pain Questionnaire which discriminates between the sensory, affective, and evaluative aspects of pain as well as giving a total pain rating index, they studied 141 successive women in active labour. The group was a representative sample of the women who gave birth in that hospital. It consisted of 87 primiparae, 61 of whom had attended prenatal classes, and 54 multiparae, of whom 30 had attended the classes.

They found the average intensity of labour pain to be extremely high, higher than for other clinical pain syndromes studied, including cancer, phantom limb, postherpetic neuralgia, and toothache. However, there was a wide range of scores, with the pain varying from 'mild' to 'excruciating'. In all dimensions of pain as well as in the total index, labour was significantly more painful for first births than for later births.

Among the primiparae, prepared childbirth training and practice were associated with lower pain scores for the sensory, affective, miscellaneous, and total pain rating measures. Similar but less marked differences were found for the multiparae. Other factors associated with lowered mean pain scores were complications during pregnancy, age, and socioeconomic status. Using multiple regression analysis to determine statistically reliable predictors of pain, they found that in the primiparae, prepared childbirth practice accounted for 8 per cent of the variance in the sensory component, 13 per cent in the affective component, and 10 per cent in the total pain index. The prepared women experienced significantly but not dramatically less pain even though they had elected to have the training, and therefore represented a self-selected sample with positive attitudes. In this study, use of epidural analgesia was extremely high, both among the prepared women (82 per cent) and the unprepared (81 per cent).

While confirming the expected negative correlation between class attendance and the use of anaesthesia, Davenport-Slack and Boylan (1974) found no correlation between class attendance and the woman's subjective report of pain during childbirth. They concluded that these unexpected and seemingly inconsistent findings may have reflected the way in which the pain was measured. The wording of the questions designed to evaluate pain is important. When women in their study were asked how painful childbirth was in comparison to other painful experiences, 97 per cent said it was the most painful experience they had ever had. Yet, when asked to describe childbirth in terms of a range from 'extremely painful' to 'not painful at all,' only 27 per cent placed childbirth in the former category.

More recently, Niven and Gijsbers (1984) studied labour pain, administering the McGill Pain Questionnaire once during the first stage of labour to describe present pain, and again 24 to 48 hours postpartum to recall the pain experienced during the first and second stages. As others have found, labour pain varied greatly among the 29 subjects, but the average level was severe. The postpartum assessments tended to be higher, suggesting that the pain of late labour was more severe than the pain experienced during first stage when the first assessment was made. The authors found no correlation between antenatal education and lowered pain scores, but did find the pain scores of those using various pain medications to be similar to those using psychoprophylaxis alone.

Lower pain scores were reported by women who had previously experienced significant levels of pain unrelated to childbirth (for example, dysmenorrhea, headache, and migraine). The authors suggest that the repetitious and long lasting nature of such pain may result in hormonal adaptations or cause the woman to establish coping strategies which she draws on during labour. They believe that women with little experience with repeating or long lasting pain are particularly vulnerable to childbirth pain, and need careful preparation and emotional support during labour.

As mentioned earlier, Copstick *et al.* (1986) questioned 80 prepared primiparae between one and four days postpartum on their assessments of labour pain as measured on a visual analogue scale of 0 to 100 (with 100 being 'the worst pain imaginable'). The mean pain rating was approximately 99, and was the same in those who received epidural blocks as in those who did not.

6 Analogues of labour pain

The search to establish the true value of antenatal classes has taken the form of testing each component of Lamaze instruction in the laboratory, in simulated pain situations. Subjects are taught various pain-coping techniques and compared with a control group for their ability to tolerate pain as created by various measurable analogues for pain: for example, plunging the forearm into ice water (the cold pressor) for a measured length of time; increasing pressure on the distal index finger (the Forgione–Barber pain stimulator), and others. Research on the analgesic effectiveness of many of the component strategies of prepared childbirth has been reviewed by Stevens (1977) and Stevens and Heide (1977). Geden *et al.* (1985) reviewed previous labour analogue research, and the problems inherent in generalizing the findings to clinical childbirth settings. The pain induced in labour analogue research is of short duration and cannot compare with that experienced in a labour of average length. The ethical requirement that subjects in analogue research be allowed to drop out at any time precludes generalization of findings to labour. Finally, the social context of pain influences perception, 'and there are obvious differences between the environment of an experimental pain laboratory and that of a labour room in a hospital'.

The motivation for finding a reliable analogue for labour pain stems from the desire to develop new labour-coping strategies and improve their effectiveness in reducing pain. Worthington (1982) tested the validity of the cold pressor as an analogue for the pain of early labour by comparing the effectiveness of Lamaze techniques and other techniques with groups of women, first with the cold pressor and later with labour pain. There was a significant correlation between the women's performances in the cold pressor test and in early labour. Lamaze classes improved performance when compared to Red Cross classes and a control group. The influence of self-selection of those in the Lamaze group was not controlled, but the matter of self-selection was addressed by testing two other groups of non-pregnant students who were randomly assigned to receive either brief Lamaze training or none. The former performed better on the cold pressor test.

In a later report using the cold pressor as the labour analogue with nulliparous women, Worthington *et al.* (1982) tested coping strategies taught in childbirth classes. They found that the combination of structured breathing, attention focal points, and coaching provided the strongest treatment. Practice under stress was also found to be more effective than imaginal practice or no practice. They found effleurage to be ineffective with the cold stressor. The external validity of this finding on effleurage may be questioned, since one's sense of touch is profoundly altered by cold in a way not at all similar to the labour situation. Relaxation as a coping strategy was not examined. Although the authors simulated childbirth preparation as closely as they could, they acknowledge differences in anxiety levels between the experimental groups and labouring women. Length of training, strength of contractions, amount of practice, and the fact that women in the experimental group could stop the pain by removing their hand from the ice water when they wished, while labouring women cannot stop contractions when they wish, all raise questions on the application of these findings to childbirth education.

Geden *et al.* (1985) tested components of Lamaze preparation (relaxation training, breathing exercises, and information) in all possible combinations, using repeated exposure over a one hour period to a pain stimulus (pressure on the distal index finger). They found the relaxation component to be the most efficacious of the three components tested. They suggest that if the less effective components of Lamaze preparation are deleted, more emphasis can then be placed on the more effective components, and on different new pain-coping strategies. A clinical trial comparing those strategies found to be most effective in the laboratory setting with standard Lamaze preparation may provide clinically relevant findings.

7 Other effects

Antenatal education has received credit for a number of other obstetrical advantages, such as decreased blood loss (Thoms and Karlovsky 1954; Miller 1961), decreased operative intervention (Yahia and Ulin 1965; Enkin *et al.* 1972; Hughey *et al.* 1978), and improved condition of the baby (Hughey *et al.* 1978). However, these findings are not confirmed by other studies, and when present are probably secondary to decreased use of medication (see Chapter 57). Some studies have reported a shortening of labour (Van Auken and Tomlinson 1953; Miller 1961; Ringrose 1966, 1976); others have found no differences (Enkin *et al.* 1972; Hughey *et al.* 1978; Patton *et al.* 1985). Scott and Rose (1976) found labour to be slightly longer in the mothers who had received the training. The best controlled study (Timm 1979) found no difference in length of labour or in birthweight, the only outcome variables measured in addition to use of medication.

While they are important, psychological variables such as an enhanced feeling of self-esteem, a sense of achievement or a positive feeling about the birth experience, are extremely difficult to measure. Roberts *et al.* (1953) stated: 'It would be a grave mistake to be guided by figures alone, because there does not appear to be any satisfactory yardstick by which we can measure the peace of mind and sense of security that mothers derive from the antenatal classes'. Morris (1960) asked: 'How can we produce statistics to show how many women emerge from labour exalted rather than demoralized, confident rather than afraid?'. Other more recent researchers (Scott and Rose 1976), daunted by the difficulty, have simply ignored the issue and restricted their study to obstetric outcome.

Kondas and Scetnicka (1972) studied two groups of 20 anxious pregnant women, as determined on Taylor's 'manifest anxiety scale'. The groups were matched for age, parity, education, and level of anxiety. One group received standard psychoprophylactic preparation, in which information about labour and delivery was given in full; the other was subject to systematic desensitization, and only spontaneous questions were answered. Both groups showed a decrease in anxiety related to childbirth, but those having systematic desensitization showed it more strongly. Slight or no pain was recorded for 68 per cent of the systematic desensitization group, compared with 21 per cent of the psychoprophylactic group. The level of anxiety and the amount of pain were assessed by the therapist, and the possibility of observer bias must be acknowledged.

Despite the difficulties involved in devising satisfactory methods of measurement, several studies have attempted to assess the impact of antenatal training on the experience of childbirth. Davenport-Slack and Boylan (1974) found childbirth training to be highly correlated with an unstructured account of childbirth by the mother as a 'positive rewarding experience.' Tanzer (1968) found that attenders at a natural childbirth class experienced a significantly higher ratio of positive to negative emotions than non-attenders. Enkin *et al.* (1972) used a rating scale applied to a series of positive and negative adjectives describing labour, delivery and the over-all experience. Compared with a control group who had requested but not received training, the women who attended the classes had a significantly more positive experience of labour and delivery; the difference between the class group and the group who had not requested classes was even greater. There was no significant difference between the two control groups.

Huttel *et al.* (1972) evaluated mothers' ratings of their delivery experience by means of a series of questions administered immediately postpartum. The answers given were recorded, transcribed verbatim, and ranked by observers who were unaware of the group to which the mother had been allocated. Significant differences were found in favour of the instructed group, specifically in their impression of birth as having been 'mastered actively' rather than 'experienced passively', and in the fact that their wish for further children tended to be enhanced rather than weakened by the delivery experience.

Mothers' attitudes to childbirth and to their babies were scored by independent raters in the study by Doering and Entwisle (1975). These authors found that antenatal preparation leads to increased awareness, and that such awareness had a larger impact on the mothers' experience and reactions than did the direct effect of the preparation itself.

In their study of psychological outcomes of antenatal education, Charles *et al.* (1978) and Norr *et al.* 1977), in two papers relating to the same study, point out that decreased pain and enjoyment in childbirth are not totally interdependent. They used independent scales to evaluate separately the subjective pain a woman felt and her enjoyment of the childbirth experience. They found that women who had taken classes experienced both less pain and more enjoyment during the birth than those who had not, but that the difference in the enjoyment index was greater than the difference in the pain index. In other words, reduction in pain was not the only factor determining the woman's enjoyment. Prepared women also had continuous bedside support from their husbands, which contributed to their enjoyment. Unfortunately, despite the use of two-way analysis of variance to allow for the effects of parity, socioeconomic status, self-confidence and some other variables, the lack of comparability between the experimental and the control groups impaired the validity of what otherwise would have been a most illuminating approach.

Humenick (1981) proposed that if pain management is the key to satisfaction in childbirth, then it logically follows that 'epidural or other analgesia is the best answer' to coping with childbirth, since it is more effective in reducing pain than relaxation, patterned breathing, and other coping techniques. She hypothesized that mastery—mobilizing inner resources, being self-reliant, independent, and self-controlled during childbirth—is the key to childbirth satisfaction.

In a study designed to test this hypothesis, Humenick and Bugen (1981) found that among 37 Lamaze prepared women, more active participation in labour and women's ratings of their birth experience were significantly correlated with increases in instrumentality scores. Instrumentality includes 'independence, activity (vs. passivity), competitiveness, decisiveness, confidence, and ability to stand up well under pressure'. The study suffered from selection bias and lack of a control group, but may demonstrate areas worthy of further research.

Felton and Segelman (1978) studied beliefs about personal control in new mothers and fathers who had had Lamaze training as compared to Red Cross training or no training. Pre-tests using Rotter's Internal External scale were administered approximately six to eight weeks before their due dates and before the trained couples took their classes. Post-tests (the same test) were administered to some after classes were finished but before the births; to others after the births of their children. Results indicated that the Lamaze-trained women who completed the post-test after the birth, and the Lamaze-trained men who completed the post-test after the classes but before the birth showed significant shifts in beliefs about personal control in the direction of greater belief in themselves as the origin of control. There were no significant differences in any of the other groups.

In discussing the differences in the Lamaze-trained men's and women's feelings about personal control before and after the birth, the authors stated that the women, before birth, were concerned about unexpected complications in labour over which they would have no control.

After birth, when those complications had not arisen, they then began to feel greater personal control. The men, before birth, perceived themselves as responsible for their partners' welfare, and thus perceived themselves as having greater personal control. But after birth, with the full impact of total responsibility for the baby's welfare, and the great unpredictable demands, they felt less in control.

In studying the effects of antenatal education on young, low-income, minority women, Masterpasqua (1982) compared an experimental group of 30 women who selected antenatal education with two control groups of 30 women each: one group chose not to take the available classes; the other had attended the clinic during the year before classes became available and thus could not take classes. There were no differences between the groups in perinatal complications, maternal behaviours or mothers' perceptions of their infants. However, when the groups were further categorized into 'at risk' (for subsequent psychiatric problems for the child) and 'no risk' groups, Masterpasqua reported significantly reduced risk among male infants and infants of multiparas in the group who received antenatal education. The psychological benefits of antenatal education in an at-risk group deserves further exploration.

Though more difficult to assess, it appears that antenatal classes may result in various types of personal growth which have little to do with obstetric outcomes, but which may have equal or greater long term significance.

8 Adverse effects

If the benefits of antenatal education are difficult to document in a systematic manner, the adverse effects and potential hazards are even more elusive. The extent to which fear is created rather than alleviated by classes, that women succumb to peer or educator pressures to conform, or refuse needed medication or intervention is completely unknown.

'Old doctors' tales' abound with anecdotes of the woman who suffered untold agony unnecessarily because she had been brainwashed by her childbirth educator into believing that all medication was bad, or the baby who was lost because a woman insisted on 'natural childbirth' and refused necessary operative intervention. There has been little documentation of such events in the literature, and we have no data on the frequency of their occurrence.

The dearth of documented cases of obstetrical ill-effects caused by childbirth education has not deterred criticism. From the earliest beginnings of consumer interest in preparation for childbirth, highly placed opponents have been numerous and vocal. Reid and Cohen (1950) were scathing in their criticism of what they called 'present day trends in obstetrics', pointing out that 'the very basis of modern obstetrics, with its fivefold decrease of maternal mortality in the past two decades' was being challenged by the concept that 'what was natural must be good'. They demonstrated the fallacies in the beliefs that childbirth among primitive peoples is always easy, and that uterine contractions are not actually painful. They went on to point out the (then) lack of evidence that any maternal medication adversely affects the newborn, or that separation of mother and newborn does any harm.

The discussion following the paper by Davis and Morrone (1962), which found neither beneficial nor adverse effects from childbirth education, was an opportunity for the acknowledged leaders of American obstetrics to voice their opinions. The concerns which they expressed indicate the degree of resistance to antenatal education at the time and which remains to some degree today: 'The elaborate programme of preparation tends to create rather than allay apprehension'; 'If there is nothing to be afraid of, why raise such a fuss about it?' 'If truly natural childbirth is to be fostered, the key figure must be a wise, kindly understanding obstetrician who generates such an atmosphere of happiness and assurance that apprehension is inevitably dispelled' (Eastman 1962). Or again: 'Some patients who give the most vocal support to childbirth without aid end up by requiring large amounts of medication'; '... In any preparation programme some patients might yield to psychological pressures to carry on their labours the way the group intended' (Evans 1962); 'The unmedicated patient limits or introduces compromise in the selection of the type of anaesthesia when it is truly indicated.' Fielding and Benjamin (1962) claimed that the truth can be stated simply: 'Natural childbirth's basic principle carries with it definite dangers to mother and child. It is a positive decision to let the destructive side of nature takes its course.' However, nowhere in their book did they give any specific examples of these hazards. They agreed, however, that there are 'no charts or statistics on "natural childbirth" failures beyond those relating to women who drop out of prenatal training programmes before completion of their courses.'

More recently, Macdonald (1983) contemptuously cited anecdotes of a woman who wished to eat her placenta; a duty registrar who asked that the senior registrar relieve him so that he could accompany his wife in labour; a father who refused medication at first on behalf of his wife. The author says, 'My professional and personal experiences of childbirth have led me to believe that far too much is made of the emotional aspects, bonding, etc., and not enough of safety.'

Two recent reports (Stewart 1982, 1985) describe psychiatric symptoms following attempted natural childbirth. Stewart's earlier report describes five women and four men whose expectations for natural childbirth were not met and who sought psychiatric treatment within 6 months of the birth. Generally the women expressed feelings of depression, inadequacy, and guilt at receiving interventions (or, in one case, refusing them) which they believed were unnecessary or harmful. Two of the women worried that their babies were brain-damaged, one after refusing non-stress testing and later delivering a postmature baby with breathing difficulties and neurologic sequelae; the other after accepting epidural anaesthesia and requiring forceps for delivery.

The men had accompanied their wives into the case room, but felt faint and anxious when there. Depression, anger at their wives, and feelings of inadequacy led them to seek psychiatric treatment. In all cases, the patients responded to psychotherapy lasting between 3 and 12 months.

The author cites childbirth classes which are inflexible and intolerant of medications and interventions as the underlying causes for these cases of depression. All the referred patients had received their antenatal training from community based organizations whose teachers' backgrounds were non-medical and whose classes emphasized natural childbirth and expected participation of the partner.

In a letter responding to Stewart's 1982 article, Campbell (1983) questioned the assumption that it was the childbirth education that caused the psychiatric symptoms. First, as Stewart had no comparison group, it is impossible to state whether parents attending natural childbirth classes are more or less likely than others to suffer postnatal psychiatric symptoms. Secondly, Stewart failed to consider other psychosocial factors which may influence one's reactions to childbirth or one's interest in attending natural childbirth classes. Finally, Campbell pointed out that nurses and doctors need to be more flexible in their care of parents, anticipating that they may have disappointment or depression if the birth is unsuccessful in their eyes. Not only childbirth educators, but obstetric staff as well, may play an important role in shaping postpartum feelings about the birth.

As if to answer Campbell's objections to her 1982 conclusions, Stewart (1985) reported that the percentage of patients seeking psychiatric treatment for symptoms related to their childbirth experience dropped precipitously after the hospital instituted its own antenatal classes in 1983. From 1972 to 1980, of 504 patients with postpartum neuroris or psychosis, only 3 attributed their symptoms to the birthing experience. By 1981 the number of community based prenatal programmes had doubled, and in 1981 and 1982, 18 of 125 patients attributed their postpartum symptoms to their birthing experience. All had taken the community based classes. In 1983 the hospital began offering and encouraging attendance at their own classes. Only 6 of 130 referrals were women attributing their postpartum symptoms to their birthing experiences. The author did not state which classes the 6 patients had taken.

Stewart offers evidence suggesting that the community based classes being offered during 1981 and 1982 may have prepared people unrealistically for the experience they would have in her hospital. The classes offered by her hospital appear to have performed that role better. One still may wonder if the lower frequency of birth-related psychiatric symptoms may have resulted from the hospital staff having become more flexible in their attitudes rather than, or along with, the changing the nature of the classes.

Sandelowski (1984) also discussed feelings of failure engendered in women whose high expectations are not met: 'The women who appear to be most susceptible to feelings of failure . . . are those who belong to what can loosely be described as the "natural childbirth culture" . . . In an important sense, the proponents of alternative childbirth have expectations that are too high or unrealistic when viewed against prevailing obstetric practice.' She pointed out that when expectations are high, change in maternity practices frequently result, but many women suffer disappointment. When expectations are lowered, women are less likely to be disappointed, but change cannot occur.

The dilemma so well described by Sandelowski illustrates the differing views toward antenatal classes and their purposes. Yet there has been little systematic evaluation of the extent to which negative feelings of anger, guilt, or inadequacy are engendered when a woman's or her partner's expectations are not met. Nor has the role of antenatal classes in creating these high expectations. Nelson (1982) found, in her study of approximately 300 women, that, 'Visions of childbirth that are most distinct from the prevailing medical model can be found among the women who remain unprepared. . . . Middle class women might well find that childbirth preparation has the unanticipated consequence of bringing their ideology into line with the established protocol of the hospital in which they are preparing to give birth.'

Hott (1980) investigated antenatal and postpartum attitudes towards self, spouse, and the 'ideal' self or spouse among 47 couples who chose the Lamaze method of childbirth. Thirty-four of the couples shared the delivery as planned; the other 13 were prevented from doing so by complications resulting in caesarean section. She found that both men and women who did not achieve their goal of a shared experience held both themselves and their various ideal concepts in lower esteem than did those whose experience went as planned. No studies comparing these concepts among trained and untrained couples have been carried out.

Hott's findings disagree with those of Christensen-Szalanski (1984), who followed 18 women's preferences regarding the use of anaesthesia in labour longitudinally, surveying them at one month before labour, during early and late labour, and again one month postpartum. His sample, taken from independent childbirth classes, expressed a rather strong desire to avoid anaesthesia one month before labour. This desire remained during early labour, but diminished from then until complete dilatation. In other words, their desire to avoid anaesthesia was strongest when they had no pain and, not unexpectedly, diminished when they had severe pain. Eleven of the 18 women received anaesthesia (8 primiparae, 3 multiparae). However, when interviewed one month later, both the women who used and those who did not use anaesthesia were shifting dramatically back toward avoiding anaesthesia in a future birth. Among those who did not receive anaesthesia, the desire to avoid it in the future was as strong as it had been one month before their due date. These findings suggest that the women's expectations and desires for future births were changed little by their actual experiences with present births.

The differences in the findings of Hott and Christensen-Szalanski are difficult to explain, but may reflect the content of classes or the quality of emotional support available to each group.

For the individual expectant mother, the benefits and risks of the prenatal class depend to a large extent on the same factors that determine the benefits and hazards of any other obstetrical intervention: the individual's or couple's needs; how appropriate the class is for the those involved; and the skill and sensitivity with which the class is conducted.

9 Wider effects of antenatal classes

As antenatal classes have become more popular, they have begun reaching, and apparently benefiting, more women from the less privileged classes (Timm 1979; Masterpasqua 1982; Nelson 1982). While antenatal classes have appealed primarily to the middle classes in years past, they are now routinely offered in many clinics, health departments, and schools for pregnant adolescent women.

Although antenatal classes are spreading to a wider audience, the interest in natural childbirth appears to remain essentially with the middle class. In a regional study of 2302 hospital birth records reviewed from 11 hospitals, Cave (1978) investigated the social characteristics of 678 'natural childbirth adopters'. She confirmed Davis and Morrone's 1962 findings that the 'adopters' were on average two years older, had more college education and a higher socioeconomic status than non-user groups. Perkins (1980), on the other hand, collected data on all the women who gave birth in a particular district over a three-month period. 72 per cent of the women said they had been offered classes, but did not differ significantly, in age, marital status or social class, from those not offered classes. A woman was more likely to be offered classes if this was her first pregnancy, and 56 per cent of those offered classes accepted. There was a relationship between attendance and social class, but the most significant factors determining attendance were first pregnancy and a previous history of only unsuccessful pregnancies. The most frequently given explanation for non-attendance was that the woman had other children to look after. Although frequently it is assumed that women in their second pregnancies have no need of classes because they would have attended the first time, only 53 per cent of women who had had previous live births had attended classes during a previous pregnancy.

The effects of a prenatal class depend not only on the characteristics of those who attend and the competence and skills of the teacher, but also to a large extent, on the underlying objectives of the programme. Some classes are taught by independent childbirth educators, some are co-ordinated by large consumer groups such as the National Childbirth Trust, the American Society of Psychoprophylaxis in Obstetrics, the American Academy for Husband Coached Childbirth, or the International Childbirth Education Association. Others are offered by official health agencies; still others by doctors for their own patients or by hospitals for the women who plan to deliver there. The curricula outlined for these classes may be similar, and there may be little difference in the information taught, or the skills imparted. Nevertheless, there may be great differences in the attitudes which are encouraged. 'Community sponsored childbirth education classes are structured to incorporate the interests of parents into the curriculum; hospital based classes are required and expected to explain existing policies to parents, not to question, nor to offer alternatives, nor to help parents decide their own birth plans' (Edwards 1980). The Nurses Association of the American College of Obstetricians and Gynecologists recently published *Guidelines for Childbirth Education* (NAACOG 1981) illustrate Edwards' point. The guidelines emphasize information, self-care, and coping techniques for labour, but place little, if any, emphasis on choices, risks, benefits, and alternatives in management.

However, it is possible that the actual existence of prenatal classes is more important than the details of what is taught; that in actuality 'the medium is the message' (McLuhan 1964). The number of women attending prenatal classes is now substantial: while few nationally collected data are available, figures from a number of communities indicate that between 30 and 70 per cent of all expectant mothers in the English-speaking world attend some form of antenatal class (Chamberlain and Chave 1977; Perkins 1980; Toronto Task Force on High Risk Pregnancy 1980; Hanvey 1984).

The full impact of childbirth education cannot be assessed solely by its effect on the individual parturient, for there may be indirect effects which engender significant changes in the ambience in which childbearing women give birth. Among such indirect effects are the proliferation of newspapers and magazine articles and books on subjects relating to pregnancy, birth, infant feeding, and childcare. The catalogue of a major mail order bookseller specializing in books on childbearing and early parenting (Birth and Life Bookstore 1986) lists approximately 850 titles. Such literature both reflects public interest and influences public thinking.

Once a critical mass of mothers becomes aware of the fact that options are available to them, major changes in obstetrical practice may ensue. This was noted as long ago as 1957, when De Watteville observed that during the two years following the introduction of psychoprophylactic preparation in his community, the proportion of women receiving chloroform for delivery dropped in his hospital from 80 per cent to 9.4 per cent. This major change occurred although only 27 per cent of the women had attended antenatal classes (De Watteville 1957).

Significant changes towards more family centred maternity care have occurred over the ensuing quarter century (McMaster 1981). One can only speculate on the extent to which these changes have resulted from the increasing use of childbirth education classes rather than from other influencing factors. The continuing impact of antenatal education on maternity care will depend on the continuing existence of independent, consumer oriented classes. If information on risks, benefits, and alternatives to conventional care remains a major focus among a significant proportion of antenatal classes, we may expect increasingly influential and well informed consumer involvement in the future patterns of childbirth practices. If, however, the ideology of classes continues shifting to reflect an acceptance of conventional obstetric practices, the group consciousness among expectant parents may fade, reducing their impact and their influence on the direction of maternity care.

10 Conclusions

The perceived need for antenatal classes arose with changes in society that weakened the extended family's role in education and support, and also increased the complexity of maternity care. Antenatal classes began as a way to restore simplicity and satisfaction to the birth experience by increasing the participation of the mother and reducing her use of pain medications. Evaluation of the effectiveness of antenatal training has been difficult, due to the difficulty in designing and conducting well-controlled trials. The attitudes conveyed in classes, the quality of instruction, and the specific techniques being taught all vary, making it impossible to generalize about the effects of antenatal classes *per se*.

The existing evidence, however, suggests that women who attend antenatal classes use somewhat less analgesic medication, and feel somewhat less pain in labour, although pain levels can still be very high. The wide variation in results from different studies may depend not only on differences in the classes, but also on the support provided by the caregivers in labour. Adverse effects of antenatal classes have not been systematically evaluated. The very existence of classes and their growing popularity appear to have contributed to significant changes in maternity care.

10.1 Implications for current practice

The widespread popularity of antenatal classes testifies to the desire of expectant parents for this form of childbirth education. As there appear to be benefits in terms of amount of analgesic medication used and in some aspects of satisfaction with childbirth, and significant adverse effects have not been demonstrated, such classes should be made available and encouraged. The objectives of the classes must be made clearly explicit to the participants; unrealistic expectations of what the classes can achieve must be avoided. A variety of different types of classes, whose goals are explicitly stated, may help women or couples choose the programme most likely to meet their needs.

10.2 Implications for future research

Antenatal classes represent a significant and widespread intervention in pregnancy care today. The need for further study of both the benefits and the risks of these classes is clear. Shearer (1983) called for a 'nation-wide system for experimentally testing the truth of claims made for various techniques and advice, and for searching out unexpected harmful effects of what we do'. When educators begin to clearly state the goals and objectives of their courses, and then systematically determine whether or not those goals and objectives have been achieved, the true place of antenatal classes as a useful form of education for childbirth and parenthood can be determined.

References

Beck NC, Hall D (1978). Natural childbirth—a review and analysis. Obstet Gynecol, 52(3): 371–379.

Beck NC, Siegel LJ (1980). Preparation for childbirth and contemporary research on pain, anxiety, and stress reduction: a review and critique. Psychosom Med, 42(4): 429–447.

Beck NC, Siegel LJ, Davidson NP, Kormeier S, Breitenstein A, Hall DG (1980). The prediction of pregnancy outcome: maternal preparation, anxiety and attitudinal sets. J Psychosom Res 24(6): 343–351.

Bing E (1967). Six Practical Lessons for an Easier Childbirth. New York: Grossop & Dunlap.

Bing E, Karmel M, Tanz A (1962). A Practical Course for the Psychoprophylactic Method of Childbirth (Lamaze Technique). New York: ASPO.

Birth and Life Bookstore (1986). Imprints, 18: 17–30.

Bonnel AM, Boureau F (1985). Labor pain assessment: validity of a behavioural index. Pain, 22: 81–90.

Bradley R (1965). Husband-coached Childbirth. New York: Harper & Row.

Brant HA (1962). Childbirth with preparation and support in labour: an assessment. NZ Med J, 61(356): 211–219.

Buxton CL (1962). A study of psychophysical methods for relief of childbirth pain. Philadelphia: WB Saunders.

Campbell A, Worthington Jr. EL (1981). A comparison of two methods of training husbands to assist their wives with labor and delivery. J Psychosom Res, 25(6): 557–563.

Campbell D (1983). Psychiatric symptoms following attempted natural childbirth (Letter). Can Med Assoc J, 128(5): 517.

Castallo M (1958). Preparing parents for parenthood. JAMA, 166: 1970–1973.

Cave C (1978). Social characteristics of natural childbirth users and nonusers. Am J Public Health, 68: 898–901.

Chamberlain G, and Chave S (1977). Antenatal education. Community Health, 9: 11–16.

Charles AG, Norr KL, Block CR, Meyering S, Meyers E (1978). Obstetric and psychological effects of psychoprophylactic preparation for childbirth. Am J Obstet Gynecol, 131(1): 44–52.

Christensen-Szalanski JJJ (1984). Discount functions and the measurement of patients' values: Women's decisions during childbirth. Med Decis Making, 4(1): 47–58.

Cogan R (1983). Variations in the effectiveness of childbirth preparation. Perinatal Press, 7(4): 51–54.

Cogan R, Hennebon W, Klopfer F (1976). Predictors of pain during prepared childbirth. J Psychosom Res, 20: 523–533.

Copstick S, Hayes RW, Taylor KE, Morris NF (1985). A test of a common assumption regarding the use of antenatal training during labour. J Psychosom Res, 29(2): 215–218.

Copstick SM, Taylor KE, Hayes R, Morris N (1986). Partner support and the use of coping techniques in labour. J Psychosom Res, 30(4): 497–503.

Davenport-Slack B, Boylan CH (1974). Psychological correlates of childbirth pain. Psychosom Med, 36: 215–223.

Davis CD, Morrone FA (1962). An objective evaluation of a prepared childbirth programme. Am J Obstet Gynecol, 84: 1196–1201.

De Watteville PH (1957). The use of obstetrical analgesia at the maternity hospital of Geneva. Am J Obstet Gynecol, 73: 473–491.

Doering SG, Entwisle DR (1975). Preparation during pregnancy and ability to cope with labor and delivery. Am J Orthopsychiatry 45(5): 825–837.

Earn AA (1962). Mental concentration—a new and effective psychological tool for the abolition of suffering in childbirth. Preliminary report. Am J Obstet Gynecol, 83: 29–36.

Eastman NJ (1962). Discussing Davis and Morrone, 1962. Am J Obstet Gynecol, 84: 1201–1202.

Edwards M (1980). The childbirth educator. Certified to represent the hospital or the parents? Birth Family J, 7: 79–80.

Enkin MW, Smith SL, Dermer SW, Emmett JO (1972). An adequately controlled study of the effectiveness of PPM training. In: Psychosomatic Medicine in Obstetrics and Gynecology. Morris N (ed). Basel: Karger.

Evans TN (1962). Discussing Davis and Morrone, 1962. Am J Obstet Gynecol, 84: 1202–1203.

Felton GS, Segelman FB (1978). Lamaze childbirth training and changes in belief about personal control. Birth Family J 5(3): 141–150.

Fielding W, Benjamin L (1962). The Childbirth Challenge. Commonsense versus 'Natural' Methods. New York: Viking Press.

Freeman RM, Macaulay AJ, Eve L, Chamberlain GVP (1986). Randomised trial of self hypnosis for labour. Br Med J, 292(6521): 657–658.

Gamper M (1971). Preparation for the Heir-minded. Hammond, Indiana: Sheffield Press.

Geden E, Beck NC, Brouder G, Glaister J, Pohlman S (1985). Self-report and psychophysiological effects of Lamaze preparation: an analogue of labor pain. Res Nurs Health 8: 155–165.

Gregg RH (1978). Biofeedback relaxation training effects in childbirth. Behav Engineering, 4: 57–61.

Gross HN, Posner NA (1963). An evaluation of hypnosis for obstetric delivery. Am J Obstet Gynecol, 87: 912–920.

Hanvey L (1984). A national review of prenatal education programs. In: Pre-pregnancy and Pregnancy Care and Education: Proceedings of the 6th Symposium on the Prevention of Handicapping Conditions, pp 188–196. Alberta: Edmonton.

Heardman H (1948). A Way to Natural Childbirth. Edinburgh: Livingstone.

Henneborn WJ, Cogan R (1975). The effect of husband participation on reported pain and probability of medication during labor and birth. J Psychosom Res, 19: 215–222.

Hott JR (1980). Best laid plans. Pre- and post-partum comparison of self and spouse in primiparous Lamaze couples who share delivery and those who do not. Nurs Res, 29: 20–27.

Hughey MJ, McElin TW, Young T (1978). Maternal and fetal outcome of Lamaze-prepared patients. Am J Obstet Gynecol, 51(6): 643–647.

Humenick SS (1981). Mastery: the key to childbirth satisfaction? A review. Birth Family J, 8(2): 79–83.

Humenick SS, Bugen LA (1981). Mastery: the key to childbirth satisfaction? A study. Birth Family J, 8(2): 84–90.

Huttel FA, Mitchell I, Fischer WM, Meyer AE (1972). A quantitative evaluation of psychoprophylaxis in childbirth. J Psychosom Res, 16: 81–93.

Karmel M (1959). Thank You, Dr. Lamaze. Philadelphia: Lippincott.

Katona CLE (1981). Approaches to antenatal education. Soc Sci Med, 15A(1): 25–33.

Kitzinger S (1962). The Experience of Childbirth. New York: Taplinger.

Kitzinger S (1978). Pain in childbirth. J Med Ethics, 4: 119–121.

Kitzinger S (1980). The Complete Book of Pregnancy and Birth. New York: Alfred A. Knopf.

Kondas O, Scetnicka B (1972). Systematic desensitization as a method of preparation for childbirth. J Behav Ther Exp Psychiatry, 3(1): 51–54.

Lamaze F (1958, 1984). Painless Childbirth: The Lamaze Method. Chicago: Contemporary Books. (Reissue of 1958 edition.)

Lamaze F, Vellay P (1952). L'accouchement sans douleur par la méthode psychophysique. Quoted in Buxton (1962).

Leonard RF (1973). Evaluation of selection tendencies of patients preferring prepared childbirth. Obstet Gynecol, 42: 371–377.

Lumley J, Astbury J (1980). Birth Rites Birth Rights: Childbirth Alternatives for Australian Parents. Sphere: Melbourne, Australia.

Macdonald R (1983). Personal view. Br Med J, 287, 1544.

Masterpasqua F (1982). The effectiveness of childbirth education as an early intervention program. Hosp Community Psychiat, 33: 56–58.

McLuhan HM (1964). Understanding Media. New York: McGraw-Hill.

McMaster University Department of Obstetrics and Gynecology (1981). Family centered maternity care. Bulletin, the Society of Obstetricians and Gynecologists of Canada. II, 3.

Melzack R, Taenzer P, Feldman P, Kinch RA (1981). Labour is still painful after prepared childbirth training. Can Med Assoc J, 125(4): 357–363.

Miller HL (1961). Education for childbirth. Obstet Gynecol, 17: 120–123.

Moore D (1983). Prepared childbirth and marital satisfaction during the antepartum and postpartum periods. Nurs Res, 32(2): 73–77.

Morgan BM (1984). The consumer's attitude toward obstetric care. Br J Obstet Gynaecol, 91: 624–628.

Morris N (1960). Human relations in obstetric practice. Lancet, 1: 913–915.

NAACOG (1981). Guidelines for Childbirth Education. Chicago: The Nurses Association of the American College of Obstetricians and Gynecologists.

Nelson MK (1982). The effect of childbirth preparation on women of different social classes. J Health Soc Behav, 23(4): 339–352.

Nettelbladt P, Fagerstrom CF, Uddenberg N (1976). The significance of reported childbirth pain. J Psychosom Res, 20(3): 215–221.

Nichols FH (1987). The psychological effects of prepared childbirth on self esteem, active participation during childbirth, and childbirth satisfaction of single adolescent mothers. J Obstet Gynecol Neonatal Nurs, May/June: 207–208.

Niven C, Gijsbers K (1984). A study of labour pain using the McGill Pain Questionnaire. Soc Sci Med, 19(12): 1347–1351.

Norr KL, Block CR, Charles A, Meyering S, Meyers E (1977). Explaining pain and enjoyment in childbirth. J Health Soc Behav, 18(3): 260–275.

Patton LL, English EC, Hambleton JD (1985). Childbirth preparation and outcomes of labour and delivery in primparous women. J Family Practice, 20(4): 375–378.

Perkins ER (1980). The pattern of women's attendance at antenatal classes: Is this good enough? Health Educ J, 39: 3–9.

Read GD (1933). Natural Childbirth. London: W. Heinemann.

Read GD (1956). Natural Childbirth Primer. New York: Harper & Row.

Reid DE, Cohen ME (1950). Evaluation of present day trends in obstetrics. J Am Med Assoc, 142: 615–623.

Ringrose CAD (1966). Quoted by Ringrose (1976).

Ringrose CAD (1976). Lamaze preparation for childbirth. New Engl J Med, 295, 453.

Roberts H, Wooton IDP, Kane KM, Harnett WE (1953). The value of antenatal preparation. J Obstet Gynecol Br Empire, 60: 404–408.

St. James-Roberts I, Chamberlain G, Haran FJ, Hutchinson CMPA (1982). Use of electromyographic and skin-conductance biofeedback relaxation training to facilitate childbirth in primiparae. J Psychosom Res, 26(4): 455–462.

Sandelowski M (1984). Expectations for childbirth versus actual experiences: the gap widens. Matern Child Nurs J, 9: 237–239.

Schultz JH, Luthe W (1959). Autogenic Training. New York: Grune & Stratton. (Quoted by Buxton 1962.)

Scott JR, Rose NB (1976). Effects of psychoprophylaxis (Lamaze preparation) on labor and delivery in primiparas. New Engl J Med, 294(22): 1205–1207.

Shearer M (1983). What we need next to progress in perinatal education (Editorial). Birth, 10(3): 149.

Stevens RJ (1976). Psychological strategies for management of pain in prepared childbirth. I: a review of the research. Birth Family J, 3(4): 157–164.

Stevens RJ, (1977). Psychological strategies for management of pain in prepared childbirth. II: A study of psychoanalgesia in prepared childbirth. Birth Family J, 4(1): 4–9.

Stevens RJ, Heide F (1977). Analgesic characteristics of prepared childbirth techniques: attention focusing and systematic relaxation. J Psychosom Res, 21(6): 429–438.

Stewart DE (1982). Psychiatric symptoms following attempted natural childbirth. Can Med Assoc J, 127: 713–716.

Stewart DE (1985). Possible relationship of post-partum psychiatric symptoms to childbirth education programmes. J Psychosom Obstet Gynecol, 4: 295–301.

Tanzer D (1968). Natural childbirth: pain or peak experience. Psychol Today, (October) 17.

Thoms H, Karlovsky E (1954). Two thousand deliveries under a training for childbirth programme. Am J Obstet Gynecol, 68: 279–284.

Timm MM (1979). Prenatal education evaluation. Nurs Res, 28(6): 338–342.

Toronto Task Force on High Risk Pregnancy (1980) Report: City of Toronto, Department of Public Health, pp 93–95.

Van Auken WB, Tomlinson DR (1953). An appraisal of patient training for childbirth. Am J Obstet Gynecol, 66: 100–105.

Velvovsky I, Platnov K, Ploticher V, Shugom E (1960). Painless Childbirth Through Psychoprophylaxis. Moscow: Foreign Languages Publishing House.

Worthington Jr. EL (1982). Labor room and laboratory: clinical validation of the cold pressor as a means of testing preparation for childbirth strategies. J Psychosom Res, 26(2): 223–230.

Worthington Jr. EL, Martin GA, Shumate M (1982). Which prepared-childbirth coping strategies are effective? J Obstet Gynecol Neonatal Nurs, 45–51.

Yahia C, Ulin PR (1965). Preliminary experience with a psychophysical program for childbirth. Am J Obstet Gynecol, 93: 942–949.

Zax M, Sameroff AJ, Farnum JE (1975). Childbirth education, maternal attitudes, and delivery. Am J Obstet Gynecol, 123(2): 185–190.

Zimmermann-Tansella C, Dolcetta G, Azzini V, Zacche G, Bertagni P, Siani R, Tansella H (1979). Preparation courses for childbirth in primipara: a comparison. J Psychosom Res, 23(4): 227–233.

21 Antenatal preparation for breastfeeding

Sally Inch

1 Introduction

Human milk has evolved over many thousands of years to meet the needs of human infants, just as the milk of all other mammals has evolved to meet the specific needs of their young. Human milk is thus uniquely intended for the human infant and superior to all other forms of nourishment. In the past in industrialized societies (and at present in many non-industrialized countries) a baby was breastfed or it died (Smith 1979; Cone 1979). Now that it is possible for a baby to be fed exclusively on non-human milk and still thrive (at least in most industrialized societies), a mother can choose not to perform this once imperative biological function.

That any woman who is physiologically capable of breastfeeding her child—as 97 per cent or more are (Morley 1974; Chetley 1986)—should elect not to do so is a monument both to the power of advertising, which has changed and shaped our cultural behaviour and values, and to the lack of regard paid by mothers and professionals to the potential adverse effects of artificial feeding, even in optimal conditions.

It may be that a woman who intends to feed her child artificially will, if pressed, acknowledge that she believes that breastfeeding is best and that bottle-feeding is second best, but she may also feel that the differences are so trivial that she can allow social factors to influence her decision (Ross *et al.* 1983). She may well be acquainted with other women who have bottle-fed their babies, and whose infants have come to no harm.

On the whole, infant formula products are probably safe enough today, and, used in accordance with the manufacturers' instructions, are probably nutritionally adequate for most babies (Minchin 1985). With any manufactured product, however, there is always the possibility of error, either in its manufacture or its use. In the case of infant formula, manufacturers have included excesses or deficiencies of essential items such as vitamins, minerals, fatty acids, and proteins, and bacterial contamination before the milk reached the customer; customers, on the other hand, have made up overconcentrated, overdiluted, and bacterially contaminated feeds (Minchin 1985).

There are problems with the methodology of all the studies that have investigated the advantages of breastfeeding over bottle feeding. The most important of these problems relates to the way in which infant feedings are measured and categorized. Most breastfed babies in most studies have had other forms of nourishment at some stage, and many bottle-fed babies were breastfed at some period (Auerbach *et al.* 1988).

Nevertheless, some general conclusions can be drawn. The more that is learned about the nutritional and immunological properties of breast milk, the more superior it appears to other available milks for human babies (Vahlquist 1976); and the more 'formula mishaps' are recorded (Minchin 1985) the more apparent it becomes that artificially feeding human infants, unless it is truly unavoidable, means exposing them to unnecessary risks.

1.1 Trends in breastfeeding

This century has seen a general decline in both the incidence and duration of breastfeeding. In Britain the decline reached its nadir in the 1970s. Mounting concern at this state of affairs culminated in the setting up of a Department of Health and Social Security working party, which recommended that babies should be breastfed for at least the first four months of their lives (Department of Health and Social Security 1974). At that time, of all the women giving birth in England and Wales, only half (51 per cent) began to feed their babies at the breast (Martin 1978). Five years later the percentage of women in England and Wales who began breastfeeding from birth had risen to 67 per cent (Martin and Monk 1982) This was interpreted by the authors of the survey as being a consequence of the increased publicity about the benefits of breastfeeding. Over the same period of time, however, there was an abrupt decline in the duration of breastfeeding among those who began feeding in this way: in 1980 and 1985 only 27 per cent and 26 per cent of women in England and Wales were still breastfeeding at four months after delivery (Department of Health and Social Security 1988).

Two problems face those who take it as axiomatic that all babies should be exclusively breastfed until they are at least four months of age: first, the difficulty of persuading all mothers to breastfeed their infants from birth; and second, the task of providing them with the help, information, and support that they need to continue to breastfeed successfully.

1.2 Influencing the decision to breastfeed

The majority of women who decide to breastfeed seem to make this decision prior to, or very early in pregnancy (Beske and Garvis 1982; Ladas 1972; Jones 1986; Lynch *et al.* 1986; Hally *et al.* 1984). Those who choose to bottle-feed tend to make up their minds later in pregnancy (Beske and Garvis 1982). Jones *et al.* (1986), who interviewed 1525 mothers at delivery and the 649 mothers who chose to breastfeed again at 12 months, found that women who considered that breastfeeding was better for the baby were likely to breastfeed for longer than those who considered that it made no difference.

That this effect was not mediated by knowledge alone was demonstrated by two earlier randomized controlled trials (Ross *et al.* 1983; Kaplowitz and Olson 1983). The latter investigators found that giving women well-designed, -written, and -illustrated information about breastfeeding, increased (or reinforced) their knowledge of the subject, but had little effect on their choice of feeding method, or on the duration of breastfeeding. The choice of feeding method and the duration of feeding seem to be more strongly influenced by socially acquired *attitudes* to breastfeeding (Kaplowitz and Olson 1983), and to the support women feel they will receive from their families and friends (Jones *et al.* 1986; Ladas 1972; Switzky *et al.* 1979), than by information alone. Furthermore, the data suggest that once a woman *has* decided how she will feed her baby, she is unlikely to change her mind subsequently (Kaplowitz and Olson 1983).

As no form of antenatal preparation of the breasts has been shown to be of benefit (see below), the common practice of asking a woman early in her pregnancy how she plans to feed her baby may not only be of little value, it may even be counterproductive if she has not already decided to breastfeed and feels pressured into making a decision before she is ready to do so.

2 Preparation of the pregnant woman

While information alone, at least in a written form, may not affect the *decision* to breastfeed, antenatal information in the form of a class given to women who have *already decided to breastfeed* does seem to be beneficial in some circumstances. Wiles (1984) found in her randomized controlled trial, that one antenatal breastfeeding class (of unspecified length) given in the last two months of pregnancy to women who intended to breastfeed had a significant positive effect, not only on the duration of breastfeeding, but also on the way in which the mother perceived herself and her infant postnatally. The class, designed by an American nurse midwife, was based on the concept of anticipatory guidance, and aimed to give the women a realistic perception of what breastfeeding and mothering might entail. It contained information on the anatomy and physiology of lactation, how to breastfeed, self-care of the breastfeeding mother, possible setbacks early in breastfeeding and how to cope with them, breastfeeding and the working mother, and how to obtain help from both professionals and voluntary breastfeeding organizations when necessary. It also reinforced the advantages of breastfeeding, but without giving this part of the class undue emphasis.

In another trial to assess the effects of providing information for women who had decided to breastfeed, no difference in breastfeeding success was detected (Kaplowitz and Olson 1983). The results of the two trials are shown in Table 21.1. The available information suggests that antenatal classes may be effective in promoting breastfeeeding in some circumstances, but more evidence is undoubtedly needed to assess which elements of the information and what kind of classes women find helpful.

Fourteen per cent of the women who had decided to breastfeed surveyed by Jones (1986) were unaware

Table 21.1 Effect of antenatal breastfeeding education on discontinuing before 1–2 months postpartum

Study	EXPT		CTRL		Odds ratio	Graph of odds ratios and confidence intervals
	n	(%)	*n*	(%)	(95% CI)	0.01 0.1 0.5 1 2 10 100
Kaplowitz *et al.* (1983)	13/18	(72.22)	17/22	(77.27)	0.77 (0.19–3.18)	
Wiles (1984)	2/20	(10.00)	14/20	(70.00)	0.09 (0.03–0.30)	
Typical odds ratio (95% confidence interval)					0.23 (0.09–0.58)	

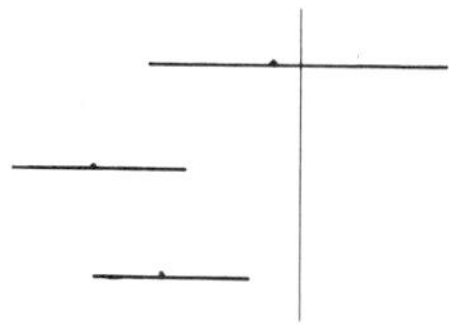

that breastfeeding was better for the baby. This group breastfed for a significantly shorter time than those who believed that breastfeeding would be beneficial. It would thus seem advisable to mention the advantages of breastfeeding in an antenatal class, but not to the exclusion of other aspects of more general value (see Chapter 20), bearing in mind what a relatively small percentage of potential breastfeeding women are likely to be in need of this information.

Putting undue emphasis on information that is of value to only a few members of the class and thus (because of limited time) excluding other aspects of breastfeeding, may have been the reason for the lack of success experienced by Ross *et al.* (1983). In this trial women were randomly allocated to receive, or not to receive a breastfeeding 'health education programme' which consisted of two half-hour sessions, the first devoted to the advantages of breastfeeding, and the second to technique. Unlike the trial conducted by Wiles (1984), none of these women had previously made clear to the researcher whether or not they intended to breastfeed. They were drawn from a population in which over 95 per cent of women attending the maternal and child health clinics had been shown, in a previous study, to start breastfeeding, but in which only about half were still fully breastfeeding at between five to eight weeks after delivery. Thus this study also was primarily concerned with increasing the duration for which the women breastfed, rather than the number who commenced breastfeeding.

The mothers were interviewed after delivery by a researcher who did not know whether or not the mother had participated in the health education programme. Within 24 weeks of delivery the women were interviewed again, this time at home. There was a statistically significant increase in the breastfeeding knowledge of the women who had received the classes when compared with those who had not, but this was not accompanied by the desired change in behaviour. At the time of the home interview 66 per cent of the mothers in the 'educated' group had introduced supplementary feeds at a mean(SD) age of 4.71(3.4) weeks, compared with 56 per cent of those in the control group who had introduced them at a mean age of 5.22(4.9) weeks. Thus the programme seemed to have had a slightly detrimental effect on feeding practices: more women who had experienced the programme introduced formula, and at an earlier age, than those in the control group.

There does not seem an easy solution to the problem of persuading women that they should breastfeed. Simply telling them that 'breast is best' is clearly not sufficient. Campaigns in the mass media and in clinics have been found to have little effect on feeding practices (Svejcar 1977; Kirk 1979; Gueri *et al.* 1979). If increased publicity did contribute to the rise in the number of women beginning to breastfeed in England and Wales between 1975 and 1980, it does not appear to have sustained many of them in their attempts (Martin and Monk 1982). The situation has not improved: women discontinued breastfeeding at the same rate in 1985 as they had done in 1980 (Department of Health and Social Security 1988). The mass media may convey information effectively, but they do not, on the whole, seem well suited to accomplishing the attitudinal and behavioural changes that are evidently required to change infant feeding practices (Kaplowitz and Olsen 1983; Switzky *et al.* 1979). This accords with the findings of others who have suggested that changes in attitudes are more likely to be brought about by personal contact (Bettinghaus 1973).

3 Preparation of the breasts

3.1 Woolwich Shells

Sore and/or cracked nipples constitute one of the commonest problems encountered in the early postnatal care of breastfeeding women (Whichelow 1982; Jones 1984). It is second only to 'insufficient milk' as the main reason for discontinuing breastfeeding altogether (Sloper *et al.* 1977; Martin and Monk 1982). Thus much of the advice pregnant women may be given on the subject of antenatal breast preparation is with the aim of preventing these two postnatal problems.

More than fifty years ago, Waller (1938) maintained that the main cause of nipple damage was that the nipple was not sufficiently far back in the baby's mouth during suckling. Indeed, he felt that there was no way to avoid damage during feeding other than by ensuring that the nipple rested between the base of the tongue and the soft palate (Waller 1938). He believed that this, in turn, was dependent on the nipple's proctractility, as determined by the 'pinch test' (Waller 1946). In this procedure the nipple is pulled gently between the thumb and forefinger. Then, with the finger and thumb placed on the areola behind the base of the nipple, light compression is applied to make the nipple protrude. For those who failed this test he advocated the wearing of glass shells, originally designed in Victorian times to collect milk that leaked from the breasts between feeds and so protect the mother's clothes. The purpose of this was to gradually stretch and loosen the non-protractile nipple from 'its attachment to the deeper structures of the breast'. The same rationale is used by advocates of the 'Hoffman technique', in which both thumbs are placed at the base of the nipple and pressure is exerted towards the breast tissue as the thumbs are pulled away from each other. This procedure is then repeated at right angles to the first attempt (La Leche League International 1985).

The relation of nipple protractility and breastfeeding difficulty is tenuous at best. Waller did not do a trial of the glass shell, but carried out a trial to assess the effectiveness of antenatal expression of colostrum. Of the 200 primigravidae recruited to his trial of the effectiveness of antenatal colostrum expression, he judged that 56 (28 per cent) had poorly protractile nipples, and treated all these women with the Woolwich Shell. Blaikeley *et al.* (1953), who repeated Waller's trial, considered that 52 (22 per cent) of the 234 primigravidae they recruited had poorly protractile nipples, and these women were all given glass shells, as recommended by Waller, to wear for the last 20 weeks of pregnancy. Despite the 'good improvement' noted in almost all of the women who wore shells (94 per cent), less than half of them (44 per cent) were deemed to have lactated successfully. There was no control series of women with poor nipples who received no treatment.

Hytten (1954) found that only 14 per cent of primigravidae in Aberdeen had 'poor nipples', and only 16 per cent of these (2 per cent overall) had difficulty in breastfeeding. Of the primigravidae considered to have normal nipples, 3.5 per cent had breastfeeding difficulties attributable to nipple problems. Thus, although the antenatal examination of the nipples might have had some predictive value, most of those considered to have poor nipples (84 per cent) had no related problems despite receiving no treatment.

In 1980, L'Esperance studied 102 breastfeeding women for the first four days following delivery in relation to the 16 factors which had been reported in the literature to have an association with nipple pain. She found a statistically significant relationship with nipple pain for only 3 of the 16 factors. Two of these showed a positive correlation with nipple pain, but one, nipple shape, showed a negative correlation; although 22.5 per cent of the women in her study were deemed to have 'poor' nipples, a smaller proportion of these mothers had pain than did women with protruding nipples.

An explanation for the inconsistency of the relationship between nipple shape and nipple problems may lie in the cineradiographic studies of Adran *et al.* (1958). These showed clearly that the baby makes a 'teat', not from the nipple alone, but from the surrounding breast tissue. This teat is about three times as long as the nipple at rest, with the nipple itself extending back as far as the junction between the hard and the soft palate. These findings have since been substantiated using ultrasound imaging of events in the baby's mouth (Weber *et al.* 1984). Compared with the importance of ensuring that the baby has an adequate 'mouthful' of breast tissue with which to form this teat, the actual shape of the nipple may be a secondary consideration.

3.2 Nipple conditioning

A popular explanation for the contrast between the high incidence of nipple pain amongst breastfeeding women in industrialized societies and the low incidence amongst those in the more 'primitive' cultures observed by Margaret Mead (Newton 1952) has been that in the former the nipple is rarely exposed and is therefore protected from abrasion, changes of temperature, and sunlight which might serve to toughen the epithelium. To those who subscribe to this view it seems logical to advocate some antenatal method of toughening the nipple in order to prepare it for its sudden hard use. Although many different methods have been suggested in attempts to accomplish this aim, they fall basically into three categories: (1) some form of nipple friction; (2) the application of some form of cream; and (3) the antenatal expression of colostrum. (The latter action is also advocated as a means of improving lactation itself.)

Several researchers have attempted to assess the efficacy of antenatal nipple 'conditioning'. Atkinson (1979) studied the effect of nipple conditioning in 22 right-handed primiparous women who acted as their own controls by conditioning one nipple and not the other. The nipple to be conditioned was assigned alternately, so that half the women prepared the right nipple and half the left. Nipple conditioning began 6 weeks prior to the expected date of delivery and consisted of: nipple rolling twice a day for two minutes at a time; providing gentle friction with a towel for 15 seconds following a daily shower; airing the nipples for two hours a day; and allowing the outer clothing to rub against the nipple. The 17 women who completed the protocol were asked to assess nipple pain on a three-point scale after each feed for the first 5 days following delivery. At the end of this time they posted their assessment sheets to the investigator. There was no attempt to assess the state of the nipples objectively. Atkinson found that the women reported significantly less overall pain on the conditioned side, but she also acknowledged that her subjects may have been biased in making their ratings, in an attempt to show that the time and energy they had expended in conditioning their nipples had not been wasted.

Brown and Hurlock (1975) also conducted a study in which women were used as their own controls. Three weeks before their expected date of delivery 57 primiparous women were randomly assigned to one of three treatment groups. The nipple to be conditioned was also chosen randomly by tossing a coin. The three treatment groups involved either nipple rolling, the application of Masse cream, or the expression of colostrum. The chosen nipple was prepared in the assigned way twice daily; the other nipple received no treatment. The breasts of each woman were examined each day while she was in hospital and every other day after she returned home, for a period of 10 days, by an examiner who did not know which nipple had been treated. In addition, the women themselves were asked to rate nipple sensitivity on a four-point scale. No statistically significant differences were found, either objectively or subjectively, between the three methods of conditioning or between the use of Masse cream, expression of colostrum or the unprepared nipple.

A number of less adequately controlled studies (Whitley 1978; L'Esperance 1980; Jones 1984; Clark 1985; Hewat and Ellis 1987) have also failed to show any effects of antenatal nipple conditioning. Furthermore, if it were true that sore or cracked nipples could be prevented by measures designed to toughen the nipple, then one would expect there to be a considerable difference in the incidence of soreness in women breastfeeding for the first time and those who have breastfed before. This difference has not been observed. Gunther (1945) found no relation between parity and soreness, although she did find that multiparae were less likely to complain about soreness and more likely to take it for granted. Nicholson (1985) found that half of the women who participated in her trial to assess different ways of managing sore nipples had previously breastfed. Likewise, Jones (1984) found a similar incidence of sore nipples in primiparae and multiparae. These observations call into question the idea that nipples need to be 'tough' to prevent them becoming damaged.

3.3 Breast massage and the expression of colostrum

When Waller first introduced the practice of teaching women to express colostrum antenatally, it was with the intention of providing them with an opportunity to master the technique in case they should need to use it postnatally. Manual expression was considered to be the appropriate response to breast engorgement, and it was felt that the interval between delivery and the start of milk secretion was too short for mothers to become proficient postnatally. He also felt that providing postnatal instruction took up too much of the time of ward staff.

The effects of a regimen of antenatal breast massage and expression of colostrum compared to a no treatment control group has been examined in three randomized controlled trials (Waller 1946; Blaikeley *et al.* 1953; Brown and Hurlock 1975) and one non-randomized cohort comparison (Ingelman-Sundberg 1958). One of the randomized trials does not present any numerical results (Brown and Hurlock 1975).

The regimens used in each of these studies differed. Waller (1946) encouraged women to express colostrum for the last three months of pregnancy. For those women in either group whose breasts became engorged postnatally, postnatal manual expression of 'the excess' was carried out. The high rate of drop-out in Waller's study (only 100 of the original 200 remained for analysis) was due to highly unusual circumstances: 'A bomb which destroyed a large part of the hospital . . . brought the work to an end'. This unfortunate occurrence seems unlikely to have introduced any systematic bias into the analysis! In the trial by Blaikeley *et al.* (1953), which was intended to replicate Waller's trial, antenatal expression of colostrum and breast massage was started at 32 to 33 weeks of gestation, and routine postnatal expression after all feeds was carried out in both groups. In both of these trials women were alternately allocated to their respective groups.

The results of these two trials are presented in Tables 21.2 and 21.3. They suggest that antenatal expression of colostrum reduces the incidence of engorgement and damaged nipples and leads to a reduction in breastfeeding failure up to at least 6 months postpartum.

In the trial conducted by Brown and Hurlock (1975), women were randomly allocated to three groups: nipple rolling; application of cream; and antenatal (but not postnatal) expression of colostrum. Women were asked to treat one breast and not the other. In the non-randomized cohort study reported by Ingelman-Sundberg (1958), women in the experimental group were treated by the investigator himself, while those in the control group were treated by his obstetric colleagues. The experimental group were advised to use massage and express colostrum from the 20th week of pregnancy; women in the control group received no such advice. Women in both groups practised routine postnatal expression of colostrum.

The results of these two studies of antenatal expression of colostrum appear to be inconsistent with the effects shown in Tables 21.2 and 21.3. Neither detected any benefit from antenatal expression of colostrum,

Table 21.2 Effect of antenatal expression of colostrum on severe engorgement

Study	EXPT n	EXPT (%)	CTRL n	CTRL (%)	Odds ratio (95% CI)	Graph of odds ratios and confidence intervals (0.01 0.1 0.5 1 2 10 100)
Blaikeley *et al.* (1953)	17/111	(15.32)	43/116	(37.07)	0.33 (0.18–0.59)	
Waller (1946)	25/100	(25.00)	58/100	(58.00)	0.26 (0.15–0.45)	
Typical odds ratio (95% confidence interval)					0.29 (0.19–0.43)	

Effect of antenatal expression of colostrum on damaged nipples

Study	EXPT n	EXPT (%)	CTRL n	CTRL (%)	Odds ratio (95% CI)	Graph
Blaikeley *et al.* (1953)	4/111	(3.60)	9/116	(7.76)	0.46 (0.15–1.42)	
Waller (1946)	12/100	(12.00)	24/100	(24.00)	0.45 (0.22–0.91)	
Typical odds ratio (95% confidence interval)					0.45 (0.25–0.83)	

Table 21.3 Effect of antenatal expression of colostrum on full breastfeeding on discharge

Study	EXPT n	EXPT (%)	CTRL n	CTRL (%)	Odds ratio (95% CI)	Graph of odds ratios and confidence intervals (0.01 0.1 0.5 1 2 10 100)
Blaikeley *et al.* (1953)	102/111	(91.89)	97/116	(83.62)	2.14 (0.97–4.72)	
Waller (1946)	97/100	(97.00)	83/100	(83.00)	4.70 (1.87–11.82)	
Typical odds ratio (95% confidence interval)					2.99 (1.64–5.44)	

Effect of antenatal expression of colostrum on full breastfeeding at 3 months

Study	EXPT n	EXPT (%)	CTRL n	CTRL (%)	Odds ratio (95% CI)	Graph
Blaikeley *et al.* (1953)	78/111	(70.27)	60/116	(51.72)	2.17 (1.27–3.69)	
Waller (1946)	87/100	(87.00)	65/100	(65.00)	3.32 (1.74–6.34)	
Typical odds ratio (95% confidence interval)					2.58 (1.71–3.88)	

Effect of antenatal expression of colostrum on full breastfeeding at 6 months

Study	EXPT n	EXPT (%)	CTRL n	CTRL (%)	Odds ratio (95% CI)	Graph
Blaikeley *et al.* (1953)	56/109	(51.38)	30/113	(26.55)	2.83 (1.65–4.86)	
Waller (1946)	83/100	(83.00)	42/100	(42.00)	5.70 (3.22–10.09)	
Typical odds ratio (95% confidence interval)					3.94 (2.66–5.83)	

although neither measured breastfeeding rates after discharge from hospital, or looked at engorgement or nipple damage.

There may be several reasons for this apparent discrepancy in the results of the four studies. First, mothers in the experimental groups in the studies by Waller and Blaikeley *et al.* had extra attention from a midwife, both antenatally and postnatally. Secondly, both these studies took place in the same hospital, which had a reputation for being particularly interested in breastfeeding. Thirdly, there was a high incidence of engorgement (15 to 37 per cent) in both the experimental and control groups in both these studies. At the time that these studies were undertaken, limitation of feeding duration was recommended in this hospital. These practices were likely to have increased the incidence of engorgement. It may be that the expression of colostrum antenatally, combined with postnatal expression is an effective method of relieving engorgement. With the more flexible feeding regimen that may have been practised by the mothers in the studies of Ingelman-Sundberg and Brown and Hurlock, such expression might not have been either necessary or helpful.

4 Conclusions

4.1 Implications for current practice

Incorporaton of information on breastfeeding in antenatal classes appears to be of value to women who have already decided to breastfeed, and this practice should be recommended.

The available information suggests that antenatal expression of colostrum will reduce the incidence of breast engorgement and sore nipples and increase the rate of breastfeeding success, but that this effect may be limited to circumstances in which the existing incidence of breast engorgement and sore nipples is already high because of inappropriate postnatal practices. None of the other commonly advocated methods of antenatal preparation for breastfeeding has been shown by adequately controlled studies to have a beneficial effect. No form of nipple conditioning which has been studied by randomized controlled trials has been shown to have any beneficial effect.

4.2 Implications for future research

Although there are no good predictors of breastfeeding success, inverted nipples continue on some occasions to present a real problem. Of particular importance is the protractility of the tissue surrounding the nipple, as it is this which determines the baby's ability to make an effective 'teat' from the breast. Studies are required to determine whether or not the Hoffman technique or the use of Woolwich Shells (glass or plastic shields) are effective. At least one such study is in progress (Alexander, personal communication).

Further, better controlled studies are required to evaluate the place of antenatal expression of colostrum as a means to prevent problems with breastfeeding.

References

Adran GM, Kemp FH, Lind J (1958). A cineradiographic study of breastfeeding. Br J Radiol, 31: 156–162.

Atkinson LD (1979). Prenatal nipple conditioning for breastfeeding. Nurs Res, 28: 267–271.

Auerbach KG, Renfrew Houston MJ, Minchin M (1988). Feeding comparisons: I and II. Acta Paediatr Scand (Suppl) (in press).

Beske EJ, Garvis MS (1982). Important factors in breastfeeding success. Matern Child Nurs, 7: 174–179.

Bettinghaus EP (1973). Persuasive communication. In: New York: Holt, Rinehart & Winston, pp 155–156.

Blaikeley J, Clarke S, MacKeith R, Ogden KM (1953). Breastfeeding—factors affecting success. J Obstet Gynaecol Br Empire, 60: 657–669.

Brown MS, Hurlock JT (1975). Preparation of the breast for breastfeeding. Nurs Res, 24: 448–451.

Chetley A (1986). The Politics of Babyfood—Successful Challenges to International Marketing Strategy. London: (Francis Pinter Ltd), in which he quotes the WHO provisional summary record of the 8th meeting of Committee A, 33rd World Health Assembly; Document No. A33/A/SR/8; Geneva 17 May 1980, p 11.

Clark M (1985). A study of 4 methods of nipple care offered to postpartum mothers. NZ Nurs J, 78: 16–18.

Cone TE (1979). History of American Paediatrics. Boston: Little, Brown, p 57.

Department of Health and Social Security (1974). Present Day Practice in Infant Feeding. London: Her Majesty's Stationery Office.

Department of Health and Social Security (1988). Present Day Practice in Infant Feeding. Third Report. London: Her Majesty's Stationery Office.

Gueri M, Jutsum P, White A (1979). Evaluation of a breastfeeding campaign in Trinidad. Bol of Sanit Panam, 86: 189–195.

Gunther M. (1945) Sore nipples: causes and prevention. Lancet, 2: 590–593.

Hally MR, Bond J, Crawley J, Gregson B, Phillips P, Russell IT (1984). Factors influencing the feeding of firstborn infants. Acta Paediatr Scand, 73: 33–39.

Hewat RJ, Ellis DJ (1987). A comparison of the effectiveness of two methods of nipple care. Birth, 14: 41–45.

Hytten FE (1954). Clinical and chemical studies in lactation. IX: Breastfeeding in hospital. Br Med J, 18 Dec: 1447–1452.

Ingelman-Sundberg A (1958). The value of antenatal massage of nipples and expression of colostrum. J Obstet Gynaecol Br Empire, 65: 448–449.

Jones D (1984). Breastfeeding problems. Nursing Times, 15 Aug: 53–54.

Jones DA (1986). Attitudes of breastfeeding mothers: a survey of 649 mothers. Soc Sci Med, 23: 1151–1156.

Jones DA, West RR, Newcombe RG (1986). Maternal characteristics associated with the duration of breastfeeding. Midwifery, 2: 141–146.

Kaplowitz DD, Olson CM (1983). The effect of an education programme on the decision to breastfeed. J Nutr Educ, 15: 61–65.

Kirk TR (1979). An evaluation of the impact of breastfeeding promotion in Edinburgh. Proc Nutr Soc 38: 77A.

La Leche League International (1985). The Womanly Art of Breastfeeding. Illinois: La Leche League International, pp 30–31.

L'Esperance CM (1980). Pain or pleasure: the dilemma of early breastfeeding. Birth Family J, 7: 21–26.

Ladas AK (1972). Breastfeeding: the less available option. Environ Child Health, 18: 316–346.

Lynch SA, Koch AM, Hislop TG, Goldman AJ (1986). Evaluating the effect of a breastfeeding consultant on the duration of breastfeeding. Can J Public Health, 77: 190–195.

Martin J (1978). Infant Feeding 1975: Attitudes and Practice in England and Wales. London: Her Majesty's Stationery Office.

Martin J, Monk J (1982). Infant Feeding 1980. London: Office of Population Censuses and Surveys (Social Survey Division).

Minchin MK (1985). Breastfeeding Matters. Melbourne: Alma Publications/Allen & Unwin Australia.

Morley D (1974). Quoted in: The Baby Killer. Muller M, London: War on Want, p 6.

Newton N (1952). Nipple pain and nipple damage. J Pediatr, 41: 411–423.

Nicholson W (1985). Cracked nipples in breastfeeding mothers—a randomized trial of three methods of management. Nursing Mothers Association of Australia, 21: 7.

Ross SM, Loening W, Van Middelkoop A (1983). Breastfeeding—evaluation of a health education programme. S Afr Med J, 64: 361–363.

Sloper KS, Elsden E, and Baum JD (1977). Increasing breastfeeding in a community. Arch Dis Child, 52: 700–702.

Smith RF (1979). The People's Health 1830–1910. Canberra: A N U Press.

Svejcar J (1977). Methodological approaches to the promotion and maintenance of breastfeeding. Klin Paediatr, 189: 333–336.

Switzky LT, Vietze P, Switzky HN (1979). Attitudinal and demographic predictors of breastfeeding and bottlefeeding behaviour by mothers of six week old infants. Psychol Rep, 45: 3–14.

Vahlquist IPA Bulletin (1976), 5: 45. Quoted in Minchin MK (1985) *op cit.*

Waller H (1938). Clinical Studies in Lactation. London: Heinemann, p 117.

Waller H (1946). The early failure of breastfeeding. Arch Dis Child, 21: 1–12.

Weber F, Woolridge MW, Baum JD (1984). An ultrasonographic analysis of sucking and swallowing in newborn infants. Pediatr Res, 18: 806.

Whichelow MJ (1982). Factors associated with the duration of breastfeeding in a privileged society. Early Hum Dev, 7: 273–280.

Whitley N (1978). Preparation of the breasts for breastfeeding. A one-year follow-up of 34 mothers. J Obstet Gynecol Neonatal Nurs, 7: 44–48.

Wiles LS (1984). The effect of prenatal breastfeeding education on breastfeeding success and maternal perception of the infant. J Obstet Gynecol Neonatal Nurs, 13: 253–257.

Part IV

Screening and diagnosis during pregnancy

22 Formal risk scoring during pregnancy

Sophie Alexander and Marc J. N. C. Keirse

1 Introduction

Since early antiquity, obstetric teaching has recognized that some women are more likely to experience poor outcome of pregnancy than others. Though the term 'risk pregnancy' was not formally used, Hippocratic writings contain many cautionary notes relating to high risk groups (Lloyd 1983). Some of the factors cited by Hippocrates, such as 'a damp mild winter . . . followed by a dry spring . . . tends to produce miscarriage on the slightest pretext in women approaching term in the spring', are no longer considered to be risk factors. Others, such as low maternal weight or bleeding in pregnancy, are still included in many contemporary risk scores. Hippocrates recognized the distinction between risk factors that are present from the beginning of pregnancy (e.g. 'pregnant women who are abnormally delicate have a fetal loss before the fetus becomes sizeable') and risk factors that arise during pregnancy (e.g. 'menstrual bleeding which occurs during pregnancy indicates an unhealthy fetus'), a distinction that, again, can be noted in most modern risk assessments. Hippocratic writings (Lloyd 1983) also recognized that the outcome of pregnancy was influenced by intrinsic as well as by external and environmental factors. The basic understanding on which current risk scoring systems are based has thus been implicit in obstetric teaching for many centuries.

At the beginning of this century, obstetric textbooks contained lists of physical and social risk factors, similar to those found in contemporary textbooks (see, for example, Fabre 1913). These lists must certainly be considered early forms of risk scoring and they reaffirm that implicit risk scoring has been in existence for millennia, and that it has been embedded in the daily routine of clinicians for decades.

More formalized risk scoring systems became popular in the 1960s, when large, computerized obstetric data banks became available. During the last 20 years, these have resulted in dozens of scoring systems, which have already been the subject of several reviews (Newcombe *et al.* 1977; Newcombe and Chalmers 1981; World Health Organization 1981; Committee assessing alternative birth settings 1982; Committee to study the prevention of low birthweight 1985; Peters and Golding 1985; Lumley 1987). The various scoring systems have also known different fates. Hobel's score (Hobel *et al.* 1973), the great favourite, has been quoted more than 300 times since its publication in 1973, while others have been quoted less than once a year. Opinions on the scores vary from optimistic claims that scoring '. . . allows earlier detection of the imperfections that should be corrected to obtain a healthy maternal environment for successful gestation' (Leon 1973), to statements of disenchantment such as 'many clinicians agree that except for the most extreme cases, such screening systems are grossly inadequate' (Grimes *et al.* 1983), or '. . . formal assessment of risk in obstetrics is doomed to failure for the immediate future' (Lilford and Chard 1983). Consensus on the use of risk scoring systems, even within one country, currently seems far off.

Identification of pregnancies that are at greater than average risk is a fundamental concept in antenatal care. In theory at least, an approach that substitutes rationally based risk scoring for the rather nebulous process of clinical impression should have distinct advantages. Such an approach should be more accurate than the less formal risk assessment that is part of daily clinical practice, just as formal scoring systems for antenatal cardiotocography have been shown to be more reproducible than informal impressions (Trimbos and Keirse 1978). As for many other tests, however, the validity and utility of risk scoring systems remain to be determined.

This chapter concentrates on evaluating scoring systems that are used throughout pregnancy and which are directed at all pregnant women without preselection. Its emphasis will be on evaluating the place of formal risk scoring as a screening test, and its potential benefits and hazards for individual babies and mothers.

2 Principles of risk scoring systems

2.1 Uses of formal risk scores

The primary purpose of a risk scoring system is to permit the classification and allocation of individual women into different categories for which different and appropriate actions can then be planned. This is not the only, and perhaps not even the most important, use of scoring systems. Issel (1979), while stating that he felt that risk scoring was of no avail to individual women, described five 'values' of scoring, and most initiators of scoring systems emphasize their value for other purposes than the care for the individual woman and baby.

Several authors have stressed the usefulness of risk scoring in medical education indicating to the student the most important markers for the prognosis of pregnancy. Others have pointed out that it provides less experienced caregivers with a useful check-list for supervising pregnancy. Papiernik (1984b), for example, who has been disappointed by the use of formal risk scoring for screening, considered these other functions to be their major benefits. Some have advocated the use of presently available risk scoring systems as the Gold Standard against which to weigh new and more sophisticated screening procedures (Hack and Breslau 1986), just as new placental function tests have been evaluated by comparing their performance to that of other, equally unvalidated, placental function tests (see Chapters 3 and 29).

Scoring has also been used to describe and characterize different obstetric populations for comparative studies between different centres or regions (Bréart *et al.* 1981; Alexander et al. 1988), and to describe and define populations, rather than individuals, in need of differing levels of care. In this context, risk scoring becomes an instrument in public health issues or, as the World Health Organization expressed it, 'risk strategy is a management tool for the organization of health care' (World Health Organization 1981). The use of scores as population-definers can then be used to target the allocation of resources and funds at high-risk populations (Jones *et al.* 1988).

These important, but secondary issues will not be addressed in this chapter, which will deal with the use of various scoring systems only from the point of view of identifying individual women and babies at risk of various adverse outcomes of pregnancy.

2.2 Scoring the risk of what?

The great variety of scores that are used in pregnancy and childbirth aim to identify, prospectively, individuals at high risk and to discriminate between levels of risk. The term 'risk' is, however, vague and undefined. To be understood, the outcomes for which the woman or baby are at risk must be specified.

Some scores have been developed for narrow and specific purposes. Examples of these include: the Bishop (Bishop 1964) and other scores for assessment of the cervix before induction of labour (see Chapter 61); the Apgar score for assessment of the newborn and neonatal wellbeing (Apgar 1953; see Chapter 83); and the Fischer score for assessment of antepartum cardiotocograms (Fischer *et al.* 1976; Trimbos and Keirse 1978).

Others have been designed more as a form of triage to allow rapid allocation of individual women to a predetermined management scheme; scores for breech delivery (Zatuchni and Andros 1967), or for preterm labour (Baumgarten and Grüber 1974; Essed *et al.* 1978) are examples. In this case the score result determines issues such as the choice between caesarean section and vaginal delivery for breech presentation, or between tocolysis or no tocolysis in preterm labour. Although such scoring systems would qualify for inclusion in the broad context of perinatal risk scoring systems, they are not discussed in this chapter as they are not as a rule applied to unselected populations of pregnant women. Other scores that are applied during labour rather than in pregnancy include, for instance, the score of Smith *et al.* (1985), which scored for the need for skilled resuscitation, defined as a one-minute Apgar score of 5 or less.

Many of the risk scoring systems that have been

adopted in clinical practice do not clearly define the outcomes which they attempt to predict, and are directed at non-specific targets such as 'poor outcome' (e.g. Hobel *et al.* 1973; Coopland *et al.* 1977), or 'poor neonatal outcome' (e.g. Edwards *et al.* 1979; Baruffi et al. 1984). Evaluation by reference to final and clear-cut measures of adverse outcome (see Chapter 3) is not always possible and some outcome measures, such as 'infants requiring more than routine neonatal care' (Coopland *et al.* 1977), are so prone to bias that the scoring system can easily become no more than a self-fulfilling prophecy.

Other scoring systems are nothing more than tautologies. Screening for the need for specialist care (Grimes *et al.* 1983; Nuovo 1985), or for the need to transfer patients to tertiary care centres (Haliday *et al.* 1980) are examples of this. Indeed, some conditions, such as insulin dependent diabetes, hypertension or multiple pregnancy, that are incorporated in the scoring system, almost automatically lead to transfer (Grimes *et al.* 1983; Nuovo 1985), so that the adverse outcome is not really an outcome, but the obligatory consequence of high-risk allocation.

The majority of the risk scoring systems that are routinely applied in pregnancy do address the risk of clear-cut and finite outcomes such as perinatal mortality, duration of gestation, and birthweight. These have been variously defined, however. Thus scoring systems for low birthweight may, as the official definition of the term suggests (FIGO News 1976; World Health Organization 1977), estimate the risk of delivering an infant weighing less than 2500 g at birth (Alberman 1974), and this will include a sizeable proportion of infants born preterm (less than 37 weeks' gestation; World Health Organization 1977; FIGO News 1976). Only a few scoring systems specifically address low birthweight at term (Adelstein and Fedrick 1978); others are confined to low birthweight preterm (e.g. Guzick *et al.* 1984); others refer to infants below 2501 g rather than to infants below 2500 g (Thalhammer *et al.* 1976; Rudelstorfer *et al.* 1976) which, due to the well-known preference for round figures, may make a considerable difference in the incidence of low birthweight (Macfarlane and Mugford 1984). Still others assume that people will intuitively know what is meant by low birthweight.

Identification and comparability of the risk that is scored for is most problematic among the various risk scoring systems for preterm birth. Many of these, including some of the most recent ones, do not even refer to preterm birth as such (World Health Organization 1977; FIGO News 1976), but to 'prematurity', an outmoded concept that was (Keirse 1979) and, in the different scoring systems still is, variously defined. Often it is not clear to what extent the risk relates to birth following spontaneous preterm labour in singleton pregnancies, elective caesarean section, or induction of labour before 37 weeks, fetal death before the onset of labour, or lethal congenital malformations, which together account for a considerable proportion of preterm births (Keirse and Kanhai 1981; see Chapter 74). When the outcome is properly defined, it does not always relate to births at less than 37 weeks, but may relate to less than 38 weeks, less than 36 weeks (e.g. Nesbitt and Aubry 1969), or to infants of less than 2500 g born before 37 weeks (e.g. Fedrick and Anderson 1976; Guzick *et al.* 1984).

2.3 Risk scoring as a screening test

When applied to a general population of pregnant women, a risk scoring system is in fact a screening test and it should conform to the criteria described elsewhere (see Chapter 3). This is not always the case, however, since many scoring systems include clinical diagnoses (e.g. diabetes, hypertension, renal disease, etc.) and diagnostic test results, (e.g. low haemoglobin, abnormal glucose tolerance, or presence of Rhesus antibodies) among the parameters from which the score is constructed. A diagnosis of severe renal disease, for example, will place a woman very high in many risk scoring systems for poor pregnancy outcome. Severe renal disease, however, is a diagnosis rather than a test result. Most obstetricians would consider a woman with that diagnosis to be at high risk whether or not they use formal risk scoring. Yet, the disease entity is entered into a scoring system, not so much as a condition that will require special attention, but as an element that will, in combination with others, form the background from which a more general risk estimate of 'poor outcome', perinatal mortality, or low birthweight is derived.

While risk scoring systems are intended as screening procedures, in practice they often combine elements of screening with elements of diagnosis. This has two consequences. First, women with a diagnosis of serious disease qualify almost automatically as being at high risk in most scoring systems. More often than not, these women would be identified equally well as being at risk without resorting to risk scoring. When incorporated in a scoring system their inclusion (because of their easy identification and obvious disease) adds unwarranted credibility to the screening system. Second, high scores almost invariably draw attention to the predominant individual components of that score, which leads to further assessment and often to further diagnostic procedures. The adjustments that result from these additional activities may then be entered into an update of the score result. Thus scoring systems often go beyond the classical screening concepts described in Chapter 3. Such scoring systems are then basically no different from case records, except for the fact that they are more formally constructed and confer predetermined weights to the observations listed.

It is noteworthy that, although the outcomes for which the screening is conducted in the various scoring systems may be quite different, there is much overlap between the elements that are incorporated in the various scoring systems as being predictive of these different outcomes (Table 22.1). As shown in Table 22.1, differences in whether or not a particular marker is included in the score are sometimes larger among scores that apparently address the same issue, for instance low birthweight in the scores of Thalhammer (Thalhammer 1973; Thalhammer *et al.* 1976) and Adelstein and Fedrick (1978), than among scores which address different outcomes, for instance low birthweight in the score of Thalhammer *et al.* (1976) and preterm delivery in the score of Creasy *et al.* (1980).

Consequently, many of the scoring systems and charts look quite similar, whatever the particular outcome of pregnancy that they attempt to predict. At the basis of this may be the assumption that reproductive calamities of all kinds accumulate as a continuum. But the degree to which this intuitive feeling is true has never actually been tested. In effect, most risk scores and the variety of markers that are incorporated in them do not circumvent, but rather reflect the problem that poor perinatal and childhood outcomes are often part of a poor social background (Chalmers I 1985). The actual type of 'poor outcome' that is experienced or addressed in the formal risk scoring systems may well be very non-specific, when considered in this context. In any event, risk markers used to screen for high-risk pregnancies also appear in the risk scores that are used in the neonatal period for prediction of the sudden infant death syndrome. Moreover, Golding and Peters (1985), for instance, examined the outcome of children who were scored to be at high risk of cot death but who did not die and found that these children had a higher incidence of pneumonia and non-accidental injury and an excess of repeated and prolonged hospital admissions.

3 Construction of risk scores

Risk scores are constructed in two steps: first, a list of empirical data is selected; then weighting is introduced, either arbitrarily, or on the basis of some kind of statistical analysis.

3.1 Data collection

Even with complex computer-generated data sets, the risk markers that are included in the scoring systems must be limited to the data that were entered in the data bank. It would be wrong to assume that these data have always been collected with a clear view of their later use and potential, and many of them are very arbitrary indeed. For instance, it has been suggested that the exact type of movements that working women have to perform is an excellent predictor for preterm birth (Mamelle *et al.* 1984), but few data sets provide the information that would allow that claim to be assessed, let alone incorporate it in a risk scoring system.

The point that needs to be made is that, irrespective of the sophistication of the methodology that went into the design of a particular risk scoring system, all of the systems contain only those markers which, for whatever reason, were considered worth recording and on which

Table 22.1 Examples of elements that are encountered as risk markers for different outcomes in formal risk scores

Authors and scoring system for	Encountered as a marker in the risk score				
	Maternal age	Parity or birth order	Single parent	Smoking	Twins
Hobel *et al.* (1973) 'Poor outcome'	YES	NO	NO	YES	YES
Haeri *et al.* (1974) Perinatal mortality	YES	YES	YES	NO	NO
Thalhammer *et al.* (1976) Birthweight <2501 g	YES	NO	YES	YES	YES
Adelstein and Fedrick (1978) Low birthweight at term	NO	YES	NO	YES	NO
Creasy *et al.* (1980) Preterm delivery	YES	NO	YES	YES	YES
Smith *et al.* (1985) 1 min Apgar 5 or less	YES	YES	NO	YES	YES
Carpenter *et al.* (1977) Sudden infant death	YES	YES	YES	YES	YES

sufficient data were available. In this sense, all scoring systems are creatures of the era during which the data source was implemented and they thus all suffer from the conceptual limitations of that time.

The risk markers that are incorporated in the various scores available vary with time: scores described before 1973 include low eosinophilic counts, low pregnandiol, maternal age above 29, increasing parity, and working mothers. Ten years later, the biological markers have changed: low eosinophilic index and pregnandiol have been replaced by inadequate plasma volume expansion (Sagen *et al.* 1984). Elements associated with an increased risk now include a low level of education (Lieberman et al. 1987), receiving welfare support (Lieberman *et al.* 1987), psychosocial stress (Newton *et al.* 1979; Newton and Hunt 1984), exposure to diethylstilboestrol (Creasy *et al.* 1980), previous termination of pregnancy (Pickering and Forbes 1985), *in vitro* fertilization (Australian In Vitro Fertilisation Collaborative Group 1985), unknown last menstrual period (Hall and Carr-Hill 1985), low haematocrit for preterm birth (Lieberman *et al.* 1987), and high haematocrit for low birthweight (Sagen *et al.* 1984). Some radical reversals have even taken place. French national survey data in 1972 and 1976, for instance, found that, within each social class, women who do not work are at increased risk of preterm birth (Goujard 1978; Mamelle *et al.* 1984; Saurel-Cubizolles *et al.* 1986), whereas scores constructed in that country (Papiernik-Berkhauer 1969; Papiernik and Kaminski 1974) and modified for the United States (Creasy *et al.* 1980; Herron et al. 1982) considered working mothers to be at higher risk of preterm birth than those who had no employment.

The elements that are incorporated in the scores are often referred to as risk factors. The tacit implication of this must be that, if only the factor could be removed or corrected, the risk of adverse outcome would no longer be present. For many of them this is certainly not true, as they are not aetiological for the outcome that they are trying to predict. At the most, they are mere markers for the likely presence of, usually unknown, aetiological mechanisms. For instance, there is no evidence that deleting a history of preterm birth in an individual woman, if at all possible, would reduce the risk in a subsequent pregnancy. In fact, the evidence points in the other way in that her own obstetric history already testifies to the fact that preterm birth occurred in the absence of a history of preterm birth. Some authors have argued that the poor performance of risk scoring systems is due precisely to the fact that too few of the risk factors are truly aetiological for the outcome that they are trying to predict (Lilford and Chard 1983; Joffe 1984). The opposite view, however, could stress that if most of the markers were truly aetiological there would be little need for elaborate risk scoring systems. Risk scoring could then better be replaced by appropriate attention to the elimination of the individual aetiological elements.

3.2 Score construction

The statistical techniques that have been employed to obtain scores have been described extensively by Peters and Golding (1985). Weighting is sometimes done on a completely arbitrary basis. The weights of all characteristics can be summed (Papiernik-Berkhauer 1969; Goodwin *et al.* 1969; Hobel *et al.* 1973; Creasy *et al.* 1980; Edwards *et al.* 1979; Smith *et al.* 1985), and the sum may then either indicate the level of risk or it may be subtracted from the perfect score result (Aubry and Nesbitt 1969).

Alternatively, weighting can depend on more or less sophisticated statistical analyses. A simple approach of this kind was used by Fedrick and Adelstein (1978). They calculated the relative risks for the various parameters from a national data set (the 1958 British Perinatal Mortality Survey; Butler and Alberman 1969). In the scoring system, the known relative risks were then multiplied to produce a composite score for each individual woman (Adelstein and Fedrick 1978). One of the possible advantages of such a system is that it allows both positive and negative points to be taken into account; for instance, women who are tall and have delivered heavy babies will see their risk score for delivering a low birthweight infant decrease below that of the population at large. This is not unlike the type of 'risk scoring' that is used by car insurance brokers and, at least in theory, it may have more potential for reducing false positive results than a system which only takes negative factors into account.

The most popular approach to weighting seems to be based on multivariate analysis techniques (Butler and Alberman 1969; Rantakalio 1969; Donahue and Wan 1973; Stembera 1977; Hobel et al. 1979; Chik and Sokol 1982; Fortney and Whitehorne 1982; Chenoweth *et al.* 1983; Guzick *et al.* 1984). Unfortunately, few of these scores have been tested prospectively and some of them are hardly usable without access to a computer on-line. However, they too have the advantage that both risk-increasing and risk-decreasing markers can be taken into account. More recent approaches have been based on the use of logistic regression models to attribute appropriate weights to the different markers (Ross *et al.* 1986), but thus far, there have been no published attempts at prospective evaluation.

3.3 Validation of the score

Not infrequently, authors of a risk scoring system have sought to validate their system by referring it back to the same set of pregnancies from which it was derived. As indicated by Newcombe and Chalmers (1981), this nearly always results in an over-optimistic assessment of its predictive power. Indeed, the parameters to be included in the score are usually chosen to maximize their discriminative power. This is bound to reflect the underlying effects and the sampling vagaries of the database from which it was constructed. Moreover, interpretation of the various 'predictive' markers (or even of the outcomes) may, as will be shown below, vary between clinicians; other individuals may thus find the instrument to be far less predictive than they were led to expect. For such scoring systems it would be more appropriate to refer to 'postdictive' markers instead of predictive factors. Unless the scoring system has been evaluated on an independent data set, the term 'validation' is also less appropriate than the term 'back-validation'. Many scoring systems have been introduced in this manner (e.g. Goodwin *et al.* 1969; Haeri *et al.* 1974; Fedrick 1976; Rumeau-Rouquette *et al.* 1974; Ross *et al.* 1986), although some have later been validated independently (Yeh *et al.* 1977; Newcombe and Chalmers 1981; Baruffi *et al.* 1984). Others (e.g. Papiernik-Berkhauer 1969; Saling 1972) were introduced before any evaluation, including back-validation, appeared to have been undertaken, and sometimes later validation primarily consisted of the introduction of updated versions with roughly the same characteristics (Giffei and Saling 1974; Klingmüller-Ahting *et al.* 1975).

4 Practical issues in the use of scoring systems

4.1 Definitions

Most scores examined include poorly defined factors. These include 'bleeding' (spotting included?; bleeding from cervix included?), 'polyhydramnios' (clinical?; on scan?; how severe?), 'low socioeconomic status' and 'very low economic status' (purely on clinical acumen?).

Further definition problems are culturally determined. 'Contractions' is the word in Francophone and German-speaking systems. In Creasy's adaptations of Papiernik's score (Papiernik-Berkhauer 1969) for the United States (Creasy *et al.* 1980) these have been replaced by 'uterine irritability'. In France, 'contractions' are found on a large scale, leading to betamimetic treatment in up to 50 per cent of all pregnancies in some centres (Bréart *et al.* 1981). It is unlikely that the physiology of the Anglo-Saxon myometrium is completely different, but highly likely that, in English-speaking countries, women who report 'contractions' are told these are tightening, niggling, etc. (Alexander and Slater 1987).

Another problem related to definitions is that of the moment and quantity (or duration) of exposure to the risk factor. Self-evident examples in pregnancy include abnormal fetal position, smoking, and drinking.

4.2 Rigidity of assigning risks

With formalized risk scoring, a woman may be assigned to the high-risk group because of rigid definitions of the risk markers, whereas a capable clinician could have assessed the situation more sensitively thanks to implicit clinical judgment. Two examples can illustrate this. In either Creasy's (Creasy *et al.* 1980; Creasy and Herron 1981) or Papiernik's (Papiernik-Berkhauer 1969; Papiernik and Kaminski 1974) scoring system for preterm delivery, a gravida 2, whose first baby was born preterm, and who experiences 'contractions' at 27 weeks, will score the same (high) risk as a gravida 4, whose first baby was born too soon, but whose two following babies were born at term, and who experiences 'contractions' at 34 weeks. Yet, clinicians will usually implicitly know that the former is at higher risk than the latter. Moreover, the longitudinal study of Bakketeig *et al.* (1979) showed that, merely on the basis of reproductive history, the first woman would have a relative risk of preterm birth that is four times as high as that of the second one.

Another example was described by JA Chalmers, as long ago as 1944, in relation to the elderly primigravida. He showed that this group, commonly listed as high-risk, could be divided in two distinct groups: those who had married young but had become elderly primigravidae because of prolonged infertility; and those who had married late in life. The first group showed the characteristics of what, at that time, was named a 'dystrophia–dystocia syndrome' including, among others, delayed onset of labour, prolonged labour, early rupture of membranes, frequent instrumental delivery and caesarean section, obesity, and toxaemia. The second group, in general, showed none of these features and instead tended to have relatively easy labours, and a low perinatal mortality in comparison to the first group.

In order to be workable, formal scoring systems need to be based on clear and sharply defined items. However, the need to dichotomize continuous variables that are as different from each other as blood pressure (how high?), smoking (how much?), and bleeding in pregnancy (how often, when and how much?), tends to impose a rigidity that will occasionally defeat the whole object of the exercise, at least with the methods that are currently employed.

4.3 Accuracy and reproducibility of scoring

As scoring systems rely heavily on past reproductive performance, socioeconomic and behavioural data, accuracy of the data is an important consideration. The quality of the data will certainly depend on the willingness of the woman to provide information on what she may consider to be sensitive issues, such as previous induced abortions, level of income, smoking, drinking habits, or housework. It will also depend on the willingness and the amount of detail with which clinicians are prepared to enquire about such sensitive issues.

There is certainly evidence that the quality of history taking may be very variable, even in departments where risk scoring is routine. A study based on Lambotte's risk score for preterm birth (Lambotte 1977), which contains several items on socioeconomic circumstances, housing conditions, etc., was conducted in Belgium by Moschert (1980). Scores were taken in a routine manner by the medical staff and subsequently by an independent 'surveyor'. The clinicians rated 6 per cent of the women as high risk, while the more thorough assessment by the surveyor classified 14 per cent of the same population as high risk. After the delivery, the surveyor went to the homes of the women who had delivered before 37 completed weeks of gestation to conduct a further assessment. At their antenatal assessment, only 15 per cent of these women had attained a very high risk score, but the retrospective scoring postpartum showed 50 per cent to belong to this category.

The under-rating was systematically related to poor recording of socioeconomic data, such as type of work, stairs in the house, hours taken to reach work, etc. This field assessment of risk scoring by Moschert (1980) is certainly in agreement with reports by Hall and Chng (1982) that experienced clinicians often fail to note significant features of obstetric histories.

4.4 Time needed for scoring

Apart from the still small number of antenatal clinics where details of each pregnant woman are referred interactively to a computer (an approach which remains unevaluated), scoring is done by a busy clinician, with pen and paper. To be feasible, there should be not too many questions, values should be restricted to integers, and addition is preferable to multiplication of risk markers, as illustrated in Table 22.2.

Fortney and Whitehorne (1982), for their score, compared addition and multiplication of the scores and found comparable predictive values for both.

Some score-inventors have specifically tried to compact their scores. Edwards *et al.* (1979), for instance, stated that the time required to complete the sheet did not exceed 20 seconds, while Hobel's scoring system required about 5 minutes and the use of a reference dictionary. Jones *et al.* (1988) compared a 47-marker score with a simplified 19-marker score, and found that the simplified tool could be used with a predictive success at least equal to that of the more complex tool.

4.5 Timing of scoring and effect of reassessment during pregnancy

There are large differences between the various scoring systems in respect of the duration of pregnancy at which they are implemented and of the number of assessments made.

From a practical point of view, an ideal scoring system should not be time-consuming and should allow assignment to a risk group in time for appropriate care to be scheduled. However, reassessment allows the inclusion of complications appearing in the current pregnancy. While alarming signs or abnormal test results allow the risk to be upgraded in some women, their non-occurrence may lead to a shading down of the level of risk in others. In the evaluation of Creasy's system (Creasy *et al.* 1980), for instance, of the 59 women who actually delivered preterm, only 26 had been classified high risk on initial evaluation, but 38 had been assigned to the high risk group by the end of the 28th week of pregnancy (Creasy *et al.* 1980). Re-

Table 22.2 Example of calculating the level of risk using different types of scoring systems

Characteristics of the woman	Marks given in the scores of		
	Fedrick (1976)	Edwards *et al.* (1979)	Lambotte (1977)
One previous stillbirth	1.1	5	–
One previous baby <2000 g	2.5	1	5
Mild hypertension	0.8	2	2
Non-smoker	0.8	–	–
Threatened miscarriage	1.7	–	4
Height 150 cm	1.5	–	3
Weight 49.5 kg	2.1	2	–
Late booking	–	2	–
Non-white	–	1	–
Total score	9.4	13	17
Score obtained by	multiplication	addition	addition
Memorization of values	difficult	easy	easy
High-risk cut-off	4	11	11

evaluation at 28 weeks thus resulted in a 45 per cent improvement in prediction. Again, little is known, in respect of other scores, about the benefits of re-evaluation; Lambotte's score (Lambotte 1977) requires re-evaluation, including cervical assessment, at each antenatal visit; at the opposite extreme, Hobel's system (Hobel *et al.* 1973) requires women to be scored only once. The utility of these arbitrary and opposite approaches needs further evaluation if scoring is to be assessed properly.

Obviously, scoring systems will perform better at least in assessing the risk, though not necessarily in offering possibilities or opportunities to influence the level of risk, if they are implemented late in pregnancy or if they allow for readjustment during pregnancy. This leads to the paradoxical situation, however, that the best and most precise risk prediction is made at a time when there is no further need for it, whereas the much more necessary early identification is notoriously imprecise.

4.6 Cut-off level

As in other tests (see Chapter 3), the clinical accuracy of the scoring system will depend on the prevalence of the condition in the population screened and on the cut-off point used. This is abundantly illustrated in Table 22.3. In Fedrick's score (Fedrick 1976), for instance, the relation is almost linear; by setting the cut-off point at 1 per cent of the population, 11 per cent of preterm low birthweight babies are detected. However, this proportion is doubled by setting the cut-off point at 3 per cent, and trebled if it is set at 6 per cent.

This concept is at the back of the term 'medium risk', which has been arbitrarily included in a few scores: e.g. those of Papiernik (Papiernik-Berkhauer 1969; Papiernik 1984a), Lambotte (1977) and Creasy *et al.* (1980). Baruffi *et al.* (1984) applied Hobel's score (Hobel *et al.* 1973) retrospectively to 1600 women in two maternity units in Baltimore, and found that adding a 'medium risk' category provided a clearer understanding of the association between risk and outcome. This is not a situation that is peculiar to risk scoring systems and it has been clearly demonstrated for several tests, including, for instance, the assessment of antepartum cardiotocography (Keirse and Trimbos 1980, 1981; see also Chapter 3).

Table 22.3 Relation between the cut-off points used (percentage of women considered to be at high risk) and the sensitivity and specificity of a scoring system for preterm birth using both simple addition of factors and logistic regression analysis (data from Ross *et al.* (1986); 6.4 per cent prevalence of preterm birth)

Type of scoring		Per cent considered high risk	Sensitivity	Specificity
Number of 'risk factors' present	1	48.1	66.6	53.1
	2	16.0	37.1	85.3
	3	4.7	16.1	96.0
	4	1.6	6.3	98.7
	5	0.4	2.0	99.7
	6	0.2	1.0	99.9
Logistic Scoring System		33.0	55.6	68.4
		22.0	46.4	79.5
		15.0	39.7	86.2

It is clear that most of the risk scoring systems currently in use aim to identify the few individuals who are likely to experience an adverse outcome of pregnancy from among the large majority of apparently healthy pregnant women. They do not, in general, try to single out those who are at the other side of the spectrum and whose chances of a good outcome of pregnancy are so excellent that they are unlikely to be improved by whatever obstetrics as a medical discipline can offer them. Although many scoring systems would allow the construction of medium risk categories, most authors do not concentrate on delineating individuals at extremely high risk from those at extremely low risk to leave a large, residual group in between for whom the score result has little, if any, predictive value. In general, they aim to predict, as well as possible, any and all occurrences of the adverse outcome under consideration. These are important qualifiers to keep in mind when judging the performance of the various risk scoring systems reported in the literature.

5 Assessment of established scoring systems

5.1 Randomized trials

Obviously, the most powerful way to test the effectiveness of formal risk scoring systems is to mount a randomized controlled trial wherein part of the pregnant population receives care of which formal risk scoring is a component, while the remainder receive the usual antenatal care without formal risk scoring. As far as we are aware, no such trials have been reported. One appears to be ongoing in Finland (Rantakallio, personal communication). Another was mounted in France, but it failed for two reasons (Bréart 1986). First, the caregivers were so convinced of the benefit of scoring that they considered it unethical to deny scoring to part of the population, a situation which is not uncommon when established clinical convictions are at stake (see Chapter 1). Secondly, most patients in high risk groups, with factors such as toxaemia, previous preterm birth, or even poor socioeconomic circumstances, were clinically identifiable without the scoring system. As the same clinicians were caring for both groups, they found themselves unintentionally scoring the control group too and automatically 'contaminating' the two experimental groups by doing so. Theoretically, this problem can be avoided by randomly allocating women not to the same clinicians administering two types of care, but to different clinicians or hospitals each administering different types of care, but there are obviously other logistic problems attached to that approach (see Chapter 1 for a more general discussion of these issues).

5.2 Other evidence

Two studies have claimed improvement in outcome after introduction of systematic scoring, apparently without the introduction of new types of intervention. Both Papiernik (Papiernik-Berkhauer 1977) in France and Lambotte (1977) in Belgium reported that, after introduction of scoring, preterm births decreased in their departments. They attributed this improvement to better selection of those women who required treatment, and to better 'systematization of interventions'.

It is important to realize, however, that the fact that no new types of intervention were introduced does not mean that intervention continued at a similar level. For instance, it has been reported that the introduction of Papiernik's formalized risk scoring resulted in an increase in the incidence of cervical cerclage from 5 up to 18 per cent of all pregnant women (Lazar *et al.* 1978, 1979). There is some evidence that other preventive interventions are also applied on a far wider scale with than without risk scoring. A comparison of practice in Belgium and The Netherlands, for instance, showed that widespread use of formal risk scoring for preterm birth in Belgium was associated with a significantly greater prophylactic use of tocolytic drugs (Keirse 1984b), although opinions about these drugs were otherwise similar in the two countries (Keirse 1984a).

Interestingly, Papiernik *et al.* (1985) attributed most of the reduction in the incidence of preterm birth that was achieved with their scoring and prevention programme to a decrease in the incidence of preterm birth among the low and medium risk rather than among the high risk women. A further factor, which they considered to be instrumental in reducing the incidence of preterm birth, was a general decrease in the incidence of strong risk factors in the population of pregnant women (Papiernik *et al.* 1985). Although the authors felt that their prevention policy had played a great part in the overall reduction of preterm birth rates, little of that was achieved in the women scored to be at high risk.

In the United States, Herron *et al.* (1982) also reported a dramatic reduction in the incidence of preterm birth following adoption of Papiernik's scoring system offering mainly telephone consultation, regular visits, adequate information, as well as constant reassurance and moral support as the added intervention. However, this claim, too, is based on comparison with historical controls in their own institution and data in an affiliated institution in which no scoring was used. It is not entirely clear what the effect of formal scoring may have been on other types of appropriate or superfluous intervention. Pavelka *et al.* (1980) claimed a 50 per cent reduction in preterm births in women on whom they used Thalammer's score. However, 61 per cent of the 121 women with a high score received outpatient 'treatment' with tocolytic drugs, 52 per cent had a cervical suture inserted, 5 per cent even had a second suture inserted, and 29 per cent were admitted to hospital for other reasons than these mentioned here. Moreover, the control group consisted of 41 women who refused the offer to attend a special clinic for that intensive prenatal care, indicating, once more, the difficulty of interpreting such results outside the clean framework of a controlled trial.

It is clear that assessment of the value of formal risk scoring in clinical practice is besieged by the problem that it is virtually never introduced as a single measure. Usually, its introduction entails a whole series of changes, particularly in the group of women considered to be at high risk of the outcome that is being screened for. This was recently emphasized by Lumley (1988),

Table 22.4 Interventions that have accompanied formal risk scoring in prevention programmes for preterm birth (adapted from Lumley 1988)

Risk assessment
Education of
  Staff
  Patients
  Public
Advice
  Reduce paid work
  Reduce housework and child care
  Reduce smoking
  Reduce stress
  Reduce travel, commuting, moving house
  Reduce/stop sexual activity
  Improve nutrition
  Bed rest at home
Self-monitoring of uterine activity
Antenatal care
  Increased frequency of contact
  Continuity of care (single caregiver)
  Facilitated access to hospital
Support systems
  Home visiting nurses/midwives
  Home help
  Family help
  Social worker assignment
  Stress management classes
Specific obstetric interventions
  Regular cervical examination
  Cervical suture
  Bed rest in hospital
Drug treatment with
  Progestogens
  Betamimetics
  Calcium antagonists

who compiled an impressive list of co-interventions that have accompanied the introduction of risk scoring for preterm birth (Table 22.4). While this level of co-intervention makes it difficult to evaluate the merits and value of the scoring system as such, the problem should not be exaggerated beyond proportion. Indeed, if scoring systems aim to confer benefit to individual women and babies, and we assume this to be their main purpose, it may be sufficient to demonstrate conclusively that the women and babies exposed to them do indeed benefit from that approach. The question of whether the same benefit could also be derived from another system of antenatal care that obviates the need for formal risk scoring is, of course, legitimate, but this would become a question of the second order, if and when formal risk scoring would have been demonstrated to be beneficial.

5.3 Test properties of the risk scores

Tables 22.5 to 22.8 review the data of various scoring systems used to screen for increased risk of perinatal mortality (Table 22.5), low birthweight (Table 22.6), preterm birth (Table 22.7), and low Apgar score at birth (Table 22.8), all as defined by the respective authors. Our aim in compiling these tables has been to present as comprehensive an account as possible of published scoring systems aimed at prospective and pragmatic use in clinical practice. The tables also include some reports of retrospective analyses, but with a lesser degree of completeness.

The tables provide data on the size of the population included in the various reports and on the prevalence of the adverse outcome(s) under consideration in that particular population. Data are also provided on the number of items included in the various scores; on the type of analysis (arbitrary, based on relative risks or other statistical analyses) that was used for weighting of the various items; on the time in pregnancy when the score was applied; and on the number of times that scores were calculated during pregnancy (single or repeat, i.e. one-time or adjusted scoring). The tables further indicate the sensitivity, specificity and positive and negative predictive values (see Chapter 3) obtained with these scores in the various populations studied.

The sensitivity of the scoring systems was strongly related to the type of outcome that was being predicted. For perinatal mortality, a rare occurrence (low prevalence), sensitivity ranged between 65 and 90 per cent, while for low birthweight and preterm birth it ranged between 10 and 90 per cent. Whatever the type of outcome, specificity was nearly always higher than sensitivity, mostly ranging between 70 and 95 per cent.

The positive predictive value, however, was generally very poor, an observation that is not uncommon in screening tests (see Chapter 3). Depending on the cut-off point and the test chosen, only between 10 and 30 per cent of the women who were allocated to the high risk group, actually experienced the adverse outcome for which the scoring system had declared them to be at high risk. On the other hand, between 20 and 50 per cent of the mothers, who delivered preterm or low birthweight infants, had low-risk scores.

5.4 Difference between arbitrary and calculated scores

The tables also show that the predictive power of the scoring systems was more or less independent of the manner in which they were constructed and, in particular, of whether weighting had been achieved by arbitrary means or by more advanced statistical analyses. Surprisingly, arbitrary scores often performed best indicating that, at least for the moment, computer-generated risk scores are not superior to those that can be created by experienced obstetricians.

The most illustrative example of this was found in the study of Ross *et al.* (1986), who used a linear logistic regression model to assign weights to the various parameters that were incorporated in their risk scoring system for 'prematurity'. Ross *et al.* (1986) believed their logistic scoring system to be optimal in assigning the appropriate weights to the various risk markers. However, when women with any two or more risk markers (identified by simple chi-square analysis) were considered to be at high risk, 16 per cent would be selected as at high risk in their population, in which the prevalence of 'prematurity' was 6.4 per cent (Table 22.3). The sensitivity and specificity with this 16 per cent cut-off was respectively 37 and 85 per cent, which is nearly identical to the 39 and 86 per cent achieved with a logistic scoring that would select 15 per cent of the women to be at high risk (Table 22.3).

The lack of marked differences between the performance of the arbitrary and the rather more sophisticated scores is in agreement with conclusions reached by Lilford and Chard (1983), who examined the possibility of using established statistical methods for the calculation of precise risk estimates for use in formal decision analysis. They concluded that there are two insuperable limitations, at least for the present. First, the current data bases are inadequate, both in the numbers of women entered and, as mentioned previously, in the choice and quantity of items entered for each pregnancy. Second, many risk markers are largely interdependent, but as the extent of the dependence is unknown, classical methods for combining risk markers are not easily applied. This problem of interdependent risk factors was also addressed by Chenoweth *et al.* (1983) with regard to the risk of preterm labour. Twenty-one variables were investigated by the mathematical technique of path analysis and nine direct and independent precursors of preterm labour were identified. Chenoweth *et al.* (1983) suggested that other

Table 22.5 Scoring systems for the prediction of perinatal mortality

Authors and year	No. of women	% Prevalence	Time of scoring*	No. of times scored	No. of items in score	Type† of score	Cut-off (% at risk)	Sensitivity	Specificity	Positive predictive value	Negative predictive value
Akthar and Seghal (1980)	1224	1.9	ANC	1	27	ARB	12	40	85	7	97
Casson and Sennett (1984)	266	1.8	ANC	1–4	27	ARB	61	40	38	1	95
Edwards *et al.* (1979)	2085	3.4	ANC	2	67	ARB	47	88	54	6	99
Goodwin *et al.* (1969)	936	15.3	NA	NA	27	ARB	14	77	97	NA	NA
Haeri *et al.* (1974)	7912	2.6	ANC	1	36	ARB	29	49	69	4	98
							22	40	78	5	98
Haliday *et al.* (1980)	1268	2.4	ANC	1	36	ARB	62	67	75	6	99
							26	49	72	5	98
Hobel *et al.* (1973)	738	3.4	ANC	4	91	ARB	34	76	67	7	99
McCarthy *et al.* (1982)	230,585	1.2	last week	1	16	SA	10	38	89	4	99
Mohapatra (1982)	396	10.6	last week	1	8	ARB	21	80	86	40	97
Morrison and Olsen (1979)	16,733	1.9	36	2	26	ARB	19	69	82	7	99
Nesbitt and Aubry (1969)	997	3.0	ANC	1	51	ARB	29	43	70	4	97
Rantakallio (1969)	11,931	2.4	24–28	1	43	SA	14	30	87	5	98
Rumeau-Rouquette *et al.* (1974)	4441	1.0	<16	1	17	SA	4	25	96	9	99
Sokol *et al.* (1977)	1275	1.8	ANC	NA	91	ARB	49	92	52	3	99
Wilson and Sill (1973)	298	17.0	ANC	1	51	ARB	50	46	50	16	82

* Weeks of gestation; ANC = at first antenatal visit; NA = not available
† Score derived arbitrarily (ARB), from relative risk calculations (RR) or by some form of statistical analysis (SA).

Table 22.6 Scoring systems for the prediction of 'low birthweight'

Authors and year	No. of women	% Prevalence	Time of scoring*	No. of times scored	No. of items in score	Type† of score	Cut-off (% at risk)	Sensitivity	Specificity	Positive predictive value	Negative predictive value
Adelstein and Fedrick (1978)	408 + 490	2.4	28–36	1	12	RR	2.6	26	98	24	98
							1.0	15	99	36	98
							12.2	58	89	11	99
Akthar and Seghal (1980)	1224	13.0	ANC	3	27	ARB	12	39	76	20	89
							26	25	90	28	89
Fedrick (1976)	468 + 490	2.8	last week	1	10	RR	26	58	89	12	99
							46	73	55	5	98
Giffei and Saling (1974)	568	8.0	ANC	1–7	38	ARB	45	61	57	11	94
Goujard (1978)	3995	4.4	<16	1	17	SA	36	63	65	8	96
Guzick *et al.* (1984)	2864	8.8	NA	1	9	SA	24	62	79	22	NA
							12	43	90	30	NA
							2	10	98	44	NA
							1	4	99	55	NA
Kaminski *et al.* (1973)	4132	4.0	<16	1	13	SA	15	39	85	10	97
Nesbitt and Aubry (1969)	993	13.0	ANC	1	51	ARB	29	43	73	20	89
Rantakallio (1969)	11,931	4.2	24–28	1	43	SA	14	41	87	12	97
Rumeau-Rouquette *et al.* (1976)	11,105	5.0	>28	1	4	SA	20	32	79	8	96
Thalhammer *et al.* (1976)	431	4.9	24	1–3	28	ARB	NA	71	78	NA	NA
Wennergen and Karlsson (1982)	611	2.3	34	1	8	SA	7	100	96	34	100

* Weeks of gestation; ANC = at first antenatal visit; NA = not available

† Score derived arbitrarily (ARB), from relative risk calculations (RR) or by some form of statistical analysis (SA).

Table 22.7 Scoring systems for the prediction of preterm birth

Authors and year	No. of women	% Prevalence	Time of scoring*	No. of times scored	No. of items in score	Type† of score	Cut-off (% at risk)	Sensitivity	Specificity	Positive predictive value	Negative predictive value
Akthar and Seghal (1980)	1224	3.1	ANC	3	27	ARB	12	32	97	8	98
Creasy *et al.* (1980)	966	6.1	<34	1	31	ARB	28	69	74	15	97
				2			32	80	71	15	98
				1			9	44	93	29	96
				2			13	64	90	30	98
Fedrick (1976)	468 + 480	2.8	last week	1	10	RR	26	58	89	12	99
							46	73	55	5	98
Goujard (1978)	3995	7.1	<16	1	17	SA	16	36	86	17	95
							32	57	70	13	96
Kaminski *et al.* (1973)	4008	8.0	<16	1	13	SA	14	30	87	17	93
							34	59	67	14	95
Kaminski and Papiernik (1974)	153 + 222	case control	32	1	30	ARB	case	54	83	NA	NA
						SA	control	66	86	NA	NA
Lambotte (1977)	300	7.0	ANC	1–9	24	ARB	22	76	82	24	93
							6	43	97	50	96
Main *et al.* (1987)	480	15.0	<18	1	25	ARB	31	26	80	18	86
Nesbitt and Aubry (1969)	1001	6.5	ANC	1	51	ARB	29	47	71	16	95
							69	78	31	7	95
Rantakallio (1969)‡	11,536	1.2	24–28	1	43	SA	NA[6]	39	86	NA	NA
Rumeau-Rouquette *et al.* (1976)	1105	8.8	>28	1	4	SA	20	34	80	14	93
Ross *et al.* (1986)	8240	6.4	Birth	1	22	SA	33	56	68	NA	NA
						SA	22	46	80	NA	NA
						SA	15	40	86	NA	NA
						RR	33	56	68	NA	NA
						RR	16	37	85	NA	NA
						RR	4.7	16	96	NA	NA

* Weeks of gestation; ANC = at first antenaval visit; NA = not available or not applicable

† Score derived arbitrarily (ARB), from relative risk calculations (RR) or by some form of statistical analysis (SA).

‡ Preterm in this study refers to less than 32 weeks' gestation.

Table 22.8 Scoring systems for the prediction of a low Apgar score at birth

Authors and year	No. of women	% Prevalence	Time of scoring*	No. of times scored	No. of items in score	Cut-off (% at risk)	Sensitivity	Specificity	Positive predictive value	Negative predictive value
Akthar and Seghal (1980)	1224	8	ANC	3	27†	12	36	90	21	95
Bompiani *et al.* (1972)	1000	NA	ANC	1	77	NA	24	94	NA	NA
Coopland *et al.* (19770	5459	NA	last week	1	24	NA	NA	NA	13	NA
Goodwin *et al.* (1985)	792	3	NA	NA	27†	8	57	93	18	99
Smith *et al.* (1985)	100	13	last week	1	28	27	68	79	41	80
Yeh *et al.* (1977)	266	NA	last week	1	27†	28	36	88	NA	NA

* All scores included in the table gave arbitrary weights to the items included in the score; ANC = at first antenatal visit; NA = not available.
† Based on the score of Goodwin *et al.* (1969).

predictive factors have their impact through one of these nine key variables (antepartum haemorrhage, poor antenatal attendance, previous delivery of a small baby, multiple pregnancy, proteinuria, grand multiparity, cervical suture, low maternal weight, and a history of bleeding before 20 weeks).

While Chenoweth *et al.* (1983) and Lilford and Chard (1983) concluded similarly that mathematical risk prediction formulae are no better than the non-formalized risk prediction of the experienced clinician, they offered opposite explanations for this. Chenoweth *et al.* (1983) believes that this is because only 9 factors are of importance (i.e. risk scores comprise too many markers), while Lilford and Chard (1983) envisage that truly massive data banks are necessary to allow computing of adequate risk scores. The paradox could be more apparent than real, if massive data banks would allow the selection of a limited but adequate number of risk markers. There is, however, no evidence as yet that this goal is in sight.

5.5 Difference in test performance in different populations

Used on an individual basis, these pregnancy risk scoring systems are thus disappointing. Yet, it is noteworthy that the same tests, when applied to different populations, showed very different results, not only in terms of predictive value, which is to be expected, but also in terms of sensitivity and specificity, which are meant to be far less influenced by prevalence. This effect is seen, for instance, in Table 22.7 with adaptations of Papiernik's original score (Papiernik-Berkhauer 1969) used by Papiernik's team (Kaminski and Papiernik 1974), Lambotte (1977), Creasy *et al.* (1980) and Main *et al.* (1987).

There are several possible explanations for this difference in the performance of scoring systems in different populations. The most obvious relates to the time in pregnancy when scoring is performed and to whether scoring is performed only once or is repeated later in pregnancy. Possible differences in the proportion of parous and nulliparous women form another explanation, particularly since most scoring systems rely heavily on past reproductive performance. Markers with the highest positive predictive value may be more prevalent in one population than in another, or alternatively the significance of a particular marker may vary among populations. For instance, Rush (1977) found that a history of a prior low birthweight infant was more predictive of delivery of a low birthweight infant in a subsequent pregnancy in white than in black women in the United States. These authors suggested that poor outcome in women of lower social status as opposed to those of higher social status is less likely to be influenced by inherent pathophysiological conditions than by environmental factors which would be less likely to remain constant throughout reproductive life.

A further possible explanation for the difference in performance in different populations is that some scoring systems may derive much of their power from distinguishing different socioeconomic or (under)privileged groups in the childbearing population. Main and Gabbe (1987) considered this as one of the main potential explanations for the discrepancy between their findings in a universally low-income group (Main *et al.* 1987) and those of others using the same scoring system in other populations (Creasy *et al.* 1980; Herron *et al.* 1982).

The difference in performance, however, may also be due to the poor reproducibility of risk scoring, discussed earlier.

5.6 Scoring in nulliparous and parous women

Where the performance of scoring systems has been presented separately for nulliparae and multiparae, scoring has been shown to be markedly more effective in multiparae. Only two exceptions have been reported. Both in Columbia and in Bangladesh, Fortney and Whitehorne (1982) retrospectively tested a score for perinatal mortality and low birthweight, after developing it from a random sample of hospitals in Columbia. They found 'remarkably little difference' between predictive values for nulliparae and multiparae. The same lack of difference between nulliparae and multiparae was observed by Main *et al.* (1987) who used Papiernik's score, developed in France, on a black urban population in Philadelphia.

The poor predictive value of the scoring systems for nulliparae is generally acknowledged and it is, at least in part, inherent in the choice of risk markers that are incorporated in the various scores. Indeed, many of these, and particularly those with the greatest weights, relate to characteristics of the past obstetric history, which, by definition, is absent in nulliparae. For scores which give an important weight to socioeconomic markers, mainly the score of Papiernik (Papiernik-Berkhauer 1969) and its modified version used by Lambotte (1977), no such comparisons between multiparae and nulliparae have been published apart from the study of Main *et al.* (1987) mentioned above. It is logical, however, to expect that the discriminant performance of the scores in nulliparae as compared to multiparae could be improved by attributing less weight to past reproductive history and more weight to such markers as can be assessed in nulliparae.

In Hobel's score (Hobel *et al.* 1973), for instance, out of the possible 309 points that a woman could score if she presented all of the risk markers, only 13 (4 per cent) are not related to obstetric history, pathology of pregnancy, or general disease. This is very different in Lambotte's score, though. Out of a maximum of 95 points, 43 (45 per cent) are not related to pathology of pregnancy or obstetric history. Thus, an unmarried girl of 16, who expects her first baby, comes from a very poor family, smokes heavily, lives on the top floor of a slum with no lift, works in a factory more than an hour's travel away from her home, weighs less than 45 kg, is shorter than 150 cm, and feels tired and unhappy, will not be regarded as at increased risk after scoring with Hobel's system. She will score 25 on Lambotte's score, which defines her as a very high risk patient indeed.

This is not to suggest that in Papiernik's and related scores, discrimination is not often better in multiparae than in nulliparae; it probably is. But, Hobel's score (Hobel *et al.* 1973) has been constructed in such a way that nulliparae without physical disease can only be rated as at high risk if they are outside the normal range for both weight and age. When used for a total population of pregnant women, it is clear that the performance of such scores will largely depend, not only on the prevalence of the target condition, but also on the proportion of nulliparous and parous women in the population.

6 Other considerations

6.1 Utility of scoring

It may be useful to the clinician to know which pregnancies under his or her care are likely to be plagued by an adverse outcome. To the individual woman the high risk identification is likely to be beneficial only when something can be done to either decrease the risk or reduce its consequences.

As mentioned earlier, most of the elements that are incorporated in the scores are mere markers indicating a statistical association with the outcome that is being scored for. They are not aetiological for the outcome nor do they usually represent the mechanisms by which (unknown) aetiological factors lead to that outcome. With few exceptions, intervening with the risk markers themselves during pregnancy is therefore not likely to significantly alter the likelihood that the outcome will actually occur. In addition, a large number of markers, such as parity, pregnancy weight, and height, and certainly the most powerful ones, such as past reproductive performance, cannot be altered by whatever intervention that may be applied. For the individual woman labelled as being at increased risk, both the threat of adverse outcome and the inability to change its markers may create or augment feelings of guilt and inadequacy. It would appear that the enhancement of such feelings is unlikely to improve pregnancy outcome.

Another problem is that current risk scores mainly address surrogate outcomes. Those that are commonly used at present are directed at either preterm birth or low birthweight. These outcomes are not by themselves of great relevance to mother or baby. They derive their importance mainly from the fact that they in turn constitute an element of risk for mortality, morbidity, and disability which are of far greater relevance to mother and baby. Risk scoring for preterm birth, for instance, estimates the likelihood that delivery will occur before 37 weeks. If delivery occurs at 36 weeks, the score will have shown adequate prediction, equally well as if delivery had occurred at 26 weeks; but the outcome for the infant is likely to be entirely different (see Chapter 74).

The consequence of this is that formal risk scoring and the co-interventions that accompany it can lower the incidence of the outcome that is addressed without having any impact whatsoever on the issues that are of real importance. For instance, a reduction in the rate of preterm birth from 8 to 5 per cent may appear to be a major achievement; if all of it is achieved at 34 to 36 weeks of gestation without lowering or even increasing the incidence of delivery before 32 weeks its impact on perinatal health is likely to be minimal. The reverse may occur, too; a scoring policy may have no influence on the incidence of the outcome addressed and yet have a major impact on outcomes that really matter. For instance, if implementation of a scoring system for preterm birth succeeds in postponing births that occur before 32 weeks up to 35 or 36 weeks, the incidence of the target adverse outcome will not have changed; yet, such system would undoubtedly have great potential for improving infant outcome. An even more complex situation could be present with regard to scoring for low birthweight. A shift in the birthweight distribution with a few hundred grams can markedly change the outlook for infants of 1500 to 2000 g or more without altering the incidence of low birthweight *per se*. In addition, it is likely that the outcome for some of these infants could be improved substantially by detection earlier in pregnancy followed by elective delivery earlier, and thence with a lower birthweight than would have been achieved without scoring.

The complexity of the issues involved indicates the near impossibility of assessing the utility of scoring systems outside the context of a clean clinical trial.

6.2 Ethics of formal risk scoring

It would be inappropriate not to draw attention to some of the ethical issues that are incumbent upon those who introduce formal risk scoring. How acceptable is it to ask women for details on their socioeconomic situation and note these in case records or scoring forms, which, of necessity, will be available to several individuals? Does the relationship between socioeconomic markers and pregnancy outcome and, in particular, the potential for modifying this relationship, warrant such intrusion into the privacy of the pregnant woman? How much tact, experience, and consideration is needed to obtain some of the information that is required without being unduly inquisitive?

Issues that are even more important concern the 'high risk' label that will be attached to some women. Can it be justified not to give precise information on the process and the results of scoring? If not, is it fair to impart the feeling that the woman is putting her pregnancy at risk because she married a husband with a low income, lives four floors up in an old apartment building without a lift, and travels for an hour every day to do a job that she really likes? Would it change the outcome of pregnancy if she were to exchange the husband for a rich widower, who owns a stately home in the country, where her activities would be limited to picking fresh flowers every day? Such issues may sound ridiculous to some, but clearly there is a lot more to pregnancy and to women's feelings about their pregnancy than a 'level of risk'.

It has been suggested that access to even apparently sensitive information may be of benefit to the woman. Reading 'heavy smoker' in the case notes or being aware of its effect in increasing the risk of adverse outcome, may be an incentive to stop or decrease smoking (see Chapter 16). It is difficult to imagine a similar scenario, however, for an unmarried, unemployed woman, who has had two late abortions and lives in poor housing conditions. She will score quite high, for instance on Lambotte's score (Lambotte 1977), but the most likely effects of her getting access to this information will be embarrassment for her caregiver and distress for herself. Could the mere effect of assigning a woman to a high risk group not doom her to become a loser?

7 Conclusions

7.1 Implications for current practice

In the final analysis, formal risk scoring appears to be a mixed blessing for the individual woman and her baby. The evidence that we reviewed indicates that such systems may be instrumental in providing a minimum level of care and attention in regions where pregnancy itself is not considered to be a sufficient reason to provide these (Heins *et al.* 1983). The evidence also indicates, however, that in other health care organizations risk scoring, for preterm delivery in particular, results in a profusion of interventions such as prophylactic drug 'treatment' with tocolytics and progestogens, cervical cerclage, and hospitalization in pregnancy.

In the early days of scoring, all of these interventions have been regarded as intrinsic to the 'success' of the new approach with little evidence in support of such claims. These beliefs have now largely, but not entirely, disappeared. Yet, evidence that is available on the effects of these interventions (see Chapters 38, 40 and 44) certainly does not support their use on so wide a scale as that seen in institutions and countries which rely heavily on the use of formal risk scoring. Currently, other interventions such as home monitoring of uterine contractility are being added to improve predictive values and to select women for treatment when necessary (Katz *et al.* 1986). Presently, it is incumbent upon those who favour such approaches to adequately evaluate such measures as and when they are introduced. One small trial of home monitoring of uterine contractility for preterm labour has been reported thus far (Morrison *et al.* 1987), but this will require replication in a larger population before firm conclusions can be reached.

The weakness of evidence in favour of formal risk scoring as a means to reduce adverse pregnancy outcomes has been emphasized by others (Main and Gabbe 1987; Lumley 1988); it is a constant feature of research in this area. Even authors whose commitment to this strategy is beyond doubt have repeatedly indicated that improvements in outcome have been more pronounced in women at low risk than in those judged to be at high risk and have been associated more with a lower prevalence of the classical risk markers among pregnant women than with improved detection of such markers (Papiernik *et al.* 1985).

When risk scoring is applied in clinical practice, there is a very real danger that a potential but highly imprecise risk of adverse outcome becomes replaced by the certain risk of dubious treatments and interventions, whose benefits have not been demonstrated and whose hazards are largely unknown.

As mentioned earlier, different risk scores also behave very differently in different populations. There are a large number of explanations for this. They range from the prevalence of the risk that is being screened for, through the prevalence and significance of the various markers in a particular population, up to the extent and type of co-interventions that accompany formal risk scoring in clinical practice. Whatever the true reasons for the discrepancies may be, they provide a strong case for not introducing formal risk scoring outside the context of a well-designed trial.

7.2 Implications for future research

There is an urgent need to know whether and for what populations risk scoring provides more benefit than harm. Such harm can result from unwarranted intrusion in women's private lives, from superfluous interventions and treatments, from creating unnecessary stress and anxiety, and from allocating scarce resources to areas where they are least needed. Potential benefits of risk scoring have been widely publicized, but the potential harm is hardly referred to in the current literature.

There is evidence from some observational studies (Pavelka *et al.* 1980) that women not infrequently refuse the interventionism that accompanies the use of scoring systems. The general assumption, however, appears to be that these women are misguided; not that the system itself is at fault. This, clearly, is misguided. Research to investigate women's feelings about risk assignments and the way in which it does or does not change their perception of pregnancy and childbirth may be of benefit to both the receivers and providers of care.

The introduction of formal risk scoring as a single measure is entirely unpractical. It is not realistic to assume that a clinician confronted with a figure that indicates an increased risk of adverse outcome will behave in exactly the same way as if no such figure had been provided. Neither is it realistic to assume that the awareness of being at higher than average risk will have no influence on behaviour and circumstances of the pregnant woman and her family. This has two important research consequences. First, there is a need to carefully distinguish the effects of the risk scoring itself from those of the co-interventions that either intentionally or unintentionally accompany its use. Second, unbiased evaluation of a scoring system can only be achieved when institutions or individual caregivers are randomly assigned to provide one or the other type of care, or when women are randomly allocated to teams using or not using formal risk scoring as part of their approach. Such research will be difficult to mount unless collaboration among various centres can be assured.

Current data from centres where formal risk scoring is part of standard antenatal care indicate that a large number of interventions are applied with a frequency that is considerably higher than that found elsewhere. In such centres there would seem to be a need for randomized comparisons in order to establish whether the same or better 'success' rates cannot be achieved with fewer procedures, fewer interventions, and less interference with the daily life of pregnant women and their families.

References

Adelstein P, Fedrick J (1978). Antenatal identification of women at increased risk of being delivered of a low birth weight infant at term. Br J Obstet Gynaecol, 85: 8–11.

Akthar J, Seghal N (1980). Prognostic value of a prepartum and intrapartum risk-scoring method. South Med J, 73: 411–414.

Alberman E (1974). Factors influencing perinatal wastage. Clin Obstet Gynaecol, 1: 1–15.

Alexander S, Slater C (1987). Laboring under linguistic delusions: The impact of linguistic factors in international studies of preterm labour. Language Communication, 7: 179–185.

Alexander S, Yudkin P, Papiernik E, Schwers J, Chalmers I (in preparation) (1988). Policy of prevention of preterm birth: Comparison of outcomes in three European hospitals.

Apgar VA (1953). A proposal for a new method of evaluation of the new born infant. Curr Res Anesth Analg, 32: 260–267.

Aubry R, Nesbitt R (1969). High risk obstetrics. I: Perinatal outcome in relation to a broadened approach to obstetric care for patients at special risk. Am J Obstet Gynecol, 105: 241–247.

Australian In Vitro Fertilisation Collaborative Group (1985). High incidence of preterm births and baby losses in pregnancy after in vitro fertilisation. Br Med J, 291: 1160–1163.

Bakketeig LS, Hoffman HJ, Harley EE (1979). The tendency to repeat gestational age and birth weight in successive births. Am J Obstet Gynecol, 135: 1086–1103.

Baruffi G, Strobino DM, Dellinger WS (1984). Definitions of high risk in pregnancy and evaluation of their predictive validity. Am J Obstet Gynecol, 148: 781–786.

Baumgarten K, Grüber W (1974). Tokolyse-index. In: Perinatale Medizin. Dudenhausen JW, Saling E (eds). Stuttgart: Thieme Verlag, pp 58–59.

Bishop EH (1964). Pelvic scoring for elective induction. Obstet Gynecol, 24: 266–268.

Bompiani A, Romanini C, Oliva GC, Palla GP, Liverani A (1972). Selezione di alcuni indici di 'alto riescho perinatale' e valutazione della loro attendibilita. Ann Ostet Ginecol Med Perinat, 43: 624–638.

Bréart G (1986). Evaluation de l'efficacité de la surveillance prénatale et d'autres actions. In: Prévention de la Naissance Prématuré. Nouveaux Objectifs et Nouvelles Pratiques des Soins Prénataux. Papiernik E, Bréart G, Spira N (eds). Paris: Editions INSERM, pp 101–116.

Bréart G, Goujard J, Blondel B, Maillard F, Chavigny C, Sureau C, Rumeau-Rouquette C (1981). A comparison of two policies of antenatal supervision for the prevention of prematurity. Int J Epidemiol, 10: 241–244.

Butler NR, Alberman ED (eds) (1969). Perinatal Problems. Edinburgh: Churchill Livingstone.

Carpenter RG, Gardner A, McWeeny PM, Emery JL (1977). Multistage scoring system for identifying infants at risk of unexpected death. Arch Dis Child, 52: 606–612.

Casson RI, Sennett ES (1984). Prenatal risk assessment and obstetric care in a small rural hospital: Comparison with guidelines. Can Med Assoc J, 130: 1311–1315.

Chalmers JA (1944). The Elderly Primigravid. University of Edinburgh: MD thesis.

Chalmers I (1985). Short, Black, Baird, Himsworth and social class differences in fetal and neonatal mortality rates. Br Med J, 2: 231–232.

Chenoweth JN, Esler EJ, Chang A, Keeping JD, Morrison J (1983). Understanding preterm labour: The use of path analysis. Austral NZ Obstet Gynaecol, 23: 199–203.

Chik I, Sokol RJ (1982). Risk—Intervention—Outcome. A model for the evaluation of an on-line computer generated running risk score for intrapartum fetal monitoring. Acta Obstet Gynecol Scand (Suppl) 109: 96–98.

Committee assessing alternative birth settings (1982). Risk

assessment. In: Research Issues in the Assessment of Birth. Washington DC: National Academy Press, pp 45–55.

Committee to study the prevention of low birth weight (1985). Screening for obstetric risk. In: Preventing Low Birthweight. Washington DC: National Academy Press, pp 76–94.

Coopland AT, Peddle LJ, Baskett TF, Rollwagen R, Simpson A, Parker E (1977). A simplified antepartum high-risk pregnancy scoring form: Statistical analysis of 5459 cases. Can Med Assoc J, 116: 999–1001.

Creasy RK, Herron MA (1981). Prevention of preterm birth. Seminars Perinatol, 5: 295–302.

Creasy RK, Gummer BA, Liggins GC (1980). System for predicting spontaneous preterm birth. Obstet Gynecol, 55: 692–695.

Donahue C, Wan T (1973). Measuring obstetric risks of prematurity: A preliminary analysis of neonatal death. Am J Obstet Gynecol, 116: 911–915.

Edwards E, Barrada I, Tatreau RW, Hakanson EY (1979). A simplified antepartum risk-scoring system. Obstet Gynecol, 54: 237–240.

Essed GGM, Eskes TKAB, Jongsma HW (1978). A randomized trial of two betamimetic drugs for the treatment of threatening early labor. Eur J Obstet Gynecol Reprod Biol, 8: 341–348.

Fabre H (1913). Traité d'Obstétrique. Paris: Masson, pp 32–39.

Fedrick J (1976). Antenatal identification of women at high risk of spontaneous preterm birth. Br J Obstet Gynaecol, 83: 351–354.

Fedrick J, Adelstein P (1978). Factors associated with low birth weight of infants delivered at term. Br J Obstet Gynaecol, 85: 1–7.

Fedrick J, Anderson ABM (1976). Factors associated with spontaneous preterm birth. Br J Obstet Gynaecol, 83: 342–350.

FIGO News (1976). Lists of gynecologic and obstetrical terms and definitions. Int J Gynaecol Obstet, 14: 570–576.

Fischer WM, Stude I, Brandt H (1976). Ein Vorschlag zur Beurteilung des antepartalen Kardiotokogramms. Z Geburtsh Perinatol, 180: 117–123.

Fortney J, Whitehorne AM (1982). The development of an index of high risk pregnancy. Am J Obstet Gynecol, 143: 501–508.

Giffei JM, Saling E (1974). First results and experiences with our prematurity and dysmaturity prevention program (PDP-Program). J Perinat Med, 2: 45–53.

Golding J, Peters TJ (1985). What else do SIDS risk prediction scores predict? Early Hum Dev, 12: 247–260.

Goodwin JW, Dunn JT, Thomas BW (1969). Antepartum identification of the fetus at risk. Can Med Assoc J, 101: 458–464.

Goujard J (1978). Discussion about risk factors. In: Perinatal Medicine, Sixth European Congress, Vienna. Thalhammer O, Baumgarten K, Pollak A (eds). Stuttgart: Georg Thieme, pp 150–153.

Grimes L, Mehl L, Mcrae J, Peterson G. (1983). Phenomenological risk screening for child birth: Successful prospective differentiation of risk for medically low risk mothers. J Nurs Midwifery, 28: 27–30.

Guzick DS, Daikoku NH, Kaltreider DF (1984). Predictability of pregnancy outcome in preterm delivery. Obstet Gynecol, 63: 645–650.

Hack M, Breslau N (1986). Very low birth weight infants: Effects of brain growth during infancy on intelligence quotient at 3 years of age. Pediatrics, 77: 196–202.

Haeri AD, South J, Naldrett J (1974). A scoring system for identifying pregnant patients with a high risk of perinatal mortality. J Obstet Gynaecol Br Commwlth, 81: 535–538.

Haliday HL, Jones PK, Jones SL (1980). Method of screening obstetric patients to prevent reproductive wastage. Obstet Gynecol, 55: 656–661.

Hall MH, Carr-Hill RA (1985). The significance of uncertain gestation for obstetric outcome. Br J Obstet Gynaecol, 92: 452–460.

Hall M, Chng PK (1982). Antenatal care in practice. In: Effectiveness and Satisfaction in Antenatal Care. Enkin M, Chalmers I (eds). London: Spastics International Medical Publications, Heinemann Medical Books, pp 60–68.

Heins HC, Miller JM, Sear A, Goodyear N, Gardner S (1983). Benefits of a statewide high-risk perinatal program. Obstet Gynecol, 62: 294–296.

Herron MA, Katz M, Creasy RK (1982). Evaluation of a preterm birth prevention program: Preliminary report. Obstet Gynecol, 59: 452–456.

Hobel CJ, Hyvarinen MA, Okada DM, Oh W (1973). Prenatal and intrapartum high risk screening: I. Prediction of the high risk neonate. Am J Obstet Gynecol, 117: 1–9.

Hobel CJ, Youkeles L, Forsythe A (1979). Prenatal and intrapartum high risk screening: II. Risk factors reassessed. Am J Obstet Gynecol, 135: 1051–1056.

Issel EP (1979). Evaluation of various scores. In: Perinatal Medicine, Sixth European Congress, Vienna. Thalhammer O, Baumgarten K, Pollak A (eds). Stuttgart: Georg Thieme, pp 126–128.

Joffe M (1984). Association of syndromes predisposing to low birth weight. Early Hum Dev, 10: 107–113.

Jones MM, Meglen MC, Heins HC, Ingram DE, Padgett S (1988). Evaluation of low birth-weight risk assessment tools in South Carolina. Med Care, 26: 504–509.

Kaminski M, Papiernik E (1974). Multifactorial study of the risk of prematurity at 32 weeks of gestation. II: A comparison between an empirical prediction and a discriminant analysis. J Perinat Med, 2: 37–44.

Kaminski M, Goujard J, Rumeau-Rouquette C (1973). Prediction of low birthweight and prematurity by a multiple regression analysis with maternal characteristics known since the beginning of the pregnancy. Int J Epidemiol, 2: 195–204.

Katz M, Newman RB, Gill PJ (1986). Assessment of uterine activity in ambulatory patients at high risk of preterm labor and delivery. Am J Obstet Gynecol, 154: 44–47.

Keirse MJNC (1979). Epidemiology of pre-term labour. In: Human Parturition. New Concepts and Developments. Keirse MJNC, Anderson ABM, Bennebroek Gravenhorst J (eds). The Hague: Leiden University Press, pp 219–234.

Keirse MJNC (1984a). A survey of tocolytic drug treatment in preterm labour. Br J Obstet Gynaecol, 91: 424–430.

Keirse MJNC (1984b). Betamimetic drugs in the prophylaxis of preterm labour: Extent and rationale of their use. Br J Obstet Gynaecol, 91: 431–437.

Keirse MJNC, Kanhai HHH (1981): An obstetrical viewpoint on preterm birth with particular reference to perinatal morbidity and mortality. In: Aspects of Perinatal Morbidity. Huisjes HJ (ed). Groningen: Universitaire Boekhandel Nederland, pp 1–35.

Keirse MJNC, Trimbos JB (1980). Assessment of antepartum cardiotocograms in high-risk pregnancy. Br J Obstet Gynaecol, 87: 261–269.

Keirse MJNC, Trimbos JB (1981). Clinical significance of suspicious antepartum cardiotocograms: A study of normal and high-risk pregnancies. Br J Obstet Gynaecol, 88: 739–746.

Klingmüller-Ahting U, Saling E, Giffei J (1975). Frühgeburt und intrauterine Mangelentwicklung. Gefahren—Vermeidung—Ergebnisse. Gynäkologe, 8: 186–197.

Lambotte R (1977). Discussion. In: Pre-term Labour. Proceedings of the Fifth Study Group of the Royal College of Obstetricians and Gynaecologists. Anderson A, Beard R, Brudenell JM, Dunn PM (eds). London: Royal College of Obstetricians and Gynaecologists, pp 40–41.

Lazar P, Dreyfus J, Papiernik E, Winisdoerfer G, Colli D, Gueguen S (1978). Prédiction de la prématurité a des fins préventives. Arch Fr Pediatr, 35: 19–26.

Lazar P, Servent B, Dreyfus J, Gueguen S, Papiernik E (1979). Comparison of two successive policies of cervical cerclage for the prevention of pre-term birth. Eur J Obstet Gynecol Reprod Biol, 9: 307–312.

Leon J (1973). High risk pregnancy: Graphic representation of the maternal and fetal risks. Am J Obstet Gynecol, 117: 497–504.

Lieberman E, Ryan KJ, Manson RR, Schoenbaum SC (1987). Risk factors accounting for racial differences in the rate of premature birth. New Engl J Med, 317: 743–748.

Lilford RJ, Chard T (1983). Problems and pitfalls of risk assessment in antenatal care. Br J Obstet Gynaecol, 90: 507–510.

Lloyd GER, (ed). (1983). Hippocratic Writings. Harmondsworth: Penguin Classics, pp 214, 224–226.

Lumley J (1987). Prediction of preterm birth. In: Prematurity. Yu VYH, Wood EC (eds). Edinburgh: Churchill Livingstone, pp 43–53.

Lumley J (1988). The prevention of preterm birth: Unresolved problems and work in progress. Austral Paediatr J, 24: 101–111.

Macfarlane A, Mugford M (1984). Birth Counts. Statistics of Pregnancy and Childbirth. London: Her Majesty's Stationery Office, pp 6–8.

Main DM, Gabbe SG (1987). Risk scoring for preterm labor: Where do we go from here? Am J Obstet Gynecol, 157: 789–793.

Main DM, Richardson D, Gabbe SG, Strong S, Weller SC (1987). Prospective evaluation of a risk scoring system for predicting preterm delivery in black inner city women. Obstet Gynecol, 69: 61–66.

Mamelle N, Laumon B, Lazar P (1984). Prematurity and occupational activity during pregnancy. Am J Epidemiol, 119: 309–322.

McCarthy BJ, Schulz KF, Terry JS (1982). Identifying neonatal risk factors and predicting neonatal deaths in Georgia. Am J Obstet Gynecol, 142: 557–562.

Mohapatra SS (1982). Simplified scoring system for identification of high risk births. Evaluation in a rural community. Indian Pediatr, 19: 913–915.

Morrison I, Olsen J (1979). Perinatal mortality and antepartum risk scoring. Obstet Gynecol, 53: 362–366.

Morrison JC, Martin JN, Maryin RW, Gookin KS, Wiser WL (1987). Prevention of preterm birth by ambulatory assessment of uterine activity. A randomized study. Am J Obstet Gynecol, 156: 536–543.

Moschert A (1980). Un bilan rétrospectif et prospectif d'utilisation du coefficient de risque d'accouchement prématuré. Mémoire de fin d'études. Université de Liège.

Nesbitt R, Aubry R (1969). High risk obstetrics. II: Value of semiobjective grading system in identifying the vulnerable group. Am J Obstet Gynecol, 103: 972–985.

Newcombe RG, Chalmers I (1981). Assessing the risk of preterm labor. In : Preterm Labour. Elder MG, Hendricks CH (eds). London: Butterworths, pp 47–60.

Newcombe R, Fedrick J, Chalmers I (1977). Antenatal identification of patients 'at risk' of pre-term labour. In: Preterm Labour. Proceedings of the Fifth Study Group of the Royal College of Obstetricians and Gynaecologists. Anderson A, Beard R, Brudenell JM, Dunn PM (eds). London: Royal College of Obstetricians and Gynaecologists, pp 17–28.

Newton RW, Hunt LP (1984). Psychosocial stress in pregnancy and its relation to low birth weight. Br Med J, 288: 1191–1194.

Newton RW, Webster PAC, Binu PS, Maskrey N, Phillips AB (1979). Psychosocial stress in pregnancy and its relation to the onset of premature labour. Br Med J, 2: 411–413.

Nuovo J (1985). Clinical application of a high risk scoring system on a family practice obstetric service. J Family Practice, 20: 139–144.

Papiernik-Berkhauer E (1969). Coefficient de risque d'accouchement prématuré (C.R.A.P.). Presse Méd, 77: 793–794.

Papiernik-Berkhauer E (1977). Discussion. In: Pre-term Labour. Proceedings of the Fifth Study Group of the Royal College of Obstetricians and Gynaecologists. Anderson A, Beard R, Brudenell JM, Dunn PM (eds). London: Royal College of Obstetricians and Gynaecologists, pp 29–39.

Papiernik E (1984a). Prediction of the preterm baby. Clin Obstet Gynaecol, 11: 315–336.

Papiernik E (1984b). Proposals for a programmed prevention policy of preterm birth. Clin Obstet Gynecol, 27: 614–635.

Papiernik E, Kaminski M (1974). Multifactorial study of the risk of prematurity at 32 weeks of gestation. I: A study of the frequency of 30 predictive characteristics. J Perinat Med, 2: 30–36.

Papiernik E, Bouyer J, Dreyfus J (1985). Risk factors for preterm births and results of a prevention policy. The Hagenau Perinatal Study 1971–1982. In: Preterm Labour and its Consequences. Beard RW, Sharp F (eds). London: Royal College of Obstetricians and Gynaecologists, pp 15–20.

Pavelka R, Riss P, Parschalk O, Reinold E (1980). Practical experiences in the prevention of prematurity using Thalhammer's score. J Perinat Med, 8: 100–108.

Peters T, Golding J (1985). Assessing risk assessment. In: Advances in Perinatal Medicine, Vol. 4. Milunsky A, Friedman EA, Gluck L (eds). New York: Plenum Medical Books, pp 235–266.

Pickering RM, Forbes JF (1985). Risks of preterm delivery and small-for-gestational age infants following abortion: A population study. Br J Obstet Gynaecol, 92: 1106–1112.

Rantakallio P (1969). Groups at risk in low birth weight infants and perinatal mortality. Acta Paediatr Scand (Suppl) 193: 5–71.

Ross MG, Hobel CJ, Bragonier JR, Bear MB, Bemis RL (1986). A simplified risk scoring system for prematurity. Am J Perinatol, 3: 339–344.

Rudelstorfer B, Kucera H, Pavelka R, Reinold E (1976). Erste Erfahrungen und Ergebnisse mit dem PDP-Programm nach Saling. Z Geburtsh Perinatol, 180: 251–257.

Rumeau-Rouquette C, Kaminski M, Goujard J (1974). Prediction of perinatal mortality in early pregnancy. J Perinat Med, 2: 196–207.

Rumeau-Rouquette C, Bréart G, Deniel M, Hennequin JF, du Mazaubrun C (1976). La notion de risque en périnatologie. Résultats d'enquètes épidémiologiques. Rev Epidemiol Santé Publique, 24: 253–276

Rush D (1977). Closing discussion. In: The Epidemiology of Prematurity. Reed D, Stanley FJ (eds). Baltimore: Urban & Schwarzenberg, pp 359–360.

Sagen N, Nilsen ST, Kim HC, Bergsjo P, Koller O (1984). Maternal hemoglobin concentrations is closely related to birthweight in normal pregnancies. Acta Obstet Gynecol Scand, 63: 245–248.

Saling E (1972). Prämaturitäts- und Dysmaturitäts-Präventionsprogramm (PDP-Programm). Z Geburtsh Perinatol, 176: 70–81.

Saurel-Cubizolles MJ, Kaminski M, Garcia J (1986). Conditions de travail des femmes enceintes et prématurité. In: Prévention de la Naissance Prématuré. Nouveaux Objectifs et Nouvelles Pratiques des Soins Prénataux. Papiernik E, Bréart G, Spira N (eds). Paris: Editions INSERM, pp 139–154.

Smith M, Stratton WC, Roi L (1985). Labor risk assessment in a rural community hospital. Am J Obstet Gynecol, 151: 569–574.

Sokol RJ, Rosen MG, Stojkov J, Chik L (1977). Clinical application of high-risk scoring on an obstetric service. Am J Obstet Gynecol, 128: 652–656.

Stembera Z (1977). Die differenzierte perinatale Betreuung der Risikoschwangerschaft. Zbl Gynäkol, 99: 1281–1285.

Thalhammer O (1973) Verhütung von Frühgeburtlichkeit und pränataler Dystrophie. I: Ein einfaches System zur Vorausberechnung des Frühgeburtsrisikos sowie des Aufwandes und Nutzens bei Ausschaltung von Risikofaktoren. Z Geburtsh Perinatol, 177: 169–177.

Thalhammer O, Coradello H, Pollak A, Scheibenreiter S, Simbruner G (1976). Prospective and retrospective examination of an easily applicable score to predict the probability of premature birth defined by weight. J Perinat Med, 4: 38–44.

Trimbos JB, Keirse MJNC (1978). Observer variability in assessment of antepartum cardiotocograms. Br J Obstet Gynaecol, 85: 900–906.

Wennergen M, Karlsson K (1982). A scoring system for antenatal identification of fetal growth retardation. Br J Obstet Gynaecol, 89: 520–524.

Wilson EW, Sill HK (1973). Identification of the high risk pregnancy by a scoring system. NZ Med J, 78: 437–440.

World Health Organization (1977). Recommended definitions, terminology and format for statistical tables related to the perinatal period and use of a new certificate for cause of perinatal deaths. Acta Obstet Gynecol Scand, 56: 247–253.

World Health Organization (1981). Public Health Practice: Risk approach for maternal and child health care. World Health Forum, 2: 413–422.

Yeh SY, Forsythe A, Lowensohn RI, Hon EH (1977). A study of the relationship between Goodwin's high-risk score and fetal outcome. Am J Obstet Gynecol, 127: 50–55.

Zatuchni GI, Andros GJ (1967). Prognostic index for vaginal delivery in breech presentation at term. Am J Obstet Gynecol, 98: 854–857.

23 Screening for genetic disease and fetal anomaly during pregnancy

Michael Daker and Martin Bobrow

1 Introduction

Over the past two decades, increasing recognition has been given to the role of genetics in the causation of human disease. Of particular interest has been the growth in prenatal screening for congenital abnormalities and genetic disorders, since the development of amniocentesis in 1969. In this chapter we describe briefly the classification of genetic diseases and discuss the ways in which they may be detected in human populations.

Genetic disease falls into three distinct categories: single gene disorders, multifactorial conditions which have both environmental and genetic components, and chromosome disorders.

1.1 Single gene disorders

Single gene disorders may be the result of an autosomal mutation where the mutant gene is located on a non-sex chromosome. The mutation may be dominant (e.g. Huntington's chorea; adult polycystic kidney disease) where an affected parent has a 50 per cent risk of passing the trait on to each child), or recessive (e.g. cystic fibrosis; phenylketonuria) where the risk of an affected child is one in four if both parents carry the mutation; where only one parent carries a recessive mutation, the risk of producing affected offspring is zero. Other single gene disorders are due to mutations of genes carried on the X chromosome. These X-linked conditions (e.g. Duchenne muscular dystrophy; haemophilia) are predominantly recessive in nature, with the condition usually manifesting only in males, females being symptomless carriers.

1.2 Multifactorial conditions

Multifactorial conditions include disorders such as diabetes mellitus and schizophrenia, as well as congenital malformations, such as spina bifida and congenital dislocation of the hip. Disorders of this type have both a genetic component that is polygenic in nature (i.e. influenced by a relatively large number of genes of similar effect) and an environmental component. Unlike the single gene disorders, where the risks remain constant for each pregnancy, the risks for future pregnancies increase with each affected child in multifactorial conditions.

1.3 Chromosomal disorders

Chromosomal disorders may be numerical in nature, where there is an extra whole chromosome present (e.g. Down's syndrome, trisomy 21) or a missing chromosomes (e.g. Turner's syndrome, females with a single X chromosome). There may also be structural chromosomal changes. These include unbalanced changes such as deletions, (e.g. *Cri-du-chat* syndrome; Prader–Willi syndrome) where there is loss of part of a chromosome arm with consequent gene loss. Balanced chromosome rearrangements include translocations and inversions where there is exchange of chromosome segments without gene loss. Individuals carrying balanced structural anomalies are normal themselves, but are at risk of producing genetically unbalanced gametes.

1.4 Frequency of genetic disease

Weatherall (1985) has suggested that the total load of genetic disease lies somewhere between 37 and 53 per 1000 births. There is, however, wide variation in the frequencies of disorders. Some recessive diseases are very rare, occurring with frequencies of the order of 0.01 per 1000 births, while other disorders such as Down's syndrome occur with a frequency greater than 1 per 1000 births. There is racial and geographical variation in the frequency of some specific genetic diseases. The autosomal recessive disorder, Tay–Sachs disease, occurs in 0.4 in 1000 births in populations of Ashkenazi Jews, while in non-Jewish populations it is very rare (0.003 in 1000 births) (Aronson and Volk 1962). Adrenogenital syndrome is relatively common in Yupik Eskimos (2 per 1000 births), but in north Europe it is less frequent (0.5 per 1000 births).

Genetic disorders of the red cells, the thalassaemias and sickle-cell anaemia, illustrate variation in frequency in relation to geographical distribution, occurring with frequencies as high as 10–20 per 1000 births in some areas. Both disorders, together with glucose 6-phosphate dehydrogenase deficiency (a red cell enzyme deficiency), are to be found across a broad belt of Africa through the Middle East to the Far East, apparently because heterozygote carriers are relatively protected against *Plasmodium falciparum* malaria. Disorders occurring at such high frequencies represent a massive health care problem, but in other countries these diseases are very rare.

1.5 Screening for genetic disease

The prime objective of all genetic screening must be to bring benefit to the individual, family or society as a whole. The nature of the benefit will differ according to circumstances. For many it will be a question of reassurance; for some a matter of counselling, with perhaps an assessment of risk; for others, it will help them to make informed decisions for example, with regard to the termination of pregnancy in which the fetus is abnormal.

The planning of a genetic screening programme involves defining those high risk populations in which screening procedures are justifiable. To do this requires careful consideration of a number of factors.

1.5.1 Prevalence

Accurate estimates of prevalence may be difficult to obtain for a variety of reasons (incomplete notification; bias of data from hospital records; condition may be under- or over-diagnosed, etc.), but the condition should occur with sufficient frequency to justify screening.

Careful monitoring is necessary to explain any unexpected discrepancies between the original estimates of frequency and the frequency data generated by the screening test. Monitoring frequency over time will indicate whether prevalence changes as the screening programme is introduced.

1.5.2 Severity of the disorder

The range of severity of genetic disorders, in terms of handicap to the affected individuals, is broad. There would, for instance seem little point in devising a screening programme for a disorder that does not lead to serious handicap unless the prevalence was very high. Conversely to screen for a disorder that normally resulted in early spontaneous abortion (see later discussion) would seem equally unprofitable. It is, of course, debatable as to what constitutes a serious condition. What is important is that screening should be directed to those disorders for which it is possible to take effective action (e.g. counselling, treatment, or pregnancy termination) when an individual who is affected or at risk of having an affected fetus has been identified.

1.5.3 Heterogeneity

Many inherited diseases are heterogeneous at the gene level. For example, retinitis pigmentosa may be autosomal dominant, autosomal recessive, or X-linked in its mode of inheritance; some cases are very probably not genetic in origin at all. The X-linked form can be diagnosed prenatally using linked DNA polymorphisms (q.v.), but these procedures would give a totally invalid result if applied to a family with an autosomal form of the disease.

1.5.4 Sensitivity

Sensitivity and specificity of available assays are obviously of critical importance. In several common assays for congenital abnormalities and genetic disorders (e.g. alpha-fetoprotein testing for neural tube defects; heterozygote testing for Tay–Sachs disease) there is no clear separation into normal and abnormal results. It is important, therefore, to know first the extent to which a test is able to discriminate between normal and affected individuals, and secondly to know the probability of an individual being affected for any given result obtained. The likelihood that an individual is affected can be expressed as a probability (the predictive value of a positive test) or as a likelihood ratio (an odds ratio of the number affected to the number unaffected amongst those with a positive result) (see Chapter 3).

In all screening tests, regular quality assessment should be carried out to ensure the maintenance of standardization of techniques.

1.5.5 Safety

Safety and acceptability to the patient require careful consideration. Risks of the procedure must be weighed against the possible benefits of screening.

1.5.6 Cost

For mass screening of large populations, the cost of the test per individual needs to be low, or the total costs may become prohibitive. More expensive tests can only be applied to defined high risk populations. Costs of testing must also be weighed against possible financial savings that the identification of affected individuals might bring in terms of treatment saved, etc.

Costs, however, are not wholely financial, and it is equally important to weigh the possible 'human costs'. Although screening programmes may bring reassurance to some who are tested, for others, screening may generate anxiety by merely raising the question of abnormality, while the undesirable results that may be generated by occasional erroneous diagnoses, must be a matter for very careful consideration.

In summary, the successful design of a genetic screening programme depends on a balance between safety, accuracy, and costs of the test, and severity and prevalence of the disease.

1.6 Principles and classification of screening for genetic disease

The prime objective of genetic screening is to reduce the overall burden of a disorder within a population, either by prevention or treatment. To do this, it is necessary in the first instance to identify those individuals whose children are at risk of having genetic disease. There are three ways of approaching the problem.

(1) The delineation of a high risk group using demographic parameters such as age or ethnic origin.
(2) The detection of heterozygote carriers by population screening.
(3) Diagnostic testing of individuals within families with a history of affected members.

In some cases, a logical sequence of events would involve (1) followed by (2). The concept of a step-by-step system of screening is an important one if good use is to be made of resources. For example, in testing for Tay–Sachs disease the following regimen offers an efficient approach. The initial screening is on the basis of ethnic origin only. This is then followed by heterozygote testing of the husband (in preference to the wife, since oral contraception or pregnancy may result in false positive results). If the husband is found to be a carrier, then the wife must be screened. Only if both are found to be carriers will a prenatal test be justifiable.

In the course of this chapter, we will be considering aspects of genetic screening under the headings set out below, basing the discussion on some of the more familiar examples of genetic disease. To accommodate unavoidable overlaps between sections, different aspects of screening for any given disorder are considered under the most appropriate heading:

A. *Adult screening*—where the aim is to prevent fetal handicap by identifying those individuals whose children are at risk of having genetic disease. Population screening of adults includes heterozygote testing to identify individual carriers of deleterious genetic traits, prior to testing during pregnancy.

(a) Autosomal heterozygote testing (e.g. for Tay–Sachs; sickle-cell disease; the thalassaemias).
(b) X-linked heterozygote testing (e.g. for glucose 6-phosphate dehydrogenase deficiency; Duchenne muscular dystrophy).

B. *Screening during pregnancy*—where the aim is to prevent handicap by identification of a disorder at an early stage, so that either treatment may be given as soon after birth as possible, or if appropriate and acceptable, the pregnancy can be terminated. (The term 'secondary prevention' is often applied to the control of congenital disorders by termination of affected pregnancies.)

(a) Morphological abnormalities
(b) Neural tube defects
(c) Chromosome disorders

2 Adult screening

In this section a number of familiar examples of recessive genetic disorders are given. For convenience, these are grouped under one of two headings; either autosomal heterozygote testing, or X-linked heterozygote testing, where the siting of the defective gene on an X chromosome raises special problems for consideration.

2.1 Autosomal heterozygote testing

2.1.1 Tay-Sachs disease

Tay–Sachs disease provides a classical example of an

autosomal recessive condition for which there are well-established screening procedures. This disorder is due to a deficiency of a lysosomal enzyme (hexosaminidase A), resulting in accumulation of ganglioside GM_2. It occurs predominantly in Ashkenazim Jews with a frequency of 0.4 per 1000 births. The carrier frequency is 1 in 30, which is approximately ten times greater than in the non-Jewish population. The disorder results in progressive neurological degeneration, the first symptoms occurring by the 5th or 6th month. A characteristic cherry red macular spot is usually visible in the retina before the age of 1 year. There is no known cure, and the condition is lethal by about 3 to 4 years of age.

Hexosaminidase A can be assayed in either serum or leukocytes. This is done by obtaining an estimate of total hexosaminidase activity, before and after heat inactivation, which destroys the HEX-A isozyme, while leaving the Hex-B isozyme intact. Various factors, such as the temperature of inactivation, affect the result, and there is a need for careful standardization of the assay. Population screening is usually carried out by the serum assay, which is relatively simple and inexpensive. There is, however, a region of overlap between carriers and non-carriers; Kaback *et al.* (1977) give a figure of 87 per cent for the proportion of obligatory carriers (parents of infants with Tay–Sachs disease) correctly identified by serum testing. The more costly leucocyte test provides a better discrimination and should be used when serum tests have proved inconclusive, or where the woman is pregnant or using oral contraception.

Since 1969, considerable effort has gone into setting up carrier detection screening programmes for Tay–Sachs disease, especially in the United States, where 210 174 individuals were tested during the 10-year period from 1969 to 1979 (Kaback 1981). Similar programmes that have been running during this period include Canada (30 307 individuals tested) and Israel (9678 individuals tested). These figures, however, must be set against the total population at risk. As Hecht and Cadien (1984) point out, figures published by Kaback in 1977 on the first seven years' experience, indicated that less than 2 per cent of the Jewish population of the United States had been screened for Tay-Sachs disease. This emphasizes the problem of all screening programmes, that of persuading individuals of the advantages to being tested.

Heterozygote testing may be possible in a number of other biochemical disorders, such as Gaucher disease type 1, which is again, relatively frequent in Ashkenazim Jews (0.4 per 1000 births). Other disorders including galactosaemia, metachromatic leucodystrophy, glycogen storage diseases, the mucopolysaccharidoses, and maple syrup urine disease, etc., are very uncommon, occurring with frequencies ranging from 0.1 to 0.001 per 1000 births. It is not practical to offer population screening for all such disorders, which means, unfortunately, that testing will be initiated only after the identification of an affected individual within a family.

2.1.2 The autosomal recessive haematological disorders

The autosomal recessive haematological disorders, the thalassaemias and sickle-cell anaemia, form a distinct group, on account of their immense numerical importance. With birth frequencies that range up to 20 per 1000 births, it has been suggested by Weatherall and Clegg (1981) that they are the commonest single gene disorders in the world population, with hundreds of millions of carrier individuals and 200 000 seriously affected homozygotes born each year.

2.1.2.1 *The thalassaemias* The thalassaemias form a heterogeneous group of disorders, all of which are typified by an abnormal haemoglobin constitution resulting from a reduced rate of production of one or more globin chains. In alpha-thalassaemias, gene deletion results in a deficiency of the alpha chains, and although the heterozygous states are more or less symptomless, affected individuals may have severe haemolytic anaemia. A total lack of alpha chains results in intrauterine death. More important clinically, are the beta-thalassaemias, where a range of molecular defects may interfere with the expression of the gene for beta-chain production, so that the effect is not shown until after birth at the time when the switch to the adult form of haemoglobin occurs. The heterozygous states are more or less symptomless, but the homozygous state results in severe haemolytic anaemia, hepatosplenomegaly, bone deformities, proneness to infection, etc., and, unless adequate transfusion is given, the disorder is usually fatal in early childhood.

Geographically, the thalassaemias are distributed in a broad band across the Mediterranean, the Middle East and South-east Asia. Beta-thalassaemia is particularly common in the Mediterranean island populations such as Cyprus and Sardinia, and in parts of Italy and Greece.

The high gene frequency in specific populations justifies heterozygote screening, particularly for beta-thalassaemia. In Sardinia, where there is a very high incidence of beta-thalassaemia, the success of screening programmes is being reflected by an apparent fall in the incidence of the disorder (from 4.69 per 1000 live births in 1976 to an estimated 1.05 per 1000 live births in 1980 (World Health Organization 1983)). With improved treatment, however, affected individuals have a greater life expectancy, so that the prevalence of the disorder continues to rise. In the Ferrara province of Italy, a screening programme aimed at identifying beta-thalassaemia heterozygotes, has been operational since 1955. The success of this programme may be measured by the large proportion of individuals identified as heterozygotes who knew of their carrier status and understood the implications. It is interesting to note, however, that the effect of such knowledge has not had any apparent influence on the choice of marriage partners (Barrai and Vullo 1980).

Standard tests for this disorder rely on the observation of microcytosis together with raised haemoglobin A_2 levels. Couples who are at risk of having an affected child can be identified and offered prenatal diagnosis. This prenatal testing can be carried out by the measuring of globin-chain synthesis in fetal blood, but there are now DNA probes available that can be used to diagnose the common haemoglobin disorders (Weatherall *et al.* 1985) and this is likely to be the method of the future (see Section 6).

2.1.2.2 *Sickle-cell disorders* Sickle-cell disorders are prevalent in people of African origin, as well as those regions of the Mediterranean and Middle East where the mutant gene (a single-base substitution in the gene for the beta-globin chain) has achieved a high frequency as a result of the selective advantage of the heterozygotes, who are conferred with a degree of resistance to malaria. In some regions of Africa, over 25 per cent of the population are heterozygotes for the mutation and 100 000 infants are born annually with the disorder (World Health Organization 1983). A similar frequency of heterozygotes is found among the oasis populations of Saudi Arabia. In the heterozygous condition (sickle-cell trait) there is very little disability, while in the homozygous state there is a wide range in variability of the disease, from severe anaemia with painful crises followed by death in early infancy, to a relatively mild form in parts of the Caribbean, and also in Saudi Arabia where it is particularly mild.

Such differences in expression are not yet fully understood, and it is necessary to learn more of the natural history of the disease. In the United States, for example, where sickle-cell disease is relatively mild, and compatible with adult life, screening among the black population met with opposition (US National Academy of Sciences, 1975).

Heterozygote testing is simple, demonstrated by the sickling of red blood cells when exposed, *in vitro*, to very low oxygen tensions. Population screening is aimed largely at pregnant women living in areas of high incidence, or who are descended from high incidence populations. Where a woman is found to be a heterozygote, haemoglobin electrophoresis should be carried out in order to detect any possible sickling variants, and in particular, haemoglobin SC, which may cause complications during pregnancy. Where the woman shows a positive reaction to sickling tests, her partner is also tested and should he also prove to be a carrier, prenatal diagnosis may be carried out, using specific probes on either chorionic villus or amniotic fluid cell samples, or, by globin-chain analysis in fetal blood. Views with regard to prenatal diagnosis differ, but Weatherall and Letsky (1984) consider that general antenatal screening with a view to offering selective termination in the case of an affected fetus cannot be justified until more is known of the natural history of sickle-cell disease. However, it is important to recognize affected infants, so that they can receive the best management during the initial, most vulnerable years of life. Where both parents are known to be heterozygous, but do not choose to undertake prenatal diagnosis, then early postnatal testing of the newborn should be carried out, so that the parents can be warned of the possible complications that might occur, particularly during the first few years of life.

2.2 X-linked heterozygote testing

Most X-linked diseases are recessive in nature, and therefore, seen almost exclusively in males. This is because the male, having only a single X chromosome, will be affected if he inherits an abnormal recessive gene on his X chromosome (he is said to be hemizygous for the gene). It follows that only females can be carriers of X-linked conditions. Only where the disorder attains a very high prevalence will homozygous females occur with any significant frequency (e.g. glucose 6-phosphate dehydrogenase deficiency in some populations).

Testing for carriers of X-linked disorders is somewhat complicated by the effects of X chromosome inactivation, a random process whereby one of the pair of X chromosomes in each cell of the female embryo becomes 'switched off'. A woman, therefore, who is heterozygous for a particular mutant gene, is in effect, a mosaic. In the case of a simple biochemical deficiency disorder, one would expect a heterozygous female to express half the amount of gene product shown by a non-affected male. However, because X inactivation is random, the numbers of cells expressing and those not expressing may not be equal, leading to overlaps between carrier and normal distributions.

This problem may be overcome by the *in vitro* culture of cells derived from single cells from a positive heterozygote female. Such cultures (clones) will have the same X chromosome inactivated in all the cells. Therefore, where a woman is heterozygous for a gene mutation on the X chromosome, some clones may be expected to express the mutant allele, others the non-mutated allele. For a number of metabolic disorders, cells of hair follicles have been used as 'natural clones', each follicle normally being derived from only about two or three cells. Hunter's disease (Yutaka *et al.* 1978; Nwokoro and Neufeld, 1979; Chase *et al.* 1986), and Lesch–Nyhan disease (Gartler *et al.* 1971) are among the disorders for which successful heterozygote testing on hair-root follicles has been carried out. Such methods, however, are costly and not suitable for population screening.

2.2.1 Glucose 6-phosphate dehydrogenase deficiency

Glucose 6-phosphate dehydrogenase (G6PD) deficiency, is the most common of the X-linked disorders apart from colour blindness, and in the newborn, up to 5 per cent of infants with glucose 6-phosphate dehydrogenase deficiency develop severe hyperbilirubinemia with the risk of kernicterus. It occurs particularly in Central Africa, where up to 30 per cent of males may be affected; in America, in the negro populations; in certain regions of Europe, especially Greece and Sardinia; and in South-east Asia. Like the thalassaemias and sickle-cell disease, the high frequency in these areas is associated with a degree of protection against malaria that this disorder apparently confers on the heterozygotes (Luzzatto *et al.* 1969).

The gene mutation in glucose 6-phosphate dehydrogenase is not a simple one, but a series of multiple alleles resulting in over 150 molecular variants of this enzyme, some of which have normal activity while others show widely differing levels of reduced activity. Affected males are usually symptomless unless exposed to specific triggers, such as the antimalarial drugs (Primaquine, etc.), sulphonamides, nitrofurantoin, chloramphenicol, etc., as well as the ingestion of broad beans (fava beans), all of which may induce haemolytic anaemia.

Although the disorder is relatively mild in its effects, because it occurs in well-defined populations, population screening programmes to identify both carriers and affected individuals could be set up. The basis of the screening test is a specific fluorescent staining technique and visual examination of red blood cells using a UV light source. Red cells from glucose 6-phosphate dehydrogenase deficient blood show little or none of the fluorescence seen when normal red blood cells are stained and examined in the same way (Beutler *et al.* 1979). Heterozygotes show intermediate levels of fluorescence. Affected individuals could be advised appropriately regarding the avoidance of certain drugs and foods. Postnatal screening is also important, in view of the risks of neonatal jaundice, which is one of the main problems with this disorder. Prenatal screening is not indicated.

2.2.2 Duchenne muscular dystrophy

Duchenne muscular dystrophy (DMD) is a serious X-linked disorder occurring with an incidence of approximately 0.3 per 1000 male births (Gardner-Medwin 1970). The onset is in early childhood, when the first signs of muscular weakness appear. This progresses until, at the age of about 10, the affected boys are confined to wheelchairs, eventually dying from respiratory infections in their late teens or twenties.

The accepted method of heterozygote testing involves estimation of the level of serum creatine phosphokinase (CPK), which is non-specifically elevated in many forms of muscle disease. It is, however, far from being satisfactory, since only about two-thirds of obligatory heterozygotes have levels that are clearly outside the normal range. Furthermore, the serum creatine phosphokinase levels are subject to many confounding artefacts, and are particularly unreliable during pregnancy. Results are usually expressed as a likelihood ratio, or as a probability that an individual with a given serum creatine phosphokinase level is a carrier. However, it is widely accepted that 20 per cent or more of obligate heterozygotes are not detected by this test. The carrier risk derived from serum creatine phosphokinase assay is then combined, using Bayesian methods, with pedigree information to give a final risk estimate for genetic counselling purposes. The calculations are greatly influenced by the fact that one-third of cases of Duchenne muscular dystrophy are probably the result of new mutations, and their mothers are not carriers of the abnormal gene.

Much current research is being directed towards exploring the use of DNA probes to identify carriers in these families (see Section 6). These techniques can also identify which of the two X chromosomes of a carrier mother bears the mutant allele, and show whether or not it has been passed on to her fetus. It is now known that the gene is located near the middle of the short arm of the X chromosome in region p21, and considerable progress has been made in identifying fairly closely linked polymorphic loci which are clinically useful (Kolata 1985). In the majority of females, the segregation of the two X chromosomes can be followed with 95–98 per cent accuracy.

2.2.3 Haemophilia

Haemophilia occurs with a frequency of about 0.2 per 1000 males in the United Kingdom. There are two forms of this disorder that are clinically indistinguishable from each other; Haemophilia A, and the less common Haemophilia B (Christmas disease) resulting from deficiencies of factors VIII and IX respectively. Severity of the bleeding is related to the level of either factor VIII or IX in the blood; total loss of one or other of these factors causes spontaneous bleeding into joints and muscles which produces severe crippling deformities.

Mass screening for the detection of heterozygote carriers of haemophilia is not feasible, but carrier detection and prenatal screening can be carried out in high risk families. As for the haemoglobinopathies, the development of techniques for fetal blood sampling opened up possibilities for prenatal diagnosis. Factor VIII levels have been measured using a bioassay which measures coagulation activity; combining these with measurement of Factor VIII related antigen, considerably improves the separation of carrier from normal. More recently, immunoradiometric assays of factor VIII related antigens added further improvements. The gene sequences for factors VIII and IX have now been largely cloned, and the method of choice for the future clearly lies with the use of recombinant DNA techniques for both the detection of carriers and for prenatal diagnosis.

3 Screening during pregnancy

Pregnancies may be screened in either the first or second trimester to detect certain specific biochemical disorders, chromosome abnormalities or some structural malformations, particularly neural tube defects. Following a short section summarizing the use of ultrasound in genetic screening, we discuss at some length the two predominant aspects of prenatal screening, neural tube defects, and chromosome abnormalities.

3.1 Diagnosis of morphological abnormalities

Many structural abnormalities of the fetus are now diagnosable directly by ultrasound or fetoscopy, and the introduction of real-time scanning has opened the way for the screening of antenatal populations (see reviews in Bennett 1984). In addition, ultrasound is an essential obstetric aid in the procedure of amniocentesis, helping the obstetrician to recognize twin pregnancies, assess fetal viability, and identify placental location. However, it has been shown in controlled trials by Levine *et al.* (1978) and Nolan *et al.* (1981) that ultrasound does not significantly reduce the failure rate of amniocentesis, the incidence of multiple needle insertions, or the proportion of blood stained samples. In chorionic villus sampling, ultrasound allows direct guidance of the cannula used for aspirating specimens.

It is well known that ultrasound is probably damaging to cells and DNA *in vitro*, but although the quality of objective information from properly controlled trials leaves much to be desired, the evidence suggests that there is no damage either to the fetus or mother, caused by the use of obstetric ultrasound (see Chapter 27).

Abnormality scanning is carried out between 16 and 22 weeks gestation, and may include a general assessment of the fetal anatomy (head, heart, stomach, bladder, kidney, and spine). Where the initial scan shows possible evidence of fetal abnormality, or in cases referred because of a specific risk of a fetal abnormality, then a more detailed examination will be required.

Ultrasound scanning is becoming the method of choice for confirmation of suspected neural tube defects. Other craniospinal defects detectable by ultrasound include hydrocephaly, encephalocele, holoprosencephaly, and microcephaly.

Ultrasound examination of the heart can be of use when a fetus is at risk for congenital heart disease, and one group (Allan *et al.* 1986) suggests a simplified approach to fetal cardiac scanning which would help in the detection of many severe defects, and which could perhaps be incorporated into routine obstetric ultrasound examination from 16 weeks of gestation onwards.

Gastrointestinal disorders that can be diagnosed with ultrasound include omphalocele, gastroschisis, diaphragmatic hernia, umbilical hernia and duodenal atresia. Renal tract anomalies detectable on screening include obstructive uropathy, infantile polycystic disease, Meckel's syndrome, and renal agenesis (Potter's syndrome). Other features of the fetus that can readily be examined with ultrasound include limb deformities, such as amelia and phocomelia, as well as the shortening of the long bones of limbs associated with achondroplasia, achondrogenesis, thanatorphoric dwarfism, etc. (Warsof and Griffin 1984).

Fetal ascites, seen very clearly with ultrasound, is most usually secondary to fetal hydrops, and therefore, an indicator of a wide range of possible disorders, including chromosome disorders, achondroplasia, tuberous sclerosis, congenital heart disease, glucose 6-phosphate dehydrogenase deficiency, haemoglobinopathies, pulmonary hypoplasia, congenital nephrosis, maternal diabetes mellitus, or intrauterine infections, etc. Nicolaides *et al.* (1986) reported on 118 pregnancies where a fetal anomaly was demonstrable by ultrasound. Of particular interest was the finding that 8 out of 12 fetuses with exomphalos showed a chromosome abnormality.

3.2 Neural tube defects

Neural tube defects are among the more common birth defects. Frequency varies according to ethnic group, being relatively common among Caucasians, less so in Mongolians, and rare in Negroes. There is also geographical, temporal and socioeconomic variation in occurrence. In the United Kingdom, where the overall incidence is high (about 5 per 1000 births) the frequency is greatest in the north-west, decreasing progressively down and across the country to the south-east. In common with all disorders showing a multifactorial mode of inheritance, the occurrence within a family of a child with a neural tube defect increases the likelihood of having further affected children in subsequent pregnancies (tenfold after the first, twentyfold after the second affected child).

Brock and Sutcliffe (1972) noted that affected pregnancies had elevated amniotic fluid alpha-fetoprotein (AFP) levels, and data from the United Kingdom Collaborative Study (1979) showed that 98.2 per cent of open lesions could be detected by this test (0.79 per cent of pregnancies not associated with open neural tube defects had positive results). The development of a gel electrophoresis assay of amniotic fluid acetylcholinesterase (AChE) (Chubb *et al.* 1979; Smith *et al.* 1979) provided a highly specific test for neural tube defects, virtually eliminating the few false positives that occur with alpha-fetoprotein testing (Collaborative Acetylcholinesterase Study 1981). In practice, acetylcholinesterase (being the more expensive of the two tests) is used as a confirmatory test in conjunction with the amniotic fluid alpha-fetoprotein assay.

Since amniocentesis is an invasive procedure, amniotic fluid alpha-fetoprotein screening is only offered to women at known increased risk of having an affected fetus. The development of serum alpha-fetoprotein screening using a radioimmune assay technique made general population screening a viable proposition, particularly where there is a high incidence of neural tube defects. Arguments have also been put forward for population screening in areas of low incidence, on the grounds that cost-effectiveness of maternal serum screening programmes should not be judged only on the basis of the number of neural tube defects (and other abnormalities) detected, but should also take into consideration the reassurance that it provides for a very large number of pregnant women (Ghosh *et al.* 1986).

Serum alpha-fetoprotein testing should be carried out at the end of the first trimester of pregnancy. The 'cut-off' point for defining a serum alpha-fetoprotein is usually taken as 2.5 multiples of the population normal median (MoM), but this may be varied; for example, where the incidence is high, a lower 'cut-off' point can be used and vice versa.

Serum alpha-fetoprotein testing is not such a discriminating test as the amniotic fluid alpha-fetoprotein assay. In the United Kingdom, using a cut-off point of 2.5 MoM, 3.3 per cent of unaffected singleton pregnancies will have a high serum alpha-fetoprotein. Conversely, 12 per cent of anencephalic pregnancies and 21 per cent of open spina bifida pregnancies will not be detected (United Kingdom Collaborative AFP Study Report 1977, 1979). However, because the test is safe and simple it can be used for screening large populations of pregnant women. As a commonly accepted strategy, where the initial result from a serum test shows an elevated level of alpha-fetoprotein, a repeat sample is requested. If the second test also shows elevated levels of alpha-fetoprotein, the woman undergoes amniocentesis to allow the more sensitive amniotic fluid alpha-fetoprotein assay to be carried out, as well as acetylcholinesterase testing.

Alpha-fetoprotein assays are diagnostically relatively non-specific, and in addition to neural tube defects, a raised alpha-fetoprotein may indicate other problems such as an omphalocele, gastroschisis, congenital nephrotic syndrome (of the Finnish type), intrauterine death, and Turner's syndrome (where there are large cystic hygromata). The acetylcholinesterase test can also be of value in experienced hands in the diagnosis of abdominal wall defects.

With increasing expertise in the use of ultrasound, most of the neural tube defects are directly detectable by this technique. Some of these abnormalities, such as anencephaly and severe spina bifida will be picked up as a result of routine scanning during early pregnancy. The smaller lesions, however, will require a more detailed examination by an experienced ultrasonographer. As a method of mass screening for neural tube defects, therefore, ultrasound has not yet been shown to be appropriate. However, in specialist centres, it is now beginning to be used as the method of choice for following-up abnormal serum alpha-fetoprotein results.

3.3 Chromosome disorders

Studies on newborn infants show a world-wide frequency of chromosome disorders of about 6 per 1000 births (Hook and Hamerton 1977). Such a figure is a minimum estimate. Advances in cytogenetic techniques have been made over the past decade, enabling smaller and more subtle abnormalities to be detected than had been possible with traditional methods of staining. The total population load of chromosome abnormalities is, however, far greater still, the majority of affected individuals miscarrying spontaneously early in pregnancy. Creasy (1982) summarizes the evidence that suggests about 50 per cent of all clinically recognizable spontaneous abortuses are chromosomally abnormal. Of these, nearly 50 per cent will be autosomal trisomies, 20 per cent female fetuses with a single X chromosome, and 15 per cent triploids. The significance of such high abnormality rates becomes evident in relation to prenatal diagnosis, and in particular, to first trimester fetal diagnosis by chorionic villus sampling.

Over the past fifteen years, we have seen a steady rise in demand for prenatal diagnosis for chromosome disorders. In our own laboratory the mean annual increase during the 5-year period from 1980 to 1985 has been over 16 per cent. A large majority of all referrals (75 per cent in our own laboratory) for prenatal chromosome diagnosis are for older women (aged 35 and over) who have an increased risk of carrying a fetus with Down's syndrome (trisomy 21) and most other chromosomal trisomies.

The association between Down's syndrome (trisomy 21) and advanced maternal age has been known for many years (Smith and Berg 1976). Although we know that the origin of the extra chromosome is most often due to maternal non-disjunction during the first meiotic division (Langenbeck *et al.* 1976; Magenis and Chamberlin 1981), we still do not understand the cause.

Analysis of accumulated data from a number of

surveys (Hook 1981) show that up to the age of about 29 there is little effect of maternal age on the frequency of Down's syndrome (the incidence ranging from approximately 0.5 to 1.0 per 1000 live births). Between the ages of 30 and 34 the incidence curve begins to rise slightly, but at 35 the incidence is of the order of 2 to 3 per 1000 live births. This rises to about 8 or 9 per 1000 at the age of 40, while for women over 45, most of the surveys show frequencies in excess of 30 per 1000 live births. Currently, many laboratories use age 35 as the cut-off point for offering prenatal diagnosis, a decision governed partly by available resources, and also because below this age, the risks of the procedure (less than 1 per cent) more or less balance the risks of a chromosomal disorder. With the exception of trisomy 16, the frequencies of other autosomal trisomies also increase with maternal age (Hassold *et al.* 1980).

At the present time, there is considerable interest in the reports by Merkatz *et al.* (1984) and Cuckle *et al.* (1984) that pregnancies resulting in babies with Down's syndrome (and other abnormal trisomies) are associated with low levels of maternal serum alpha-fetoprotein (AFP). Such observations clearly have important implications with regard to possible improvements in screening for Down's syndrome, and Cuckle *et al.* (1984, 1987) suggest a sliding scale of reduced cut-off concentrations of maternal serum alpha-fetoprotein with decreasing maternal age. Murday and Slack (1985) have tested this type of strategy and shown it to be effective for women of 32 and older whose risk of having a baby with Down's syndrome, after taking account of the maternal serum alpha-fetoprotein level, is less than one in 200. Such strategies could possibly also result in reduction of cytogenetic studies on older women who have normal levels of maternal serum alpha-fetoprotein (Martin and Liu 1986).

Other chromosome abnormalities include the Fragile-X syndrome (Martin Bell syndrome), a chromosome abnormality associated with a particular form of X-linked mental retardation. Herbst and Miller (1980) suggest that it is the most common cause of mental retardation after Down's syndrome; Bundey *et al.* (1985) found a prevalence of 9 per cent in a community-based study of 156 boys with idiopathic, severe mental retardation. The genetics of the disorder is complicated by the fact that transmission may sometimes be through a non-affected male, and also because the female carriers, who may themselves show a degree of retardation, do not always show the fragile site.

The chromosome abnormality, which usually appears as a small gap near the tip of the long arm of the X chromosome, is seen in varying proportions of cells (from 2 to 70 per cent). Furthermore, expression of the fragile X is folate sensitive, so that special culture media must be used which are low in folic acid. For this reason mass prenatal screening for fragile X cannot be carried out using routine chromosome preparations of amniotic fluid cells. However, where fragile X mental retardation has been established within a family, prenatal testing should always be carried out on fetuses at risk. It is possible to do this successfully using amniotic fluid cells (Shapiro *et al.* 1982), but currently fetal blood sampling is the method of choice. In the near future, it is anticipated that prenatal testing will also include studies of restriction fragment length polymorphisms close to the fragile site to identify the X chromosome carrying the abnormality.

3.3.1 *Techniques for prenatal diagnosis of chromosome disorders*

The techniques in current use for the prenatal diagnosis of chromosome disorders are, amniocentesis, fetal blood sampling, and chorionic villus sampling. Each aspect is considered in turn with particular emphasis on the problems associated with cell culture, and the difficulties that may arise over the interpretation of results.

3.3.1.1 *Amniotic fluid sampling* The overall safety of early second trimester amniocentesis has been well established from several large studies, including those from the USA, Canada, and Great Britain (Rodeck 1984). The chief concern with amniocentesis has been the abortion rate associated with the procedure; Rodeck (1984) suggests that many would accept that an uncomplicated amniocentesis carries only a 0.5 per cent risk of fetal loss. This is lower than the 1.5 per cent excess fetal loss reported by the large British Medical Research Council study (1978), but it is felt that problems over the selection of controls may have influenced the result of the Medical Research Council report. However, the only fully randomized controlled trial of amniocentesis is the study by Tabor *et al.* (1986), who report a 1.0 per cent increase in miscarriage rate.

Amniotic fluid cell chromosome studies are carried out by culturing the few viable cells present in the fluid. These are grown in culture for two to three weeks until their numbers have increased sufficiently to allow for chromosome studies. An optimal specimen should be between 10–20 ml in volume and a clear straw colour in appearance. On centrifuging there should be a small white precipitate of cells in the bottom of the tube. With good samples, success rates should be of the order of 99 per cent; a failure rate of more than 5 per cent indicates a culture problem that requires urgent investigation. Where the specimens are suboptimal, success rate may certainly be expected to fall and reporting times are likely to be delayed.

Although results have been obtained from as little as 1 ml, a small volume usually decreases the chance of success because of the reduced number of viable cells present. Similarly, fluids of adequate volume, but with a very small precipitate of cells, may take longer to establish as viable cultures, or fail completely. It is not unknown to receive samples of maternal urine in the laboratory, but these can be readily detected before culture is attempted.

Discoloured fluids are likely to give poor growth. Those stained with fresh blood are not necessarily at a disadvantage, but where it is very heavy, and a Kleihauer test shows that the blood is mainly fetal, it may be helpful to set up some of the fluid as a short term blood culture. If chromosome analysis subsequently indicates a male fetus, one can use the result with confidence. Infection is another cause of culture failure, which is most likely to be introduced at the time of sampling.

Apart from culture failure, the most common reason for requesting a repeat amniocentesis is because of mosaicism, the finding of a mixture of normal and abnormal cells. This is sometimes due to maternal cell contamination, a situation that is normally only detectable when the fetus is male. To eliminate the possibility of maternal cell contamination in the case of a female fetus requires the use of special staining techniques on fetal and parental chromosomes, in order to compare chromosome variants (small, clinically unimportant structural differences between individual chromosomes). This is too costly to be performed on all samples. Estimates of the frequency of maternal cell contamination vary from 1 per 1000 (Therkelsen 1979) to 3 per 1000 (Hamerton *et al.* 1980) and 5 per 1000 (Benn and Hsu 1983). Our own data suggest a figure of 1.5 per 1000.

The mosaic situation may sometimes be a true reflection of the fetal chromosome constitution (true mosaicism) which has been estimated to occur with a frequency of 2.5 per 1000 (Simpson *et al.* 1982). More often, however, these represent cases of pseudomosaicism, (occurring with a frequency of 59 per 1000 (Simpson *et al.* 1982)) the aberrant cell being derived from one of the fetal membranes, or originating during culture. Such pseudomosaicism is not of clinical significance, but differentiating the various causes of amniotic fluid chromosome mosaicism is a common and serious laboratory problem.

Normally, two or more cell cultures are set up from each fluid. If an abnormal cell line is found in all the cultures, it is more likely to be true mosaicism. If, on the other hand, the abnormal cells are found in only one culture, it is likely to be a pseudomosaic. Certain abnormalities arise quite frequently as *in vitro* artefacts, particularly trisomies of chromosomes 2 and 20. On the other hand, trisomy 20 can be also be found as a true mosaic (Djalali *et al.* 1985).

Marker chromosomes are small chromosomes additional to the normal complement. They occur with a frequency of approximately 1 per 1000 individuals in the general population (Buckton *et al.* 1985). Some are genetically inert (heterochromatic) and of no clinical significance. Others containing active chromatin (euchromatic) may be associated with mental retardation. Special staining techniques indicate whether there is euchromatin present, and therefore, whether they are likely to produce detrimental clinical effects. Where the same chromosome abnormality is present in a normal, healthy parent, it is highly likely (but not entirely certain) that the marker in the fetus will also be benign.

Although chromosome studies on amniotic fluid cell cultures are primarily for the detection of trisomies, unexpected structural abnormalities are occasionally detected. If the abnormality has been inherited in a balanced form from one of the parents, then there is no cause for concern, but if it has arisen *de novo*, even if apparently balanced, there is a risk of mental retardation. Funderburk *et al.* (1977) concludes from pooled data that balanced reciprocal translocations are five times more frequent among mentally retarded individuals than in a population of consecutive newborns. Warburton (1984), in a review of 66 apparently balanced *de novo* rearrangements found at amniocentesis, reported evidence of phenotypic abnormality in 5, while Gosden (1984) suggests that the risk of mental retardation in the case of balanced *de novo* reciprocal translocations may be as high as 1 in 8.

Mosaicism and maternal cell contamination will inevitably lead to the occasional diagnostic error; indeed, many of the reported errors have been normal babies of the 'wrong' sex, and probably largely due to maternal contamination. Transcription errors at the report stage and mislabelling of specimen bottles at source have undoubtedly contributed to the overall error rate, which is reported as approximately 0.3 per cent (Berry *et al.* 1981). Errors of serious clinical consequence, such as the misdiagnosis of Down's syndrome, are fortunately very rare indeed (we would suggest a figure in the order of 10^{-4} to 10^{-5}), and are most likely to occur through attempting to analyse preparations of very poor quality. Knowing when to ask for a repeat sample is extremely important, and requires experience.

Amniotic fluid cell chromosome studies have two major drawbacks. First, it usually takes from two to three weeks from the time the sample is taken, until the result is given out. Many women find this long wait in itself to be distressing, but the second point is that amniocentesis is not normally carried out until the 16th week of pregnancy, so that should termination be indicated, it will have to be carried out at a relatively late stage in pregnancy. Culture failure occurs in about 2 per cent of samples. In these cases a repeat sample becomes necessary, and the pregnancy is likely to be very near to the legal limit for termination before the result is finally available.

3.3.1.2 *Fetal blood sampling* Fetal blood sampling is

becoming a useful alternative to a repeat amniocentesis for chromosome studies. This may be carried out under direct vision using a fetoscope, the best site being the placental insertion of the cord (Rodeck and Campbell 1979), or by needle insertion under ultrasound guidance. Short term lymphocyte cultures are set up and the cells harvested after two or three days. The procedure, however, is by no means universally available, requiring considerable expertise on the part of the obstetrician, and the risks of fetal loss are greater than for amniocentesis; probably between 2 and 5 per cent, as compared with the 1 per cent increase in miscarriage rate associated with amniocentesis (Tabor *et al.* 1986).

3.3.1.3 *Chorionic villus sampling* Chorionic villus sampling (CVS) could become an attractive alternative to amniocentesis or fetal blood sampling, since it can be performed in the first trimester.

CVS involves the use of a cannula (or biopsy forceps) under ultrasound guidance, to take a small biopsy (10 to 40 mg) of villi, from the chorion frondosum. A majority of obstetricians take samples by a transcervical route; some advocate a transabdominal approach on the grounds that this is less likely to cause intrauterine infections. A recent randomized study by MacKenzie *et al.* (1986) set up to compare three different types of cannula used for transcervical chorionic villus sampling, showed that the design of the cannula is important with regard to the ease of insertion and condition of the specimens after aspiration.

The advantages of first trimester diagnosis are obvious, but there are still certain problems, both obstetric and cytogenetic, that need to be resolved. The relatively low early fetal loss rate is encouraging, although to some extent it probably reflects careful selecting-out of cases which the obstetrician is not prepared to biopsy. The precise safety of the technique, however, and all questions relating to possible long term effects on the developing fetus, require further investigation, and several randomized trials are currently being undertaken in various countries, which should provide objective information on the subject over the next few years.

In the cytogenetic analysis of chorionic villi, there is a choice to be made as to whether the tissue is cultured (for a period of two to three weeks) or whether it is processed directly, relying on the presence of actively dividing cells at the time of collection, the so-called 'direct preparation method'. The latter method, enables the diagnosis to be made in a day or two as opposed to weeks. However, it has certain drawbacks. The mitotic index is often very low, metaphase spreads are frequently broken and chromosome morphology is usually poor. Given time, the quality of direct chromosome preparations will undoubtedly improve, but for the present, it is of concern to cytogeneticists that they are required to make decisions on preparations that are often far from satisfactory. Aneuploidy and gross structural changes should be detectable, but more subtle changes such as small deletions (which are nevertheless clinically significant) may well be overlooked. Where a laboratory is relying on the analysis of direct preparations it is important that women undergoing chorionic villus sampling for advanced maternal age should be advised that it is primarily a test to detect Down's syndrome and abnormalities of a similar chromosomal nature, and that it does not guarantee the fetus will be chromosomally normal.

Currently many laboratories set up cultures as well as making direct preparations, providing a reassuring back-up. Chromosome preparations from cultured material can be expected to be of good quality, and suitable for detailed analysis.

Although Blakemore *et al.* (1985) have shown that dividing maternal cells may be present in direct preparations of first trimester decidua, maternal cell contamination is very much less likely to occur than when material is cultured. This fact, in itself, is a good reason for adopting the direct method.

Apart from technical difficulties, there are other important aspects of prenatal diagnosis by chorionic villus sampling that require consideration. Reference has already been made to the high level of chromosomally unbalanced conceptuses that are miscarried spontaneously in early pregnancy, so that a significant proportion of the chromosomally abnormal fetuses that are detected through chorionic villus sampling may have been destined to miscarry spontaneously by the time that amniocentesis would have been carried out.

It has also been suggested that abnormal cell lines occur more frequently in the fetal membranes than in the fetus itself, although the evidence for this is inconclusive. Kalousek and Dill (1983) found 2 out of 45 term pregnancies where mosaicism was restricted to the membranes, while Brambati *et al.* (1985) reported two cases where apparently normal fetuses were terminated because chromosome studies of preparations of chorionic villi had indicated a trisomy. These last two cases prompted Brambati to suggest that it would seem prudent to confirm such abnormal findings of first trimester sampling by a follow-up amniocentesis at 16 weeks. However, this not only defeats the object of making early termination possible, but also subjects the woman to a second invasive investigation, creates an extended period of anxious waiting for her, and effectively doubles the cost of the procedure. Disadvantages of CVS, as compared with amniocentesis, have also been pointed out by Mantingh *et al.* (1986), who suggests that if it becomes necessary to confirm abnormal karyotypes found on CVS by amniocentesis, then it may mean that CVS will have to be thought of as a screening test rather than a diagnostic procedure.

At the present time, not all laboratories are sufficiently competent to accept chorionic villus specimens, and of those who do, most would admit that the procedures are far from streamlined, each sample requiring considerable individual attention. At the present time, one cytogeneticist can handle about six amniotic fluid cultures a week, but probably not more than three chorion biopsies. This makes prenatal diagnosis by this method more labour intensive, and hence, more costly than by amniocentesis. Chorionic villus sampling is proving equally important in other areas of prenatal diagnosis including biochemical enzyme analysis and diagnosis using DNA probes.

4 Testing with gene probes

The principle of testing with gene probes relies on the use of enzymes (restriction enzymes) that recognize specific sequences in the DNA and cut the strand into fragments at these points. A change in the base sequence of the DNA may cause loss of an existing recognition site or create a new one. In either case, the fragment's length will be changed and this can be detected by electrophoretic separation. These differences detected between normal individuals are known as RFLPs (restriction fragment length polymorphisms). In alpha-thalassaemia, deletion of a large number of bases within the gene results in an alteration of fragment length, thus allowing diagnosis by a direct 'assay' of the gene. In most disorders, such as Duchenne muscular dystrophy or cystic fibrosis (q.v.), diagnosis is possible by identifying restriction enzyme sites that are very close (i.e. tightly linked) to the gene. The further apart they are, the greater the likelihood that the linkage will be broken by the occurrence crossing over between the paired homologous chromosomes during meiosis, in the region between the gene and the restriction enzyme site. The linked RFLP marker allows the individual chromosome carrying the disease-causing mutation to be recognized from its homologue; the 'disease' gene can, therefore, be traced through the family and identified if it should be present in a fetal sample.

5 Genetic screening and ethics

The prevention and treatment of genetic disease is still very much a new branch of medicine. In many medical schools it is only within the last few years that 'genetics' has achieved sufficient respectability to be included in the preclinical curriculum in its own right, while teaching at the clinical level is often very inadequate or virtually lacking. Nevertheless, genetic counselling is becoming an increasingly important component of health care. The list of disorders that are amenable to screening continues to grow and there is already strong evidence that the era of DNA probes will accelerate expansion of this field of medicine. It is to be hoped that support for the implementation of new developments will keep pace with the inevitable demands that physicians will make on behalf of their patients.

Counselling prior to prenatal testing is universally regarded as important. The central issue is, of course, one of risk—what is the risk of producing an abnormal child? It is clear, however, that one individual may interpret risk figures very differently from another (Wertz *et al.* 1986). Moreover, as Lippman-Hand and Fraser (1979a,b) have suggested, parental decisions may depend, not only on the actual level of risk, but on whether or not they could imagine handling the consequences of having an abnormal child. There is still a regrettable dearth of good quality psychological and sociological research into the field of prenatal diagnosis.

As a matter of practical concern, it is quite usual for women undergoing amniocentesis to be scheduled for counselling on the same day that the procedure is carried out, but Lorenz *et al.* (1985) have suggested that it is preferable for counselling to be given before the day of the planned amniocentesis, to allow time for couples to think carefully and without the feeling of being pressured to reach their decision. This policy, however, is not free of problems, and many patients may find it unduly disruptive to have to make an additional hospital visit where this involves substantial amounts of travelling.

Action taken as a result of a screening test should be the decision of the individuals themselves, after they have been made thoroughly aware of the situation, and any screening programme must have built into it adequate provision of time to allow for full counselling where it is required. Fitzsimmons (1987) points out the need to be particularly aware of emotional, psychological, and social problems that may be involved in prenatal diagnosis. The same is true for other areas of genetic counselling; Huntington's chorea, for example (a late onset dominant condition), is a case in point. Now that gene probes are available for this disease, the element of ignorance that existed in the past over whether or not an individual was a carrier, can be removed. For some, the knowledge that they are carriers would be more stressful than the state of ignorance. Farrer (1986) discusses the relatively high suicide and attempted suicide rates among sufferers from Huntington's chorea, and stresses the need for thorough psychological testing and extensive patient support following exposure to screening for this disorder.

Personal or religious beliefs will influence whether screening is undertaken at all. For example, there would seem little point in carrying out prenatal diagnosis for chromosome studies when the couple would refuse a termination under any circumstances. However, no-one should be made to feel that once they have undergone screening, they are bound to follow a rigid course of action. The couple should feel free to exercise whatever options they choose.

For a small number of couples, for whom the risk of producing an abnormal child is unacceptably high, artificial insemination by donor may provide a possible alternative. The extent to which potential donors themselves can be screened for genetic disease is limited, but chromosome studies at least should be carried out on all individuals before they are used as donors. Madan *et al.* (1984) reported a paracentric inversion in a donor, while more recently, Selva *et al.* (1986) reported on the screening of 676 donors of whom 18 were excluded on cytogenetic grounds. Our own experience includes a reciprocal translocation detected at amniocentesis, the fetus having been conceived using a donor carrying the translocation.

Genetic screening tests often yield information that is relevant to other family members. Usually there is no barrier to a free exchange of information within the family, but occasionally individuals will wish to keep the results of tests to themselves. This puts the counsellor in a difficult position. He must preserve confidentiality, but at the same time, there may be relatives at risk of genetic disease who should be traced and tested.

Confidentiality of genetic test results is a matter of concern in a much broader sense. In the United States the Office of Technology Assessment published a report in 1983 on the role of genetic testing in the prevention of genetic disease (see review by Kolata 1986). This indicated a growing number of companies who were screening their workers for genetic disorders. It would appear that the test most frequently carried out was for sickle-cell trait—one wonders why. It is possible that we will see an increase in such practices as the scope broadens of disorders that can be detected using gene probes. The problem, however, is complex. It could be fairly convincingly argued, for example, that it is in the best interests of individuals with alpha 1-antitrypsin deficiency (a condition that predisposes to lung disease) that they should be protected from jobs which expose them to dust, etc. On the other hand individuals with predisposition to disorders such as Alzheimer's disease or Huntington's chorea might well find themselves a target for discrimination, not only with regard to their job prospects, but also by insurance companies. As Berg and Fletcher (1986) point out, there is an urgent need for legislation over the disclosure of the results of screening tests.

The possible misuse of genetic screening by eugenicists may give rise to some concern. However, apart from the moral issues, arguments against the marriage of individuals with similar disorders are often ill-founded scientifically. Assortative mating among the blind, as discussed by Polani and Berry (1982), in response to a paper by Philips *et al.* (1982) provides a good example. Those affected with such handicaps frequently consider them to be much less of a burden than sighted individuals. Moreover, with blindness, ignoring the fact that over half the forms of blindness are due to 'acquired' changes, it has been estimated that there are between 50 and 70 mutations involved at different loci that result in blindness. Half of these are of the autosomal recessive type. The probability that two individuals having identical recessive genotypes will meet is very small. The net effect is that the great majority of children from marriages involving two blind people are normally sighted.

6 The future of genetic screening

The use of gene probes will undoubtedly increase rapidly over the next decade, expanding widely the range of genetic disorders that can be detected and allowing accurate prediction of risks in many cases. These techniques, however, are likely to remain relatively time-consuming and, therefore, costly. In some cases it is possible that molecular research will soon give us knowledge of the gene products, and from this it may well be possible to devise cheaper and more effective biochemical methods of screening.

Ultrasound and fetal blood sampling are both relatively new techniques that are being improved all the time, and one would expect increasing sophistication in these areas. Chorion villus sampling, already an acceptable method for prenatal diagnosis of biochemical disorders and for DNA probe work, may largely replace amniocentesis for prenatal screening for chromosome disorders. Automation of karyotyping is already becoming available, and offers the possibility of increasing laboratory output in the future.

Current interest in *in vitro* fertilization is building and now that the techniques have been shown to be successful, the demand for their use can be expected to rise accordingly. Already there are reports of chromosome studies on pre-embryos (Angell *et al.* 1986, and Watt *et al.* 1987), and although at present, embryos chosen for reimplantation are selected by their gross physical appearance alone, it is potentially possible to remove a single cell prior to reimplantation, with a view to culturing and examining the genetic constitution of the pre-embryo.

In all this activity directed towards the identification of genetic disease, it is to be hoped that appropriate measures for legislation will be taken to ensure that information gained through screening programmes is not used to the detriment of the individual. It is also essential that, in concentrating effort towards the detection of abnormality, sight is not lost of the need to develop aspects of therapy, possibly working towards the ultimate goal of 'gene' therapy.

References

Allan LD, Crawford DC, Chita SK, Tynan MJ (1986). Prenatal screening for congenital heart disease. Br Med J, 292: 1717–1719.

Angell RR, Templeton AA, Aitken RJ (1986). Chromosome studies in human *in vitro* fertilization. Hum Genet, 72: 333–339.

Aronson SM, Volk BW (1962). Genetic and demographic consideration concerning Tay–Sachs disease. In: Cerebral Sphingolipidoses. Aronson SM, Volk BW (eds). New York: Academic Press, pp 372–394.

Barrai I, Vullo C (1980). Genetic counselling in beta thalassaemia in Ferrara. J Genet Hum, 28: 97–104.

Benn PA, Hsu LYF (1983). Maternal cell contamination of amniotic fluid cell cultures: Results of a U.S., nationwide survey. Am J Med Genet, 15: 297–305.

Bennett MJ (1984). Ultrasound in Perinatal Care. Chichester: John Wiley.

Berg K, Fletcher J (1986). Ethical and legal aspects of predictive testing. Lancet, 1: 1043.

Berry AC, Blunt S, Daker MG (1981). Problems arising from amniocentesis for the detection of chromosome abnormalities. In: Recent Advances in Prenatal Diagnosis: Proceedings of the First International Symposium of Recent Advances in Prenatal Diagnosis, Bologna, September 1980. Orlandi C, Polani PE, Bovicelli L (eds). Chichester: John Wiley, pp 151–161.

Beutler KG, Blume JC, Kaplan DW, Löme AW, Ramot B, Valentine, WN (1979). International committee for standardization in haematology: Recommended screening test for glucose 6-phosphate dehydrogenase (G6PD) deficiency. Br J Haematol, 43: 465–467.

Blakemore KJ, Samuelson J, Breg WR, Mahoney MJ (1985). Maternal metaphases on direct chromosome preparation of first trimester decidua. Hum Genet, 69: 380.

Brambati B, Simoni G, Danesino C, Oldrini A, Ferrazzi E, Romitti L, Terzoli G, Rossella F, Ferrari M, Fraccaro M (1985). First trimester fetal diagnosis of genetic disorders: Clinical evaluation of 250 cases. J Med Genet, 22: 92–99.

Brock DJH, Sutcliffe RG (1972). Alpha-fetoprotein in the antenatal diagnosis of anencephaly and spina bifida. Lancet, 2: 197–199.

Buckton KE, Spowart G, Newton MS, Evans HJ (1985). Forty-four probands with an additional 'marker' chromosome. Hum Genet, 69: 353–370.

Bundey S, Webb TP, Thake A, Todd J (1985). A community study of severe mental retardation in the West Midlands and the importance of the fragile X chromosome in its aetiology. J Med Genet, 22: 258–266.

Chase DS, Morris AH, Ballabio A, Pepper S, Giannelli F, Adinolfi M (1986). Genetics of Hunter syndrome: Carrier detection, new mutations, segregation and linkage analysis. Ann Hum Genet, 50: 349–360.

Chubb IW, Pilowsky PM, Springell HJ, Pollard AC (1979). Acetylcholinesterase in human amniotic fluid: An index of fetal neural development? Lancet, I: 688–690.

Collaborative Acetylcholinesterase Study (1981). Amniotic fluid acetylcholinesterase electrophoresis as a secondary test in the diagnosis of anencephaly and open spina bifida in early pregnancy. Lancet, 2: 321–324.

Creasy MR (1982). Chromosome aberrations as a cause of prenatal death. In: Paediatric Research: A Genetic Approach. Festschrift for Paul Polani. Clinics in Developmental Medicine No. 83. Adinolfi M, Benson P, Giannelli F, Seller M (eds). London: Spastics International Medical Publications, William Heinemann Medical Books, pp 122–135.

Cuckle HS, Wald NJ, Lindenbaum RH (1984). Maternal serum alpha-fetoprotein measurements: A screening test for Down syndrome. Lancet, 1: 926–929.

Cuckle HS, Wald NJ, Thompson SG (1987). Estimating a woman's risk of having a pregnancy associated with Down's syndrome using her age and serum alpha-fetoprotein level. Br J Obstet Gynaecol, 94: 337–402.

Djalali M, Steinbach P, Schwinger E, Schwartz G, Tettenborn U, Wolf FM (1985). On the significance of true trisomy 20 mosaicism in amniotic fluid culture. Hum Genet, 69: 321–326.

Farrer LA (1986). Suicide and attempted suicide in Huntington disease: Implications for preclinical testing of persons at risk. Am J Med Genet, 24: 305–311.

Fitzsimmons JS (1987). Counselling in prenatal diagnosis. In: Chorion Villus Sampling. Liu DTY, Symonds EM, Golbus MS (eds). London: Chapman & Hall.

Funderburk SJ, Spence MA, Sparkes R S (1977). Mental retardation associated with 'balanced' chromosome rearrangements. Am J Med Genet, 29: 136–141.

Gardner-Medwin D (1970). Mutation rates in Duchenne type muscular dystrophy. J Med Genet, 7: 334–337.

Gartler SM, Scott RC, Goldstein JL, Campbell B, Sparkes R (1971). Lesch–Nyhan syndrome: Rapid detection of heterozygotes by use of hair follicles. Science, 172: 572–574.

Ghosh A, Tang MHY, Tai D, Nie G, Ma HK (1986). Justification of maternal serum alpha fetoprotein screening in a population with low incidence of neural tube defects. Prenat Diagn, 6: 83–87.

Gosden CM (1984). The recognition of clinically significant chromosome abnormalities in prenatal diagnosis: Problem cases. In: Prenatal Diagnosis. Rodeck CH, Nicolaides KH (eds). London: Royal College of Obstetricians and Gynaecologists, pp 65–84.

Hamerton JL, Boué A, Cohen MM, de la Chapelle A, Hsu LY, Lindsten J, Mikkelsen M, Robinson A, Stengel-Rutkowski D, Webb T, Willey A, Worton R (1980). Chromosome disease. Prenat Diagn (Special issue).

Hassold T, Jacobs P, Kline J, Stein Z, Warburton D (1980). Effect of maternal age on autosomal trisomies. Ann Hum Genet, 44: 29–36.

Hecht F, Cadien JD (1984). Tay–Sachs disease and other fatal metabolic disorders. In: Antenatal and Neonatal Screening. Wald NJ (ed). Oxford: Oxford University Press, pp 128–154.

Herbst DS, Miller JR (1980). Non-specific X-linked mental retardation. II: The frequency in British Columbia. Am J Med Genet, 7: 461–469.

Hook EB (1981). Down syndrome: Frequency in human populations and factors pertinent to variation in rates. In: Trisomy 21 (Down Syndrome) Research Perspectives. De la Cruz FF, Gerald PS (eds). Baltimore: University Park Press, pp 3–67.

Hook EB, Hamerton JL (1977). The frequency of chromosome abnormalities detected in consecutive newborn studies: Differences between studies. Results by sex and by severity of phenotypic involvement. In: Population Cytogenetics: Studies in Humans. Proceedings of a Symposium on Human Population cytogenetics, New York, October 1975. Hook EB, Porter IH (eds). New York: Academic Press, pp 63–80.

Jackson L (1986). CVS Newsletter 6th March, 1986. Philadelphia: Jefferson Medical College.

Kaback MM (1981). Heterozygote screening and prenatal diagnosis in Tay–Sachs disease: A worldwide update. In: Lysosomes and Lysosomal Storage Diseases. Callahan JW, Lowden JA (eds). New York: Raven Press, pp 331–342.

Kaback MM, Shapiro LJ, Hirsch P, Roy C (1977). Tay–Sachs disease heterozygote detection: A quality control study. In: Progress in Clinical and Biological Research, Vol 9. Based on the First International Conference on Tay–Sachs Disease, Palm Springs, California. Kaback MM (ed). New York: Alan Liss, pp 267–279.

Kalousek DK, Dill FJ (1983). Chromosomal mosaicism confined to the placenta in human conceptions. Science, 221: 665–667.

Kolata G (1985). Closing in on the muscular dystrophy gene. Science, 230: 307–308.

Kolata G (1986). Genetic screening raises questions for employers and insurers. Science, 232: 317–319.

Langenbeck U, Hansmann I, Hinney B, Hönig V (1976). On the origin of the supernumary chromosome in autosomal trisomies, with special reference to Down's syndrome. A bias in tracing non-disjunction by chromosomal and biochemical polymorphisms. Hum Genet, 33: 89–102.

Levine SC, Filly RA, Golbus MS (1978). Ultrasonography for guidance of amniocentesis in genetic counselling. Clin Genet, 14: 133–138.

Lippman-Hand A, Fraser FC (1979a). Genetic counselling: The post-counselling period. I: Parents' perceptions of uncertainty. Am J Med Genet, 4: 51–71.

Lippman-Hand A, Fraser FC (1979b). Genetic counselling: The post-counselling period. II: Making reproductive choices. Am J Med Genet, 4: 73–87.

Lorenz RP, Botti JJ, Schmidt CM, Ladda RL (1985). Encouraging patients to undergo prenatal genetic counselling before the day of amniocentesis. J Reprod Med, 30: 933–935.

Luzzatto L, Usanga EA, Reddy S (1969). Glucose 6-phosphate dehydrogenase deficient red cells: Resistance to infection by malarial parasites. Science, 164: 839–842.

MacKenzie WE, Homes DS, Webb T, Whitehouse C, Newton JR (1986). A randomized study of three cannulas for transcervical chorionic villus sampling. Am J Obstet Gynecol, 154: 34–39.

Madan K, Seabright M, Lindenbaum RH, Bobrow M (1984). Paracentric inversions in man. J Med Genet, 21: 407–412.

Magenis RE, Chamberlin J (1981). Parental origin of nondisjunction. In: Trisomy 21 (Down Syndrome) Research Perspectives. De la Cruz FF, Gerald PS (eds) Baltimore: University Park Press, pp 77–93.

Mantingh A, Breed ASPM, Bodgert A, Govaerts LCP (1986). The other side of the CVS coin. Eur J Epidemiol, 2: 324–325.

Martin AO, Liu K (1986). Implications of 'low' maternal serum alpha-fetoprotein levels: Are maternal age risk criteria obsolete? Prenat Diagn, 6: 243–247.

Medical Research Council (1978). An assessment of the hazards of amniocentesis. Br J Obstet Gynaecol, 85: (Suppl 2).

Merkatz IR, Nitowsky HM, Macri JN, Johnson WE (1984). An association between low maternal serum alpha-fetoprotein and fetal chromosome abnormalities. Am J Obstet Gynecol, 14: 886–892.

Murday V, Slack J (1985). Screening for Down's syndrome in the North East Thames Region. Br Med J, 291: 1315–1318.

Nicolaides KH, Rodeck CH, Gosden CM (1986). Rapid karyotyping in non-lethal fetal malformations. Lancet, 1: 283–287.

Nolan GH, Schmickel RD, Chantaratherakitti P, Knickerbocker C, Hamman J, Louwsma G (1981). The effect of ultrasonography on midtrimester genetic amniocentesis complications. Am J Obstet Gynecol, 140: 531–534.

Nwokoro N, Neufeld EF (1979). Detection of Hunter heterozygotes by enzymatic analysis of hair roots. Am J Hum Genet, 31: 42–49.

Philips CI, Newton MS, Gosden CM (1982). Procreatic instinct as a contributory factor to prevalence of hereditary blindness. Lancet, 1: 1169–1172.

Polani PE, Berry AC (1982). Genetic counselling for the blind. Lancet, 2: 106 -107.

Rodeck CH (1984). Obstetric technique in prenatal diagnosis. In: Prenatal Diagnosis. Rodeck CH, Nicolaides KH (eds). London: Royal College of Obstetricians and Gynaecologists, pp 15–28.

Rodeck CH, Campbell S (1979). Umbilical cord insertion as source of pure fetal blood for prenatal diagnosis. Lancet, 1: 1244–1245.

Selva J, Leonard C, Albert M, Auger J, David G (1986). Genetic screening for artificial insemination by donor (AID): Results of a study on 676 semen donors. Clin Genet, 29: 389–396.

Shapiro LR, Wilmot PL, Brenholz P, Leff A, Martino M, Harris G, Mahoney MJ, Hobbins JC (1982). Prenatal diagnosis of fragile X chromosome. Lancet, 1: 99–100.

Simpson JL, Martin AO, Verp MS, Elias S, Patel VA (1982). Hypermodal cells in amniotic fluid cultures: Frequency, interpretation and clinical significance. Am J Obstet Gynecol, 143: 250–258.

Smith AD, Wald NJ, Cuckle HS, Stirrat GM, Bobrow M, Lagercrantz H (1979). Amniotic fluid acetylcholinesterase as a possible diagnostic test for neural tube defects in early pregnancy. Lancet, 1: 685–688.

Smith GF, Berg JM (1976). Down's Anomaly (2nd edn). Edinburgh: Churchill Livingstone.

Tabor A, Madsen M, Obel EB, Philip J, Bang J, Norgaard-Pedersen B (1986). Randomized controlled trial of genetic amniocentesis in 6406 low-risk women. Lancet, 1: 1287–1293.

Therkelsen A (1979). Group report on cell culture and cytogenetic technique. In: Proceedings of the Third European Conference on Prenatal Diagnosis. Murken JD, Stengel-Rutkowski S, Schwinger E (eds). Stuttgart: Enke, pp 258–270.

United Kingdom Collaborative Study on Alpha-fetoprotein in Relation to Neural Tube Defects (1977). Maternal serum alpha-fetoprotein measurement in antenatal screening for anencephaly and spina bifida in early pregnancy. Lancet, 1: 1323–1332.

United Kingdom Collaborative Study on Alpha-fetoprotein in Relation to Neural Tube Defects (1979). Amniotic fluid alpha-fetoprotein measurement in antenatal diagnosis of anencephaly and open spina bifida in early pregnancy. Lancet, 2: 651–662.

US National Academy of Sciences (1975). Genetic screening: Programs, principles and research. Washington: National Academy of Sciences, 116–129.

Warburton D (1984). Outcome of cases of *de novo* structural rearrangements diagnosed at amniocentesis. Prenat Diagn, 4: 68–70.

Warsof SL, Griffin D (1984). The diagnosis of fetal abnormalities. In: Ultrasound in Perinatal Care. Bennett MJ (ed). Chichester: John Wiley.

Watt JL, Templeton AA, Messing I, Bell L, Cunningham P, Duncan RO (1987). Trisomy 1 in an eight cell human preembryo. J Med Genet, 24: 60–64.

Weatherall DJ (1985). The New Genetics and Clinical Practice. Oxford: Oxford University Press.

Weatherall DJ, Clegg JB (1981). The Thalassaemia Syndromes (3rd edn). Oxford: Blackwell Scientific Publications.

Weatherall DJ, Letsky EA (1984). Genetic haematological disorders. In: Antenatal and Neonatal Screening. Wald NJ (ed). Oxford: Oxford University Press, pp 155–192.

Weatherall DJ, Old JM, Thein SL, Wainscoat JS, Clegg JB (1985). Prenatal diagnosis of the common haemoglobin disorders. J Med Genet, 22: 422–430.

Wertz DC, Sorenson JR, Heeren TC (1986). Clients' interpretation of risks provided in genetic counselling. Am J Hum Genet, 39: 253–264.

World Health Organization (1983). Report on the community control of hereditary anaemias. Memorandum from a World Health Organization meeting. Bull WHO, 61: 63–80.

Yutaka T, Fluharty AL, Stevens RL, Kihara H (1978). Idurate sulfatase analysis of hair roots for identification of Hunter syndrome heterozygotes. Am J Hum Genet, 30: 575–582.

24 Detecting hypertensive disorders of pregnancy

Henk C. S. Wallenburg

1 Introduction

Hypertensive disorders in pregnancy comprise at least two aetiologically different entities. One is a disorder induced by pregnancy. It is a disease mainly, but not exclusively, of nulliparae, that appears in the course of pregnancy and is reversed by delivery. The other condition is pre-existing hypertension, unrelated to but coinciding with pregnancy, which may be detected for the first time in pregnancy and does not regress after delivery. To complicate matters further, the two conditions of pregnancy-induced and pregnancy-associated hypertensive disorders may occur together in the same woman.

Hypertensive disorders in pregnancy may be associated with minor problems or with severe emergencies such as eclampsia. They are now a leading cause of maternal death in the United States (Kaunitz *et al.* 1985) and in England and Wales (Department of Health and Social Security 1986), and an important cause of fetal and neonatal morbidity and mortality (Chamberlain *et al.* 1978; MacGillivray 1983).

Eclampsia has been known since Hippocrates' time as a convulsive disease occurring in pregnant women, but it was not distinguished from epilepsy until the nineteenth century. The proteinuria of eclampsia was discovered in the 1840s. In 1896 Scipione Riva Rocci described the technique of indirect measurement of arterial blood pressure using an arm occluding cuff with a mercury sphygmomanometer, a method that has not been greatly changed to this day (Riva Rocci 1896). Riva Rocci used palpation to detect arterial pulsations, but in 1905 Korotkoff recognized the occurrence of sounds during deflation of the cuff, and introduced the auscultatory method of blood pressure measurement (Laher and O'Brien 1982). These methods of blood pressure detection were rapidly applied in pregnant women, and in the first decades of the twentieth century hypertension and proteinuria became generally accepted as indicative of obstetric pathology and as warning signs of eclampsia (Chesley 1978). Since that time, screening for elevated arterial blood pressure and urinalysis for protein has become standard practice in antenatal care.

The terminology and definitions used to classify the hypertensive disorders of pregnancy have been—and still are—inconsistent and confusing, which makes comparison of the results of epidemiologic and clinical studies difficult and often impossible (Chesley 1978). More than 60 names in English and over 40 in German have been applied to these conditions (Rippmann 1969); a variety of terms such as 'toxaemia', 'toxicosis', and 'gestosis' are still used in many countries. In different ways, most definitions emphasize four features that may occur alone or in combination: hypertension, oedema, proteinuria, and convulsions (Chesley 1978). Of these, an elevation of blood pressure is essential to define the disorder as hypertensive. The threshold between normotension and hypertension has been set at various and largely arbitrarily chosen levels, and the same is true for the definitions of pathologic proteinuria. The diagnosis of convulsions will cause little difficulty, but the recognition and assessment of oedema is highly subjective.

The signs of pregnancy-induced hypertensive disease become apparent at a relatively late stage in pregnancy, usually in the course of the late-second or the third trimester; maternal symptoms may occur even later or not at all. However, the fundamental problem of a misalliance of fetal trophoblast with maternal tissue, which is thought to be the underlying cause of the disturbed maternal circulatory adaptation, appears to occur much earlier in pregnancy, between 8 and 18 weeks' gestation (Wallenburg 1988b). For that reason, it seems logical to search for earlier indicators of pregnancy-induced hypertensive disease than hypertension and proteinuria. A multitude of tests have been proposed to predict the later development of the disease (Chesley 1978).

This chapter will first discuss the problems associated with definition and diagnosis of hypertensive disorders in pregnancy. After assessing the use of standard methods of antenatal care in the diagnosis and prediction of pregnancy-induced hypertensive disorders, it will then review several biochemical and biophysical markers and various tests that have been proposed to predict the development of hypertensive disease in pregnancy and evaluate their relative importance.

2 The conventional defining signs

Since the aetiology of the pregnancy-induced hypertensive syndrome is not understood, definition and diagnosis are based on the signs that are conventionally considered to be most characteristic: hypertension, proteinuria, and oedema. These signs, of which the presence of an elevated blood pressure is a prerequisite, constitute secondary features of an underlying circulatory disorder. As signs they are non-specific; they can be induced by pregnancy itself, as well as by a variety of conditions unrelated to, but coinciding with pregnancy. Hypertension and proteinuria are usually asymptomatic and must be detected by screening.

2.1 Hypertension

The term hypertension denotes an abnormally high arterial blood pressure. Arterial blood pressure can be measured easily, which makes it an attractive variable for screening. But what does it mean? Blood pressure is a continuous haemodynamic variable which, in association with cardiac output and peripheral vascular resistance, characterizes the systemic circulation. The pumping action of the heart converts energy into pressure, which produces flow. The relationship between pressure and flow can be expressed as 'flow' = 'pressure divided by resistance of the vascular system' which in turn mainly depends on vessel diameter (Wallenburg 1988a). Although this Poiseuille-Hagen equation represents a gross simplification of haemodynamics it serves to illustrate an important principle. The key function of the circulatory system: to deliver flow for the exchange of water, gases, substances, and heat, cannot be assessed by measuring blood pressure alone. An increase in cardiac output may be accompanied by a rise, a fall, or no change in arterial blood pressure, depending on the change in resistance.

The 40 per cent increase in maternal blood volume and cardiac output that normally occurs in the first trimester and is sustained throughout pregnancy, is haemodynamically accommodated by a decrease in peripheral vascular resistance due to vasodilatation (de Swiet 1980; Wallenburg 1988a). Usually peripheral resistance decreases somewhat more than required to maintain pressure, and arterial blood pressure tends to fall. The decrease is mostly in the diastolic pressure and is maximal in midpregnancy. Blood pressure levels tend to rise again to about non-pregnant values in the course of the third trimester (MacGillivray 1969; Christianson 1976; Friedman 1976; Chesley 1978). The diastolic midpregnancy dip was not found in some studies (Margulies *et al.* 1987). The physiological vasodilatation in pregnancy is associated with a marked attenuation of the pressor effects of vasoactive substances such as angiotensin II (Chesley *et al.* 1965), perhaps through local prostanoid activity (Wallenburg 1981; Ylikorkala and Mäkilä 1985).

A host of theories has been advanced to explain the impressive maternal circulatory changes in pregnancy (Longo 1983), but the underlying mechanisms remain obscure. It may be presumed that they are associated with the complex interaction of fetal with maternal tissue that, among others, leads to the known vascular adaptations in the uteroplacental bed (Robertson and Khong 1987). Because so little is understood about the physiological mechanisms, it is not known why some healthy pregnant women, usually nulliparae, fail to exhibit or maintain a proper circulatory response to the presence of trophoblast.

One of the first signs of circulatory maladaptation appears to be the development, in the second half of pregnancy, of an increased sensitivity to angiotensin II, which may be followed by vasoconstriction and an abnormal rise in blood pressure (Gant *et al.* 1973). The diagnosis of 'hypertension' is made only when blood pressure passes a predefined threshold. Many pregnancies develop normally in spite of the raised blood pressure, which indicates that adequate uteroplacental and maternal organ flows are maintained. A certain degree of hypertension may very well be beneficial to maintain perfusion pressures in the face of an elevated vascular resistance. Sometimes, however, cardiac output falls and the circulation in various maternal target organs may suffer. The widespread but variable involvement of different organ systems may lead to a broad spectrum of clinical, biochemical, and biophysical signs and symptoms (Table 24.1).

The hypertensive expression of the maternal circulatory maladaptation syndrome in pregnancy differs fundamentally from chronic hypertension, which is a long term problem coinciding with pregnancy. Chronic hypertension is caused by essential hypertension or renal disease, and by rare conditions such as pheochromocytoma, coarctation of the aorta, Cushing's or Conn's syndrome (MacGillivray 1983; Lindheimer and Katz 1983). The differential diagnosis of pregnancy-induced hypertension and pregnancy associated with chronic hypertension causes much confusion. In comparison with the usually nulliparous women with pregnancy-induced hypertension or pre-eclampsia, women with chronic hypertension tend to be older and parous (MacGillivray 1983; Lindheimer and Katz 1983). Many women with essential or renal hypertension show an even greater physiologic fall in blood pressure during the first half of pregnancy than do normotensive women, with an exaggerated rise in the third trimester (Chesley 1978). This makes it difficult to make a clinical distinction between pregnancy-induced hypertension and pregnancy-associated chronic hypertension in a woman with unknown prepregnancy blood pressure values who is first seen and found to be normotensive in midpregnancy, and who subsequently exhibits a rise in blood pressure above the predefined threshold. In this case one must reassess blood pressure at a remote time after delivery to make a reasonably reliable diagnosis in retrospect. The earlier in pregnancy that hypertension is noted, the more likely it is to be chronic hypertension (MacGillivray 1983; Davey and MacGillivray 1988).

If a parous woman develops what seems to be pregnancy-induced hypertension it is probable that she has an underlying vascular or renal problem. In his classic long term follow-up study of surviving eclamptic women Chesley (1977) clearly demonstrated an increased prevalence of underlying hypertension and renal disease in the multiparous group, which led to a significantly larger number of remote deaths in this group compared to both primigravid eclamptic women and normotensive women. The results of a study in which the cause of hypertension complicating pregnancy was assessed by means of renal biopsy indicated underlying subclinical renal disease in 50 per cent of parous women as compared with 15 per cent of nulliparae (Fisher *et al.* 1981). On the other hand, a follow-up study of 84 women with (proteinuric) pre-eclampsia diagnosed between 20 and 37 weeks' gestation showed renal abnormalities as frequently in primiparae (67 per cent) as in multiparae (63 per cent) (Ihle *et al.* 1987). This study, however, included only about half of the women with pre-eclampsia before 37 weeks of gestation who were delivered at that hospital, and a selection bias may have been present.

Table 24.1 Signs of maternal system involvement in pregnancy-induced hypertensive disorders

Vascular system	Increased sensitivity to angiotensin II (Gant *et al.* 1973) Raised blood pressure Raised peripheral resistance (Groenendijk *et al.* 1984) Reduced plasma volume (Hays *et al.* 1985) Reduced cardiac output (Groenendijk *et al.* 1984) Haemolysis (Weinstein 1982)
Renal system	Reduced uric acid clearance (Redman 1976a) Reduced renal blood flow (Chesley and Duffus 1971) Reduced glomerular function (Chesley and Duffus 1971) Glomerular capillary endotheliosis (Spargo *et al.* 1959)
Hepatic system	Elevated liver enzymes (Weinstein 1982)
Platelet-coagulation system	Reduced platelet count (Redman et al. 1978) Reduced platelet life span (Wallenburg and Rotmans 1982) Reduced antithrombin III (Weiner and Brandt 1982) Elevated factor VIII R : AG (Thornton and Bonnar 1977)

Chronic hypertension is a major predisposing factor for pre-eclampsia ('superimposed pre-eclampsia') (Redman 1980; Sibai and Anderson 1986; Guzick *et al.* 1987). The maternal and fetal risks of chronic hypertension in pregnancy seem to be mainly attributable to the development of superimposed pre-eclampsia; the majority of chronically hypertensive women who do not develop pre-eclampsia have a normal perinatal outcome (Redman 1980; Sibai and Anderson 1986).

2.2 Proteinuria

Renal protein excretion increases in normal pregnancy (Lopez-Espinoza *et al.* 1986), and proteinuria is not considered abnormal until it exceeds 300 mg per 24 hours (McEwan 1968; Lindheimer and Katz 1977). Protein excretion exhibits diurnal variation; there is a trend for peak protein excretion between 2 and 8 pm (McEwan 1987), and factors such as posture, physical activity, cold, and stress may considerably influence protein excretion (Lindheimer and Katz 1977). An increase in protein output will usually but not always lead to higher concentrations in random urine samples. The volume and concentration of urine will affect protein concentration and may give rise to erroneously high or low results of tests on random urine specimens (Davey and MacGillivray 1988).

Proteinuria may be a temporary phenomenon due to pregnancy-induced renal lesions, or it may be an expression of pre-existing renal disease coinciding with pregnancy (MacGillivray 1983; Lindheimer and Katz 1983). In the first case it should disappear at some time after delivery; in the latter it will remain present.

Proteinuria is a late sign of pregnancy-induced hypertension, but it is associated with a marked increase in the incidence of poor fetal outcome (Friedman and Neff 1976; Page and Christianson 1976a; Chamberlain *et al.* 1978; MacGillivray 1983). For this reason, pregnancy-induced hypertension associated with proteinuria is considered to be a more severe state of disease and is commonly referred to as pre-eclampsia. This terminology will be used throughout this chapter. The overall correlation between the degree of elevation of blood pressure and the occurrence of proteinuria is weak (McEwan 1987). On the other hand, the magnitude of protein loss correlates positively with the severity of renal lesions (Fisher *et al.* 1981).

In conclusion, the presence of pathologic proteinuria in pregnancy-induced hypertension indicates a severe maternal circulatory disturbance with an increased risk of poor fetal outcome. Thus urine testing is a vital part in the screening process for hypertensive disorders in pregnancy.

2.3 Oedema

Moderate oedema has been reported to occur in 50 (Thomson *et al.* 1967) to 80 per cent (Robertson 1971) of healthy normotensive pregnant women. This physiologic oedema of pregnancy is often confined to the lower limbs, but it may also occur in other sites such as the fingers or face, or as generalized oedema (Thomson *et al.* 1967; Robertson 1971). Indeed, most pregnant women note that the rings on their fingers become tight in the course of the third trimester. Physiologic oedema usually develops gradually, and is associated with a smooth rate of weight-gain. The finding that pregnant women with generalized oedema without hypertension or proteinuria have larger babies than women without obvious oedema (Thomson *et al.* 1967) strongly suggests that oedema is a part of the normal maternal adaptation to pregnancy.

Oedema affects approximately 85 per cent of women with pre-eclampsia (Thomson *et al.* 1967). It may appear rather suddenly and may be associated with a rapid rate of weight-gain. However, it cannot be differentiated clinically from oedema in normal pregnancy. In Robertson's (1971) prospective study, pregnant women without oedema, and with early or late onset oedema, all had a similar incidence of hypertension.

Data from the large prospective Collaborative Perinatal Project show that the combination of hypertension and oedema, or hypertension and increased maternal weight-gain, is associated with a somewhat lower fetal death rate than is hypertension alone (Friedman and Neff 1976). Pre-eclampsia without oedema ('dry pre-eclampsia') has long been recognized as a dangerous variant of the condition, with a higher maternal and fetal mortality than pre-eclampsia with oedema (Eden 1922; Vosburgh 1976).

Clinical assessment of oedema is subjective. For this reason the rate of weight-gain in pregnancy has been used as a measurable index of fluid retention and has in the past been made part of some definitions of pre-eclampsia (Nelson 1955; Hughes 1972), even in the absence of hypertension (Rippmann 1969). The assessment of studies on weight gain in pregnancy is complicated by the fact that over the past 50 years or so pregnant women in developed countries have frequently been put on restricted diets (see Chapter 18).

As oedema in pregnancy is common and does not define a group at risk, it should not be used as a defining sign of hypertensive disorders in pregnancy.

2.4 Other signs and symptoms

A number of additional signs and symptoms have been described as suggestive, predictive, or even diagnostic of hypertensive disorders in pregnancy. These include visual symptoms (blurring of vision, diplopia, scotomas, or flashes of light), headache, epigastric or upper quadrant abdominal pain, oliguria or anuria, and pulmonary oedema or cyanosis (MacGillivray 1983). These signs and symptoms are relatively rare and non-specific, but when they occur during established pregnancy-induced hypertensive disease they suggest widespread involvement of various maternal organs and thus severe disease.

3 Terminology, definitions, and diagnosis

3.1 Terminology

The term 'toxaemia' was introduced in the middle of the nineteenth century, and covered a broad spectrum of diseases thought to be caused by circulating toxins, including acute yellow atrophy of the liver, vomiting of pregnancy, and 'nephritic and preeclamptic toxaemia' and eclampsia (Chesley 1978). No circulating toxin has ever been demonstrated and the aetiological terms 'toxaemia', 'toxicosis', or 'pre-eclamptic toxaemia' have now largely been replaced by descriptive terms based on the hypertensive and proteinuric manifestations of the disease.

Gestational (Hughes 1972; Davey and MacGillivray 1988), or pregnancy-induced (Gant and Worley 1980; Wallenburg 1988a) hypertension are terms used to describe hypertension caused by pregnancy itself. The term pre-eclampsia is often used as an equivalent of pregnancy-induced hypertension (Nelson 1955), with proteinuria (Hughes 1972). Since the occurrence of proteinuria increases the risk of perinatal death about twofold (Page and Christianson 1976a; MacGillivray 1983; Chamberlain *et al.* 1978) it seems appropriate to reserve the term pre-eclampsia for the combination of pregnancy-induced hypertension and proteinuria as is done in this chapter (although eclampsia can still occur in the absence of proteinuria (Sibai *et al.* 1981). The term EPH-gestosis (Edema, Proteinuria, Hypertension) (Rippmann 1969) is used in Germany. 'Chronic hypertension' or 'chronic hypertensive disease' is the term which describes the condition of pre-existing hypertension with or without proteinuria (Hughes 1972; Davey and MacGillivray 1988). 'Superimposed pre-eclampsia' describes the occurrence of pregnancy-induced pre-eclampsia in a pregnant woman with pre-existing, chronic hypertension.

3.2 Definitions and diagnosis

The definition and diagnosis of hypertensive disorders in pregnancy is based on the level of arterial blood pressure and the degree of proteinuria, in relation to gestational age. As discussed before, oedema should not be used as a defining criterion.

3.2.1 Measurement of blood pressure

Direct measurement of arterial blood pressure using a catheter inserted into an artery and connected to a pressure transducer is the most accurate technique; however, it carries real risks and is much too invasive for general use (Raftery 1978). For screening purposes indirect methods are used, based on compression of a peripheral artery with a cuff and detection of the vibrations transmitted as the cuff is deflated (Raftery and Ward 1968). The vibrations are generated by the turbulence of the flow through the partially occluded artery, and can be heard by means of a stethoscope or a microphone as the Korotkoff sounds, or they can be detected by Doppler-shift signals or oscillometry (Raftery 1978; Hunyor *et al.* 1978).

The errors of blood pressure measurement, attributable to the instrument and to the observer, have been reviewed in depth (Conceiçao *et al.* 1976; Hunyor *et al.* 1978; O'Brien *et al.* 1985; Murnaghan 1987). Even when cuff size and speed of descent of the mercury column are standardized, and the cuff is at the reference level of the left atrium, there is a large observer error. The accuracy of the indirect blood pressure measurement is limited when compared with intra-arterial readings as the gold standard, with important differences between various types of sphygmomanometers (Hunyor *et al.* 1978). The aneroid gauge is subject to many more potential errors than the simple mercury manometer (Murnaghan 1987; O'Brien *et al.* 1985). The automated Doppler and oscillometric devices have no observer error, but they may produce grossly erroneous readings (Hunyor *et al.* 1978).

Phase I of the Korotkoff sounds identifies systolic blood pressure. There is now increasing agreement that in pregnancy the diastolic pressure should be determined at phase 4, the 'muffling' of the sounds (Wichman *et al.* 1984; Davey and MacGillivray 1988). In situations of high cardiac output and low peripheral resistance, such as pregnancy and exercise, Korotkoff sounds may not disappear at all, and taking phase 5 diastolic pressure readings may be grossly misleading (Raftery and Ward 1968; Wichman *et al.* 1984). In both normotensive (Ginsburg and Duncan 1969) and in hypertensive (Hovinga *et al.* 1978) pregnancies, sphygmomanometry gives higher systolic and diastolic readings than does direct measurement of arterial pressure (Wallenburg 1988a). Even more important than the difference between directly and indirectly measured blood pressure values is the poor correlation between the two (O'Brien *et al.* 1985). The relevant point is that virtually all studies reported in the literature and all clinical correlations between hypertensive disorders and outcome of pregnancy refer to readings obtained by indirect blood pressure measurement.

The position of the arm on which the blood pressure is taken has a marked influence on the readings (Webster *et al.* 1984). An important methodologic error occurs when blood pressure is taken on the right arm of a pregnant woman lying on her left side. In that position the right and uppermost brachial artery will be at a distance of 15–20 cm above the left atrium. Since each centimetre of vertical height above or below the level of the heart is the equivalent of a difference in hydrostatic pressure of 0.7 mm Hg, the blood pressure measured in the uppermost arm will be approximately 10–14 mm Hg lower than the true pressure at the level of the heart.

In addition to the technical, methodologic, and observer errors associated with indirect blood pressure measurement, sampling errors may also occur due to blood pressure variability. Many factors cause marked variability in blood pressure between individuals (e.g. age, parity, race) and within the same pregnant woman, such as time of day, level of activity, sleep, emotions, and posture (MacGillivray *et al.* 1969; Christianson 1976; Redman 1984). Measurements by doctors or nurses in antenatal clinics are usually higher than those obtained at home ('white coat hypertension', O'Brien *et al.* 1985).

Blood pressure behaviour is altered in hypertensive pregnant women. In normotensive pregnant women blood pressure follows a circadian rhythm similar to that of the non-pregnant state. The highest blood pressures occur at midmorning, followed by a progressive fall throughout the rest of the day, a nadir at about 3 a.m., and a subsequent slow rise (Ruff *et al.* 1982). In hypertensive pregnant women these circadian rhythms may be deranged and reversed, with peak blood pressure values occurring around midnight (Redman *et al.* 1976b; Ruff *et al.* 1982).

Although determination of blood pressure is the mainstay of screening, diagnosis, and decision-making in pregnant women, the inherent technical and sampling errors, whether by auscultation or by automatic devices, constitute an important limitation of the accuracy and precision of this measurement. The sampling error can be reduced by averaging a large number of blood pressure readings taken under standardized conditions (Redman 1984). In practice and in most clinical studies, the number of blood pressure readings per day is limited, and a diagnosis of hypertension is usually based on two measurements obtained with a certain time interval (Hughes 1972; Davey and MacGillivray 1988) or even on a single reading (Davey and MacGillivray 1988).

Systolic blood pressure is more affected by changes in cardiac output due to exercise, stress, or posture than is diastolic pressure (de Swiet 1980). The systemic diastolic blood pressure, in particular, reflects peripheral vascular resistance (Guyton 1986), which is where the primary circulatory problem in pregnancy-induced hypertensive disorders appears to lie (Wallenburg 1988a). High levels of systolic blood pressure are associated with increased rates of fetal death, but only when they occur in conjunction with a high diastolic pressure (Friedman and Neff 1976). High levels of diastolic blood pressure, on the other hand, are associated with an adverse fetal outcome even when systolic levels are within the normal range. Both systolic and diastolic blood pressure are indicators of risk, but measurement of systolic pressure does not add to the information obtained by measuring diastolic blood pressure alone (Davey and MacGillivray 1988).

Page and Christianson (1976b) have advocated the use of mean arterial pressure, defined as systolic blood pressure plus twice the diastolic pressure divided by three, for the definition of hypertension in pregnancy. From a haemodynamic point of view, mean arterial pressure may indeed be a better measure of systemic perfusion pressure than diastolic blood pressure alone. However, there is no evidence that it is a better predictor of fetal outcome than diastolic blood pressure (Friedman and Neff 1976). Moreover, mean arterial pressure is not measured directly, but is calculated on the basis of systolic and diastolic blood pressure readings, each with their inherent errors of measurement. The calculation will increase the total error and further decrease reliability.

In conclusion, there are good reasons to base the clinical definitions and diagnosis of hypertension in pregnancy on diastolic blood pressure values alone (Davey and MacGillivray 1986), taken at phase 4 of the Korotkoff sounds.

How should hypertension in pregnancy be defined? This question can be approached in at least two ways, statistically or clinically. The statistical approach is based on the observation that values of diastolic blood pressure will follow a certain distribution. If the distribution is known, a cut-off level can be chosen (e.g. 2 or 3 standard deviations above the mean) to identify a fraction of the population at the extreme upper end of the diastolic pressure distribution; these women may then be called hypertensive. This approach has several important disadvantages (see Chapter 3). First, the actual distribution of diastolic blood pressure levels has been studied in only a few well-defined populations of pregnant women (Christianson 1976; MacGillivray *et al.* 1969; Chesley 1976; Redman 1984; Redman and Jefferies 1988). Second, blood pressure in pregnancy is not in a steady state; the mean values of the diastolic pressure distributions in early and midpregnancy are lower than those at term. In Chesley's (1976) study of 1400 white American primigravidae, a diastolic blood pressure of 90 mm Hg or more (a level often used to define hypertension) identified about 5 per cent of the population in the first half of pregnancy, and approximately 20 per cent at term. These figures are supported by results of later studies (MacGillivray *et al.* 1969; Redman 1984).

In view of the physiologic changes in blood pressure that occur in the course of pregnancy, hypertension may also be defined as an abnormal increment in blood pressure, rather than as an absolute value. In a serial study of blood pressure, taken both sitting and lying, in 226 primigravidae, MacGillivray *et al.* (1969) showed that the average increase in diastolic blood pressure is about 5 mm Hg between weeks 24 and 30, and approximately 15 mm Hg between weeks 30 and 40. A rise in diastolic blood pressure of 20 mm Hg or more, from the lowest level, occurred in 57 per cent of these primigravid women (MacGillivray *et al.* 1969). In Redman's (1984) study of 6790 women with singleton pregnancies in Oxford, 32 per cent of primiparae showed an increment in diastolic pressure of 11–20 mm Hg between booking and maximum antenatal blood pressures; in 19 per cent the increment was more than 20 mm Hg. To define hypertension in pregnancy reliably on the basis of an abnormal rise in diastolic blood pressure, at least two readings taken in the course of pregnancy are needed, and their difference should be related to the distribution of differences in the pregnant population at large.

In the clinical approach to defining hypertension in pregnancy, the outcome of the pregnancy is considered. Pregnant women with a diastolic blood pressure between 90 and 100 mm Hg in the second half of pregnancy, experienced an increased incidence of proteinuria and perinatal death (Friedman and Neff 1976; Page and Christianson 1976a; MacGillivray 1983). For that reason, a diastolic blood pressure level somewhere between 90 and 100 mm Hg may be considered to be a threshold between women at low risk and women with an increased risk of pregnancy complications. A diagnosis of hypertension so defined, is not a diagnosis of a disease, but a marker of an increase in risk and an indication for careful monitoring of mother and fetus. It is clinically important to realize that, in view of the physiological blood pressure changes in pregnancy, a diastolic blood pressure of 90 mm Hg in midpregnancy is more abnormal than it is when it occurs for the first time at term.

There is limited epidemiologic data on the clinical importance of increments in diastolic blood pressure. The results of two studies suggest that the absolute level of blood pressure is far more important than the rise, both in relation to the occurrence of proteinuria and in terms of prognosis (MacGillivray 1961; Page and Christianson 1976a). However, a recent detailed study indicates that a combination of a first diastolic reading of less than 90 mm Hg, a subsequent increase of at least 25 mm Hg, and a maximum reading of at least 90 mm Hg may be better for identifying a group of pregnant women with pre-eclamptic features than either measurement alone (Redman and Jefferies 1988).

Finally, the period of gestation in which hypertension develops is of significance with respect to definition and classification. Many authors agree that, in the absence of trophoblastic disease, pregnancy-induced hypertensive disorders rarely occur before 20 weeks' gestation (MacGillivray 1983; Chesley 1978; Lindheimer and Katz 1983). Hypertension and/or proteinuria diagnosed before 20 weeks will usually be due to pre-existing chronic hypertension or renal disease. Hypertension may also be diagnosed for the first time during labour; such hypertension will often be transitory, due to effort and/or anxiety. Only one of the usual definitions or classifications makes a distinction between hypertension diagnosed in pregnancy and during labour (Davey and MacGillivray 1988), and most studies provide no information as to whether or not women who develop hypertension for the first time during labour were included. One study showed that inclusion of women who developed hypertension for the first time in labour raised the incidence of pregnancy-induced hypertension from 10 to 30 per cent (Knutzen and Davey 1977).

3.2.2 Measurement of proteinuria

In practice, screening for proteinuria is usually done with reagent strips or 'dipstick' tests, which will start detecting protein (albumin) concentrations of approximately 50 mg/l. The semi-quantitative colour reactions of trace, +, + +, + + +, and + + + + correspond to urinary protein concentrations of approximately 0.3 to 0.5, 1, 3, and 20 g per litre, respectively. The method is quite specific for albumin but does not detect abnormal globulins (e.g. Bence–Jones protein), a shortcoming that is not very important in antenatal screening (Lindheimer and Katz 1977). False positive reactions may occur with alkaline urine, or if specimens are contaminated with quaternary ammonium compounds or chlorhexidine. Protein concentrations depend on urine volume and specific gravity. Thus, when urine volume is high and specific gravity is low, abnormal proteinuria exceeding 300 mg/24 hr may remain undetected by screening of random urine samples (Lindheimer and Katz 1977). Simultaneous determination of specific gravity—also by means of a dipstick—may improve the reliability of the detection of proteinuria in random urine samples. Dipsticks may give up to 25 per cent false positive results with a trace reaction, and 6 per cent false positive results with a one + reaction on testing of random specimens from women with normal 24-hour total protein excretion (Shaw *et al.* 1983).

The definitive test for proteinuria in pregnancy is determination of total protein excretion in a 24-hour urine collection, using a reliable quantitative method (e.g. Esbach's). This should be performed whenever significant proteinuria is detected on screening of a random urine specimen, but it is too complicated to be used for screening of pregnant women on an outpatient basis. Even in the hospital, collection of complete 24-hour urine specimens presents considerable problems. Alternative approaches to the measurement of 24-hour protein excretion, such as determination of the protein/creatinine index in random urine specimens

(Shaw *et al.* 1983), await validation. Concentrations of protein measured in random samples must be considered acceptable for purposes of screening. To be certain that the proteinuria is of renal origin and not due to contamination, the urine tested should be either a clean-catch midstream or a catheter specimen.

3.3 Recommendations

Of the many definitions and classifications that have been proposed (Hughes 1972; Nelson 1955; Rippmann 1969), the recommendations of the International Society for the Study of Hypertension in Pregnancy (Davey and MacGillivray 1988) fit in best with the general considerations presented above. Table 24.2 gives a summary of the definitions and the classification based on them. The definition of hypertension is based on a single cut-off level of diastolic blood pressure of 90 mm Hg established on two occasions. However, when diastolic blood pressure is markedly elevated, one cannot delay treatment in order to repeat the measurement after an interval of several hours; hence the arbitrarily chosen cut-off level of 110 mm Hg or more for a single observation.

Pathologic proteinuria is defined as a total protein excretion of 300 mg or more per day, but protein concentrations determined in random samples are also considered, taking into account specific gravity. The classification based on these definitions is simple and entirely clinical; it may be revised after delivery or even in the puerperium, until 6 weeks after delivery. In this classification the term 'gestational hypertension' is used instead of 'pregnancy-induced hypertension', the term

Table 24.2 Summary of the definition and classification of hypertensive disorders in pregnancy, as recommended by the International Society for the Study of Hypertension in Pregnancy (Davey and MacGillivray 1988)

DEFINITIONS	
Hypertension	1. One indirect measurement of diastolic blood pressure (Korotkoff 4) of 110 mm Hg or more, or 2. Two consecutive indirect measurements of DBP of 90 mm Hg or more, 4 hours or more apart.
Proteinuria	1. Total protein excretion of 300 mg or more per 24 hours. 2. Two random clean-catch or catheter urine samples collected 4 hours or more apart, with (a) †† (1 g/l) or more on reagent strip if SG is more than 1030 or (b) + (0.3 g/l) or more if SG is less than 1030.
CLASSIFICATION	
Gestational hypertension or proteinuria†	Hypertension or proteinuria developing after the 20 weeks of pregnancy in a previously normotensive nonproteinuric woman.
Gestational proteinuric hypertension (pre-eclampsia)†	Hypertension in combination with proteinuria developing after 20 weeks' gestation in a previously normotensive non-proteinuric woman.
Chronic hypertension or chronic renal disease†	Hypertension and/or proteinuria in pregnancy in a woman with chronic hypertension or chronic renal disease diagnosed before or during, or persisting after pregnancy.
Chronic hypertension with superimposed pre-eclampsia	Proteinuria developing for the first time during pregnancy in a woman with chronic hypertension.
Unclassified hypertension and/or proteinuria	Hypertension and/or proteinuria found at first antenatal examination after 20 weeks' gestation. May be classified after delivery.
Eclampsia	The occurrence of generalized convulsions during pregnancy, labour, or within 7 days of delivery, and not caused by epilepsy or other convulsive disorders.

†Further subdivided according to development during pregnancy, labour, or the puerperium.

used in this chapter because it more clearly expresses the nature of the disorder.

It should be noted that no attempt has been made to classify conditions according to severity, which would greatly increase the complexity of the classification.

4 Identification of pregnancy-induced hypertension

4.1 Standard methods of antenatal care

Antenatal visits are conventionally arranged monthly until 28 weeks, 2-weekly up to 36 weeks, and weekly thereafter until delivery. These visits are dominated by a check of blood pressure and urine, and by the determination of weight-gain. How do these routines contribute to the prediction or early diagnosis of hypertensive disorders?

Whether the development of pregnancy-induced hypertension may be predicted on the basis of the standard variables that are determined in antenatal care—blood pressure, proteinuria, and weight-gain—has been addressed in several retrospective and some prospective studies. The use of the term 'prediction' in this context is debatable. If it is accepted that the signs of pregnancy-induced hypertension are a relatively late expression of a fundamental problem of circulatory maladaptation that begins early in pregnancy, then the search is for an early diagnosis, rather than for ways to predict the development of the disorder.

Of the prospective, controlled investigations, Gallery's (1977) study dealt with 42 nulliparae and 40 multiparae, all of whom were initially normotensive. Standardized blood pressure readings were obtained monthly from 16 weeks' gestation onwards, using a mercury random-zero sphygmomanometer. Of these 82 women, 9 nulliparae and 6 multiparae developed hypertension, defined as systolic pressures above 135 mm Hg and/or diastolic pressures above 85 mm Hg in late pregnancy, presumably without proteinuria. The blood pressures in this group of women did not show the fall in diastolic blood pressure between 17 and 20 weeks' gestation that occurred in women who remained normotensive. Of the 15 women who became hypertensive later in pregnancy, 10 had diastolic blood pressure values of 75 mm Hg or more at 17 to 20 weeks' gestation, as compared with 6 of 67 women who remained normotensive (Gallery *et al.* 1977).

A larger prospective study in 808 nulliparous and 175 parous women with singleton pregnancies was reported by Moutquin *et al.* (1985). The investigators used an automatic oscillometric sphygmomanometer and started their blood pressure readings between 9 and 12 weeks' gestation. A total of 7800 blood pressure readings were obtained at intervals of 4 weeks. The results were not withheld from physicians or women, but no particular intervention was suggested for any blood pressure reading. Of 734 initially normotensive nulliparae 46, (6 per cent) developed pre-eclampsia as defined by the authors (blood pressure at or above 140/90 mm Hg, oedema and/or proteinuria after 20 weeks).

A mean diastolic blood pressure of over 80 mm Hg at 17 to 20 weeks gestation had a sensitivity of 32 per cent, a specificity of 91 per cent, and a positive predictive value of only 18 per cent of identifying women who would subsequently develop pre-eclampsia. Using 85 mm Hg as the cut-off point, the sensitivity dropped to 16 per cent, the specificity increased to 97 per cent, and the positive predictive value rose to a modest 27 per cent.

Mean arterial pressure values in the second trimester (18 to 26 weeks) have also been used in the prediction of the development of pre-eclampsia later in pregnancy. Page and Christianson (1976b) presented data on the outcome of pregnancy based on a prospective study of 14 833 single births. They found that when the averaged mean arterial pressure in the middle trimester was 90 mm Hg or greater, there was a significant increase in the frequency of pregnancy-induced hypertension, proteinuria, fetal growth retardation and stillbirths.

Moutquin *et al.* (1985) found that a mean arterial pressure of 85 mm Hg or more at 17 to 20 weeks had a sensitivity of 86 per cent, a specificity of 50 per cent and a positive predictive value of less than 10 per cent for the prediction of subsequent pre-eclampsia (which had a prevalence of 5 per cent in their population). A cut-off point of 90 mm Hg arterial pressure dropped the sensitivity to 68 per cent, with a specificity of 75 per cent, and a positive predictive value of 14 per cent, which is little different from the predictive values found using diastolic pressures alone.

Two additional smaller studies (Quaas *et al.* 1982; Öney and Kaulhausen 1983) using more than 90 mm Hg mean arterial pressure found sensitivities of 93 and 63 per cent, specificities of 66 and 89 per cent and positive predictive values of 32 and 58 per cent for the prediction of pregnancy-induced hypertension with prevalences of 29 and 20 per cent respectively.

Reviewing the reports on standard blood pressure measurements as a means to predict pre-eclampsia or pregnancy-induced hypertension at an early stage, one is struck by the fact that very few investigators state whether or not the results of these measurements were revealed to the physicians who make management decisions. As measurements were usually part of routine antenatal care and will therefore have been recorded in the patients' charts, it is unlikely that the diagnosis was made without knowledge of the test results. This can lead to serious biases in the assessment of test results (see Chapter 3).

In a recent investigation in 100 pregnant women of mixed parity attending a high risk antenatal clinic,

Lopez-Espinoza *et al.* (1986) studied microalbuminuria using a sensitive radioimmunoassay to determine whether an increasing loss of albumin would predict the occurrence of proteinuric pre-eclampsia. No evidence was found that gross proteinuria is preceded by a gradual increase in microalbuminuria, and the authors conclude that there is no value in using precise techniques of detecting proteinuria to predict pre-eclampsia.

Weight-gain is of no value for the prediction of subsequent pre-eclampsia. This subject has been fully addressed elsewhere in this book (see Chapter 18).

4.2 Biochemical and biophysical tests

A number of tests have been devised to demonstrate the presence or absence of an abnormal vascular responsiveness before the clinical onset of pregnancy-induced hypertension. Most of these tests are of historical value only and will be mentioned only briefly.

4.2.1 Cold pressor test

The cold pressor test was devised more than 50 years ago (Hines and Brown 1933) to test the hypothesis that an exaggerated blood pressure response to immersion of the hand in ice-cold water for 1 to 2 minutes could predict the later development of hypertension or pre-eclampsia (Dieckmann *et al.* 1938; Reid and Teel 1938; Chesley and Chesley 1939; Chesley and Valenti 1958). The general conclusion of these studies was that the test is unreliable and cannot be used to predict the onset of pregnancy-induced hypertension or to differentiate it from chronic hypertension.

4.2.2 Flicker fusion test

The nitroglycerine flicker fusion threshold test was first described by Krasno and Ivy (1950). Following some enthusiastic reports on the reliability with which the test performed in early pregnancy could predict the development of pre-eclampsia later in pregnancy (Brill *et al.* 1952; Marty and Hardy 1952), subsequent investigators have found the test to be worthless (Gillim 1954; Rugart 1953; Gardiner and Herdan 1957).

4.2.3 Isometric exercise test

Degani *et al.* (1985) proposed that the diastolic blood pressure response to an isometric handgrip exercise, which is known to increase systemic arterial blood pressure (Lind and McNicol 1967), might reflect vascular reactivity in pregnant women, and might thus be useful for detecting vascular hyperreactivity and for predicting pregnancy-induced hypertension. One hundred healthy primigravidae performed an isometric handgrip exercise test between 28 and 32 weeks' gestation (Degani *et al.* 1985). The published data, if taken at face value, suggest that this test could be useful. In these women the prevalence of pregnancy-induced hypertension was 16 per cent and the test showed a sensitivity of 81 per cent, a specificity of 96 per cent, and a positive predictive value of 81 per cent. These results are highly suspect as a roll-over test conducted on the same women reported a prevalence of pregnancy-induced hypertension of 9 per cent which is patently incompatible with the 16 per cent noted in these women with the other test.

4.2.4 Roll-over test

During their angiotensin infusion studies, Gant *et al.* (1973) noted that many nulliparous, normotensive pregnant women who were sensitive to angiotensin II demonstrated an increase in diastolic blood pressure of 20 mm Hg or more when they turned from their left sides onto their backs. Thus the roll-over or supine pressor test came into being. They performed the test between 28 and 32 weeks of pregnancy with the woman lying on her left side until the diastolic blood pressure was stabilized (Gant *et al.* 1974). The woman was then turned on her back, and diastolic blood pressure was again recorded; a rise of 20 mm Hg or more defined a positive test. The first study comprised 50 healthy primigravid women but pregnancy outcome was given for only 38 of them. Fifteen of the 16 women with a positive roll-over test developed pregnancy-induced hypertension compared to 2 of 22 with a negative roll-over test. The prevalence of pregnancy-induced hypertension (blood pressure 140/90 mm Hg or above and/or a rise in diastolic blood pressure of 20 mm Hg or more) in this allegedly unselected sample of primigravidae was 45 per cent, which must be one of the highest prevalences anywhere in the world.

Since this report many investigators have studied the validity of the roll-over test in their own institutions (Table 24.3). Studies in which a positive test result led to some form of intervention (Thompson and Mueller-Heubach 1978; Spinapolice *et al.* 1983) are not included. The high sensitivity and specificity of the roll-over test reported by Gant *et al.* (1974) have not been confirmed by most of the other studies. Various factors may explain the marked disparity in results of this relatively simple test. Although all investigators define an increase in diastolic blood pressure of at least 20 mm Hg as a positive test, there is considerable variation among investigators in the methodology of the test (Poland *et al.* 1980). The definition of pregnancy-induced disorders shows the usual inconsistencies: it is usually not stated whether or not elevations of blood pressure occurring for the first time during labour or in the early postpartum period are included; in most studies pre-eclampsia is not distinguished from non-proteinuric hypertension. All authors, with only a few exceptions (Campbell 1978; Kuntz 1980) fail to identify the arm used to record blood pressure. This is of great importance, since turning from the left side on the back with blood pressure recorded from the right (superior)

Table 24.3 Validity of the roll-over test in reported studies

Authors	Number of patients	Parity	Pregnancy-induced hypertension Definition*	Prevalence %	Sensitivity %	Specificity %	p.v.+† %	p.v.−† %
Gant *et al.* (1974)	38	0	⩾140/90 DBP↑⩾20	45	88	95	93	91
Phelan *et al.* (1977)	207	?	⩾140/90 DBP↑⩾20	13	78	82	39	82
Karbhari *et al.* (1977)	178	0	?	21	71	99	93	93
Marshall and Newman (1977)	100	0	⩾140/90 DBP↑⩾20	28	75	94	84	91
Gusdon *et al.* (1977)	60	0	⩾140/90 DBP↑⩾20	22	77	79	50	93
Verma *et al.* (1980)	130	?	⩾140/90 DBP↑⩾15	23	63	62	51	88
Campbell (1978)	85	0	DBP⩾90	53	4	97	66	48
Kuntz (1980)	65	0	⩾140/90	38	60	68	54	73
Thurnau *et al.* (1983)	75	?	⩾140/90	37	73	35	37	71
Didolkar *et al.* (1979)	39	0	⩾140/90 DBP↑⩾30	20	41	81	35	85
Poland *et al.* (1980)	139	0	⩾140/90 DBP↑⩾20	32	42	62	34	69
Kassar *et al.* (1980)	74	0	⩾140/90	27	60	35	25	70
Öney and Kaulhausen (1983)	188	0	⩾140/90	14	63	75	30	92
Degani *et al.* (1985)	100	0	⩾140/90 DBP↑⩾20	9	67	57	13	95
Marx *et al.* (1980)	78	0	?	22	88	51	33	94
Tunbridge (1983)	100	0	DBP⩾95	19	10	90	20	81

*Main blood pressure criteria for diagnosis of pregnancy-induced hypertensive disorders. DBP↑⩾20 = increase in diastolic blood pressure of
20 mm Hg or more.
†Predictive value of a positive/negative test.
?Not reported.

arm will result in a predictable increase in diastolic pressure of approximately 10–15 mm Hg due to the increase in hydrostatic pressure relative to the level of the heart. Indeed, subjects with the cuff on the left (inferior) arm showed a fall in diastolic pressure after rolling over (Sobel *et al.* 1980). Biologic variability in blood pressure due to exercise, talking, and anxiety may further contribute to the variability of the test results. Moreover, serial roll-over tests performed weekly in the same primigravid women showed very poor reproducibility (O'Grady *et al.* 1977).

Although it is stated in a few publications (Gusdon *et al.* 1977; Phelan *et al.* 1977; Kassar *et al.* 1980; Verma *et al.* 1980) that the results of the tests were not revealed to the physicians or to the women, in most cases it is not mentioned whether the diagnosis of pregnancy-induced hypertensive disorders was made with or without knowledge of the test results.

4.2.5 *Infusion of catecholamines*

The pressor effects of adrenaline infused in physiologic (Nisell *et al.* 1985) and pharmacologic (Zuspan *et al.* 1964; Raab *et al.* 1956) doses appear to be greater in women with (mild) pregnancy-induced hypertension than in normotensive pregnant women. Raab *et al.* (1956) investigated the pressor effects of two doses of adrenaline in 163 normotensive pregnant women between 28 and 34 weeks' gestation. They noted a higher increase in systolic blood pressure in women who later became hypertensive than in women who remained normotensive. However, there was extreme variability in response and considerable overlap between the responses of normotensive and hypertensive women. The pressor response to noradrenaline also appears to be greater in hypertensive pregnant women than in normotensive pregnant women (Talledo *et al.* 1968; Nisell *et al.* 1985). No further attempts have been made to use the pressor effects of catecholamines as a test to predict the development of pregnancy-induced hypertension.

4.2.6 *Infusion of vasopressin*

Half a century ago two independent groups reported an increased vascular sensitivity to extracts of the posterior pituitary gland (Dieckmann and Michel 1937; Schockaert and Lambillon 1937) in pre-eclamptic women. Marked rises in blood pressure were noted, sometimes accompanied by oliguria and even precipitation of convulsions, but later investigations found the responses to vasopressin to be extremely variable, both in normotensive and in hypertensive pregnant women. Infusion of vasopressin in pregnant women is a hazardous procedure and cannot be used for prediction or early diagnosis of hypertensive disease in pregnancy.

4.2.7 Infusion of angiotensin II

Abdul-Karim and Assali (1961) reported that intravenous infusion of angiotensin II ('angiotonin') caused a smaller rise in blood pressure in pregnant women than in non-pregnant individuals. The relative refractoriness to the pressor effects of angiotensin II in normal pregnancy was later confirmed in several studies (Chesley *et al.* 1965; Talledo 1966; Schwarz and Retzke 1971) and, in addition, it was found that this refractoriness is much less in pre-eclamptic women (Chesley 1966; Talledo *et al.* 1968). Gant *et al.* (1973) used the determination of the sensitivity to infused angiotensin II to predict the development of pregnancy-induced hypertension.

They studied the effect of infused angiotensin II on diastolic blood pressure sequentially throughout pregnancy in 192 young (13 to 17 years old) and apparently healthy primigravidae, measuring the amount of angiotensin II per kilogram of bodyweight per minute needed to raise the diastolic blood pressure (Korotkoff 5) by 20 mm Hg. The average so-called effective pressor dose (Kaplan and Silah 1964) was found to be about 8 ng/kg/min in non-pregnant individuals and in early (7 to 10 weeks) pregnancy; it increased approximately two-fold to 15 ng/kg/min by 28 weeks, and fell gradually thereafter to a level of 11–12 ng/kg/min at term. Up to about 20 weeks' gestation, all pregnant women showed refractoriness to the pressor effects of angiotensin II. In women who ultimately developed pregnancy-induced hypertension (blood pressure of 140/90 or higher and/or a rise in diastolic pressure of 20 mm Hg or more), the refractoriness gradually decreased. Between 28 and 32 weeks the effective pressor dose had returned to nonpregnant values. Forty-five of the 58 women with a positive test (an effective pressor dose of less than 8 ng/kg/min) between the 28th and 32nd week of pregnancy subsequently developed pregnancy-induced hypertension, compared to 5 of 95 with a negative test.

The validity of this complicated and time-consuming test in predicting pregnancy-induced hypertension has been assessed in clinical investigations (Morris *et al.* 1978; Orozco *et al.* 1979; Öney and Kaulhausen 1982; Nakamura *et al.* 1986). As shown in Table 24.4, the number of women included in these studies is small and the definitions of a positive test and of pregnancy-induced hypertension varied.

The angiotensin sensitivity test is too complicated and time consuming to be used as a screening procedure. It may, however, be useful for research purposes to define groups of women at high or low risk of developing pregnancy-induced hypertension (Wallenburg *et al.* 1986).

4.3 Haematological and biochemical tests

Concentrations of a large number of constituents of blood and urine, including hormones, have been shown to change in pregnancy-induced hypertensive disorders (see Chapter 29). Some of these have been proposed for the prediction or early diagnosis and will be discussed in the following paragraphs.

4.3.1 Plasma volume, haemoglobin concentration, haematocrit

Plasma volume rises progressively during pregnancy,

Table 24.4 Validity of the angiotensin sensitivity test in reported studies

Authors	EPD*	Number of patients	Duration of gestation (wks)	Parity 0/M	Pregnancy-induced hypertension: Definition†	Pregnancy-induced hypertension: Prevalence %	Sensitivity %	Specificity %	p.v. + ‡ %	p.v. − ‡ %
Morris *et al.* (1978)	< 8§	26	29–32	0	DBP ≥ 90	12	33	39	7	82
	< 10§				DBP↑ ≥ 15		67	30	11	87
Nakamura *et al.* (1986)				0:30	≥ 140/90 SBP↑ ≥ 30					
	< 8	48	30	M:18	DBP↑ ≥ 15	21	20	97	75	82
	< 10						80	82	53	94
	< 12						100	74	50	100
Öney and Kaulhausen (1982)	< 10	231	28–32	0	≥ 140/90	15	76	83	45	95
Orozco *et al* (1979)	< 8§	33	28–32	0:15 M:18	≥ 120/80	27	89	79	62	95

*Effective pressor dose (ng/kg/min) below which test was considered positive.
†Main blood pressure criteria for diagnosis of pregnancy-induced hypertensive disorders. DBP↑ ≥ 15 = increase in diastolic blood pressure of 15 mm Hg or more.
‡Predictive value of a positive/negative test.
§At least one positive test in serial testing

and is accompanied by a proportionally much smaller rise in red cell mass which causes the haemoglobin concentration to fall (Letsky 1980). Many authors have reported that the average plasma volume is reduced in women with pregnancy-induced hypertension and particularly more so in pre-eclampsia (MacGillivray 1983; Chesley 1972). Plasma volume contraction sometimes precedes the blood pressure rise in pre-eclampsia (Blekta *et al.* 1970; Gallery et al. 1979; Hays *et al.* 1985); the number of women studied is small, and there is considerable overlap between values of plasma volume in normal and abnormal groups. In addition, dye-dilution techniques for estimating plasma volume are unreliable (Campbell and MacGillivray 1980) and too complicated to be used as a screening procedure.

The contraction of plasma volume that is often observed in pre-eclampsia may be reflected in a rise in haemoglobin concentration or haematocrit (Sagen *et al.* 1982). In a retrospective study of over 54 000 singleton pregnancies, Murphy *et al.* (1986) showed a highly significant correlation in both nulliparae and multiparae between haemoglobin concentration at first booking and the incidence of hypertensive disorders. Determination of the haematocrit is a relatively easy and cheap procedure. More detailed investigation of the relationship between midtrimester haematocrit values and the subsequent course of pregnancy may be worthwhile.

4.3.2 Uric acid

In 1925, Stander *et al.* reported raised serum uric acid levels in women with pre-eclampsia. Many investigators have confirmed this finding and demonstrated a positive correlation between serum uric acid levels and the clinical severity of pregnancy-induced hypertension (Lancet and Fisher 1956; Thurnau *et al.* 1983) and perinatal outcome (Redman *et al.* 1976a; Schuster and Wepelmann 1981; Liedholm *et al.* 1984). On the basis of the results of a prospective but not blinded study in 332 hypertensive pregnant women of mixed parity, Redman *et al.* (1976a) concluded that plasma uric acid levels constitute a better indicator of fetal prognosis than blood pressure.

In a study in which the nature of the hypertensive disorder in pregnancy was established by renal biopsy, women with pregnancy-induced pre-eclampsia were found to have marked hyperuricemia, whereas uric acid levels were normal in pregnant women with chronic hypertension without pre-eclampsia (Pollak and Nettles 1960). However, an association between hyperuricemia, chronic hypertension, and early nephrosclerosis in non-pregnant individuals has also been reported (Messerli *et al.* 1980). It is not clear whether or not uric acid levels can usefully distinguish between pregnancy-induced hypertension and chronic hypertensive disease.

Hyperuricemia is non-specific. It may result from various metabolic or erythrocyte disorders, impaired renal function, and drugs (e.g. diuretics) (Messerli *et al.* 1980). The cause of the hyperuricemia in pregnancy-induced hypertension is not well understood (Wallenburg and Van Kreel 1978).

The results of many (Redman *et al.* 1977; Gallery *et al.* 1980; Riedel *et al.* 1981), but not of all studies (Fay *et al.* 1985), in normotensive pregnant women suggest that serum uric acid levels may begin to rise before the appearance of hypertension and proteinuria. Women studied include nulliparous as well as parous women, some of them with proven renal disease or treated chronic hypertension (Redman *et al.* 1977), and the way the data are presented does not allow a reliable evaluation of the results. Moreover, the predictive value of uric acid determinations was not assessed without prior knowledge of the test results.

Thus, there is insufficient evidence to warrant the use of uric acid levels as a screening test to predict the later development of pregnancy-induced hypertension. In women with established pre-eclampsia, serum uric acid levels appear to reflect fetal prognosis. For that reason uric acid levels can be used in the management of women with a pregnancy-induced hypertensive disorder to monitor the course of the disease.

4.3.3 Calcium excretion

Recently, Taufield *et al.* (1987) reported that established pre-eclampsia is associated with hypocalciuria. The authors investigated a group of 40 pregnant women—20 nulliparae and 20 multiparae—in the third trimester of pregnancy; 10 were normotensive, 5 had transient hypertension, 6 had chronic hypertension, 7 had chronic hypertension with superimposed pre-eclampsia, and 12 had pre-eclampsia. The authors used a very broad definition of pre-eclampsia, and although none of the women received diuretics during the study, it is not stated whether or not other kinds of therapy were used.

Urinary calcium excretion was significantly lower in women with pre-eclampsia than in normotensive women. Women with pre-eclampsia had much lower levels of 42 ± 29 (mean ± SD) mg per 24 hours compared to levels of 313 ± 140 in normotensive women. Levels in women with chronic or transient hypertension were similar to those in normotensive women. The mechanism of hypocalciuria in pre-eclampsia is not known. Further prospective studies are needed to support or refute these findings, and to determine whether a decrease in urinary calcium excretion could be used as an early predictor of the disease.

4.3.4 Enzymes and hormones

Concentrations of various enzymes in serum or plasma have been studied in women with hypertensive disorders, mainly to assess placental function (see Chapter 29). Following a brief period of clinical enthusiasm, none of these enzymes has been shown to be of use as a predictor of hypertensive disease in pregnancy, or as a biochemical measure of its severity. As an extension of earlier studies (Redman *et al.* 1977; Williams and Jones 1975), recent investigators have shown that serum levels of deoxycytidylate deaminase increase in pre-eclampsia, but not in chronic hypertension (Williams and Jones 1982). The latter investigators performed at least two determinations of deoxycytidylate deaminase, one at booking and one in the third trimester, in serum of 2460 pregnant women, the parity of whom is not reported. A total of 133 women (5.4 per cent) developed pregnancy-induced hypertension or pre-eclampsia. Of 187 women with raised deoxycytidylate deaminase levels, 125 (67 per cent) had pregnancy-induced hypertension or pre-eclampsia compared to 8 of 2273 (0.4 per cent) with levels that were within the normal range. It should be emphasized that the majority of these women already had clinical signs of hypertensive disease at the time of determination of deoxycytidylate deaminase values. No abnormally elevated levels were found before 24 weeks' amenorrhea, and very few (4) before 28 weeks. Moreover, the results were known to the physicians and women were admitted to the hospital and treated for the sole reason of having abnormally high deoxycytidylate deaminase levels. Further properly designed studies are required to determine the value of the estimation of deoxycytidylate deaminase—and of the closely related enzyme cytidine deaminase (Jones *et al.* 1982)—in normotensive and hypertensive pregnancies.

It has been claimed (Hughes *et al.* 1980; Toop and Klopper 1981) that the levels of the placental protein hormone termed pregnancy-associated plasma protein A are raised towards the end of the second trimester in women who are likely to develop pre-eclampsia, but the usefulness of this test for the prediction of pre-eclampsia has not been evaluated.

The rate at which the placenta clears maternal blood of isotope-labelled dehydroisoandrosterone sulphate for oestradiol synthesis has been postulated to reflect uteroplacental perfusion (Gant *et al.* 1971). A longitudinal study of the metabolic clearance rate of dehydroisoandrosterone sulphate in women who developed pregnancy-induced hypertension later in pregnancy showed that placental perfusion during the first half to two-thirds of pregnancy was similar to or even above that in women who remained normotensive. The metabolic clearance rate began to fall 2–4 weeks before hypertension was detected, by which time it was only 35–50 per cent of normal (Worley *et al.* 1978). These results have not been confirmed by others. In addition, the late fall in the metabolic clearance rate of dehydroisoandrosterone sulphate and the important inter-individual variation make it unlikely that this test would be useful for the prediction or early diagnosis of hypertensive disease in pregnancy.

4.3.5 Coagulation factors and platelets

Evidence for the occurrence of abnormal coagulation processes and platelet activation was originally based on the finding as early as 1893 of fibrin deposits and thrombi in vessels of various organs of women who died of eclampsia (Schmorl 1893). In later years, factors of the extrinsic and intrinsic coagulation system have been studied extensively in women with hypertensive disorders in pregnancy, and a complicated coagulation index has been proposed to predict the clinical progress of pre-eclampsia (Howie *et al.* 1976). These studies have recently been reviewed (Wallenburg 1987b); the results are generally equivocal and do not suggest that marked consumption of coagulation factors is a consistent feature in pregnancy-induced hypertensive disorders. The most frequently occurring haemostatic abnormalities in women with pregnancy-induced hypertension or pre-eclampsia are a rise in the factor VIII related antigen level, and a reduced antithrombin III concentration.

There appears to be a particularly good correlation between plasma factor VIII related antigen activity and the occurrence of fetal growth retardation, with or without maternal hypertension (Fournie *et al.* 1981; Whigham *et al.* 1980; Scholtes *et al.* 1983; Boneu *et al.* 1977).

Decreased levels of antithrombin III have been demonstrated in a majority of women with pre-eclampsia, but not in pregnant women with chronic hypertension (Weiner and Brandt 1982; Weenink *et al.* 1984). Exacerbations and remissions of the disease were reflected in fluctuations of antithrombin III levels, and low antithrombin III concentrations appear to be associated with placental infarction and poor fetal outcome (Weenink *et al.* 1984). However, none of the coagulation studies have thus far been shown to be useful for the early prediction of pregnancy-induced hypertension or pre-eclampsia.

Recently, attention has been focused on plasma levels of fibronectin, a glycoprotein involved in coagulation, platelet function, tissue repair, and the vascular endothelial basement membrane. Fibronectin levels were found to be markedly elevated in pre-eclamptic women (Stubbs *et al.* 1984; Graninger *et al.* 1985; Saleh *et al.* 1987) and correlated with low antithrombin III levels and with the degree of proteinuria (Graninger *et al.* 1985; Saleh *et al.* 1987). Lazarchick *et al.* (1986) published a prospective blinded study in a group of apparently normotensive out-patients, but as the number of women involved in the study and their parities were not reported, no valid conclusion can be derived. High fibronectin levels have earlier been reported in non-pregnant women with nephrotic syndrome and cholestasis (Stathakis *et al.* 1981).

Many reports in the literature indicate that women with pregnancy-induced hypertension on average have lower platelet counts than normotensive women (Gibson *et al.* 1982; Giles and Inglis 1981), and that thrombocytopenia may occur as an early (Redman *et al.* 1978) but also as a relatively late (Fay *et al.* 1985) feature of the disorder. Thrombocytopenia is not common in pregnant women with chronic hypertension without superimposed pre-eclampsia (Gibson *et al.* 1982; Giles and Inglis 1981). However, platelet behaviour in women with a pregnancy-induced hypertensive disorder is extremely variable (Wallenburg 1987b), and reduced platelet counts are not found in all cases, even of eclampsia (Pritchard *et al.* 1976; Sibai *et al.* 1982). Results of various large studies suggest that approximately 20 per cent of women with a pregnancy-induced hypertensive disorder develop thrombocytopenia, varying from 7 per cent in mild pregnancy-induced hypertension to 50 per cent in severe pre-eclampsia and eclampsia (Giles and Inglis 1981).

Platelet counts can easily be obtained and repeat counts are an important aid in the clinical management of established hypertensive disease in pregnancy. As yet there are no studies on the predictive value of platelet counts in pregnancy.

In conclusion, the determination of factor VIII related antigen activity, plasma antithrombin III concentrations, and platelet counts may be of value in the management of hypertensive disorders in pregnancy. At present there is no convincing evidence that these determinations or that of fibronectin are of any value for prediction or very early diagnosis of the disease.

4.4 Doppler-ultrasound techniques

As mentioned earlier, the most likely underlying cause of the maternal circulatory maladaptation must be sought in a misalliance of fetal trophoblast with maternal tissue in the uteroplacental bed. This misalliance is thought to block the second wave of cytotrophoblast invasion into the myometrial portions of the spiral arteries, which normally occurs between 16 and 20 weeks' gestation. Spiral arteries bypassed by migratory trophoblast are left with an undisturbed non-pregnant architecture and fail to dilate (for review see Robertson and Khong 1987).

The development of continuous wave and pulsed range-gated Doppler-ultrasound systems has made it possible to study the perfusion of deep-lying vessels such as the arcuate arteries and other branches of the uterine vasculature (Campbell *et al.* 1983; Griffin *et al.* 1983; Cohen-Overbeek *et al.* 1985; Trudinger *et al.* 1985; Campbell *et al.* 1986; Schulman 1987). Because of the as yet inevitable errors in the measurement of volume flow (Griffin *et al.* 1983) most emphasis has been put on the quantitative examination of flow velocity waveforms. The velocity waveforms in the branches of the uterine arteries in normal pregnancy show an increase in end-diastolic flow velocity between 14 and 20 weeks; there appears to be no further change in this pattern of low pulsatility and high diastolic velocity until term (Campbell *et al.* 1983; Cohen-Overbeek *et al.* 1985; Trudinger *et al.* 1985). Since the velocities in end diastole are thought to reflect vascular resistance, the change in flow velocity profile observed in the arcuate arteries in the first half of normal pregnancy concurs with the secondary wave of trophoblast invasion in the wall of the spiral arteries followed by vasodilatation.

In their first study in women with an established pregnancy disorder, Campbell *et al.* (1983) observed arcuate artery waveform patterns with reduced end-diastolic velocities suggestive of an elevated uteroplacental vascular resistance in 14 of 31 women with complicated pregnancies. Of these 14 women, 10 had proteinuric hypertension and 8 were eventually delivered of an infant with low birthweight for gestational age. Of the 17 women with normal arcuate artery flow velocity waveforms, only 4 had proteinuric hypertension, and 6 of the fetuses were of low weight for gestational age. A later article dealing with the same study states that the clinicians who cared for these pregnancies had no knowledge of the results (Cohen-Overbeek *et al.* 1985) but it cannot be excluded that the investigators were aware of the clinical severity of the pregnancy complication, which may have biased the results. The results of this study were subsequently confirmed in a larger non-blinded study of uterine arterial waveforms in 91 women with complicated pregnancies (Trudinger *et al.* 1985).

To date the only prospective study on the predictive value of abnormal arcuate artery waveforms in the second trimester of pregnancy has been reported by Campbell *et al.* (1986). A group of 149 unselected pregnant women was investigated. Of these 149 women, 17 were delivered elsewhere and records were incomplete for 6 of them. Of the remaining 126 women 41 were nulliparous. Arcuate artery waveforms were determined between 16 and 18 weeks' gestation and the clinicians who cared for the women were not informed about the results. Of the 76 women with normal waveforms 5 developed pregnancy-induced hypertension, one with fetal growth retardation, and 5 pregnancies were complicated by isolated fetal growth retardation. Of the 50 women with abnormal waveforms 10 developed pregnancy-induced hypertension, 2 of which were complicated by fetal growth retardation, and 10 pregnancies were complicated by fetal growth retardation alone. There was one fetal death in a hypertensive patient. The sensitivity of the test for the prediction of pregnancy-induced hypertension and/or fetal growth retardation is 68 per cent; specificity is 69 per cent. The predictive value of a positive test is 42 per cent, of a negative test 87 per cent. The authors do not present an explanation for the remarkable incidence of 40 per cent abnormal waveforms in an unselected sample of pregnant women, or for the high incidence (24 per cent) of complicated pregnancies.

Measurement of arcuate artery blood flow velocities between 16 and 18 weeks' gestation may diagnose impaired trophoblast invasion of the spiral arteries and may therefore have great potential in predicting pregnancies destined to become complicated by a hypertensive disorder and/or fetal growth retardation. The method may also be useful to monitor the course of the hypertensive disorder and the effects of treatment. However, the errors of measurement (Griffin *et al.* 1983) and the many possible sampling errors (Wallenburg 1987a) need further analysis and assessment. Judgement on the validity of these methods awaits the results of further well-designed and carefully executed prospective clinical studies.

5 Conclusions

5.1 Implications for current practice

Hypertension and pre-eclampsia are usually asymptomatic; screening and diagnosis depend mainly on careful determination of blood pressure and proteinuria. The occurrence of pregnancy-induced hypertension is relatively rare before 28 weeks of pregnancy, but when it occurs it frequently leads to pre-eclampsia with its associated high rate of perinatal morbidity and mortality (Sibai *et al.* 1985). On the other hand, pregnancy-induced hypertension occurs much more frequently late in the third trimester, when antenatal visits are usually increased in frequency, but the maternal and fetal risks of late-onset disease are much smaller. Therefore, although routine antenatal screening for hypertensive disorders before 28 weeks' gestation may have a low productivity in terms of the number of positive diagnoses per visit (Hall *et al.* 1980), it has a high potential in terms of prevention of maternal and fetal morbidity and mortality. For that reason the number of antenatal visits of nulliparae in the second trimester should certainly not be reduced, but may even be increased to once per 3 weeks; such visits may be confined to a brief discussion and measurement of blood pressure and urinalysis for protein.

Simple blood pressure measurement remains an integral part of antenatal care; it should be performed in a standardized fashion by a skilled midwife or nurse, or by the attending physician. Errors in blood pressure measurement cannot be abolished by spending money on automated equipment. In the hands of the individual nurse or doctor, the old-fashioned mercury sphygmomanometer and a stethoscope are still compatible with good antenatal care, and this will most likely remain so in the foreseeable future.

The appearance of proteinuria in a previously non-proteinuric woman with pregnancy-induced or pre-existing hypertension is associated with a marked increase in maternal and fetal risk. For that reason, screening for proteinuria using a dipstick should be carried out routinely. In pregnant women with established hypertensive disease, quantitative measurement of protein concentration in 24-hour urine collections can be recommended.

None of the other tests advocated for screening, prediction and early diagnosis of pregnancy-induced hypertensive disease has been shown to be clinically useful. Determination of haematocrit values, serum uric acid concentrations, platelet counts and, to a lesser extent, plasma antithrombin III concentration and factor VIII related antigen may be of value in monitoring the progress of established hypertensive disorders in pregnancy.

5.2 Implications for future research

The first prerequisite for useful research on hypertensive disorders in pregnancy is the use of clearly defined and reproducible criteria. It is disturbing to note that such criteria for the diagnosis of hypertension are often not stated in publications on hypertensive disorders in pregnancy.

The search should continue for a simple screening test that can be carried out early in pregnancy to predict the later development of pregnancy-induced hypertensive disorders in normotensive women and in women with pre-existing hypertension. Doppler-ultrasound studies of perfusion patterns in uterine arterial branches in the early second trimester of pregnancy may be a promising avenue for research (see Chapter 27). Such studies should be properly designed, involving a sufficient number of individuals.

References

Abdul-Karim R, Assali NS (1961). Pressor response to angiotonin in pregnant and nonpregnant women. Am J Obstet Gynecol, 82: 246–51.

Blekta M, Hlavaty V, Trnkov M, Bendl J, Bendova L, Chytil M (1970). Volume of whole blood and absolute amount of serum proteins in the early stage of late toxemia of pregnancy. Am J Obstet Gynecol, 106: 10–13.

Boneu B, Bierme R, Fourni A, Pontonnier G (1977). Factor VIII complex, fetal growth retardation and toxemia. Lancet, 1: 263.

Brill HM, Long JS, Klawans AH, Golden M, Seaman I (1952). The nitroglycerin flicker infusion threshold test in toxemia of pregnancy. Am J Obstet Gynecol, 64: 1201–1207.

Campbell DM (1978). The effect of posture on the blood pressure in pregnancy. Eur J Obstet Gynecol Reprod Biol, 8: 263–268.

Campbell DM, MacGillivray I (1980). Evans blue disappearance rate in normal pregnancy and preeclampsia. In: Pregnancy Hypertension. Bonnar J, MacGillivray I, Symonds EM (eds). Lancaster: MTP Press, pp 191–195.

Campbell S, Griffin DR, Pearce JM, Diaz-Recasens J, Cohen-Overbeek TE, Willson K, Teague MJ (1983). New Doppler technique for assessing uteroplacental blood flow. Lancet, 1: 675–677.

Campbell S, Pearce JMF, Hackett G, Cohen-Overbeek T, Hernandez C (1986). Qualitative assessment of uteroplacental blood flow: early screening test for high-risk pregnancies. Obstet Gynecol, 68: 649–653.

Chamberlain G, Philipp E, Howlett B, Masters K (1978). British Births 1970, Vol 2, Obstetric Care. London: Heinemann, pp 80–107.

Chesley LC (1966). Vascular reactivity in normal and toxemic pregnancy. Clin Obstet Gynecol, 9: 871–881.

Chesley LC (1972). Plasma and red cell volumes during pregnancy. Am J Obstet Gynecol, 112: 440–449.

Chesley LC (1976). Proposal for classification. In: Blood Pressure, Edema, and Proteinuria in Pregnancy. Friedman EA (ed). New York: Alan Liss, p 251.

Chesley LC (1977). The remote prognosis of eclamptic women. Am Heart J, 93: 407–408.

Chesley LC (1978). Hypertensive Disorders in Pregnancy. New York: Appleton-Century-Crofts.

Chesley LC, Chesley ER (1939). The cold pressure test in pregnancy. Surg Gynecol Obstet, 69: 436–440.

Chesley LC, Duffus GM (1971). Preeclampsia, posture and renal function. Obstet Gynecol, 38: 1–5.

Chesley LC, Valenti C (1958). The evaluation of tests to differentiate pre-eclampsia from hypertensive disease. Am J Obstet Gynecol, 75: 1165–1173.

Chesley LC, Talledo OE, Bohler CS, Zuspan FP (1965). Vascular reactivity to angiotensin II and norepinephrine in pregnant and nonpregnant women. Am J Obstet Gynecol, 91: 837–842.

Christianson RE (1976). Studies in blood pressure during pregnancy. I. Influence of parity and age. Am J Obstet Gynecol, 125: 509–513.

Cohen-Overbeek T, Pearce JM, Campbell S (1985). The antenatal assessment of utero-placental and feto-placental blood flow using Doppler ultrasound. Ultrasound Med Biol, 11: 329–339.

Conceiçao S, Ward MK, Kerr DNS (1976). Defects in sphygmomanometers: An important source of error in blood pressure recording. Br Med J, 1: 886–888.

Davey DA, MacGillivray I (1988). The classification and definition of the hypertensive disorders of pregnancy. Am J Obstet Gynecol, 158: 892–898.

Degani S, Abinader E, Eibschitz I, Oettinger M, Shapiro I, Sharf M (1985). Isometric exercise test for predicting gestational hypertension. Obstet Gynecol, 65: 652–654.

Department of Health and Social Security (1986). Reports on Confidential Enquiries into Maternal Deaths in England and Wales, from 1952–54 to 1979–81. London: Her Majestys' Stationery Office.

de Swiet M (1980). The cardiovascular system. In: Clinical Physiology in Obstetrics. Hytten F, Chamberlain G (eds). Oxford: Blackwell Scientific Publications, pp 3–42.

Didolkar SM, Sampson MB, Johnson WL, Petersen LP (1979). Predictability of gestational hypertension. Obstet Gynecol, 54: 224–225.

Dieckmann WJ, Michel HL (1937). Vascular-renal effects of posterior pituitary extracts in pregnant women. Am J Obstet Gynecol, 33: 131–137.

Dieckmann WJ, Michel HL, Woodruff PW (1938). The cold pressure test in pregnancy. Am J Obstet Gynecol, 36: 408–412.

Eden TW (1922). Eclampsia: a commentary on the reports presented to the British Congress of Obstetrics and Gynaecology. J Obstet Gynaecol Br Empire, 29: 386–401.

Fay RA, Bromham DR, Brooks JA, Gebski VJ (1985). Platelets and uric acid in the prediction of preeclampsia. Am J Obstet Gynecol, 152: 1038–1039.

Fisher KA, Luger A, Spargo BH, Lindheimer MD (1981). Hypertension in pregnancy: clinico-pathological correlations and late prognosis. Medicine, 60: 267–276.

Fournié A, Monrozies M, Pontonnier G, Boneu B, Bierme R (1981). Factor VIII complex in normal pregnancy, pre-eclampsia and fetal growth retardation. Br J Obstet Gynaecol, 88: 250–254.

Friedman EA (1976). Blood pressure relationships. In: Blood Pressure, Edema and Proteinuria in Pregnancy. Friedman EA (ed). New York: Alan Liss, pp 123–151.

Friedman EA, Neff RK (1976). Pregnancy outcome as related to hypertension, edema and proteinuria. In: Hypertension in Pregnancy. Lindheimer MD, Katz AI, Zuspan FP (eds). New York: John Wiley, pp 13–22.

Gallery EDM, Hunyor SN, Ross M, Györy AZ (1977). Predicting the development of pregnancy-associated hypertension. The place of standardised blood-pressure measurement. Lancet, 1: 1273–1275.

Gallery EDM, Hunyor SN, Györy AZ (1979). Plasma volume contraction: a significant factor in both pregnancy-associated hypertension (pre-eclampsia) and chronic hypertension in pregnancy. Qtrly J Med, 48: 593–602.

Gallery EDM, Saunders DM, Boyce ES, Gyry AZ (1980). Relation between plasma volume and uric acid in the development of hypertension in pregnancy. In: Pregnancy Hypertension. Bonnar J, MacGillivray I, Symonds EM (eds). Lancaster: MTP Press, pp 175–179.

Gant NF, Worley RJ (1980). Hypertension in Pregnancy. Concepts and Management. New York: Appleton-Century-Crofts.

Gant NF, Hutchinson HT, Siiteri PK, MacDonald PC (1971). Study of the metabolic clearance rate of dehydroisoandrosterone sulfate in pregnancy. Am J Obstet Gynecol, 111: 555–563.

Gant NF, Daley GL, Chand S, Whalley PJ, MacDonald PC (1973). A study of angiotensin II pressor response throughout primigravid pregnancy. J Clin Invest, 52: 2682–2689.

Gant NF, Chand S, Worley RJ, Whalley PJ, Crosby UD, MacDonald PC (1974). A clinical test useful for predicting the development of acute hypertension in pregnancy. Am J Obstet Gynecol, 120: 1–7.

Gardiner J, Herdan G (1957). A statistical evaluation of the nitroglycerin flicker-fusion threshold test and the 'weight-gain sign' in the prediction of the clinical syndrome of pre-eclampsia. J Obstet Gynaecol Br Empire, 64: 691–699.

Gibson B, Hunter D, Neame PB, Kelton JG (1982). Thrombocytopenia in preeclampsia and eclampsia. Semin Thromb Haemost, 8: 234–247.

Giles C, Inglis TCM (1981). Thrombocytopenia and macrothrombocytosis in gestational hypertension. Br J Obstet Gynaecol, 88: 1115–1119.

Gillim DL (1954). Evaluation of flicker fusion photometry. Obstet Gynecol 4: 264–269.

Ginsburg J, Duncan SLB (1969). Direct and indirect blood pressure measurements in pregnancy. J Obstet Gynaecol Br Commwlth, 76: 705–710.

Graninger W, Tatra G, Pirich K,. Nasz F (1985). Low antithrombin III and high fibronectin in pre-eclampsia. Eur J Obstet Gynecol Reprod Biol, 19: 223–229.

Griffin D, Cohen-Overbeek T, Campbell S (1983). Fetal and uteroplacental blood flow. Clin Obstet Gynecol, 10: 565–602.

Groenendijk R, Trimbos JBMJ, Wallenburg HCS (1984). Hemodynamic measurements in preeclampsia: preliminary observations. Am J Obstet Gynecol, 150: 232–236.

Gusdon JP, Anderson SG, May WJ (1977). A clinical evaluation of the "roll over test" for pregnancy-induced hypertension. Am J Obstet Gynecol, 127: 1–3.

Guyton AC (1986). Textbook of Medical Physiology. Philadelphia, W B Saunders.

Guzick DS, Klein VR, Tyson JE, Lasky RE, Gant NF, Rosenfeld CR (1987). Risk factors for the occurrence of pregnancy-induced hypertension. Clin Exp Hypertens—Hypertension in Pregnancy B6: 281–287.

Hall MH, Chng PK, MacGillivray I (1980). Is routine antenatal care worthwhile? Lancet, 1: 78–80.

Hays PM, Cruikshank DP, Dunn LJ (1985). Plasma volume determination in normal and preeclamptic pregnancies. Am J Obstet Gynecol, 151: 958–966.

Hines EA, Brown GE (1933). A standard test for measuring the variability of blood pressure; its significance as an index of the prehypertensive state. Ann Intern Med, 7: 209–217.

Hovinga G, Aarnoudse JG, Huisjes HJ (1978). The effect of supine and lateral positions on intra-arterial pressure in hypertensive pregnancies. Am J Obstet Gynecol, 131: 233–238.

Howie PW, Begg CB, Purdie DW, Prentice CRM (1976). Use of coagulation tests to predict the clinical progress of pre-eclampsia. Lancet, 2: 323–325.

Hughes EC (1972). Obstetric–Gynecologic Terminology. Philadelphia: FA Davis, 422–423.

Hughes G, Bischof P, Wilson G, Smith R, Klopper A (1980). Tests of fetal wellbeing in the third trimester of pregnancy. Br J Obstet Gynaecol, 87: 650–656.

Hunyor SN, Flynn JM, Cochineas C (1978). Comparison of performance of various sphygmomanometers with intra-arterial blood-pressure readings. Br Med J, 2: 159–162.

Ihle BU, Long P, Oats J (1987). Early onset pre-eclampsia: recognition of underlying renal disease. Br Med J, 294: 79–81.

Jones DD, Bahijri S, Roberts EL, Williams GF (1982). Activity of serum cytidine deaminase during pregnancy. Br J Obstet Gynaecol, 89: 314–317.

Kaplan NM, Silah JG (1964). The effect of angiotensin II on the blood pressure in humans with hypertensive disease. J Clin Invest, 43: 659–669.

Karbhari D, Harrigan JT, LaMagra R (1977). The supine hypertensive test as a predictor of incipient preeclampsia. Am J Obstet Gynecol, 127: 620–622.

Kassar NS, Aldridge J, Quirk B (1980). Roll over test. Obstet Gynecol, 55: 411–413.

Kaunitz AM, Hughes JM, Grimes DA, Smith JC, Rochat RW, Kafrissen ME (1985). Causes of maternal mortality in the United States. Obstet Gynecol, 65: 605–612.

Knutzen VK, Davey DA (1977). Hypertension in pregnancy: perinatal mortality and causes of fetal death. S Afr Med J, 51: 675–679.

Krasno LR, Ivy AC (1950). The response of the flicker fusion threshold to nitroglycerin and its potential value in the diagnosis, prognosis, and therapy of subclinical and clinical cardiovascular diseases. Circulation, 1: 1267–1276.

Kuntz WD (1980). Supine pressor (roll-over) test: An evaluation. Am J Obstet Gynecol, 137: 764–768.

Laher M, O'Brien E (1982). In search of Korotkoff. Br Med J, 285: 1796–1798.

Lancet M, Fisher IL (1956). The value of blood uric acid levels in toxaemia of pregnancy. J Obstet Gynaecol Br Empire, 63: 116–119.

Lazarchick J, Stubbs TM, Romein L. Van Dorsten JP, Loadholt CB (1986). Predictive value of fibronectin levels in normotensive gravid women destined to become pre-eclamptic. Am J Obstet Gynecol, 154: 1050–1052.

Letsky E (1980). The haematological system. In: Clinical Physiology in Obstetrics. Hytten F, Chamberlain G (eds). Oxford: Blackwell Scientific Publications, pp 43–78.

Liedholm H, Montan S, Aberg A (1984). Risk grouping of 113 patients with hypertensive disorders during pregnancy, with respect to serum urate, proteinuria and time of onset of hypertension. Acta Obstet Gynecol Scand (Suppl), 118: 43–48.

Lind AR, McNicol GW (1967). Circulatory responses to sustained hand-grip contractions performed during other exercise, both rhythmic and static. J Physiol, 192: 595–607.

Lindheimer MD, Katz AI (1977). Kidney Function and Disease in Pregnancy. Philadelphia: Lea & Febiger.

Lindheimer MD, Katz AI (1983). Hypertension and Pregnancy. In: Hypertension (2nd edn). Genest J, Kuchel O, Pavel H, Cantin M, (eds). New York: McGraw-Hill, pp 889–913.

Longo LD (1983). Maternal blood volume and cardiac output during pregnancy: a hypothesis of endocrinologic control. Am J Physiol, 245: R720–729.

Lopez-Espinoza I, Dhar H, Humphreys S, Redman CWG (1986). Urinary albumin excretion in pregnancy. Br J Obstet Gynaecol, 93: 176–181.

MacGillivray I (1961). Hypertension in pregnancy and its consequences. Br J Obstet Gynaecol, 68: 557–569.

MacGillivray I (1983). Pre-eclampsia. The Hypertensive Disease of Pregnancy. London: WB Saunders.

MacGillivray I, Rose GA, Rowe B (1969). Blood pressure survey in pregnancy. Clin Sci, 37: 395–407.

Margulies M, Voto LS, Fescina R, Lastra L, Lapidus AM, Schwarcz R (1987). Arterial blood pressure standards during normal pregnancy and their relation with mother–fetus variables. Am J Obstet Gynecol, 156: 1105–1109.

Marshall GW, Newman RL (1977). Roll over test. Am J Obstet Gynecol, 127: 623–625.

Marty JP, Hardy JA (1952). Flicker fusion thresholds in pregnancy. Am J Obstet Gynecol, 64: 1149–1153.

Marx GF, Husain FJ, Shiau HF (1980). Brachial and femoral blood pressures during the prenatal period. Am J Obstet Gynecol, 136: 11–13.

McEwan HP (1968). Investigation of proteinuria in pregnancy by immunoelectro-phoresis. Br J Obstet Gynaecol, 75: 289–294.

McEwan HP (1987). Nature of proteinuria in hypertension in pregnancy. In: Hypertension in Pregnancy. Sharp F, Symonds EM (eds). Ithaca, NY: Perinatology Press, pp 63–67.

Messerli FH, Frohlich ED, Dreslinski GR, Suarez DH, Aristimmo GG (1980). Serum uric acid in essential hypertension: an indicator of renal vascular involvement. Ann Intern Med, 93: 817–821.

Morris JA, O'Grady JP, Hamilton C, Davidson EC (1978). Vascular reactivity to angiotensin II infusion during gestation. Am J Obstet Gynecol, 130: 379–384.

Moutquin JM, Rainville C, Giroux L, Raynauld P, Amyot G, Bilodeau R, Pelland N (1985). A prospective study of blood pressure in pregnancy: prediction of preeclampsia. Am J Obstet Gynecol, 151: 191–196.

Murphy JF, Newcombe RG, O'Riordan J, Coles EC, Pearson JF (1986). Relation of haemoglobin levels in first and second trimesters to outcome in pregnancy. Lancet, 1: 992–994.

Murnaghan GA (1987). Methods of measuring blood pressure and blood pressure variability. In: Hypertension in Pregnancy. Sharp F, Symonds EM (eds). Ithaca NY: Perinatology Press, pp 19–28.

Nakamura T, Ito M, Matsui K, Yoshimura T, Kawasaki N, Maeyama M (1986). Significance of angiotensin sensitivity test for prediction of pregnancy-induced hypertension. Obstet Gynecol, 67: 388–394.

Nelson TR (1955). A clinical study of pre-eclampsia. J Obstet Gynaecol Br Empire, 62: 48–66.

Nisell H, Hjemdahl P, Linde B (1985). Cardiovascular responses to circulating catecholamines in normal pregnancy and in pregnancy-induced hypertension. Clin Physiol, 5: 479–493.

O'Brien E, Fitzgerald D, O'Malley K (1985). Blood pressure measurement: current practice and future trends. Br Med J, 290: 729–734.

O'Grady JP, Hamilton C, Morris JA, Davidson EC (1977). Sequential evaluation of the supine hypertension or "roll-over" test in a high risk population. Gynecol Invest, 8: 282–287.

Öney T, Kaulhausen H (1982). The value of the angiotensin sensitivity test in the early diagnosis of hypertensive disorders in pregnancy. Am J Obstet Gynecol, 142: 17–20.

Öney T, Kaulhausen H (1983). Risiko- und Früherkennung hypertensiver Schwangerschaftskomplikationen. In: Schwangerschaftsbedingte Hypertonie. Kaulhausen H, Schneider J (eds). Stuttgart: Georg Thieme Verlag, pp 138–148.

Orozco JZ, Pinsker VS, Hernandez J, Karchmer S (1979). Valor de la prueba de la angiotesina II y del "roll over test" como metodos predictivos de la enfermedad hipersentiva aguda del embarazo (preeclampsia/eclampsia). Ginecol Obstet Mex, 46: 235.

Page EW, Christianson R (1976a). Influence of blood pressure with and without proteinuria upon outcome of pregnancy. Am J Obstet Gynecol, 126: 821–833.

Page EW, Christianson R (1976b). The impact of mean arterial blood pressure in the middle trimester upon the outcome of pregnancy. Am J Obstet Gynecol, 125: 740–746.

Phelan JP, Everidge GJ, Wilder TJ, Newman C (1977). Is the supine pressor test an adequate means of predicting acute hypertension in pregnancy? Am J Obstet Gynecol, 128: 173–176.

Poland ML, Mariona F, Darga L, Laurent D, Lucas CP (1980). The roll-over test in healthy primigravid subjects. In: Pregnancy Hypertension. Bonnar J, MacGillivray I, Symonds M (eds). Lancaster, England: MTP Press, pp 113–118.

Pollak VE, Nettles JA (1960). The kidney in toxemia of pregnancy. A clinical and pathologic study based on renal biopsies. Medicine, 39: 469–526.

Pritchard JA, Cunningham FG, Mason RA (1976). Coagulation changes in eclampsia: their frequency and pathogenesis. Am J Obstet Gynecol, 124: 855–859.

Quaas L, Robrecht D, Kaltenbach FJ (1982). The mean arterial pressure versus roll-over test as predictors of hypertension in pregnancy. In: Pregnancy Hypertension. Sammour MB, Symonds EM, Zuspan FP, El-Tomi N (eds). Cairo: Ain Shams University Press, pp 145–149.

Raab W, Schroeder G, Wagner R, Gigee W (1956). Vascular reactivity and electrolytes in normal and toxemic pregnancy. J Clin Endocrinol, 16: 1196–1216.

Raftery EB (1978). The methodology of blood pressure recording. Br J Clin Pharmacol, 6: 193–201.

Raftery EB, Ward AP (1968). The indirect method of recording blood pressure. Cardiovasc Res, 2: 210–218.

Redman CWG (1980). Treatment of hypertension in pregnancy. Kidney Int, 18: 267–278.

Redman CWG (1984). The Definition of Pre-eclampsia. Scand J Clin Lab Invest, 169: 7–14.

Redman CWG, Jefferies M (1988). Revised definition of pre-eclampsia. Lancet, 1: 809–812.

Redman CWG, Beilin LJ, Bonnar J, Wilkinson RH (1976a). Plasma-urate measurement in predicting fetal death in hypertensive pregnancy. Lancet, 1: 1370–1373.

Redman CWG, Beilin LJ, Bonnar J (1976b). Variability of blood pressure in normal and abnormal pregnancy. In: Hypertension in Pregnancy. Lindheimer MD, Katz AI, Zuspan FP (eds). New York: John Wiley, pp 53–59.

Redman CWG, Williams GF, Jones DD, Wilkinson RH (1977). Plasma urate and serum deoxycytidylate deaminase measurements for the early diagnosis of preeclampsia. Br J Obstet Gynaecol, 84: 904–908.

Redman CWG, Bonnar J, Beilin LJ (1978). Early platelet consumption in preeclampsia. Br Med J, 1: 467–469.

Reid DE, Teel HM (1938). A study of the 'cold test' in normal and in toxemic pregnancy . Am J Obstet Gynecol, 35: 305–309.

Riedel H, Bahlmann J, Eisenbach GM (1981). Results of a prospective study of toxemia of pregnancy. Contrib Nephrol, 25: 137–144.

Rippmann ET (1969). Präeklampsie oder Schwangerschaftsgestose? Gynaecologia, 167: 478–490.
Riva Rocci S (1896). Un sfigmomanometro nuovo. Gaz Med Torino, 47: 981–996.
Robertson EG (1971). The natural history of oedema during pregnancy. J Obstet Gynaecol Br Commwlth, 78: 520–529.
Robertson WB, Khong TY (1987). Pathology of the uteroplacental bed. In: Hypertension in Pregnancy. Sharp F, Symonds EM (eds). Ithaca, NY: Perinatology Press, pp 101–118.
Ruff SC, Mitchell RH, Murnaghan GA (1982). Long-term variations of blood pressure rhythms in normotensive pregnancy and preeclampsia. In: Pregnancy Hypertension. Sammour MB, Symonds EM, Zuspan FP, El-Tomi N (eds). Cairo: Ain Shams University Press, pp 129–133.
Rugart KF (1953). Flicker fusion threshold (FFT) during pregnancy. Obstet Gynecol, 1: 564–570.
Sagen N, Koller O, Haram K (1982). Haemoconcentration in severe pre-eclampsia. Br J Obstet Gynaecol, 89: 802–805.
Saleh AA, Bottoms SF, Welch RA, Ali AM, Mariona FG, Mammen EF (1987). Preeclampsia, delivery, and the hemostatic system. Am J Obstet Gynecol, 157: 331–336.
Schmorl G (1893). Pathologisch-anatomische Untersuchungen über Puerperal-Eklampsie. Leipzig: FCW Vogel.
Schockaert JA, Lambillon J (1937). Un nouveau test permittant le diagnostic précoce et differentiel des états preéclamptiques. Bruxelles-Méd, 17: 1468–1474.
Scholtes MCW, Gerretsen G, Haak HL (1983). The factor VIII ratio in normal and pathological pregnancies. Eur J Obstet Gynecol Reprod Biol, 16: 89–95.
Schulman H (1987). The clinical implications of Doppler ultrasound analysis of the uterine and umbilical arteries. Am J Obstet Gynecol, 156: 889–893.
Schuster E, Wepelmann B (1981). Plasma urate measurements and fetal outcome in preeclampsia. Gynecol Obstet Invest, 12: 162–167.
Schwarz R, Retzke U (1971). Cardiovascular response to infusion of angiotensin II in pregnant women. Obstet Gynecol, 38: 714–718.
Shaw AB, Risdon P, Lewis-Jackson JD (1983). Protein creatinine index and Albustix in assessment of proteinuria. Br Med J, 287: 929–932.
Sibai BM, Anderson GD (1986). Pregnancy outcome of intensive therapy in severe hypertension in first trimester. Obstet Gynecol, 67: 517–522.
Sibai BM, McCubbin JH, Anderson GD, Lipshitz J, Dilts PV (1981). Eclampsia I: Observations from 67 recent cases. Obstet Gynecol, 58: 609–613.
Sibai BM, Anderson GD, McGubbin JH (1982). Eclampsia II. Clinical significance of laboratory findings. Obstet Gynecol, 59: 153–157.
Sibai BM, Taskini MT, Abdella TN, Brooks TF, Spinnato JA, Anderson GD (1985). Maternal and perinatal outcome of conservative management of severe pre-eclampsia in midtrimester. Am J Obstet Gynecol, 152: 32–37.
Sobel B, Laurent D, Ganguly S, Favro L, Lucas C (1980). Hydrostatic mechanisms in the roll-over test. Obstet Gynecol 55: 285–290.
Spargo B, McCartney CP, Winemiller R (1959). Glomerular capillary endotheliosis in toxemia of pregnancy. Arch Pathol, 68: 593–599.
Spinapolice RX, Feld S, Harrigan JT (1983). Effective prevention of gestational hypertension in nulliparous women at high risk as identified by the rollover test. Am J Obstet Gynecol, 146: 166–168.
Stander HJ, Duncan EE, Sisson WE (1925). Chemical studies in toxaemias of pregnancy. Bull Johns Hopkins Hosp, 36: 411–427.
Stathakis N, Fountas A, Tsianos E (1981). Plasma fibronectin in normal subjects and in various disease states. J Clin Pathol, 34: 504–508.
Stubbs TM, Lazarchick J, Horger III EO (1984). Plasma fibronectin levels in preeclampsia: A possible biochemical marker for vascular endothelial damage. Am J Obstet Gynecol, 150: 885–889.
Talledo OE (1966). Renin–angiotensin system in normal and toxemic pregnancies. I. Angiotensin infusion test. Am J Obstet Gynecol, 96: 141–143.
Talledo OE, Chesley LC, Zuspan FP (1968). Renin-angiotensin system in normal and toxemic pregnancies. III Differential sensitivity to angiotensin II and norepinephrine in toxemia of pregnancy. Am J Obstet Gynecol, 100: 218–221.
Taufield PA, Ales KL, Resnick LM, Druzin ML, Gartner JM, Laragh JH (1987). Hypocalciuria in preeclampsia. New Engl J Med, 316: 715–718.
Thomson AM, Hytten RE, Billewicz WZ (1967). The epidemiology of oedema during pregnancy. J Obstet Gynaecol Br Commwlth, 74: 1–10.
Thompson DS, Mueller-Heubach E (1978). Use of supine pressor test to prevent gestational hypertension in primigravid women. Am J Obstet Gynecol, 131: 661–664.
Thornton CA, Bonnar J (1977). Factor VIII related antigen and factor VIII coagulant activity in normal and preeclamptic pregnancy. Br J Obstet Gynaecol, 84: 919–923.
Thurnau GR, Dyer A, Depp OR, Martin AO (1983). The development of a profile scoring system for early identification and severity assessment of pregnancy-induced hypertension. Am J Obstet Gynecol, 146: 406–416.
Toop K, Klopper A (1981). Concentrations of pregnancy-associated plasma protein A (PAPP-A) in patients with preeclamptic toxaemia. Placenta, Suppl 3: 167–173.
Trudinger BJ, Giles WB, Cook CM (1985). Uteroplacental blood flow velocity-time waveforms in normal and complicated pregnancy. Br J Obstet Gynaecol, 92: 39–45.
Tunbridge RDG (1983). Pregnancy-associated hypertension, a comparison of its prediction by "roll-over test" and plasma noradrenaline measurement in 100 primigravidae. Br J Obstet Gynaecol, 90: 1027–1032.
Verma UL, Tejani NA, Chatterjee S, Weiss RR (1980). Screening for SGA by the roll-over test. Obstet Gynecol, 56: 591–594.
Vosburgh GJ (1976). Blood pressure, edema and proteinuria in pregnancy. 5. Edema relationships. Prog Clin Biol Res, 7: 155–168.
Wallenburg HCS (1981). Modulation and regulation of utero-placental blood flow. Placenta Suppl 1: 45–64.
Wallenburg HCS (1987a). Uteroplacental circulation: physiology and pathophysiology. J Drugther Res 12: 22–23.
Wallenburg HCS (1987b). Changes in the coagulation system and platelets in pregnancy-induced hypertension and pre-eclampsia. In: Sharp F. Symonds EM (eds). Hypertension in Pregnancy. Ithaca NY: Perinatology Press, pp 227–244.

Wallenburg HCS (1988a). Hemodynamics in hypertensive pregnancy. In: Handbook of Hypertension, Vol 10, Hypertension in Pregnancy. Rubin P (ed). Amsterdam: Elsevier, pp 66–101.

Wallenburg HC (1988b). Prevention of hypertensive disorders in pregnancy. Clin Exp Hypertens – Hypertension in Pregnancy, B7: 121–137.

Wallenburg HCS, Van Kreel BK (1978). Transfer and dynamics of uric acid in the pregnant rhesus monkey. I. Transplacental and renal uric acid clearances. Eur J Obstet Gynecol Reprod Biol, 8: 211–217.

Wallenburg HCS, Rotmans N (1982). Enhanced reactivity of the platelet thromboxane pathway in normotensive and hypertensive pregnancies with insufficient fetal growth. Am J Obstet Gynecol, 144: 523–528.

Wallenburg HCS, Dekker GA, Makovitz JW, Rotmans P (1986). Low dose aspirin prevents pregnancy-induced hypertension and pre-eclampsia in angiotensin sensitive primigravidae. Lancet, 1: 1–3.

Webster J, Newnham D, Petrie JC, Lovell HG (1984). Influence of arm position in measurement of blood pressure. Br Med J, 288: 1574–1575.

Weenink GH, Treffers PE, Vijn P, Smorenberg-Schoorl ME, ten Cate JW (1984). Antithrombin III levels in preeclampsia correlate with maternal and fetal morbidity. Am J Obstet Gynecol, 148: 1092–1097.

Weiner CP, Brandt J (1982). Plasma antithrombin III activity: an aid in the diagnosis of preeclampsia—eclampsia. Am J Obstet Gynecol, 142: 275–281.

Weinstein L (1982). Syndrome of hemolysis, elevated liver enzymes, and low platelet count: A severe consequence of hypertension in pregnancy. Am J Obstet Gynecol, 142: 159–167.

Whigham KAE, Howie PW, Shah MM, Prentice CRM (1980). Factor VIII related antigen/coagulant activity ratio as a predictor of fetal growth retardation: A comparison with hormone and uric acid measurements. Br J Obstet Gynaecol, 87: 797–803.

Wichman K, Rydn G, Wichman M (1984). The influence of different positions and Korotkoff sounds on the blood pressure measurements in pregnancy. Acta Obstet Gynecol Scand, 118: 25–28.

Williams GF, Jones DD (1975). Deoxycytidylate deaminase in pregnancy. Br Med J, 11: 10–12.

Williams GF, Jones DD (1982). Serum deoxycytidylate deaminase as an index of high-risk pregnancy. Br J Obstet Gynaecol, 89: 309–313.

Worley RJ, Everett RB, Madden JD (1978). Fetal considerations: metabolic clearance rate of maternal dehydroisoandrosterone sulfate. Seminars Perinatol, 2: 15–18.

Ylikorkala O, Mäkilä U-M (1985). Prostacyclin and thromboxane in gynecology and obstetrics. Am J Obstet Gynecol, 152: 318–324.

Zuspan FP, Nelson GH, Ahlquist RP (1964). Epinephrine infusions in normal and toxemic pregnancy. I. Nonesterified fatty acids and cardiovascular alterations. Am J Obstet Gynecol, 90: 88–96.

25 Gestational diabetes

David J. S. Hunter and Marc J. N. C. Keirse

'It is better to have absolutely no idea where one is than to believe confidently that one is where one is not'

Cesar Francois Cassini de Thury,
eighteenth-century French Surveyor

1 Introduction

Gestational diabetes is defined by the working party of the National Diabetes Data Group (1979) as glucose intolerance appearing during pregnancy. The clinical characteristics of this disease include an association with increased perinatal morbidity and mortality and an increased risk of progress to diabetes within 5 to 10 years. The diagnosis is based on an abnormal oral glucose tolerance test as defined by O'Sullivan and Mahan (1964), although parts of the world other than North America may use different criteria (Hadden 1985; Abell and Beischer 1975; Persson *et al.* 1985). Because of the stated association with increased perinatal mortality and morbidity, the National Diabetes Data Group (1979) recommended that gestational diabetes merits a separate category in the classification of diabetes; a recommendation that was adopted by the World Health Organization Expert Committee on Diabetes (1980). Based on the summary and recommendations of two international workshops on gestational diabetes (Anonymous 1980, 1985), The American Diabetes Association (1987) has recently published a position statement that advocates routine screening of all pregnant women for glucose intolerance.

As it is clear that the primary motivation for making the diagnosis of gestational diabetes is concern for the fetus, this chapter will examine the evidence that associates an abnormal oral glucose tolerance test with increased perinatal mortality and morbidity, and the therapeutic strategies that may be expected to influence the outcome of pregnancy if the diagnosis is made.

2 The glucose tolerance test

There evolved through the 1940s and 1950s the concept of prediabetes, which held that much of the pathology associated with overt diabetes develops before the appearance of insulin dependency. Prediabetes was also felt to make a significant contribution to perinatal mortality (Herzstein and Dolger 1946; Gilbert and Dunlop 1949; Hagabard 1958). The glucose tolerance test became the mainstay of this diagnosis as it was felt to uncover a defect in glucose homeostasis which was only demonstrated after a glucose challenge. As an abnormal glucose tolerance test has also become the diagnostic criterion for gestational diabetes, its performance as a test bears close scrutiny.

The test was developed in two forms, the oral and the intravenous glucose tolerance test. The intravenous glucose tolerance test primarily measures glucose disposal, and avoids the unpredictable step of alimentary absorption that is present in the oral glucose tolerance test. It is highly reproducible (Billis and Rastogi 1966) and provides a simple numerical expression for comparative purposes. It is generally held however, that the test is unphysiological, as the intravenous route of administration of glucose bypasses the enterohepatic circulation. Furthermore the numerical expression is difficult to apply clinically. Because of these factors, and the rather cumbersome nature of the test, together with the need for a physician to administer the glucose, the intravenous glucose tolerance test is not widely used.

The oral glucose tolerance test on the other hand is still widely used. It is considered to be more physiological, and is easy to administer. However, it suffers seriously from lack of reproducibility. McDonald *et al.* (1965) administered a 100 g oral glucose tolerance test on six occasions two months apart to 334 healthy male volunteers. Using the Public Health Service criteria, 29 (9 per cent) of these volunteers had one abnormal test. Of these 29 men, 15 (52 per cent) had five and 22 (76 per cent) had four subsequently normal tests. It appears from this study, therefore, that more than half of the asymptomatic persons with an abnormal glucose tolerance test will have normal test results if the test is repeated a further five times. McDonald *et al.* (1969) repeated the study in 101 female volunteers, administering four tests at monthly intervals. Of six women who had positive tests by Public Health Service criteria, four were negative on more than one occasion when subsequently tested, and only one of the six women had a positive test on all four occasions. The authors were convinced therefore that one positive glucose tolerance test could not predict diabetes, an observation supported by the study of O'Sullivan and Mahan (1968), who tested 1113 young adults with a 100 g glucose tolerance test and found that over 70 per cent of the 389 persons with a positive test had a normal result on subsequent testing.

3 The glucose tolerance test and gestational diabetes

Prior to the work of O'Sullivan and Mahan (1964) there was much confusion and disagreement on the criteria that defined an abnormal oral glucose tolerance test, particularly during pregnancy. These authors obtained fasting blood glucose values and values at one, two, and three hours after oral administration of a 100 g glucose load to an unselected population of 752 pregnant women at the Boston City Hospital between 1956 and 1957. Forty per cent of the women with two values more than three standard deviations above the mean subsequently developed diabetes, as did 16 per cent of the women with two values more than two standard deviations above the mean. Feeling that a cut-off point of three standard deviations above the mean was likely to miss a significant number of women with prediabetes during pregnancy, the authors decided that two values more than two standard deviations above the mean would be considered as an abnormal test. These levels, measured in whole blood, are shown in Table 25.1. The levels recommended by the National Diabetes Data Group (1979) to define gestational diabetes, which are now entrenched in the obstetric literature (Pritchard and MacDonald 1980), refer to plasma levels and are derived from these values by applying a 15 per cent correction to adjust for the red cell mass.

Two points should be noted about this important study and the values it proposed. First, the definition of abnormality was linked to the later appearance of diabetes and not to the presence of gestational diabetes. Although this was appropriate in the design of a test for 'prediabetes', it did not establish an association of this diagnosis with perinatal mortality or other pregnancy outcomes. Second, the correction factor of 15 per cent is theoretical and does not take into account the variation in red cell mass seen in pregnancy (Letsky 1980).

4 Gestational diabetes and perinatal mortality

4.1 The nature of the association

It was not until 1973 that O'Sullivan *et al.* (1973) attempted to link an abnormal glucose tolerance test to perinatal mortality. All pregnant registrants between 1962 and 1970 were screened with a blood glucose estimation two hours after a 50 g oral glucose load. Those with a blood glucose value greater than 130 mg per 100 ml were tested with a 3-hour 100 g oral glucose tolerance test. From January 1967 to April 1968, a normal control group was established by selecting every tenth registrant and determining that the 3-hour oral glucose tolerance test was normal.

Four (1.5 per cent) of the 259 women with a normal oral glucose tolerance test had a perinatal loss compared to 12 (6.4 per cent) of 187 women with an abnormal glucose tolerance test ($p < 0.01$, Fisher's exact test; relative risk: 4.3). However, when the authors analysed perinatal mortality according to age, weight, and glucose tolerance, they noted that increased perinatal mortality in the presence of a positive glucose tolerance test was confined to women aged 25 years or more (Table 25.2). It is quite possible, however, that increased risk

Table 25.1 Upper limits of normal in the 100 g oral glucose tolerance test as defined by O'Sullivan and Mahan (1964) and by the National Diabetes Data Group (1979)

Time of testing (hours after glucose load)	Upper limits of normal in mg/dl and (mmol/l)			
	Blood glucose O'Sullivan and Mahan (1964)		Plasma glucose National Diabetes Data Group (1979)	
Fasting	90	(5.0)	105	(5.8)
1 hour	165	(9.0)	190	(10.5)
2 hours	145	(8.0)	165	(9.0)
3 hours	125	(6.9)	145	(8.0)

Table 25.2 Perinatal mortality according to age and relative weight and the result of the oral glucose tolerance test (GTT) (after O'Sullivan *et al.* 1973)

Age in years	Per cent relative weight	Perinatal death — numbers and (per cent)			
		Positive GTT		Negative GTT	
<25	<120	0/40	(0.0)	2/138	(1.4)
	>120	0/13	(0.0)	1/33	(3.0)
>or = 25	<120	4/54	(7.4)	0/54	(0.0)
	>120	8/80	(10.0)	1/34	(2.9)
All patients		12/187	(6.4)*	4/259	(1.5)*

Fisher's exact test: $*p = 0.007$.

of perinatal mortality is predicted as much by the indication for glucose tolerance testing, as by the test result itself. Sutherland and Stowers (1975) reported the results of 1800 intravenous glucose tolerance tests done on 1600 women during pregnancy with various indicators suggestive of diabetes (Table 25.3). It can be seen in Table 25.3 that the rate of fetal loss increases eightfold ($p < 0.001$) as the number of indications for glucose tolerance testing increases from one to four, and that the risk of fetal death for each indication is not revised significantly by the presence or absence of glucose intolerance. Hadden (1975) has also shown that certain indications for glucose tolerance testing are associated with increased perinatal mortality, in particular previous perinatal loss or fetal anomaly, which carries a fetal death rate of 7 per cent to 9.8 per cent compared to a rate of between 6.5 and 4.5 per cent in the hospital population during the same time period (1963–71).

Further circumstantial evidence linking an abnormal glucose tolerance test to perinatal mortality was provided by the study of Abell and Beischer (1975). They reviewed 2000 consecutive women who had a 3-hour 50 g oral glucose tolerance test in the third trimester of pregnancy. An abnormal test was associated with a perinatal mortality of 31.7 per 1000 as compared to 9.5 per 1000 if the glucose tolerance test was negative ($p < 0.001$; relative risk: 3.3). Although this study is important in that it is population-based and thus allows calculation of the sensitivity (0.38) and specificity (0.85) of this particular test for perinatal mortality, it is not possible to determine whether or not perinatal mortality is linked to the indication for performing the glucose tolerance test. It would be interesting to re-analyse these results and establish the risk of perinatal mortality that is predicted by other variables and to what extent the presence of glucose tolerance revises that risk.

It is likely that glucose intolerance is simply a marker for other underlying conditions that adversely influence perinatal outcome. Nevertheless, even if it is only a marker for increased perinatal mortality, it could still be a useful indicator of risk. In view of the previously cited recommendations to screen all pregnant women for glucose tolerance, it is important to determine the impact that such a programme could have on perinatal mortality.

The probability of perinatal death in the presence of a

Table 25.3 Incidence of stillbirth in relation to the number of indications for intravenous glucose tolerance testing, irrespective of and according to the test result (after Sutherland and Stowers 1975)

No. of indications	Stillbirths — numbers and (per cent)					
	All women		Positive GTT		Negative GTT	
1	19/949	(2.0)*	3/93	(3.2)	16/356	(1.9)
2	20/561	(3.6)	6/97	(6.2)	14/464	(3.0)
3	8/187	(4.3)	2/45	(4.4)	6/142	(4.2)
4	5/30	(16.6)*	4/23	(17.4)	1/7	(14.3)
Total	52/1727	(3.0)	15/258	(5.8)†	37/1469	(2.5)†

Fisher's exact test: $*p < 0.001$; $†p < 0.01$.

positive glucose tolerance test (post-test likelihood) can be calculated from the likelihood ratio which is derived from the sensitivity and specificity (see Chapter 3). From the data of Abell and Beischer (1975) with a sensitivity of 0.38 and specificity of 0.85, a likelihood ratio of 2.53 can be calculated and applied to, for instance, all births in Ontario, Canada. In 1983 there were just over 120 000 births in Ontario with a perinatal mortality rate of 11.7 per thousand. Based on an incidence of perinatal death of 0.0117 (11.7 per 1000) and a likelihood ratio of 2.53, a post-test likelihood of 29 per 1000 is obtained. The true incidence of gestational diabetes in Ontario is unknown. However, if it is assumed that the prevalence is 2 per cent (Hadden 1985), 2400 women would have gestational diabetes in one year. With a post-test likelihood of 0.029, these women would contribute 70 perinatal deaths to the total of 1404 (4.9 per cent).

The criteria of Abell and Beischer (1975) for an abnormal glucose tolerance test are much lower than those of O'Sullivan *et al.* (1973), however, and applying more stringent criteria would reduce the number of positive tests as well as the number of perinatal deaths associated with a positive test. Nevertheless, if we accept the criteria of Abell and Beischer (1975), and assume that a screening programme for gestational diabetes would be 100 per cent effective, and that (an even more unlikely eventuality) every death associated with the condition is avoidable, the screening programme would be expected, at the very best, to reduce the perinatal mortality in Ontario from 11.7 to 11.1 per thousand. This may seem to be a worthy objective, but the question remains unanswered whether or not identification and treatment of women with gestational diabetes can prevent some of the associated perinatal deaths.

4.2 Can treatment reduce perinatal mortality?

There is little, if any, purpose in making a diagnosis if one cannot improve the prognosis by treating the condition that is diagnosed. If we are to derive any value from making the diagnosis of gestational diabetes, therefore, there must be a recognized treatment or set of treatments that will improve the outcome.

O'Sullivan (1975) randomly allocated women with an abnormal glucose tolerance test to insulin therapy or diet. Women with blood sugars in excess of 300 mg/dl (16.5 mmol/l) at any time were excluded, as were gestational diabetics who registered after the 36th week of pregnancy; 328 women who had normal glucose tolerance acted as controls. There were six (1.8 per cent) perinatal deaths in the control group. Of 308 women with a positive glucose tolerance test, who were treated with diet alone, 15 (4.9 per cent) had a perinatal loss, and of 307 women with a positive glucose tolerance test treated with insulin, 13 (4.2 per cent) had a perinatal loss. None of these differences are statistically significant.

Subgroup analysis of these data suggests that insulin may reduce perinatal mortality when used in women over 25 years of age with an abnormal glucose tolerance test. O'Sullivan found that only two of 109 women in this age group so treated (1.8 per cent) had a perinatal loss as compared to 12 of 146 (8.2 per cent) in the control group ($p < 0.001$). Such subgroup analyses, however, can be seriously misleading.

Two other commonly cited studies also claim that treatment of gestational diabetes reduces perinatal mortality. Roversi *et al.* (1980) treated over 200 women with abnormal glucose tolerance tests in pregnancy with maximum doses of insulin three times a day. Two-thirds of the women had a fasting plasma glucose of less than 105 mg/dl (5.8 mmol/l), the remainder had levels between 105 and 129 mg/dl (7.1 mmol/l). After treatment, mean glucose concentrations were less than 100 mg/dl (5.5 mmol/l). There were no control subjects and the comparison made was with perinatal mortality in previous pregnancies. Gabbe *et al.* (1977) identified and treated 261 gestational diabetic women (defined as normal fasting glucose with abnormal glucose tolerance test). Perinatal mortality was 19 per thousand for the gestational diabetics compared to 32 per thousand for the hospital population as a whole during the same time period (1970–72).

The improved perinatal mortality in the gestational diabetics in these two series was ascribed by the authors to their identification and clinical management. However, in neither study was there a true control group. From Roversi's study one cannot tell whether or not a similar improvement did not occur in women with a previous perinatal loss and normal glucose tolerance; and in Gabbe's study the hospital population had a high perinatal mortality possibly because of the referral nature of its practice. Studies of this design provide no evidence whatsoever that the investigations and interventions applied to these women were in any way responsible for the outcome.

At present therefore, there is no reasonable or convincing evidence that treatment of women with gestational diabetes will reduce perinatal mortality.

5 Gestational diabetes and perinatal morbidity

5.1 The nature of the association

Although it has been suggested that gestational diabetes is associated with an increased risk of congenital anomalies, the study by Chung and Myrianthopoulous (1975) from the Boston collaborative project demonstrated convincingly that there is in fact no increased risk of congenital anomaly in this condition.

Neonatal hypoglycaemia appears to be most uncommon even in macrosomic infants. Philipson *et al.* (1985) found only 4 infants with hypoglycaemia out of 158 pregnancies with an abnormal glucose tolerance test, compared to two of 158 controls. Persson *et al.* (1985) found no increase in C-peptide levels in the cord blood of 76 gestational diabetics treated by diet and insulin as compared to 81 treated by diet alone and 196 controls. Although Gabbe *et al.* (1977) reported a 7 per cent incidence of hypoglycaemia in the infants of 261 Class A diabetics, approximately 25 per cent of these women were delivered before 38 weeks and the contribution made by low birthweight or preterm delivery was not defined.

Similarly there is no evidence that infants of mothers with gestational diabetes are at increased risk from neonatal jaundice (Table 25.4). Although it is possible that the recognition and treatment of gestational diabetes prevented an increase that would otherwise have occurred, the design of the reported studies cannot support this hypothesis.

The adverse outcome most frequently associated with gestational diabetes is fetal macrosomia. Up to 30 per cent of infants of mothers with an abnormal glucose tolerance test have a birthweight of more than 4000 g (Philipson *et al.* 1985; Gabbe *et al.* 1977; Coustan and Lewis 1978).

However, Spellacy *et al.* (1985) found that only 29 of 574 infants (5.1 per cent) with a birthweight over 4500 g were born to women with gestational diabetes. As the background incidence of infants over 4500 g was 1.7 per cent, the relative risk of macrosomia with gestational diabetes was 3.0. By comparison, 44 per cent of the macrosomic infants were born to women weighing more than 90 kg (relative risk: 25.8), and 10.8 per cent to women beyond 42 weeks of gestation (relative risk: 6.4). This report and the relative risks derived from it certainly suggest that a heavy mother and post-term pregnancy are much more closely associated with fetal macrosomia than is gestational diabetes.

Oats *et al.* (1980) reviewed the results of a 50 g 3-hours oral glucose tolerance test performed in 137 women who delivered an infant weighing more than 4540 g. Only 32 (23 per cent) had an abnormal glucose tolerance test.

Of 127 consecutive glucose tolerance tests done at McMaster University Medical Centre in 1980, 68 were for suspected large for gestational age infants. Of these 68 women, 24 delivered a baby over 4000 g, but none of them had an abnormal test. The only woman with an abnormal test delivered a baby of normal weight. Clinical judgment would appear to be more predictive of fetal macrosomia than the glucose tolerance test, as also suggested by Boyd *et al.* (1983), who were able to predict 32 per cent of macrosomic infants born to 2851 mothers based on assessment of prepregnant weight, weight-gain, and a pregnancy past 42 weeks without any reference to glucose tolerance.

It would appear, therefore, that wide application of a glucose tolerance test to pregnant women would be of limited value in identifying those women at increased risk of fetal macrosomia. Maternal size, parity, clinical assessment of fetal size, and prolonged pregnancy are better criteria for identification, although the limitations of clinical assessment of fetal weight are well known (Persson *et al.* 1986; see also Chapter 26).

The main clinical implication of fetal macrosomia is birth injury and shoulder dystocia. Gabbe *et al.* (1977) noted that 10 per cent (5/49) of infants weighing more than 4000 g suffered serious birth trauma (fractured bones or peripheral nerve injury) compared to 2 per cent of normally sized infants born to mothers with gestational diabetes. This background incidence, although similar to a recent report from Montreal (1.3 per cent; Cyr *et al.* 1984), and the University of Cincinnati clinic (1.2 per cent; Levine *et al.* 1984) would appear to be high. Acker *et al.* (1985) reported on 22 269 deliveries at the Beth Israel Hospital from Janu-

Table 25.4 Comparison of incidence of neonatal jaundice between gestational diabetics and matched controls (Philipson *et al.* 1985; Widnes *et al.* 1985), and between gestational diabetics treated with diet and those treated with diet and insulin (Persson *et al.* 1985; Landon and Gabbe 1985)

Authors	Hyperbilirubinaemia			
	Definition (mg/dl)	Incidence in		
		Study	Control	p-value
Philipson *et al.* (1985)	>3.5 and <6.5	46/96	34/62	not significant
Widnes *et al.* (1985)	>12.5	3/10	5/13	not significant
Persson *et al.* (1985)	'Treated'	8/40	6/30	not significant
Landon and Gabbe (1985)	>12.0	2/28	12/69	not significant

ary 1975 to December 1982. The incidence of similar trauma was 0.37 per cent. Among 12 848 deliveries in the Hamilton hospitals between April 1981 and March 1983, there were 33 birth injuries as defined above; an incidence of 0.26 per cent.

Although one of the recent recommendations is to deliver excessively large infants by caesarean section in order to avoid birth trauma and shoulder dystocia, it can be appreciated from the preceding discussion that part of the difficulty lies in precisely defining infants of excessive size before birth. Gabbe *et al.* (1977), for example, were only able to identify 6 of 16 infants weighing more than 4000 g prior to delivery in women with gestational diabetes despite serial ultrasonography from 28 weeks' gestation onwards. Even if all large infants could be identified before birth and delivered by caesarean section, the reduction in the number of infants suffering birth trauma would be limited (see Chapter 25).

5.2 Can treatment reduce morbidity?

There seems to be little doubt that treating women who have gestational diabetes with insulin can reduce the incidence of macrosomia.

O'Sullivan (1975) in his randomized study of insulin therapy in gestational diabetics was able to reduce the incidence of macrosomia (birthweight of 4000 g or more) from 13 per cent in those treated with diet to 4.2 per cent in those treated with insulin. The incidence of macrosomia in women with a negative glucose tolerance test was 3.7 per cent.

Coustan and Lewis (1978) randomly treated 72 women with gestational diabetes with either insulin and diet, diet alone, or neither. Of the 27 women treated with insulin and diet, 2 (7 per cent) had babies weighing more than 8.5 lb (3860 g). Of 11 treated with diet alone, 4 (36.4 per cent) had babies weighing more than 8.5 pounds, and of 34 treated with neither diet nor insulin 17 (50 per cent) had babies weighing more than 8.5 lb. Randomization was not strictly adhered to, however, as the first 20 women admitted to the study were treated according to gestational age at the time of diagnosis. Women diagnosed prior to 36 weeks were given insulin and those beyond 35 weeks acted as controls. Only the subsequent 52 women were randomized to diet, diet and insulin, or no treatment; the method of randomization is not described and the number of women allocated to each of the three groups varies considerably. Accepting these deficiencies, the incidence of macrosomia in the insulin-treated group differed significantly ($p < 0.005$) from the other two groups. The authors were disappointed to find, however, that despite this reduction in macrosomia there was no parallel reduction in the incidence of caesarean section or midforceps delivery. In a later study, that was not randomized, Coustan and Imarah (1984) reported a reduction in the incidence of both macrosomia and operative delivery in women treated with insulin in their university clinic as compared to women with gestational diabetes managed predominantly by diet alone in private physicians' offices. As yet, this is the only group that has reported a reduction in the operative delivery rate as a result of reducing birthweight with insulin therapy, and as it was non-randomized there is considerable potential for bias.

Further evidence that insulin therapy reduces the incidence of macrosomia is provided by Metzger *et al.* (1980) who divided women with gestational diabetes into three groups according to the fasting plasma glucose level at the time of diagnosis: those with a fasting plasma glucose < 105 mg/dl were treated with diet alone, whereas those with a fasting plasma glucose > 105 mg/dl were treated either with insulin or with diet alone. The mean birthweight of infants in the group treated with insulin exceeded 4000 g and was significantly higher than that in both other groups. It was concluded that insulin therapy significantly reduced the incidence of macrosomia.

More recently, Goldberg *et al.* (1986) compared the incidence of macrosomia in a cohort of gestational diabetics, who monitored blood glucose levels after each meal with home glucose monitors, with a cohort of gestational diabetics who were followed by less intensive biochemical surveillance. Insulin was used more frequently in the home monitored series than in the laboratory monitored group (50 per cent vs. 21 per cent); the incidence of macrosomia (more than 4000 g) was 24 per cent in the control group and 9 per cent in the home monitored group ($p < 0.005$). The authors felt that intensive monitoring resulted in a greater frequency of insulin usage with a concomitant reduction in the incidence of macrosomia.

Two trials from the same unit (Maresh *et al.* 1985; Gillmer *et al.* 1986) compared metabolic profiles and some infant outcomes for women with abnormal glucose tolerance detected at routine screening in the third trimester, alternately treated with insulin plus diet (10 and 8) or diet alone (10 and 7), and with normal controls (10 and 8). Diet alone did not achieve as great a reduction of plasma glucose concentrations as did treatment with insulin. However, the diet alone group still remained in the upper range of normal. As the mean percentile birthweights and neonatal skinfold thickness were the same in the treated and control groups, the relevance of this finding is questionable. There were 2 infants with hypoglycaemia in the insulin-treated group, 4 in the group treated with diet alone, and 1 in the control group.

Recently, Li *et al.* (1987) randomly assigned 209 women with an abnormal 100 g oral glucose tolerance test to a diet or no treatment group. Unfortunately, there is a large potential for bias in the study, since 51

(24 per cent) of the women randomized were excluded from the analysis. However, the two groups had near identical caesarean section and induction rates, and none of the infants in either group experienced birth trauma or neonatal hypoglycaemia, and none died. There was a slight, though not significant, excess of heavy babies (more than 4000 g) in the control group (5 of 75) as compared to the treatment group (3 of 85).

In conclusion, one has to agree with Persson *et al.* (1985) that there is as yet no evidence to suggest that treating gestational diabetes with insulin reduces the incidence of neonatal jaundice or hypoglycaemia. It seems likely, however, that the increased incidence of fetal macrosomia can be reduced by insulin therapy. Nevertheless, as 10 per cent of normal women will deliver a baby weighing more than 4000 g at term (Thomson *et al.* 1968), one should be concerned, first, about a programme that could potentially reduce this incidence below its normal level, and, secondly, about the effects of manipulating fetal growth in all women with an abnormal glucose tolerance test, the majority of whom will have babies of normal weight.

6 Conclusions

The diagnosis of gestational diabetes, as currently defined, is based on an abnormal glucose tolerance test. This test is not reproducible at least 50 to 70 per cent of the time and the increased risk of perinatal mortality and morbidity said to be associated with this 'condition' has been considerably overemphasized. No clear improvement in perinatal mortality has been demonstrated with insulin treatment for gestational diabetes, and screening of the pregnant population with glucose tolerance testing is unlikely to make a significant impact on perinatal mortality.

An abnormal glucose tolerance test is associated with a two- to threefold increase in the incidence of macrosomia, but the majority of macrosomic infants will be born to mothers with a normal glucose tolerance test. Thus far, no improvement in neonatal outcome has been demonstrated from insulin treatment for gestational diabetes, nor has there been any demonstrated benefit to the mother or infant from reducing the incidence of macrosomia by insulin therapy.

There is, however, a great potential to do more harm than good. A positive test labels the woman as having some kind of diabetes. This is an unpleasant label to have under any circumstances, particularly when repeat testing will not confirm the diagnosis in up to 70 per cent of cases. Pregnancy is likely to be transformed into a high risk situation, invoking an extensive and expensive programme of tests and interventions of unproven benefit. Women who had a less than perfect outcome of pregnancy and who had not been screened for gestational diabetes, may unfairly accuse their physicians of negligence, while the large amount of money and resources that are tied up in diagnosing and treating this 'condition' could be diverted to areas where they might be more effective. A negative glucose tolerance test, on the other hand, also has a potential for harm by falsely reassuring the physician and the woman that the risk, engendered by the indication for the test, has been removed.

Except for research purposes, all forms of glucose tolerance testing should be stopped. As suggested by Lind (1984) and Schwartz and Brenner (1982), it is more appropriate to study those women in whom diabetes is suspected with repeat random blood glucose estimations throughout pregnancy. In the meantime, there is a need for population-based research to establish the true risk, if any, associated with sub-diabetic degrees of hyperglycaemia during pregnancy. Once the degree of risk is appropriately identified, therapies designed to reduce that risk must be investigated by rigorous, randomized trials before being introduced into clinical practice.

References

Abell DA, Beischer NA (1975). Evaluation of the three hour oral glucose tolerance test in detection of significant hyperglycaemia and hypoglycaemia in pregnancy. Diabetes, 24: 874–880.

Acker DB, Sachs BP, Friedman EA (1985). Risk factors for shoulder dystocia. Obstet Gynecol, 66: 762–768.

American Diabetes Association (1987). Position statement on gestational diabetes mellitus formulated by the American Diabetes Association, Inc. Am J Obstet Gynecol, 156: 488–489.

Anonymous (1980). Summary and recommendations of the Workshop-Conference on Gestational Diabetes. Diabetes Care, 3: 499–501.

Anonymous (1985). Summary and Recommendations of the Second International Workshop Conference on Gestational Diabetes Mellitus. Diabetes, 34: 123–126.

Billis A, Rastogi GK (1966). Studies in methods of investigating carbohydrate. Diabetologia, 2: 169–177.

Boyd M, McLean F, Usher RH (1983). Fetal macrosomia, predictions, risks, proposed management. Obstet Gynecol, 61: 715–722.

Chung CS, Myrianthopoulos NC (1975). Factors affecting risks of congenital malformations. II Effect of maternal diabetes. Birth Defects, 11: No.10.

Coustan DR, Lewis SB (1978). Insulin therapy for gestational diabetes. Obstet Gynecol, 51: 306–310.

Coustan DR, Imarah J (1984). Prophylactic insulin treatment of gestational diabetes reduces the incidence of macrosomia, operative delivery, and birth trauma. Am J Obstet Gynecol, 150: 836–842.

Cyr RM, Usher RH, McLean FH (1984). Changing patterns of birth asphyxia and trauma over 20 years. Am J Obstet Gynecol, 148: 490–498.

Gabbe SG, Mestman JH, Freeman RK, Anderson GV, Lowensohn RI (1977). Management and outcome of class A diabetes mellitus. Am J Obstet Gynecol, 127: 465–469.

Gilbert JAL, Dunlop DM (1949). Diabetic fertility maternal mortality and fetal low rate. Br Med J, 1: 48–51.

Gillmer MDG, Maresh M, Beard RW, Elkeles RS, Alderson C, Bloxham B (1986). Low energy diets in the treatment of gestational diabetes. Acta Endocrinol, Suppl 277: 44–49.

Goldberg JD, Franklin B, Lasser D, Jornsay DL, Hausknecht RU, Ginsberg-Fellner F, Berkowitz RL (1986). Gestational diabetes: Impact of home glucose monitoring on neonatal birth weight. Am J Obstet Gynecol, 154: 546–550.

Hadden DR (1975). Glucose tolerance tests in pregnancy. In: Carbohydrate Metabolism in Pregnancy and the Newborn. Sutherland HW, Stowers JM (eds). Edinburgh: Churchill Livingstone, pp 19–39.

Hadden DR (1985). Geographic, ethnic, and racial variations in the incidence of gestational diabetes mellitus. Diabetes, 34: 8–11.

Hagabard L (1958). The prediabetic period from an obstetric point of view. Acta Obstet Gynecol Scand, 37: 497–518.

Herzstein J, Dolger H (1946). The fetal mortality in women during the prediabetic period. Am J Obstet Gynecol, 51: 420–422.

Landon MB, Gabbe SG (1985). Antepartum fetal surveillance in gestational diabetes mellitus. Diabetes, 34: 50–54.

Letsky E (1980). The haematological system. In: Clinical Physiology in Obstetrics. Hytten FE, Chamberlain G (eds). Oxford: Blackwell Scientific Publications, pp 43–78.

Levine MG, Holroyde J, Woods JR, Siddiqi TA, Scott M, Miodovnik, M (1984). Birth trauma: Incidence and predisposing factors. Obstet Gynecol, 63: 792–795.

Li DFH, Wong VCW, O'Hoy KMKY, Yeung CY, Ma HK (1987). Is treatment needed for mild impairment of glucose tolerance in pregnancy? A randomized controlled trial. Br J Obstet Gynaecol, 94: 851–854.

Lind T (1984). Antenatal screening for diabetes mellitus. Br J Obstet Gynaecol, 91: 833–834.

Maresh M, Gillmer MDG, Beard RW, Alderson CS, Bloxham BA, Elkeles RS (1985). The effect of diet and insulin on metabolic profiles of women with gestational diabetes mellitus. Diabetes, 34, Suppl 2: 88–93.

McDonald GW, Fisher GF, Burnham C (1965). Reproducibility of the oral glucose tolerance test. Diabetes, 14: 473–480.

McDonald GW, Burnham CE, Lewish FW (1969). Reproducibility of glucose tolerance in 101 nondiabetic women. Public Health Reports 84: No. 4.

Metzger BE, Phelps RL, Freinkel N, Navickas IA (1980). Effects of gestational diabetes on diurnal profiles of plasma glucose, lipids, and individual amino acids. Diabetes Care, 3: 402–409.

National Diabetes Data Group (1979). Classification and diagnosis of diabetes mellitus and other categories of glucose intolerance. Diabetes, 28: 1039–1057.

O'Sullivan JB (1975). Prospective study of gestational diabetes and its treatment. In: Carbohydrate Metabolism in Pregnancy and the Newborn. Sutherland HW, Stowers JM (eds). Edinburgh: Churchill Livingstone, pp 195–204.

O'Sullivan JB, Mahan CM (1964). Criteria for the oral glucose tolerance test in pregnancy. Diabetes, 13: 278–285.

O'Sullivan JB, Mahan CM (1968). Prospective study of 352 patients with chemical diabetes. New Engl J Med, 278: 1038–1041.

O'Sullivan JB, Charles, D, Mahan CM, Dandrow RV (1973). Gestational diabetes and perinatal mortality rate, Am J Obstet Gynecol, 116: 901–904.

Oats JN, Abell DA, Beischer NA, Broomhall GR (1980). Maternal glucose tolerance during pregnancy with excessive size infants. Obstet Gynecol, 55: 184–186.

Persson B, Stangenberg M, Hansson U, Nordlander E (1985). Gestational diabetes mellitus: Comparative evaluation of two treatment regimens, diet, versus insulin and diet. Diabetes, 34: 101–105.

Persson B, Stangenberg M, Lunell NO (1986). Prediction of size of infants at birth by measurement of symphysis fundus height. Br J Obstet Gynaecol, 93: 206–211.

Philipson EH, Satish CK, Rosen MG, Edelberg TG, Riha MM (1985). Gestational diabetes mellitus. Is further improvement necessary ? Diabetes, 34: 55–60.

Pritchard JA, MacDonald PC (eds) (1980). Williams Obstetrics. New York: Appleton-Century-Crofts, p 741.

Roversi GD, Gargiulo M, Nicolini U, Ferrazzi E, Pedretti E, Gruft L, Tronconi G (1980). Maximal tolerated insulin therapy in gestational diabetes. Diabetes Care, 3: 489–494.

Schwartz ML, Brenner WE (1982). The need for adequate and consistent diagnostic classifications for diabetes mellitus diagnosed during pregnancy. Am J Obstet Gynecol, 143: 119–124.

Spellacy WN, Miller S, Winegar A, Peterson PQ (1985). Macrosomia—Maternal Characteristics and infant complications. Obstet Gynecol, 66: 158–161.

Sutherland HW, Stowers JM (1975). The detection of chemical diabetes during pregnancy using the intravenous glucose tolerance test. In: Carbohydrate Metabolism in Pregnancy and the Newborn. Sutherland HW, Stowers JM (eds). Edinburgh: Churchill Livingstone, pp 153–166.

Thomson AM, Billewicz WZ, Hytten FE (1968). The assessment of fetal growth. J Obstet Gynaecol Br Commwlth, 75: 903–916.

Widnes JA, Cowett RM, Coustan DR, Carpenter MW, Oh W (1985). Neonatal morbidities in infants of mothers with glucose intolerance in pregnancy. Diabetes, 34: 61–65.

World Health Organization Expert Committee on Diabetes Mellitus (1980). Second report. Technical Report Series, No. 646. Geneva: World Health Organization.

26 Assessment of fetal size and fetal growth

Douglas G. Altman and Frank E. Hytten

1 Introduction

In any approach to the assessment of fetal size or fetal growth two questions should be considered. First, with what success does the technique used detect the small or badly growing fetus? And second, does the successful detection of the small fetus lead to more effective care during pregnancy?

An attempt to answer the first question is made by most studies, usually by comparing the intrauterine measurement with birthweight or birthweight for gestational age centile. That the detection of a relatively small fetus should predict a relatively small newborn infant is, however, neither surprising nor necessarily useful. The second question demands a better measure of outcome: if the technique could detect the poorly growing and compromised fetus who would be safer outside the uterus than remaining within it, then the clinical value would be obvious. Yet, despite the fact that a great deal of obstetric intervention stems from clinical anxiety about what is perceived to be impaired fetal growth, there is little information that would help to answer the question.

2 What is meant by fetal growth?

Fetal size and fetal growth are often confused in clinical practice: it is common to see 'birthweight-for-gestational age' standards described as 'fetal growth charts', and a weight-for-gestation below some arbitrary centile referred to as 'intra-uterine growth retardation'. Apart from the fact that *birth*weights at a given length of gestation may not be a good reflection of *fetal* weights at the same gestation, this definition of intrauterine growth retardation is based on weight alone. Infants below a particular centile may be 'light-for-gestational age' without necessarily being 'growth retarded'. The confusion between 'light-for-gestational age' (often called 'small-for-gestational age', or SGA) and fetal or 'intrauterine growth retardation' (IUGR) is illustrated by contrasting the views of Wilcox (1983), who wrote that 'There is little doubt that SGA and IUGR are not identical' with those of both Birnholz (1986), who claimed that 'IUGR and SGA are identical conceptually', and Seeds (1984) who stated that 'it is small fetal size that constitutes the problem of impaired fetal growth.'

The last of these views is plainly wrong. As Richard Asher (1972) wrote: 'The words used in clinical medicine have a tremendous influence on the subject they describe or purport to describe. They perpetuate illnesses, syndromes and signs whose existence is doubtful, they deny recognition to others whose existence is beyond question and, moreover, they distort text-book descriptions to conform to the chosen word.' It is essential to maintain the distinction between 'light-for-gestational age' and 'intrauterine growth retardation', just as it is to distinguish low birthweight from 'light-for-gestational age'. Yet, most authors use the term 'intrauterine growth retardation' to mean that the baby's birthweight falls below a certain centile of weight for gestational age. As Lin and Evans (1984) have observed: 'Currently, the most widely accepted definition for IUGR is a birthweight below the 10th percentile for a given gestational age'. Deter is unusual in having commented on the lack of any justification for this cut-off (Deter *et al.* 1982a; Deter 1986b).

The distinction between size and growth is critical. Growth cannot be estimated from less than two measurements of size, and the argument that size at some time in late pregnancy and a presumed zero size at conception can represent those two measurements is both philosophically dubious and clinically unhelpful. What the clinician would like to know is whether the fetal growth has deviated from its normal progression.

An estimate of fetal size in early pregnancy can be valuable in estimating or confirming the duration of the pregnancy (see Chapter 27), but a single estimate of fetal size in late pregnancy is of little or no clinical help to the obstetrician. The arbitrary categorization of all babies estimated to be below the 10th or 5th centile for gestational age as 'growth retarded' is highly misleading. If a single estimate of fetal size in late pregnancy suggests an unusually small baby, then the clinician might assume that some pathological interference with fetal growth has occurred; but the size alone does not prove it. It must not be forgotten that in any population of fetuses some 10 per cent will, by definition, have a weight below the 10th centile, and it is absurd to define in advance the proportion of babies that will suffer from 'intra-uterine growth retardation' (see Chapter 3). Further, there is increasing evidence that the birthweights of babies born at a particular gestational age are lower than the fetal weights at the same gestational age (Ott and Doyle 1982; Secher *et al.* 1987; Yudkin *et al.* 1987).

Some authors have made inferences about fetal growth by taking differences between cross-sectionally derived estimates of mean or median birthweight at consecutive weeks of gestation. This approach is grossly misleading and often leads to the inference that fetuses shrink beyond term. For example, Fig. 26.1 from Williams *et al.* (1982) presents curves of the difference between median birthweights at successive weeks of gestation. Although the figure is correctly, if confusingly, labelled as 'birthweight gain per week', the authors incorrectly described the curves as 'median growth rate (velocity) curves'. They used the Figure to make inferences about weight loss and intrauterine growth retardation that are completely unjustified. We stress again, inferences about growth cannot be drawn from cross-sectional data.

'Intrauterine growth retardation' cannot be diagnosed from birthweight and gestational age alone (Thomson and Billewicz, 1976). The term 'intrauterine growth retardation' should be restricted to those fetuses

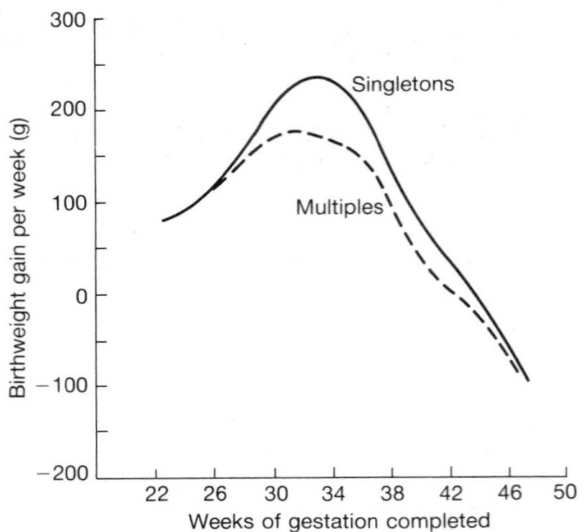

Fig. 26.1 'Median growth rate (velocity) curves' for single and multiple births in California, 1970–76 (Williams *et al.* 1982).

where there is definite evidence that growth has faltered, or to instances where clinical evidence points to loss of fetal weight *in utero*. Such infants may not necessarily be particularly 'light-for-gestational age' (Daikoku *et al.* 1979); a fetus whose weight falls from the 90th centile to the 30th in a short period of gestation is almost certainly in greater peril than a fetus who has maintained a position on the 5th centile. These may be seen to correspond to two different types of intrauterine growth retardation, often referred to as asymmetric (or disproportional, or late-flattening), and symmetric (or proportional, or low profile) (Campbell 1974; Rosso and Winick 1974). Asymmetric growth retardation is characterized by a rapid slowing of growth near term, whereas symmetric growth retardation indicates consistent suboptimal growth.

In this chapter we will emphasize the estimation of growth rather than size because the object of antenatal surveillance is to anticipate or demonstrate clinical problems which can be helped by appropriate action. Establishing that a fetus is small does not expose a clinical problem; only the demonstration of impaired growth can do that. This basic point is recognized by those studying child growth (Brook *et al.* 1986) but, in general, not by those studying fetal growth. Even when longitudinal data are available, the definition of intrauterine growth retardation remains problematic; but at least any cut-off chosen will be related to the directly relevant assessment of growth, rather than to size alone.

There are other considerations which must be addressed. How accurately can fetal size, and hence growth, be assessed? How well does that assessment relate to clinical hazards for the fetus? And what is the effect of taking that information into account in providing care during pregnancy? These issues are discussed below for clinical and ultrasound measurements, but first it is necessary to consider some more general issues.

3 Diagnosis of fetal growth retardation

The use of fetal measurements to assess fetal wellbeing may be considered in the general framework of all diagnostic tests (see Chapter 3). There is a problem here, however, in that it is not clear precisely what one is trying to predict. For example, a single fetal measurement below, say, the fifth centile of the expected distribution at that stage of pregnancy may be taken as diagnostic of growth retardation; but there is no absolute postnatal judgement of growth retardation that can be used to assess the validity of the 'test'. In the absence of an appropriate outcome measure, authors frequently use some measure of 'relatively low' birthweight, such as being below the 10th centile of weight for gestational age. Villar and Belizan (1986) have reviewed the literature of such studies. Unfortunately they took the definition of intrauterine growth retardation that was given in the original papers, and did not describe variability in how intrauterine growth retardation was defined. Partly for this reason, and partly because the selection of individuals for the studies was based on widely differing criteria, the 55 publications reviewed showed variation in the prevalence of intrauterine growth retardation (however defined) from 2.3 per cent to 60.9 per cent. While the sensitivity and specificity of a test are important, from the clinical point of view only the positive and negative predictive values of a diagnostic test are important, and these will depend upon the observed prevalence of intrauterine growth retardation in the population studied (see Chapter 3). Villar and Belizan (1986) demonstrated a positive correlation between the positive predictive value and the prevalence of intrauterine growth retardation across the studies reviewed. Despite selection of high risk samples, the majority of the studies they reviewed had a positive predictive value of less than 50 per cent, with important implications in terms of the consequences of blanket intervention.

Many factors are known to be related to fetal size, birth weight, and neonatal morbidity and mortality. Knowledge of such epidemiological associations is important, but few of them are strong enough to help the clinician directly. Thus knowledge that a clinical or fetal measurement is associated with subsequent outcome is not helpful unless the association is strong, with high sensitivity, specificity, and positive predictive value. The available tests do not fulfil this requirement, so that predicting whether or not a baby will be below a certain centile of birthweight for gestational age is of limited value. This is especially so as low birthweight is not really the most important outcome, and there is no justification for selecting a particular centile (usually the 10th) as a cut-off. Trying to predict birthweight itself is rather less sensible, especially before the last trimester.

The concept underlying the diagnostic test approach is that there is a clear dichotomy between 'normal' and 'abnormal' fetuses, and one is trying to find a perfect way of uncovering this dichotomy. While such dichotomization of continuous measurements to define disease is common in clinical practice (for example, in defining hypertension and anaemia), it may be counterproductive. Risk increases in a continuous (although not necessarily linear) manner with decreasing size, however measured. It does not suddenly occur below some arbitrarily defined threshhold. It is thus sensible to consider using three categories rather than two, with a 'buffer zone' of uncertainty between apparently normal and apparently abnormal fetuses (Campbell and Dewhurst 1971).

There is a further danger in the use of a single estimate of 'size-for-gestational age': it depends not only on the estimate of fetal size, which is bound to have an inherent degree of uncertainty, but also on gestational age, the estimation of which is subject to major errors. In particular, if the gestational age is overestimated by two weeks (or more), which is not uncommon, the fetus may well be considered light-for-gestational age throughout the pregnancy; conversely, a poorly growing fetus may be missed if the gestational age is underestimated.

Many of the same problems relate to the assessment of growth from two or more measurements. The difference is that one may reasonably infer that a growth rate below a certain centile is indicative of retarded growth *per se*, so that it is not necessary to demonstrate a strong association with birthweight, which is, in any case, only a proxy measure of growth. In addition, errors in dating are much less critical when considering growth rather than size. The direct use of centiles for growth emphasizes the variability in growth, and that risk is not simply either 'present' or 'absent'.

4 Construction and use of fetal growth standards

4.1 Fetal size

Most standards for fetal measurements or birthweight are constructed in one of two ways. The mean and standard deviation of the measurement can be obtained for each week of gestational age and the values of particular centiles estimated from these by assuming that the data have a Normal distribution. For example, the values mean 1.645 SD give the 10th and 90th centiles. (Most measurements relevant to this discussion are reasonably Normally distributed.) The alternative approach is based on taking the centiles of interest (e.g. 10th and 90th) directly from the observed data at each week of gestation. This empirical method has the advantage that no distributional assumptions are made, but the disadvantage that the centiles obtained are rather less precise estimates of the population values when the data are approximately Normally distributed. Whichever method is used, it is highly desirable that the centiles should be smoothed in some way over gestational age. It makes no sense to have irregular curves depicting the mean or particular centiles of the distribution across gestational ages.

Another very important aspect of the derivation of standards for size or growth is the selection of the sample. There is a tendency in such studies to be overselective, resulting in the standards being derived from a 'supernormal' population. Obviously one needs to exclude twins (which merit special studies), women with uncertain dates, and perhaps a few gross abnormalities, but it is certainly not reasonable to exclude cases on the basis of subsequent birthweight, and debatable whether any information not available at the stage of gestation in question should be considered (for example, fetal or neonatal morbidity and mortality). A further consideration is that the standards used should be appropriate for local use, in that they should describe the size of fetuses in the geographical area of interest apppropriately.

An additional worry about most published studies is that the number of observations made on each individual varies enormously. Apart from the usual statistical worries about the non-independence of the data, there must be some likelihood that the number of observations may be related to the perceived well-being of the mother and fetus. In a study where some women were seen once and others five or more times we may well suspect that the latter, whose data dominate, have been investigated more deeply because of some clinical concern.

4.2 Fetal growth

Standards for growth (perhaps better termed 'velocity') are constructed in the same basic way as those for size, and are subject to the same worries about the selection of the sample and the variation in the number of measurements per individual. In addition, there is a problem about how to make use of the multiple measurements on each individual. Clearly, one needs at least two measurements of size to estimate growth, and the average weekly growth can be calculated by dividing the change in size by the number of weeks between the measurements. Standards can be constructed from the distribution of such changes, relating these either to the midpoint of the time period concerned, or to the average of the two observed sizes. Both approaches were used in relation to biparietal diameter by Campbell and Newman (1971), whose two charts look very similar. The second approach was also used by Sholl *et al.* (1982). When plotting growth rate by gestational age, any error in the assessment of gestational age will be unimportant unless massive, because the average growth rate is fairly constant until late pregnancy; but plotting by size is preferable because it is unaffected by any error in dating. This is conceptually appealing and is very similar to the use of weight-for-height charts for studying growth in children.

For individuals with more than two observations there will be two or more estimates of growth rate. There should be an upper limit to the time span of such estimates, and it is probably unwise to use every pair of measurements to give an estimate of growth, restricting the data to the changes between consecutive measures of size. So, for example, four measurements of fetal size would provide three estimates of fetal growth, not six.

In estimating fetal growth the benefits of independence from dating inaccuracies are somewhat offset by the problem that measurement error will be greater for an estimate of growth than for one of size, because growth is calculated from two estimates of size. Thus it has been suggested that growth arrest should be observed over at least a two- to three-week period to be clinically significant (Crane *et al.* 1977).

Problems of construction of both cross-sectional and longitudinal standards could be alleviated by designing studies carefully, rather than taking those measurements that happen to be available.

5 Estimation of fetal size and growth

5.1 Clinical measurement

The oldest clinical method of estimating fetal size—abdominal palpation—is so inaccurate as to be little better than a blind guess. For example, Loeffler (1967) found that 20 per cent of such assessments made just prior to delivery were not within 450 g of the actual birthweight, and that the errors were worse at the extremes of the range, where the information is most needed. Similarly, Beazley and Kurjak (1973) found that 25 per cent of predictions after 36 weeks' gestation were more than 500 g in error.

Whether fetal growth is, or is not, occurring satisfactorily has in the past frequently been inferred from indirect measurements: in particular maternal weight-gain is often used clinically as an index of the well-being of the pregnancy and hence of fetal growth. To the extent that part of the weight gain is fetus, and some of the remainder—growth of the uterus and placenta, and the expansion of the maternal blood volume—is related to fetal weight, this can be justified. But the relation between fetal weight-gain and maternal weight-gain is weak (Eastman and Jackson 1968; Singer *et al.* 1968). In the last 10 weeks of pregnancy, when assessment of fetal growth is clinically most useful, fetal weight-gain is less than half of the total weight gained by the mother. It may be that there is an association between maternal weight-gain and fetal growth, but it is overstating the case to suggest that 'maternal weight gain significantly influenced birthweight' (Abrams and Laros 1986).

Apart from the looseness of the relation, there is considerable uncertainty in the maternal bodyweight itself, with day to day variation in which the standard deviation of the fluctuation is about 0.5 per cent of the mean weight (Hytten 1981). Such variation can swamp the weekly change in weight during late pregnancy and only a regression on a succession of daily weights obtained under standard conditions could establish the extent of weight-change with any degree of certainty. To base any clinical decision related to fetal growth on such a fallible piece of evidence would hardly seem sensible.

A marginally more direct approach is to measure the increase in size of the maternal abdomen which must, at least to some extent, reflect uterine growth. The two most widely practised techniques are the measurement of 'fundal height', the distance along the abdominal wall between the upper border of the symphysis pubis and the uterine fundus, and the measurement of abdominal girth at the level of the umbilicus.

There have been several studies of fundal height as an indicator of fetal size, but little investigation of the potential of this measurement for assessing growth. This is understandable, given the not inconsiderable inter- and intra-observer variation in measuring fundal height (Calvert *et al.* 1982). Nevertheless several studies have shown quite good sensitivity and specificity of fundal height for predicting low birthweight for gestation (Belizan *et al.* 1978; Quaranta *et al.* 1981; Mathai *et al.* 1987; Pearce and Campbell 1987), but others have found fundal height to be a poor predictor (Wladimiroff and Laar 1980; Rosenberg *et al.* 1982; Persson *et al.* 1986). As discussed below, the ability to predict low birthweight is not the same as the ability to detect growth retardation, but fundal height may be useful as a screening test for further investigation. Mathai *et al.* (1987) found fundal height to be superior to abdominal girth in predicting low birthweight. Especially in countries where ultrasound is not available, measurement of the fundal height may be the best way to alert the physician to the possibility of impaired fetal growth. Pearce and Campbell (1987) found that the diagnosis of low birthweight based on fundal height was nearly as good as that based on ultrasound measurement of the abdominal circumference. This was a rare longitudinal study, but serial fundal height data were not presented.

5.2 Hormone estimations

An almost equally indirect reflection of fetal growth is the production by the fetus, or the fetoplacental unit, of hormones. Again there is an undoubted statistical relation between hormone production, as reflected in maternal serum concentration or urinary output, and the size and well-being of the fetus (see Chapter 29), but the association is too loose to be useful.

5.3 Ultrasonography

Finally, there is the most direct approach to the assessment of fetal growth yet available: the measurement of an image of the fetus obtained by ultrasound. Now that the use of X-rays is no longer acceptable, the only method that can be said to offer a size estimate of any validity is measurement of fetal dimensions on an ultrasonic image.

Recent reviews have found such methods wanting as predictors of 'low-birthweight-for-gestation'. Deter (1986b) observed that 'the major problem with the current methods is the large number of false-positive results', and Benson *et al.* (1986) concluded that proposed ultrasound measurements 'do not allow one to diagnose IUGR with confidence.' These views, however, are based on the concept that one should evaluate ultrasound measurements by their ability to predict babies which will be 'light-for-gestational age'. As already pointed out, this is not really what we are interested in. We would not expect measurements of fetal dimensions or area to agree exactly with weight, so some lack of predictive ability should not be used as a criticism of ultrasound measurement. Thus, ultrasonographically derived fetal measurements, rather than 'birthweight-for-gestational age', should be considered to be the 'gold standards' for measuring fetal size and growth.

There is an extensive literature on ultrasound measurement of fetal size, which has recently been reviewed by Deter *et al.* (1986). Numerous authors have produced cross-sectional standards (often wrongly called 'growth curves') for ultrasound measurements of different parts of the fetus, notably biparietal diameter, abdominal circumference, crown–rump length, and femur length. Several authors have looked at serial measurements, but most have analysed the data as a sequence of points on cross-sectional 'growth' charts rather than looking at changes in fetal measurements over time (Queenan *et al.* 1976; Crane *et al.* 1977). These standards are valuable for estimating fetal size at a given point in pregnancy, provided that one knows the gestational age accurately, but they are not really suitable for assessing fetal growth between two points in the pregnancy.

There has been very little research aimed at producing true growth curves based on longitudinal measurements. Such information would provide a far sounder basis for assessing fetal growth, and is arguably the only valid approach for detecting growth retardation. One of the first studies presenting longitudinal ultrasound measurements was that of Campbell and Newman (1971). They produced unsmoothed centiles for the growth rate in biparietal diameter, both in relation to gestational age and also to the biparietal diameter itself. Sholl *et al.* (1982) also produced this latter type of chart for changes in biparietal diameter. Figure 26.2, taken from their paper, illustrates how one may detect fetal growth retardation more quickly by considering growth directly than by studying several estimates of size. They emphasized the usefulness of this approach when gestational age is unknown or uncertain.

A different approach was taken by Deter *et al.* (1982b) who, in a small study of several fetal measurements, fitted mathematical growth curve models to each individual's data. This method requires several observations per fetus, but Deter and Rossavik (1987) have shown good results using just two measurements per fetus. The clinical value of this approach remains to be demonstrated, but it has definite potential.

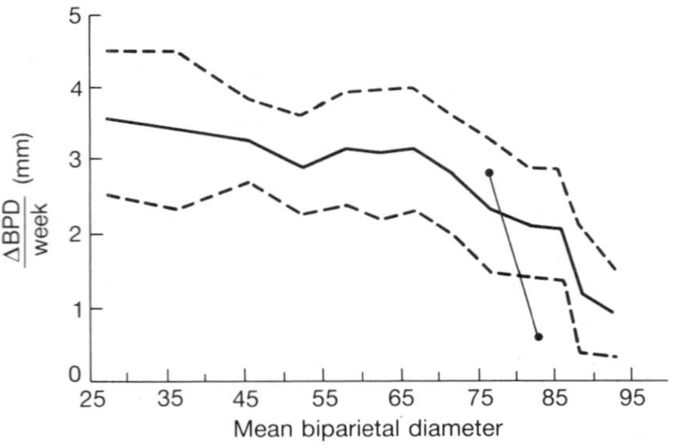

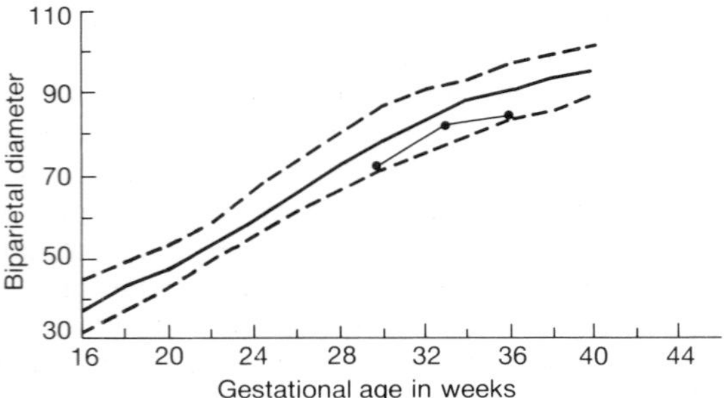

Fig. 26.2 Illustration of usefulness of serial measures of fetal size in conjunction with charts for change in biparietal diameter (from Sholl *et al.* 1982).

As mentioned earlier, two different types of growth retardation have been identified—symmetric and asymmetric. While there is no doubt that different forms of growth retardation exist, it remains uncertain how clear the distinction is between these two, and, if such a distinction exists, whether it has any implications for clinical practice. There is agreement, however, that in asymmetric retardation the brain is spared from the worst effects, so that the biparietal diameter is probably not the best fetal measurement for detecting growth retardation (Seeds 1984). In contrast, the liver is highly vulnerable, so that the abdominal circumference may be expected to give a better indication of fetal well-being. Further, it is reasonable to suppose that the ratio of head to abdomen size may be a good indicator of fetal growth problems, especially of asymmetric growth retardation. Several authors have studied this and similar ratios.

Campbell and Thoms (1977) produced cross-sectional centile charts for the ratio of head circumference to abdominal circumference. Deter *et al.* (1982) collected serial measurements of the same ratio, but they did not study serial changes. Other ratios and products have been reviewed by Deter (1986a). As yet, there is not enough information on any of them to establish clinical usefulness. One ratio of particular interest is that of femur length to abdominal circumference, as this was found to be constant in normal pregnancies from 21 weeks to term (Hadlock *et al.* 1983).

The simultaneous measurement of two or more fetal dimensions should in principle give more reliable information about fetal growth than any single measurement, but few studies have collected such data, and few of these have analysed the data longitudinally.

There may be indications of malnutrition from clinical examination of the neonate, and these may represent prior growth retardation. Body fat can be assessed by the ponderal index (Miller and Hassanein 1971), a measure of weight for height, or skinfold thickness (Oakley *et al.* 1977), and it has been shown that 'light-for-gestational age' infants have a faster body-water turnover than 'normal' infants (MacLennan *et al.* 1981). Postnatal clinical assessments should be able to distinguish between symmetric and asymmetric growth retardation, but they have not been adequately validated by relating them to fetal ultrasound measurements of growth.

Another reason for not concentrating on trying to predict 'light-for-gestational age' babies is that these are not necessarily at greatest risk. Hellier and Goldstein (1979) showed that perinatal mortality risk was related to both birthweight and gestation, especially birthweight, and that birthweight for gestational age is inferior for this purpose. Studies are needed to relate ultrasound diagnoses of growth retardation to perinatal and long term risks of mortality and morbidity.

6 Conclusions

The clinical methods of assessing fetal size and growth—maternal weight-gain, fundal height, abdominal girth—are relatively imprecise. It is possible that the use of some measure such as fundal height could be used as a screening device for referral of women to a specialist for further assessment; but these techniques are crude, many small fetuses will be missed, and many perfectly well grown fetuses will be considered worryingly small.

Ultrasound techniques have the capacity to detect abnormalities of fetal growth but have not been effectively exploited (Keirse 1984). There is a need for prospective studies to examine the differential growth of fetal parts, say head, abdomen, and femur, in large samples to see whether patterns of growth that are associated with fetal compromise and later infant morbidity can be defined. Such studies should be carried out with scheduled repeated measurements. It is particularly crucial that some sound measures of outcome should be defined. Intervention based on assessments of size or growth should be evaluated in randomized trials before they are implemented in general obstetric practice.

References

Abrams BF, Laros RK (1986). Prepregnancy weight, weight gain, and birth weight. Am J Obstet Gynecol, 154: 503–509.

Asher R (1972). Richard Asher Talking Sense. London: Pitman, p 25.

Beazley JM, Kurjak A (1973). Prediction of foetal maturity and birthweight by abdominal palpation. Nursing Times, 14 June: 763–765.

Belizan JM, Villar J, Nardin JC, Malamud J, de Vicuna LS (1978). Diagnosis of intrauterine growth retardation by a simple clinical method: measurement of uterine height. Am J Obstet Gynecol, 131: 643–646.

Benson CB, Doubilet PM, Saltzman DH (1986). Intrauterine growth retardation: predictive value of US criteria for antenatal diagnosis. Radiology, 160: 415–417.

Birnholz JC (1986). Biological foundations for fetal growth studies. In: Quantitative Obstetrical Ultrasonography. Deter RL, Harrist RB, Birnholz JC, Hadlock FP (eds). New York: John Wiley, p 57.

Brook CGD, Hindmarsh PC, Healy MJR (1986). A better way to detect growth failure. Br Med J, 293: 1186.

Calvert JP, Crean EE, Newcombe RG, Pearson JF (1982). Antenatal screening by measurement of symphysis–fundus height. Br Med J, 285: 846–849.

Campbell S (1974). Assessing size at birth. In: Size at Birth. Ciba Foundation Symposium 27. Amsterdam: Elsevier, pp 275–293.

Campbell S, Dewhurst CJ (1971). Diagnosis of the small-for-dates fetus by serial ultrasonic cephalometry. Lancet, ii: 1002–1006.

Campbell S, Newman GB (1971). Growth of the fetal biparietal diameter during normal pregnancy. J Obstet Gynaecol Br Commwlth, 78: 513–519.

Campbell S, Thoms A (1977). Ultrasound measurement of the fetal head to abdomen circumference ratio in the assessment of growth retardation. Br J Obstet Gynaecol, 84: 165–174.

Crane JP, Kopta MM, Welt SI, Sauvage JP (1977). Abnormal fetal growth patterns. Ultrasonic diagnosis and management. Obstet Gynecol, 50: 205–211.

Daikoku NH, Johnson JWC, Graf C, Kearney K, Tyson JE, King TM (1979). Patterns of intrauterine growth retardation. Obstet Gynecol, 54: 211–219.

Deter RL, Harrist RB, Hadlock FP, Carpenter RJ (1982a). The use of ultrasound in the detection of intrauterine growth retardation: a review. J Clin Ultrasound, 10: 9–16.

Deter RL, Harrist RB, Hadlock FP, Poindexter AN (1982b). Longitudinal studies of fetal growth with the use of dynamic image ultrasonography. Am J Obstet Gynecol, 143: 545–554.

Deter RL (1986a). Evaluation of studies of normal growth. In: Quantitative Obstetrical Ultrasonography. Deter RL, Harrist RB, Birnholz JC, Hadlock FP (eds). New York: John Wiley, pp 65–111.

Deter RL (1986b). Detection of fetal growth abnormalities. In: Quantitative Obstetrical Ultrasonography. Deter RL, Harrist RB, Birnholz JC, Hadlock FP (eds). New York: John Wiley, pp 123–140.

Deter RL, Harrist RB, Birnholz JC, Hadlock FP (eds), (1986). Quantitive Obstetrical Ultrasonography. New York: John Wiley.

Deter RL, Rossavik IK (1987). A simplified method for determining individual growth curve standards. Obstet Gynecol, 70: 801–806.

Eastman NJ, Jackson E (1968). Weight relationships in pregnancy. Obstet Gynecol Surv, 23: 1003–1010.

Hadlock FP, Deter RL, Harrist RB, Roecker E, Park SK (1983). A date-independent predictor of intrauterine growth retardation: femur length/abdominal circumference ratio. Am J Radiol, 141: 979–984.

Hellier JL, Goldstein H (1979). The use of birthweight and gestation to assess perinatal mortality risk. J Epidemiol Community Health, 33: 183–185.

Hytten FE (1981). Weight gain in pregnancy—30 years of research. S Afr Med J, 60: 15–19.

Keirse MJNC (1984). Epidemiology and aetiology of the growth retarded baby. Clin Obstet Gynaecol, 11: 415–436.

Lin C-C, Evans MI (1984). Intrauterine growth retardation. New York: McGraw-Hill, p 4.

Loeffler FE (1967). Clinical foetal weight prediction. J Obstet Gynaecol Br Commwlth, 74: 675–677.

MacLennan AH, Millington G, Grieve A, McIntosh JEA, Seamark RF, Cox LW (1981). Neonatal body water turnover: a putative index of perinatal morbidity. Am J Obstet Gynecol, 139: 948–952.

Mathai M, Jairaj J, Muthurathnam S (1987). Screening for light-for-gestational-age infants: a comparison of three simple measurements. Br J Obstet Gynaecol, 94: 217–221.

Miller HC, Hassanein K (1971). Diagnosis of impaired fetal growth in newborn infants. Pediatrics 48, 511–522.

Oakley JR, Parsons RJ, Whitelaw AGL (1977). Standards for skinfold thickness in British newborn infants. Arch Dis Child, 52: 287–290.

Ott WJ, Doyle S (1982). Normal ultrasonic fetal weight curve. Obstet Gynecol, 59: 603–606.

Pearce JM, Campbell S (1987). A comparison of symphysis-fundal height and ultrasound as screening tests for light-for-gestational age infants. Br J Obstet Gynaecol, 94: 100–104.

Persson B, Stangenberg M, Lunell NO, Brodin U, Holmberg NG, Vaclavinkova V (1986). Prediction of size of infants at birth by measurement of symphysis fundus height. Br J Obstet Gynaecol, 93: 206–211.

Quaranta P, Currell R, Redman CWG, Robinson JS (1981). Prediction of small-for-dates infants by measurement of symphysial–fundal-height. Br J Obstet Gynaecol, 88: 115–119.

Queenan JT, Kubarych SF, Cook LN, Anderson GD, Griffin LP (1976). Diagnostic ultrasound for detection of intrauterine growth retardation. Am J Obstet Gynecol, 124: 865–872.

Rosenberg K, Grant JM, Hepburn M (1982). Antenatal detection of growth retardation: actual practice in a large maternity hospital. Br J Obstet Gynaecol, 89: 12–15.

Rosso P, Winick M (1974). Intrauterine growth retardation. A new systematic approach based on the clinical and biochemical characteristics of this condition. J Perinat Med, 2: 147–160.

Secher NJ, Kern Hansen P, Thomsen BL, Keiding N (1987). Growth retardation in preterm infants. Br J Obstet Gynaecol, 94: 115–120.

Seeds JW (1984). Impaired fetal growth: ultrasonic evaluation and clinical management. Obstet Gynecol, 64: 577–584.

Sholl JS, Woo D, Rubin JM, Lin C-C, Moawad AH (1982). Intrauterine growth retardation risk detection for fetuses of unknown gestational age. Am J Obstet Gynecol, 144: 709–714.

Singer JE, Westphal M, Niswander K (1968). Relationship of weight gain during pregnancy to birthweight and infant growth and development in first years of life. Report from collaborative study of cerebral palsy. Obstet Gynecol, 31: 417–422.

Thomson AM, Billewicz WZ (1976). The concept of the 'light for dates' infant. In: The Biology of Human Fetal Growth. Roberts DF, Thomson AM (eds). London: Taylor & Francis, pp 69–79.

Villar J, Belizan JM (1986). The evaluation of methods used in the diagnosis of intrauterine growth retardation. Obstet Gynecol Surv, 41: 187–199.

Wilcox AJ (1983). Intrauterine growth retardation: beyond birthweight criteria (Editorial). Early Hum Dev, 8: 189–193.

Williams RL, Creasy RK, Cunningham GC, Hawes WE, Norris FD, Tashiro M (1982). Fetal growth and perinatal viability in California. Obstet Gynecol, 59: 624–632.

Wladimiroff JW, Laar J (1980). Ultrasonic measurement of fetal body size. A randomized controlled trial. Acta Obstet Gynaecol Scand, 59: 177–179.

Yudkin PL, Aboualfa M, Eyre JA, Redman CWG, Wilkinson AR (1987). The influence of elective preterm delivery on birthweight and head circumference standards. Arch Dis Child, 62: 24–29.

27 Ultrasound in pregnancy

Jim Neilson and Adrian Grant

1 Introduction

Ultrasound may be defined as mechanical vibration occurring at frequencies above the range of human hearing. The history of its development as a medical diagnostic tool has been charted by Kratochwil (1978) and by Donald (1980). An Austrian neurologist, Dussik, was the first to use ultrasound in medicine, although his attempts during the 1930s, to produce images of the adult brain failed because of the high acoustic impedance of skull bone. Refinements in ultrasound instrumentation prompted by World War II encouraged Howry in Denver to experiment with the technology as a diagnostic imaging technique. Later, with Holmes, he produced images of reasonable quality of upper abdominal organs. However, these were only obtainable by immersing the subject in a bath of water. This important practical disadvantage was overcome by Donald and Brown who, working in Glasgow, produced the first contact ultrasound scanner.

As Donald was a professor of midwifery, early diagnostic work concentrated on imaging in obstetrics and gynaecology, although ultrasound also became widely used in ophthalmology, cardiology and in the investigation of many abdominal organs. Donald's team, in a series of publications, described the use of ultrasound in the differential diagnosis of pelvic masses (Donald *et al.* 1958), the diagnosis of hydatidiform mole (Donald and Brown 1961) and the detection of blighted ova, twin pregnancies, and placenta praevia (Donald and Abdulla 1967). During the early days, development was further encouraged by the observation that there had been an increased incidence of childhood malignancy after fetal exposure to X-rays (Stewart *et al.* 1956; 1958). An undoubted advantage of ultrasonography has been that irradiation of the fetus is seldom performed today. Because of its soft-tissue imaging capabilities and its usefulness in performing accurate measurements, the applications of ultrasound in pregnancy rapidly outstripped those of X-rays.

Technique has evolved from the simple linear display of echoes reflected back to the equipment from tissue interfaces (A-mode) through a two-dimensional static image (B-mode) to the real-time systems with two-dimensional 'moving' images, which are particularly useful for the study of a continuously moving fetus. The improvement in resolution and quality of imaging of ultrasound equipment has been so rapid that progress from the first detection of the gross abnormality of anencephaly (Campbell *et al.* 1972) to current sophisticated diagnoses of many relatively subtle fetal anomalies (Campbell and Pearce 1983) has taken only a few years. This rapid evolution has two consequences. First, unless evaluation is done promptly and on a large scale it is rendered irrelevant by advances in technology. Second, the results obtained by a group of enthusiasts on any particular aspect of diagnosis, may not be applicable to all ultrasonographers.

As ultrasound scanning became more widely used, it came to be used as a screening technique (Grennert *et al.* 1978). Whether or not routine ultrasonography is warranted has been a source of recent controversy. A consensus panel of the National Institutes of Health (1984) in the United States concluded that the available evidence did not justify routine use. In a report published during the same year in Britain, a working party of the Royal College of Obstetricians and Gynaecologists (1984) reached the opposite conclusion from the same evidence.

There is a clear difference between selective and routine use of ultrasound. The time taken, the detail inspected and perhaps the status of the investigator will vary with the reason for the examination. To identify fetal presentation, for example, takes seconds and can be carried out by a minimally trained technician. To investigate thoroughly the cause of raised alphafetoprotein levels may necessitate considerable time and expertise. Routine examinations must be accomplished quickly for practical reasons, and some fetal malformations are therefore less likely to be detected than they would be if there are specific reasons to anticipate their presence. The selective examination should be tailored to answer a specific question posed by the person who requests the examination.

In this chapter we will discuss within broad categories, first, the extent to which ultrasound examination can answer specific questions and, second, the evidence as to whether such information has an impact on management and outcome. In addition to diagnostic ultrasonography, we shall also consider the use of Doppler ultrasound in the study of uteroplacental and fetoplacental blood flow, an area of great current interest. The chapter concludes with discussions of women's views of ultrasonography in pregnancy, and of studies that are relevant in assessing its safety.

2 Specific indications for ultrasound

2.1 Confirmation of fetal life

Ultrasound has the ability not only to establish rapidly and accurately whether or not a fetus is alive or dead, but also to predict whether a pregnancy is likely to continue after threatened miscarriage (Stabile *et al.* 1987). Ultrasonography has thus rationalized the management of threatened abortion in early pregnancy. Using Donald's full bladder technique, the uterus may be studied while it remains entirely within the maternal pelvis. The gestational sac can be visualized by 6 weeks menstrual age and the fetus by 7 weeks. As soon as the fetus can be demonstrated with ultrasound, it can be measured (Robinson 1973) and its viability confirmed by detection of heart movement (Robinson 1972). Fetal life is confirmed by observation of heart pulsation, and death by its absence. Apart from very early pregnancy, there should not be any doubt about the diagnosis (Levine and Filly 1977).

Assessing fetal viability is a major indication for ultrasound examination during the first trimester. In most pregnancies that miscarry spontaneously before the 14th week, development of the fetus has been arrested at an early stage, frequently in association with chromosomal abnormality. There is usually an interval of weeks between developmental arrest and miscarriage, during which time the experienced ultrasonographer can predict outcome with such certainty that the uterus may be confidently evacuated when the pregnancy is demonstrably nonviable (Robinson 1975).

Blighted ova, which constitute the largest group of early pregnancy failures, are diagnosed by the failure to detect a fetus on careful examination although, when small, the anembryonic pregnancy has to be differentiated by a repeat ultrasound examination from the normal, very early pregnancy. Missed abortion should, in contrast, always be diagnosable on a single scan by absence of heart movement. The small group of 'live' miscarriages cannot be predicted with certainty by ultrasound. These constitute 14 per cent of the total number of abortions (Robinson 1975) and there are no specific ultrasound features, although a reduction in amniotic fluid volume (Robinson 1975), diminished fetal activity, or the presence of large intrauterine haematomas (Mantoni and Pederson 1981) suggest a poor prognosis.

The characteristic ultrasound features of hydatidiform mole have long been recognized, although a similar picture may be seen in long-standing missed abortion with hydropic trophoblastic changes and in degenerating fibroids. In patients with suspected ectopic pregnancy, the main contribution of ultrasound is in detecting, or excluding, intrauterine pregnancy. While demonstration of an adnexal mass or fluid in the pouch of Douglas may contribute to the diagnosis and, on occasion, an intact pregnancy may be identified outside the uterus, ultrasound is associated with significant false positive and false negative rates in diagnosing ectopic pregnancy. Weckstein and colleagues (1985) found that only 50 per cent of ectopic pregnancies were associated with ultrasound demonstration of peritoneal fluid and 38 per cent with an adnexal mass. Interpretation of the ultrasound findings together with assay of human chorionic gonadotrophin improves diagnostic accuracy (Kadar *et al.* 1981; Weckstein *et al.* 1985).

2.2 Assessment of gestational age

The use of ultrasound to assess duration of gestation is based on the assumption that, in early pregnancy, fetal growth is rapid, that there is little biological variation in size, and that pathological growth retardation is uncommon. Gestational age can then be estimated from measurements of the fetal size. During the first trimester, measurement of the fetal crown–rump length (Robinson 1973) is reported as being accurate to within 5 days in 95 per cent of cases in estimating gestational age (Robinson and Fleming 1975). After 13 weeks, varying flexion of the fetal trunk makes this measurement less reliable, but measurement of the biparietal diameter before 18 weeks predicts the date of delivery to within 2 weeks in 89 per cent of pregnancies (Campbell 1976). Measurement of femoral length appears to be of similar accuracy to measurement of the biparietal diameter (O'Brien *et al.* 1981). Measurement of the fetus is of no value whatsoever in assessing gestational age after 30 weeks.

Estimation of gestational age is one of the areas of obstetric ultrasonography in which it has been difficult to identify a suitable 'gold standard' against which to test the validity of the technique. Previously, data have been compared with assessment of gestational age based on an 'ideal' menstrual history, alternative ultrasound techniques, or the onset of labour. None of these approaches is ideal and there remained scope for study of pregnancies in which the date of ovulation was accurately known. This has now been done (MacGregor *et al.* 1987) and has shown estimates derived using ultrasonography to be within 9 per cent of the known duration of gestation. This compares favourably with alternative means of assessment, including clinical examinations (Beazley and Underhill 1970); the date of quickening (Grennert *et al.* 1978), or radiological evaluation in late pregnancy (Robinson *et al.* 1979). The date of delivery can be reliably predicted from the menstrual history in only between 75 per cent (Grennert *et al.* 1978) and 85 per cent of pregnancies (Kloosterman 1979). Since it is not possible to identify all the women in whom an accurate knowledge of gestational age may become essential later in pregnancy, there exists a case for routine early ultrasonography and this will be discussed later. When selective ultrasonography is preferred, it would seem sensible to scan women in whom elective delivery is likely to be indicated, those with 'high risk' pregnancies, or with uncertain dates.

2.3 Fetal malformation

Ultrasound may be employed in three ways to assist the identification of fetal malformations: to visualize the malformation; to facilitate other diagnostic techniques, such as amniocentesis and chorion villus sampling; and to allow fetal measurement.

A large number of abnormalities can now be detected by modern ultrasound imaging; these have been well-reviewed elsewhere (Campbell and Pearce 1983; Warsof and Griffin 1984; Neilson and McNay 1988; see Chapter 23), and will not be considered in detail here. Some defects, such as anencephaly, are easily identified; some, such as spina bifida, are moderately difficult to detect; and some, such as certain cardiac anomalies, may be very difficult to identify. The presence of one defect may suggest the presence of others and/or of chromosomal abnormality (Platt *et al.* 1986). Detection rates may vary with the quality of the equipment and expertise of the ultrasonographer and with whether the examination has been performed because of high risk features (such as a previously malformed baby or raised alphafetoprotein levels) or is part of a screening examination, when less time (and possibly expertise) would be available.

The role of ultrasound to facilitate the performance of amniocentesis has been considered in detail by Ager and Oliver (1986) who have reviewed 28 studies of second trimester amniocentesis published between 1977 and 1985. No correlation could be found between fetal loss rate and the use of ultrasound (see chapter by Daker and Bobrow), although a clear trend over time towards universal use of ultrasonography was evident. The use of ultrasound during amniocentesis certainly seems logical to minimize the chances of placental and/or fetal contact during the insertion of the needle into the amniotic cavity. In addition, the presence of multiple pregnancies may be identified, fetal life confirmed and gestational age estimated. Both the pregnant woman and the operator may be reassured by seeing that the fetus appears unaffected by the procedure. A recent study of over 7200 genetic amniocenteses performed under ultrasound guidance revealed a twofold increase in subsequent miscarriage if the placenta was perforated or if a blood stained sample was obtained (Kappel *et al.* 1987). Romero and colleagues (1985) describe fewer blood-stained samples if the insertion of the needle is continuously monitored with ultrasound, although this conclusion is based on comparison with a historical control group.

The use of ultrasound improves the chances of successful transcervical sampling of chorionic villi for diagnostic purposes during the first trimester (Brambati and Oldrini 1986). Transabdominal chorionic villus sampling and fetal umbilical cord blood sampling (Daffos *et al.* 1985) require the simultaneous use of ultrasound.

Possible applications of information derived from ultrasound diagnosis of fetal malformations include termination of pregnancy; appropriate timing and mode of delivery; delivery in close proximity to a neonatal surgical unit; fetal therapy; and psychological preparation of the parents.

Termination of pregnancy will obviously be acceptable to many couples when the fetus has a lethal abnormality such as anencephaly, or a defect likely to result in major handicap such as spina bifida with hydrocephalus (see Chapter 66). Difficulties can arise when defects have less predictable sequelae and also because diagnostic errors may occur. Prior consultation with surgical colleagues should give more accurate prognoses and help to reduce unnecessary elective early delivery (and the consequent morbidity resulting from iatrogenic immaturity) of babies with conditions that will not benefit from early surgery (Murphy *et al.* 1984; Brereton 1984; Hutson *et al.* 1985; Griffiths and Gough 1985).

Decisions about optimal timing, method, and place of delivery are bedevilled by a lack of satisfactorily controlled data. To arrange for delivery to occur close by a specialist neonatal surgical unit could be advantageous under certain circumstances. It is clearly undesirable to use caesarean section to deliver a baby with a lethal malformation; so that the ultrasound diagnosis of, for example, a baby with renal agenesis may be of great value. In some conditions, early delivery may be beneficial to allow treatment to avoid progressive deterioration in function of an organ system. The place of fetal therapy, for example to drain an obstructed urinary tract or hydrocephalus, remains controversial (Harrison 1983).

An undoubted advantage of ultrasound is the demonstration to women who have previously had a malformed baby, that their current fetus does not share the defect. Diagnosis of a malformation may also help parents to prepare for the birth of an impaired child. However, the impact on parents of a diagnosis of fetal malformation, rather than help psychological preparation for the birth, may sometimes be to cause prolonged and devastating upset (Hutson *et al.* 1985; *Lancet* 1985). When the malformation is real and important, this anguish may be an inevitable consequence of conveying important information to those who will be most closely affected by it. But as Furness (1987) has noted, rapid technological advance has meant that each machine update reveals features of the fetus never recognized before, necessitating a reappraisal of the range of normal at each stage of pregnancy, and adding to an already extensive repertoire of artefacts and red herrings. She suggests that these dilemmas present a strong case for being highly selective, at least temporarily, when giving information to the parents.

2.4 Assessment of fetal growth

Discussion of the role of ultrasound measurements in assessment of fetal growth necessitates consideration of the complexities of establishing suitable endpoints for study (see Chapter 26).

Ultrasound techniques have, by and large, been designed to assess either fetal *size* at a point in time or fetal *growth* over a period of time. In both cases, the validity of the technique has usually been evaluated by its ability to predict babies which are of low weight-for-gestation ('light-for-dates') at birth. Much useful information on the nature and detection of fetal growth retardation instead of weight for gestation has been lost by this method (see Chapter 26).

Campbell and Dewhurst (1971) showed that up to 73 per cent (sensitivity) of 'light-for-dates' fetuses would be identified by repeated measurement of the biparietal diameter, with a specificity of 88 per cent. For many years this parameter was the standard for ultrasound assessment of fetal growth. Accurate measurement of the biparietal diameter may be difficult and sometimes impossible, especially during late pregnancy, when the fetal head is in a direct occipito-anterior or occipito-posterior position, or is low in the pelvis. It is also a relatively insensitive technique because of so-called 'brain-sparing'. If the organ weights of 'light-for-dates' infants are compared with those of controls of either similar birth weight or similar gestational age, it is found that the organs most diminished in weight are the thymus, spleen, and liver (Gruenwald 1974). In contrast, brain weight is relatively much less reduced. Thus, in performing cephalometry, the ultrasonographer was measuring an index of the size of the fetal organ least affected by growth retardation.

The fetal thymus and spleen are not readily measured, but the liver can be identified. Rather than attempting the time-consuming measurement of its volume, most workers have measured the cross-sectional dimensions of the fetal abdomen or trunk (henceforth described as trunk) at the level of the liver. Techniques vary, but measurements are generally effected on a cross-sectional image of the fetal trunk at right angles to the long axis of the fetal aorta and including the umbilical vein, which is used as a marker for the correct section (Campbell and Wilkin 1975; Hansmann 1978. In the correct plane, a short segment of the umbilical vein is usually visualized, although a longer segment may be seen in a hyperflexed fetus (e.g. small-for-dates or twin fetus or one lying transversely). Linear trunk measurements can be made, but trunk circumference and/or area measurements are preferable.

Neilson *et al.* (1980) studied 474 patients at between 34 and 36 weeks gestation and compared the effectiveness of several different fetal measurements, singly and in combination, in predicting babies that were 'light-for-dates' at birth (Table 27.1). Trunk measurements

Table 27.1 Sensitivity and specificity of various ultrasonographically derived fetal measurements, single and in combination, for predicting the birth of babies that were 'light-for-dates'

Measurement	Sensitivity (%)	Specificity (%)
Biparietal diameter	58	90
Head area	59	90
Head circumference	56	92
Trunk area	81	89
Trunk circumference	83	90
Transverse trunk diameter	61	88
Crown–rump length	69	88
Crown–rump length × trunk area	94	88
Head area/trunk area	44	91

were better predictors than head measurements, and these have been generally adopted as the best single parameter although there remains little published information on their serial use to assess growth rather than to assess size on a single measurement . Measurement of total intrauterine volume was prompted by the fact that 'light-for-dates' fetuses tend also to have small placentae and less amniotic fluid (Gohari *et al.* 1977), and this was widely used in the USA. When measured accurately using a complex and time-consuming planimetric system (Geirsson *et al.* 1984) total intrauterine volume predicts 'light-for-dates' fetuses with similar sensitivity and specificity to the much simpler trunk area (Geirsson *et al.* 1985). There is interest in alternative measurements, including femoral length and thigh circumference, but there are indications that femoral length measurements will not prove to be especially useful (Gennser and Persson 1986).

As discussed elsewhere, (see Chapter 26) 'light-for-dates' fetuses form a heterogeneous group within which individual fetal risk varies greatly. Attempts have therefore been made to analyse patterns of growth in the hope of shedding light on the underlying pathogenesis and of providing an estimate of the risk to the individual fetus. The first attempt to do this was by dividing 'light-for-dates' fetuses into two groups (Garrett and Robinson 1971; Campbell 1974): the first showing arrest of previously normal biparietal diameter growth (Campbell's 'late-flattening' pattern); the second showing early departure from normal limits of biparietal diameter growth that continues until delivery (the 'low-growth profile' pattern). Campbell (1974) attributed the first of these patterns to 'uteroplacental insufficiency', and the latter to low growth potential. This group includes infants that are abnormal (especially chromosomally abnormal), some that have suffered a major insult (e.g. by rubella) during the critical period of organogenesis, and some that are small because of their genetic endowment. Comparative measurements of the fetal head and trunk (Campbell and Thoms 1977; Hansmann 1978) have been suggested as a means to further differentiate these two groups. While there was a higher incidence of intrapartum fetal distress and operative delivery in the asymmetrical growth group, the perinatal mortality and incidence of low Apgar scores were similar and high in both groups (Campbell and Thoms 1977).

The significance of ultrasonically detected patterns of fetal growth requires further study (Deter *et al.* 1986) and seeking correlations with the results of Doppler studies (see later) would be of interest. Thus far, the available evidence indicates that trunk measurements are superior to head measurements in predicting 'light-for-dates' babies, but little is known about serial measurements and particularly their relationship to intrauterine growth patterns. We are not aware of any controlled study to evaluate the effect of ultrasonography on the outcome of pregnancies at high risk of fetal growth retardation. The controlled studies that have been performed have evaluated ultrasound measurements as screening techniques and will be discussed later.

2.5 Examination of the placenta

Ultrasound is the best available method for locating placental position. This is of particular importance prior to chorion villus sampling and amniocentesis, and in cases of antepartum haemorrhage, fetal malpresentation, or other clinical situations that suggest the possibility of placenta praevia. The placenta is easily visualized with ultrasound, although the woman needs to have a full bladder if the lower pole of the uterus is to be satisfactorily visualized. The lower margins of posteriorly sited placentae are more difficult to identify than those of anterior placentae, both because of acoustic shadowing from the fetus and because of a less clearly defined anatomical reference point. The exact margins of the lower uterine segment cannot be identified ultrasonically and therefore ultrasound cannot achieve 100 per cent accuracy in identifying or excluding placenta praevia.

The phenomenon of placental 'migration', first described by King (1973), is now well-recognized: a placenta that appears low earlier in pregnancy may, with formation of the lower uterine segment, appear to have risen on repeat ultrasound examination and thus no longer seem praevia. Thus Rizos and colleagues (1979) found, in a study of over 1000 women undergoing genetic amniocentesis during midpregnancy, that 5 per cent had ultrasound evidence of a low placenta at 16 to 18 weeks, but in only 10 per cent of this 5 per cent (that is, 0.5 per cent overall) was the placenta actually praevia at delivery. Comeau *et al.* (1983), in a retrospective study, found that only 5.6 per cent of women in whom the placenta appeared to cover the cervix at ultrasound examination during the second trimester, had placenta praevia at the time of delivery. Thus only a small proportion of patients with a low-lying placenta in mid-pregnancy will have placenta praevia at delivery.

The ultrasound appearances in placental abruption are usually undramatic, the fresh retroplacental haematoma having acoustic features similar to those of placental tissue. Examination is of limited value in clinical care, although it may be useful in follow-up of consolidation of small abruptions that have been visualized.

'Texture' of the placenta on ultrasound examination has been graded and correlated with fetal pulmonary maturation as assessed by the lecithin: sphingomyelin ratio in the amniotic fluid (Grannum *et al.* 1979). This has not been confirmed in subsequent studies. Advanced grades may appear at earlier gestational ages in pregnancies complicated by hypertensive disease or intrauterine growth retardation (Proud and Grant 1987).

2.6 Miscellaneous indications

The National Institutes of Health report (1984), while not recommending routine (screening) ultrasonography, did compile an extensive list of clinical situations in which ultrasound examination was considered useful although not necessarily mandatory. We have previously condensed and categorized the list (Neilson 1986) and will consider here those applications not discussed elsewhere in the chapter.

(1) *Investigation of raised maternal serum alpha-fetoprotein.* Raised maternal serum alpha-fetoprotein may indicate multiple pregnancy, miscalculated gestational age, intrauterine death, and various fetal anomalies, especially open neural tube and anterior abdominal wall defects. These conditions may be identified by ultrasound examination.

(2) *Suspected multiple pregnancy.* This is an important indication for ultrasound examination. Multiple pregnancy is discussed further under 'routine ultrasonography'.

(3) *Assessment of amniotic fluid volume.* Polyhydramnios or oligohydramnios may be associated with lethal fetal abnormalities (such as anencephaly and renal agenesis) as well as non-lethal malformations. These may be diagnosed with ultrasound and the information may influence subsequent management. A semi-quantitative assessment of amniotic fluid volume is part of the biophysical profile (see Chapter 30) and provides some prognostic information (Chamberlain *et al.* 1984).

(4) *Estimated fetal weight in preterm labour.* Fetal weight estimation may be of value in deciding appropriate management, although this estimation is imprecise. Gestational age, however, appears to be a better predictor of outcome than is birthweight (Verloove-Vanhorick *et al.* 1985), at least in babies under 32 weeks of gestation and in those who weigh less than 1500 g at birth.

(5) *Fetal presentation.* When fetal presentation is in doubt, ultrasound will readily resolve that doubt. This may be of particular value in determining the position of the second twin during labour.

(6) *Pelvic mass.* An ovarian cyst may be readily distinguished from a fibroid by ultrasound examination.

(7) *Adjunct to external cephalic version.* There is no evidence that ultrasonography improves the chances of successful external cephalic version (see Chapter 31) but ultrasound examination may assist detection of predisposing factors for malpresentation such as fetal abnormality, placenta praevia, and uterine anomalies.

(8) *Adjunct to cervical cerclage.* The value of ultrasound in conjunction with cervical cerclage is doubtful (see Chapter 40).

(9) *Suspected uterine abnormalities.* During pregnancy uterine abnormalities are very difficult to diagnose accurately with ultrasound. Assessment of the uterine cavity in the early puerperium may be more useful for this purpose.

(10) *Location of intrauterine contraceptive device.* The identification of an intrauterine device, even when it cannot be removed, is useful as this will alert attendants to seek it at the time of delivery.

(11) *Gestational age assessment in late attenders.* Gestational age cannot be estimated with acceptable accuracy by ultrasound in late pregnancy.

3 Routine ultrasonography

The greatest controversy surrounding obstetric ultrasound has been whether there are benefits outweighing the costs of extending its use from specific indications to either early (usually 16–19 weeks, but sometimes earlier) or late (usually 32–36 weeks) routine screening of all pregnant women. Most claims of benefit for routine scanning are based on the assumption that clinical action taken on the results of the examination improve clinical outcome. These assumptions can only be tested adequately by randomized controlled trials, but few of these have been conducted. The six trials that have been conducted are of varying design and quality, have assessed a variety of scanning regimens, and not all have used the same measures of outcome. Nevertheless, they provide the best evidence that is currently available. The main features of the trials are summarized in Table 27.2. Two non-randomized cohort studies of contrasting policies of routine ultrasonography, one comparing two obstetric specialists (Cochlin 1984) and the other two health insurance schemes (Hughey 1984) had broadly similar results to the randomized trials and will not be considered further here.

3.1 Routine early ultrasonography

It has been proposed that early scans performed at 16–20 weeks gestation may improve pregnancy outcome through clinical action prompted by earlier identification of multiple pregnancies or congenital malformations, or because of more accurate estimation of gestational age. If the screening examination is performed even earlier in pregnancy, some clinically unsuspected non-viable pregnancies (e.g. blighted ova and hydatidiform moles), may be detected. However, a satisfactory inspection of fetal anatomy to detect malformation cannot be performed before 16 weeks and if inspection of the heart is to be included, as has recently been suggested (Allan *et al.* 1986), examination closer

Table 27.2 Controlled trials of routine ultrasonography in pregnancy

	Screening regimen	Control regimen
1 IN EARLY PREGNANCY		
1.1 Bennett *et al.* (1982)		
Numbers studied	836	735
Nature of regimen	At 16 wks, BPD made available for care	At 16 wks, BPD withheld
Application	Not known	Withheld throughout pregnancy for only 20% of sample
2 IN EARLY AND LATE PREGNANCY		
2.1 Bakketeig *et al.* (1984)		
Numbers studied	510	499
Nature of regimen	At 19 and 32 wks, BPD, abdominal diameter, placental location	Scanned only on clinical indication
Application	89% of sample had early scan	90% had no scan during pregnancy
2.2 Eik-Nes *et al.* (1984)		
Numbers studied	809	819
Nature of regimen	At 18 and 32 wks, BPD, abdominal diameter, placental location, structural abnormalities	Scanned only on clinical indication
Application	Not known	86% had no scan during pregnancy
3 IN LATE PREGNANCY		
3.1 Neilson *et al.* (1984)		
Numbers studied	433	444
Nature of regimen	At 34–36 wks (after routine early scan), crown–rump length × trunk area made available for care	Information withheld
Application	As planned	As planned
3.2 Secher *et al.* (1986)		
Number studied	96	88
Nature of regimen	At 32 and 37 wks (after routine early scan), if estimated fetal weight $<85\%$ of espected mean and no clinical suspicion of growth retardation, clinician notified	Information withheld
Application	As planned	Information withheld in only 68%
3.3 Proud and Grant (1987)		
Number studied	1000	1000
Nature of regimen	At 30–32 and 34–36 wks, placental grading made available for care	Information withheld
Application	As planned	As planned

to 20 weeks may be necessary. Some or all of these diagnoses may prompt clinical actions that improve fetal and maternal outcome. Indices of maternal morbidity, such as the frequency of antenatal hospitalization and inductions of labour, or indices of fetal outcome, such as perinatal death, low Apgar score, and admission to a special care nursery, might be affected by clinical actions based on more than one aspect of these examinations.

An early scan was evaluated as a component of the routine scanning regimen in 3 of the 6 trials of routine ultrasonography in pregnancy (in 2 of these, a routine late scan was also part of the experimental regimen). The main effects on fetal diagnosis and obstetric management are shown in Table 27.3. The information provided in an early scan led to a reduction in the prevalence of undiagnosed twins at 26 weeks' gestation and undiagnosed major fetal anomalies, but the differences were not statistically significant. Routine early scanning was, however, associated with a statistically significant reduction in the use of induction for so-called 'post-term' pregnancy. Furthermore, it is worth noting that in the trial by Eik-Nes *et al.*(1984), four of the control group infants who had been delivered

Table 27.3 Effect of routine ultrasonography in early pregnancy on twins undiagnosed at 26 weeks

Study	EXPT		CTRL		Odds ratio	Graph of odds ratios and confidence intervals
	n	(%)	*n*	(%)	(95% CI)	0.01 0.1 0.5 1 2 10 100
Bakketeig *et al.* (1984)	1/6	(16.67)	1/4	(25.00)	0.63 (0.03–12.58)	
Bennett *et al.* (1982)	0/6	(0.00)	2/5	(40.00)	0.09 (0.00–1.63)	
Typical odds ratio (95% confidence interval)					0.23 (0.03–1.86)	

Effect of routine ultrasonography in early pregnancy on major fetal anomalies remaining undiagnosed

Study	EXPT		CTRL		Odds ratio	Graph
Eik-Nes *et al.* (1984)	1/3	(33.33)	2/2	(100.0)	0.11 (0.00–2.84)	
Typical odds ratio (95% confidence interval)					0.11 (0.00–2.84)	

Effect of routine ultrasonography in early pregnancy on induction for 'post-term' pregnancy

Study	EXPT		CTRL		Odds ratio	Graph
Bakketeig *et al.* (1984)	14/510	(2.75)	19/499	(3.81)	0.71 (0.36–1.43)	
Eik-Nes *et al.* (1984)	15/809	(1.85)	64/819	(7.81)	0.28 (0.18–0.43)	
Typical odds ratio (95% confidence interval)					0.37 (0.25–0.53)	

following induction for 'post-term' pregnancy were judged to be preterm by paediatricians, and also, that infants in the routinely scanned group spent fewer days in special care nursery because of hyperbilirubinaemia.

It is difficult to come to any firm conclusions about whether the overall effects of routine ultrasonography in early pregnancy on fetal diagnosis and obstetric care were reflected in improved outcomes overall, because the few differences that emerged could easily be simply a reflection of the play of chance (Table 27.4). The incidence of low Apgar scores was actually higher in the routinely scanned groups in all three trials, and when the trials are considered together, the confidence interval of the odds ratio only just includes unity. There were no detectable effects on the rate of admission to special care nurseries. There were too few perinatal deaths to permit a useful estimate of any effect routine scanning in early pregnancy may have on the risk of perinatal mortality.

3.2 Routine late ultrasonography

3.2.1 For fetal anthropometry

The main purpose of routine scanning in late pregnancy is to identify growth-retarded fetuses who may benefit from elective delivery. A variety of anthropometric indices have been used to make a diagnosis of fetal growth retardation and those used in the controlled trials included comparisons of biparietal diameter with values derived from examinations made in early pregnancy; the relationship between head size and abdominal diameter; the product of crown–rump length and trunk area; and an estimate of fetal weight less than 85 per cent of the expected mean fetal weight.

A routine late scan for fetal anthropometry was a component of the routine scanning regimen in 4 of the 6 trials of routine ultrasonography in pregnancy (in 2 of these, a routine early scan was also part of the experimental regimen). The main effects on obstetric management are shown in Table 27.4. There was no consistent pattern of effect on the chances of a woman being admitted to hospital during pregnancy or on the use of elective delivery for indications other than 'post-term' pregnancy. The data presented in Table 27.5 show that there were no detectable effects of routine scanning in late pregnancy for fetal anthropometry on the risks of low Apgar score, admission to the special care nursery or perinatal mortality.

3.2.2 For placentography

The results of the only trial to assess the value of routine ultrasonography in late pregnancy to obtain information about placental grading are presented in Table 27.6. Although provision of information about placental grading did not affect the rate of hospital admission during pregnancy, it did prompt an increased use of both antenatal cardiotocography and

Table 27.4 Effect of routine ultrasonography in early pregnancy on low Apgar score

Study	EXPT *n*	EXPT (%)	CTRL *n*	CTRL (%)	Odds ratio (95% CI)	Graph of odds ratios and confidence intervals (0.01 0.1 0.5 1 2 10 100)
Bakketeig *et al.* (1984)	34/510	(6.67)	23/499	(4.61)	1.47 (0.86–2.51)	
Eik-Nes *et al.* (1984)	41/809	(5.07)	35/819	(4.27)	1.20 (0.75–1.89)	
Bennett *et al.* (1982)	172/836	(20.57)	142/785	(18.09)	1.17 (0.92–1.50)	
Typical odds ratio (95% confidence interval)					1.22 (0.99–1.49)	

Effect of routine ultrasonography in early pregnancy on admission to special care nursery

Study	EXPT *n*	EXPT (%)	CTRL *n*	CTRL (%)	Odds ratio (95% CI)	Graph of odds ratios and confidence intervals
Bakketeig *et al.* (1984)	21/510	(4.12)	25/499	(5.01)	0.81 (0.45–1.47)	
Eik-Nes *et al.* (1984)	68/809	(8.41)	66/819	(8.06)	1.05 (0.74–1.49)	
Typical odds ratio (95% confidence interval)					0.98 (0.72–1.33)	

Effect of routine ultrasonography in early pregnancy on perinatal death

Study	EXPT *n*	EXPT (%)	CTRL *n*	CTRL (%)	Odds ratio (95% CI)	Graph of odds ratios and confidence intervals
Bakketeig *et al.* (1984)	5/510	(0.98)	5/499	(1.00)	0.98 (0.28–3.40)	
Eik-Nes *et al.* (1984)	3/809	(0.37)	8/819	(0.98)	0.41 (0.12–1.33)	
Bennett *et al.* (1982)	8/836	(0.96)	7/785	(0.89)	1.07 (0.39–2.97)	
Typical odds ratio (95% confidence interval)					0.78 (0.40–1.50)	

Table 27.5 Effect of routine fetal anthropometry in late pregnancy on antenatal hospital admission

Study	EXPT *n*	EXPT (%)	CTRL *n*	CTRL (%)	Odds ratio (95% CI)	Graph of odds ratios and confidence intervals (0.01 0.1 0.5 1 2 10 100)
Bakketeig *et al.* (1984)	104/510	(20.39)	58/499	(11.62)	1.92 (1.37–2.68)	
Eik-Nes *et al.* (1984)	184/809	(22.74)	269/819	(32.84)	0.60 (0.49–0.75)	
Neilson *et al.* (1984)	43/433	(9.93)	46/444	(10.36)	0.95 (0.62–1.48)	
Typical odds ratio (95% confidence interval)					0.86 (0.73–1.02)	

Effect of routine fetal anthropometry in late pregnancy on labour induction (overall/not post-term)

Study	EXPT *n*	EXPT (%)	CTRL *n*	CTRL (%)	Odds ratio (95% CI)	Graph of odds ratios and confidence intervals
Bakketeig *et al.* (1984)	18/510	(3.53)	19/499	(3.81)	0.92 (0.48–1.78)	
Neilson *et al.* (1984)	129/433	(29.79)	129/444	(29.05)	1.04 (0.78–1.39)	
Secher *et al.* (1986)	39/96	(40.63)	13/88	(14.77)	3.55 (1.87–6.75)	
Typical odds ratio (95% confidence interval)					1.22 (0.96–1.56)	

Table 27.5 Effect of routine fetal anthropometry in late pregnancy on low Apgar score

Study	EXPT		CTRL		Odds ratio	Graph of odds ratios and confidence intervals
	n	(%)	*n*	(%)	(95% CI)	0.01 0.1 0.5 1 2 10 100
Bakketeig *et al.* (1984)	34/510	(6.67)	23/499	(4.61)	1.47 (0.86–2.51)	
Eik-Nes *et al.* (1984)	41/809	(5.07)	35/819	(4.27)	1.20 (0.75–1.89)	
Neilson *et al.* (1984)	37/433	(8.55)	40/444	(9.01)	0.94 (0.59–1.51)	
Secher *et al.* (1986)	8/96	(8.33)	10/88	(11.36)	0.71 (0.27–1.88)	
Typical odds ratio (95% confidence interval)					1.12 (0.86–1.46)	

Effect of routine fetal anthropometry in late pregnancy on admission to special care nursery

Study	EXPT *n*	(%)	CTRL *n*	(%)	Odds ratio (95% CI)	Graph
Bakketeig *et al.* (1984)	21/510	(4.12)	25/499	(5.01)	0.81 (0.45–1.47)	
Eik-Nes *et al.* (1984)	68/809	(8.41)	66/819	(8.06)	1.05 (0.74–1.49)	
Secher *et al.* (1986)	8/96	(8.33)	8/88	(9.09)	0.91 (0.33–2.53)	
Typical odds ratio (95% confidence interval)					0.97 (0.73–1.30)	

Effect of routine fetal anthropometry in late pregnancy on perinatal death excl. lethal malformation

Study	EXPT *n*	(%)	CTRL *n*	(%)	Odds ratio (95% CI)	Graph
Bakketeig *et al.* (1984)	5/510	(0.98)	5/499	(1.00)	0.98 (0.28–3.40)	
Eik-Nes *et al.* (1984)	3/809	(0.37)	7/819	(0.85)	0.45 (0.13–1.57)	
Neilson *et al.* (1984)	0/433	(0.00)	0/444	(0.00)	1.00 (1.00–1.00)	
Secher *et al.* (1986)	0/96	(0.00)	0/88	(0.00)	1.00 (1.00–1.00)	
Typical odds ratio (95% confidence interval)					0.67 (0.28–1.60)	

urinary oetrogen estimation for further investigation of fetuses with abnormal placentography. The rate of elective delivery because of a diagnosis of fetal compromise was higher in the group in which information about placentography had been supplied to the clinicians. Although there was no difference in the rate of low Apgar scores in the two groups at 1 minute after birth, babies whose care had included the provision of information on placental grading were less likely to pass meconium during labour; to have low Apgar scores 5 minutes after birth; to be admitted to the special care nursery; and to have neonatal seizures or die from causes other than lethal malformations.

4 Doppler studies

Doppler ultrasound has been used for a number of years to identify and record fetal heart pulsation and, in adults, to assess blood flow in compromised vessels (*Lancet* 1986). In 1977, Fitzgerald and Drumm described the use of the technique to demonstrate blood velocity waveforms in the fetal umbilical artery, and Stuart and colleagues (1980) described the changes that occur in these as pregnancy advances. Since these reports, various other fetal vessels have been studied including umbilical vein and artery, fetal aorta and internal carotid artery, as well as branches of the maternal uterine artery. The optimal method of waveform analysis remains uncertain, as does the clinical significance of abnormal patterns. Most workers now concentrate on methods of wave form analysis that are independent of angle of insonation, vessel diameter, and fetal size. The most popular are the A/B ratio (Stuart *et al.* 1980) and the Pulsatility Index (Gosling and King 1975).

Currently, the most popular object of study is the umbilical artery, which has a characteristic waveform that is readily obtained with simple continuous wave equipment. Early experience suggests that alterations in fetal umbilical blood flow may occur as an early event in conditions of fetal compromise. In theory, Doppler studies could provide important information on the pathophysiology of compromised pregnancies (and especially of fetal growth retardation), and possibly provide a useful technique for evaluating fetal well-being in high risk pregnancies (Griffin *et al.* 1983; Neilson and Whittle 1988).

Trudinger and colleagues (1985), employing a broad definition of adverse outcome (neonatal death, or 5-minute Apgar score less than 7, or birthweight less than the 10th percentile) in a study of 172 high risk pregnancies, found that umbilical artery A/B ratios predicted adverse outcome with a sensitivity of 62 per cent and specificity of 79 per cent. Equivalent figures for maternal uterine artery studies were 38 per cent and 84 per cent. Comparison with alternative methods of biophysical assessment of fetal well-being requires further study but it has been suggested that flow changes precede abnormal cardiotocographic findings (Trudinger *et al.* 1986).

Although other published studies have concentrated on predicting infants who will be light-for-dates at birth, this would not seem to be an important goal as this prediction could be achieved with the use of conventional ultrasound techniques. It would seem that the main contribution, if any, of Doppler studies should be to elucidate the pathogenic mechanism of intrauterine growth retardation and to predict adverse outcomes early enough to allow useful intervention.

Thus far only one controlled trial on the utility of Doppler ultrasound has been reported (Trudinger *et al.* 1987). Doppler ultrasound study of the fetal umbilical artery was performed in 300 patients admitted to hospital for various antepartum complications. Women were allocated either to an experimental group (for which A/B ratios were reported to clinicians) or to a control group (for which this information was withheld),

Table 27.7 Effect of routine ultrasound placentography in late pregnancy on antenatal hospital admission

Study	EXPT		CTRL		Odds ratio	Graph of odds ratios and confidence intervals
	n	(%)	*n*	(%)	(95% CI)	0.01 0.1 0.5 1 2 10 100
Proud and Grant. (1987)	312/1000	(31.20)	304/1000	(30.40)	1.04 (0.86–1.26)	
Typical odds ratio (95% confidence interval)					1.04 (0.86–1.26)	

Effect of routine ultrasound placentography in late pregnancy on antenatal cardiotocography

Study	EXPT n	(%)	CTRL n	(%)	Odds ratio (95% CI)	Graph
Proud and Grant. (1987)	813/1000	(81.30)	800/1000	(80.00)	1.09 (0.87–1.36)	
Typical odds ratio (95% confidence interval)					1.09 (0.87–1.36)	

Effect of routine ultrasound placentography in late pregnancy on urinary oestrogen estimation

Study	EXPT n	(%)	CTRL n	(%)	Odds ratio (95% CI)	Graph
Proud and Grant. (1987)	268/1000	(26.80)	208/1000	(20.80)	1.39 (1.13–1.71)	
Typical odds ratio (95% confidence interval)					1.39 (1.13–1.71)	

Effect of routine ultrasound placentography in late pregnancy on elective delivery for fetal compromise

Study	EXPT n	(%)	CTRL n	(%)	Odds ratio (95% CI)	Graph
Proud and Grant. (1987)	123/1000	(12.30)	99/1000	(9.90)	1.28 (0.96–1.69)	
Typical odds ratio (95% confidence interval)					1.28 (0.96–1.69)	

Effect of routine ultrasound placentography in late pregnancy on meconium-stained liquor in labour

Study	EXPT		CTRL		Odds ratio	Graph of odds ratios and confidence intervals
	n	(%)	*n*	(%)	(95% CI)	0.01 0.1 0.5 1 2 10 100
Proud and Grant. (1987)	70/989	(7.08)	101/988	(10.22)	0.67 (0.49–0.92)	
Typical odds ratio (95% confidence interval)					0.67 (0.49–0.92)	

Effect of routine ultrasound placentography in late pregnancy on Apgar score <4 at 1 minute

Study	EXPT *n*	(%)	CTRL *n*	(%)	Odds ratio (95% CI)
Proud and Grant. (1987)	30/1014	(2.96)	29/1011	(2.87)	1.03 (0.62–1.73)
Typical odds ratio (95% confidence interval)					1.03 (0.62–1.73)

Effect of routine ultrasound placentography in late pregnancy on Apgar score <7 at 5 minutes

Study	EXPT *n*	(%)	CTRL *n*	(%)	Odds ratio (95% CI)
Proud and Grant. (1987)	12/1014	(1.18)	25/1011	(2.47)	0.49 (0.25–0.93)
Typical odds ratio (95% confidence interval)					0.49 (0.25–0.93)

Effect of Routine ultrasound placentography in late pregnancy on admission to special care nursery

Study	EXPT *n*	(%)	CTRL *n*	(%)	Odds ratio (95% CI)
Proud and Grant. (1987)	48/1014	(4.73)	60/1011	(5.93)	0.79 (0.54–1.16)
Typical odds ratio (95% confidence interval)					0.79 (0.54–1.16)

Effect of routine ultrasound placentography in late pregnancy on neonatal seizures

Study	EXPT *n*	(%)	CTRL *n*	(%)	Odds ratio (95% CI)
Proud and Grant. (1987)	1/1014	(0.10)	2/1011	(0.20)	0.51 (0.05–4.92)
Typical odds ratio (95% confidence interval)					0.51 (0.05–4.92)

depending on whether they opened an envelope with an odd or an even number. In the light of this method of allocation, it is surprising that there was a 20 per cent difference in the size of the experimental groups in the report (133 vs. 167). The main results are presented in Table 27.7. No difference in the overall rate of elective delivery was observed, but the group for which A/B ratios had been reported were less likely to experience intrapartum fetal distress, and less likely to receive oxygen therapy and assisted ventilation during the neonatal period, although all of these differences may be a reflection of the play of chance. There was no suggestion of any difference in low Apgar scores, admission rates to the special care nursery between the two groups, but the confidence interval surrounding the estimates of difference are wide. There were only two deaths from causes other than malformations in the whole study population; both of these were in the control group. The available evidence does not, at the present time, support the use of Doppler ultrasound in clinical obstetric practice (Neilson 1987).

5 Women's reactions to ultrasound in pregnancy

An ultrasound examination has the potential to be a fascinating and happy experience for prospective parents. But, as already noted, real or mistaken diagnosis of fetal abnormality using ultrasound can also lead to psychological devastation. Women's reactions to ultrasonography during pregnancy have not, however, received the systematic attention from researchers which they deserve (Stewart 1986). We have been unable to locate any research other than case reports which investigates the psychological impact of commu-

Table 27.8 Effect of ultrasound assessment of umbilical artery wave-form in high risk pregnancies on elective delivery

Study	EXPT *n*	EXPT (%)	CTRL *n*	CTRL (%)	Odds ratio (95% CI)	Graph of odds ratios and confidence intervals
Trudinger *et al.* (1987)	82/127	(64.57)	107/162	(66.05)	0.94 (0.58–1.53)	
Typical odds ratio (95% confidence interval)					0.94 (0.58–1.53)	

Effect of ultrasound assessment of umbilical artery wave-form in high risk pregnancies on fetal distress in labour

Study	EXPT *n*	EXPT (%)	CTRL *n*	CTRL (%)	Odds ratio (95% CI)	Graph
Trudinger *et al.* (1987)	3/127	(2.36)	11/162	(6.79)	0.38 (0.13–1.13)	
Typical odds ratio (95% confidence interval)					0.38 (0.13–1.13)	

Effect of ultrasound assessment of umbilical artery wave-form in high risk pregnancies on Apgar score <4 at 1 minute

Study	EXPT *n*	EXPT (%)	CTRL *n*	CTRL (%)	Odds ratio (95% CI)	Graph
Trudinger *et al.* (1987)	9/127	(7.09)	11/162	(6.79)	1.05 (0.42–2.61)	
Typical odds ratio (95% confidence interval)					1.05 (0.42–2.61)	

Effect of ultrasound assessment of umbilical artery wave-form in high risk pregnancies on Apgar score <6 at 5 minutes

Study	EXPT *n*	EXPT (%)	CTRL *n*	CTRL (%)	Odds ratio (95% CI)	Graph
Trudinger *et al.* (1987)	6/127	(4.72)	8/162	(4.94)	0.95 (0.32–2.81)	
Typical odds ratio (95% confidence interval)					0.95 (0.32–2.81)	

Effect of ultrasound assessment of umbilical artery wave-form in high risk pregnancies on admission to special care nursery

Study	EXPT *n*	EXPT (%)	CTRL *n*	CTRL (%)	Odds ratio (95% CI)	Graph
Trudinger *et al.* (1987)	27/127	(21.26)	38/162	(23.46)	0.88 (0.51–1.54)	
Typical odds ratio (95% confidence interval)					0.88 (0.51–1.54)	

Effect of ultrasound assessment of umbilical artery wave-form in high risk pregnancies on use of oxygen therapy

Study	EXPT *n*	EXPT (%)	CTRL *n*	CTRL (%)	Odds ratio (95% CI)	Graph
Trudinger *et al.* (1987)	17/127	(13.39)	31/162	(19.14)	0.66 (0.35–1.23)	
Typical odds ratio (95% confidence interval)					0.66 (0.35–1.23)	

Effect of ultrasound assessment of umbilical artery wave-form in high risk pregnancies on use of ventilatory support

Study	EXPT *n*	EXPT (%)	CTRL *n*	CTRL (%)	Odds ratio (95% CI)	Graph
Trudinger *et al.* (1987)	6/127	(4.72)	15/162	(9.26)	0.51 (0.21–1.25)	
Typical odds ratio (95% confidence interval)					0.51 (0.21–1.25)	

Effect of ultrasound assessment of umbilical artery wave-form in high risk pregnancies on perinatal death (excluding lethal malformation)

Study	EXPT *n*	EXPT (%)	CTRL *n*	CTRL (%)	Odds ratio (95% CI)	Graph
Trudinger *et al.* (1987)	0/127	(0.00)	2/162	(1.23)	0.17 (0.01–2.74)	
Typical odds ratio (95% confidence interval)					0.17 (0.01–2.74)	

Graph scale: 0.01 0.1 0.5 1 2 10 100

nicating true and false positive reports and false negative reports of fetal abnormalities to parents. Not surprisingly, the small amount of research available relates to women whose pregnancies were normal.

A majority of the women interviewed in these studies valued ultrasonography in early pregnancy because it confirmed the reality of the baby for them, and because the examination was often followed by a reduction in anxiety and an increase in confidence (Kohn *et al.* 1980; Milne and Rich 1981; Hyde 1986). The anticipation of reassurance provided by ultrasonography, and probably the felt need for it, however, depend on the circumstances in which a woman is receiving care. A comparison of two samples of women drawn from two hospitals in Manchester, England, only one of which used ultrasonography routinely, found that unscanned women in the hospital in which ultrasonography was used selectively were less likely to think that a scan would be additionally reassuring, and less likely to believe that ultrasonography should be used routinely during pregnancy (Hyde 1986). By way of contrast, a study conducted in the United States found that American women feel that nearly half the value of ultrasonography in an uncomplicated pregnancy pertains to uses outside the realm of medical decisions, such as knowing the sex of the child or having an early picture to show their children. On average, the women studied alleged that they would be willing to pay over $200 for this information (Berwick and Weinstein 1986).

Women's views on the desirability of routine ultrasonography during pregnancy, in addition to being influenced by what is actually available, also vary between individuals who may be influenced not only by differing perceptions of the potential benefits, but also by concerns about the possible adverse effects of ultrasound (Beech *et al.* 1985). The only generalization that can be based on the results of the available research into women's views about the indications for ultrasonography is that considerable variation exists. The obvious implication for practice is that it is important for

Table 27.9 Effect of high vs. low feedback to mother at fetal ultrasonography on feeling negative about examination

Study	EXPT		CTRL		Odds ratio	Graph of odds ratios and confidence intervals
	n	(%)	*n*	(%)	(95% CI)	0.01 0.1 0.5 1 2 10 100
Reading and Platt (1985)	0/11	(0.00)	2/8	(25.00)	0.08 (0.00–1.45)	
Campbell *et al.* (1982)	2/67	(2.99)	14/62	(22.58)	0.17 (0.06–0.47)	
Cox *et al.* (1987)	0/50	(0.00)	6/50	(12.00)	0.12 (0.02–0.63)	
Typical odds ratio (95% confidence interval)					0.14 (0.06–0.34)	

Effect of high vs. low feedback to mother at fetal ultrasonography on feeling neutral about examination

Study	EXPT *n*	(%)	CTRL *n*	(%)	Odds ratio (95% CI)
Reading and Platt (1985)	2/11	(18.18)	2/8	(25.00)	0.68 (0.08–5.96)
Campbell *et al.* (1982)	15/67	(22.39)	41/62	(66.13)	0.17 (0.09–0.34)
Cox *et al.* (1987)	26/50	(52.00)	40/50	(80.00)	0.29 (0.13–0.66)
Typical odds ratio (95% confidence interval)					0.23 (0.14–0.38)

Effect of high vs. low feedback to mother at fetal ultrasonography on feeling positive about examination

Study	EXPT *n*	(%)	CTRL *n*	(%)	Odds ratio (95% CI)
Campbell *et al.* (1982)	50/67	(74.63)	7/62	(11.29)	12.79 (6.39–25.56)
Reading and Platt (1985)	9/11	(81.82)	4/8	(50.00)	4.04 (0.60–27.17)
Cox *et al.* (1987)	24/50	(48.00)	4/50	(8.00)	7.13 (2.99–17.00)
Typical odds ratio (95% confidence interval)					9.51 (5.65–16.01)

ultrasonographers to take this variation into account when dealing with individuals.

Another important message with practical implications which flows from the results of a number of studies is that the subjective experience of actually having a scan, even if the findings are normal, can be an unpleasant experience because of uncommunicativeness on the part of the ultrasonographer (Stewart 1986; Smith 1985; Hyde 1986). In practice, some ultrasonographers, in particular radiographers and technicians, may be put under professional constraint so that they cannot communicate freely with the women they are examining. But whether it is as a result of these constraints, or for other reasons, uncommunicativeness can eliminate the potentially beneficial psychological effects of the examinations.

The value of good communication between ultrasonographers and pregnant women has been demonstrated in four randomized trials (Campbell *et al.* 1982 [also reported in Reading and Cox 1982; Reading *et al.* 1984a, Reading *et al.* 1984b, Reading *et al.* 1988]; Field *et al.* 1985; Reading and Platt 1985; Cox *et al.* 1987). Women undergoing routine early pregnancy ultrasonography were randomly divided into two groups. In one, the 'high feedback' group, the monitor screen was visible and the ultrasonographer pointed out the fetus and its movement; in the other group ('low feedback') the screen was not visible. Women in the high feedback group were less likely to feel negative (nervous, worried, frightened, unsteady, disappointed) and far more likely to feel positive about the examination than those in the low feedback group (Table 27.8). The results of the randomized comparison of high and low feedback by Field *et al.* (1985) also suggested that high feedback can attenuate increases in anxiety during pregnancy. In one of the trials there was some suggestion that the women in the high feedback group were more likely to reduce cigarette and alcohol consumption in the short term (Reading *et al.* 1984). However, the modest differences that existed were not detectable later in pregnancy (Reading and Cox 1984), nor were they reported in either of the other two trials.

6 Potential hazards of obstetric ultrasound

6.1 Introduction

Any consideration of the use of diagnostic ultrasound in obstetric practice must weigh potential benefits against potential risks. It is not our intention to provide a detailed review of research on possible hazards of obstetric ultrasound (for this the reader is referred elsewhere: National Institutes of Health 1984; Hill and ter Haar 1982; Mole 1986; British Institute of Radiology Working Party 1987) but in the following section we have attempted to provide a summary in a brief review.

Whenever ultrasonic energy passes through biological tissues part of its energy is converted into heat. (This is one mechanism by which ultrasound treatment may be an effective physiotherapy for soft-tissue injuries.) The size of any temperature increase depends on a variety of physical and tissue properties including the intensity of the ultrasound beam. At the level of intensity used for diagnostic ultrasound scanning in pregnancy the fluctuations in temperature are unlikely to be much greater than those that occur naturally and it seems very unlikely that the rise in tissue temperature could have any damaging effect on a mammalian fetus (Kremkau 1983). The intensities of some pulsed Doppler machines are nearer the physiotherapy range, however, and the conclusions should be more cautious for this modality.

Another mechanism relates to cavitation, because there are small volumes of gas in solution in all tissues. Vibration in microscopic bubbles caused by ultrasound is non-linear and gas is acquired from surrounding tissue. The bubble or cavity resonates and the ultrasound energy is converted into mechanically more damaging forms. It may lead to 'shearing' as fluid around the bubble moves unusually rapidly. Bubbles may collapse, generating high temperatures leading to ionization of the gas with the generation of free radicals. For cavitation to occur the tissue must be in a liquid state with dissolved gas present and the exposure must be of sufficient intensity and duration. Greater energy is required to induce cavitation from micronuclei of dissolved gas than when gas bubbles already exist within the tissues. Most plant and insect tissues contain gas bubbles of a size that are most likely to start resonating. This is one reason why the phenomenon of cavitation has been most extensively studied in plants. It remains uncertain, however, whether it can occur in mammalian tissues; but ter Haar and colleagues (1982) have recently reported that insonation of a guinea-pig leg was associated with the development of significantly more bubbles than was observed in controls. Theoretically, cavitation could cause fracture of DNA, cell disintegration and damage to cell membranes affecting ion pumping and membrane permeability.

Other biophysical phenomena caused by ultrasound have also been reported which do not seem to relate to either heating or cavitation. These include 'streaming', radiation pressure effects, and standing wave effects which lead to 'banding' or clumping of red cells with possible damage to the surface of blood vessels (Hill and ter Haar 1982).

6.2 *In vitro* and animal studies

Death of isolated cells or micro-organisms in suspension after ultrasound exposure is almost invariably associated with cavitation. There is no evidence of subsequent change in the pattern of cell proliferation (similar to that seen following exposure to ionizing radiation) when cavitation was prevented by very short pulse duration (Hill and ter Haar 1982). There is, however, some evidence of sublethal changes in plasma membranes (Chapman 1974). Electron microscopy has also suggested damage to intracellular organelles such as mitochondria and lysosymes (Hill and ter Haar 1982). Abnormal cell behaviour and motility have also been reported after ultrasound exposure (Liebeskind *et al.* 1982).

There appears to be little, if any, good evidence linking ultrasound to adverse genetic effects such as mutation or chromosome breakage (Thacker 1985). If ultrasound exposure were to cause chromosome breakage, the likely effect would be death of the cell. Much of the controversy about possible chromosomal damage caused by ultrasound exposure has centred on studies of 'sister chromatid exchange'. This is thought to be a more sensitive index of chromosomal damage than chromosome breakage but its biological significance is unknown. Sister chromatid exchanges have been observed after insonation in only 3 out of 14 studies in which they have been sought (Goss 1984), but the possibility that ultrasound exposure causes chromosome damage as evidenced by an increased rate of sister chromatid exchange cannot be ruled out.

Most of the animal research has been conducted on fruit flies (Drosophila) and on mice. Even when the ultrasound exposure had been sufficient to kill some fruit flies, no excess of lethal mutations or chromosomal disjunction has been observed (Thacker and Baker 1976), and no chromosome aberrations attributable to ultrasound exposure have been detected in the studies involving mice and rats.

Evidence derived from animal studies about other possible adverse effects is conflicting (Hill and ter Haar 1982; National Institutes of Health 1984). Suggestions that exposure may reduce fertility and or fetal survival rates remain unconfirmed. Reports of a reduction in fetal weight are more persuasive (Pizzarello *et al.* 1978; O'Brien 1983), but again the research results are not consistent (Child *et al.* 1984; Smith 1984). At least 28 studies have assessed the effects of fetal exposure to ultrasound on fetal weight in either rats or mice. Exposure of one horn of a pregnant rats' uterus to diagnostic levels of ultrasound was associated with fetal weight reduction in one study (Pizzarello *et al.* 1978) but not in another (Carstenson and Gates 1983). In studies in mice, an effect has been observed in one strain but not in another (O'Brien 1984). Animal experimentation has also suggested that ultrasound exposure may compromise the immune system, the nervous system and gonadal tissues, but again, these studies are either unconfirmed or unrepeated (National Institutes of Health 1984; British Institute of Radiology Working Party 1987).

6.3 Human studies

There has been surprisingly little well-organized research to evaluate possible adverse effects of ultrasound exposure on human fetuses. Early case series (Bernstine 1969; Hellman *et al.* 1970, Serr *et al.* 1971) ruled out a major teratogenic effect but they are of limited value due to the lack of an appropriate control group.

Two apparently well-designed and well-conducted case-control studies have sought a relationship between ultrasound exposure and childhood malignancy (Kinnear Wilson and Waterhouse 1984; Cartwright *et al.* 1984). These included 1731 and 555 children with cancer respectively, of whom 665 and 149 had leukaemia. Both were reassuring, with one possible caveat: neither study showed any difference in exposure between the cases and controls up to the age of 5, but children dying of leukaemia or cancer over the age of 5 were more likely than controls to have been exposed to ultrasound as fetuses in one of the studies (Kinnear Wilson and Waterhouse 1984). This difference was not seen in the other, statistically more powerful study, in which all cases of leukaemia or cancer (alive and dead) were compared with controls (Cartwright *et al.* 1984).

Evidence from cohort studies is very limited. Scheidt and colleagues (1978) compared the outcome of pregnancy in retrospectively-derived groups of pregnancies managed with ultrasound and amniocentesis (303), amniocentesis alone (679), or neither (970). Babies exposed to ultrasound as fetuses were more likely than controls to have abnormal grasp and tonic neck reflexes but were comparable in respect of 122 other parameters.

Stark and his colleagues (1984) attempted to follow up two cohorts of children characterized by ultrasound exposure (or lack of it) in pregnancy. A total of 1450 exposed and 1450 unexposed, matched controls were identified from three Denver hospitals. Of these children, Stark and his colleagues were able to trace and examine only 425 exposed and 381 unexposed children at 7 to 12 years of age. Many outcomes were examined and no association with ultrasound exposure was found for the majority of them. One potentially important exception concerned dyslexia which was associated with exposure to ultrasound in the matched cohorts derived from all three hospital groups. This could either have been the result of chance (it was not statistically significant in conventional terms), or of bias from inadequate matching. It is difficult to see, however, why selection bias should apply to this one outcome measure, in all three hospitals, but not to the many other outcomes studied.

These two non-randomized studies and the randomized trials have been used to investigate the effect on birthweight suggested by the animal studies. Again, they have been reassuring, providing little evidence that *in utero* exposure reduces birthweight.

The randomized controlled trials conducted to date have been far too small to have a reasonable chance of identifying an effect of ultrasound exposure on a rare adverse outcome; nor can they provide a useful upper limit of any possible effect for the same reason. A large-scale randomized trial of about 20 000 women to assess possible adverse effects of ultrasound was planned by the British Medical Research Council in the early 1970s, but was cancelled at the last moment (Mole 1986). The main reasons for this decision were that hypothetical risks were not clearly defined and many of the possible outcomes were thought to be too infrequent for even a trial of this size to have been useful. A counter view is that the existence of two prospectively defined randomized cohorts of 10 000 exposed and 10 000 unexposed offspring would have been useful to rule out major adverse effects when the possibility of these (for example, dyslexia) was suggested by other research. The much smaller cohorts of children who participated as fetuses in the Norwegian randomized trials of ultrasound are currently being examined to test some of the hypotheses about potential adverse effects that have arisen from observational studies (Bakketeig, personal communication).

7 Conclusions

7.1 Implications for current practice

Any evaluation of the effects of ultrasonography in pregnancy must make the distinction between its selective use for specific indications and its routine use as a screening procedure.

The contribution of ultrasonography in specific clinical situations has not, in general, been quantified systematically. Nevertheless, the available information suggests that it can be valuable in a number of specific situations in which the diagnosis remains uncertain after a clinical history has been ascertained and a physical examination has been performed. These include confirmation of fetal life (after threatened miscarriage or other complications of pregnancy); diagnosis of multiple pregnancy; detection of a variety of fetal malformations (and facilitation of other prenatal diagnostic techniques); location of placental position (when placenta praevia is suspected); investigation of pelvic masses; and establishing fetal presentation. In addition, fetal anthropometric measurements allow estimation of gestational duration in early pregnancy, and of fetal growth rate and fetal weight in late pregnancy. Assessment of amniotic fluid volume and placental texture may give additional prognostic information when fetal growth retardation is suspected.

In contrast, the available information does not provide a basis for recommending routine use of ultrasonography for screening in either early or late pregnancy. The overriding limitation of the available controlled trials is their small sample size. The largest trial so far reported suggests that routine assessment of placental texture in late pregnancy may prompt clinical action leading to a reduction in the risk of fetal death. Other trials of routine ultrasound have concentrated on fetal measurement (in early pregnancy, late pregnancy, or both). Although induction of labour for apparent 'post-term' pregnancy is less frequent after routine early assessment of gestational duration, larger randomized controlled trials are needed if the decision about routine ultrasound scanning in pregnancy is to be based on sound scientific evidence.

There is currently no evidence to justify the use of Doppler ultrasonography to assess patterns of fetal and uteroplacental blood flow, except in the context of properly controlled studies.

Women's views about the indications for ultrasound during pregnancy vary, and it is important that ultrasonographers take this variation into account in their dealings with individual women. The value of good communication, with 'high feedback' of the results of the examination, has been demonstrated in a number of controlled trials.

So far, there is no evidence that ultrasonography in human pregnancy has any harmful biological or physical effects.

7.2 Implications for future research

Improvement in the quality of ultrasound imaging is so rapid that evaluation of any aspect of ultrasonography requires prompt assessment to avoid seeming irrelevant. These problems should not, however, be used as an excuse for failure to conduct the studies that are required.

There is still a need for further investigation of the accuracy of ultrasonographic estimation of gestational duration using pregnancies for which the actual duration (date of conception) is known. Such investigations must ensure that the ultrasonographers are unaware of duration of pregnancy at the time they make their ultrasound examination, and that intra-observer and inter-observer variation is assessed.

The significance of some of the subtle dysmorphic features that have been observed in the fetus using modern high resolution equipment requires elucidation. Some of these could prove useful as indicators of major chromosomal problems; others may be of no pathological significance and their detection may simply cause unwarranted anxiety.

Continued concentration on ultrasonographic identification of fetuses that are subsequently born 'light-for-dates' is unlikely to be useful. There is a need to research patterns of actual fetal growth using serial ultrasound assessments, and to document the neonatal correlates of the fetal growth patterns observed in this way.

The possible merits and disadvantages of routine use of ultrasonography for screening in early and late pregnancy require assessment in large controlled trials. Well-designed observational studies are also required to assess the diagnostic accuracy of ultrasonography for a range of structural abnormalities.

Doppler ultrasound study of fetal and maternal haemodynamics is an interesting and potentially useful technique. However, there is a need for better understanding of its pathophysiological basis, and its place in clinical practice should be based on the results of randomized controlled trials of sufficient size.

There is a general consensus that there is a continuing need for more laboratory and human research into the possible bioeffects of fetal exposure to ultrasound. Research in this field is complicated by the fact that there is no satisfactory way to measure ultrasound exposure and that the dose–response model may be inappropriate. Furthermore, most studies have used ultrasound intensities beyond the range of diagnostic ultrasound and have usually employed continuous wave ultrasound rather than short pulses which may have extremely high intensities. These issues will have to be borne in mind in the design of future research in this area.

References

Ager RP, Oliver RWA (1986). The Risks of Midtrimester Amniocentesis. Salford: University of Salford.

Allan LD, Crawford DC, Chita SK, Tynan MJ (1986). Prenatal screening for congenital heart disease. Br Med J, 292: 1717–1719.

Bakketeig LS, Eik-Nes SH, Jacobsen G, Ulstein MK, Brodtkorb CJ, Balstad P, Eriksen BC, Jorgensen NP (1984). Randomized controlled trial of ultrasonographic screening in pregnancy. Lancet, 2: 207–211.

Beazley JM, Underhill RA (1970). Fallacy of the fundal height. Br Med J, 4: 404–406.

Beech BA, Green M, Rodgers C, Squire J (1985). A commentary on the Report of the RCOG Working Party on Routine Ultrasound Examination In Pregnancy. Association for Improvements in the Maternity Services.

Bennett MJ, Little G, Dewhurst J, Chamberlain G (1982). Predictive value of ultrasound measurement in early pregnancy: a randomized controlled trial. Br J Obstet Gynaecol, 89: 338–341.

Bernstine RL (1969) Safety studies with ultrasonic Doppler technique. Obstet Gynecol, 34: 707–709.

Berwick DM, Weinstein MC (1985). What do patients value? Willingness to pay for ultrasound in normal pregnancy. Med Care, 23: 881–893.

Brambati B, Oldrini A (1986). Methods of chorionic villus sampling. In: Chorionic Villus Sampling. Brambati B, Simoni G, Fabro S (eds). New York: Dekker, pp 73–97.

Brereton RJ (1984). Importance of surgical consultation after ultrasonic diagnosis. Br Med J, 289: 1618–1619.

British Institute of Radiology Working Group (1987). The safety of diagnostic ultrasound. Br J Radiol, Suppl 20.

Campbell S (1974). Fetal growth. Clin Obstet Gynaecol, 1: 41–65.

Campbell S (1976). Fetal growth. In: Fetal Physiology and Medicine. Beard RW, Nathanielsz PW (eds). London: Saunders, pp 271–301.

Campbell S, Dewhurst CJ (1971). Diagnosis of the small-for-dates fetus by serial ultrasonic cephalometry. Lancet, 2: 1002–1006.

Campbell S, Pearce JM (1983). The prenatal diagnosis of fetal structural anomalies by ultrasound. Clin Obstet Gynaecol 10: 475–506.

Campbell S, Thoms A (1977). Ultrasonic measurement of the fetal head to abdomen circumference ratio in the assessment of growth retardation. Br J Obstet Gynaecol, 83: 165–174.

Campbell S, Holt EM, Johnson FD, May P (1972). Anencephaly: early ultrasonic diagnosis and active management. Lancet, 2: 1226–1227.

Campbell S, Wilkin D (1975). Ultrasonic measurement of fetal abdomen circumference in the estimation of fetal weight. Br J Obstet Gynaecol, 82: 689–697.

Campbell S, Reading AE, Cox DN, Sledmere CM, Mooney R, Chudleigh P, Beedle J, Ruddick H (1982). Ultrasound scanning in pregnancy: the short-term psychological effects of real-time scans. J Psychosom Obstet Gynaecol, 1: 5761.

Carstensen EL, Gates AH (1984) The effect of pulsed ultrasound on the fetus. J Ultrasound Med, 3: 145–147.

Cartwright RA, McKinney PA, Birch JM, Hartley AL, Mann JR, Waterhouse JAH, Johnston HE, Draper GJ, Stiller C (1984). Ultrasound exposure in pregnancy and childhood cancer. Lancet, ii: 999–1000.

Chamberlain PF, Manning FA, Morrison I, Harman CR, Lange IR (1984). Ultrasound evaluation of amniotic fluid, volume I. The relationship of marginal and decreased amniotic fluid volumes to perinatal outcome. Am J Obstet Gynaecol, 150: 245–249.

Chapman IV (1974) The effect of ultrasound on the potassium content of rat thymocytes *in vitro*. Br J Radiol, 47: 411–415.

Child SZ, Carstensen EL, Davis H (1984). A test of the effect of low-temporal-average-intensity pulsed ultrasound on the rat fetus. Exp Cell Biol, 52: 207–210.

Cochlin DL (1984). Effects of two ultrasound scanning regimens on the management of pregnancy. Br J Obstet Gynaecol, 91: 885–890.

Comeau J, Shaw L, Marcell CC, Lavery JP (1983). Early placenta praevia and delivery outcome. Obstet Gynecol, 61: 577–580.

Cox DN, Wittmann BK, Hess M, Ross AG, Lind J, Lindahl S (1987). The psychological impact of diagnostic ultrasound. Obstet Gynecol, 70: 673–676.

Daffos F, Capella-Pavlovsky M, Forester F (1985). Fetal blood sampling during pregnancy with use of a needle guided by ultrasound: a study of 606 consecutive cases. Am J Obstet Gynecol, 153: 655–660.

Deter RL, Rossavik IK, Harrist RB, Hadlock FP (1986). Mathematic modeling of fetal growth: development of individual growth curve standards. Obstet Gynecol, 68: 156–161.

Donald I (1980). In: Recent Advances in Ultrasound Diagnosis 2. Kurjak A (ed). Amsterdam: Excerpta Medica, pp 4–20.

Donald I, Abdulla U (1967). Ultrasonics in obstetrics and gynaecology. Br J Radiol, 40: 604–611.

Donald I, Brown TG (1961). Demonstration of tissue interfaces within the body by ultrasonic echo sounding. Br J Radiol, 34: 539–546.

Donald I, MacVicar J, Brown TG (1958). Investigations of abdominal masses by pulsed ultrasound. Lancet, 1: 1188–1194.

Eik-Nes SH, Okland O, Aure JC, Ulstein M (1984). Ultrasound screening in pregnancy: a randomized controlled trial. Lancet, 1: 1347.

Field T, Sandberg D, Quetel TA, Garcia R, Rosario M (1985). Effects of ultrasound feedback on pregnancy anxiety, fetal activity, and neonatal outcome. Obstet Gynecol, 66: 525–528.

Fitzgerald DE, Drumm JE (1977). Non-invasive measurement of human fetal circulation using ultrasound: a new method. Br Med J, 22: 1450–1451.

Furness ME (1987). Reporting obstetric ultrasound. Lancet, 1: 675–676.

Garrett WJ, Robinson DE (1971). Assessment of fetal size and growth rate by ultrasonic echography. Obstet Gynecol, 38: 525–534.

Geirsson RT, Patel NB, Christie AD (1984). *In-vivo* accuracy of ultrasound measurements of intrauterine volume in pregnancy. Br J Obstet Gynaecol, 91: 37–40.

Geirsson RT, Patel NB, Christie AD (1985). Intrauterine volume, fetal abdominal area and biparietal diameter measurements with ultrasound in the prediction of small-for-dates babies in a high-risk obstetric population. Br J Obstet Gynaecol, 92: 936–940.

Gennser G, Persson P-H (1986). Biophysical assessment of placental function. Clin Obstet Gynaecol, 13: 521–552.

Gohari P, Berkowitz RL, Hobbins JC (1977). Prediction of intrauterine growth retardation by determination of total intrauterine volume. Am J Obstet Gynecol, 127: 255–260.

Gosling RG, King DH (1975). Ultrasonic angiography. In: Arteries and Veins. Hascus AW, Adamsons L (eds). Edinburgh: Churchill Livingstone, pp 61–98.

Goss SA (1984) Sister chromatid exchange and ultrasound. J Ultrasound Med, 3: 463–470.

Grannum PA, Berkowitz RL, Hobbins JC (1979). The ultrasonic changes in the maturing placenta and their relation to fetal pulmonary maturity. Am J Obstet Gynecol, 133: 915–922.

Grennert L, Persson PH, Gennser G (1978). Benefits of ultrasonic screening of a pregnant population. Acta Obstet Gynecol Scand (Suppl), 78: 5–14.

Griffin S, Cohen-Overbeek T, Campbell S (1983). Fetal and utero-placental blood flow. Clin Obstet Gynaecol, 10: 565–602.

Griffiths DM, Gough MH (1985). Dilemmas after ultrasonic diagnosis of fetal abnormality. Lancet, 1: 623–624.

Gruenwald P (1974). Pathology of the fetus and its supply line. Ciba Foundation symposium: Size at birth. Amsterdam: Associated Scientific Publishers, pp 3–19.

Hansmann M (1978). Measurements of fetal age, growth and nutrition. In: The Current Status of Fetal Heart Rate Monitoring and Ultrasound in Obstetrics. Beard RW, Campbell S (eds). London: Royal College of Obstetricians and Gynaecologists, pp 165–189.

Harrison MR (1983). Perinatal management of the fetus with a correctable defect. In: Ultrasonography in Obstetrics and Gynecology. Callen PW (ed). Philadelphia: WB Saunders, pp 177–192.

Hellman LM, Duffus GM, Donald I, Sunden R (1970) Safety of diagnostic ultrasound in obstetrics. Lancet, i: 1133–1135.

Hill CR, ter Haar G (1982) Ultrasound. In: Nonionising Radiation Protection. Suess MJ (ed). Geneva: WHO regional publication, European series No. 10, World Health Organisation, pp 199–228.

Hughey MJ (1984). Routine ultrasound for detection and management of the small-for-gestational age fetus. Obstet Gynecol, 64: 101–107.

Hutson JM, McNay MB, MacKenzie JR, Whittle MJ, Young DG, Raine PAM (1985). Antenatal diagnosis of surgical disorders by ultrasonography. Lancet, 1: 621–623.

Hyde B (1986). An interview study of pregnant women's attitudes to ultrasound scanning. Soc Sci Med, 22: 587–592.

Kadar N, DeVore G, Romero R (1981). Discriminatory HCG zone: its use in the sonographic evaluation for ectopic pregnancy. Obstet Gynecol, 58: 156–161.

Kappel B, Neilson J, Hansen KB, Mickelsen M, Therkelsen AAJ (1987). Spontaneous abortion following mid-trimester amniocentesis. Clinical significance of placental perforation and blood stained amniotic fluid. Br J Obstet Gynaecol, 94: 50–54.

King DL (1973). Placental migration demonstrated by ultrasonography. Radiology, 109: 167–170.

Kinnier Wilson LM, Waterhouse JAH (1984) Obstetric ultrasound and childhood malignancy. Lancet, 2: 997–999.

Kloosterman GJ (1979). Epidemiology of postmaturity. In: Human Parturition. Keirse MJNC, Anderson ABM, Bennebroek Gravenhorst J (eds). The Hague: Leiden University Press, pp 247–261.

Kohn CL, Nelson A, Wiener S (1980). Gravidas' responses to real-time ultrasound fetal image. J Obstet Gynaecol Neonatal Nurs, March/April: 77–80.

Kratochwil A (1978). History of ultrasound. In: Handbook of Clinical Ultrasound. De Vlieger M, Holmes JG, Kratochwil A, Kazner E, Kraus R, Kossoff G, Poujol J, Strandness DE (eds). New York: John Wiley, p 111–112.

Kremkau FW (1983) Biological effects and possible hazards. Clin Obstet Gynecol, 10: 395–405.

Lancet (1985). When ultrasound shows fetal abnormality. Lancet, 1: 618–619.

Lancet (1986). Duplex ultrasound: vision on, sound on. Lancet, 2: 137–138.

Levine SC, Filly RA (1977). Accuracy of real-time sonography in the determination of fetal viability. Obstet Gynecol, 49: 475–477.

Liebeskind D, Padawer J, Wolley R, Bases R (1982) Diagnostic ultrasound: time-lapse and transmission electron microscopic studies of cells insonated *in vitro*. Br J Cancer, 45, Suppl V: 176–186.

MacGregor SN, Tamura RK, Sabbagha RE, Minogue JP, Gibson ME, Hoffman DI (1987). Underestimation of gestational age by conventional crown–rump length dating curves. Obstet Gynecol, 70: 344–348.

Mantoni M, Pedersen JF (1981). Intrauterine haematoma: an ultrasonic study of threatened abortion. Br J Obstet Gynecol 88: 47–51.

Milne LS, Rich OJ (1981). Cognitive and affective aspects of the responses of pregnant women to sonography. Matern Child Nurs J 10: 15–39.

Mole R (1986). Possible hazards of imaging and Doppler ultrasound in obstetrics. Birth, 13: 29–37.

Murphy S, Das P, Grant DN, Hayward R (1984). Importance of neurosurgical consultation after ultrasonic diagnosis of fetal hydrocephalus. Br Med J, 289: 1212–1213.

National Institutes of Health Consensus Statement (1984). Diagnostic Ultrasound Imaging in Pregnancy. US Department of Health and Human Sciences, Washington DC.

Neilson JP (1986). Indications for ultrasonography in obstetrics. Birth, 13: 16–19.

Neilson JP (1987). Doppler ultrasound. Br J Obstet Gynaecol, 94: 929–934.

Neilson JP, McNay MB (1988). Obstetric ultrasound. In: Practical Ultrasound. Lerski R (ed). Oxford: IRL Press. pp 85–101.

Neilson JP, Whittle MJ (1988). Doppler blood flow studies in fetal growth retardation. In: Fetal and Neonatal Growth. Cockburn F (ed). Chichester: John Wiley, pp 79–91.

Neilson JP, Whitfield CR, Aitchison TC (1980). Screening for the small-for-dates fetus: a two stage ultrasonic examination schedule. Br Med J, 280: 1203–1206.

Neilson JP, Munjanja SP, Whitfield CR (1984). Screening for small-for-dates fetuses: a controlled trial. Br Med J, 289: 1179–1182.

O'Brien WD (1983). Dose-dependent effect of ultrasound on fetal weight in mice. J Ultrasound Med, 2: 1–8.

O'Brien WD (1984). Ultrasonic bioeffects: a view of experimental studies. Birth, 11: 149–157.

O'Brien GD, Queenan JT, Campbell S (1981). Assessment of gestational age in the second trimester by real-time ultrasound measurement of the femur length. Am J Obstet Gynecol, 139: 540–545.

Pizzarello DJ, Vivino A, Madden B, Wolsky A, Keegan AF, Becker M (1978) Effect of pulsed low-power ultrasound on growing tissues. 1. Developing mammalian and insect tissue. Exp Cell Biol, 46: 179–191.

Platt LD, DeVore GR, Lopez E, Herbert W, Falk R, Alfi O (1986). Role of amniocentesis in ultrasound-detected fetal malformation. Obstet Gynecol, 68: 153–155.

Proud J, Grant A (1987). Third trimester placental grading by ultrasonography as a test of fetal wellbeing. Br Med J, 294: 1641–1644.

Reading AE, Cox DN (1982). The effects of ultrasound examination on maternal anxiety levels. J Behav Med, 5: 237–247.

Reading AE, Platt LD (1985). Impact of fetal testing on maternal anxiety. J Reprod Med, 30: 907–910.

Reading AE, Campbell S, Cox DN, Sledmere CM (1982). Health beliefs and health care behaviour in pregnancy. Psychol Med, 12: 379–383.

Reading AE, Cox DN, Sledmere CM, Campbell S (1984a). Psychological changes over the course of pregnancy: a study of attitudes towards the fetus/neonate. Health Psychol, 3: 211–221.

Reading AE, Campbell S, Cox DN, Sledmere CM (1984b). Health beliefs and health care behaviour in pregnancy. Psychol Medicine, 12: 379–383.

Reading AE, Cox DN, Campbell S (1988). A controlled, prospective evaluation of the acceptability of ultrasound in prenatal care. J Psychosom Obstet Gynaecol, 8: 191–198.

Rizos N, Miskin M, Benzie RJ, Ford JA (1979). Natural history of placenta praevia ascertained by diagnostic ultrasound. Am J Obstet Gynecol, 133: 287–291.

Robinson HP (1972). Detection of fetal heart movement in first trimester of pregnancy using pulsed ultrasound. Br Med J, 4: 466–468.

Robinson HP (1973). Sonar measurement of the fetal crown–rump length as means of assessing maturity in first trimester of pregnancy. Br Med J, 4: 28–31.

Robinson GP (1975). The diagnosis of early pregnancy failure by sonar. Br J Obstet Gynaecol, 82: 849–857.

Robinson HP, Fleming JEE (1975). A critical evaluation of 'crown–rump length' measurements. Br J Obstet Gynaecol, 82: 702–710.

Robinson HP, Sweet EM, Adam AH (1979). The accuracy of radiological estimates of gestational age using early fetal crown–rump length measurements by ultrasound as a basis for comparison. Br J Obstet Gynaecol, 86: 525–528.

Romero R, Jeanty P, Reece EA, Grannum P, Bracken M, Berkowitz K, Hobbins JC (1985). Sonographically monitored amniocentesis to decrease intraoperative complications. Obstet Gynecol, 65: 426–430.

Royal College of Obstetricians and Gynaecologists (1984). Report of the Working Party on Routine Ultrasound Examinations in Pregnancy. London: Royal College of Obstetricians and Gynaecologists.

Scheidt PD, Stanley F, Bryla DA (1978) One-year follow-up of infants exposed to ultrasound *in utero*. Am J Obstet Gynecol, 121: 742–748.

Secher NJ, Hansen PK, Lenstrup C, Eriksen PS, Morsing G (1987). A randomised study of fetal abdominal diameter and fetal weight estimation for detection of light-for-gestation infants in low-risk pregnancies. Br J Obstet Gynaecol, 94: 105–109.

Serr DM, Padeh B, Zakut H, Shaki R, Mannor SM, Kalner B (1971). Studies on the effects of ultrasonic waves on the fetus. Huntingford PJ (ed). Basel: Karger, pp 302–307.

Smith CB (1984). Birth weight of fetuses exposed to diagnostic ultrasound. J Ultrasound Med, 3: 395–396.

Smith B (1985). NCT ultrasound survey—results. New Generation 4: 5.

Stabile I, Campbell S, Grudzinskas JG (1987) Ultrasonic assessment of complications during the first trimester of pregnancy. Lancet, 2: 1237–1240.

Stark CR, Orleans M, Haverkamp AD, Murphy J (1984) Short- and long-term risks after exposure to diagnostic ultrasound *in utero*. Obstet Gynecol, 63: 194–200.

Stewart A, Webb J, Hewitt D (1956). Malignant disease in childhood and diagnostic irradiation *in utero*. Lancet, 2: 447.

Stewart A, Webb J, Hewitt D (1958). A survey of childhood malignancies. Br Med J, 1: 1495–1508.

Stewart N (1986). Women's views of ultrasonography in obstetrics. Birth 13 (Suppl): 39–43.

Stuart B, Drumm J, Fitzgerald DE, Duignan NM (1980). Fetal blood velocity waveforms in normal pregnancy. Br J Obstet Gynaecol, 87: 780–785.

ter Haar GR, Daniels S, Eastaugh KC, Hill CR (1982). Ultrasonically induced cavitation *in vivo*. Br J Cancer, 45, suppl V: 151–155.

Thacker J (1985). Investigations into genetic and inherited changes produced by ultrasound. In: Biological Effects of Ultrasound. Nyborg WL, Ziskin MC (ed). New York: Churchill Livingstone, pp 67–76.

Thacker J, Baker NV (1976). The use of Drosophila to estimate the possibility of genetic hazard from ultrasound irradiations. Br J Radiol, 49: 367–371.

Trudinger BJ, Giles WB, Cook CM (1985). Flow velocity waveforms in the maternal uteroplacental and fetal umbilical placental circulations. Am J Obstet Gynecol, 152: 155–160.

Trudinger BJ, Cook CM, Giles WB (1986). A comparison of fetal heart rate monitoring and umbilical artery waveforms in the recognition of fetal compromise. Br J Obstet Gynaecol, 93: 171–175.

Trudinger BJ, Cook CM, Giles WB, Connelly A, Thompson RS (1987). Umbilical artery flow velocity waveforms in high-risk pregnancy: randomised controlled trial. Lancet, 1: 188–190.

Verloove-Vanhorick SP, Verwey RA, Brand R, Bennebroek Gravenhorst J, Keirse MJNC, Ruys JH (1986). Neonatal mortality risk in relation to gestational age and birthweight. Lancet 1: 55–57.

Warsof SL, Griffin D (1984). The diagnosis of fetal anomalies. In: Ultrasound in Perinatal Care. Bennett MJ (ed). Chichester: John Wiley, pp 75–102.

Weckstein LN, Boncher AR, Tucker H, Gibson D, Rettenmaier MA (1985). Accurate diagnosis of early ectopic pregnancy. Obstet Gynecol, 65: 393–397.

28 Fetal movement counting to assess fetal well-being

Adrian Grant and Diana Elbourne

1 Introduction

Reduction or cessation of fetal movements may precede fetal death by a day or more (Sadovsky and Yaffe 1973). In theory at least, recognition of such a reduction, followed by appropriate action to confirm jeopardy and expedite delivery, could prevent fetal death. This is the basis for using counts of fetal movements as a test of fetal well-being. The idea is not a new one: over a century ago Playfair recommended the 'induction of premature labour on the mother feeling that the movements of the child are becoming less strong' (Playfair 1884).

2 The epidemiology of antepartum stillbirth

Renewed interest in fetal movement counting as a possible means of identifying fetuses at high risk of late fetal death reflects the increasing importance of unexplained antepartum late fetal death as a component of perinatal mortality. Data from the Scottish Perinatal Mortality Surveys (McIlwaine *et al.* 1979, 1983, 1984) and Scottish Stillbirth and Neonatal Death Reports (Scottish Health Services Agency Reports for 1983, 1984 and 1985) illustrate the contrasting changes in the rates of antepartum, intrapartum, and early neonatal death of normally formed singletons (Table 28.1). When the period 1977 to 1981 is compared with the period 1982–85 the intrapartum and early neonatal death rates fell by more than 30 per cent, whereas the antepartum death rate fell by only 6 per cent. The proportion of perinatal deaths which has occurred before the onset of labour has therefore increased from 44 per cent to 50 per cent.

2.1 Gestational age and antepartum late fetal deaths

About 60 per cent of antepartum late fetal deaths are delivered before 37 completed weeks, while only 2 per cent are delivered after 42 weeks gestation (second column of Table 28.2). (It should be noted when considering late fetal death in relation to gestational age that these statistics refer to gestation at delivery; death had actually occurred at a variable time before delivery.) The timing of antepartum late fetal death as judged by the gestational age at delivery has implications for the use of fetal movement monitoring as a test of fetal well-being. Gestational-age-specific antepartum late fetal death rates are very high before 37

Table 28.1 Antepartum late fetal, intrapartum late fetal, and early neonatal death rates (per 1000) for normally formed singletons

Year	77	78	79	80	81	82	83	84	85	Proportional fall 77–81 to 82–85
Antepartum death	4.8	NA	4.0	3.7	3.7	3.6	3.7	4.1	3.9	6
Intrapartum death	1.5	NA	1.2	1.2	1.1	1.0	0.9	0.7	0.7	34
Early neonatal death	5.2	NA	4.0	3.5	3.2	3.3	2.6	2.6	2.5	31

(From McIlwaine *et al.* 1979, 1983, 1984, and Scottish Information Services Division reports for 1983, 1984, and 1985.)

Table 28.2 The relationship between gestational age at delivery and the number, rate, and risk of (a) all antepartum late fetal death (APLFD), (b) unexplained antepartum late fetal death, and (c) all other antepartum late fetal deaths

	(a) All antepartum deaths			(b) Unexplained antepartum deaths			(c) Other antepartum deaths		
Gestational age	Number (% all APLFD)	Rate per 1000 births	Risk per 1000 pregnancy—weeks	Number (% all unexplained APLFD)	Rate per 1000 births	Risk per 1000 pregnancy—weeks	Number (% all other APLFD)	Rate per 1000 births	Risk per 1000 pregnancy—weeks
28–31	228 (20)	120.3	0.22	111 (17)	58.5	0.11	117 (24)	61.7	0.11
32–36	437 (39)	38.1	0.35	230 (36)	20.1	0.18	207 (42)	18.1	0.17
37–39	315 (28)	3.7	0.51	189 (30)	2.2	0.31	126 (26)	1.5	0.20
40–41	125 (11)	0.8	0.67	95 (15)	0.6	0.55	30 (6)	0.2	0.18
42+	23 (2)	2.7	2.66	15 (2)	1.7	1.73	8 (2)	0.9	0.93

(From McIlwaine *et al.* 1984.)

weeks and lowest around term (third column of Table 28.2). This statistic, however, is potentially misleading, because it expresses antepartum late fetal deaths in relation to *births* during a gestational period. A much more appropriate denominator would be the number of women pregnant during the gestational age period, because it is their fetuses which are at *risk* of death before the onset of labour (Yudkin *et al.* 1987, Grant 1987). Risk expressed in these terms (fourth column of Table 28.2) gives a very different picture; compared with fetuses at 28 to 31 weeks of gestation, fetuses at 40–41 weeks are at threefold greater risk, and those at 42 or more weeks are at a twelvefold greater risk of an antepartum death. Because unexplained antepartum late fetal deaths tend to occur later in pregnancy than other antepartum deaths (Table 28.2) these relative risks are greater for unexplained antepartum late fetal deaths (5 and 16, respectively). These considerations present something of a conundrum when considering the timing of routine fetal movement monitoring: women who are still pregnant at relatively advanced gestational ages, in particular after 42 weeks, are at special risk of an antepartum stillbirth; nevertheless, these stillbirths constitute only a minority of all such perinatal deaths.

Risk expressed in these terms is therefore a function of the gestational age at delivery of antepartum deaths and the gestational age of all births. But it is impossible to know in advance when a particular pregnancy will end. For this reason the risk *over the remainder of pregnancy* for those (still) pregnant at a particular gestation age (Table 28.3) is more relevant when considering the gestational age at which to begin screening. These risks are highest at 28 weeks, fall steadily until term and then rise again post-term. Although the risk does rise after 42 weeks, these stillbirths constitute only a minority of all such perinatal deaths.

Table 28.3 Risk of normally formed, singleton antepartum late fetal death (APLFD) during remainder of pregnancy for those pregnant at various gestational ages

Gestational age in completed weeks	Risk of APLFD during remainder of pregnancy for those still pregnant per 1000
28	4.3
32	3.5
37	1.9
40	0.9
42	2.7

(From McIlwaine *et al.* 1984.)

2.2 Subgroups of normally formed antepartum late fetal deaths

As implied by the subdivision into unexplained and other deaths, not all antepartum late fetal deaths are potentially preventable by fetal movement monitoring. Some late fetal deaths are not preceded by a reduction in fetal movements; for others there may be insufficient time between the reduction and fetal death to allow clinical action. About 15 per cent of normally formed antepartum late fetal deaths are ascribed to abruption of the placenta (McIlwaine *et al.* 1979). In many of these cases placental separation occurs very suddenly and occasionally there may even be a transient flurry of fetal movements rather than a reduction (Sadovsky 1983). Complications of the cord (to which about 2 per cent of normally formed antepartum deaths are ascribed) may also come into these categories.

Other late fetal deaths may have associated conditions that are recognizable in their own right: about 12 per cent are preceded by pre-eclampsia and 7 per cent by maternal conditions such as essential hypertension. In these cases fetal movement counting may be theoretically useful as a supplement to other, hospital-based tests of fetal well-being.

There is no obvious 'cause' for the remaining 50–60 per cent of antepartum late fetal deaths. Overall rates of these deaths have changed little in Scotland between 1981 and 1985 (the years for which these data are available), although the gestational age at delivery tended to be somewhat older in the deaths surveyed during 1985 (Table 28.4). Most of these deaths are unpredictable and therefore the extent to which they can be prevented by current forms of antenatal care is very limited. Screening by fetal movement counting, because it can be performed each day, has theoretical advantages over other tests of fetal well-being, all of which are either difficult or impossible to perform daily for practical reasons. It is the possibility that these unexplained deaths may be preventable that is the basis for screening all pregnancies by fetal movement counting.

Table 28.4 Numbers and rates (per 1000 normally formed singletons) of unexplained normally formed late fetal deaths by birthweight

		1981	1983	1985
Normal birthweight	No.	45	52	61
	0/00	0.7	0.8	0.9
Low birthweight	No.	101	88	92
	0/00	1.5	1.4	1.4

(From McIlwaine 1983, Information Services Division reports for 1983 and 1985.)

2.3 Intrauterine growth retardation and antepartum late fetal deaths

Babies who die in late pregnancy tend to be small for their gestational age at birth. This association is much stronger when there has been a complication of pregnancy, such as hypertension, than when the pregnancy has been uncomplicated. Some of the association may be artefactual: there may be a delay between death and delivery, and maceration may result in loss of fetal weight. Also (see Chapter 26), the supposition that a particular baby which is of low birthweight for its gestational age has necessarily suffered growth retardation may be unfounded. Nevertheless, an association is consistent with a chronic condition leading to many stillbirths. As discussed later, a reduction or generally low level of fetal movements is associated with suspected intrauterine growth retardation (Bekedam *et al.* 1985) and with low birthweight for gestational age at delivery, particularly if relatively severe (Mathews 1975; Sadovsky *et al.* 1983; Rayburn 1982; Jarvis and MacDonald 1979).

2.4 Major malformations and antepartum late fetal deaths

About 10 per cent of all antepartum late fetal deaths are judged to have died because of a lethal malformation. Although this proportion is low in comparison with both intrapartum fetal deaths and early neonatal deaths (lethal malformations cause about one-third of each of these) lethal malformations do present particular problems for antenatal fetal movement monitoring.

The worry is that recognition of a reduction in the movements of a malformed fetus may lead to inappropriate interventions unless steps are first taken to check fetal morphology with ultrasound. These fetuses are also more likely to have abnormal fetal heart rate patterns (Sadovsky *et al.* 1981a) (see Chapter 30).

3 Fetal movements in late pregnancy

The mean number of movements per hour felt in late pregnancy has been variously estimated as 30 (Rayburn 1982) and 60 (Valentin *et al.* 1984) but these summary statistics hide fluctuations from time to time within individual pregnancies (Sadovsky 1985) and also the very wide range of normal variation between individuals (Benhamou and Tournaire 1981). The number of maternally perceived movements per '12-hour' day varies from 10 to 1000 for the majority of normal fetuses; but counts below 10 per 12-hour day have also been recorded for some apparently uncompromised fetuses (Rayburn 1982).

It is useful to separate this wide normal variation into four components: variation in the activity of an individual fetus; variation in the perception of her baby's movements by an individual mother; variation in activity between different babies; and variation in perception between different mothers.

3.1 Variation in the activity of an individual fetus

Timor-Tritsch and her colleagues (1978) demonstrated by ultrasound that fetuses pass through active and quiet phases. Active phases of body movement on average last 40 minutes, while quiet phases, which are characterized by absent body and extremity movements, last an average of 23 minutes. Patrick and his colleagues (1982) found that only 1 per cent of quiet phases lasted longer than 45 minutes. Of greater practical importance is Timor-Tritsch's opinion that quiet phases which last longer than 60 minutes are abnormal. The timing of this cycle of activity is largely random, so this source of variation can be reduced by prolonged or repeated measurement.

There is conflicting evidence about the extent to which non-random variation may be introduced by extrinsic factors such as maternal smoking and medication (Wood *et al.* 1979), meals (Miller *et al.* 1978; Aledjem *et al.* 1979; Gelman *et al.* 1980; see also Birkenfeld *et al.* 1981; Patrick *et al.* 1982), maternal posture (Zimmer *et al.* 1982), maternal physical activity (Rayburn 1982; Platt et al. 1983), gestational age (Pearson and Weaver 1976; Roberts et al. 1979, 1980; Birger *et al.* 1980; Ehrstrom 1984), time of day (Patrick *et al.* 1982; Ehrstrom 1984), sound and light stimulation (Sadovsky 1978; Grimwade *et al.* 1971) and uterine palpation (Rosen *et al.* 1979). It is possible to standardize conditions for monitoring movements to eliminate the potentially biasing effects of some of these, but because they represent relatively small components of the total variation, such standardization is probably not worth the effort. However, individualizing each mother and her fetus, as discussed below, does eliminate the effects of a number of these.

3.2 Variation in the perception of a baby's movements by an individual mother

In addition to the true differences in movement exhibited by a fetus, a mother's perception of her baby's movements may vary both randomly and systematically. The majority of women are consistent over time in the proportion of movements which they feel and record, but about 25 per cent may show wide day-to-day variation (Grant and Hepburn 1984). Both distraction and prolonged periods of counting reduce the proportion of movements perceived. Hence, while prolonged counting may reduce random errors, it may introduce systematic ones.

3.3 Variation in activity between different fetuses

Prolonged recording of fetal movements with ultrasound and electronic monitors has demonstrated that fetuses have inherent, individual rates of activity, which may differ considerably from one fetus to another (Ehrstrom 1979, Wood *et al.* 1979). Some fetuses are consistently vigorous and others consistently sluggish (Sadovsky *et al.* 1974). In addition, as a group, fetuses with malformations are more likely to have reduced movements than normally formed fetuses (Sadovsky *et al.* 1981a; Rayburn and Barr 1982, Valentin and Marsal 1987). In a series of 58 cases of major fetal malformation (Rayburn and Barr 1982), 16 (28 per cent) had reduced movements. Abnormalities associated with reduced movements included bilateral hip dislocation (3/3), bilateral renal agenesis (2/2), anomalies of the gastrointestinal (4/9) and central nervous systems (5/21), and fetuses with multiple anomalies (2/5); none of the 3 fetuses with trisomies or 9 fetuses with cardiac abnormalities had reduced movements.

3.4 Variation in perception between different women

Mothers differ widely in their ability to perceive movements (Hertogs *et al.* 1979; Hertogs *et al.* 1981); some notice nearly all of their baby's movements, others only a proportion, and some apparently none at all (Biale and Mazor 1985), although as described above, most are consistent in the proportion which they feel and record. There are differences of opinion about whether perception of fetal movements is altered by placental site (Neldam 1982; Hertogs *et al.* 1979) and/or maternal weight or obesity (Gettinger *et al.* 1978; Hertogs *et al.* 1979; Leader and Baillie 1979; Schmidt *et al.* 1984). The association of fewer reported movements with parity may be due to the distractions of other children rather than to parity itself (Gettinger *et al.* 1978; Hertogs *et al.* 1979; Neldam 1982; Schmidt *et al.* 1984).

Differences in the patterns of movements felt by different women provide a combined estimate of variations between babies in their activity and variations between women in their abilities to feel movements. Although, as mentioned above, most women individually report a consistent pattern, rates of perceived activity vary more than tenfold from one woman to another (Grant and Hepburn 1984). These differences between women are the major source of variation in fetal movements (Hertogs *et al.* 1981; Valentin 1986). Because they are systematic they are not reduced by prolonged observation. The attraction of using an individualized approach with each mother and fetus combination acting as their own control and looking for changes in fetal movements rates within each combination is that it totally eliminates these sources of variation. This is discussed further later in this chapter.

4 Methods of maternal fetal movement counting

Apart from informal noting of fetal movement patterns, two basic approaches to the investigation of maternally perceived fetal movements have been suggested: either the mother counts for a fixed length of time (the limit of normality being defined as a fixed, minimum number of movements in that time period); or she may be advised to count a fixed number of movements, the limit of normality then being defined by a fixed maximum time to record them.

A wide variety of fixed-time periods has been tried. The earliest proponents used 12 hours, but it proved impractical to ask mothers to count for such prolonged periods of time. Twelve-hour rates were subsequently calculated from counts made over shorter periods of time (e.g. Jarvis and MacDonald 1979). More recently, kick counts have been expressed as hourly rates, commonly after counting for an hour, although some routines use shorter (Valentin *et al.* 1984) or longer (Debdas *et al.* 1984) time periods. Some suggest repeating the count two (Birger *et al.* 1980), three (Sadovsky *et al.* 1974), or four (Leader *et al.* 1981) times each day. To reduce the chances that a diminution in movements is due to random fluctuations (e.g. a prolonged quiet phase) some authors advocate that these relatively short fixed-time periods be repeated only if the rate falls below a lower limit (e.g. Sadovsky *et al.* 1974; Neldam 1983). Even with this safeguard a high false positive alarm rate remains the chief potential drawback of fixed-time periods that are sufficiently short to be feasible in practice (Grant and Hepburn 1984, Thompson and Wheeler 1985). An individualized lower limit partially overcomes this problem (Valentin and Marsal 1986).

Fixed-number counting took a stage further the reasoning behind repeat counts when movements are few. The Cardiff 'count-to-ten' system (Pearson 1979) is the best known example of this approach. It is theoretically attractive because mothers with vigorous fetuses count for minimum lengths of time, whereas mothers with quiet fetuses will count longer. Its drawback, however, is that recording becomes less accurate with longer periods of counting, and an important minority of women with normal fetuses feel relatively few movements; these women must consistently count for long periods of time (Grant and Hepburn 1984). To overcome this problem, Grant and Hepburn (1984) suggested the use of an individualized fixed-number which takes into account variation both between fetuses and in maternal perception. An individualized hourly (or probably better, half-hourly) count is first calculated for each woman on the basis of ten days' recordings of counts for an hour; then the time taken to record this number is recorded each day for the remainder of pregnancy.

The new system did appear to result in substantially fewer 'false-alarms' (defined as the standard count taking more than 12 hours in the presence of a healthy fetus) than did the system of counting for one hour and continuing for a second hour if the level is low. In comparison with the Cardiff count-to-ten method the amount of time spent counting each day was more uniform and was halved overall. The drawback of this system is that it is more elaborate and requires two antenatal contacts to implement.

5 Definitions of normal and abnormal fetal movement counts

The choice of an appropriate cut-off point for any of these counting schemes is not easy. It reflects a tension between the need to identify 'true positives' (sensitivity) and the need to avoid 'false positives' (specificity). The balance between these competing considerations also depends on the condition being sought. Most people use the formalized kick counts to identify fetuses at increased risk of death *in utero*, others claim that it should also be used to screen for intrauterine growth retardation. By and large, a more lenient cut-off is used to increase the sensitivity for intrauterine growth retardation (Jarvis and MacDonald 1979), and this invariably results in a corresponding fall in specificity and a rise—possibly to an intolerable level—in the number of false positives. Many of the schemes have been developed for use by women at relatively high risk of antepartum late fetal death with little apparent recognition that a stricter definition of abnormality may be more appropriate for lower risk women (see Chapter 3 for a discussion of the effects of prevalence of outcome on the performance of a test).

The early use of 12-hour daily rates stemmed from Sadovsky's observations (Sadovsky and Yaffe 1973) that 'fetal movements are significantly reduced up to cessation' for at least 12 hours before fetal death. Recently, Sadovsky has defined significant reduction as 3 movements or less per hour over 12 hours (Sadovsky *et al.* 1981b). Pearson and Weaver (1976) used a statistical approach to define their lower limit of normal of 10 movements over 12 hours. They studied 61 mothers who had recorded the number of fetal movements occurring daily between 9 a.m. and 9 p.m. from 32 weeks until delivery and who subsequently delivered vigorous infants with a weight above the 25th centile for gestational age, corrected for sex and parity: 2.5 per cent of counts 'at each period of gestation' fell below 10 per 12 hours. This level was used as a 'lower limit of normal for clinical purposes'. In fact, Pearson asks his patients to contact the hospital if there is complete cessation of movement on a single day or counts below 10 on two successive days (Pearson, personal communication). For the reasons alluded to above, this stricter definition of a reduced count makes sense when the scheme is used by women at no apparent increased risk of stillbirth. Like Pearson and Weaver's definitions, most definitions of normal and abnormal counts are fixed to limit the false positives to a reasonable number. In a low risk population any more than about 5 women in every 100 with false alarms is probably unacceptable in terms of the maternal anxiety caused and the unnecessary medical intervention which this might precipitate.

Rayburn and colleagues (1980) also used a statistical definition of normality for the women under their care, who counted for an hour a day. A critical value (4 movements per hour) was retrospectively calculated such that 5 per cent of all women fell below it on two successive days at some time during late pregnancy. More pragmatically, 4 per cent of the mothers in Neldam's practice (who counted for a second hour when the first hour's count was below 4) contacted the hospital during late pregnancy because of reduced movements (Neldam 1983). Leader and others (1981) used a computer analysis of a preliminary study to find a definition of abnormally reduced movements which best separated good and poor neonatal outcome. They then validated their system in a subsequent series of women (see Table 28.5).

The upper time-limit of 12 hours for Pearson's count-to-ten approach was an extrapolation from his lower limit of 10 movements per 12 hours described above for fixed-time counting. Neldam (personal communication) has also used the count-to-ten approach but his upper limit is 3 hours—again an extension of his fixed-time, 4 movements per hour, lower limit. It is likely that this would be associated with a large number of false positives. The counter-argument, of course, is that it should improve the sensitivity and result in a better pick up of true positives. The rarity of antepartum late fetal death, however, makes this claim difficult to substantiate. As is illustrated below, the estimation of sensitivity is very imprecise because it is based on only a handful of cases. This also explains why little account can be taken of the true positives when deciding on the definition of an alarm.

Individualized limits have been defined for both the fixed-time and fixed-number approach. Valentin and colleagues (1984) calculate individualized normal levels from 5 days' recordings for 15 minutes each day and set a lower limit at 30 per cent of this figure. This corresponded to two standard deviations below the mean. As many as 11 per cent of women will, however, notice fetal movement below that level at some stage during pregnancy. Hertogs and his colleagues (1981) use the count-to-ten approach and set their danger point at 'twice the time usually needed to count-to-ten'. Unpublished work in which the authors have recently been involved has demonstrated that an approach using a number determined individually for each woman can have a stricter limit (shorter upper time period) than the standard Cardiff count-to-ten method, while maintaining the same specificity.

6 Validity of fetal movement counting as a test of fetal well-being

The reciprocal relation between sensitivity and specificity is illustrated in Table 28.5. Despite its statistical infrequency, one reference standard against which to assess the performance of a formalized fetal movement count is 'all antepartum late fetal deaths' (see top of Table 28.5). High specificity tends to be associated with low sensitivity and vice versa. Although not all such deaths are preceded by a reduction in fetal movements (Payne *et al.* 1980), there is still a clear association between reduced counts and antepartum death. Although it is not always possible to exclude the presence of lethal malformations in clinical practice, when judging the potential of the test it is reasonable to exclude deaths due to lethal malformations from the reference standard. First, it is not the aim to identify these cases by fetal movement counting; and second, it is important to realize that prediction of normally formed antepartum late fetal deaths appears to be somewhat better than prediction of all antepartum deaths (section ii, Table 28.5). Less extreme outcomes, such as low Apgar scores (section iii), 'intrauterine growth retardation' (section iv), or a combination of measures (section v) may also be predicted. If the results of the fetal movement counts are available to the clinician and the baby is delivered on the basis of low count plus a 'diagnostic' cardiotocogram trace, the surrogate outcome of the abnormal trace (section vi) may be the only one available to judge the validity of fetal movement counting, (because of the effects of intervention on later outcomes—see Chapter 3).

7 Compliance with formalized fetal movement counting

Another consideration underlying the choice of both the count method and the normal limits, is the extent to which women are prepared to follow the instructions. There are two aspects of this: first, whether women monitor fetal movements regularly as advised; and second, whether they contact those responsible for their

Table 28.5 Fetal movement counting as a predictor of various categories of outcome

Outcome category	Author (date)	Method	Lower limit normal	Outcome measure	Prevalence %	No. subjects	Sensitivity %	Specificity %	PPV* %	NPV† %	Clinicians' knowledge of results?
(i) All antepartum late fetal deaths	Rayburn (1982)	One or more convenient hour	3 or less per hour	Antepartum late fetal deaths	2	1161	70	97	35	99	Yes(?)
	Leader *et al.* (1981)	30 min 4 times per day	Complete cessation for 1 day or less than 10 in 2 hours on 2 successive days	All antepartum late fetal deaths	6	264	100	90	38	100	No
	Pearson and Weaver (1976)	12-hour daily count	Less than 10 in 12 hours	All antepartum late fetal deaths	4	122	100	92	36	100	No(?)
	Sadovsky *et al* (1981b)	30–60 min 3 times per day—extended if <3 per hour	Less than 10 in 12 hours	All antepartum late fetal deaths	1.5	212	67	92	12	99	Yes
	Koistinen *et al.* (1986)	1 hour repeated if count low	Less than 10 movements per hour in 2 successive hours	All antepartum stillbirths	0.3	403	50	96	3	100	Yes
(ii) Normally formed stillbirths	Leader *et al.* (1981)	as above	as above	Normally formed late fetal deaths	6	264	100	90	38	100	No
	Pearson and Weaver (1976)	as above	as above	Normally formed late fetal deaths	3	122	100	92	29	100	No(?)
	Koistinen *et al.* (1986)	as above	as above	Normally formed late fetal deaths	0.2	2103	40	96	2	100	Yes
(iii) Low Apgar scores	Rayburn (1982)	as above	as above	Apgar $\leqslant 6$ at 5 min	6	1138	12	97	27	95	Yes(?)
	Leader *et al.* (1981)	as above	as above	Apgar $\leqslant 6$ at 5 min + feto–maternal arterial base deficit difference of 5 mEq/1	2	247	50	91	12	99	No
	Pearson and Weaver (1976)	as above	as above	Apgar $\leqslant 6$ at 1 min	20	122	34	96	71	82	No(?)
	Mathews (1975)	Mother's impression		Apgar $\leqslant 6$ at 5 min	10	50	100	80	36	100	Yes
	Koistinen *et al.* (1986)	as above	as above	Apgar $\leqslant 6$ at 5 min	2	2103	24	96	9	99	Yes

(iv) Intra-uterine growth retardation	Rayburn (1982)	as above	as above	bwt < 5th centile	4	1161	29	97	28	97	Yes(?)
	Jarvis and MacDonald (1979)	Same 3 hours each day multiplied by 4 for daily 12-hour rate	Less than 12 per 12 hours	bwt > 2 standard deviations below mean for gestational age (Aberdeen scale)	14	90	77	86	48	96	No
	Koistinen *et al.* (1986)	as above	as above	bwt < 10th centile	5	2103	8	96	9	96	Yes
(v) Mixed outcomes	Rayburn (1982)	as above	as above	Late fetal death + abnormal intrapartum FHR trace + caesarean section for fetal distress + Apgar ⩽6 at 5 min + bwt ⩽5th centile	11	1161	20	98	54	91	Yes
	Leader *et al.* (1981)	as above	as above	Antepartum fetal death Apgar ⩽6 + base deficit difference	8	262	86	91	46	99	No
(vi) Antepartum cardiotocography	Rayburn *et al.* (1980)	as above	as above	Suspicious or positive CST‡ or Abnormal NST$ (if CST contraindicated)	6	349	50	97	56	97	No
	Harper *et al.* (1981)	3 1-hour periods per day	Cessation over a day	Non-reactive NST	4	91	15	99	75	99	No
	O'Leary and Adrinopoulos (1981)	3 30-min periods per day	< 5 movements for each period in a day	Non-reactive NST	5	237	15	82	5	94	No
	Liston *et al.* (1982)	Count to 10	Less than 10 in 12 hours	Non-reactive NST	7	133	60	97	67	96	Yes
	Koistinen *et al.* (1986)	as above	as above	Non-reactive NST	3	2100	16	96	12	97	Yes

* Positive predictive value
† Negative predictive value
‡ Contraction stress test
$ Non-stress test

antenatal care when fetal movements are sufficiently reduced to constitute an alarm signal. One difficulty in interpreting statistics about compliance is that they all refer to chart completion rather than monitoring of movements *per se*. Some completed charts may not be returned after delivery. More importantly, some 'non-compliers' may make a mental note of their babies' movements even if the movements are not formally recorded, whereas other 'non-compliers' may take no notice of movements at all; and some women who do not count may fill in the chart to please the doctor or midwife.

The fact that it is the mother rather than the doctor who assumes responsibility when fetal movements are being monitored is an attraction of this method of surveillance, but it has implications for compliance. Variation in compliance with completing fetal movement charts is associated with a variety of factors. Multiparae, teenagers, and women over the age of 35, (Valentin and Marsal 1986), women of lower social class, and women who receive charts that are not printed in a language with which they are familiar, for example, seem less likely to complete a chart. These women are often at higher than average risk of late fetal death. On the other hand, women with, or admitted to hospital because of, an antepartum complication are probably more likely to comply.

The attitudes to fetal movement counting of those providing antenatal care are also likely to be very important. Valentin and her colleagues (1986) found significant differences in compliance rates in groups of women supervised by twelve different midwives. Unless the staff are convinced that fetal movement counting is useful they are unlikely to motivate women fully. Time needs to be set aside to teach women how to count and record movements; at subsequent antenatal consultations interest must be taken in the entries on the chart even if they suggest a perfectly normal fetus.

The counting procedure used is also likely to affect compliance with regular recording of movements. The longer during a day that women record movements the less reliable the recording becomes (Sadovsky *et al.* 1974; Wood *et al.* 1979, Rayburn and McKean 1980). For this reason shorter fixed-time periods (for example, Valentin *et al.* 1984) and individualized fixed-numbers (Grant and Hepburn 1984) have been recommended. Counting during the daytime can be unpopular because women are preoccupied with other things at this time. A higher proportion of movements are perceived if women stop other activities: perception may also be improved by lying down (Minors and Waterhouse 1979). For these reasons some protocols recommend that women count fetal movements in the evening. But there are obvious drawbacks to this if movements are reduced: counting may go on late into the night; if movements are abnormally reduced, women may delay seeking advice or it may be difficult to make contact with doctors or midwives; diagnostic tests such as cardiotocography and obstetric ultrasound may not be available; and facilities for emergency delivery and neonatal resuscitation may be more limited.

Estimates of compliance rates are usually between 70 and 80 per cent (Henrion and Heard 1979; Harper *et al.* 1981; Neldam 1980 and 1983; Valentin *et al.* 1984; Valentin 1986) but both higher (Draper *et al.* 1986) and lower rates (Fischer *et al.* 1981; Thompson and Wheeler 1985) have been reported. There have been too few studies to assess reliably which of the various counting methods is associated with the best compliance. The only formal comparison was conducted by Valentin and her colleagues (1984). Two-thirds of the women in their study preferred a 15-minute count in the evening to a daily 'count-to-ten' in the morning.

The other facet of compliance is whether women contact those responsible for their antenatal care when movements are reduced. It is well known that women with low counts often do not seek help and there are anecdotal reports of this in the literature (Fischer *et al.* 1981; Beach *et al.* 1983). Valentin and her colleagues (1986) studied this systematically and found that 31 per cent of women failed to consult the hospital about a decrease in the fetal movement count; repeated 'alarms' were most likely to be disregarded. A related issue is contacts made because of worries about fetal movements even though the movement pattern does not fulfill the criterion for 'alarm'. In Valentin's series (Valentin *et al.* 1986) these contacts were made by only 2 per cent of women, but represented 30 per cent of all calls to the hospital about fetal movements.

8 Do clinical actions taken on the basis of fetal movement counting improve fetal outcome?

Demonstration that a reduction in fetal movements is predictive of antepartum late fetal death and other measures of adverse outcome still leaves the two most crucial questions unanswered. First, does it predict adverse outcome at a time when it would be possible to avert or moderate the outcome? Even though there is often a delay between a reduction in movements and poor outcome recognized at delivery, it is possible that the pathological process may be too far advanced to be altered. Second, is there a suitable treatment available to effect this improvement? Early intervention prompted by a reduction in fetal movements might lead to the delivery of a baby who dies intrapartum or neonatally rather than in the antepartum period, or who survives with a severe handicap.

Few studies have addressed the question of whether clinical actions taken on the basis of fetal movement counting do improve fetal outcome. To the best of our knowledge, only two randomized controlled trials have been completed, both conducted in Copenhagen.

The earlier trial was conducted by Steen Neldam (Neldam 1980, 1983). All women who booked for delivery in the Rigshospitalet in Copenhagen between August 1978 and May 1980 were included in the trial. By alternation, half were allocated to the counting group and half to the control group, the allocation being organized by a secretary. Women in the treatment group (even numbers) counted movements for an hour, two hours after meals, once a week until 30 weeks, and then three times a week thereafter. Counts below three were repeated over a second hour. If they remained three per hour or less after two hours counting, the mother was instructed to contact the hospital immediately.

Dynamic ultrasound was then used to see whether the fetus was motionless or moving normally. A cardiotocogram was performed and serum oestriol and human placental lactogen were measured. If the fetus was motionless and did not respond to external maternal stimulation, and the cardiotocograph tracing indicated the possibility of intrauterine asphyxia in a mother who was not taking a sedative, a caesarean section was performed as soon as possible. If during the scan the fetal movement rate was less than 50 per cent of normal for that fetus, the mother was admitted to hospital for 24 hours' observation. If after this, the fetus was still moving less than normal, but cardiotocography, oestriol, and human placental lactogen were normal, the patient was examined weekly as an out-patient, with repeated oestriol, human placental lactogen, and biophysical profile determinations, until normal fetal activity was established. If the cardiotocography or hormone values were abnormal, delivery was induced within 24 hours. Women who noticed a diminution of fetal movements, but not to less than 50 per cent of normal, had cardiotocograph and hormone analyses performed. If these were satisfactory, they were sent home.

The control group (odd numbers) were tested according to the normal procedure in the hospital. They were not given specific fetal movement counting instructions, but at every antenatal visit were asked if they were feeling fewer fetal movements. If they reported a reduced frequency of fetal movements, hormone analyses and cardiotocographs were performed and the obstetrician in charge decided on treatment (Neldam 1980, 1983).

After excluding 104 women in the counting group and 117 in the control group who either miscarried or moved from the region, a total of 1562 women had been allocated to count fetal movements and 1549 to the control group. Three hundred and forty-one (22 per cent) of those allocated to count did not complete their charts. Sixteen refused to participate in the study; for 22 it proved impossible because of language problems; and the remainder failed to comply with the counting instructions. For a further 124 women (8 per cent), no completed chart was available at the end of the trial, either because the chart had been lost or because none had been given to the mother during her pregnancy. Nevertheless, all of these women were included in the final analysis.

About 4 per cent of the formal counting group contacted the hospital because of reduced movements (but so did a similar number in the control group, who were worried about fetal movements in a more general way). Half of these were reassured by simple clinical evaluation, the other half required further assessment with ultrasound, cardiotocography, and hormone analysis. Thirteen babies were delivered (10 by emergency caesarean section) because these supplementary tests 'confirmed' fetal compromise. Prior to the reduction in fetal movements, 5 of these mothers were apparently normal, five had pre-eclampsia (2 with associated intrauterine growth retardation), 1 had diabetes mellitus, 1 had low oestriol and human placental lactogen estimations, and in 1 there was suspected intrauterine growth retardation alone.

There were 12 antepartum deaths of normally formed babies weighing more than 1500 g in the control group (7 in apparently normal pregnancies, 3 in diabetic pregnancies, 1 after premature rupture of the membranes, and 1 following placental abruption), compared with only 3 in the counting group (2 in apparently normal pregnancies and 1 following placental abruption). Neldam pointed out that 1 case in the control group had not received any antenatal care at the hospital and 1 case in the counting group had delivered within a month of the start of allocation and had not received any instruction or fetal movement chart.

The striking difference in normally formed antepartum late fetal deaths observed by Neldam must, however, be qualified. First, after the onset of labour there were two more deaths in the counting group than in the control group (11 vs. 9) so part of the difference in antepartum deaths may have been as a consequence of a delay in the timing of death. Second, the trial was not primarily designed to identify a reduction in the risk of antepartum stillbirth; its main purpose was to assess the feasibility and acceptability of a programme of formal fetal movement counting. Third, the difference observed in the antepartum death rates is only just significant at the 5 per cent level. The 95 per cent confidence limit for the true effect is compatible with a true reduction of only 8 per cent. Neldam's trial is clearly too small to give a sufficiently precise estimate of the true effect of fetal movement counting. Despite these limitations it should be pointed out that no other screening test of fetal well-being has been shown in a well conducted randomized trial to be of such promise.

The more recently conducted randomized controlled trial was mounted at Herlev Hospital, Copenhagen, and compared routine fetal movement counting with routine human placental lactogen and oestriol estimation. It has not yet been formally reported. There was, however, no clear difference between the two groups in the antepartum late fetal death rate (Legarth and Weber, personal communication), although this is not surprising when the low risk of such deaths is taken into consideration.

Lobb and his colleagues in Liverpool (Lobb *et al.* 1985) compared two concurrently cared for groups of women, one of which was given the Cardiff count-to-ten chart while the other acted as control. A few women in the control group who were deemed to be at high risk of stillbirth were given charts, otherwise formal fetal movement monitoring was not used. The allocation to counting or control group was not random, but was based on the specialist under whose care a woman was booked to have antenatal care: the two academic unit consultants introduced counting for all women under their care, while the other four consultants did not. The two study groups were considered to be similar except for an excess of women with severe rhesus isoimmunization in the control group, reflecting a special interest of the control consultants. The women in the two groups were of similar age and parity. Over the 5-year period 1978–82 there were just over 20 000 deliveries. Overall the antepartum late fetal death rate was 1 per 1000 lower in the counting group (5.3 per 1000 vs. 6.3 per 1000, Table 28.6). However, 60 per cent of this difference was explained by a greater number of deaths attributed to severe rhesus isoimmunization in the control group. Furthermore, the remaining 0.4 per 1000 difference observed in the types of antepartum death which were thought to be preventable by fetal movement counting (bottom two lines of Table 28.6), was restricted to births weighing less than 1500 g.

Table 28.6 Results of the Liverpool cohort study of daily fetal movement counting (Lobb *et al.* 1985)

	Counting 6597 (0/00)	Control 13705 (0/00)
Total antepartum late fetal deaths	35 (5.3)	86 (6.3)
Antepartum deaths attributed to lethal malformations, rhesus isoimmunization, abruptio placentae, or one of twins	18 (2.7)	45 (3.3)
Other antepartum deaths		
Total	17 (2.6)	4 (3.0)
> 1500 g	13 (2.0)	26 (1.9)
< 1500 g	4 (0.6)	15 (1.1)

(From Lobb *et al.* 1985.)

These deaths would seem less likely to be preventable by fetal movement counting than deaths of heavier babies because many would occur before formal counting conventionally begins at about 28 weeks. The movement patterns are known for 8 of the 13 intrauterine deaths in the counting group which weighed more than 1500g; 2 showed no cessation of movements, 1 showed cessation for less than 12 hours, and 5 had cessation for more than one day. It seems telling that 'one of these five mothers received advice from a neighbour that cessation of movements before labour was a normal event. A second mother took no action. A third mother attended her general practitioner who heard the fetal heart and no further action was taken. A fourth mother attended the hospital because she had felt reduced fetal movements and a cardiotocograph was not reactive. No action was taken and 2 days later an intrauterine death was diagnosed at the antenatal clinic. The baby of the fifth mother had a terminal cardiotocograph but died before action could be taken' (Lobb *et al.* 1985). Despite the fact that 20 000 women were studied, the estimate of the effect of routine fetal movement counting is not very precise: the 95 per cent confidence limits of the observed relative risk of the groups of stillbirths which are thought to be preventable (0.86), are 0.49 and 1.51. There are also worries that the management of the two groups may have differed importantly in other respects, or that the groups may have differed more fundamentally other than in the prevalence of severe rhesus isoimmunization. Nevertheless, the results of this study should be taken seriously.

Westgate and Jamieson (1986) conducted a historical control study. Perinatal mortality in the 20 months prior to the introduction of fetal movement count-to-ten charts was compared with mortality in the 20 months following their introduction. The potential for such studies to be misleading is well known (Doll and Peto 1980; and see Chapter 54). Little weight should be given to this study even though when taken at face-value, it suggests an important reduction in unexplained stillbirth as a result of fetal movement counting.

9 Wider implications of a policy of maternal fetal movement counting

There are wider implications of formal fetal movement counting than fetal outcome which must also be taken into account when considering formalized fetal movement counting. Health service resources are required to train women in the counting procedures and to respond to reports of reduced movements. This has never been accurately quantified. Counting and acting on reduced movements is also time-consuming for the mothers and there is a possibility that this may induce stress and anxiety (McIlwaine *et al.* 1980). On the other hand the formalized focusing of a mother on her fetus *in utero* may strengthen the mother–infant bond after delivery. The provision of a formal channel of communication between mothers and hospital personnel, combined with clear guidelines about when to make contact, may decrease stress and anxiety. Feedback to women of information about their fetuses has been shown in other contexts of antenatal care to reduce anxiety, to increase confidence and positive feelings towards the fetus, to enhance compliance with other health-related advice (Campbell *et al.* 1982; Reading *et al.* 1982), to increase feelings of control and to improve communication with staff (Elbourne *et al.* 1987). These wider implications apply to all women and not just to those with reduced movements. They are particularly important in the context of a test which, at most, will alter the obstetrical outcome in only a small minority of cases.

Draper and her colleagues (1986) have recently examined some of these issues in a study of antenatal care in Cambridge. Out of 132 women who used Cardiff count-to-ten charts, 55 per cent were reassured by filling in the chart, many equating fetal movements with fetal well-being. But 23 per cent were worried by formal counting. These worries were of two broad types: first, those resulting from lack of knowledge about normal variations in fetal movement patterns both within and between pregnancies, and second, those caused by episodes of perceived reductions in movement. Valentin (1986) and Koistinen and her colleagues (1986) reported broadly similar findings.

10 Conclusions

Where does this leave us? Antepartum late fetal death is the component of perinatal mortality that has shown greatest resistance to change over recent years. In part this reflects its relative unpredictability; in part it reflects the relatively long period of time over which it can occur. Close surveillance is possible during the intrapartum and early neonatal period in a way in that it is not possible during the entire last trimester of pregnancy. Most tests of fetal well-being during pregnancy are hospital-based and this, among other factors, limits the number of times that they can be performed. If antepartum deaths only occurred in a group of pregnancies which were at identifiable high risk this would be less of a problem, but this is not the case. More than 50 per cent are unexplained and many of the others appear to be either unpredictable or belong to identifiable 'higher-risk' groups which, in statistical terms, are not at very high risk. This latter consideration is the basis for selective use of fetal movement counting; for example, in cases of essential or pregnancy-induced hypertension, rhesus isoimmunization, diabetes mellitus, suspected intrauterine growth retardation, or when there is a past obstetric history of antepartum late fetal death.

The question of main importance is whether the addition of fetal movement counting to other tests of fetal well-being leads to an improvement in fetal outcome. Selective screening with fetal movement counting is also sometimes recommended on the basis of prolonged pregnancy. The risk over the remainder of pregnancy for those still pregnant falls during the third trimester until a late rise after 42 weeks (Table 28.3). On this basis it seems most sensible either to advise women to start counting at the beginning of the third trimester or to restrict advice to count to those who go past term. Post-term pregnancies are undoubtedly at higher risk, but they contribute only a small proportion of all antepartum late fetal deaths. The risk *at a particular gestational age* for those still pregnant increases with advancing gestation, however (Table 28.2), hence if counting is started early, its value is likely to increase as pregnancy advances.

Taking all these arguments together there is certainly a case for considering the screening of all pregnancies to try to prevent antepartum late fetal death. However, only one in a thousand women might benefit in terms of prevention of late fetal death. It is for this reason that the wider medical, social, psychological and economic implications must be taken into account. What are the implications for the women who are asked to count? On balance, is counting reassuring or anxiety-generating? Does it lead to unnecessary medical intervention? What are the consequences for the medical services and for those providing those services? And what are the cost implications of introducing such screening?

The fundamental question remains whether the policy of formal maternal recording of fetal movement counting does, indeed, prevent antepartum late fetal death. There is a good basis for thinking that it might, but also worries that theory may not be reflected in reality. There is often a period of reduced movements before fetal death, but will this reduction be recognized and if so, will it be acted on sufficiently quickly to improve outcome?

All these questions are currently being addressed in a large-scale international collaborative trial of routine fetal movement counting (Grant and Elbourne 1985; Grant *et al.* 1986, 1987). About 69 000 women are being randomly allocated in groups (clusters) either to antenatal care which includes a policy of formal fetal movement counting using a modification of the count-to-ten approach, or to antenatal care which does not routinely include formal counting. The 66 groups characterized by the specialist giving care or by the clinic or hospital providing care, were first matched into 33 pairs on the basis of the past antenatal late fetal death rate and other characteristics. One member of each pair was randomly allocated to each policy. To a large extent, this design overcomes the potential for 'contamination' caused by women in the two trial groups attending the same antenatal clinic. In addition to the medical implications of the two policies, a subsample of women was asked for their views. The trial involves obstetricians from Great Britain, Belgium, Sweden, Ireland, and the United States. Recruitment to the study ended in early 1988. This trial should be free of selection bias and yet have the statistical power to address some of the many questions about fetal movement counting which are still outstanding.

10.1 Implications for current practice

Maternal monitoring of fetal movements is a simple and inexpensive test of fetal well-being that can be performed daily. If used, it should be used as a screening test which prompts other, diagnostic tests, rather than more definitive obstetric intervention. The possibility of congenital malformation should be considered before delivery is expedited.

There is a good basis for selective screening of subgroups of women identified as being at increased risk of antepartum late fetal death on the basis of past obstetric history, medical problems in the current pregnancy, and prolonged pregnancy. About 50 per cent of antepartum late fetal deaths are not associated with any recognizable risk factor, however, and this is the rationale for screening all pregnancies in late pregnancy. If this practice is adopted, fetal movement counting should start before the third trimester begins, and should continue with increasing vigilance until delivery.

One attraction of fetal movement counting as a method of screening for fetal well-being is that it is the mother rather than her medical attendants who takes responsibility for monitoring her pregnancy, and she decides for herself whether or not she wants to perform the test. The professional, however, still has a major responsibility. The likelihood that a woman will comply with advice to record fetal movements and report reduced movements is to a large extent dependent on the attitude of those providing her antenatal care. Furthermore, benefits will only accrue from fetal movement counting if reports of reduced movements prompt appropriate action, and there are reasons to believe that this does not always occur.

There are advantages and disadvantages to all the methods of formalized fetal movement counting, and no one method is clearly the best. As a general principle, the length of the counting time should be kept to the minimum that will avoid confusion by physiological rest periods.

There are good theoretical reasons, and there is some empirical evidence, to suggest that daily fetal movement counting can lead to clinical actions which, on balance, improve fetal outcome. This cannot, however, be considered an established fact, and furthermore, there are wider medical, social, psychological, and economic implications that must also be taken into account.

10.2 Implications for future research

Many questions about formalized fetal movement counting still remain unanswered. Very large randomized controlled trials are required if the effects of either routine or selective screening by fetal movement counting on fetal mortality and major neonatal morbidity, are to be assessed with any precision. One such trial is underway but replication could only strengthen it.

Uncertainties about the wider implications of formal fetal movement counting, both for the women counting and for the health services which provide antenatal care, are also addressed most satisfactorily in (less large) randomized controlled trials. There is an urgent need to clarify these issues given that, potentially, they apply to such large numbers of women.

There is still scope for improving the techniques used for monitoring fetal movements. Probably more important is research into the practical arrangements for teaching the techniques, encouraging compliance, and responding to reports of reduced movements. This would maximize the chances that any theoretical benefits of fetal movement counting are translated into real benefits for mothers and their babies.

References

Aladjem S, Feria A, Rest J, Gull K, O'Connor M (1979). Effect of maternal glucose load on fetal activity. Am J Obstet Gynecol, 134: 276–280.

Beach PR, Duff PW, Everett MT (1983). Use of fetal movement chart. J R Coll Gen Pract, 33: 424–430.

Bekedam DJ, Visser GHA, de Vries JJ, Prechtl HFR (1985). Motor behaviour in the growth retarded fetus. Early Hum Dev, 12: 155–165.

Benhamou M, Tournaire M (1981). Le compte des mouvements actifs du foetus. J Gynecol Obstet Biol Reprod, 10: 449–458.

Biale Y, Mazor M (1985). Absence of fetal movements and normal infants. Eur J Obstet Gynecol Reprod Biol, 19: 133–136.

Birger M, Homburg R, Insler V (1980). Clinical evaluation of fetal movements. Int J Gynaecol Obstet, 18: 377–382.

Birkenfeld A, Laufer N, Sadovsky E (1981). Diurnal variation of fetal activity. Obstet Gynecol, 55: 417–419.

Campbell S, Reading AE, Cox DN, Sledmore CM, Mooney R, Chudleigh P, Beedle J, Ruddick H (1982). Ultrasound scannning in pregnancy: the short-term psychological effects of early real-time scans. J Psychosom Obstet Gynaecol, 1: 57–61.

Debdas AK, Kaur T, Menon H (1984). Monitoring high-risk pregnancy by maternal counting of foetal movements. J Indian Med Assoc, 82: 57–59.

Draper J, Field S, Thomas H, Hare MJ (1986). Women's views on keeping fetal movement charts. Br J Obstet Gynaecol, 93: 334–338.

Doll R, Peto R (1980). Randomized controlled trials and retrospective controls. Br Med J, 280: 44.

Ehrstrom C (1979). Fetal movement monitoring in normal and high-risk pregnancies. Acta Obstet Gynecol Scand, Suppl 80.

Ehrstrom C (1984). Circadian rhythm of fetal movements. Acta Obstet Gynecol Scand, 63: 539–541.

Elbourne D, Richardson M, Chalmers I, Waterhouse I, Holt E (1987). Newbury Maternity Care Study: a randomized controlled trial to evaluate a policy of women holding their own obstetric records. Br J Obstet Gynaecol, 94: 612–619.

Fischer S, Townsend-Fullerton J, Trezise L (1981). Fetal movement and fetal outcome in a low-risk population. J Nurs Midwifery, 26: 24–30.

Gelman SR, Spellacy WN, Wood S, Birk SA, Buhi WC (1980). Fetal movements and ultrasound: effect of maternal intravenous glucose administration. Am J Obstet Gynecol, 137: 459–461.

Gettinger A, Roberts AB, Campbell S (1978). Comparison between subjective and ultrasound assessments of fetal movement. Br Med J, 2: 88–90.

Grant A (1987). Risk of unexplained stillbirth at different gestational ages. Lancet, ii: 43–44.

Grant A, Elbourne D (1985). Compliance and maternal fetal movement counting. Lancet, 2: 1304.

Grant A, Hepburn M (1984). Merits of an individualized approach to fetal movement counting compared with fixed-time and fixed-number methods. Br J Obstet Gynaecol, 91: 1087–1090.

Grant A, Elbourne D, Ward S (1986). Multicentre Fetal Movements Trial. First progress report. Medical Research Council Fetal Movements Trial, June 1986. Oxford: National Perinatal Epidemiology Unit.

Grant A, Elbourne D, Ward S, Targett R (1987). Multicentre Fetal Movements Trial. Second progress report. Medical Research Council Fetal Movements Trial, January 1987. Oxford: National Perinatal Epidemiology Unit.

Grimwade J, Walker D, Bartlett M, Gordon S, Wood C (1971). Human fetal heart rate change and movement in response to sound and vibration. Am J Obstet Gynecol, 109: 86–90.

Harper RG, Greenberg M, Farahani G, Glassman I, Kierney CMP (1981). Fetal movements, biochemical and biophysical parameters, and the outcome of pregnancy. Am J Obstet Gynecol, 141: 39–42.

Henrion R, Heard I (1979). Surveillance du foetus *in utero* grace au compte des mouvements actifs. Nouv Presse Med, 8: 3113–3116.

Hertogs K, Roberts AB, Cooper D, Griffin DR, Campbell S (1979). Maternal perception of fetal motor activity. Br Med J, 2: 1183–1185.

Hertogs K, Roberts A, Campbell S (1981). Do fetal movements reflect fetal well-being? Br Med J, 282: 1153–1154.

Jarvis GJ, MacDonald HN (1979). Fetal movements in small-for-dates babies. Br J Obstet Gynaecol, 86: 724–727.

Koistinen E, Saarikoski S, Salmi A (1986). Liikkeiden laskenta sikion hyvinvoinnin seurantana. Suomen Laakarilehti, 41: 698–703.

Leader LR, Baillie P (1979). The accuracy of maternal observation of fetal movements. S Afr Med J, 55: 836–837.

Leader LR, Baillie P, van Schalkwyk DB (1981). Fetal movements and fetal outcome: a prospective study. Obstet Gynecol, 57: 431–436.

Liston RM, Cohen AW, Mennuti MT, Gabbe SG (1982). Antepartum fetal evaluation by maternal perception of fetal movement. Obstet Gynecol, 60: 424–426.

Lobb MO, Beazley JM, Haddad NG (1985). A controlled study of daily fetal movement counts in the prevention of stillbirths. J Obstet Gynaecol, 6: 87–91.

McIlwaine GM, Howat RCL, Dunn FH, MacNaughton MC (1979). Scotland 1977 Perinatal Mortality Survey. University of Glasgow.

McIlwaine GM, Howat RCL, Dunn FH, MacNaughton MC (1980). Perinatal practice and compensation for handicap. Br Med J, 281: 1067.

McIlwaine GM, Howat RCL, Dunn FH, MacNaughton MC (1983). Perinatal Mortality Statistics—Scotland 1981. University of Glasgow.

McIlwaine GM, Dunn FH, Howat RCL, Smalls M, Wyllie MM, Macnaughton MC (1984). The Scottish Perinatal Mortality Survey 1977–1981. University of Glasgow.

Mathews DD (1975). Maternal assessment of fetal activity in small-for-dates infants. Obstet Gynecol, 45: 488–493.

Miller FC, Skiba H, Klapholz H (1978). The effect of maternal blood sugar levels on fetal activity. Obstet Gynecol, 52: 663–665.

Minors DS, Waterhouse JM (1979). The effect of maternal posture, meals and time of day on fetal movements. Br J Obstet Gynaecol, 86: 717–723.

Neldam S (1980). Fetal movements as an indicator of fetal well-being. Lancet, 1: 1222–1224.

Neldam S (1982). Fetal movements. A comparison between maternal assessment and registration by means of dynamic ultrasound. Dan Med Bull, 29: 197–199.

Neldam S (1983). Fetal movements as an indicator of fetal well-being. Dan Med Bull, 30: 274–280.

O'Leary JA, Andrinopoulos GC (1981). Correlation of daily fetal movements and the nonstress test as tools for assessment of fetal welfare. Am J Obstet Gynecol, 139: 107–108.

Patrick J, Campbell K, Carmichael L, Natale R, Richardson B (1982). Patterns of gross fetal body movements over 24 hours observation intervals during the last 10 weeks of pregnancy. Am J Obstet Gynecol, 142: 363–371.

Payne PA, Gordon AN, Johnson TRB (1980). Fetal death without preceding movement. New Engl J Med, 303: 1419–1420.

Pearson JF (1979). Fetal movement recording: a guide to fetal well-being. Nursing Times, 75: 1639–1641.

Pearson JF, Weaver JB (1976). Fetal activity and fetal well-being: an evaluation. Br Med J, 1: 1305–1307.

Platt LD, Artal R, Semel J, Sipos L, Kammula RK (1983). Exercise in pregnancy II. Fetal responses. Am J Obstet Gynecol, 147: 487–491.

Playfair WS (1884). A Treatise on the Science and Practice of Midwifery, Vol. II (5th edn). London: Smith Elder.

Rayburn WF (1982). Antepartum fetal assessment: fetal activity monitoring. Clin Perinatol, 9: 231–252.

Rayburn WF, Barr M (1982). Activity patterns in malformed fetuses. Am J Obstet Gynecol, 142: 1045–1047.

Rayburn WF, McKean HE (1980). Maternal perception of fetal movement and perinatal outcome. Obstet Gynecol, 56: 161–164.

Rayburn WF, Zuspran F, Motley ME, Donaldson M (1980). An alternative to antepartum fetal heart rate testing. Am J Obstet Gynecol, 138: 223–226.

Reading AE, Campbell S, Cox DN, Sledmore CM (1982). Health beliefs and health care behaviour in pregnancy. Psychol Med, 12: 379–383.

Roberts AB, Little D, Cooper D, Campbell S (1979). Normal patterns of fetal activity in the third trimester. Br J Obstet Gynaecol, 86: 4–9.

Roberts AB, Griffin D, Mooney R, Cooper DJ, Campbell S (1980). Fetal activity in 100 normal third trimester pregnancies. Br J Obstet Gynaecol, 87: 480–484.

Rosen MG, Hertz RH, Dierker LJ, Zador I, Timor-Tritsch I (1979). Monitoring fetal movements. Clin Obstet Gynecol, 58: 325–334.

Sadovsky E (1978). What do movements of the fetus tell about its well-being? Contemporary OB/GYN, 12: 59.

Sadovsky E (1983). Antepartum monitoring of fetal movements. In: Modern Management of High-Risk Pregnancy. Lauerson NH (ed). Plenum Publishing Company, New York, pp 325–346.

Sadovsky E (1985). Monitoring fetal movement: a useful screening test. Contemporary OB/GYN, April: 1–6.

Sadovsky E, Yaffe H (1973). Daily fetal movement recording and fetal prognosis. Obstet Gynecol, 41: 845–850.

Sadovsky E, Yaffe H, Polishuk WZ (1974). Fetal movement monitoring in normal and pathologic pregnancy. Int J Gynaecol Obstet, 12: 75–79.

Sadovsky E, Rabinowitz R, Yaffe H (1981a). Decreased fetal movements and fetal malformations. J Fetal Med, 1: 62–64.

Sadovsky E, Weinstein D, Evin Y (1981b). Antepartum fetal evaluation by assessment of fetal heart rate and fetal movements. Int J Gynecol Obstet, 19: 21–26.

Sadovsky E, Ohel G, Harazeleth H, Steinwell A, Penchas S (1983). The definition and the significance of decreased fetal movements. Acta Obstet Gynecol Scand, 62: 409–413.

Schmidt W, Csch I, Hara K, Kubli F (1984). Maternal perception of fetal movements and real-time ultrasound findings. J Perinat Med, 12: 313–318.

Scottish Health Services Agency, Information Services Division. Perinatal Mortality Survey 1983. Edinburgh.

Scottish Health Services Agency, Information Services Division. Perinatal Mortality Survey 1984. Edinburgh.

Scottish Health Services Agency, Information Services Division. Scottish Stillbirth and Neonatal Death Report 1985. Edinburgh.

Thompson SL, Wheeler T (1985). Compliance and maternal fetal movement counting. Lancet, 2: 1122.

Timor-Tritsch IE, Dierker LJ, Hertz RH, Deagan NC, Rosen MG (1978). Studies of antepartum behavioural state in the human fetus at term. Am J Obstet Gynecol, 132: 524–528.

Valentin L (1986). Fetal movements in late pregnancy—detection of fetal jeopardy by objective recording and maternal counting. Doctoral dissertation, University of Lund, Sweden.

Valentin L, Marsal K (1986). Subjective recording of fetal movements. II. Screening of a pregnant population; methodological aspects. Acta Obstet Gynecol Scand, 65: 639–644.

Valentin L, Marsal K (1987). Pregnancy outcome in women perceiving decreased fetal movements. Eur J Obstet Gynecol Reprod Biol, 24: 23–32.

Valentin L, Lofgren O, Marsal K, Gullberg B (1984). Subjective recording of fetal movements. I. Limits and acceptability in normal pregnancies. Acta Obstet Gynecol Scand, 63: 223–228.

Valentin L, Marsal K, Wahlgren L (1986). Subjective recording of fetal movements. III. Screening of a pregnant population; the clinical significance of decreased fetal movement counts. Acta Obstet Gynecol Scand, 65: 753–758.

Westgate J, Jamieson M (1986). Stillbirths and fetal movements. NZ Med J, 99: 114–116.

Wood C, Gilbert M, O'Connor A, Walters WAW (1979). Subjective recording of fetal movements. Br J Obstet Gynaecol, 86: 836–842.

Yudkin PL, Wood L, Redman CWG (1987). Risk of unexplained stillbirth at different gestational ages. Lancet, i: 1192–1194.

Zimmer EZ, Peretz BA, Marcovici R, Goldstein I, Eyal A, Paldi E (1982). Correlation of fetal movements with maternal posture. J Obstet Gynaecol, 3: 85–86.

29 Biochemical assessment of fetal well-being

Sophie Alexander, Rosalind Stanwell-Smith, Pierre Buekens, and Marc J. N. C. Keirse

'I have no clear idea what I am looking for, but in ordering this test I feel in a vague way (like Mr Micawber) that something might turn up'

Richard Asher (1954).

1 Introduction

A wide range of biochemical tests of fetal well-being have been introduced during the last 50 years, but there is little agreement on their usefulness. Preferences for one biochemical test or another have changed to encompass a variety of substances, such as steroids, protein hormones, enzymes, and fetal and placental proteins. In sharp contrast to other branches of medicine, where tests of liver function, for instance, have not markedly changed in 30 years, biochemical tests for 'placental function' or 'fetal well-being' have changed radically over this period of time. In 1965, Greene *et al.* (1965) listed more than 20 biochemical tests of placental function, including maternal serum proteins, alkaline phosphatase, diamine oxidase, and Rose–Waaler titres. Only two of these (human chorionic gonadotrophin and oestriol) were still found on a similar list compiled by Chard and Klopper (1982) 17 years later.

In addition to the difference in the tests used over time, there is a wide variation in the frequency of their use from country to country and from institution to institution. In some countries their use continues unabated; in others they have largely been replaced by biophysical tests of fetal well-being (see Chapter 30).

The concept underlying all of these tests has remained remarkably similar throughout the years, in that 'accurate measurement of . . . metabolic changes should logically be useful in the determination of the fetal status . . . and could help reduce perinatal mortality and morbidity and contribute to the solution of problems of mental retardation, cerebral palsy and congenital malformation' (Greene *et al.* 1965). Many authors also felt confident that such tests would allow not only evaluation of the fetal condition at the time of the test, but also the prediction of complications later on. As far back as 1933, Smith and Smith reported that 'total oestrogenic proportion of blood and urine fails to rise, or decreases over a 3 to 8 week period before clinical signs of toxemia . . . ' (see Chapter 38).

The range of tests currently available, and the theoretical bases for using them, has been well-described elsewhere (MacNaughton 1967; Diczfalusy 1974; Goebelsman 1979; Tulchinsky 1980; Chard and Klopper 1982; Fuchs and Klopper 1983; Grudzinskas *et al.* 1986; Westergaard *et al.* 1986). These tests have increased our knowledge and understanding of fetal and placental physiology and endocrinology. This does not necessarily mean that the use of these tests in clinical practice confers any benefit to the individual women and babies on whom they are performed.

If, in reviewing commonly used biochemical tests of fetal well-being, we were to restrict attention to the tests that have been evaluated by randomized trials the subject would be rapidly covered. Indeed, only two such trials (Spellacy *et al.* 1975; Duenhoelter *et al.* 1976) have been published. For that reason we will examine the available data on the basis of the general principles outlined in Chapter 3, limiting our attention to those tests that are still in reasonably common use. A large proportion of the clinical research on biochemical tests used for assessment of fetal well-being does not provide data in a form that allows construction of 2×2 tables (see Chapter 3) from which the test properties, and the predictive values in particular, can be calculated. For each of these tests for which appropriate categorical data were available we have constructed sets of 2×2 tables for some of the outcome measures studied. In the construction of these tables we used the numbers of subjects for whom data were reported in the results section of the papers. On occasions, these may therefore differ somewhat from the numbers stated by the authors in the methods or summary sections of their papers.

In general, biochemical tests have been used for screening, for diagnostic follow-up, and for deciding on the need for intervention. The purposes of biochemical screening procedures range from the detection of abnormalities that are already present (e.g. alpha-fetoprotein screening for neural tube defects), to the prediction of anomalies that may subsequently occur (e.g. urinary oestrogens for low Apgar scores; Gerhard *et al.* 1986). A large number of outcomes has been screened for or addressed by the various tests. It has often been difficult to determine to what extent the tests were used for each of these purposes, or for which outcome measures. Most published reports refer to several of these aspects at the same time, and frequently it is quite impossible to subdivide them.

2 Oestrogens

The formation and metabolism of oestrogens in pregnancy has been extensively investigated (for review see Lauritzen and Klopper 1983). Several oestrogens (total oestrogen, oestriol, oestriol conjugates, oestetrol, etc.) have been proposed as markers of fetal well-being and/or feto-placental function. Theoretically, oestetrol should have advantages over most other compounds for assessment of fetal well-being, because it is produced solely by the fetus (Tulchinsky *et al.* 1975). The clinical studies, on the other hand, indicate that the information provided by oestetrol assays is not markedly different from that provided by the more widely used oestriol measurements (Heikkilä and Luukkainen 1971; Tulchinsky *et al.* 1975; Notation and Tagatz 1977). Oestriol has been the most widely investigated oestrogen in pregnancy, although before the advent of the radioimmunoassay most studies dealt with total urinary oestrogen. In our review of the available literature we have not been able to discover marked differences in terms of clinical utility between these measures. Therefore this section deals mainly with the measurement of oestriol in pregnancy; data on total oestrogen measurements are added to complete the picture.

2.1 Variables affecting oestrogen levels and their measurement

Most precursors of oestriol are formed by the fetal adrenal. Oestriol production is thus profoundly reduced in case of fetal adrenal hypoplasia, a condition that can occur in isolation or in association with fetal anencephaly (Ostergard 1973). Suppression of adrenal function by maternal ingestion of high doses of corticosteroids also reduces oestriol production (Bolognese *et al.* 1972).

An essential step in the biosynthesis of oestriol in the placenta is the hydrolysis of steroid sulphates derived from the fetus. Placental sulphatase deficiency will reduce plasma concentrations of oestriol to 5 per cent or less of its mean value (Harkness *et al.* 1983). This condition is associated with X-linked ichthyosis and delayed onset of labour. It occurs in 1 per 2000 to 6000 pregnancies and can be diagnosed by the dehydroepiandrosterone sulphate loading test (Bradshaw and Carr 1986). This test has formerly been advocated as a dynamic measure of feto-placental function (Lauritzen 1967) but its value for this purpose has not withstood the test of time (Korda *et al.* 1975; Fraser *et al.* 1976).

The maternal liver and kidney influence oestriol conjugation and excretion. Liver failure, modification of renal plasma flow, decreased renal clearance and altered tubular excretion can modify oestriol concentrations (Ostergard 1973). Variations over time in circulating oestriol levels have been described even in normal pregnancies, but the evidence for a circadian rhythm has been conflicting (Houghton *et al.* 1983). Various drugs, most notably antibiotics, depress oestrogen levels during pregnancy (Van Look *et al.* 1981) and it is accepted that this depression results from interference with the normal enterohepatic cycle of steroids. A similar interference has been found in vegetarian women (Adlercreutz *et al.* 1986). Administration of frequently used drugs, such as phenobarbitone (Hardy and Basalammah 1981) and aspirin (Castellanos *et al.* 1975) can also influence urinary oestriol excretion.

Another important issue is the choice between urine and blood for the measurement of oestriol. Several studies compared concurrent use of blood and urine. Some (e.g. Miller *et al.* 1977) claimed a strong correlation between the two, whereas others did not (Aickin *et al.* 1974; Katagiri *et al.* 1976). The difference in performance between blood and urinary measurements appears to relate more to differences in laboratory technique and experience than to which of the two measurements is clinically superior. This is true also for differences in the collection and assay techniques that are used. The determination of unconjugated oestriol in blood does not appear to offer clinical advantages over the simpler determination of total oestriol (Perry *et al.* 1984; Nielsen *et al.* 1985). In urine, the case for early morning urine vs. 24-hour urine specimens remains to be proven, though it should be noted that 24-hour collection of urine seriously interferes with the daily activity of pregnant women. Seibel *et al.* (1982) found little correlation between the single first morning specimen and one collected over 24 hours; but Aubry *et al.* (1975) found 'excellent correlation' in the oestriol/creatinine ratio between a random early morning urine sample and the 24-hour specimen. Neither of these studies examined test performance with regard to outcome of pregnancy and good comparison between these methods in terms of pregnancy outcome are not available. Salivary total oestriol measurements reflect the concentrations of serum oestriol and could be an alternative to urine or blood assays (Vining *et al.* 1983; Cusick *et al.* 1986), but again, their clinical utility remains unevaluated.

2.2 Test characteristics

The large majority of the studies on oestrogen measurements that have been reported in the last 40 years, do not provide data in a form that allows assessment of the test properties in 2 × 2 tables. Most of the studies that allow construction of 2 × 2 tables deal with oestrogen measurement in high risk populations, studying women with hypertension, diabetes, poor obstetric history, and clinically suspected intrauterine growth retardation. The number of women in these studies ranged from less than 10, to 1000. To compare this wide range of studies, tables were constructed for various outcome measures, the commonest being perinatal mortality, intrauterine growth retardation (generally defined as birth weight for gestational age below the 10th centile), and fetal distress (usually defined as low Apgar score at delivery, abnormal fetal heart rate patterns, or the presence of meconium). Other outcome measures have also been considered by some authors; for instance, Stovall *et al.* (1985) suggested that a serum oestriol higher than 15 mg/ml was a good predictor of pulmonary maturity.

2.2.1 Perinatal mortality

Ten of the 15 studies listed in Table 29.1 showed a perinatal mortality rate that was at least twice as high in

Table 29.1 Test properties of oestriol and total oestrogen measurements for prediction of perinatal mortality

Authors	No. of women	No. high risk	% Prevalence	Range of gestation (weeks)	No. of samples	Sensitivity	Specificity	Positive predictive value	Negative predictive value
Greene and Touchstone (1963)	32	32	31	?	2+	100	36	42	100
Hausknecht (1967)	122	122	13	35–40	3+	93	72	34	99
Macleod *et al.* (1967)	103	103	7	14–42	1+	100	76	23	100
Beischer and Brown (1968)	597	—	—	13–42+	4+	44	89	8	99
Corson and Bolognese (1968)	81	81	5	?	1–4	75	62	7	98
Heys *et al.* (1968)	403	403	4	⩾26	2+	78	41	24	88
Heys *et al.* (1969)	42	42	17	?	?	86	46	24	94
Frandsen *et al.* (1970)	1001	–	7	?	1–6+	60	94	42	97
Watney *et al.* (1970)	180	180	5	?	3+	64	—	—	—
Hoag (1971)	194	194	7	33–37	1–2+	88	100	100	94
Campbell and Kurjak (1972)	284	284	5	?	3+	64	—	—	—
Targett *et al.* (1973)	1000	—	2	30–36	1–4	50	87	8	99
Aickin *et al.* (1974)	285	166	5	15–45	4	67	79	15	98
Trudinger *et al.* (1979)	60	60	2	⩾33	?	29	88	64	—
Khouzami *et al.* (1981)	677	677	1	⩾42	2+	67	92	7	100

women with low oestrogens (post-test probability) than in the total population studied (pre-test probability). It is therefore easy to understand the enthusiasm for oestrogen assays that prevailed in the 1960s and 1970s, which led to statements such as 'Now that the test has been shown to be a valuable guide in the management of pregnancy, the next step is to set up the measurement as a routine procedure . . .' (Macleod *et al.* 1967).

Yet, any attempt to synthesize the data in Table 29.1 is unrealistic because of the heterogeneity of the studies, which can easily be appreciated from the table. Although 12 of the 15 reports purported to relate to high-risk populations, the prevalence of perinatal death in the population at risk ranged from 10 to 310 per 1000. When a wide range of gestational ages was studied, the population sometimes included women with diagnoses of hydatidiform mole and lethal malformations. Often little attention was given to gestational age, or to whether single or multiple determinations were made. The possibility of an intervention effect (see Chapter 3) was present in all studies since only one of them (Macleod *et al.* 1967) specifically stated that results were 'generally ignored in the management of pregnancy'.

Studies of plasma oestriol (Aickin *et al.* 1974; Bashore and Westlake 1977; Gabbe and Hagerman 1978; Hagerman 1979; Lindberg *et al.* 1974; Isouard 1979; Trudinger *et al.* 1979) produced estimates of sensitivity, specificity and predictive values which were similar to those found for urinary oestrogens. Specificity was generally higher than sensitivity. In all of the studies the positive predictive value was low, ranging from 3 to 22 per cent, with the exception of the study by Trudinger *et al.* (1979), which gave a positive predictive value of 83 per cent.

2.2.2 *Low birthweight and low birthweight for gestational age*

The prediction of low birthweight for gestational age by oestrogen measurement was examined in a large number of studies. Most investigators defined low birthweight for gestational age as a birthweight below the 10th centile of weight for gestation in a defined standard population. In the studies dealing with urinary oestrogen assays (Table 29.2) sensitivity varied between 14 per cent (Gerhard *et al.* 1986) and 86 per cent (Low *et al.* 1973), although some reported a higher sensitivity in subgroup analyses. Michie (1967), for instance, reported a sensitivity of 100 per cent in a subgroup of 38 women with mild to moderate pre-eclampsia, but in 14 women with severe pre-eclampsia the sensitivity was only 67 per cent, which indicates the fallacies inherent in subgroup analyses. Specificity ranged from 63 per cent (Petrucco *et al.* 1973) to 94 per cent (Beischer *et al.* 1969). The test properties of the plasma and serum assays (Table 29.3) were comparable to those of urinary assays. In the majority of the studies, the incidence of low weight for gestational age was twice the population value. As with the studies on perinatal mortality, the assays were done at a wide range of gestational ages and the measurements were usually serial rather than a single estimation. In only one (Nielsen 1983) of the studies listed in Tables 29.2 and 29.3, was it reported that the clinicians caring for

Table 29.2 Test properties of urinary oestriol and total oestrogen measurements for prediction of low birthweight and low weight for gestational age

Authors and year	No. of women	No. high risk	% Prevalence	Range of gestation (weeks)	No. of samples	Sensitivity	Specificity	Positive predictive value	Negative predictive value
Michie (1967)	130	130	21	35–42	?1	67	90	64	91
Fliegner *et al.* (1969)	80	80	28	≥35	?	64	83	58	86
Beischer *et al.* (1969)	195	195	73	14–44	2+	68	94	86	85
Heys *et al.* (1969)	290	290	10	?	?	50	90	38	94
Frandsen *et al.* (1970)	823	—	14	?	1–6	41	92	46	88
Watney *et al.* (1970)	168	168	26	?	2+	67	85	60	88
Campbell and Kurjak (1972)	284	284	31	?	2+	53	83	58	80
Dickey *et al.* (1972)	563	80	11	26–40	1–2+	59	90	43	95
Low *et al.* (1973)	423	423	15	≥34	3–9	86	90	55	97
Petrucco *et al.* (1973)	17	17	35	28–35	3+	67	63	50	78
	59	59	37	34–40	3+	86	76	68	90
Targett *et al.* (1973)	1000	—	12	30–36	1–4	30	89	27	90
Aickin *et al.* (1974)	285	166	15	15–45	4	55	82	36	91
Kunz and Keller (1976a)	83	83	18	28–40	10	67	—	—	—
Laatikainen and Peltonen (1980)	12	12	29	33–41	1	50	—	—	—
Gerhard *et al.* (1986)	654	?	?	28–34	1	19	92	—	—
	397	?	?	35–41	1+	14	94	—	—

Table 29.3 Test properties of plasma and serum oestriol assays for prediction of low birthweight and low weight for gestational age

Authors and year	No. of women	No. high risk	% Prevalence	Range of gestation (weeks)	No. of samples	Sensitivity	Specificity	Positive predictive value	Negative predictive value
Aickin *et al.* (1974)	285	166	15	15–45	4	66	72	30	92
Linberg *et al.* (1974)	88	88	15	⩾35	?	31	67	29	88
Hagerman (1974)	169	169	14	29–44	2+	42	79	24	90
Edwards *et al.* (1976)	369	369	23	⩾35	1+	57	93	71	88
Nielsen *et al.* (1985)	800	0	5	37–43	1+	15	96	15	96
	242	242	11	?	1+	27	98	58	92
Gerhard *et al.* (1986)	869	?	?	28–34	1	23	91	—	—
	423	?	?	35–41	1+	31	85	—	—
Sagen *et al.* (1984b)	74	74	34	31–41	1+	55	82	79	61
Chard *et al.* (1985)	392	147	10	⩾36	1	28	91	26	92
					3	33	91	30	93

these pregnancies had no knowledge of the assay results.

2.2.3 Fetal/neonatal morbidity

Several of the studies that we reviewed related oestrogen assays to fetal or neonatal morbidity. Some used urinary oestrogen (Beischer and Brown 1968; Beisher *et al.* 1969; Campbell and Kurjak 1972; Dooley *et al.* 1984; Fliegner *et al.* 1969; Greene and Touchstone 1963; Keller *et al.* 1971), some used plasma or serum measurements (Bashore and Westlake 1977; Hagerman 1979; Persson *et al.* 1980; Sagen *et al.* 1984b; Yeh and Read 1983), and one used both urinary and serum assays (Gerhard *et al.* 1986). No two studies, however, used the same criteria for defining fetal or neonatal morbidity. Where low Apgar score was taken as the endpoint, the definition of abnormality ranged from a score of less than 3 at 2 minutes after birth (Fliegner *et al.* 1969), to less than 9 at 1 minute after birth (Gerhard *et al.* 1986). Hagerman (1979) used neonatal 'asphyxia' or development of respiratory distress syndrome as the outcome measure. The outcome measure reported by Yeh and Read (1983) was dysmaturity, the latter being defined as the presence of one of the following criteria: oligohydramnios with meconium-stained amniotic fluid; neonatal examination indicating signs of dysmaturity; Roher's ponderal index—100 × weight in grams divided by length in cm^3—of less than 2.3 associated with meconium-stained amniotic fluid. As these examples indicate, the studies are so heterogeneous that any attempt to synthesize the results would be meaningless.

2.3 Evidence of clinical usefulness

2.3.1 Randomized trial

Over a hundred studies conducted in 15 countries during the last 40 years were consulted for this review. Only one of these was a randomized trial (Duenhoelter *et al.* 1976). In that study the authors set out to demonstrate whether perinatal mortality could be reduced with knowledge of the results of plasma oestriol. A series of 622 women with high-risk pregnancy (hypertension, diabetes, suspected fetal growth retardation, previous history of fetal wastage, post-maturity, and other complications) between 28 and 40 weeks of gestation were randomly assigned to two groups on the basis of their chart numbers. Plasma oestriol was serially measured in both groups but in only one group were the results reported to the clinician. In the group for whom results were reported a special notice was also issued when results were consistently low or falling. A total of 4678 samples were measured, which amounts to an average of 7.5 per pregnancy. Yet, the analysis (Table 29.4) shows that knowledge of oestriol levels did not result in any detectable effect on either perinatal mortality or the rate of elective delivery (whether by caesarean section or by induction of labour).

2.3.2 Studies using historical controls

Similar conclusions have been reached from studies using historical controls in which pregnancy outcomes were compared within the same institution in two consecutive periods. General care during pregnancy was believed to have been similar for the comparison groups, except that oestrogen assays were no longer used in the second period. Two such studies have been published (Chamberlain 1984; Sharf *et al.* 1984). One study (Chamberlain 1984) reported on a total hospital population during a period of systematic use of oestrogen assays for hospitalized women and during the period after the test was abandoned. A perinatal mortality rate of 23 per 1000 was found in the period when oestrogen assays were routinely used, and a rate of 17 per 1000 after they were abandoned. Sharf *et al.* (1984) studied the outcome of 306 hypertensive pregnancies;

Table 29.4 Effect of serial plasma oestriol measurements in high risk pregnancies on elective delivery

Study	EXPT		CTRL		Odds ratio	Graph of odds ratios and confidence intervals
	n	(%)	*n*	(%)	(95% CI)	0.01 0.1 0.5 1 2 10 100
Duenhoelter *et al.* (1976)	141/315	(44.76)	142/307	(46.25)	0.94 (0.69–1.29)	
Typical odds ratio (95% confidence interval)					0.94 (0.69–1.29)	

Effect of serial plasma oestriol measurements in high risk pregnancies on perinatal death (excluding congenital malformation)

Study	EXPT		CTRL		Odds ratio	Graph of odds ratios and confidence intervals
Duenhoelter *et al.* (1976)	6/312	(1.92)	8/305	(2.62)	0.73 (0.25–2.10)	
Typical odds ratio (95% confidence interval)					0.73 (0.25–2.10)	

154 were managed with serum oestriol assays and 152 without. There were no differences detected in perinatal mortality or in any of the indices of fetal and neonatal morbidity investigated.

2.4 Conclusion

On the basis of the available studies, there is little evidence to support earlier optimistic statements that 'the value of oestrogen assay is well established' (Dickey *et al.* 1972). It would seem that oestriol assays may occasionally be helpful, for instance when there is a need to rule out or confirm conditions such as placental sulphatase deficiency or fetal adrenal hypoplasia. On the whole, however, they contribute little if anything to effective care in pregnancy.

3 Human placental lactogen

Human placental lactogen, previously known as human chorionic somatomammotrophin, was first identified in 1955 (Gemzell *et al.* 1955) and was introduced on a large scale as a test of fetal well-being in the early 1970s (for extensive review see Josimovich 1983).

3.1 Variables affecting human placental lactogen levels and their measurement

Serum levels of human placental lactogen vary with the time of day and with the onset of labour (Pavlou *et al.* 1972). Variations are more marked with long fasting (Tyson *et al.* 1971) or hypoglycaemia (Gaspard *et al.* 1974). A very small number of pregnancies with total absence of human placental lactogen and a normal outcome have been reported (Barbieri *et al.* 1986). When compared to oestrogens, human placental lactogen has the theoretical advantage that it does not undergo complex metabolic transformations that may complicate interpretation of the data.

3.2 Test characteristics

A number of studies have documented the use of human placental lactogen in a manner that allows

Table 29.5 Test properties of human placental lactogen measurements for prediction of the outcome of theratened abortion

Authors and year	No. of women	% Prevalence	Range of gestation (weeks)	No. of samples	Sensitivity	Specificity	Positive predictive value	Negative predictive value
Gartside and Tindall (1975	191	48	<20	1	96	89	88	89
Kunz and Keller (1976b)	65	66	6–20	1	79	64	81	61
Hertz (1984)	173	46	6–19	1	?	?	90	74
				serial	?	?	100	90
Westergaard *et al.* (1985)								
All women	108	39	7–20	1	17	67	24	56
				serial	21	71	32	59
Fetal heart positive	77	14	7–20	1	18	92	29	87
				serial	36	92	44	89

Table 29.6 Test properties of human placental lactogen measurements for prediction of low birthweight for gestational age

Authors and year	No. of women	No. high risk	% Prevalence	Range of gestation (weeks)	No. of samples	Sensitivity	Specificity	Positive predictive value	Negative predictive value
England *et al.* (1974)	438	—	2	38–42	?	56	93	14	99
Edwards *et al.* (1976)	383	383	22	≥35	1+	78	83	58	93
Harrigan *et al.* (1976)	53	—	9	37–42	?	80	96	67	98
	47	47	36	37–42	?	94	90	84	96
Kunz and Keller (1976a)	83	83	18	28–40	6	53	68	38	87
Hensleigh *et al.* (1977)	58	58	36	≥20	±9	71	49	44	75
Gohari et al. (1978)	111	111	34	?	?	37	90	67	62
Zlatnik* *et al.* (1979)	806	242	2	34–43	1+	17	95	7	98
Morrison *et al.* (1980)	148	148	15	30–40	≤12	41	84	31	89
Persson *et al.* (1980)	93	—	11	16–42	8–11	10	100	100	89
Nielsen *et al.* (1981)	1050	244	6	20–40	2+	13	98	33	95
	263	263	12	20–40	2+	25	96	47	90
Odendaal *et al.* (1981)	77	77	57	?	?	81	57	69	68
Obiekwe and Chard (1983)	522	—	10	36–40	1	25	91	27	90
Sagen *et al.* (1984b)	74	74	54	?	twice weekly	70	82	82	70
Westergaard *et al.* (1984a)	208	?	16	20	1	39	89	32	87
	325	?	10	30	1	36	89	28	93
	392	?	7	35	1	54	90	28	96

*In the study of Zlatnik *et al.* results were not reported to the clinician before delivery.

Table 29.7 Test properties of human placental lactogen measurements for prediction of a variety of 'poor outcome' measures

Authors and year	No. of women	No. high risk	% Prevalence	Range of gestation (weeks)	No. of samples	Sensitivity	Specificity	Positive predictive value	Negative predictive value
Letchworth and Chard (1972)	333	133	8	≥33	serial	52	87	52	94
England *et al.* (1974)	547	—	12	42		29	93	36	91
Harrigan *et al.* (1976)	94	41	19	37–42	?	74	81	48	93
Letchworth *et al.* (1978)	972	951	2	32–40	serial	76	95	25	95
Gordon *et al.* (1978)	1029	104	10	20–40	?	18	91	18	91
Trudinger *et al.* (1979)	60	60		≥33	?	42	89	71	—
Zlatnik *et al.* (1979)	806	242	13	≥34	1+	6	94	13	87
Leader and Baillie (1980)	135	135	6	30–42	weekly	63	86	22	97
Persson *et al.* (1980)	93	—	17	16–42	8–11	6	100	100	84
Nielsen *et al.* (1981)	806	0	2	26–35	3+	44	75	3	99
	244	0	3	26–35	3+	88	67	8	99
	263	263	7	26–35	3+	53	66	10	95
Obiekwe and Chard (1983)	421	—	7	36–40	1	17	89	9	—
Gerhard and Runnebaum (1984)	844	—	12	8–16	1	62	64	18	—
Sagen *et al.* (1984b)	74	74	54	?	twice weekly	68	79	79	68

assessment of test properties and these are shown in Tables 29.5, 29.6, and 29.7.

3.2.1 Miscarriage

Studies on women admitted with threatened abortion have shown positive predictive values with single measurements of human placental lactogen of between 81 and 90 per cent, and negative predictive values ranging from 61 to 89 per cent (Table 29.5). Although this may appear promising, the study of Westergaard *et al.* (1985) showed that there was a marked difference in the test properties when applied to pregnancies with a live or dead fetus on ultrasound. This information can now be readily obtained with accuracy, and human placental lactogen measurements must be regarded as pointless in the presence of a dead fetus. One study (Gerhard and Runnebaum 1984) examined the value of human placental lactogen measurements, in the absence of bleeding, between 8 and 16 weeks in a population of 844 women. Twelve per cent of them subsequently miscarried. With a cut-off point for normality set at the 5th centile, these authors obtained a specificity of 62 per cent and a sensitivity of 64 per cent. As the positive predictive value was 18 per cent this implies that the likelihood of miscarriage with a human placental lactogen level below the 5th centile was 18 per cent compared with 12 per cent in the entire group of women irrespective of human placental lactogen results.

3.2.2 Low birthweight and low birthweight for gestational age

Human placental lactogen assay has been used to predict low birthweight for gestational age in several studies (Table 29.6). The results are similar to those discussed for oestrogen assays and neither test appears to be very effective in predicting this outcome. Again, the wide gestational range, the heterogeneity of the women studied, and the differing definitions of low birthweight or low weight for gestational age limit the possibilities for drawing any conclusions about the usefulness of human placental lactogen measurements in this respect.

3.2.3 Other measures of poor fetal or neonatal outcome

Human placental lactogen measurements have been utilized in the hope of predicting a variety of poor outcomes (Table 29.7). In only 4 of the studies mentioned in Table 29.7 were the results of the assays withheld until the pregnancy had ended, and in the study of Nielsen *et al.* (1981), this applied only to the group of women with apparently normal pregnancies. In the high-risk pregnancies human placental lactogen results were always disclosed and used in management (Nielsen and Schioler 1981). The study of Persson *et al.* (1980) also compared measurement with other monitoring tests in a sample of 93 'randomly chosen' women. The authors commented that human placental lactogen performed less well than measurement of the fetal biparietal diameter by ultrasound and alpha-fetoprotein measurements in distinguishing 'normal outcome' from 'poor outcome', which in this study also included 'prematurity' as well as 'birth asphyxia'.

The wide disparity of outcomes, populations studied, and cut off-levels of normality is such that no two studies are alike. As with oestrogen determinations, no valid conclusions can be derived from such comparisons as reported in Table 29.7.

3.3 Evidence of clinical usefulness

There has been only one randomized intervention study of human placental lactogen measurement (Spellacy *et al.* 1975). This study was mounted after a retrospective survey of perinatal deaths in a 6-year period had suggested that low human placental lactogen levels had preceded over half of the fetal deaths reviewed. A total of 2733 women with high risk pregnancies were assigned to two different groups on the basis of the last digit of their hospital chart number. Human placental lactogen measurements were performed at each visit in all women, but in half of them (the control group) the results were not reported to the clinician before the pregnancy had ended. In the experimental group abnormal human placental lactogen values were reported promptly to a perinatology fellow who then tagged the woman's case record, reviewed her notes and recalled her for a control visit and a repeat human placental lactogen determination. If the fetus was considered to be mature and the repeat measurement was also low, action was undertaken to expedite delivery.

The results shown in Table 29.8 suggest, on first inspection, that revealing the results of human placental lactogen measurements to a clinician armed with a predetermined intervention programme statistically significantly reduced fetal and perinatal mortality. These data, however, relate only to the 8 per cent (4 per cent in each group) of pregnancies that had abnormal human placental lactogen values. Data on the large majority of pregnancies (92 per cent) that did not belong to that category were not reported and are no longer available (Spellacy, personal communication 1988).

The data thus indicate that, when abnormal human placental lactogen values are obtained, it is better to

Table 29.8 Effect of routine human placental lactogen measurements in high-risk pregnancies on perinatal death

Study	EXPT		CTRL		Odds ratio	Graph of odds ratios and confidence intervals
	n	(%)	*n*	(%)	(95% CI)	0.01 0.1 0.5 1 2 10 100
Spellacy *et al.* (1975)	4/117	(3.42)	17/113	(15.04)	0.25 (0.10–0.61)	
Typical odds ratio (95% confidence interval)					0.25 (0.10–0.61)	

Table 29.9 Effect of revealing placental function test result on perinatal morality when test is abnormal

Study	EXPT		CTRL		Odds ratio	Graph of odds ratios and confidence intervals
	n	(%)	*n*	(%)	(95% CI)	0.01 0.1 0.5 1 2 10 100
Duenhoelter *et al.* (1976)	4/52	(7.69)	8/53	(15.09)	0.48 (0.15–1.60)	
Spellacy *et al.* (1975)	4/117	(3.42)	17/113	(15.04)	0.25 (0.10–0.61)	
Typical odds ratio (95% confidence interval)					0.32 (0.15–0.65)	
Effect of revealing placental function test result on perinatal morality when test is normal						
Duenhoelter *et al.* (1976)	4/263	(1.52)	2/254	(0.79)	1.89 (0.38–9.46)	
Typical odds ratio (95% confidence interval)					1.89 (0.38–9.46)	
Effect of revealing placental function test result on perinatal mortality—all pregnancies						
Duenhoelter *et al.* (1976)	8/315	(2.54)	10/307	(3.26)	0.77 (0.30–1.98)	
Typical odds ratio (95% confidence interval)					0.77 (0.30–1.98)	

reveal them to the clinician than to conceal them. They do not indicate, however, whether the provision of normal human placental lactogen measurements results in false clinical reassurance with possible harmful effects to the women and babies concerned. Although the data of this trial are often believed to indicate that human placental lactogen measurements are beneficial for the surveillance of high risk pregnancy, one cannot exclude the possibility that the benefits found in pregnancies with abnormal values were counterbalanced or outweighed by negative effects in pregnancies with normal values. Sub-analyses, like the one found in this trial, which report outcomes for only 8 per cent of the women entered, have the potential for suggesting differences that do not, in fact, exist. For instance, if the data of Duenhoelter *et al.* (1976) referred to earlier (Table 29.4) had been reported in a similar way, i.e. giving data only on pregnancies with abnormal test results, this trial too would have suggested the biochemical test to be useful in reducing perinatal mortality, as illustrated in Table 29.9

3.4 Conclusion

Despite the unsatisfactory evidence concerning its usefulness as a screening procedure or as a diagnostic test, human placental lactogen measurements have acquired great popularity. In part, this can be attributed to the infectious enthusiasm and optimism exuded by proponents of this test. In part, it relates to the easily remembered single cut-off point of 4 mg/ml that was popularized early on, and that appeared to have proved its usefulness in the only randomized controlled trial that was ever reported on this subject (Spellacy *et al.* 1975).

4 Alpha-fetoprotein

Alpha-fetoprotein is a specific fetal protein that was reported for the first time by Bergstrand and Csar in 1956. It is secreted by the fetal liver and is one of the two major proteins in the fetal circulation. Its concentration in various maternal biological compartments depends both on fetal liver secretion and on its rate of escape from the fetal circulation to glomeruli, fetal urine, amniotic fluid, and finally to the maternal circulation. Any form of increased leakage can lead to abnormally high levels of maternal serum alpha-fetoprotein. This metabolic characteristic has been used widely for antenatal screening of neural tube defects and other congenital malformations (see Chapter 23). Later, investigators became interested in the outcome of pregnancies that had abnormal alpha-fetoprotein levels and no detectable malformation. It was observed that low birthweight occurred more frequently in this group of pregnancies (Brock *et al.* 1977; Wald *et al.* 1977) and interest was generated in the assay as a predictor of fetal well-being.

4.1 Variables affecting alpha-fetoprotein levels and their measurement

Alpha-fetoprotein levels increase rapidly during the

16th to 20th week of pregnancy, the time when routine screening is performed. This means that an error in gestational age will have a great influence on whether the test is truly or only seemingly abnormal. Roberts *et al.* (1979) suggested that 10 per cent of abnormal results could be reversed to normal by a change of as little as one week in the estimate of gestational age. A short term variation has been described by Houghton *et al.* (1983). This variation within the same individual is in the order of about 10 per cent; it shows no diurnal pattern and cannot be solely attributed to inter-assay variation. This variation may explain why an 'abnormal' alpha-fetoprotein level frequently reverts to 'normal' on second sampling. In multiple gestation, alpha-fetoprotein levels, like all other biochemical markers of fetal well-being, are increased. In twin pregnancies, monozygous pairs produce a significantly higher maternal alpha-fetoprotein level than dizygous pairs (Wald *et al.* 1979).

Amniocentesis leads to a rise in alpha-fetoprotein level in 7 per cent of women (Lachman *et al.* 1977), while a rise over 40 per cent could be detected in 75 per cent of women undergoing chorionic villus sampling (Mariona *et al.* 1986).

4.2 Usefulness as a screening test for fetal well-being

4.2.1 General considerations

Alpha-fetoprotein screening has mainly been validated for neural tube defects. From early on, attention was drawn to the outcome of women with a high alpha-fetoprotein level but whose baby had no neural tube defect. Associations between high alpha-fetoprotein and 'poor fetal outcome' have been described since 1977 (Chard *et al.* 1986). Unfortunately, most authors have concentrated on demonstrating the association between pregnancy complications and abnormal alpha-fetoprotein levels, rather than on evaluating the effects of using alpha-fetoprotein assays as a screening test. Many authors have presented comparisons between women with high alpha-fetoprotein levels and others (Evans and Stokes 1984; Hamilton *et al.* 1985; Walters *et al.* 1985), or between women who deliver low birthweight babies and others (Smith 1980). Other investigators have simply described an association between increased alpha-fetoprotein levels and low birthweight (Brock *et al.* 1979a; Corry and Whyler 1984).

Another difficulty in interpreting results is the variety of cut-off points used; these include 2, 2.5, or 3 multiples of the median; 2 standard deviations above the mean; and the 90th or 95th centile. Finally, all except one of the studies for which 2 × 2 tables can be made originate from the United Kingdom.

4.2.2 Prediction of low birthweight or low birthweight for gestational age

Only a few studies (Table 29.10) in singleton pregnancies allow calculation of sensitivity, specificity and predictive values (Brock *et al.* 1982; Gordon *et al.* 1978; Gordon *et al.* 1979; Persson *et al.* 1980; Wald *et al.* 1980; Chard *et al.* 1986). All except the Swedish study (Persson *et al.* 1980) showed a positive predictive value below 35 per cent for low birthweight or low weight for gestational age. In these studies alpha-fetoprotein was assayed once, or twice at the most, and between 520 and

Table 29.10 Test properties of alpha-fetoprotein measurements for prediction of low birthweight or low weight for gestational age

Authors and year	No. of women	% Prevalence	Range of gestation (weeks)	No. of samples	Cut-off point†	Sensitivity	Specificity	Positive predictive value	Negative predictive value
Low birthweight (< 2500 g)									
Brock *et al.* (1979a)	15481	?	15–22	1	2 MoM	—	—	9.1	—
					4 MoM	—	—	8.7	—
Gordon *et al.* (1979)	828	4.3	16–22	1–2	P_{95}	11	91	5	96
Wald *et al.* (1980)	4198	5.4	16–18	1	2 MoM	14	95	13	95
Brock *et al.* (1982)	520	7.0	18–20	1	2 MoM	19	97	33	93
Evans and Stokes (1984)	4864	?*	16–18	2	?	—	—	14	95
Hamilton *et al.* (1985)	10885	?*	16–20	2	2.5 MoM	—	—	27	95
Chard *et al.* (1986)	887	5.5	15–18	1	P_{90}	16	91	9	95
Low birthweight for gestational age									
Gordon *et al.* (1978)	835	10.5	16–24	1–2	P_{95}	6	90	6	89
Persson *et al.* (1980)	93	10.0	16–20	serial	2 SD	70	93	58	96
Hamilton *et al.* (1985)	10885	?*	16–20	2	2.5 MoM	—	—	18	77
Chard *et al.* (1986)	887	9.4	15–18	1	P_{90}	14	91	14	91

* Compared with control group.
†MoM = multiples of the median; P_{95} = 95th percentile.

4198 women were screened. The study of Persson *et al.* (1980) followed only 93 women with serial alpha-fetoprotein measurements (and ultrasound scan and other biochemical tests) every 3 weeks until term. The higher sensitivity (70 per cent) and positive predictive value (58 per cent) in that study may be due to chance (small numbers), to repeat assays, or even to more accurately defined gestational ages in a carefully selected population. It is unlikely to be due to the choice of different gestational ages for screening, because Brock *et al.* (1982) showed in serial measurements that the likelihood of finding an association between elevated maternal plasma alpha-fetoprotein and low birthweight was highest before 20 weeks of gestation. Apart from the study by Persson *et al.* (1980), only one of the studies listed in Table 29.10 found the probability of low birthweight or low weight for gestational age in women with an abnormal test result to be at least twice as high as in all women tested. In one of the studies (Gordon *et al.* 1978), the probability of having an infant of low weight for gestational age after an abnormal test result was even lower than the probability in the entire population screened! From these data it does not appear that alpha-fetoprotein screening is a reliable predictor of low birthweight or low weight for gestation.

The test does not appear to perform any better when applied in high-risk populations. Twin pregnancies were examined by Brock *et al.* (1979b), who found positive predictive values that were roughly of the same order of magnitude as the prevalence (Table 29.11). One can therefore only conclude that the validity of the test is very poor.

4.2.3 Screening for other conditions

An association of abnormal alpha-fetoprotein with poor fetal outcome has been sought since neural tube defect screening was introduced and since associations with twin pregnancy (Knight *et al.* 1981), proteinuric pre-eclampsia (Walters *et al.* 1985), early pregnancy loss (Bennett *et al.* 1978), and 'poor outcome' (Garoff 1976) were observed. None of these studies allow satisfactory evaluation because the data usually do not allow the construction of 2 × 2 tables and because they virtually never relate to the entire population tested but to specific test results or specific outcomes. When either sensitivity or positive predictive value could be determined, these were always below 20 per cent. If one considers that twin pregnancy can be diagnosed by ultrasonography with a sensitivity of about 95 per cent, that 'poor outcome' has no clear definition, and that proteinuric pre-eclampsia too is variously defined (see Chapter 24), the validity of alpha-fetoprotein screening for conditions other than neural tube defects seems to be very poor indeed.

An exception should be made for low alpha-fetoprotein levels. In 1984, Merkatz *et al.* and Cuckle *et al.* reported lower alpha-fetoprotein concentrations in pregnancies in which the fetus was affected by Down's syndrome; an observation that has subsequently been confirmed by many authors (see Chapter 23).

While low alpha-fetoprotein concentrations can certainly not be considered as diagnostic for Down's syndrome, there is no doubt that the combination of maternal age and alpha-fetoprotein levels is more precise in estimating the likelihood of Down's syndrome than is maternal age alone (Cuckle *et al.* 1987; Tabor *et al.* 1987).

A follow-up of infants without neural tube defect born to mothers with elevated maternal serum alpha-fetoprotein levels was conducted by Burton and Dillard (1986). They examined 380 children at 1 and 12 months of age and found their developmental, mental and psychomotor scores to be similar to those of controls.

5 Human chorionic gonadotrophin

Human chorionic gonadotrophin is a glycoprotein secreted in large quantities by the trophoblast. It can be described as one of the ancestors of reproductive endocrinology, having been named as early as 1920 and assayed in 1927 by the classical Asheim and Zondek pregnancy test. More recently, as assays have become more sensitive, detection of lower concentrations has been possible, demonstrating production of the glycoprotein in non-trophoblastic sites. It is now known that

Table 29.11 Test properties of a single alpha-fetoprotein measurement at 15 to 22 weeks gestation for the prediction of low birthweight in twin pregnancy (data from Brock *et al.* 1979b)

No. of women	Outcome of twins predicted	% Prevalence	Cut-off point*	Sensitivity	Specificity	Positive predictive value	Negative predictive value
64	at least one <2500 g	56	2 MoM	44	64	62	47
			2.5 MoM	25	79	60	45
64	both <2500 g	35	2 MoM	56	68	50	74
			2.5 MoM	34	83	53	69

*MoM = multiples of the median.

human chorionic gonadotrophin is a ubiquitous substance produced not only by the trophoblast, but also by fetal tissues (McGregor *et al.* 1983), pre-implantation embryos (Fishel *et al.* 1984), many neoplasms (Odell *et al.* 1977), and some bacteria (Acevedo *et al.* 1985). It is secreted in a pulsatile fashion, probably from the pituitary in all normal adults (Odell and Griffin 1987).

The introduction of highly sensitive human chorionic gonadotrophin assays has had a direct impact on clinical practice, allowing early diagnosis of ectopic pregnancy and follow-up of *in vitro* fertilization. Human chorionic gonadotrophin assays have also proved useful in the diagnosis and management of trophoblastic disease (Dawood *et al.* 1977; Berkowitz *et al.* 1985).

The subject has been extensively reviewed by Saxena (1983) and Van Leusden (1976). The physiological role of human chorionic gonadotrophin is still poorly understood, though it is noteworthy that in contrast to human placental lactogen, pregnancies without human chorionic gonadotrophin have never been observed.

5.1 Variables affecting human chorionic gonadotrophin levels and their measurement

Like alpha-fetoprotein, human chorionic gonadotrophin increases very sharply in early pregnancy. This characteristic has been used for the estimation of gestational age in case of uncertain dates (Chervenak *et al.* 1986). Conversely, the possibility of erroneous data on gestational age renders serial rather than single human chorionic gonadotrophin measurement almost indispensable for a correct interpretation of the test results when used for any other purpose than the diagnosis of pregnancy (Schwers *et al.* 1986).

Further technical problems in interpretation relate to the non-linearity of the exponential rise of serum human chorionic gonadotrophin in normal pregnancy before the 6th to 7th week of gestation (Pittaway *et al.* 1985). Other problems relate to the type of antibody used in radioimmunoassays; in some cases, the antibody may cross-react with luteinizing hormone, creating difficulties when the level of luteinizing hormone is as high as it is at the time of ovulation. Values obtained in these circumstances may be in the same range found in ectopic pregnancy. Such problems can be largely avoided through use of the beta subunit assay techniques. Like other biochemical markers in pregnancy, human chorionic gonadotrophin levels are well above the normal range in multiple pregnancy.

Since the 1950s, there have been descriptions of 'hyperplacentosis': situations where a large placenta coexisted with an elevated level of human chorionic gonadotrophin. This hyperplacentosis has been described in pre-eclampsia (Crosignani *et al.* 1974) and in pruritus of pregnancy (Goodlin *et al.* 1985).

5.2 Test properties and clinical usefulness

Human chorionic gonadotrophin has mainly been used as a pregnancy test and for assessment of bleeding or anomalies of early pregnancy, such as threatened abortion, ectopic pregnancy and molar pregnancy. The same difficulties in assessing its value are present as with other tests discussed in this chapter. Many studies present mean values and do not allow 2×2 tables to be constructed; other studies vary in the cut-off points used; above all, not all authors state whether 'abnormal human chorionic gonadotrophin' means abnormal at the beginning of symptoms or at any time during pregnancy. Furthermore, only the relatively recent papers refer to results that are commensurate with current laboratory practice.

Although routine screening of all early pregnancies with human chorionic gonadotrophin assay has been advocated (Dhont *et al.* 1978; Dhont *et al.* 1982), the benefit of such a policy has never been assessed. On the other hand, there are many studies of human chorionic gonadotrophin in bleeding of early pregnancy. In the

Table 29.12 Test properties of human chorionic gonadotrophin for diagnosis of non-viable pregnancy.

Authors and year	No. of women	% Prevalence	Range of gestation (weeks)	No. of samples	Sensitivity	Specificity	Positive predictive value	Negative predictive value
Kunz and Keller (1976b)	65	66	6–20	1	88	55	78	71
Jouppila *et al.* (1979)	188	50	6–20	1	59	94	91	71
Dhont *et al.* (1982)	471	67	5–14	?	93	94	97	87
Hertz (1984)	63	46	6–19	1+	?	?	100	88
				serial	?	?	96	89
Westergaard *et al.* (1985)								
All women	108	39	7–20	1	62	94	87	80
				serial	14	61	19	53
Fetal heart positive	77	14	7–20	1	0	94	0	85
				serial	9	92	17	86

absence of ultrasound scanning, human chorionic gonadotrophin performs satisfactorily for the diagnosis of non-viable pregnancies (Table 29.12). The positive predictive value is always higher than 90 per cent and when the estimate of gestational age is correct, abnormally low human chorionic gonadotrophin levels correlate well with poor outcome. The reverse is not true, in that up to 30 per cent of women with normal human chorionic gonadotrophin levels still experience a pregnancy failure, mainly because the presence of a blighted ovum is not infrequently associated with human chorionic gonadotrophin levels that are within the normal range.

In clinical practice, however, one may question the utility of human chorionic gonadotrophin assays in threatened abortion. Ultrasound scanning will usually provide an instant and accurate diagnosis of embryonic death. Westergaard *et al.* (1985) subdivided their series of women with bleeding in early pregnancy according to the results of ultrasound scanning. Among 77 pregnancies with evidence of fetal heart activity and bleeding in early pregnancy, 11 aborted but only one of these had a human chorionic gonadotrophin level below the 10th centile.

A few studies in later pregnancy have focused on the correlation between so-named hyperplacentosis and pre-eclampsia (Crosignani *et al.* 1974). Said *et al.* (1984) assayed human chorionic gonadotrophin in women with excessive weight-gain between 20 and 30 weeks and found that all women who subsequently developed pre-eclampsia had human chorionic gonadotrophin levels above 6000 international units. No reports of systematic screening for pre-eclampsia in this manner have been reported although there is little reason to believe that this measure would be inferior to other currently proposed methods such as antithrombin III and fibronectin (see Chapter 24).

Relating human chorionic gonadotrophin to birthweight, Rhesus sensitization, diabetes, and Apgar score seems to be a disappointing exercise. More than 20 such reports were reviewed by Van Leusden (1976), but the presentation of the data generally does not allow the construction of 2×2 tables. These can be constructed for the data of Obiekwe and Chard (1983), which showed that abnormal human chorionic gonadotrophin levels in late pregnancy predicted 15 per cent of light-for-dates babies and 13 per cent of instances of fetal distress. This prediction is hardly better than a clinical guess, but better than the results reported by Persson *et al.* (1980) in which none of the women with poor outcome had abnormal human chorionic gonadotrophin levels.

Thus, where ultrasound scanning is available, there is little place for the use of human chorionic gonadotrophin in established intrauterine pregnancy, whether early or late.

6 Placental proteins

In addition to human placental lactogen and human chorionic gonadotrophin, which may be described as placental protein hormones, several proteins of placental origin have been described since the 1970s and new ones are regularly being reported. Extensive reviews of recognized placental proteins have been published, which address both the physiology and the clinical use of these substances (Klopper 1982; Grudzinskas *et al.* 1982; Chard and Klopper 1982; Rosen 1986). These reviews are fairly comprehensive and often consider the tests in terms of sensitivity, specificity, and predictive values.

Placental proteins have never gained the popularity enjoyed by oestrogens, human placental lactogen, alpha-fetoprotein, or human chorionic gonadotrophin as markers for healthy pregnancy, nor has there been much pressure to use placental protein measurements on a large scale. They have been applied more for research. Their value in clinical practice is still somewhat experimental. For all these reasons only a brief summary on the use of these biochemical tests for the surveillance of pregnancy will be presented.

6.1 Pregnancy-associated plasma protein A

Pregnancy-associated plasma protein A was first described by Lin *et al.* in 1974. It is a large molecule with a molecular weight that is more than 10 times that of human chorionic gonadotrophin or human placental lactogen. Much interest has been directed to its potential physiological role for immunosuppression in early pregnancy, complement inhibition, and coagulation changes (Bischof *et al.* 1982a; Bischof *et al.* 1983). Although this protein was first described as a placental protein, there has been much discussion as to its origin. It can be found in plasma of non-pregnant women and men. Undoubtedly levels of pregnancy-associated plasma protein A are much higher in pregnancy. They rise throughout pregnancy even after 36 weeks (Bischof *et al.* 1982b), but whether the source is placental, decidual, or both remains a source of controversy.

It has been suggested that pregnancy-associated plasma protein A is the only satisfactory predictor of poor outcome in first trimester bleeding when ultrasound scanning shows a live embryo (Westergaard *et al.* 1985). The small study on which this proposition was based (77 women with threatened abortion and a live embryo, 11 of whom subsequently had a miscarriage), certainly needs to be replicated. Even if the data can be confirmed, however, the benefit of this type of prediction can be questioned. What is the benefit to an individual woman of knowing that the prospects for her pregnancy are grim, or conversely that she may be optimistic? The effect of such knowledge is unclear since threatened abortion is a condition for which there is no effective treatment to date (see Chapter 38).

In ectopic pregnancies in which human chorionic gonadotrophin levels were within the normal range, Chemnitz *et al.* (1984), Sinosich *et al.* (1985) and Grudzinskas *et al.* (1986) found that levels of pregnancy-associated plasma protein A levels were always outside the normal range. If these observations can be confirmed on larger numbers of women, laparoscopy for suspected ectopic pregnancy, which is undoubtedly more hazardous, could become less frequent and be reserved for instances when levels of pregnancy-associated plasma protein A are abnormal.

Only one woman in whom pregnancy-associated plasma protein A was undetectable during an otherwise unremarkable pregnancy has been mentioned in the literature: the fetus was affected with the Cornelia de Lange syndrome (Westergaard *et al.* 1983).

A few studies are available in late pregnancy. There have been reports that pregnancy-associated plasma protein A levels are reduced in diabetic pregnancy (Barnea *et al.* 1986; Sutcliffe *et al.* 1982), but the published data do not allow the construction of 2 × 2 tables. In pre-eclampsia, data are conflicting. Lin *et al.* (1977), Klopper and Hughes (1980), Hughes *et al.* (1980a,b) and Toop and Klopper (1981) found increased pregnancy-associated plasma protein A levels, while Westergaard *et al.* (1984b) and Barnea *et al.* (1986) found levels in pre-eclamptic women to be similar to those in the normal pregnant population. In the few studies (Hughes *et al.* 1980a,b; Salem *et al.* 1981b; Toop and Klopper 1981; Pledger *et al.* 1984; Westergaard *et al.* 1984a) dealing with a variety of outcomes for which 2 × 2 tables could be constructed, positive predictive values never attained a level that indicated a doubling of the likelihood of detecting an abnormal outcome by comparison with a blind guess.

It seems, therefore, that pregnancy-associated plasma protein A is an interesting protein, with characteristics that are definitely different from those of other placental proteins. At present, there is no place for its use in obstetric care.

6.2 Schwangerschaftsprotein-1

This protein was originally described by Bohn in 1971. Its physiological role is unknown. It is now apparent that at least two different proteins cross-react with antisera to Schwangerschaftsprotein-1: Schwangerschaftsprotein-1a and Schwangerschaftsprotein-1b. The ratio of these two proteins varies from one pregnant woman to another (Ahmed *et al.* 1982) and, within individual women, with gestational age (Huttenmoser *et al.* 1987). The practical implication is that until parallel dose–response curves can be achieved for all variants, results must be treated with reserve (Schultz-Larsen *et al.* 1979; Rosen 1986). As an illustration of this, Decoster and Vassart (1984) reported on over 900 women screened routinely with a commercial kit for Schwangerschaftsprotein-1; 32 had exceptionally low values for gestational age, while human placental lactogen and oestriol were in the normal range. Clinical outcome was normal in all of these women. In addition, Schwangerschaftsprotein-1 levels are significantly altered by administration of glucose or insulin.

Early claims suggested that Schwangerschaftsprotein-1 could be useful for early pregnancy testing (especially in women treated with human chorionic gonadotrophin); diagnosis of dead or ectopic pregnancy in the presence of first trimester bleeding; as a marker of gestational age; and for early diagnosis of multiple pregnancy. All of these indications have since been superseded by ultrasonography.

Despite the serious assay problems, people have attempted to use Schwangerschaftsprotein-1 as a marker of fetal well-being in late pregnancy. As a predictor of low birthweight for gestational age the data are as conflicting as they are for human placental lactogen, oestriol, and alpha-fetoprotein. Two studies

Table 29.13 Test properties of Schwangerschaftsprotein–1 measurements for prediction of low birthweight or low weight for gestational age

Authors and year	No. of women	% Prevalence	Range of gestation (weeks)	No. of samples	Sensitivity	Specificity	Positive predictive value	Negative predictive value
Gordon *et al.* (1977)	180	15	31–40	?	74	88	54	95
Chapman *et al.* (1981)	605	10	31–34	1	64	NA	17	NA
Karg *et al.* (1981)	823	14	32–40	2–6	62	89	50	93
Salem *et al.* (1981b)	254	7	16	1	27	92	26	93
Obiekwe and Chard (1983)	522	53	36–40	?	15	90	15	90
Pledger *et al.* (1984)*	118	32	?	?	10	88	10	88
Westergaard *et al.* (1984a)	208	16	20	1	21	90	29	86
	320	9	30	1	21	90	20	91
	392	7	35	1	32	90	20	95

*Retrospective analysis; NA = not available.

which have assayed Schwangerschaftsprotein-1 in apparently comparable, unselected populations found low weight for gestational age in approximately half of the women with low Schwangerschaftsprotein-1 levels (Gordon *et al.* 1977; Karg *et al.* 1981). Others, however, (Chapman *et al.* 1981; Obiekwe and Chard 1983; Pledger *et al.* 1984) found that less than 20 per cent of the women with low Schwangerschaftsprotein-1 levels gave birth to infants with low birthweight or low weight for their gestational age (Table 29.13). In studies that compared the performance of Schwangerschaftsprotein-1 with that of human placental lactogen for the prediction of low weight for gestational age (Westergaard *et al.* 1984a; Pledger *et al.* 1984), results were consistently in favour of human placental lactogen.

All of this indicates that Schwangerschaftsprotein-1 assays have no value in obstetrical care. From a biochemical point of view, the protein is a mixture of different compounds; there are many technical problems related to the assay; it has none of the specific characteristics of pregnancy-associated plasma protein A; and the clinical evidence tends to show that it is inferior to many other tests.

6.3 Other placental proteins

The few available data relating to placental protein-5, suggest that it may be associated with coagulation and it shows unique modification in the presence of pregnancy coagulation disorders (Salem *et al.* 1981a). More research may be warranted to understand its relation to coagulation disorders in pregnancy, but presently this compound is not a marker for, nor a predictor of, fetal well-being. Any suggestion that placental protein-5 could be of use for prediction of low birthweight seems to be dispelled by studies of Obiekwe *et al.* (1980) and Salem *et al.* (1981b) who found positive predictive values of respectively 9 and 0 per cent!

One study has been published (Howell *et al.* 1985) in which 501 women were routinely screened in late pregnancy with human placental lactogen and placental protein-12 measurements. Cut-off points for normality were less than the 10th centile for human placental lactogen and more than the 90th centile for placental protein-12. Sensitivity and predictive values were better for placental protein-12 than for human placental lactogen. No other assessment of placental protein-12 in the clinical care for pregnancy has been reported.

It may be that there is some scope for further research in the field of placental proteins, but there are no indications as yet that any of these are of current clinical use.

7 Miscellaneous biochemical tests

Various other hormones, enzymes, and other substances have generated interest, although such interest has often been short-lived. For many of them there is an abundant literature, but published data are usually expressed in such a way that 2×2 tables cannot be constructed. It is quite possible that some of these biochemical markers, had they had more eloquent protagonists, would have turned out to be as widely applied and acclaimed as oestriol or human placental lactogen measurements. A few will be briefly listed here.

7.1 Oxytocinase (cystoaminopeptidase)

Oxytocinase is a placental enzyme, the physiological role of which is unclear, although it was previously thought to have a role in the inhibition of the biological activity of oxytocin (Fekete 1932). Its levels increase exponentially during pregnancy and many early reports claimed it to be useful for the assessment of abnormal pregnancies. Fifteen papers on the clinical use of oxytocinase measurements were reviewed by Kleiner and Brouet-Yager (1973), but as results were expressed as means, no further analysis can be made. Advantages claimed by the protagonists include the technical ease of the assay, the absence of maternal metabolic interference with the levels of this substance, and the possibility to use one and the same marker throughout pregnancy.

There are too few published data for which 2×2 tables can be constructed, so that it is unclear whether oxytocinase is superior, inferior, or equal to more popular tests. Giussi *et al.* (1979a,b) compared oxytocinase to oestriol and human placental lactogen, and found it to be the least sensitive in screening for low birthweight. This assertion is not supported by Hensleigh *et al.* (1977), who also used low birthweight as an outcome and found oxytocinase to be superior to human placental lactogen.

7.2 Alkaline phosphatase (thermostable and leucocyte)

Levels of alkaline phosphatase increase greatly with advancing gestation, mainly because of placental secretion, but liver secretion is modified as well (Okpere *et al.* 1985). It is only a fraction of the total amount of alkaline phosphatase that was measured as a marker of pregnancy well-being; mostly it was the thermostable fraction, although, to a lesser extent, the leucocyte alkaline phosphatase has also been used. A general review of this subject can be found in Shane and Suzuki (1974).

When the properties of this test are assessed in 2×2 tables based on the available data, it performs similarly to other biochemical tests such as oestriol and human placental lactogen, which have acquired a far larger following. Kunz and Keller (1976b) prospectively compared oestriol, human placental lactogen, pregnandiol, and heat-stable alkaline phosphatase in 83 high risk pregnancies; the positive predictive value of alkaline phosphatase measurements was similar to that of the other tests. Brock and Barron (1988) recently compared placental alkaline phosphatase with alpha-fetoprotein levels for the prediction of low birthweight and found that both performances afforded a roughly equal prediction of low birthweight. Levels of placental alkaline phosphatase and alpha-fetoprotein above twice the median value indicated respectively a 3.8 times and a 4.7 times higher incidence of low birthweight than that in the population at large (Brock and Barron 1988). Despite this, alkaline phosphatase measurements, whether as thermostable or as leucocyte fractions, virtually disappeared from the obstetrical armentarium long before ultrasound scanning had become the competitive tool that it now is. More recently, the availability of monoclonal antibodies specific for placental alkaline phosphatase which do not cross-react with the isoenzyme from liver or kidney (McLaughlin *et al.* 1983; Travers and Bodmer 1984) has revived interest in this parameter as an indicator of pregnancy outcome (Brock and Barron 1988).

7.3 Progestogens

Pregnandiol and progesterone aroused much interest in the early days of biochemical testing and there are a large number of studies dealing with these measurements in pregnancy. However, none of these present data in a way that allows compilation of 2 × 2 tables.

8 Haemoglobin

All the biochemical tests thus far discussed were introduced because the substances measured were thought to reflect the adequacy of fetal or placental function, although most of them are also influenced by a variety of maternal factors. Since successful outcome of pregnancy depends as much on maternal as on fetal or placental function, assessment of maternal physiological adaptation to pregnancy could serve as an equally useful marker for prognosis of pregnancy.

One of the important physiological adaptations is the increase in blood, and especially in plasma, volume, with its resultant haemodilution (see Chapter 19). Adequate expansion of plasma volume has been shown to correlate well with birthweight and good outcome of pregnancy (Mau 1977; Koller *et al.* 1979; Garn *et al* 1981; Sagen *et al.* 1984a; Campbell and MacGillivray 1985). Hence, measurement of haemoglobin or haematocrit, which reflects haemodilution, might serve as a useful marker of the adequacy of this adaptation.

Blood sampling for haemoglobin is performed almost routinely as a component of antenatal care in industrialized countries. The usual aim of this test is to screen for maternal anaemia, which is systematically found as a risk factor for poor pregnancy outcome in most textbooks and risk scoring systems (see Chapter 22). In the late 1970s it was observed that, contrary to expectations, when maternal haemoglobin concentration and haematocrit were high, there was an increased risk of the pregnancy ending in the birth of a light-for-dates infant (Dunlop *et al.* 1978; Mau 1977; Koller *et al.* 1979). It is worth pointing out, though, that the line of thought at that time was also contrary to earlier opinions that bloodletting was a remedy for most disorders of pregnancy. High haemoglobin levels have not, in practice, been applied in the same way as other biochemical markers, such as oestriol or human placental lactogen determinations, to predict fetal outcome. As data are available, however, we felt it to be worthwhile to examine the test properties of this simple and economical test in the same manner as that used to evaluate the classical biochemical markers of fetal well-being.

When categorical data were available, 2 × 2 tables were compiled in the same manner as was done for the other tests reported (Table 29.14). High haemoglobin levels were related to low birthweight or to low weight

Table 29.14 Test properties of high haemoglobin levels for prediction of low birthweight or low weight for gestational age

Authors and year	No. of women	% Prevalence	Range of gestation (weeks)	No. of samples	Sensitivity	Specificity	Positive predictive value	Negative predictive value
Mau (1977)	4690	10	28–40	1	14	92	16	90
Koller *et al.* (1979)	120	—†	37	1	88	96	60	99
Bissenden *et al.* (1981)	25	20	20–37	4	100	80	55	100
	15	33	20–37	4	60	80	60	80
Sagen *et al.* (1984a)*	847	25	28–36	1	62	79	49	86
Sagen *et al.* (1984b)	74	54	last week	1	60	82	80	80
Knottnerus *et al.* (1986)	494	5	30–32	1	33	89	13	96

*Outcome studied was birthweight <25th centile of weight for gestation.
†7 with birthweight <2.5th centile of weight for gestation, and 113 controls.

for gestation, an outcome measure that is frequently used to evaluate the performance of hormone assays in pregnancy. It is clear that the test properties shown in Table 29.14 compare favourably with those of the hormonal and placental protein assays previously discussed.

9 Conclusions

The development and deployment of biochemical tests of fetal well-being has contributed greatly to current understanding of the endocrinology and physiology of pregnancy. The indirect benefits of this for effective care in pregnancy have, with few exceptions, not been matched by any direct benefits. Apart from early pregnancy and screening for fetal (including chromosomal) abnormalities (see Chapter 23), biochemical tests of fetal well-being are of disappointingly little value for the general care of individual women and their babies.

In spite of this, the use of these tests persists, albeit at remarkably different levels from one country to another. In France for instance, Lewin (1983) managed a *tour de force* of non-commitment in his recommendations for routine antenatal care when he stated that 'It is legitimate to ask for some ultrasound scans and two or three hormone assays. The efficacy and cost of other tests has not yet been established with sufficient precision so that one cannot affirm that they are mandatory in all pregnancies. Nevertheless it is desirable that such tests be widely used . . .' (Lewin 1983).

None of the biochemical tests that were and still are employed in obstetric care have been demonstrated to be of benefit for screening purposes in the second half of pregnancy. The generally poor predictive power of all these tests has led clinicians to combine a number of them together in the hope that the use of several of these imprecise instruments may prove to be better than just one used alone.

In view of the high costs involved, such policies need to be either abandoned or adequately assessed, not only in terms of test properties (see Chapter 3) but also in terms of the health benefits that are alleged to accrue from their use.

As discussed above, there is obviously a place for some of these biochemical tests in early pregnancy, either for the diagnosis or pregnancy, for screening for fetal abnormality (including Down's syndrome), or in the differential diagnosis of intrauterine and extrauterine pregnancy. In the second half of pregnancy there may be rare occasions on which one of these tests may be useful, for example, when there is a suspicion of adrenal hypoplasia. For the large majority of potential indications, however, current evidence suggests that use of biochemical tests of fetal well-being is a waste of scarce resources.

References

Acevedo HF, Campbell-Acevedo E, Kloos WE (1985). Expression of human choriogonadotrophin-like material in coagulase-negative staphylococcus species. Infect Immunol, 3: 860–868.

Adlercreutz T, Fotsis C, Bannwart E (1986). Urinary estrogen profile determination in young Finnish vegetarian and omnivorous women. J Steroid Biochem, 24: 289–296.

Ahmed AG, Bremmer R, Nisbet A, Horne CH, Klopper A (1982). Measurement of SP1 in samples with varying SP1alpha : SP1beta ratios. Clin Chim Acta, 121: 217–224.

Aickin DR, Smith MA, Brown JB (1974). Comparison between plasma and urinary oestrogen measurements in predicting fetal risk. Austral NZ J Obstet Gynaecol, 14: 59–76.

Asher R (1954). The dangers of going to bed. Quoted in: Talking Sense. Avery-Jones F (ed) (1972). London: Pitman Medical.

Aubry RH, Rouke JE, Cuenva VG, Marshall LD (1975). The random urine estrogen/creatinine ratio. A practical and reliable index of fetal welfare. Obstet Gynecol, 46: 64–68.

Barbieri E, Boticeli A, Consarino R, Genazzani AR, Velpe A (1986). Failure of placenta to produce HPL in an otherwise uneventful pregnancy: A case report. Biol Res Pregnancy Perinatol, 7: 131–133.

Barnea ER, Bischoff P, Page C, DeCherney AH, Herrmann W, Naftolin F (1986). Placental and circulating pregnancy-associated plasma protein A concentrates in normal and pathological term pregnancies. Obstet Gynecol, 68: 382–385.

Bashore RA, Westlake J (1977). Plasma unconjugated estriol values in high-risk pregnancy. Am J Obstet Gynecol, 128: 371–379.

Beischer NA, Brown JB (1968). The significance of high urinary oestriol excretion during pregnancy. J Obstet Gynaecol Br Commnwlth, 75: 622–628.

Beischer NA, Brown JB, Smith MA, Townsend L (1969). Studies in prolonged pregnancy. Clinical results and urinary estriol excretion in prolonged pregnancy. Am J Obstet Gynecol, 103: 483–495.

Bennett MJ, Grudzinskas JG, Gordon YB, Turnbull AC (1978). Circulating levels of alpha-fetoprotein and pregnancy specific β_1 glycoprotein in pregnancies without an embryo. Br J Obstet Gynaecol, 85: 348–350.

Bergstrand CZ, Czar B (1956). Demonstration of new protein fraction in serum from human fetus. Scand J Clin Lab Invest, 8: 174–179.

Berkowitz RS, Goldstein DP, Bernstein MR (1985). Natural history of partial molar pregnancy. Obstet Gynecol, 66: 677–681.

Bischof P, DuBerg SG, Schindler AM (1982a). Is PAPP-A an immunomodulator during human pregnancy? Placenta, Suppl 4: 93–102.

Bischof P, Duberg S, Herrmann W, Sizonenko PC (1982b). Amniotic fluid and plasma concentrations of pregnancy-associated plasma protein-A (PAPP-A) throughout pregnancy: Comparison with other fetoplacental products. Br J Obstet Gynaecol, 89: 358–363.

Bischof P, Meisser A, Haenggeli L (1983). Pregnancy associated plasma protein A inhibits thrombin induced coagulation of plasma. Thrombosis Res, 32: 45–55.

Bissenden JG, Scott PH, Hallum J, Mansfield HN, Scott P, Wharton BA (1981). Racial variations in tests of fetoplacental function. Br J Obstet Gynaecol, 88: 109–114.

Bohn H (1971). Nachweis und Charakteriserung von Schwangerschaftsproteinen in der menslichen Placenta sowie ihre quantitative immunologische Bestimmung im Serum schwangeren Frauen. Arch Gynecol, 210: 440–457.

Bolognese RJ, Corson SL, Touchstone JC (1972). Factors affecting the yield of urinary estriol. Obstet Gynecol, 39: 683–687.

Bradshaw KD, Carr BR (1986). Placental sulfatase deficiency: Maternal and fetal expression of steroid sulfatase deficiency and X-linked ichthyosis. Obstet Gynecol Surv, 41: 401–413.

Brock DJ, Barron L (1988). Measurement of placental alkaline phosphatase in maternal plasma as an indicator of subsequent low birthweight outcome. Br J Obstet Gynaecol, 95: 79–83.

Brock DJH, Barron L, Jelen P, Watt M, Scrimgeour JB (1977). Maternal serum alpha-fetoprotein measurements as an early indicator of low birth weight. Lancet, 2: 267–268.

Brock DJH, Barron L, Duncan P, Scrimgeour JB, Watt M (1979a). Significance of elevated mid-trimester maternal plasma-alpha-fetoprotein values. Lancet, 1: 1281–1282.

Brock DJH, Barron L, Watt M, Scrimgeour JB (1979b). The relation between maternal plasma alpha-fetoprotein and birth weight in twin pregnancies. Br J Obstet Gynaecol, 86: 710–712.

Brock DJH, Barron L, Watt M, Scrimgeour JB, Keay AI (1982). Maternal plasma α-fetoprotein and low birth weight: A prospective study throughout pregnancy. Br J Obstet Gynaecol, 89: 348–351.

Burton BK, Dillard RG (1986). Outcome in infants born to mothers with unexplained elevations of maternal serum α-fetoprotein. Pediatrics, 77: 582–586.

Campbell S, Kurjak A (1972). Comparison between urinary oestrogen assay and serial ultrasonic cephalometry in assessment of fetal growth retardation. Br Med J, 4: 336–340.

Campbell DM, MacGillivray I (1985). The importance of plasma volume expansion and nutrition in twin pregnancy. Obstet Gynecol Surv, 40: 144–145.

Castellanos JM, Aranda M, Cararach J, Cararach V (1975). Effects of aspirin on oestriol excretion in pregnancy. Lancet, 1: 859.

Chamberlain GV (1984). An end to antenatal oestrogen monitoring. Lancet, 1: 1171–1172.

Chapman MG, O'Shea RT, Jones WR, Hillier R (1981). Pregnancy-specific β_1-glycoprotein as a screening test for at risk pregnancies. Am J Obstet Gynecol, 141: 499–502.

Chard T, Klopper A (1982). Placental Function Tests. Berlin: Springer-Verlag.

Chard T, Sturdee J, Cokrill B, Obiekwe BC (1985). Which is the best placental function test? A comparison of placental lactogen and unconjugated oestriol in the prediction of intrauterine growth retardation. Eur J Obstet Gynecol Reprod Biol, 19: 13–17.

Chard T, Rice A, Kitau MJ, Hird V, Grudzinskas JG, Nysenbaum AM (1986). Mid-trimester levels of alpha-fetoprotein in the screening of low birthweight. Br J Obstet Gynaecol, 93: 36–38.

Chemnitz J, Tornehave D, Teisner B, Poulsen HKS, Westergaard JG (1984). The localisation of pregnancy proteins (HPL, SPI and PAPP-A) in intra- and extra-uterine pregnancies. Placenta, 5: 489–494.

Chervenak FA, Brightman RC, Thornton J, Berkowitz GS, David S (1986). Crown-rump length and serum human chorionic gonadotrophin as predictors of gestational age. Obstet Gynecol, 67: 210–213.

Corry I, Whyler D (1984). Outcome of pregnancies associated with raised serum and normal amniotic fluid α-fetoprotein concentrations. Br Med J, 288: 1836.

Corson SL, Bolognese RJ (1968). Urinary estriol in the management of obstetric problems. Am J Obstet Gynecol, 101: 633–637.

Crosignani PG, Trojsi L, Attanasio AEM, Finzi GCL (1974). Value of HCG and HCS measurement in clinical practice. Obstet Gynecol, 44: 673–681.

Cuckle HS, Wald NJ, Lindenbaum RH (1984). Maternal serum alpha-fetoprotein measurement. A screening test for Down's syndrome. Lancet, 1: 926–929.

Cuckle HS, Wald NJ, Thompson SC (1987). Estimating a woman's risk of having a pregnancy associated with Down's syndrome using her age and serum alpha-fetoprotein level. Br J Obstet Gynaecol, 94: 387–402.

Cusick PE, Alston WC, Truran PL, Read GF (1986). Sub-hourly variations in salivary estriol concentrations in the last trimester of pregnancy. Acta Obstet Gynecol Scand, 65: 435–438.

Dawood MY, Saxena BBG, Landesman R (1977). Human chorionic gonadotropin and its subunits in hydatidiform mole and choriocarcinoma. Obstet Gynecol, 50: 172–181.

Decoster C, Vassart G (1984). Pitfall in the use of commercial kits for evaluating pregnancy-specific β_1-glycoprotein (SP1). Clin Chem, 30: 1881.

Dhont M, Serreyn R, Vandekerckhove D, Thiery M (1978). Serum-chorionic-gonadotropin assay and ectopic pregnancy. Lancet, 1: 559.

Dhont M, Thiery M, Vandekerckhove D (1982). Human chorionic gonadotrophin (HCG) assay in the diagnosis and management of early pregnancy disorders. J Obstet Gynaecol, 2: 134–139.

Dickey RP, Grannis GF, Hanson FW, Schumacher A, Ma S (1972). Use of the estrogen/creatinine ratio and the 'estrogen index' for screening of normal and 'high-risk' pregnancy. Am J Obstet Gynecol, 113: 880–886.

Diczfalusy E (1974). Fetoplacental hormones and human gestation. Basic Life Sci, 4: 385–402.

Dooley SL, Depp R, Socol ML, Tamura RK, Vaisrub N (1984). Urinary estriols in diabetic pregnancy: A reappraisal. Obstet Gynecol, 64: 469–475.

Duenhoelter JH, Whalley PJ, MacDonald PC (1976). An analysis of the utility of plasma immunoreactive estrogen measurements in determining delivery time of gravidas with a fetus considered at high risk. Am J Obstet Gynecol, 125: 889–898.

Dunlop W, Furness C, Hill LM (1978). Maternal haemoglobin concentration, haematocrit and renal handling of urate in pregnancies ending in the births of small-for-dates infants. Br J Obstet Gynaecol, 85: 938–940.

Edwards R, Diver MJ, Davis JC, Hipdin LJ (1976). Plasma oestriol and human placental lactogen measurements in patients with high risk pregnancies. Br J Obstet Gynaecol, 83: 229–237.

England P, Lorrimer D, Fergusson JC, Moffat AM, Kelly AM (1974). Human placental lactogen: The watchdog of fetal distress. Lancet 1: 5–7.

Evans J, Stokes IM (1984). Outcome of pregnancies associated with raised serum and normal amniotic fluid fetoprotein concentrations. Br Med J, 288: 1494.

Fekete K (1932). Gibt es während der Schwangerschaft ein aktives Hypophysen-Hinterlappenhormon im Blute? Endokrinologie, 10: 16–23.

Fishel SB, Edwards RG, Evans CJ (1984). Human chorionic gonadotropin secreted by preimplantation embryos cultured in utero. Science, 223: 816–818.

Fliegner JH, Renou P, Wood C, Beischer NA, Brown JB (1969). Correlation between urinary estriol excretion and fetal acidosis in high-risk pregnancies. Am J Obstet Gynecol, 105: 252–256.

Frandsen V, Jorgensen A, Svenstrup B (1970). The adventures of 1001 obstetrical patients assessed by oestriol excretion. Ann Clin Res, 2: 354–364.

Fraser IS, Leask R, Drife J, Bacon L, Michie E (1976). Plasma estrogen response to dehydroepiandrosterone sulphate injection in normal and complicated late pregnancy. Obstet Gynecol, 47: 152–158.

Fuchs F, Klopper A, (eds) (1983). Endocrinology of Pregnancy (3rd edn). Philadelphia: Harper & Row.

Gabbe SG, Hagerman DD (1978). Clinical application of estriol analysis. Clin Obstet Gynecol, 21: 353–362.

Garn SM, Keating MT, Falkner F (1981). Hematological status and pregnancy outcomes. Am J Clin Nutr, 34: 115–117.

Garoff L (1976). Prediction of fetal outcome by urinary estriol, maternal serum placental lactogen, and alpha-fetoprotein in diabetes and hepatosis of pregnancy. Obstet Gynecol, 48: 659–666.

Gartside MW, Tindall VR (1975). The prognostic value of human placental lactogen levels in threatened abortion. Br J Obstet Gynecol, 82: 303–309.

Gaspard U, Sandront H, Luyckx A (1974). Glucose-insulin interaction and the modulation of human placental lactogen (HPL) during pregnancy. J Obstet Gynaecol Br Commnwlth, 81: 201–209.

Gemzell CA, Heijkenskjold F, Strom L (1955). A method for demonstrating growth hormone activity in human plasma. J Clin Endocrinol Metab, 15: 537–546.

Gerhard I, Runnebaum B (1984). Predictive value of hormone determinations in the first half of pregnancy. Eur J Obstet Gynecol Reprod Biol, 17: 1–17.

Gerhard I, Fitzer C, Klinga K, Rahman N, Runnebaum B (1986). Estrogen screening in evaluation of fetal outcome and infant's development. J Perinat Med, 14: 279–291.

Giussi, G, Ballejo, G, Marinho E, Xercavina J, Vinacur J, Nieto F, Roca P, Rieppi G (1979a). HCS, estriol and oxytocinase in maternal serum and neonatal condition in high risk pregnancies. J Perinat Med, 7: 243–249.

Giussi G, Vinacur J, Ballejo G, Garafalo EG, Martino I (1979b). Human chorionic somatomammotropin, estriol and oxytocinase as indexes of fetal growth. J Perinat Med, 7: 235–242.

Goebelsman U (1979). Protein and steroid hormones in pregnancy. J Reprod Med, 23: 166–177.

Gohari P, Hobbins JC, Berkowitz R (1978). Use of HPL in the diagnosis of intrauterine growth retardation. Obstet Gynecol, 52: 127–128.

Goodlin RC, Anderson JC, Skiles TL (1985). Pruritus and hyperplacentosis. Obstet Gynecol, 66 (Suppl 3): 36S–38S.

Gordon YB, Grudzinskas JG, Jeffrey D, Chard T (1977). Concentrations of pregnancy-specific β_1-glycoprotein in maternal blood in normal pregnancy and in intrauterine growth retardation. Lancet, 1: 331–332.

Gordon YB, Grudzinskas JG, Kitau MJ, Usherwood M McD, Letchworth AT, Chard T (1978). Fetal wastage as a result of an alpha-fetoprotein screening programme. Lancet, 1: 677–678.

Gordon YB, Lewis JD, Leighton M, Kitau MJ, Clarke PC, Chard T (1979). Maternal serum alpha-fetoprotein levels as an index of fetal risk. Am J Obstet Gynecol, 4: 422–424.

Greene JW, Touchstone JC (1963). Urinary estriol as an index of placental function. Am J Obstet Gynecol, 85: 1–9.

Greene JW Jr, Duhring JL, Smith K (1965). Placental function tests. A review of methods available for assessment of the fetoplacental complex. Am J Obstet Gynecol, 92: 1030–1058.

Grudzinskas JG, Teisner B, Seppälä M, eds. (1982). Pregnancy Proteins. Sydney: Academic Press.

Grudzinskas JG, Westergaard JG, Teisner B (1986). Biochemical assessment of placental function. Clin Obstet Gynaecol, 13: 553–569.

Hagerman DD (1979). Clinical use of plasma total estriol measurements in late pregnancy. J Reprod Med, 4: 179–184.

Hamilton MPR, Abdalla HI, Whitfield CR (1985). Significance of raised maternal serum α-fetoprotein in singleton pregnancies with normally formed fetuses. Obstet Gynecol, 65: 465–470.

Hardy MJ, Basalammah AH (1981). Effect of phenobarbitone on serum unconjugated oestriol levels in pregnancy: A case report. J Obstet Gynaecol, 2: 25–26.

Harkness RA, Taylor NF, Crawfurd MA (1983). Recognising placental steroid sulphatase deficiency. Br J Obstet Gynaecol, 287: 2–3.

Harrigan JT, Langer A, Hung CT, Pelosi MA, Washington E (1976). Predictive value of human placental lactogen determinations in pregnancy. Obstet Gynecol, 47: 443–445.

Hausknecht RU. (1967). Estriol and fetal health. Obstet Gynecol, 30: 639–645.

Heikkilä J, Luukkainen T (1971). Urinary excretion of estriol and 15a-hydroxyestriol in complicated pregnancies. Am J Obstet Gynecol, 110: 509–521.

Hensleigh PA, Cheatum SG, Spellacy WN (1977). Oxytocinase and human placental lactogen for prediction of intrauterine growth retardation. Am J Obstet Gynecol, 15: 675–678.

Hertz JB (1984). Diagnostic procedures in threatened abortion. Obstet Gynecol, 64: 223–229.

Heys RF, Oakey RE, Scott JS, Stitch SR (1968). Urinary oestrogen and late pregnancy. Lancet, 1: 328–330.

Heys RP, Scott JS, Oakey RE, Stitch SR (1969). Estriol excretion in abnormal pregnancy. Obstet Gynecol, 33: 390–396.

Hoag RW (1971). Use of urinary estriol determinations in high risk pregnancy in the community hospital. Am J Obstet Gynecol, 110: 203–209.

Houghton DJ, Perry LA, Newnham JP, Chard T (1983). Nyctohemeral variation in the level of 'unconjugated' oestriol in maternal serum. J Obstet Gynaecol, 3: 221–224.

Howell RJS, Perry LA, Choglay NS, Dohn H, Chard T (1985). Placental protein 12 (PP12): A new test for the prediction of the small-for-gestational-age infant. Br J Obstet Gynaecol, 92: 1141–1144.

Hughes G, Bischof P, Wilson G, Klopper A (1980a). Assay of a placental protein to determine fetal risk. Br Med J, 280: 671–672.

Hughes G, Bischof P, Wilson G, Smith R, Klopper A (1980b). Tests of fetal wellbeing in the third trimester of pregnancy. Br J Obstet Gynaecol, 87: 650–656.

Huttenmoser JL, Weil-Franck C, Bischof P (1987). The disappearance rate of Schwangerschaftsprotein-1 in normal and pathological pregnancies. Br J Obstet Gynaecol, 94: 420–424.

Isouard G (1979). Value of total serum oestriol and human placental lactogen in the assessment of fetal-placental function. Austral NZ J Obstet Gynaecol, 16: 69–76.

Josimovich JB (1983). Placental lactogen and pituitary prolactin. In: Endocrinology of Pregnancy. Fuchs F, Klopper A (eds). Philadelphia: Harper & Row, pp 144–160.

Jouppila P, Tapanainen J, Huhtaniemi I (1979). Plasma HCG levels in patients with bleeding in the first and second trimesters of pregnancy. Br J Obstet Gynaecol, 86: 343–349.

Karg NJ, Csaba JF, Than GN, Arany AA, Szabo DG (1981). The prognosis of the possible foetal and placental complications during delivery by measuring maternal serum levels of pregnancy-specific beta 1-glycoprotein (SP1). Arch Gynecol, 231: 69–73.

Katagiri H, Distler W, Freeman RK, Goebelsmann U (1976). Estriol in pregnancy IV: Normal concentrations, diurnal and/or episodic variations and day-to-day changes of unconjugated and total estriol in late pregnancy plasma. Am J Obstet Gynecol, 124: 272–280.

Keller PJ, Baertschi U, Bader P, Gerber C, Scmid J, Saltermann R, Kopper E (1971). Biochemical detection of fetoplacental distress in risk pregnancies. Lancet, 2: 729–731.

Khouzami VA, Ginsburg DS, Daikoku NH, Johnson JW (1981). Urinary estrogens in postterm pregnancy. Am J Obstet Gynecol, 141: 205–211.

Kleiner, H, Brouet-Yager, M. (1973). Activité de la L-cystinyl-di-beta-naphtylamide hydrolase ('oxytocinase') sérique dans la grossesse normale, mesurée par une méthode chimique rapide. Clin Chim Acta, 48: 299–309.

Klopper A (1982). Newly discovered pregnancy-associated plasma proteins. Br J Obstet Gynaecol, 89: 687–693.

Klopper A, Hughes G (1980). The new placental proteins: Some clinical applications of their measurements. In: The Human Placenta: Proteins and Hormones. Klopper A, Geneazzani A, Grossipnani P (eds). London: Academic Press, pp 17–25.

Knight GJ, Kloza EM, Smith DE, Haddow J (1981). Efficency of human placental lactogen and alpha-fetoprotein measurement in twin pregnancy detection. Am J Obstet Gynecol, 141: 585–586.

Knottnerus JA, Delgado L, Knipschild PG (1986). Maternal haemoglobin and pregnancy outcome. Lancet, 2: 282.

Koller O, Sagen N, Ulstein M, Vaula D (1979). Fetal growth retardation associated with inadequate haemodilution in otherwise uncomplicated pregnancy. Acta Obstet Gynecol Scand, 58: 9–13.

Korda AR, Challis JJ, Anderson ABM, Turnbull AC (1975). Assessment of placental function in normal and pathological pregnancies by estimation of plasma oestradiol levels after injection of dehydroepiandrosterone sulphate. Br J Obstet Gynaecol, 82: 656–661.

Kunz J, Keller PJ (1976a). Ultrasound and biochemical findings in intrauterine growth retardation. J Perinat Med, 4: 85–94.

Kunz J, Keller PJ (1976b). HCG, HPL, oestradiol, progesterone and AFP in serum in patients with threatened abortion. Br J Obstet Gynaecol, 83: 640–644.

Laatikainen TS, Peltonen JI (1980). Amniotic fluid estriol, estriol precursors and pregnandiol in intrauterine growth retardation. J Steroid Biochem, 13: 265–269.

Lachman E, Hingley SM, Bates G, Ward AM, Stewart CR, Duncan SLB (1977). Detection and measurement of fetomaternal haemorrhage: Serum alpha-fetoprotein. Br Med J, 1: 1377–99.

Lauritzen CH (1967). A clinical test for placental functional activity using DHEA-sulphate and ACTH injections in the pregnant woman. Acta Endocrinol, Suppl 119: 188.

Lauritzen CH, Klopper A (1983). Estrogens and androgens. In: Endocrinology of Pregnancy. Fuchs F, Klopper A (eds). Philadelphia: Harper & Row, pp 73–91.

Leader LR, Baillie P (1980). Comparison of fetal movements and human placental lactogen as predictors of fetal outcome. S Afr Med J, 58: 609–610.

Letchworth AT, Chard T (1972). Placental lactogen levels as a screening test for fetal distress and neonatal asphyxia. Lancet, 1: 704–706.

Letchworth AT, Slattery M, Dennis KJ (1978). Clinical application of human-placental-lactogen values in late pregnancy. Lancet, 1: 955–957.

Lewin D (1983). Consultation prénatale. In: Traité d'Obstétrique. Vokaer R (ed). Paris: Masson, p 386.

Lin TM, Halbert SP, Kiefer D, Spellacy W, Gall S (1974). Characterization of four human pregnancy-associated plasma proteins. Am J Obstet Gynecol, 118: 223–236.

Lin TM, Halbert SP, Spellacy W, Berne BH (1977). Plasma concentration of four pregnancy proteins in complications of pregnancy. Am J Obstet Gynecol, 128: 808–810.

Lindberg S, Johansson E, Nilsson A (1974). Plasma levels of non conjugated oestradiol 17 and oestriol in high risk pregnancies. Acta Obstet Gynecol Scand (Suppl), 28: 38.

Low JA, Galbraith RS, Boston RW (1973). Maternal urinary estrogen patterns in intrauterine growth retardation. Obstet Gynecol, 42: 325–329.

McLaughlin PJ, Gee H, Johnson PM (1983). Placental-type alkaline phosphatase in pregnancy and malignancy plasma: Specific estimation using a monoclonal antibody in a solid phase enzyme immunoassay. Clin Chim Acta, 130: 199–209.

Macleod SC, Brown JB, Beischer NA (1967). The value of urinary oestriol measurment during pregnancy. Austral NZ J Obstet Gynaecol, 7: 25–27.

MacNaughton MC (1967). Hormone excretion as a measurement of fetal growth and development. Am J Obstet Gynecol, 27: 998–1019.

Mariona FG, Bhatia R, Syner FN, Koppitch F (1986). Chorionic villi sampling changes maternal serum alpha-fetoprotein. Prenat Diagn, 6: 69–73.

Mau G (1977). Hemoglobin changes during pregnancy and growth disturbances in the neonate. J Perinat Med, 5: 172–177.

McGregor WG, Kuhn RW, Jaffe RB (1983). Biologically active chorionic gonadotropin: Synthesis by the human fetus. Science, 220: 306–308.

Merkatz IR, Nitowsky HM, Maori JN, Johnson WE (1984). An association between low maternal serum alpha-fetoprotein and fetal chromosome abnormalities. Am J Obstet Gynecol, 148: 886–891.

Michie EA (1967). Urinary oestriol excretion in pregnancies complicated by suspected retarded intrauterine growth, toxaemia or essential hypertension. J Obstet Gynaecol Br Commnwlth, 74: 896–901.

Miller CA, Fetter MC, Boguslaski RC, Heiser EW (1977). Maternal serum unconjugated estriol and urine estriol concentration in normal and high risk pregnancy. Obstet Gynecol, 49: 287–292.

Morrison I, Green P, Oomen B (1980). The role of human placental lactogen assays in antepartum fetal assessment. Am J Obstet Gynecol, 136: 1055–1060.

Nielsen PV, Egebo K, Find C, Olsen CE (1981). Prognostic value of human placental lactogen (HPL) in an unselected obstetrical population. Acta Obstet Gynecol Scand, 60: 469–474.

Nielsen PV, Schioler V (1981). Ratio of human placental lactogenic hormone in amniotic fluid/maternal serum. Acta Obstet Gynecol Scand, 60: 9–12.

Nielsen PV, Schultz-Larsen P, Schioler V (1985). Screening in pregnancy with unconjugated estriol compared with total estriol. Acta Obstet Gynecol Scand, 64: 297–301.

Notation AD, Tagatz GE (1977). Unconjugated estriol and 15α-hydroxyestriol in complicated pregnancies. Am J Obstet Gynecol, 128: 747–756.

Obiekwe BC, Chard T (1983). A comparative study of the clinical use of four placental proteins in the third trimester. J Perinat Med, 11: 121–126.

Obiekwe BC, Grudzinskas JG, Chard T (1980). Circulating levels of placental protein 5 in the mother: Relation to birthweight. Br J Obstet Gynaecol, 87: 302–340.

Odell WO, Griffin J (1987). Pulsatile secretion of human chorionic gonadotropin in normal adults. New Engl J Med, 317: 1688–1691.

Odell WD, Wolfsen A, Yoshimoto Y, Weitzmann R, Fischer D, Hirose F (1977). Ectopic peptide synthesis: A universal concomitant of meoplasia. Trans Assoc Am Phys, 90: 204–227.

Odendaal HJ, Malan C, Oosthuizen T. (1981). Hormonal placental junctions and intra uterine growth retardation in patients with positive contraction stress tests. S Afr Med J, 59: 979–981.

Okpere E, Okorodudu AO, Gbinigie AO (1985). Fall in the heat-labile alkaline phosphatase isoenzyme levels during pregnancy in healthy Nigerians. Br J Obstet Gynaecol, 92: 1134–1136.

Ostergard DR (1973). Estriol in pregnancy. Obstet Gynecol Surv, 28: 215–231.

Pavlou C, Chard T, Letchworth AT (1972). Circulatory levels of human chorionic somatomammotrophin in late pregnancy: Disappearance from the circulation after delivery, variation during labour and circadian variation. J Obstet Gynaecol Br Commnwlth, 79: 629–634.

Perry L, Fattah D, Cochrane G, Obiekwe BC, Chard T (1984). Assays for blood oestriol in the assessment of fetal well-being: Is an extraction step necessary? J Obstet Gynaecol, 4: 154–156.

Persson PH, Grennert L, Gennser G, Eneroth P (1980). Fetal biparietal diameter and maternal plasma concentrations of placental lactogen, chorionic gonadotrophin, oestriol and alpha-fetoprotein in normal and pathological pregnancies. Br J Obstet Gynaecol, 87: 25–32.

Petrucco OM, Cellier K, Fishtall A (1973). Diagnosis of intrauterine fetal growth retardation by serial serum oxytocinase, urinary oestrogen and serum heat stable alkaline phosphatase (HSAP) estimations in complicated and hypertensive pregnancies. J Obstet Gynaecol Br Commnwlth, 80: 499–507.

Pittaway DE, Reish RI, Wentz AC (1985). Doubling times of human chorionic gonadotrophin increase in early viable intrauterine pregnancies. Am J Obstet Gynecol, 152: 299–302.

Pledger DR, Belfield A, Calder AA (1984). The predictive value of three pregnancy-associated proteins in the detection of the light-for-dates baby. Br J Obstet Gynaecol, 91: 870–874.

Roberts CJ, Hibbard BM, Evans DR, Evans KT, Lawrence KM, Hode M, Roberts E, Ennis WP (1979). Precision in estimating gestational age and its influence on sensitivity of alpha-fetoprotein screening. Br Med J, 1: 981–983.

Rosen SW (1986). New placental proteins: Chemistry, physiology and clinical use. Placenta, 7: 575–594.

Sagen N, Nilsen ST, Kim HC, Bergsjo P, Koller O (1984a). Maternal hemoglobin concentration is closely related to birth weight in normal pregnancies. Acta Obstet Gynecol Scand, 63: 245–248.

Sagen N, Nilsen ST, Kim HC, Koller O, Bergsjo P (1984b). The predictive value of total estriol, HPL and Hb on perinatal outcome in severe pre-eclampsia. Acta Obstet Gynecol Scand, 63: 603–608.

Said ME, Campbell DM, Azzam ME, MacGillivray I (1984). Beta-human chorionic gonadotrophin levels before and after the development of pre-eclampsia. Br J Obstet Gynaecol, 91: 772–775.

Salem HT, Westergaard JG, Hindersson P, Seppälä M, Chard T (1981a). Placental protein 5 (PP5) in placental abruption. Br J Obstet Gynaecol, 80: 500–503.

Salem HT, Lee JN, Seppälä M, Vaara L, Aula P, Al-Ani ATM, Chard T (1981b). Measurement of placental protein 5, placental lactogen and pregnancy specific β_1 glycoprotein in mid-trimester as a predictor of outcome of pregnancy. Br J Obstet Gynaecol, 88: 371–374.

Saxena BB (1983). Human chorionic gonadotrophin. In:

Endocrinology of Pregnancy. Fuchs F, Klopper A (eds). Philadelphia: Harper & Row, pp 50–72.

Schultz-Larsen, P, Sizaret Ph, Martel N, Hinderson P (1979). Differences in the slopes of dose–response curves measuring pregnancy specific Beta1-glycoprotein (SP1) by means of radioimmunoassay. Clin Chim Acta, 95: 347–351.

Schwers J, Hubinont C, Thomas C, Markowicz E (1986). The rate of increase of serum human chorionic gonadotrophin in normal intrauterine pregnancy. Am J Obstet Gynecol, 155: 255.

Seibel MM, Levesque LA, Seidenber EJ, Ransil BJ (1982). Serial first morning estriol determinations in evaluating the high risk obstetric patient. Obstet Gynecol, 59: 27–32.

Shane JM, Suzuki K (1974). Placental alkaline phosphatase: A review and re-evaluation of its applicability in monitoring fetoplacental function. Obstet Gynecol Surv, 29: 97–105.

Sharf M, Eibschitz I, Hakim M, Degani S, Rosner B (1984). Is serum free estriol measurement essential in the management of hypertensive disorders during pregnancy. Eur J Obstet Gynecol Reprod Biol, 17: 365–375.

Sinosich MJ, Ferrier A, Teisner B, Porter R, Westergaard JG, Saunders DM (1985). Circulating pregnancy-associated plasma protein A and its tissue concentration in tubal ectopic gestation. J Clin Reprod Fertil, 3: 311–317.

Smith ML (1980). Raised maternal serum alpha-fetoprotein levels and low birthweight babies. Br J Obstet Gynaecol, 87: 1099–1102.

Smith GV, Smith OW (1933). Excessive anterior-pituitary like hormone and variations in oestrin in toxemias of late pregnancy. Proc Soc Exp Biol Med, 30: 918–919.

Spellacy WN, Buhi WC, Birk SA (1975). The effectiveness of human placental lactogen measurements as an adjunct in decreasing perinatal deaths. Results of a retrospective and a randomized controlled prospective study. Am J Obstet Gynecol, 15: 835–844.

Stovall WS, Dashow EE, Read JA (1985). Serum unconjugated estriol level as a predictor of pulmonary maturity. Am J Obstet Gynecol, 153: 568–569.

Sutcliffe RG, Kukulska-Langlands BM, Horne CH, Maclean AB, Jandial V, Sutherland HW, Gibb S, Bowtian AW (1982). Studies on the concentration of PAPP-A during normal and complicated pregnancy. Placenta, 3: 71–80.

Tabor A, Larsen SO, Nielsen J, Nielsen J, Philip J, Pilgaard B, Videbech P, Norgaard-Pedersen B (1987). Screening for Down's syndrome using an iso-risk curve based on maternal age and serum alpha-fetoprotein level. Br J Obstet Gynaecol, 94: 636–642.

Targett CS, Gunesee H, McBride F, Beischer N (1973). An evaluation of the effects of smoking on maternal oestriol excretion during pregnancy and on fetal outcome. J Obstet Gynaecol Br Commnwlth, 80: 815–821.

Toop K, Klopper A (1981). Concentration of pregnancy-associated plasma protein A (PAPP-A) in patients with pre-eclamptic toxaemia. In: Placenta: Receptors, Pathology and Toxicology. Miller RK, Thiede H (eds). London: Saunders, pp 167–171.

Travers P, Bodmer WF (1984). Preparation and characterisation of monoclonal antibodies against placental alkaline phosphatase and other human trophoblast-associated determinants. Int J Cancer, 33: 633–641.

Trudinger BJ, Gordon YB, Grudzinskas JG, Hull MRG, Lewis PJ (1979). Fetal breathing movements and other tests of fetal well-being: A comparative evaluation. Br Med J, 2: 577–579.

Tulchinsky D (1980). Use of biochemical indices in the management of high risk obstetric patients. Clin Perinatol, 7: 413–421.

Tulchinsky D, Frigoletto FD, Ryan KJ, Fischman J (1975). Plasma estetrol as an index of fetal well-being. J Clin Endocrinol Metab, 40: 560–567.

Tyson JE, Austin KL, Favinholt JW (1971). Prolonged nutritional deprivation in pregnancy: Changes in human chorionic somatomammotrophin and growth hormone secretion. Am J Obstet Gynecol, 109: 1080–1082.

Van Leusden HA (1976). Chorionic gonadotrophin in pathological pregnancy. In: Plasma Hormone Assays in Evaluation of Fetal Well-being. Klopper A (ed). Edinburgh: Churchill Livingstone.

Van Look PFA, Top-Huisman M, Gnodde HP (1981). Effect of ampicillin or amoxycillin administration on plasma and urinary estrogen levels during normal pregnancy. Eur J Obstet Gynecol Reprod Biol, 12: 225–233.

Vining RF, McGinley RA, Symons RG (1983). Hormones in saliva: Mode of entry and consequenct implications for clinical interpretation. Clin Chem, 29: 1752–1756.

Wald NJ, Cuckle H, Stirrat GM, Bennett MJ, Turnbull AC (1977). Maternal serum alpha-fetoprotein and low birthweight. Lancet, 2: 208–209.

Wald NJ, Cuckle HS, Peck S, Stirrat GM, Turnbull AC (1979). Maternal serum alpha fetoprotein in relation to zygosity. Br Med J, 1: 455.

Wald NJ, Cuckle HS, Boreham J, Turnbull AC (1980). Maternal serum alpha-fetoprotein and birthweight. Br J Obstet Gynaecol, 87: 860–863.

Walters BNJ, Lao T, Smith V, De Swiet M (1985). Alpha-fetoprotein elevation and proteinuric pre-eclampsia. Br J Obstet Gynaecol, 92: 341–344.

Watney RJM, Hallum J, Ladell D, Scott P (1970). The relative usefulness of methods of assessing placental junction. J Obstet Gynaecol Br Commnwlth, 77: 301–311.

Westergaard JG, Chemnitz J, Teisner B, Poulsen HK, Ipsen L, Besck B (1983). Pregnancy associated plasma protein A: A possible marker in the classification and diagnosis of Cornelia de Lange syndrome. Prenat Diagn, 3: 225–232.

Westergaard JG, Teisner B, Hau J, Grudzinskas JG (1984a). Placental protein measurements in complicated pregnancies. I: Intrauterine growth retardation. Br J Obstet Gynaecol, 91: 1216–1223.

Westergaard JG, Teisner B, Hau J, Grudzinskas JG (1984b). Placental protein measurements in complicated pregnancies. II: Pregnancy-related hypertension. Br J Obstet Gynaecol, 91: 1224–1229.

Westergaard JG, Teisner B, Sinosich MJ, Madsen LT, Grudzinskas SG (1985). Does ultrasound examination render biochemical tests obsolete in the prediction of early pregnancy failure. Br J Obstet Gynaecol, 92: 77–83.

Westergaard JG, Teisner B, Grudzinskas JG (1986). Biochemical assessment of placental function. Late pregnancy. Clin Obstet Gynaecol, 13: 571–591.

Yeh SY, Read JA (1983). Plasma unconjugated estriol as an indicator of fetal dysmaturity in post-term pregnancy. Obstet Gynecol, 62: 22–25.

Zlatnik FJ, Varner MW, Hauser KS (1979). Human placental lactogen: A predictor of perinatal outcome. Obstet Gynecol, 54: 314–317.

30 Biophysical assessment of fetal well-being

Patrick Mohide and Marc J. N. C. Keirse

1 Introduction

Biophysical methods of monitoring both high and low risk pregnancies have largely replaced biochemical tests of endocrine function of the fetoplacental unit, such as oestrogens and human placental lactogen which were popularized in the 1970s (see Chapter 29). Biophysical methods have identified measures of fetal function that provide indirect information about the integrity and functional state of neurological, neuromuscular, and excretory function.

This chapter will address some of the most widely used of these methods: cardiotocography (stressed and non-stressed) and the biophysical profile and some of its components. Other biophysical methods of assessing fetal well-being, including fetal movement counting (see Chapter 28) and Doppler measurement of blood flow (see Chapter 27), are discussed elsewhere in this book. Although the continuation of adequate fetal growth (see Chapters 26 and 27) is also a measure of continuing fetal health, it is a long term measure and could not be expected to detect relatively sudden changes in fetal status occurring over days, or even one or two weeks. It is in this area that biophysical methods show most promise. No known method of fetal assessment is likely to predict or prevent the consequences of sudden events such as rupture of the membranes with cord prolapse or abruptio placentae.

Events that may be detectable over short time-spans include antepartum stillbirth; decreases in amniotic fluid volume leading to umbilical cord compression and fetal hypoxia (particularly in post-term pregnancy or intrauterine growth failure; see Chapter 26); deterioration of placental function (due to partial placental abruption, severe pregnancy induced hypertension (see Chapter 33), other maternal cardiovascular disease); and fetal disease (such as severe anaemia due to isoimmunization (see Chapter 35) or fetal–maternal haemorrhage, infections, or fetal malformations).

It is hoped and believed that these methods of antenatal detection, combined with prompt intervention, will prevent some undesirable outcomes such as antepartum or intrapartum stillbirth, fetal distress in labour, asphyxia at birth (as measured by low Apgar score and/or cord blood gases), neonatal death, neonatal morbidity (as measured by the occurrence of specific neonatal events); and long term outcomes such as mental retardation, cerebral palsy, or learning disabilities. Few of these outcomes, except death, are free from problems of reproducibility in their measurement. Also, some women may experience more than one of these outcomes.

What, then, is the standard against which we should measure the success or failure of a programme of antenatal monitoring? Considering only mortality carries the risk of grossly underestimating the value of a test. Including all the other outcomes carries the risk of overestimating its clinical effects. Some authors have used measures (indices) that combine adverse perinatal events (Kaar 1980).

What useful measures are available when abnormalities in antenatal biophysical monitoring are detected?

Only a few pathologies affecting the fetus can be potentially reversed or relieved by known interventions, and none of these has been validated in clinical trials. These may include pharmacotherapy for correction of fetal cardiac irregularities, surgical correction of fetal abnormalities, and other intrauterine therapy, such as exchange transfusion for severe isoimmunization (see Chapter 35). General measures such as enforced bed rest in hospital (see Chapter 39) have not proved to be beneficial in the conditions for which they were used.

The most commonly used therapy is to move the fetus to what is believed to be a safer environment, the neonatal nursery. This can be achieved by induction of labour or caesarean section.

Much has been made of the effectiveness of these tests in providing reassurance to the physician, midwife, and pregnant woman about the continuing normality of the pregnancy. This reassurance may, in fact, alter caregiver behaviour, and reduce the number of other interventions, reduce the length of antenatal hospital stay, and allow women to continue as outpatients (Flynn *et al.* 1982). Although claims to this effect may or may not be valid, the reduction of 'unnecessary' interventions has become a major goal for the providers and consumers of perinatal care and for those involved in funding it (governments, insurers, consumers, and the taxpayer). It may therefore be considered an important and useful secondary outcome of antenatal screening.

Two general types of evidence have been put forward to support the contention that antenatal biophysical monitoring is clinically useful. These can be summarized into assertions that, first, these methods can detect or predict adverse perinatal events and that, second, when used with appropriate obstetrical interventions, they can reduce the frequency or severity of adverse perinatal events.

The evaluations which follow are based on published data that compared test results of non-stress antepartum cardiotocography and of biophysical profile scoring with the occurrence of adverse perinatal events. Only reports that displayed sufficient data to permit calculation of test properties were included, and only the stable test properties (sensitivity, specificity, and likelihood ratios) have been compared.

Only six randomized or quasi-randomized studies were identified in which alternative test strategies were compared prospectively. (Brown *et al.* 1982; Flynn *et al.* 1982; Kidd *et al.* 1985; Lumley *et al.* 1983; Manning *et al.* 1984; Platt *et al.* 1985). The most common form of investigative report was the 'case series', reporting results of tests used in hospital out-patient or in-patient settings. In virtually all studies, results were not blinded but were available to the physicians and used in clinical decision-making. This may have led, therefore, to distortions in the predictive properties of tests (see Chapter 3).

Reporting of target conditions varied greatly and included stillbirth, neonatal death or both, anomalies, fetal distress or abnormal fetal heart rate patterns in labour, low Apgar score, light for dates, and neonatal morbidity. Some reported combined outcomes of one or more adverse perinatal events.

Rates of clinical intervention such as caesarean section for fetal distress, and admission to neonatal units were reported in a few studies. In most studies, the number of cases included in the analysis of test results was either unclear or stated to be restricted to the 'last test' performed before delivery. This means that for studies where two or more tests were performed per woman, the majority of test results were not included in calculations of test properties. More important, this retrospective viewpoint does not reflect the perspective of the clinician who does not yet know the timing of delivery and must nevertheless consider the test result at hand. It does not help us to determine, for instance, the probability that an abnormal or equivocal test result will return to normal if no clinical action is taken.

Very little account has been taken of the longitudinal development of fetal function with gestational age. Druzin *et al.* (1985) has shown a clear relationship between the frequency of 'non-reactive' antenatal cardiotocograms and gestational age. Bottoms *et al.* (1986) identified the physiological variance in the measurement of amniotic fluid volume with gestational age. Rarely have other sources of variation in function or behavioural states, or of the timing and duration of observation (Brown and Patrick 1981) been evaluated. The reproducibility within and between observers has been assessed for some tests (Trimbos and Keirse 1978a) but not for others, such as biophysical scoring, which incorporates multiple potential sources of variation in measurement, or for Doppler flow measurement (see Chapter 27).

The various biophysical assessments of the fetus, have been evaluated with respect to a number of perinatal outcomes. The most clear-cut and unequivocally measured is perinatal death. Indices of morbid outcome, such as low Apgar score, are of particular interest since pregnant women, physicians, and society as a whole are concerned with the quality of survival. More important than the prediction of any particular outcome is the prediction that *any* adverse outcome might occur; that is, the likelihood of fetal *or* neonatal death *or* fetal asphyxia at birth *or* neonatal morbidity *or* long term handicap. Although some studies have used such combinations as a measure of poor outcome, no comprehensive index is as yet widely accepted. The use of individual measures, on the other hand, will tend to result in underestimates of the true predictive powers of tests.

2 Methods of biophysical assessment

2.1 Antepartum fetal heart rate monitoring (cardiotocography)

2.1.1 Contraction stress testing

Continuous recording of fetal heart rate and uterine activity was first developed for use in labour in an attempt to identify the fetus at risk of death or morbidity due to intrapartum asphyxia (see Chapter 54). Because many fetal deaths occur prior to the onset of labour, Pose *et al.* (1969) proposed the stimulation of contractions with oxytocin for short periods of time in pregnancies at risk, to allow observation of the fetal heart rate for evidence of deceleration patterns under labour-like conditions. This technique, which subsequently became known as the 'oxytocin challenge test' or 'contraction stress test', suffers from a number of disadvantages. It is time-consuming, requires an intravenous infusion and has the potential to harm the fetus. Indeed, its use is contraindicated in some pregnancies at risk; for example, when there is antepartum bleeding, placenta praevia, a history of preterm labour, or preterm rupture of membranes. Some have substituted prostaglandins for oxytocin to avoid the need for infusion, but the same concerns remain.

The nipple stimulation stress test is similar in purpose to, and has been directly compared with (Lipitz *et al.* 1987), the oxytocin challenge test. The pregnant woman is encouraged to stimulate her nipples with her fingers, palms, warm moist washcloth, or a heating pad, directly or through her clothing (Hill *et al.* 1986a,b; Moenning and Hill 1986; Curtis *et al.* 1986; Moenning and Hill 1987). Contractions can be stimulated effectively but the mechanism, previously assumed to be oxytocin release, remains unknown (Ross *et al.* 1986). Placebo also produces an equivalent contractile response in 20 per cent of women (Curtis *et al.* 1986). The nipple stimulation stress test has some of the same disadvantages as the oxytocin challenge test with the additional problem that, while stimulation is easily discontinued, there is a time lag of more than 3 minutes between stimulation and peak uterine response (Moenning and Hill 1986, 1987). Also, excessive uterine activity occurs in as many as 55 per cent of women and hyperstimulation with fetal bradycardia in 7 to 14 per cent (Hill *et al.* 1984; Moenning and Hill 1986, 1987). Hill *et al.* (1986a,b) and Schellpfeffer *et al.* (1985) have also reported cases of severe uterine tetany associated with fetal heart rate abnormalities. Because of these concerns, and because it offers no clear advantages over other techniques, the nipple stimulation stress test should probably be relegated to the history books.

2.1.2 Non-stress testing

The evaluation of fetal heart rate patterns without the added stress of induced contractions was first proposed by Kubli *et al.* (1969) and Hammacher (1969). This 'non-stress test' has been widely incorporated into antenatal care as a screening and as a diagnostic test.

How reproducible is this test? To answer this question we must examine the three major sources of error that may cause interference with reproducible results: 'the examination, the examined, and the examiner'.

There is no universally accepted technique for performing non-stress antepartum testing. Various durations and frequencies of monitoring are used, and these can have a powerful influence on the predictive properties of the test (Brown and Patrick 1981). Additional manoeuvres, such as abdominal stimulation, sound stimulation (Smith *et al.* 1986), glucose infusions (Devoe *et al.* 1987a), post-prandial repeat tests and follow-up oxytocin challenge tests for suspected abnormal records, have been suggested or used (Miller *et al.* 1978; Paul and Keegan 1979; Barrett *et al.* 1981). Like the contraction stress test, the non-stress test requires sophisticated equipment which may occasionally malfunction. Ultrasound transducers are prone to physical damage and may present artefactual information to the monitor circuitry. Fetal and maternal movements may also produce artefacts since ultrasound detects movement rather than sound; however, the results of at least one study suggest that ambulation with telemetry does not interfere with non-stress testing (Devoe *et al.* 1987b). If the ultrasound beam is misdirected, flow in maternal blood vessels may be sufficient to be counted, and the record (especially if the mother has a tachycardia) may be indistinguishable from a fetal heart rate. The microprocessor circuitry within the fetal monitor may occasionally err in computing heart rate, and display a value that is half or double the true rate.

Maternal obesity, polyhydramnios, the presence of an active or mobile fetus, or a very small or preterm fetus, may result in an unsatisfactory record. Fetal cardiac arrhythmias frequently make satisfactory recording difficult or impossible. When all these factors are taken into consideration, as many as 10–15 per cent of all records may be unsatisfactory for interpretation (Lyons *et al.* 1979; Keirse and Trimbos 1980). During fetal rest periods, which not uncommonly last for more than 30 minutes, normal physiological reduction in heart rate variability may be confused with pathological change (Trimbos and Keirse 1978b; Visser *et al.* 1981). Medications taken by the mother are often transferred to the fetus, and, particularly in the case of drugs with a sedative effect on the central nervous system, may in themselves produce heart rate patterns that can be interpreted as abnormal. Likewise the gestational age of the fetus has a strong influence on the frequency of false positive non-reactive tests (Bishop 1981), with 'abnormal' patterns being more frequently described in the preterm fetus (Dawes *et al.* 1982).

A variety of methods for interpreting non-stress cardiotocograms have been described, all of which include evaluation of some or all of the following characteristics: baseline fetal heart rate; various interpretations of short- and long-term fetal heart rate variability; accelerations of fetal heart rate associated with spontaneous and/or stimulated movements of the fetus; and decelerations associated with spontaneous uterine contractions. The more complicated systems assign scores to some or all of these parameters (e.g. Fischer *et al.* 1976; Pearson and Weaver 1978), sometimes subsequently grouping the scores (e.g. Trimbos and Keirse 1978a). The most commonly used method is to divide traces into reactive (normal) and non-reactive (abnormal), based on the presence or absence of adequate baseline heart rate variability and heart rate accelerations with fetal movement (e.g. Schifrin *et al.* 1981; Flynn and Kelly 1977).

In a study of 300 consecutive high risk cases, Flynn *et al.* (1982) used four different methods for reporting traces, and demonstrated that identical traces could have prompted different clinical managements depending on the approach used. Trimbos and Keirse (1978a) examined the interpretation of 'difficult' 20-minute traces by five experienced observers. When the visual assessment of these observers was compared with their assessments using the computed total Fischer scores, the latter method yielded more consistent agreement (82 vs. 71 per cent). The improvement when the score was used was small for the differentiation between 'good' and 'moderate' traces and most marked for the clinically more important distinction between 'moderate' and 'bad'. Using visual assessment, 10 per cent of traces were considered bad on one occasion and not on the other, whereas with the Fischer score the figure was less than 2 per cent. The likely practical implications of this are illustrated by a study conducted by Krebs and Petres (1978). They correlated test interpretations using scored and unscored methods for 253 women with adverse pregnancy outcome (perinatal deaths plus neonatal morbidity) and demonstrated an improved test specificity with a consequent reduction in false positive results with scoring (Table 30.1).

Table 30.1 Comparison of unscored and scored assessment of antepartum cardiotocography

	Death or morbidity	Healthy
Unscored		
Non-reactive	18	16
Reactive	15	204
Scored		
Score <9	18	3
Score <9	15	217
	Unscored reactive/non-reactive (%)	**Scored (Fischer) (%)**
Sensitivity	54.5	54.5
Specificity	92.7	98.6
Likelihood ratios:		
Abnormal	7.5	38.9
Normal	0.5	0.5
Positive predictive value	52.9	85.7
Negative predictive value	93.2	93.2
Accuracy	87.7	92.9
Cohen's Kappa	0.47	0.63

(Data from Krebs and Petres 1978.)

Even when a fixed method is used, interpretation of a trace may vary when an individual observer 'reads' the same trace at different times or when the same trace is 'read' by different observers. Trimbos and Keirse (1978a) found that for the five parameters of the Fischer score (Fischer *et al.* 1976), intra-observer agreement ranged from 99 to 73 per cent, and inter-observer agreement from 97 to 34 per cent. Agreement was best for basal heart rate and worst for accelerations (although after redefinition of 'acceleration', agreement greatly improved).

As can be seen in Tables 30.2 to 30.7, perinatal death, fetal distress, Apgar scores, cord pH, newborn morbidities, and combined assessments of these outcome events have all been used. The non-stress test is a relatively good predictor of adverse outcome when morbidities and mortalities are combined (Table 30.7) although the biophysical profile is considerably better.

Kaar (1980) collected four types of antenatal test results on the same group of women and evaluated them against the same outcome, a combined mortality and morbidity index. The comparison showed that the non-stress test (scored) and oxytocin challenge test were twice as sensitive as and not less specific than oestriol excretion and human placental lactogen measurements (Table 30.8).

In the majority of these studies clinicians have not been 'blinded' to the test results. Clinical action based on the results clearly could have altered the outcome. Using perinatal mortality as an example, a death that would otherwise have occurred might have been prevented by appropriate action; conversely, a death that would not otherwise have occurred might have resulted from, for example, unwarranted elective delivery preterm. In such cases, the outcome would not accurately reflect the validity or predictive power of the test result: in the first instance, a positive test would appear to have been a false positive; in the second, what would have been a false positive would appear to have been true.

In screening, it has been suggested that the non-stress test is more useful for its negative predictive

Table 30.2 Antepartum cardiotocography and biophysical profile: test properties for the outcome perinatal death

Author	Year	Sensitivity	Specificity	Likelihood ratio for test result	
				Positive	Negative
Non-stress cardiotocography					
Baskett *et al.*	1984	0.64	0.90	6.1	0.4
Beischer *et al.*	1983	0.53	0.90	5.4	0.5
Devoe	1980	0.33	0.79	1.6	0.8
Flynn and Kelly	1977	1.00	1.00	N.C.	N.C.
Keane *et al.*	1981	0.33	0.81	1.8	0.8
Kubli *et al.*	1977	0.54	0.93	8.3	0.5
Lyons *et al.*	1979	0.76	0.94	12.0	0.3
Manning FA *et al.*	1980	0.71	0.77	3.1	0.4
Manning FD *et al.*	1984	0.75	0.84	4.6	0.3
Mendenhall *et al.*	1980	0.80	0.83	4.8	0.2
Phelan	1981	0.64	0.81	3.4	0.5
Platt *et al.*	1983	0.50	0.91	5.6	0.6
Pratt *et al.*	1979	0.0	0.96	0.0	1.0
Rayburn *et al.*	1980	0.67	0.96	17.6	0.4
Rochard *et al.*	1976	1.00	0.70	3.3	0.0
Vintzileos *et al.*	1983	1.00	0.88	8.6	0.0
Biophysical profile					
Baskett et al.	1984	0.64	0.97	21.7	0.4
Manning FA et al.	1980	0.60	0.79	2.9	0.5
Manning FD et al.	1984	0.50	0.94	8.8	0.5
Manning FA et al.	1985	0.33	0.99	45.8	0.7
Platt et al.	1983	0.50	0.95	9.4	0.5
Platt et al.	1985	0.67	0.97	23.1	0.3

N.C. = Not calculable, division by zero.

Table 30.3 Antepartum cardiotocography and biophysical profile: test properties for the outcome fetal distress in labour

Author	Year	Sensitivity	Specificity	Likelihood ratio for test result	
				Positive	Negative
Non-stress cardiotocography					
Baskett *et al.*	1984	0.23	0.90	2.3	0.9
Flynn and Kelly	1977	0.89	0.86	6.5	0.1
Keane *et al.*	1981	0.55	0.88	4.5	0.5
Lenstrup and Haase	1985	0.79	0.84	5.1	0.2
Manning FA *et al.*	1979	0.68	0.98	30.3	0.3
Manning FA *et al.*	1980	0.48	0.78	2.1	0.7
Mendenhall *et al.*	1980	0.47	0.84	2.9	0.6
Phelan	1981	0.41	0.82	2.3	0.7
Platt *et al.*	1983	0.57	0.93	8.2	0.5
Pratt *et al.*	1979	0.06	0.97	2.0	1.0
Rayburn *et al.*	1980	0.63	0.97	19.2	0.4
Vintzileos *et al.*	1983	1.00	0.90	9.6	0.0
Biophysical profile					
Baskett *et al.*	1984	0.13	0.97	5.1	0.9
Manning FA *et al.*	1980	0.74	0.85	4.8	0.3
Platt *et al.*	1983	0.36	0.96	8.1	0.7
Platt *et al.*	1985	0.31	0.98	15.2	0.7

Table 30.4 Antepartum cardiotocography and biophysical profile: test properties for the outcome low Apgar score

Author	Year	Sensitivity	Specificity	Likelihood ratio for test result	
				Positive	Negative
Non-stress cardiotocography					
Baskett *et al.*	1984	0.33	0.90	3.2	0.7
Beischer *et al.*	1983	0.19	0.91	2.2	0.9
Chew *et al.*	1985	0.43	0.79	2.1	0.7
Flynn and Kelly	1977	0.59	0.85	3.8	0.5
Keane *et al.*	1981	0.54	0.87	4.1	0.5
Lenstrup and Haase	1985	0.44	0.81	2.3	0.7
Manning FA *et al.*	1979	0.53	0.78	2.4	0.6
Manning FA *et al.*	1980	0.58	0.79	2.7	0.5
Manning FD *et al.*	1984	0.53	0.85	3.5	0.5
Pratt *et al.*	1979	0.12	0.97	4.5	0.9
Rayburn *et al.*	1980	0.14	0.96	3.7	0.9
Biophysical profile					
Baskett *et al.*	1984	0.27	0.97	9.1	0.8
Manning FA *et al.*	1980	0.68	0.83	4.0	0.4
Manning FD *et al.*	1984	0.76	0.97	27.4	0.2
Platt *et al.*	1983	0.14	0.94	2.5	0.9
Platt *et al.*	1985	0.25	0.97	8.5	0.8

Table 30.5 Antepartum cardiotocography and biophysical profile: test properties for the outcome low umbilical cord pH

Author	Year	Sensitivity	Specificity	Likelihood ratio for test result	
				Positive	Negative
Non-stress cardiotocography					
Chew *et al.*	1985	0.38	0.77	1.6	0.8
Kubli *et al.*	1977	0.20	0.94	3.5	0.9
Lenstrup and Haase	1985	0.36	0.81	1.9	0.8
Vintzileos *et al.*	1987	1.00	0.72	3.6	0.0
Biophysical profile					
Vintzileos *et al.*	1987	0.90	0.96	23.4	0.1

Table 30.6 Antepartum cardiotocography and biophysical profile: test properties for the outcome neonatal morbidity as defined by the respective authors

Author	Year	Sensitivity	Specificity	Likelihood ratio for test result	
				Positive	Negative
Non-stress cardiotocography					
Hann *et al.*	1987	0.13	0.95	2.6	0.9
Keane *et al.*	1981	0.53	0.88	4.3	0.5
Rochard *et al.*	1976	0.74	0.87	5.8	0.3
Biophysical profile					
Hann *et al.*	1987	0.13	0.95	2.6	0.9

Table 30.7 Antepartum cardiotocography and biophysical profile: test properties for combined adverse outcomes grouped by the authors

Author	Year	Sensitivity	Specificity	Likelihood ratio for test result	
				Positive	Negative
Non-stress cardiotocography					
Baskett *et al.*	1984	0.20	0.91	2.2	0.9
Devoe	1980	0.52	0.82	2.9	0.6
Keirse and Trimbos	1980	0.70	0.87	5.6	0.3
Krebs+ (scored)	1978	0.55	0.99	40.0	0.5
Krebs+ (unscored)	1978	0.55	0.93	7.5	0.5
Lenstrup and Haase	1985	0.52	0.89	4.6	0.5
Mendenhall *et al.*	1980	0.55	0.85	3.6	0.5
Platt *et al.*	1983	0.43	0.94	7.4	0.6
Pratt *et al.*	1979	0.07	0.98	2.1	1.0
Rayburn *et al.*	1980	0.29	0.97	10.3	0.7
Rochard *et al.*	1976	0.83	0.87	6.5	0.2
Biophysical profile					
Baskett *et al.*	1984	0.12	0.99	14.6	0.9
Platt *et al.*	1983	0.32	0.97	10.4	0.7
Platt *et al.*	1985	0.32	0.99	60.1	0.7

Table 30.8 Comparison of various antenatal tests for prediction of perinatal mortality and morbidity

Test	Positive predictive value (%)	Sensitivity (%)
Urinary estriol	65	20
Human placental lactogen	49	22
Non-stress test (scored)	41	42
Oxytocin challenge test (scored)	48	53

(Data from Kaar 1980; n = 292, prevalence = 26%)

value than for positive diagnosis and can be safely used to screen all pregnant women. Given the current statistically low risk of adverse outcome, this is almost certainly not true (Trimbos and Keirse 1978b). With the perinatal mortality rate in the general population at its current level (approximately 10 per 1000) one would be correct in guessing, without any test data whatsoever, that a fetus or neonate would have a 99 per cent chance of survival. In order to demonstrate a statistically significant improvement on that prediction, an enormous sample size would be needed. Even if such a small difference could be demonstrated statistically it would have little clinical significance. Even in high risk populations, where the prevalence of abnormal outcome is higher, negative test results do not alter post-test likelihood enough to be clinically useful.

The inclusion of lethal congenital abnormalities in the 'gold standard' presents special problems. They are more often associated with abnormal than with normal test results (10 per cent vs. 0.32 per cent, Varma 1981; 13 per cent vs. 0.4 per cent, Lyons *et al.* 1979). Including babies with congenital abnormalities in the 'gold standard' tends therefore to overestimate the value of the test. If action is taken to deliver a baby with a severe congenital abnormality on the basis of an abnormal tracing, not only will the mother run all the risks of the intervention, but there is clearly a possibility that the baby may still succumb or be rescued only to survive with a serious impairment. Proponents of routine ultrasound screening and biophysical profile scoring claim that their methods can differentiate the normal from the malformed fetus.

There are several real dangers in using the non-stress test to screen women in whom the likelihood of the fetus being in difficulty is small. The more frequently non-stress tests are performed, the greater will be the proportion which are of unsatisfactory quality (Pearson 1981). Screening a group of women with a low probability of adverse outcome will result in a higher proportion of positive test results that are false positive. Intervention based on the results of a 'positive' non-stress test in a low-risk group of women will often do more harm than good. Take, for example, a woman with a one per cent risk of poor perinatal outcome. When we review Table 30.7 we see that all but one report demonstrate likelihood ratios for abnormal results between 2.1 and 10.3. Let us assume likelihood ratio of 6 for an abnormal non-stressed result. What will happen to this woman's probability of poor outcome if her test result is abnormal?

pre-test probability = 1% = 0.01
pre-test odds = 0.01:(1–0.01) = 0.01:0.99

Table 30.9 Effect of changes in definition of normality on performance of non-stress tests

Abnormal scores	Positive predictive (%)	Negative predictive (%)	Sensitivity (%)	Specificity (%)	Likelihood ratios	
					Low score	High score
0–2	100	76	8	100	N.C.	0.9
0–3	100	76	12	100	N.C.	0.9
0–4	85	77	14	99	14	0.9
0–5	76	77	17	98	9	0.8
0–6	59	78	26	94	4	0.8
0–7	43	80	45	79	2	0.7
0–8	36	85	72	55	2	0.5
0–9	29	88	93	18	1	0.4

N.C. = not calculable, division by zero.
*Data derived from Kaar 1980; n = 292, prevalence = 26% (perinatal mortality/morbidity index).

post-test odds = 6 × 0.01:0.99 = 0.06:0.99
post-test probability = 0.06/(0.06 + 0.99) = 0.057 = 5.7%

Her post-test probability is still only 5.7 per cent; that is, there is still a greater than 94 per cent chance of the test result being false positive.

Other questions remain even when non-stress tests are performed and scored meticulously. If a test result (for example, a Fischer score), can have a value between 0 and 10, where should the cut-off between normal and abnormal be set? The nearer a score is to the extreme of the range the greater the confidence with which a prediction of outcome can be made. Keirse and Trimbos (1980) found that Fischer scores between 0 and 5 were good predictors of adverse outcome, and scores between 8 and 10 were predictive of good outcome, but that the 15 per cent of traces which scored 6 or 7 were 'too unreliable predictor(s) to be of real clinical value'. The manner in which results in this 'grey zone' are assigned to normal or abnormal categories has major implications for the performance of the test overall (Keirse and Trimbos 1981). All the test properties are influenced by the choice of threshold (Table 30.9) and they reach optimal values at different levels of cut-off. The final choice must be based on a value judgement which takes into account the level of risk in the women being tested (if the prevalence of adverse outcome is low, the cut-off should be higher) and the extent of likely benefits and hazards that may result from any action based on these results. Alternatively, it can be argued that the intermediate group should be managed clinically with serial non-stress tests to try to assign them to the clearly normal and clearly abnormal group. As has been described (before see Chapter 3), likelihood ratios offer an advantage over sensitivity and specificity in quantifying the predictive power of diagnostic and screening tests when test results can or must be expressed in more than two categories of results. The likelihood ratios for each category will provide a guide to assigning appropriate intervention (or non-intervention) strategies.

2.2 Fetal biophysical profile

In 1980, Manning reported on a prospective, blinded study of 216 pregnancies with a variety of high risk factors including post dates, hypertension, diabetes and suspect intrauterine growth retardation. He followed all pregnancies with serial ultrasounds and antenatal cardiotocography (non-stress test) and he identified five biophysical 'variables': fetal movement, tone, reactivity, breathing, and qualitative amniotic fluid volume (Table 30.10). Combining these assessments into a score he was able to reduce the incidence of false positive and false negative results compared to non-stress test alone.

These variables are not independent. Four out of the five variables depend on the presence of fetal movement of one type or another. The fifth measure, amniotic fluid volume, may be influenced by very different physiological and pathological processes, but may also, in its more severe form, directly affect the other measures in the biophysical score by restricting movement.

How reproducible is this test? There are no published data that consider this aspect of the biophysical score. It is reasonable to suggest that because of their subjective nature, some of the variables may be subject to considerable variation in measurement. The problems associated with the non-stress test, which is incorporated into the biophysical score, have already been reviewed. Fetal breathing movements can be influenced by a variety of factors; for example, maternal blood glucose levels (Boylan and Lewis 1980; Devoe *et al.* 1986; Nijhuis *et al.* 1986; Devoe *et al.* 1987a,b). The assessment of fetal breathing, fetal tone, and amniotic fluid volume movements may be subject to considerable inter-observer error. Clearly there is a need for assessment of the reproducibility of the biophysical score and its component variables.

Table 30.10 Fetal biophysical scoring

Variable	Score 2
Fetal breathing movements	The presence of at least 30 sec of sustained fetal breathing movements in 30 min of observation
Fetal movements	Three or more gross body movements in 30 min of observations. Simultaneous limb and trunk movements counted as a single movement
Fetal tone	At least one episode of motion of a limb from a position of flexion to extension and a rapid return to flexion
Fetal reactivity	Two or more fetal heart rate accelerations of at least 15 sec and associated with fetal movement in 40 minutes
Qualitative ámniotic fluid volume	A pocket of amniotic fluid that measures at least 1 cm in two perpendicular planes

One additional claim made for the biophysical profile is that it permits assessment of the possibility of major congenital anomalies. This may well be important. Whether or not this is an advantage remains to be proven. The detection of a serious anomaly may, on occasion, prevent major interventions such as caesarean section where the baby is clearly abnormal. Decision-making about care in the case of antenatally identified non-lethal malformations is often difficult. The temptation to 'get on with delivery' may sometimes result in a surviving infant with additional problems associated with being born unnecessarily early. In addition, the emotional effects on parents should be considered. Early knowledge without the power to influence outcome may not be a benefit but rather an additional burden to them. Grief, guilt, frustration, and depression may be sequelae suffered as a result of early awareness combined with the impotence of not being able to alter the course of events.

In fact, one of the major issues that goes hand in hand with ultrasound and other types of imaging is the 'baggage' that comes along with it. Other features, beyond the five biophysical variables, will be observed. The effects of recognizing fibroids, variations in fetal growth, polyhydramnios, congenital anomalies, malpresentations, and other features of the ultrasound image may be difficult to separate from the effects of the biophysical score itself on improvements in patient outcomes. Their recognition may stimulate interventions which affect the outcome either positively or negatively.

Comparisons of the biophysical test score with the non-stress test properties (Tables 30.2 to 30.7) show that, although there is considerable variation, for most outcomes the biophysical profile score appears to offer higher specificity and likelihood ratio for abnormal results than the non-stress test. Because it is a relatively high cost, high technology test it is better used as a 'diagnostic test' than as a screening test. The role of the non-stress test as either a diagnostic or a screening test seems questionable because of its relative high cost and poor predictive properties. Perhaps a combination of fetal movement counting as a screening test (see Chapter 28) and biophysical assessment as a diagnostic test will offer the greatest efficiency in screening for fetal health. This strategy has not yet been evaluated in controlled clinical trials.

3 Evidence from controlled clinical trials

While some antenatal screening tests may be shown to be predictive of various outcomes, it cannot be concluded that prediction will result in improvement in these outcomes. For this improvement to occur, treatment must be available and undertaken, and the value of the improvement must outweigh any direct or indirect complications of either the test or the treatment. Since the clinical effects of tests are achieved indirectly, the size of clinical trials to demonstrate their effects will need to be very large. Only a few randomized clinical trials have been carried out in antenatal biophysical assessment, and most have involved small numbers of women. Thus little evidence is as yet available to assess the effect of biophysical testing on outcome.

3.1 Antepartum fetal heart rate monitoring

Four randomized controlled clinical trials have been completed in which the non-stress test was evaluated as a diagnostic test (Brown *et al.* 1982; Kidd *et al.* 1985; Flynn *et al.* 1982; Lumley *et al.* 1983). All four trials were of the 'management' type, assessing the benefit accruing from the additional information supplied by the non-stress test; other 'diagnostic' tests were available to both groups and no attempt was made to standardize their use.

Details of the trials are outlined in Table 30.11. All pregnancies studied were considered to be at high risk. In each of the four trials, fetal heart rate abnormalities during labour (Table 30.12) and perinatal deaths from causes other than malformations (Table 30.13) were more common in the groups in which clinicians had access to the test results ('revealed') than in the control ('concealed') groups (Table 30.12). A detailed analysis of the case records of the deaths has shown that the difference in death rates is largely explained by differences in rate of asphyxial conditions during labour (Grant 1984). In only one of these cases did false reassurance of a 'normal' cardiotocograph trace seem likely to have been implicated. There was no demonstrable effect on caesarean section rates (Table 30.14), the incidence of low Apgar scores (Table 30.15), abnormal neonatal neurological signs (Table 30.16), or admission to special care nurseries (Table 30.17). At the very least, these analyses provide little support for non-stress cardiotocography as used in these studies as a supplementary diagnostic test of fetal compromise; yet they remain the best data currently available with which to assess the value, if any, of this time consuming and expensive activity.

3.2 Fetal biophysical profile

Only two controlled trials of biophysical profile testing have been performed (Manning *et al.* 1984; Platt *et al.* 1985). Both were conducted in women referred to units specialized in fetal biophysical assessment. Manning *et*

Table 30.11 Randomized trials of non-stress antepartum cardiotocography: study design

	Brown *et al.* (1982)	Flynn *et al.* (1982)	Lumley *et al.* (1983)	Kidd *et al.* (1985)
No. of women	353	300	530	396
'Treatment'	Revealed non-stress test, 182	Revealed non-stress test, 144	Monitored 271	Revealed non-stress test, 198
'Control'	Concealed non-stress test, 171	Concealed non-stress test, 156	Not monitored 259	Concealed non-stress test, 198
Type of women entered	2 university clinics selected high risk	Women 'at risk' in-and out-patients	Admission to antenatal ward	Admissions to antenatal ward
Time of entry	32–36 weeks	Variable	26–41 weeks	Variable
Frequency of tests	Weekly	At least weekly	Weekly	Daily
Allocation of manoeuvre	True randomization	Odd or even registration	True randomization	Odd or even date of birth
Test performed by	Research technician	Research staff	Members fetal intensive care unit	Midwife
Assessment of non-stress test	Scored by authors	Reactive or non-reactive (with description) by authors	2 consultants	Open, but assessed independently by authors
No. of non-stress test traces per woman	4: mode 1–9: range	2: mean	4: mean	5: mean 1–27: range
Tests included for associations	Last	Last	All	All
Other tests for fetal well-being	Yes	Yes	Yes, many	Yes

Table 30.12 Effect of antenatal cardiotocography on intrapartum fetal heart rate abnormality

Study	EXPT		CTRL		Odds ratio	Graph of odds ratios and confidence intervals
	n	(%)	*n*	(%)	(95% CI)	0.01 0.1 0.5 1 2 10 100
Brown *et al.* (1982)	69/182	(37.91)	51/171	(29.82)	1.43 (0.92–2.22)	
Lumley *et al.* (1983)	59/271	(21.77)	48/259	(18.53)	1.22 (0.80–1.87)	
Flynn *et al.* (1982)	16/144	(11.11)	16/156	(10.26)	1.09 (0.53–2.27)	
Kidd *et al.* (1985)	53/198	(26.77)	48/198	(24.24)	1.14 (0.73–1.79)	
Typical odds ratio (95% confidence interval)					1.24 (0.98–1.58)	

Table 30.13 Effect of antenatal cardiotocography on perinatal death (excluding lethal malformation)

Study	EXPT		CTRL		Odds ratio	Graph of odds ratios and confidence intervals
	n	(%)	*n*	(%)	(95% CI)	0.01 0.1 0.5 1 2 10 100
Brown *et al.* (1982)	2/182	(1.10)	0/171	(0.00)	6.99 (0.44–99.99)	
Lumley *et al.* (1983)	7/271	(2.58)	4/259	(1.54)	1.67 (0.50–5.49)	
Flynn *et al.* (1982)	2/144	(1.39)	0/156	(0.00)	8.09 (0.50–99.99)	
Kidd *et al.* (1985)	3/198	(1.52)	0/198	(0.00)	7.46 (0.77–72.18)	
Typical odds ratio (95% confidence interval)					3.01 (1.19–7.62)	

Table 30.14 Effect of antenatal cardiotocography on delivery by caesarean section

Study	EXPT		CTRL		Odds ratio	Graph of odds ratios and confidence intervals
	n	(%)	*n*	(%)	(95% CI)	0.01 0.1 0.5 1 2 10 100
Brown *et al.* (1982)	38/182	(20.88)	29/171	(16.96)	1.29 (0.76–2.19)	
Lumley *et al.* (1983)	73/271	(26.94)	70/259	(27.03)	1.00 (0.68–1.46)	
Flynn *et al.* (1982)	14/144	(9.72)	16/156	(10.26)	0.94 (0.44–2.00)	
Kidd *et al.* (1985)	57/198	(28.79)	53/198	(26.77)	1.11 (0.71–1.72)	
Typical odds ratio (95% confidence interval)					1.08 (0.85–1.37)	

Table 30.15 Effect of antenatal cardiotocography on low Apgar score

Study	EXPT		CTRL		Odds ratio	Graph of odds ratios and confidence intervals
	n	(%)	*n*	(%)	(95% CI)	0.01 0.1 0.5 1 2 10 100
Brown *et al.* (1982)	18/182	(9.89)	20/171	(11.70)	0.83 (0.42–1.62)	
Lumley *et al.* (1983)	57/271	(21.03)	52/259	(20.08)	1.06 (0.70–1.62)	
Flynn *et al.* (1982)	13/144	(9.03)	17/156	(10.90)	0.81 (0.38–1.73)	
Kidd *et al.* (1985)	10/198	(5.05)	12/198	(6.06)	0.83 (0.35–1.95)	
Typical odds ratio (95% confidence interval)					0.94 (0.69–1.27)	

Table 30.16 Effect of antenatal cardiotocography on abnormal neonatal neurological signs

Study	EXPT		CTRL		Odds ratio	Graph of odds ratios and confidence intervals
	n	(%)	*n*	(%)	(95% CI)	0.01 0.1 0.5 1 2 10 100
Brown *et al.* (1982)	3/182	(1.65)	0/171	(0.00)	7.03 (0.73–68.13)	
Lumley *et al.* (1983)	22/271	(8.12)	23/259	(8.88)	0.91 (0.49–1.67)	
Flynn *et al.* (1982)	4/144	(2.78)	3/156	(1.92)	1.45 (0.32–6.50)	
Typical odds ratio (95% confidence interval)					1.09 (0.63–1.88)	

Table 30.17 Effect of antenatal cardiotocography on admission to special care nursery

Study	EXPT		CTRL		Odds ratio	Graph of odds ratios and confidence intervals
	n	(%)	*n*	(%)	(95% CI)	0.01 0.1 0.5 1 2 10 100
Brown *et al.* (1982)	24/182	(13.19)	19/171	(11.11)	1.21 (0.64–2.30)	
Lumley *et al.* (1983)	79/271	(29.15)	70/259	(27.03)	1.11 (0.76–1.62)	
Flynn *et al.* (1982)	21/144	(14.58)	27/156	(17.31)	0.82 (0.44–1.51)	
Typical odds ratio (95% confidence interval)					1.06 (0.79–1.41)	

al. (1984) allocated women by 'coin flip' and Platt by odd and even sequential study numbers. It is unfortunate that neither author chose to use a blinded method of true randomization. While in Manning's study this did not lead to an evident allocation bias, in Platt's study it did. First, it is surprising, to say the least, for an odd or even number strategy to lead to enrolment of 279 in one group and 373 in the other. Second, there is a difference in the pattern of indications for testing in the two groups with 43 per cent post dates in the biophysical profile group and 34 per cent in the non-stress test group (difference significant at $p = 0.023$).

Both compared management based on biophysical score result vs. management according to non-stress test result following a management algorithm. In Platt's study, any persistently abnormal result of either test was followed by contraction stress testing, whereas, Manning's protocol recommended delivery without further testing.

A number of outcomes were measured, including perinatal death, fetal distress in labour, low Apgar score, and low birthweight for gestational age. As can be seen in Table 30.18, neither statistical nor clinically important differences were found.

Both authors examined the residual predictive properties of the tests (Table 30.19). In both studies the biophysical profile score was a better predictor of low 5-minute Apgar scores than the non-stress test (Manning *et al.* 57 per cent vs. 13 per cent; Platt *et al.* 25 per cent vs. 20 per cent). In Platt's study the biophysical profile was both more sensitive (32 per cent vs. 14 per cent) and more specific (99.5 per cent vs. 32 per cent) for overall abnormal outcome than the non-stress test.

One additional randomized trial (Arias 1987) compared the value of weekly ultrasound plus non-stress test with weekly non-stress test alone after 40 weeks gestation, in 243 private patients all of whom had one or more ultrasound examinations during pregnancy. No differences in outcomes were noted, and no useful data could be gleaned from this study.

How should we interpret this contrast between good predictive properties and lack of impact on perinatal outcome? Many explanations are possible, including biased allocation because of unblinded quasi-randomization, unintentional revelation of the results of the biophysical profile in non-stress test managed women, lack of physician or patient compliance with the study management algorithms, and lack of efficacy of the

Table 30.18 Controlled trials of biophysical profile vs. non-stress antepartum cardiotocography

	Manning *et al.* (1985) (n = 735)		Platt *et al.* (1985) (n = 625)	
	Non-stress test	Biophysical profile	Non-stress test	Biophysical profile
Number of women	360	375	373	279
Number of tests—total	–	–	960	668
—per woman	–	–	2.6	2.4
Delivery >7 days	–	–	97 (26%)	68 (24%)
Perinatal deaths	4	4	3	3
Congenital anomalies	3	4	–	–
Low weight for gestation	–	–	14 (4%)	6 (2%)
Fetal distress in labour	–	–	16	13
Low 5-minute Apgar	15	17	9	8
One or more bad outcomes	–	–	35 (10%)	22 (8%)

Table 30.19 Comparison of 'residual test properties' from controlled trials of biophysical profits vs. non-stress antepartum cardiotocography

	Manning *et al.* (1985)				Platt *et al.* (1985)			
	Non-stress cardiotocography		Biophysical profile scoring		Non-stress cardiotocography		Biophysical profile scoring	
	Sensitivity	Specificity	Sensitivity	Specificity	Sensitivity	Specificity	Sensitivity	Specificity
Perinatal death	75	84	50	94	33	95	67	97
Low weight for gestation	–	–	–	–	21	95	67	98
Fetal distress in labour	–	–	–	–	13	95	31	98
Low Apgar at 5 minutes	57	85	77	97	33	96	25	97
Overall abnormal outcome	–	–	–	–	14	96	32	99

*Data are derived from diagnostic impact studies and therefore represent *residual* test properties, the benefits and risks of intervention(s) having been provided.

major intervention, 'delivery', in altering perinatal outcome. Also, change in some of the outcomes may have been an unreasonable expectation. For instance, the 64 women referred because of clinically identified intrauterine growth failure could not be expected to show differences in subsequent growth pattern based on the described management plans prompted by biophysical profile or non-stress test. Certainly, delivery could not be expected to produce a difference other than by delivering the women in one group sooner or later than in the other.

Another possibility is that the failure of these studies to demonstrate differences is a chance finding, related to small sample sizes, or to methodologic flaws in design and execution of the trials. It is worthwhile to remember the history of randomized trials of intrapartum fetal monitoring. Early trials were inconclusive. A pooled analysis of these trials suggested that a beneficial effect might have been missed due to insufficient numbers of women studied (Chalmers 1979). Based on this, the large Dublin trial was performed demonstrating some benefit (MacDonald *et al.* 1985; and see Chapter 54). It is worth noting here that a low technology method of fetal biophysical assessment, maternal fetal movement counting, is an equally effective predictor of adverse fetal outcome (see Chapter 28).

4 Conclusions

4.1 Implications for current practice

At the present time, biophysical tests have largely replaced the biochemical tests of fetal well-being that were popular some years ago. They are employed today with the same enthusiasm that characterized biochemical testing in the past. While biochemical tests have greatly increased our understanding of fetal physiology and the endocrinology of pregnancy, it is now generally recognized that they have little to offer to the care of the individual women (see Chapter 29). It is similarly evident that biophysical tests have greatly increased our understanding of fetal behaviour and development, but the use of these tests has not been demonstrated to confer benefits in the care of an individual woman. For this reason, despite their widespread clinical use, biophysical tests of fetal well-being should be considered of experimental value only, rather than as validated clinical tools. Prudence would dictate that they be acknowledged as such, and that, at the very least, further extension of their clinical use should be curtailed until or unless they can be demonstrated to be of benefit in improving the outcome for mother or baby.

4.2 Implications for future research

There is a need for careful reassessment of current knowledge, and for well-conducted trials to evaluate whether or not these tests do indeed confer the benefits that the medical profession has been led to expect from them.

References

Arias F (1987). Predictability of complications associated with prolongation of pregnancy. Obstet Gynecol, 70: 101–106.

Barrett JM, Salyer SL, Boehm FH (1981). The nonstress test: an evaluation of 1000 patients. Am J Obstet Gynecol, 141: 153–157

Baskett TF, Gray JH, Prewett SJ, Young LM, Allen EC. (1984). Antepartum fetal assessment using a fetal biophysical profile score. Am J Obstet Gynecol, 148: 630–633.

Beischer NA, Drew JH, Ashton PW, Oats JN, Gaudrey E, Chew FTK. Parkinson P (1983). Quality of survival of infants with critical fetal reserve detected by antenatal cardiotocography. Am J Obstet Gynecol, 146: 662–670.

Bishop EH (1981). Fetal acceleration test. Am J Obstet Gynecol, 141: 905–909.

Bottoms SF, Welch RA, Zador IE, Sokol RJ, (1986). Limitations of using maximum vertical pocket and other sonographic evaluations of amniotic fluid volume to predict fetal growth: technical or physiologic? Am J Obstet Gynecol, 155: 154–158.

Boylan P, Lewis PJ (1980). Fetal breathing in labor. Obstet Gynecol, 56: 35–38.

Brown R, Patrick J (1981). The non-stress test: how long is enough? Am J Obstet Gynecol, 141: 646–651.

Brown VA, Sawers RS, Parsons RJ, Duncan SLB, Cooke ID (1982). The value of antenatal cardiotocography in the management of high-risk pregnancy: a randomized controlled trial. Br J Obstet Gynaecol, 89: 716–722.

Chalmers I (1979). Randomized controlled trials of fetal monitoring 1973–1977. In: Perinatal Medicine. Thalhammer O, Baumgarten K, Pollak A (eds). Stuttgart: Georg Thieme, pp 260–265.

Chew FT, Drew JH, Oats JN, Riley SF, Beischer NA (1985). Nonstressed antepartum cardiotocography in patients undergoing elective cesarean section: Fetal outcome. Am J Obstet Gynecol, 151: 318–321.

Curtis P, Evens S, Resnick J, Rimer R, Lynch K, Carlson JR (1986). Uterine responses to three techniques of breast stimulation. Obstet Gynecol, 67: 25–28.

Dawes GS, Houghton CRS, Redman CWG, Visser GHA (1982). Pattern of the normal human fetal heart rate. Br J Obstet Gynaecol, 89: 276–284.

Devoe LD (1980). Clinical implications of prospective antepartum fetal heart rate testing. Am J Obstet Gynecol, 137: 983–990.

Devoe LD, Castillo RA, Searle NS, Searle JR (1986). Maternal dietary substrates and human fetal biophysical activity. I. The effects of tryptophan and glucose on fetal breathing movements. Am J Obstet Gynecol, 155: 135–139.

Devoe LD, Searle N, Castillo RA, Searle J (1987a). Fetal biophysical testing. The effects of prolonged maternal fasting and the oral glucose tolerance test. J Reprod Med, 32: 563–568.

Devoe LD, Arthur M, Searle N (1987b). The effect of maternal ambulation on the nonstress test. Am J Obstet Gynecol, 157: 240–244.

Druzin ML, Fox A, Kogut E, Carlson C (1985). The relationship of the nonstress test to gestational age. Am J Obstet Gynecol, 153: 386–389.

Fischer WM, Stude I, Brandt H (1976). Ein vorschlag zur beurteilung des antepartalen kardiotokograms. Z Geburtsh Perinatol, 180: 117–123.

Flynn AM, Kelly J (1977). Evaluation of fetal well-being by antepartum fetal heart rate monitoring. Br Med J, 1: 936–939.

Flynn AM, Kelly J, Mansfield H, Needham P, O'Conor M, Viegas O (1982). A randomized controlled trial of non-stress antepartum cardiotocography. Br J Obstet Gynaecol, 89: 427–433.

Grant A (1984). Principles for clinical evaluation of methods of perinatal monitoring. J Perinat Med, 12: 227–233

Hammacher K (1969). The clinical significance of cardiotocography. In: Perinatal Medicine. Huntingford PS, Huter EA, Saling E (eds). New York: Academic Press, pp 80–93.

Hann L, McArdle C, Sachs B (1987). Sonographic biophysical profile in the postdate pregnancy. J Ultrasound Med, 6: 191–195.

Hill WC, Moenning RK, Katz M, Kitzmiller JL (1984). Characteristics of uterine activity during breast stimulation stress test. Obstet Gynecol, 64: 489–492.

Hill C, Krohn V, Russel JA (1986a). Stimulation of the bare or covered nipple to obtain contractions for the breast stimulation stress test. Proceedings of the Annual Meeting of the Society of Perinatal Obstetricians, January 1986.

Hill C, Hicks J, Krohn V (1986b). The uterine activity produced by nipple preparation for breastfeeding. Proceedings of the Annual Meeting of the Society of Prenatal Obstetricians, January 1986.

Kaar K (1980). Antepartal cardiotocography in the assessment of fetal outcome. Acta Obstet Gynecol Scand (Suppl) 94.

Keane MWD, Horger III EO, Vice L (1981). Comparative study of stressed and nonstressed antepartum fetal hear rate testing. Obstet Gynecol, 57: 320–324.

Keirse MJNC, Trimbos JB (1980). Assessment of antepartum cardiotocograms in high-risk pregnancy. Br J Obstet Gynaecol, 87: 261–269.

Keirse MJNC, Trimbos JB (1981). Clinical significance of suspicious antepartum cardiotocograms: a study of normal and high-risk pregnancies. Br J Obstet Gynaecol, 88: 739–746.

Kidd LC, Patel NB, Smith R (1985). Non-stress antenatal

cardiotocography—a prospective randomized clinical trial. Br J Obstet Gynaecol, 92: 1156–1159.

Krebs HB, Petres RE (1978). Clinical application of a scoring system for evaluation of antepartum fetal heart rate monitoring. Am J Obstet Gynecol, 130: 765–772.

Kubli F, Kaeser O, Hinselmann M (1969). Diagnostic management of chronic placental insufficiency. In: The Fetoplacental Unit. Pecile A, Finci C (eds). Amsterdam: Exerpta Medica.

Kubli F, Boos R, Ruttgers H, Hagens CV, Vanselow H (1977). Antepartum fetal heart rate monitoring. In: Current Status of Fetal Heart Rate Monitoring and Ultrasound in Obstetrics. Beard RW, Campbell S (eds). London: Royal College of Obstetricians and Gynaecologists, pp 28–45.

Lenstrup C, Haase N (1985). Predictive value of antepartum fetal heart rate non-stress test in high-risk pregnancy. Acta Obstet Gynecol Scand, 64: 133–138.

Lipitz S, Barkai G, Rabinovici J, Mashiach S (1987). Breast stimulation test and oxytocin challenge test in fetal surveillance: a prospective randomized study. Am J Obstet Gynecol, 157: 1178–1181.

Lumley J, Lester A, Anderson I, Renou P, Wood C (1983). A randomized trial of weekly cardiotocography in high-risk obstetric patients. Br J Obstet Gynaecol, 90: 1018–1026.

Lyons ER, Blysma-Howell M, Shamsi S, Towell ME (1979). A scoring system for nonstressed antepartum fetal heart rate monitoring. Am J Obstet Gynecol, 133: 242–246.

MacDonald D, Grant A, Sheridan-Pereira M, Boylan P, Chalmers I (1985). The randomized controlled trial of intrapartum fetal heart rate monitoring. Am J Obstet Gynecol, 152: 524–539.

Manning FA, Platt LD, Sipos L, Keegan KA (1979). Fetal breathing movements and the non-stress test in high-risk pregnancies. Am J Obstet Gynecol, 135: 511–515.

Manning FA, Platt LD, Sipos L (1980). Antepartum fetal evaluation: development of a fetal biophysical profile. Am J Obstet Gynecol, 136: 787–795.

Manning FA, Morrison I, Lange IR, Harman CR, Chamberlain PF (1985). Fetal assessment based on fetal biophysical profile scoring: experience in 12 620 referred high-risk pregnancies. Am J Obstet Gynecol, 151: 343–350.

Manning FD, Lange IR, Morrison I, Harman CR (1984). Fetal biophysical profile score and the non-stress test: a comparative trial. Obstet Gynecol, 64: 326–331.

Mendenhall HW, O'Leary J, Phillips KO (1980). The nonstress test: the value of a single acceleration in evaluating the fetus at risk. Am J Obstet Gynecol, 136: 87–91.

Miller FC, Skiba H, Klapholz H (1978). The effect of maternal blood sugar levels on fetal activity. Obstet Gynecol, 52: 662–665.

Moenning RK, Hill WC (1986). Comparison of the wet and dry methods of performing the breast stimulation test. Proceedings of the Annual Meeting of the Society of Perinatal Obstetricians, January 1986.

Moenning RK, Hill WC (1987). A randomized study comparing two methods of performing the breast stimulation stress test. J Obstet Gynecol Neonatal Nurs July/August: 253–257

Nijhuis JG, Jongsma HW, Crijns IJMJ, de Valk IMGM, van der Velden JWHJ (1986). Effects of maternal glucose ingestion on human fetal breathing movements at weeks 24 and 28 of gestation. Early Hum Dev, 13: 183–188.

Paul RH, Keegan KA (1979). Nonstress antepartum fetal monitoring. Clinics in Obstetrics and Gynecology, 6: 351–358.

Pearson JF (1981). The value of antenatal fetal monitoring. In: Progress in Obstetrics and Gynecology, Vol. 1. Studd J (ed). London: Churchill Livingstone.

Pearson JP, Weaver JB (1978). A six-point scoring system for antenatal cardiotocographs. Br J Obstet Gynaecol, 85: 321–327.

Phelan JP (1981). The non-stress test: a review of 3000 tests. Am J Obstet Gynecol, 139: 7–10.

Platt LD, Eglinton GS, Sipos L, Broussard PM, Paul RH (1983). Further experience with the fetal biophysical profile. Obstet Gynecol, 61: 480–485.

Platt LD, Walla CA, Paul RH, Trujillo ME, Loesser CV, Jacobs ND, Broussard PM (1985). A prospective trial of the fetal biophysical profile versus the nonstress test in the management of high-risk pregnancies. Am J Obstet Gynecol, 153: 624–33.

Pose SV, Castillo JB, Mora-Rojas EO, Soto-Yances A, Caldeyro-Barcia R (1969). Test of fetal tolerance to induced uterine contractions for the diagnosis of chronic distress. In: Perinatal Factors Affecting Human Development. Pan American Health Organization, Scientific publication No. 185: pp 96–104.

Pratt D, Diamond F, Yen H, Bieniarz J, Burd J (1979). Fetal stress and non-stress tests: an analysis and comparison of their ability to identify fetal outcome. Obstet Gynecol, 54: 419–423.

Rayburn W, Greene J, Donaldson M (1980). Non-stress testing and perinatal outcome. J Reprod Med, 24: 191–196.

Rochard F, Schifrin BS, Goupil F, Legrand H, Blottiere J, Sureau C (1976). Nonstressed fetal heart rate monitoring in the antepartum period. Am J Obstet Gynecol, 126: 699–706.

Ross MG, Ervin MG, Leake RD (1986). Breast stimulation contraction test: Uterine contractions in the absence of oxytocin release. Am J Perinatol, 3: 35–37.

Schellpfeffer MA, Hoyle D, Johnson JWC (1985). Antepartal uterine hypercontractility secondary to nipple stimulation. Obstet Gynecol, 65: 588–591.

Schifrin BS, Guntes V, Gergely RC, Eden R, Roll K, Jacobs J (1981). The role of realtime scanning in antenatal fetal surveillance. Am J Obstet Gynecol, 140: 525–530.

Smith CV, Phelan JP, Platt LD, Broussard P, Paul RH (1986). Fetal acoustic stimulation testing. II. A randomized clinical comparison with the nonstress test. Am J Obstet Gynecol, 155: 131–134.

Trimbos JB, Keirse MJNC (1978a). Observer variability in assessment of antepartum cardiotocograms. Br J Obstet Gynaecol, 85: 900–906.

Trimbos JB, Keirse MJNC (1978b). Significance of antepartum cardiotocography in normal pregnancy. Br J Obstet Gynaecol, 85: 907–913.

Varma TR (1981). Clinical experience in non-stressed antepartum cardiotocography in high-risk pregnancies. Int J Gynaecol Obstet, 19: 433–439.

Vintzileos AM, Campbell WA, Ingardia CJ, Nochimson DJ

(1983). The fetal biophysical profile and its predictive value. Obstet Gynecol, 62: 271–278.

Vintzileos AM, Campbell WA, Nochimson DJ, Weinbaum PJ (1987). The use and misuse of the fetal biophysical profile. Am J Obstet Gynecol, 156: 527–533.

Visser GHA, Dawes GS, Redman CWG (1981). Numerical analysis of the normal human antenatal fetal heart rate. Br J Obstet Gynaecol, 88: 792–802.

31 Suspected fetopelvic disproportion

G. Justus Hofmeyr

1 Introduction

Fetopelvic disproportion exists when the capacity of the birth canal is insufficient for the safe vaginal delivery of the fetus. Antenatal strategies to diagnose fetopelvic disproportion have received considerable attention in the past, the objective being early induction of labour or delivery by planned caesarean section should disproportion be diagnosed.

The value of such strategies will differ with various obstetric situations. It is important to distinguish between the risk of disproportion related to the presenting fetal part and that related to a non-leading part of the fetus, because of the special hazards of obstructed labour to the partly born fetus. Obstruction following birth of the head is unusual except in the presence of fetal macrosomia, particularly in association with maternal diabetes mellitus (Acker *et al.* 1985). Obstruction of the aftercoming head is unusual in breech presentation, provided that the thighs are flexed on the trunk (frank or complete breech), the head is not extended, and the fetus is of at least average weight.

Although pelvic dimensions may occasionally change with time because of lumbo-sacral subluxation, the most reliable predictor of pelvic adequacy remains the history of the uncomplicated birth of a baby of similar or greater birthweight than that estimated for the current pregnancy. The remainder of this chapter pertains largely to the care of women without such a history.

2 Clinical diagnosis of cephalopelvic disproportion

Attempts to predict the occurrence of cephalopelvic disproportion have included measurement of maternal height and shoe size, and clinical and X-ray pelvimetry. Several studies have found maternal height to be of limited predictive value in this respect (Cox 1963; Philpott and Castle 1972; Stewart *et al.* 1979; Naeye *et al.* 1977). Others have found a significant correlation of maternal height with caesarean section rate (Mati *et al.* 1983a; Everett 1975; Yudkin and Redman 1986) and perinatal mortality (Mati *et al.* 1983b). Liljestrand *et al.* (1985) found a history of perinatal loss among 717 Mozambican women to be significantly more frequent in those measuring less than 150 cm. Of 45 women delivered by caesarean section for cephalopelvic disproportion, 36 per cent were below 150 cm, compared with only 4 per cent in a group of 50 women who underwent caesarean section for other reasons and 9 per cent in a group of 107 women delivered vaginally.

Frame *et al.* (1985) studied 351 singleton births in London, England. Caesarean section rates varied significantly with shoe size, from 21 per cent in women whose shoe size was below size 4½, to 10 per cent in women whose shoe size was from 4½ to 6, and 3 per cent in women whose shoe size was above 6. Maternal height correlated poorly with caesarean section rate, but significantly with the use of rotational forceps.

The statistical significance of correlations between maternal height or shoe size and cephalopelvic disproportion is of limited clinical use because of the large overlap in the obstetrical outcome between women with small and large dimensions. While these measurements may be the only feasible screening method for cephalopelvic disproportion in situations where selection for hospital delivery is necessary, their lack of discriminatory power must be recognized.

There are divergent opinions concerning the accuracy of clinical pelvimetry. Kaltreider (1954) found clinical assessment of the intertuberous diameter to be unreliable, whereas Holmberg (1966) found that outlet obstruction could be predicted by clinical evaluation of intertuberous and sagittal outlet diameters. Floberg *et al.* (1986) found a significant correlation between clinical and radiological assessment of pelvic outlet contracture and measurement of intertuberous diameter, but not of the sagittal diameter. Radiologically diagnosed borderline or contracted pelvic outlet was detected clinically with a sensitivity of 25 per cent and specificity of 90 per cent. Parsons and Spellacy (1985) found agreement between clinical and radiological pelvimetry in 77 per cent of cases. Fine *et al.* (1980) studied 100 selected cases and concluded that X-ray pelvimetry was not significantly more accurate than clinical pelvimetry in predicting the outcome of labour.

The effects of clinical pelvimetry have not, apparently been evaluated by randomized studies.

The meaning of non-engagement of the fetal head near term as an indicator of cephalopelvic disproportion is not well established. In black primigravidae, in whom such non-engagement commonly occurs, Briggs (1981) found it to be associated with longer labours, but not with increased maternal or fetal morbidity or with operative interference.

3 X-ray pelvimetry

The widespread use of X-ray pelvimetry to predict cephalopelvic disproportion has come under critical scrutiny since the reports of an association between prenatal irradiation and childhood leukaemia (Stewart *et al.* 1956; MacMahon 1962). As a general principle, irradiation that is not likely to benefit mother or baby should be avoided. The use of ultrasound for pelvimetry has been reported (Kratochwil and Zeibekis 1972; Vaclavinkova 1973) but it has not been widely adopted.

There is wide variation among individuals and institutions in the use of X-ray pelvimetry (Kelly *et al.* 1975). Its utility has been questioned because of its poor predictive value as a screening test for cephalopelvic disproportion, and the infrequency with which the results influence management (Joyce *et al.* 1975; Varner *et al.* 1980; Laube *et al.* 1981). Radomsky and Radomsky (1980) found that 19 of 69 women (28 per cent) with radiologically average pelvic dimensions were delivered by caesarean section, while 29 of 59 women (49 per cent) with radiologically borderline pelves delivered vaginally. Fine *et al.* (1980) evaluated 100 X-ray pelvimetry examinations retrospectively. The rate of vaginal delivery following the diagnosis of disproportion was 29 per cent and 23 per cent for the Thorn and Ball radiological methods respectively, and 27 per cent for women in whom cephalopelvic disproportion was diagnosed by manual pelvimetry.

The results of two prospective randomized studies of X-ray pelvimetry are summarized in Tables 31.1, 31.2, and 31.3. Crichton (1962) found a decrease in neonatal 'asphyxia' (13 per cent vs. 20 per cent) and perinatal mortality when X-ray pelvimetry was used in the management of intrapartum complications. Parsons and Spellacy (1985), on the other hand, found that the

Table 31.1 Effect of X-ray pelvimetry in cephalic presentations on caesarean section/symphysiotomy

Study	EXPT		CTRL		Odds ratio	Graph of odds ratios and confidence intervals
	n	(%)	*n*	(%)	(95% CI)	0.01 0.1 0.5 1 2 10 100
Crichton (1962)	63/151	(41.72)	49/154	(31.82)	1.53 (0.96–2.43)	
Parsons and Spellacy (1985)	29/102	(28.43)	18/98	(18.37)	1.75 (0.91–3.35)	
Typical odds ratio (95% confidence interval)					1.60 (1.10–2.33)	

Table 31.2 Effect of X-ray pelvimetry in cephalic presentations on 'Asphyxia'

Study	EXPT		CTRL		Odds ratio	Graph of odds ratios and confidence intervals
	n	(%)	*n*	(%)	(95% CI)	0.01 0.1 0.5 1 2 10 100
Crichton (1962)	20/151	(13.25)	31/154	(20.13)	0.61 (0.34–1.11)	
Typical odds ratio (95% confidence interval)					0.61 (0.34–1.11)	

Table 31.3 Effect of X-ray pelvimetry in cephalic presentations on perinatal mortality

Study	EXPT		CTRL		Odds ratio	Graph of odds ratios and confidence intervals
	n	(%)	*n*	(%)	(95% CI)	0.01 0.1 0.5 1 2 10 100
Crichton (1962)	5/151	(3.31)	8/154	(5.19)	0.63 (0.21–1.91)	
Parsons *et al.* (1985)	0/102	(0.00)	0/98	(0.00)	1.00 (1.00–1.00)	
Typical odds ratio (95% confidence interval)					0.63 (0.21–1.91)	

use of X-ray pelvimetry prior to induction of labour was associated with an increase in the number of caesarean sections (not statistically significant), and a statistically significant decrease in mean 5-minute Apgar scores and in the forceps delivery rate. X-ray pelvimetry prior to augmentation of labour was associated with an increase in caesarean sections, but a difference of this size could have arisen by chance. In the subgroup with borderline clinical pelvimetry findings, the caesarean section rate was statistically significantly increased when X-ray pelvimetry was used (Table 31.4). Parsons and Spellacy (1985) concluded that the use of X-ray pelvimetry did not confer any advantages to the fetus when electronic fetal monitoring was used routinely during labour. Improved methods of fetal surveillance and intervention may well account for the difference in findings between the two trials.

Neither X-ray nor clinical pelvimetry have been shown to predict cephalopelvic disproportion with sufficient accuracy to justify elective caesarean section for cephalic presentations. Cephalopelvic disproportion is best diagnosed by a carefully monitored trial of labour (Philpott 1982), and X-ray pelvimetry should seldom if ever be necessary. The use of height, shoe size, and clinical pelvimetry should largely be limited to the selection of women for special monitoring during labour, or in countries or rural areas where referral may be necessary for delivery in a centre with operating facilities.

4 Previous caesarean section

In a review of the literature between 1950 and 1980, Lavin *et al.* (1982) found that many authors recommended X-ray pelvimetry in the evaluation of patients for trial of labour after caesarean section, but they found little evidence that its use improved outcome. The suggestion that scar dehiscence is more common after caesarean section for cephalopelvic disproportion (O'Sullivan *et al.* 1981) is contradicted by data presented by Lavin *et al.* (1982) and Tahilramaney *et al.* (1984). Both of these studies actually found that dehiscence occurred less frequently after caesarean section for cephalopelvic disproportion than after caesarean section for other reasons, possibly because the well-formed lower uterine segment in these women allows the uterine incision to be well within the lower segment. Recent studies have shown an acceptable rate of vaginal delivery when trial of labour is allowed after previous caesarean section for cephalopelvic disproportion (See Chapter 71).

Davey *et al.* (1987) found no correlation between scar dehiscence and either small pelvic inlet dimensions or cephalopelvic disproportion having been the indication for the primary caesarean section. In their population, however, women with a true conjugate below 10.5 cm were not allowed a trial of labour. Richards *et al.* (1985) randomly allocated 102 women with singleton cephalic presentation and a history of lower segment caesarean

Table 31.4 The effect of X-ray pelvimetry on operative delivery rates

	Caesarean section		Forceps delivery	
	Exptl	Control	Exptl	Control
Total patients (%)	29/102 (28.4)	18/98 (18.4)	6/102 (5.9)	14/98 (14.3)
Subgroups:				
Induced labour	15/56 (26.8)	11/54 (20.4)	2/56 (3.6)	10/54* (18.5)
Augmented labour	14/46 (30.4)	9/44 (20.4)	4/46 (8.7)	4/44 (9.1)
Borderline clinical pelvimetry	13/25 (52.0)	2/24† (8.3)	2/25 (8.0)	4/24 (16.6)

(Parsons and Spellacy 1985) *$p<.01$; †$p<.05$.

section to undergo X-ray pelvimetry before or after delivery. Of 52 women with antenatal X-ray pelvimetry, 15 (28 per cent) delivered vaginally compared with 26/50 (52 per cent) of the women who had postnatal pelvimetry. Of the women in the latter group who delivered vaginally, 12/26 (46 per cent) were found to have a true conjugate of less than 10.5 cm. Only one scar dehiscence ocurred in each group and in both cases the women had adequate pelvic dimensions. The two fetal deaths in the control group occurred before labour.

The antenatal diagnosis of relative cephalopelvic disproportion in women with previous caesarean section has in practice not been shown to be useful for predicting the outcome of labour or the occurrence of scar dehiscence.

5 Breech presentation

Cephalopelvic disproportion is perilous in a breech presentation because of the risk of entrapment of the aftercoming head. However, no trials have been conducted to assess the value of X-ray pelvimetry for breech delivery. Early retrospective studies reported unacceptably high perinatal mortality and morbidity rates when vaginal delivery was attempted in the presence of reduced or borderline pelvic dimensions (Todd and Steer 1963; Dunn *et al.* 1965; Beischer 1966). O'Leary (1979) compared the outcome in 81 uncomplicated term breech presentations managed in a teaching department according to a protocol that included X-ray pelvimetry, to that of 69 women managed without such a protocol in a non-teaching setting (Table 31.5). The caesarean section rates were 33/81 (41 per cent) and 14/69 (20 per cent), perinatal mortality 0/81 (0 per cent) and 2/69 (2.8 per cent), breech extractions 1/81 (1.2 per cent) and 10/69 (14 per cent), low Apgar scores (0–3) 1/81 (1.2 per cent) and 8/69 (12 per cent), and birth injuries 1/81 (1.2 per cent) and 4/69 (6 per cent) respectively.

Several recent studies have confirmed the safety of vaginal breech delivery in women carefully selected to exclude cephalopelvic disproportion using X-ray pelvimetry, and usually estimation of fetal weight, assessment of neck flexion, and exclusion of double footling presentation (Table 31.6). Such studies in no way establish that X-ray pelvimetry contributes significantly to the selection of women for either vaginal or abdominal delivery. To do so, a randomized trial comparing women with and without pelvimetry would be required.

The rare condition of deflexion of the head with a breech presentation may add additional risk to vaginal delivery (Ballas and Toaff 1976). Ultrasound examina-

Table 31.5 Comparison of outcomes in breech presentations with X-ray pelvimetry in a teaching department to those without X-ray pelvimetry in a non-teaching setting

	Teaching department		Non-teaching setting	
	n/N	(%)	*n*/N	(%)
Caesarean section	33/81	(41.0)	14/69	(20.0)
Perinatal mortality	0/81	(0.0)	2/69	(2.8)
Breech extractions	1/81	(1.2)	10/69	(14.0)
Low Apgar scores (0.3)	1/81	(1.2)	8/69	(12.0)
Birth injuries	1/81	(1.2)	4/69	(6.0)

(O'Leary 1979).

Table 31.6 Vaginal delivery rates in term breech presentations with 'adequate' X-ray pelvimetry

Authors	Pelvimetries	'Adequate'	Vaginal delivery
Westin (1977)	224	169	158 (93%)
Collea *et al.* (1980)	112	60	49 (82%)
Jaffa *et al.* (1981)	321	277	260 (94%)
Gimovsky *et al.* (1983)	70	47	31 (66%)
Capeless and Mann (1985)	107	86	51 (59%)
Kopelman *et al.* (1986)	32	17	14 (82%)
Barlov and Larsson (1986)	226	125	102 (82%)
Total	1092	781	665 (85%)

tion in early labour can lead to rapid diagnosis or exclusion of the condition (Confino *et al.* 1985).

Computed tomographic pelvimetry, which greatly reduces the radiation exposure to the fetus, has been found in two small studies to be easier to perform (Kopelman *et al.* 1986) and in the measurement of a model pelvis, probably more accurate (Gimovsky *et al.* 1985) than conventional X-ray pelvimetry.

There is no reason to expect that X-ray pelvimetry should be more accurately predictive of cephalopelvic disproportion for breech than for cephalic presentations. In breech presentations, however, it is usual to avoid vaginal delivery when pelvic dimensions are even slightly reduced, in an attempt to ensure exclusion of all potential cases of cephalopelvic disproportion. Careful assessment of fetopelvic relationships should be possible even in advanced labour, with the use of beta-stimulants to temporarily delay the progress of labour (Gimovsky 1985).

6 Shoulder dystocia

Shoulder dystocia is an obstetric emergency associated with considerable risk of fetal trauma. If a high likelihood of the condition could be predicted antenatally this would enable prevention by the performance of caesarean section.

Acker *et al.* (1985) in a retrospective study found shoulder dystocia to occur significantly more often in fetuses when birthweight was above 4500 g (23 per cent), or above 4500 g with an arrest of progress in labour (55 per cent), or above 4000 g and accompanied by maternal diabetes mellitus (31 per cent). As the great majority of post-term pregnancies were not affected, they could not agree with Johnstone (1979) that induction of all post term pregnancies to avoid shoulder dystocia is justified. The authors recommend that elective caesarean section should be performed for diabetic women with fetal weight estimated to be above 4000 g, and that the operation should be considered for non-diabetic women in whom the fetal weight is estimated to be above 4500 g and there is abnormal progress of labour. Such a policy has not been subjected to prospective evaluation, and even if fetal weight estimation were accurate, this would prevent only 11 per cent of potential cases of shoulder dystocia, while 68 per cent of the operations would be unnecessary (see also Chapter 36). Indeed, some 47 per cent of cases of shoulder dystocia occur in infants weighing less than 4000 g (Acker *et al.* 1986).

Modanlou *et al.* (1982) have suggested that body configuration rather than weight alone, is predictive of shoulder dystocia. Elliot *et al.* (1982) found that when the fetal chest diameter minus biparietal diameter was more than 1.4 cm, that shoulder dystocia was more likely to occur during delivery of diabetic women. Use of such measurements when ultrasound estimation of fetal weight exceeds 4000 g has been suggested by Gross *et al.* (1987), but not validated prospectively.

There is at present no reliable method of antenatal prediction of shoulder dystocia, and efforts to reduce the problem should be directed towards ensuring that birth attendants are skilled in the management of this condition. Recent reports of novel methods of management require further evaluation. These include squatting (Carter 1986), symphysiotomy (Hartfield 1986), and cephalic replacement using a beta-stimulant followed by caesarean section (Sandberg 1985).

7 Conclusions

No reliable methods are available for accurate prediction of fetopelvic disproportion before labour. Labour is the best test of pelvic adequacy in cephalic presentations. Areas of research that might be worth exploring include the use of ultrasound for pelvimetry.

References

Acker DB, Sachs BP, Friedman EA (1985). Risk factors for shoulder dystocia. Obstet Gynecol, 66: 762–768.

Acker DB, Sachs BP, Friedmann EA (1986). Risk factors for shoulder dystocia in the average weight infant. Obstet Gynecol, 67: 614–618.

Ballas S, Toaff R (1976). Hyperextension of the fetal head in breech presentation. Radiological evaluation and significance. Br J Obstet Gynaecol, 83: 201–204.

Barlov K, Larsson G (1986). Results of a five-year prospective study using a feto–pelvic scoring system for term singleton breech delivery after uncomplicated pregnancy. Acta Obstet Gynecol Scand, 65: 315–319.

Beischer NA (1966). Pelvic contraction in breech presentation. J Obstet Gynaecol Br Commwlth, 73: 421–427.

Briggs ND (1981). Engagement of the fetal head in the negro primigravida. Br J Obstet Gynaecol, 88: 1086–1089.

Capeless EL, Mann LI (1985). A vaginal delivery protocol for the term breech infant utilising Ball pelvimetry. J Reprod Med, 30: 545–548.

Carter V (1986). Another technique for resolution of shoulder dystocia. Am J Obstet Gynecol, 154: 964.

Collea JV, Chein C, Quilligan EJ (1980). The randomized management of term frank breech presentation. Am J Obstet Gynecol, 137: 235–244.

Confino E, Gleicher N, Elrad H, Ismajovich B, David MP (1985). The breech dilemma. A review. Obstet Gynecol Surv, 40: 330–337.

Cox ML (1963). Contracted pelvis in Nigeria. J Obstet Gynaecol Br Commnwlth, 70: 487–494.

Crichton D (1962). The accuracy and value of cephalopelvimetry. J Obstet Gynaecol Br Cmmnwlth, 69: 366–78.

Davey MR, Moodley J, Hofmeyr GJ (1987). Labour after caesarean section: the problem of scar dehiscence. S Afr Med J, 71: 766–768.

Dunn LJ, van Voorhis L, Napier J (1965). Term breech presentations: A report of 499 consecutive cases. Obstet Gynaecol, 25: 170–176.

Elliot JP, Garite TJ, Freeman RK, McQuown DS, Patel JM (1982). Ultrasonic prediction of fetal macrosomia in diabetic patients. Obstet Gynecol, 60: 159–162

Everett VJ (1975). The relationship between maternal height and cephalopelvic disproportion in Dar es Salaam. East Afr Med J, 52: 251–256.

Fine EA, Bracken M, Berkowitz RL (1980). An evaluation of the usefulness of X-ray pelvimetry: Comparison of the Thorns and modified Ball methods with manual pelvimetry. Am J Obstet Gynecol, 137: 15–20.

Floberg J, Belfrage P, Carlsson M, Ohlsen H (1986). The pelvic outlet. Acta Obstet Gynecol Scand, 65: 321–326.

Frame S, Moore J, Peters A, Hall D (1985). Maternal height and shoe size as predictors of pelvic disproportion: an assessment. Br J Obstet Gynaecol, 92: 1239–1245.

Gimovsky ML (1985). Short-term tocolysis adjunctive to intrapartum term breech management (Letter). Am J Obstet Gynecol, 153: 233.

Gimovsky ML, Wallace RL, Schifrin BS, Paul RH (1983). Randomized management of the nonfrank breech presentation at term: a preliminary report. Am J Obstet Gynecol, 146: 34–40.

Gimovsky ML, Willard K, Neglio M, Howard T, Zerne S (1985). X-ray pelvimetry in a breech protocol: a comparison of digital radiography and conventional methods. Am J Obstet Gynecol, 153: 887–888.

Gross SJ, Shime J, Farine D (1987). Shoulder dystocia; predictors and outcome. A five year review. Am J Obstet Gynecol, 156: 334–336.

Hartfield VJ (1986). Symphysiotomy for shoulder dystocia. Am J Obstet Gynecol, 155: 228.

Holmberg NG (1966). Clinical evaluation of the pelvic outlet. Acta Obstet Gynecol Scand, 45: 377–382.

Jaffa AJ, Peyser MR, Ballas S, Toaff T (1981). Management of term breech presentation in primigravidae. Br J Obstet Gynaecol, 88: 721–724.

Johnstone NR (1979). Shoulder dystocia: A study of 47 cases. Austral NZ J Obstet Gynaecol, 19: 28–31.

Joyce DN, Giwa-Osagie F, Stevenson GW (1975). Role of pelvimetry in the active management of labour. Br Med J, 4: 505–507.

Kaltreider D (1954). The prediction and management of outlet dystocia. Am J Obstet Gynecol, 67: 1049–1056.

Kelly KM, Madden DA, Arcarese JS, Barnett M, Brown RF (1975). The utilisation and efficacy of pelvimetry. Am J Roentgenol Radium Ther Nucl Med, 125: 66–74.

Kopelman JN, Duff P, Karl RT, Schipul AH, Read JA (1986). Computed tomographic pelvimetry in the evaluation of breech presentation. Obstet Gynecol, 68: 455–458.

Kratochwil A, Zeibekis N (1972) Ultrasonic pelvimetry. Acta Obstet Gynecol Scand, 51: 357–362.

Laube DW, Varner MW, Cruikshank DP (1981). A prospective evaluation of X-ray pelvimetry. JAMA, 246: 2187–2188.

Lavin JP, Stephens RJ, Miodovnik M, Barden TP (1982). Vaginal delivery in patients with a prior cesarean section. Obstet Gynecol, 59: 135–148.

Liljestrand J, Bergstrom S, Westman S (1985). Maternal height and perinatal outcome in Mozambique. J Trop Pediatr, 31: 306–310.

MacMahon B (1962). Prenatal X-ray exposure and childhood cancer. J Natl Cancer Inst, 28: 1173–1191.

Mati JKG, Aggarwal VP, Lucas S, Corkhill R (1983a). The Nairobi birth survey III. Labour and delivery. J Obstet Gynaecol East Centr Afr, 2: 47–56.

Mati JKG, Aggarwal VP, Lucas S, Sanghvi HCG, Corkhill R (1983b). The Nairobi birth survey IV. Early perinatal mortality rate. J Obstet Gynaecol East Centr Afr, 2: 129–133.

Modanlou HD, Komatsu G, Dorchester W, Freeman RK, Bosu SK (1982). Large for gestational age neonates; anthropometric reasons for shoulder dystocia. Obstet Gynecol, 60: 417–423.

Naeye RL, Dozor A, Tafari N, Ross SM (1977). Epidemiological features of perinatal death due to obstructed labour in Addis Ababa. Br J Obstet Gynaecol, 84: 747–750.

O'Leary JA (1979). Vaginal delivery of the term breech. A preliminary report. Obstet Gynecol, 53: 341–343.

O'Sullivan MJ, Fumia F, Holsinger K, McLeod AG (1981). Vaginal delivery after cesarean section. Clin Perinatol, 8: 131–143.

Parsons MT, Spellacy WN (1985). Prospective randomized study of X-ray pelvimetry in the primigravida. Obstet Gynecol, 66: 76–79.

Philpott RH (1982). The recognition of cephalopelvic disproportion. Clin Obstet Gynaecol, 9: 609–624.

Philpott RH, Castle WM (1972). Cervicographs in the management of labour in primigravidae. I. The alert line for detecting abnormal labour. J Obstet Gynaecol Br Commnwlth, 79: 592–598.

Radomsky JW, Radomsky NA (1980). Efficacy of pelvimetry. J Can Assoc Radiol, 31: 43–44.

Richards A, Strang A, Moodley J, Philpott RH (1985). Vaginal delivery following a previous caesarean section—does this affect perinatal mortality? Proceedings of the Fourth Annual Conference on Priorities in Perinatal Care in South Africa, Drakensburg, 12–15 March: 62–65.

Sandberg EC (1985). The Zavanelli manouver: A potentially revolutionary method for the resolution of shoulder dystocia. Am J Obstet Gynecol, 152: 479–484.

Stewart A, Webb J, Giles D, Hewitt D (1956). Malignant disease in childhood and diagnostic irradiation *in utero*. Lancet, 2: 447.

Stewart RS, Cowan DB, Philpott RH (1979). Pelvic dimensions and the outcome of trial labour in Shona and Zulu primigravidas. S Afr Med J, 55: 847–851.

Tahilramaney MP, Boucher M, Eglinton GS, Beall M, Phelan JP (1984). Previous caesarean section and trial of labor. Factors related to uterine dehiscence. J Reprod Med, 29: 17–21.

Todd WD, Steer CM (1963). Term breech: Review of 1006 term breech deliveries. Obstet Gynecol, 22: 583–595.

Vaclavinkova V (1973). A method of measuring the interspinous diameters by an ultrasonic technique. Acta Obstet Gynecol Scand, 52: 161–165.

Varner MW, Cruikshank DP, Laube DW (1980). X-ray pelvimetry in clinical obstetrics. Obstet Gynecol, 56: 296–300.

Westin B (1977). Evaluation of a feto-pelvic scoring system in the management of breech presentations. Acta Obstet Gynecol Scand, 56: 505–508.

Yudkin PL, Redman CWG (1986). Caesarean section dissected 1978–1983. Br J Obstet Gynaecol, 93: 135–144.

Part V

Specific elements of care during pregnancy

32 Symptoms in pregnancy: nausea and vomiting, heartburn, constipation, and leg cramps

Michael Bracken, Murray Enkin, Hubert Campbell, and Iain Chalmers

1 Introduction

Although an uneventful pregnancy is generally considered to be a state of health rather than disease, it is frequently accompanied by symptoms that at other times or in other circumstances might be thought to be signs of illness. Nausea and vomiting, heartburn, constipation, and leg cramps are neither life-threatening nor, in themselves, hazardous to mother or baby. Nevertheless, they can be the cause of significant discomfort and unpleasantness and, understandably, their alleviation is an important aspect of antenatal care. It is disturbing, however, that pharmacological agents of unproven benefit or safety are so often the first, or even only, method used.

Hill (1973) found that, on average, the women he surveyed took more than 10 different medications during pregnancy, the range being from 3 to 29. Forfar and Nelson (1973) found that 97 per cent of the women in their sample received prescribed drugs during pregnancy. More recent studies suggest a reduction in the number of prescription drugs used in pregnancy, perhaps because of increasing concern and public awareness about their safety. In Glasgow during 1982–84, 93.3 per cent of women reported no drug use in the 1st trimester, and 65.2 per cent reported that they had not used drugs at any time during pregnancy (Rubin *et al.* 1986). Over the same time period in New Haven, Connecticut, 69.1 per cent of pregnant women used a drug in pregnancy, but there has been a marked reduction in prescription drugs, only 21.6 per cent of all women (31.2 per cent of drug users) taking prescribed drugs (Bracken 1984). Many of these drugs are used for symptomatic purposes only; for example, Oakley (1979) reported that 43 per cent of her sample took medication for indigestion, 38 per cent took laxatives, 16 per cent took painkillers, and 13 per cent took sleeping pills. The extent of this drug usage is indicative both of the frequency of the symptoms and of the readiness with which doctors prescribe, or women resort to, medication for their relief. In New Haven, 61.4 per cent of non-prescription drugs and 27.6 per cent of prescription drugs were analgesics. The second largest category of non-prescription drugs was antacids (10.5 per cent of non-prescription drugs), and tranquillizers (17.0 per cent) were the second largest category of prescription drugs (Bracken 1984).

It took four years of extensive use before the hazards of thalidomide, a major teratogen, were recognized (McBride 1961), and over 20 years before the hazards of diethylstilboestrol were appreciated (Herbst *et al.* 1971). No drug taken during pregnancy can ever be proven to be absolutely safe, although epidemiological studies may provide considerable reassurance that the risks of using a drug, if they exist at all, are so small that they are of no practical importance. As a minimum requirement, however, a drug should at least be proven effective for the purpose for which it is prescribed.

2 Nausea and vomiting

Nausea and vomiting is the most frequent, the most characteristic, and perhaps the most troublesome symptom of early pregnancy. The prevalence of reported nausea has been highly uniform at about 70 per cent (Speert and Guttmacher 1954; Medalie 1957; Petitti 1986). The prevalence of vomiting ranges from 37 per cent to 58 per cent (Coppen 1959; Semmens 1968; Klebanoff *et al.* 1985). Nausea and vomiting are more likely to occur in young, primiparous women (Klebanoff *et al.* 1985; Petitti 1986) and in heavier women (Klebanoff *et al.* 1985). Women who smoke are less likely to vomit in pregnancy (Klebanoff *et al.* 1985) and are less likely to have used Debendox (Gibson *et al.* 1981; Eskenazi and Bracken 1982; Morelock *et al.* 1982). Nausea and vomiting tend to be associated with a more favourable pregnancy outcome: those pregnancies associated with nausea and vomiting are less likely to end in miscarriage or ectopic pregnancy (Klebanoff *et al.* 1985; Petitti 1986), but the evidence is more equivocal for stillbirths, preterm delivery, low birthweight, and congenital malformations.

The aetiology of nausea in pregnancy is unknown, and the multitude of treatments which have been recommended reflect the various theories as to the underlying cause. In the second century AD, Soranus, a Greek physician working in Rome, observed that nausea started around the 40th day and persisted for about four months. Initial treatment was to fast for one day and on the second day 'one ought to give a rubdown with ointment, but should give little and easily digested food, like a soft boiled egg or a porridge, and some not very fat fowl, as well as water to drink, not much, but if customary cold, so that the abundance of fluids in the stomach may be checked' (Soranus, undated, p 50). All of this still seems an appropriately conservative form of treatment, much more so than that advocated by some later authors. Smellie (1779), for instance, considered it to be 'the fullness of the vessels of the uterus owing to the obstructed catamenia, the whole quantity of which cannot be as yet employed in the nutrition of the embryo'. Quite logically, he concluded that 'the complaint is best relieved by bleeding'. More recently the basis of the symptom has been thought to be endocrine, neurotic (see Chapter 86), or allergic, and treatment has been advocated accordingly. Fairweather (1968) lists studies (many of them uncontrolled) on 30 different treatments, including various hormones, vitamins, amphetamines, phenothiazines, and antihistamines.

As might be expected in a self-limiting condition, uncontrolled trials have yielded rather spectacular, if spurious, results. For example, Finch (1940) found that 91 per cent of patients were relieved by desensitization with corpus luteum extracts. Hawkinson (1938) reported essentially the same benefit with oestrogens, and Shute (1941) achieved an 80 per cent rate of cure with testosterone. With diethylstilboestrol, Smith *et al.* (1944) reported marked improvement in 96 per cent and complete cure in 70 per cent of patients.

In contrast to the results obtained in the uncontrolled trials, those from controlled trials have not been quite so impressive. King (1955) compared methamphetamine, meclozine, and placebo. To improve and measure compliance he gave each patient 'a package of pills with

Table 32.1 Effect of antihistamines for nausea in pregnancy on nausea and vomiting with placebo control

Study	EXPT		CTRL		Odds ratio	Graph of odds ratios and confidence intervals
	n	(%)	*n*	(%)	(95% CI)	0.01 0.1 0.5 1 2 10 100
Cartwright (1951)	16/39	(41.03)	20/38	(52.63)	0.63 (0.26–1.54)	
Erez *et al.* (1971)	18/100	(18.00)	39/50	(78.00)	0.08 (0.04–0.16)	
Lask (1953)	7/60	(11.67)	53/60	(88.33)	0.05 (0.02–0.10)	
King (1955)	7/60	(11.67)	8/40	(20.00)	0.52 (0.17–1.60)	
Conklin and Nesbitt (1958)	1/32	(3.13)	3/11	(27.27)	0.06 (0.01–0.63)	
Diggory and Tomkinson (1962)	3/76	(3.95)	37/63	(58.73)	0.07 (0.03–0.15)	
Fitzgerald (1955)	17/58	(29.31)	43/56	(76.79)	0.15 (0.07–0.31)	
Typical odds ratio (95% confidence interval)					0.12 (0.09–0.16)	

the explanation that these were something very new and of proven (*sic*) efficacy', but that they were 'so expensive that any unused pills were to be returned'. He found no evidence of a beneficial effect in the active preparations. His 'improvement or cure' rate was 22/32 (68 per cent) with methamphetamine, 53/60 (88 per cent) with meclozine, and 48/58 (83 per cent) in the two placebo groups combined.

In a double-blind trial of meclozine and pyridoxine compared with pyridoxine alone, the General Practitioner Research Group (Baum *et al.* 1963) found these two treatments to have virtually identical effects: 27/40 (68 per cent) of women obtained relief with the pyridoxine–antihistamine combination and 25/36 (69 per cent) with pyridoxine alone. The authors correctly conclude that 'it would be of interest to compare pyridoxine with a placebo', but unfortunately no such comparison has ever been carried out.

A number of trials have demonstrated antihistamines to be better than placebo (Table 32.1). Lask (1953) compared the effects of two antihistamine preparations, mepyramine maleate ('Antisan'), and promethazine-8-chlorotheophyllinate ('Avomine'), with placebo. Overall 53/60 (88 per cent) of the antihistamine groups and 7/60 (12 per cent) of the control group were improved. However, there is no evidence in the study that the groups were randomly selected, or that evaluations were blind. In a double-blind trial, Conklin and Nesbitt (1958) compared two antihistamines (buclizine and meclozine) with vitamin B_{12} and with placebo. Satisfactory results were obtained in 31/32 (97 per cent) of the women treated with antihistamines, and in 8/11 (73 per cent) of those treated with placebo or B_{12}. In a similar trial (Winters 1961), trimethobenzamide ('Tigan') helped 169/199 (85 per cent) of patients while only 75/195 (38 per cent) benefited from the placebo. Diggory and Tomkinson (1962) allocated patients with nausea and vomiting alternately to treatment with meclozine, meclozine plus pyridoxine, placebo, or dietary instructions alone. Improvement was noted in 10/29 (34 per cent) of women given dietary advice alone, 26/63 (41 per cent) of those taking placebo, 40/41 (98 per cent) of those taking meclozine, and 33/35 (94 per cent) of those receiving meclozine and pyridoxine. In a double-blind study of hydroxyzine hydrochloride, Erez *et al.* (1971) reported partial or complete relief in 82/100 (82 per cent) of patients receiving the medicine, compared to 11/50 (22 per cent) of those taking placebo. Newlinds (1964) reported on a double-blind trial in which non-compliers were excluded from the analysis. He found that 53/93 (57 per cent) of the patients treated with the phenothiazine thiethylperazine achieved complete relief of symptoms, compared with only 26/87 (30 per cent) of those given a placebo.

Simple antihistamines, although they sometimes provoke troublesome side-effects such as drowsiness and blurring of vision, are generally considered to be safe during pregnancy.

In summary, the bulk of evidence would seem to indicate that simple antihistamines are of benefit in the alleviation of nausea and vomiting during pregnancy. No serious doubts have been raised about their safety, although few large epidemiological studies have been conducted. The frequency with which they are used, however, may be excessive. As nausea and vomiting during pregnancy tends to be self-limiting, and frequently seems to respond to such innocuous measures as small, frequent meals, the avoidance of stale or unpleasant odours, and of cooking smells generally (Lennane and Lennane 1973) there may be scope for reducing the extent of antiemetic medication.

2.1 Debendox (Bendectin)

By far the most widely presented drug used to treat nausea in pregnancy was, until recently, Debendox (marketed as Bendectin in the United States, and Lenotan in some other countries). Indeed, Debendox was the most widely used prescription drug of any kind taken in pregnancy (Bracken 1984). In 1978, doctors in the United States wrote 3.4 million prescriptions for the preparation—an average of one prescription for almost every pregnant women, although only about 40 per cent of these prescriptions appear to have been used (Check 1979).

In June 1983 Debendox was removed from the market as a direct result of litigation, brought against the manufacturers, claiming that the drug had caused congenital malformations in the offspring of women who had used it. The litigation was brought despite overwhelming evidence *against* Debendox being a teratogen (Kolata 1980) and has almost certainly led to an increased use of alternative medications for treating nausea and vomiting, about which, for any single product, much less human research has been conducted. Since Debendox is another example of a growing number of medications where litigation has led to the removal of treatments despite evidence of their safety, a review of the evidence is timely.

Debendox, at the time of its recall, had been used by over 30 million women world-wide, and in many countries between a quarter and a third of all pregnant women used Debendox. When Debendox is used to treat nausea it is usually in the first trimester, during embryological development. Indeed, because of concern about the teratogenic risks of other drugs, Debendox was often the only prescription drug used in pregnancy. If we assume an overall congenital malformation incidence rate of 3.5 per cent at delivery, then exposure to Debendox will have occurred in over one million babies born with a congenital malformation *purely by chance alone*. In the inevitable search for what may have produced her child's malformations, it is not surprising that many mothers implicated Debendox and, perhaps prompted by over-eager lawyers, some chose to sue.

Let us now review the scientific studies concerning Debendox, first the trials of efficacy and then the epidemiological studies of safety.

2.1.1 Efficacy of Debendox

We have been able to identify only 3 controlled trials of Debendox. This is a surprisingly small number of controlled trials for such a widely used drug. Indeed, only 241 women were entered into all three trials for a drug eventually used by millions of women. The results of the trials are shown in Table 32.2. In the first trial, by Geiger *et al.* (1959), 49/53 (92 per cent) of women obtained complete or partial relief in the Debendox group compared with 37/57 (65 per cent) of women treated with placebo. McGuinness and Binns (1971) reported that 29/41 (71 per cent) of women randomly assigned to Debendox reported a reduction in symptoms compared with 22/40 (55 per cent) of those using placebo. Wheatley (1977) found that only 6/24 (25 per cent) reported a total absence of nausea and vomiting after Debendox, but this was higher than the 1/26 (4 per cent) reporting relief after using pyridoxine alone. The overview of these three small trials provides strong evidence that Debendox provides considerable relief for nausea and vomiting in pregnancy (typical odds ratio = 0.30, 95 per cent confidence interval 0.16–0.54).

2.1.2 Safety of Debendox

Animal studies are not able to resolve questions concerning the safety of drug use in humans. Thalidomide, for example, despite being highly teratogenic in humans, does not affect many animal species (Mellin and Katzenstein 1962), and corticosteroids have not been shown to affect the human fetus adversely, although they are teratogenic in many animal species (Lewis *et al.* 1985). Clinical trials designed to test a drug's efficacy are far too small to demonstrate teratogenic effects on the offspring. Investigation of the safety of drug use in pregnancy, therefore, usually depends on epidemiological studies conducted after the drug has entered widespread use.

The 19 epidemiological studies of Debendox and congenital malformations in offspring are shown in Table 32.3. The studies represent both case-control and prospective designs, vary considerably in size, and use either the mother's own report or prescription notes to ascertain Debendox use. The Debendox was almost equally divided between the 2-component product (doxylamine succinate and pyridoxine) and the older, 3-component product, which included dicyclomine hydrochloride. In choosing controls some investigators elected to use healthy newborns, whereas others used newborns with malformations other than those being studied (Bracken and Berg 1983).

In spite of the wide variety of populations studied and methods employed, there is widespread agreement among the studies that Debendox is *not* associated with an increased risk of congenital malformations in offspring. One study found an association between the 2-ingredient product and oesophageal atresia among a large number of associations examined (Cordero *et al.* 1981); another found an association with cleft lip and palate (Golding *et al.* 1983), and a third an association with genital malformations in males but not for 9 other reproductive outcomes studied (Gibson *et al.* 1981). None of these observations was replicated in other larger studies. Of all the malformations studied, only pyloric stenosis has been found to be associated with Debendox in two studies (Eskenazi and Bracken 1982; Aselton *et al.* 1984, 1985), but a third study found no relation (Mitchell *et al.* 1983), and none of these investigators claim that a causal relationship has been documented.

The power of studies to detect positive relationships is always a question when statistically significant relationships are not observed. The Debendox studies include some very large ones. Case-control studies with over 1400 cases and 3000 controls have the same power

Table 32.2 Effect of Debendox (Bendectin) for nausea in pregnancy on nausea and vomiting

Study	EXPT		CTRL		Odds ratio	Graph of odds ratios and confidence intervals
	n	(%)	*n*	(%)	(95% CI)	0.01 0.1 0.5 1 2 10 100
McGuiness and Binns (1971)	12/41	(29.27)	18/40	(45.00)	0.51 (0.21–1.26)	
Geiger *et al.* (1959)	4/53	(7.55)	20/57	(35.09)	0.20 (0.08–0.50)	
Wheatley (1977)	18/24	(75.00)	25/26	(96.15)	0.18 (0.04–0.87)	
Typical odds ratio (95% confidence interval)					0.30 (0.16–0.54)	

Table 32.3 Epidemiological studies of Debendox (Bendectin) and congenital malformations in offspring

				Debendox		Measure of association		
Authors and year	Type of study[1]	No. cases studied	Exposure measure[2]	Formula[3]	Use in controls	Estimate[4]	95% CI	Comment[5]
Milkovich and Van den Berg (1976)	Pr	153	P	3	6.2	0.5	NE	All malformations Healthy controls
Shapiro *et al.* (1977)	Pr	'At least 500'	SR/P	Doxylamine	NE	1.1	NE	Major malformations
				Dicyclomine	NE	1.1	NE	Healthy controls Heavy exposure
Mitchell *et al.* (1981)	CC	98 CP 221 CP + CPL 122 HD	SR	Mostly 2	21.0	0.9 0.6 1.0	0.5, 1.5 0.4, 0.8 0.6, 1.6	Cleft palate, Cleft lip + palate Heart malformations Other malformations Controls
Cordero *et al.* (1981)	CC	1231	SR	3 & 2	9.5	NE	NE	All malformations Only oesophageal atresia (3 ingred.) and encephalocoele (2 ingred.) $p < 0.05$
Gibson *et al.* (1981)	Pr		SR	3	22.2	1.1	NE ($p > 0.25$)	All malformations, Genital malformations ($p < 0.05$). CNS, cardiac, skeletal, IUGR, prematurity, and neonatal death NS
Jick *et al.* (1981)	Pr	80	P	Mostly 2	33.0	0.9	NE	All malformations Healthy controls
Eskenazi and Bracken (1982)	CC	1427	SR	3	4.6	1.4	1.0, 2.1	All malformations, Healthy controls Pyloric stenosis OR = 4.3 (1.8, 10.8)
Morelock *et al.* (1982)	Pr	163	SR	2	22.2	1.1	NE	All malformations Healthy controls
Aselton and Jick (1983)	Pr	6	P	2	26.0	1.4	0.3, 7.7	Limb defects Healthy controls
Bracken and Berg (1983)	CC	10	SR	3	6.6	1.6	0.2, 12.4	Diaphragmatic hernia Healthy controls
Golding *et al.* (1983)	CC	196	P	3	2.2	2.8	NE ($p = 0.02$)	Cleft lip + palate Healthy controls
Mitchell *et al.* (1983)	CC	325	SR	Mostly 2	20.0	0.9	0.6, 1.2	Pyloric stenosis Other malformation Controls
Aselton *et al.* (1984)	Pr/CC	26	P	2	28.7	2.5	1.2, 5.2	Pyloric stenosis Healthy controls
McCredie *et al.* (1984)	CC	155	SR	3	25.0	1.1	0.8, 1.5	Limb defects Healthy controls
Aselton *et al.* (1985)	Pr	105	P	2	23.0	1.2	0.8, 1.9	All malformations Healthy controls
Elbourne *et al.* (1985)	CC	93	P	3	9.0	0.65	0.3, 3.3	Cleft lip + palate Healthy controls

Table 32.3—*continued* Epidemiological studies of Debendox (Bendectin) and congenital malformations in offspring

Authors and year	Type of study[1]	No. cases studied	Exposure measure[2]	Debendox: Formula[3]	Debendox: Use in controls	Measure of association: Estimate[4]	Measure of association: 95% CI	Comment[5]
McKinney *et al.* (1985)	CC	555	SR/P	3	8.9	1.0	NE	Transplacental cancer Healthy controls
Zierler and Rothman (1985)	CC	298	SR/P	2	16.6	1.1	0.8, 1.5[6]	Heart malformations Healthy controls
Porter *et al.* (1986)	CC	9	P	2	30.6	1.8	0.5, 7.0[6]	Stillbirth
		13			34.6	0.6	0.2, 1.8[6]	Placental disorders
		17			20.6	0.8	0.2, 2.6[6]	Cord problems

[1] Pr = Prospective, CC = Case control
[2] P = Prescription, SR = Self-report
[3] Formula 3 = Dicyclomine hydrochloride, Doxylamine succinate, Pyridoxine
Formula 2 = Doxylamine and Pyridoxine
[4] For case-control studies the odds ratio; for prospective studies, relative risk.
[5] For prospective studies 'controls' refers to newborns without malformation.
[6] 90% confidence interval
NE = Not estimable NS = $p > 0.05$

as prospective studies of 50 000 births. Moreover, the confidence intervals shown in Table 32.3 rarely exclude 1.0. The existing epidemiologic studies, therefore, provide very strong evidence as to the safety of Debendox. Other, less well controlled studies, also support this conclusion (Correy and Newman 1981; David 1982).

The abrupt withdrawal of Debendox from the market has provided a unique further test of its safety. Despite the reduction in use of Debendox, from use in about one-third of pregnancies to use in none, there has been no correlated reduction in ventricular septal defects (Brent 1985) or, indeed any other malformation group as judged by their incidence reports (e.g. Center for Disease Control Congenital Malformation Surveillance Reports; Office of Population Censuses and Surveys). If Debendox doubled the risk of a specific malformation which occurred in unexposed pregnancies at a rate of 1.5 per 1000, the drop in exposure from 30 per cent to 0 per cent would lead to a 23 per cent decline in incidence. That this has not occurred provides additional evidence that Debendox is not associated with increased risks of malformation.

This type of 'ecological' correlation is not, in itself, one that is usually given much credence in determining the safety of a drug although, in the present context, it provides strong supportive evidence. There are no other drugs used in pregnancy which have dropped so rapidly from such a high exposure rate to non-use.

With the withdrawal of the most widely studied antiemetic, Debendox, from the market, nausea in pregnancy is being treated by antihistamines which appear to be efficacious, as evidenced by the early trials, but whose safety has not been studied extensively.

3 Heartburn

Heartburn affects about two-thirds of all women at some stage of pregnancy (Atlay *et al.* 1973). It is another so-called 'minor' disorder of pregnancy, but it causes more discomfort and distress than do many more serious conditions. It is commonly associated with eating, stooping, or lying down. The most clear-cut precipitating factor is posture (Hart 1978).

Self-medication with proprietary antacids is the most commonly employed treatment. There appears to be little evidence of differences in efficacy between the various available preparations. In a double-blind crossover trial, Briggs and Hart (1972) found a proprietary preparation, 'Alcin' (anhydrous sodium aluminium salicylate and basic magnesium aluminate), to be more effective in relieving heartburn than was aluminium hydroxide BP; both afforded relief in over 90 per cent of episodes. However, patients rated the proprietary preparation as significantly more pleasant and acceptable.

Shaw (1978) tested the relative efficacy of an antacid gel compared with a neutral gel of pectin agar ('active placebo') in a double-blind randomized trial. Overall, 50/60 (83 per cent) of women receiving the active preparation and 42/60 (70 per cent) of those taking neutral gel found the preparations sufficiently acceptable to complete the 7-day trial. There was some evidence that the active preparation was more effective, but the degree of benefit tended to decrease with increasing initial levels of discomfort.

Bower (1961) studied 100 women who failed to obtain relief from heartburn with antacids, testing prostigmine (0.5 mg intramuscularly) against placebo in a double-blind trial; 38/50 (76 per cent) of women were helped by the prostigmine, compared with only 20/50 (40 per cent) who were helped by placebo.

Based on the suggestion from their earlier work (Atlay *et al.* 1973) that better management of heartburn might be achieved by directing efforts toward counteracting the effects of regurgitated bile on the stomach and oesophagus than by concentrating on reducing the acidity of the stomach, Atlay *et al.* (1973) randomly allocated 55 women to initial treatment with dilute hydrochloric acid, sodium bicarbonate, or placebo. Symptoms disappeared or improved in 26/47 (55 per cent) with alkali; 31/45 (69 per cent) with acid; and 20/49 (41 per cent) with placebo. Both acid and alkali were statistically significantly better than placebo. An important feature of the trial was its crossover design. This enabled comparison of secondary lines of treatment, which showed that women who had not obtained relief from their symptoms with alkali were likely to obtain relief from acid, and vice versa. In this way they found a 98 per cent probability that one or other of these treatments would be efficacious.

No treatment is entirely free of hazard. Sodium bicarbonate presents the potential for sodium overload and systemic alkalosis. Magnesium preparations may lead to severe diarrhoea; calcium carbonate to hypercalcaemia, impairment of renal function, and stimulation of gastric secretion; and aluminium hydroxide (when taken in large doses) to phosphate depletion (Morrissey and Barreras 1974). However, there does not appear to be any hazard from the occasional use of any of the agents we have discussed. After a crossover randomized trial of four antacid preparations, Jacyna *et al.* (1984) concluded that individuals should be allowed to choose among different preparations, since therapeutic compliance will be increased when the product is found to be palatable. Of the available antacids, the magnesium salts would appear to be the safest option for longer term use. In situations where simple and sensible measures such as avoiding fatty or spicy foods and minimizing bending or lying flat after eating have failed, the evidence suggests that alkalis should be prescribed initially. If symptoms fail to respond to alkalis, dilute hydrochloric acid or prostigmine may be tried.

4 Constipation

Constipation is a troublesome problem for many women during pregnancy, particularly during the last trimester. Women who are habitually constipated usually become more so during pregnancy (Burgess 1972). The frequency of constipation among pregnant women will reflect their dietary habits, fluid intake, and pattern of physical exercise. In one report (Greenhalf and Leonard 1973) nearly a third of the women studied were troubled by constipation. Another report noted that 85 per cent of parous women first experienced anorectal symptoms during their first pregnancy or immediately after the birth of their first child (Marks and Thiele 1955).

Management of constipation using physiological approaches (alterations in diet, fluid intake, or exercises) has been found to bring relief in at least a third of cases (Greenhalf and Leonard 1973); nevertheless, laxatives are required by many women.

An extensive review of therapeutic agents for constipation (Godding 1972) states that 'laxative drugs in current use constitute a medley of substances with most diverse actions, and often with little rationale to support them'. The treatment used often depends upon the particular whim and fancy of the doctor or midwife in charge (Greenhalf and Leonard 1973).

Laxatives are usually classified by their mode of action. Saline cathartics (magnesium, sodium, and potassium salts) and lubricants (such as mineral oils) are contraindicated in pregnancy, the former because of the danger of inducing electrolyte disturbances, the latter because they interfere with absorption of fat-soluble vitamins, tend to seep through the anal sphincter and cause pruritis, and occasionally cause lipoid pneumonia and paraffinomas (Godding 1972).

Hydrophilic bulking agents (polysaccharide and/or cellulose derivatives) and detergent stool-softeners (the dioctylsulphosuccinates) are relatively free of adverse effects because they are inert and not absorbed (Bishop 1978).

A variety of laxatives operate by their irritant action on the intestine. These include the diphenylmethanes (for example, bisacodyl and phenolphthalein), the antraquinones (aloe, cascara, and senna), and castor oil. These irritant laxatives are all absorbed systemically to some extent. Most of them probably cross the placenta, but there is little information about possible effects on the fetus. The most common side-effects include cramping or griping and increased mucous secretion and excessive catharsis with resultant fluid loss. Chronic use can result in loss of normal bowel function and laxative dependence (Bishop 1978).

We have only been able to find two randomized trials of laxative use during pregnancy. Greenhalf and Leonard (1973) compared two bulking agents ('Normacol standard' and 'Normacol special'), standardized senna, and a combination of an irritant laxative and stool softener ('Normax'). The two preparations containing irritant laxatives were more effective in relieving constipation than the bulking agents, but this benefit was accompanied by a high incidence of side-effects which included abdominal pain, diarrhoea, discoloration of the urine, and nausea. Interestingly, investigation of patient acceptability of the different treatments failed to reveal any differences. There were no detectable differences between agents in the rate at which normal bowel function was restored.

The only other controlled trial of laxative use in pregnancy also compared a bulking agent (psyullium hydrophilic mucilloid) with irritant laxatives (Fianu and Vaclavinkova 1975). No significant differences were observed.

More recent interest has focused on using modest supplemental intake of dietary fibre to reduce constipation. In a randomized trial comparing dietary supplement with wheat or corn bran with no intervention, women in both fibre-supplemented groups increased their number of bowel movements (statistically significantly so in the corn-bran-supplemented group) and experienced less constipation than the untreated women (Anderson and Whichelow 1985). The dietary fibre supplement for corn-based biscuits was 10 g daily and 23 g daily for wheat bran. A similar study has shown that wheat and corn bran supplements reduce constipation in the general population (Graham *et al.* 1982) and is in accord with advice given to pregnant women in Italy to increase their dietary fibre to 13 g daily (Sculati 1980).

In summary, in attempts to prevent and treat constipation in pregnancy, modification of the diet, including improving dietary fibre intake and increased fluid intake, should be considered before resorting to laxatives. Both bulking agents and stool softeners are safe for long term use in pregnancy. If these preparations fail to relieve symptoms, irritant laxatives (for example, standardized senna or bisacodyl) should be used on a short term basis. Saline cathartics and lubricant oils should not be used at all.

5 Leg cramps

Leg cramps (painful spasms of the calf muscles) are experienced to some extent by almost half of all pregnant women, particularly in the later months of pregnancy. The symptom tends to occur at night and may recur repeatedly for weeks or months, causing considerable distress (Salvatore 1961). The cause and mechanism of these cramps are still not clear. Sometimes based on rather astonishing analogies, unsupported hypotheses, and uncontrolled studies, a number of drugs have been widely prescribed for treatment and prophylaxis.

Quinine has been recommended as a treatment (Shervington 1974), on the basis of an uncontrolled trial by Moss and Herrmann (1940), who found the drug to be useful in elderly patients suffering from similar symptoms caused by poor circulation. Naide (1950) argued that 'this condition can usually be prevented by administration of quinine', but failure of one patient to respond led him to try diphenhydramine hydrochloride ('Benadryl') because of its presumed effectiveness in Parkinson's disease (Budnitz 1948). Naide (1950) found that 'Benadryl' prevented cramps in 17 patients, and suggested that it might be useful, as 'obstetricians may hesitate to prescribe quinine for relief of leg cramps in pregnancy, whereas diphenhydramine is commonly administered antepartum'.

The superficial resemblance of the cramps to tetany, together with the finding of lowered serum calcium in late pregnancy, led some to believe that calcium deficiency was the cause of the cramps (e.g. Mendenhall and Drake 1934). Thus, vitamin D and either dicalcium phosphate or an increased milk intake were recommended for both prophylaxis and treatment.

Hardy (1956) selected 50 patients in the 3rd trimester of pregnancy. To 10 women (the control group) he gave no dietary supplement; 3 of these had leg cramps and 2 of these recovered spontaneously. A second group of 10 women, given 'conventional prenatal supplements' containing dicalcium phosphate, all developed leg cramps. The third group of 10 initially all had cramps and were treated with calcium lactate: 'all but one were relieved at the end of the week, a 90 per cent cure rate'. The fourth group contained 20 patients, 18 of whom had leg cramps: these women were given a supplement containing oyster-shell calcium carbonate, and all were stated to be cured within three weeks.

Although these studies were totally devoid of any scientific merit, the reports were capitalized on commercially. Within a period of 3 years, nine pharmaceutical companies had produced and publicized prenatal vitamin-mineral supplements containing calcium lactate instead of dicalcium phosphate: one company introduced a supplement containing aluminium hydroxide, another the oyster-shell calcium carbonate product endorsed by Hardy (Abrams and Aponte 1958). These preparations became widely prescribed with the aim of preventing leg cramps.

To test the prophylactic potential of these preparations, Abrams and Aponte (1958) divided women who had registered for prenatal care prior to the 22nd week into three groups, on the basis of the type of medication to be administered. Women in the first group were given supplements devoid of calcium, phosphorous, or vitamin D; 4 of the 10 patients developed leg cramps. Women in the second group were given supplements with dicalcium phosphate; 2 out of 8 developed cramps. In the third group given supplements containing calcium lactate and vitamin D, an unfortunate 8 out of 10 women developed leg cramps. They took a careful dietary history from these women, and, in addition, from 19 other women who registered for care after the

22nd week, complained of leg cramps, but had been given no medication. In addition to finding no benefit from calcium lactate, they found no relation of leg cramps to intake of dairy products.

Robinson (1947) studied 198 pregnant women with leg cramps, allocating them alternately to treatment with calcium lactate, saccharine as a placebo, sodium chloride, or an untreated control group. The cramps ceased before the end of pregnancy in 44 per cent of the women given saccharine tablets, in 47 per cent of the women given no treatment, in 48 per cent of those given calcium lactate, and in 88 per cent of those who took the sodium chloride.

A randomized trial (Hammar *et al.* 1981) apparently demonstrated diminution of leg cramps following the use of a phosphate-free calcium supplement. No effect was demonstrated on ionized serum calcium levels. Unfortunately, failure to use placebo controls or to double-blind the study, leaves placebo effect as a reasonable explanation of the results. A more recent and more effectively controlled trial conducted by the same investigators (Hammar *et al.* 1987) failed to show any improvement in symptoms among women who took 1 g of calcium twice daily for three weeks (a finding similar to that in the placebo-controlled trial reported by Odendaal (1974).

Calcium salts are still widely prescribed for the syndrome of nocturnal calf-cramps in pregnancy, despite the weakness of the evidence from any controlled trials that they have any benefit beyond that of a placebo. Unfortunately, no further trials of the efficacy of increased sodium intake appear to have been carried out. It is probable that the observed benefits may be restricted to patients who are sodium-deficient. Massage, and putting the affected muscles on the stretch, is stated to afford relief during an attack (Shervington 1974), and these innocuous measures are surely worth trying.

6 Conclusions

Our review of the available methods for managing some of the symptoms commonly experienced during pregnancy indicates that often these will be amenable to relief by using simple and physiological approaches. Where medication is deemed to be necessary, simple antihistamines appear to be the drugs of choice in the management of nausea and vomiting, although no single product has been satisfactorily tested for efficacy in enough trials and few studies are available to inform us about possible teratogenic risks. Unfortunately, Debendox—the antinauseant for which efficacy and safety have been documented—is no longer available.

When symptoms of heartburn are troublesome, antacids should be taken, and dilute hydrochloric acid if these fail to bring relief. Bulking agents, if necessary combined with stool softeners, should be used in the management of constipation; irritant laxatives (such as standardized senna) should be reserved for short term use in refractory cases. No pharmaceutical treatment for leg cramps has yet been firmly based on scientific evidence.

It is surprising how the most prevalent and discomforting symptoms of pregnancy have received such little study in properly controlled trials. The most distressing of these symptoms is nausea, which is not a psychological condition, and which is amenable to treatment. New trials are urgently needed to identify efficacious therapy and to study the safety of those antihistamines which appear, at the present time, to be most efficacious.

References

Abrams J, Aponte GE (1958). The leg cramp syndrome during pregnancy. The relationship to calcium and phosphorus metabolism. Am J Obstet Gynecol, 76: 432–437.

Anderson AS, Whichelow MJ (1985). Constipation during pregnancy: Dietary fibre intake and the effect of fibre supplementation. Human Nutrition: Applied Nutrition 39A: 202–207.

Aselton P, Jick H (1983). Additional follow-up of congenital disorders in relation to Bendectin use. JAMA, 250: 33–34.

Aselton P, Jick H, Chentow SJ, Perera DR, Hunter JR, Rothman KJ (1984). Pyloric stenosis and maternal Bendectin exposure. Am J Epidemiol, 120: 251–256.

Aselton P, Jick H, Milunsky A, Hunter JR, Stergachis A (1985). First trimester drug use and congenital disorders. Obstet Gynecol, 65: 451–455.

Atlay RD, Gillison EW, Horton AL (1973). A fresh look at pregnancy heartburn. J Obstet Gynaecol Br Commnwlth, 80: 63–66.

Baum G, Boxer EI, Davidson JH, Lawrence N, Lewis JBR, Morgan DJR, Stowell TES (1963). Meclozine and pyridoxine in pregnancy sickness. Practitioner, 190: 251–253.

Bishop C (1978). Nonprescription drugs: A guide to the pregnant patient. Can Pharm J, 111: 385–388.

Bower D (1961). The use of prostigmine in the heartburn of pregnancy. Br J Obstet Gynaecol, 68: 846–847.

Bracken MB (1984). Methodologic issues in the epidemiologic investigation of drug-induced congenital malformations. In: Perinatal Epidemiology. Bracken MB (ed). New York: Oxford University Press, pp 423–449.

Bracken MB, Berg A (1983). Bendectin (Debendox) and congenital diaphragmatic hernia. Lancet, 1: 586.

Brent RL (1985). Bendectin and interventricular septal defects. Teratology, 32: 317–318.

Briggs DW, Hart DM (1972). Heartburn of pregnancy. A continuation study. Br J Clin Pract, 26: 167–169.

Budnitz J (1948). The use of Benadryl in Parkinson's disease. New Engl J Med, 238: 874–875.

Burgess DE (1972). Constipation in obstetrics. In: Management of Constipation. Avery Jones Sir F, Godding EW (eds). Oxford: Blackwell.

Cartwright EW (1951). Dramamine in nausea and vomiting of pregnancy. West J Surg, 59: 216–234.

Check WA (1979). CDC study: No evidence for teratogenicity of Bendectin. JAMA, 242: 2518.

Conklin FJ, Nesbitt REL (1958). Buclizine hydrochloride for nausea and vomiting of pregnancy. Obstet Gynecol, 11: 214–219.

Coppen AJ (1959). Vomiting of early pregnancy: Psychological factors and body build. Lancet, 1: 172.

Cordero JF, Oakley GP, Greenberg F, James LM (1981). Is Bendectin a teratogen? JAMA, 245: 2307–2310.

Correy FJ, Newman NM (1981). Debendox and limb reduction deformities. Med J Austral, 1: 417–418.

David TJ (1982). Debendox does not cause the Poland anomaly. Arch Dis Child, 57: 479–480.

Diggory PLC, Tomkinson JS (1962). Nausea and vomiting in pregnancy. A trial of meclozine dihydrochloride with and without pyridoxine. Lancet, 2: 370–372.

Elbourne D, Mutch L, Dauncey M, Campbell H, Samphier M (1985). Debendox revisited. Br J Obstet Gynaecol, 92: 780–785.

Erez S, Schifrin BS, Dirim O (1971). Double-blind evaluation of hydroxyzine as an antiemetic in pregnancy. J Reprod Med, 7: 35–37.

Eskenazi B, Bracken MB (1982). Bendectin (Debendox) as a risk factor for pyloric stenosis. Am J Obstet Gynecol, 144: 919–924.

Fairweather DVI (1968). Nausea and vomiting in pregnancy. Am J Obstet Gynecol, 102: 135–175.

Fianu S, Vaclavinkova V (1975). Comparison between a bulk laxative and irritant laxatives in obstetrical and gynecological departments. (Swedish) Opuscula Medica, 20: 167–171. (Cited by Bishop C 1978).

Finch JW (1940). The nausea and vomiting of pregnancy due to allergic reaction. A study of 192 cases. Am J Obstet Gynecol, 40: 1029–1036.

Fitzgerald JPB (1955). The effect of promethazine in nausea and vomiting of pregnancy. NZ Med J, 54: 215–218.

Forfar JO, Nelson MN (1973). Epidemiology of drugs taken by pregnant women: Drugs that may affect the fetus adversely. Clin Pharmacol Ther, 14: 632–642.

Geiger CJ, Fahrenbach DM, Healey FJ (1959). Bendectin in the treatment of nausea and vomiting in pregnancy. Obstet Gynecol, 14: 688–690.

Gibson GT, Colley DP, McMichael AJ, Hartshorne JM (1981). Congenital anomalies in relation to the use of Doxylamine/Dicylcomine and other antenatal factors. An ongoing prospective study. Med J Austral, 1: 410–414.

Godding EW (1972). Therapeutic agents. In: Management of Constipation. Avery Jones Sir F, Godding EW (eds). Oxford: Blackwell.

Golding J, Vivian S, Baldwin JA (1983). Maternal antinauseants and clefts of lip and palate. Hum Toxicol, 2: 63–73.

Graham DY, Moser SE, Estes MK (1982). The effects of bran on bowel function in constipation. Am J Gastroenterol, 7: 599–603.

Greenhalf JO, Leonard HS (1973). Laxatives in the treatment of constipation in pregnant and breastfeeding mothers. Practitioner, 210: 259–263.

Hammar M, Larsson L, Tegler L (1981). Calcium treatment of leg cramps in pregnancy. Effect on clinical symptoms and total serum and ionized serum calcium concentrations. Acta Obstet Gynecol Scand, 60: 345–347.

Hammar M, Berg G, Solheim F, Larsson L (1987). Calcium and magnesium status in pregnant women. A comparison between treatment with calcium and vitamin C in pregnant women with leg cramps. Int J Vitam Nutr Res, 57: 179–183.

Hardy JA (1956). Blood calcium levels in pregnancy. Obstet Gynecol, 8: 565–568.

Hart DM (1978). Heartburn in pregnancy. J Int Med Res, 6 (Suppl 1): 1–5.

Hawkinson LF (1938). Estrogens in vomiting of pregnancy. JAMA, 111: 1235.

Herbst AL, Ulfelder H, Poskanzer DC (1971). Adenocarcinoma of the vagina. Association of maternal stilbestrol therapy with tumor appearance in young women. New Engl J Med, 284: 878–881.

Hill RM (1973). Drugs ingested by pregnant women. Clin Pharmacol Ther, 14: 654–659.

Jacyna MR, Boyd EJS, Wormsley KG (1984). Comparative study of four antacids. Postgrad Med J, 60: 592–596.

Jick H, Holmes LB, Hunter JR, *et al.* (1981). First trimester drug use and congenital disorders. JAMA, 246: 343–346.

King AG (1955). The treatment of pregnancy nausea with a pill. Obstet Gynecol, 6: 332–338.

Klebanoff MA, Koslowe PA, Kaslow R, Rhoads GG (1985). Epidemiology of vomiting in early pregnancy. Obstet Gynecol, 66: 612–616.

Kolata GB (1980). How safe is Bendectin? Science, 210: 518–519.

Lask S (1953). Treatment of nausea and vomiting of pregnancy with antihistamines. Br Med J, 1: 652–653.

Lennane KJ, Lennane RJ (1973). Alleged psychogenic disorders in women—a possible manifestation of sexual prejudice. New Engl J Med, 288: 288–292.

Lewis JH, Weingold AB, Committee on FDA Related Matters, American College of Gastroenterology (1985). The role of gastrointestinal drugs during pregnancy and lactation. Am J Gastroenterol, 80: 912–923.

Marks MM, Thiele GH (1955). Management of proctologic disease in pregnant and parous women. Am J Surg, 90: 826–833.

McBride WG (1961). Thalidomide and congenital abnormalities. Lancet, 2: 1358.

McCredie J, Kricker A, Elliott J, Forrest J (1984). The innocent bystander. Doxylamine/dicyclomine/pyridoxine and congenital limb defects. Med J Austral, 140: 525–527.

McGuinness BW, Binns DT (1971). 'Debendox' in pregnancy sickness. J R Coll Gen Pract, 21: 500–503.

McKinney PA, Cartwright RA, Stiller CA, Hopton PA, Mann JR, Birch JM, Hartley AL, Waterhouse JAH, Johnston HE (1985). Inter-regional epidemiological study of childhood cancer (IRESCC): Childhood cancer and consumption of Debendox and related drugs in pregnancy. Br J Cancer, 52: 923–929.

Medalie JH (1957). Relationship between nausea and/or vomiting in early pregnancy and abortion. Lancet, 2: 298–299.

Mellin GW, Katzenstein M (1962). The saga of thalidomide. New Engl J Med, 267: 1184–1192, 1238–1244.

Mendenhall AM, Drake JC (1934). Calcium deficiency in pregnancy and lactation: A clinical investigation. Am J Obstet Gynecol, 27: 800–807.

Milkovich L, van den Berg B (1976). An evaluation of the teratogenicity of certain antinauseant drugs. Am J Obstet Gynecol, 125: 244–248.

Mitchell AA, Rosenberg L, Shapiro S, Slone D (1981). Birth defects related to Bendectin use in pregnancy. JAMA, 245: 2311–2314.

Mitchell AA, Schwingl PJ, Rosenberg L, Louik C, Shapiro S (1983). Birth defects in relation to Bendectin use in pregnancy. II: Pyloric Stenosis. Am J Obstet Gynecol, 147: 737–742.

Morelock S, Hingson R, Kayne H, Dooling E, Zuckerman B, Day N, Alpert JJ, Flowerdew G (1982). Bendectin and fetal development. Am J Obstet Gynecol, 142: 209–213.

Morrissey JF, Barreras RF (1974). Drug therapy: Antacid therapy. New Engl J Med, 290: 550–554.

Moss HK, Herrmann LG (1940). Use of quinine for relief of 'night cramps' in the extremities. Preliminary report. JAMA, 115: 1358–1359.

Naide M (1950). Diphenhydramine (Benadryl) for nocturnal leg cramps. JAMA, 142: 1140.

Newlinds JS (1964). Nausea and vomiting in pregnancy. Med J Austral, 51: 234–236.

Oakley A (1979). Becoming a Mother. Oxford: Martin Robertson.

Odendaal HJ (1974). Evaluation of the aetiology and therapy of leg cramps during pregnancy. S Afr Med J, 48: 780–781.

Petitti DB (1986). Nausea and pregnancy outcome. Birth, 13: 223–226.

Porter JB, Hunter-Mitchell J, Jick H, Walker AM (1986). Drugs and stillbirth. Am J Public Health, 76: 1428–1431.

Robinson M (1947). Cramps in pregnancy. J Obstet Gynaecol Br Empire, 54: 826–829.

Rubin PC, Craig GF, Gavin K, Sumner D (1986). Prospective survey of use of therapeutic drugs, alcohol, and cigarettes during pregnancy. Br Med J, 292: 81–83.

Salvatore CA (1961). Leg cramp syndrome in pregnancy. Obstet Gynecol, 17: 634–639.

Sculati O, Fichera D, Setti M, (1980). High fibre diet in the prevention and treatment of constipation in pregnancy. Minerva Dietol Gastroenterol, 26: 27–33.

Semmens JP (1968). Hyperemesis gravidarum: Diagnosis and treatment. Obstet Gynecol, 32: 587.

Shapiro S, Heinonen OP, Siskind V, Kaufman OW, Monson RR, Slone D (1977). Antenatal exposure to doxylamine succinate and dicyclomine hydrochloride (Bendectin) in relation to congenital malformation, perinatal mortality rate, birthweight, and intelligence quotient score. Am J Obstet Gynecol, 128: 480–485.

Shaw RW (1978). Randomized controlled trial of Syn-Ergel and an active placebo in the treatment of heartburn of pregnancy. J Int Med Res, 6: 147–151.

Shervington PC (1974). Common pregnancy disorders and infections. In: Obstetric Therapeutics. Clinical Pharmacology and Therapeutics in Obstetric Practice. Hawkins DF (ed). London: Ballière Tindall, pp 231–273.

Shute E (1941). Hormone management of the nausea and vomiting of early pregnancy. Am J Obstet Gynecol, 42: 490–492.

Smellie W (1779). Treatise on the Theory and Practice of Midwifery, Book 2. London: Wilson.

Smith OW, Smith GV, Schiller S (1944). Cited in Fairweather DVI (1968). Nausea and vomiting in pregnancy. Am J Obstet Gynecol, 102: 135–175.

Soranus. Gynecology. Translated by Temkin O. Baltimore: Johns Hopkins University Press, 1956.

Speert H, Guttmacher AF (1954). Frequency and significance of bleeding in early pregnancy. JAMA, 155: 711–715.

Wheatley D (1977). Treatment of pregnancy sickness. Br J Obstet Gynaecol, 84: 444–447.

Winters HS (1961). Antiemetics in nausea and vomiting of pregnancy. Obstet Gynecol, 18: 753–756.

Zierler S, Rothman KJ (1985). Congenital heart disease in relation to maternal use of Bendectin and other drugs in early pregnancy. New Engl J Med, 313: 347–352.

33 Pharmacological prevention and treatment of hypertensive disorders in pregnancy

Rory Collins and Henk C. S. Wallenburg

1 Introduction

Two aetiologically distinct entities account for most hypertensive disorders in pregnancy: one is a pregnancy-induced disorder, and the other is associated with chronic hypertension.

The pregnancy-induced disorder that leads to elevated blood pressure and its sequelae, is believed to be due to inadequate adaptation of the maternal circulation to the presence of trophoblast. This clinical expression of 'circulatory maladaptation disease' occurs most commonly in nulliparae and generally resolves rapidly following delivery. Many hypotheses have been advanced to explain the aetiology of pregnancy-induced hypertensive disease (Gant and Worley 1980), yet its underlying cause (other than the presence of trophoblast) remains obscure (see Chapter 24). The only known aetiologically-based treatment of pregnancy-induced hypertension is removal of the trophoblast by terminating the pregnancy. All other treatment (with the possible exception of antithrombotic treatment; see later) is primarily symptomatic, aimed at prolonging pregnancy, in the hope that this will result in improvements in maternal and perinatal morbidity and mortality.

The second pathologic entity that accounts for most of the remaining hypertensive disease in pregnancy arises from chronic hypertension, most commonly in multiparae. In addition, since chronic hypertension is an important predisposing factor to pregnancy-induced hypertensive disease, a combination of the two fundamental pathological conditions may occur, and this is referred to as 'superimposed pre-eclampsia'.

In this review of the results of randomized controlled trials of pharmacological approaches to the prevention and treatment of pregnancy-induced hypertension and pre-eclampsia, the definitions reported by the study investigators have been used in the overviews. In discussing the results, however, the term 'pre-eclampsia' has generally been reserved for the combination of pregnancy-induced hypertension *and* proteinuria.

There are surprisingly few population-based studies of the frequency with which hypertensive disorders occur in pregnancy. There is also little information on the magnitude of the risk of pre-eclampsia developing in a woman with pregnancy-induced hypertension. The incidence of pre-eclampsia occurring prior to delivery in 339 consecutively diagnosed pregnant women with an initial diagnosis of pregnancy-induced hypertension is shown in Table 33.1. These data suggest that the risk of developing pre-eclampsia decreases after 33 weeks' gestation, both in nulliparae and in multiparae. Of

Table 33.1 Incidence of the development of proteinuric pre-eclampsia following an initial diagnosis of pregnancy-induced hypertension (PIH) in 339 untreated pregnant women at Dijkzigt Hospital, Erasmus University, Rotterdam

Duration of amenorrhea at diagnosis of PIH (weeks)	Nulliparae ($n=235$)			Multiparae ($n=104$)		
	No. of patients with diagnosis of PIH*	No. with eventual development of pre-eclampsia†		No. of patients with diagnosis of PIH*	No. with eventual development of pre-eclampsia†	
	n	*n*	%	*n*	*n*	%
<29	27	9	33.3	17	5	29.4
29–30	16	4	25.0	6	0	0
31–32	15	5	33.3	11	2	18.2
33–34	28	2	7.1	21	4	19.0
35–36	51	5	9.8	14	3	21.4
37–38	64	2	3.1	23	0	0
39–40	24	1	4.2	10	0	0
41–43	10	0	0	2	0	0

* Two consecutive measurements of diastolic blood pressure of 90 mm Hg or more, 4 hours or more apart.
† PIH and proteinuria of 500 mg per 24 hours or more.

women who became hypertensive *before* 33 weeks, 31 per cent of nulliparae and 21 per cent of multiparae eventually developed pre-eclampsia. In contrast, of those who became hypertensive *after* 33 weeks' gestation, only 6 per cent and 10 per cent of women, respectively, developed pre-eclampsia. In primigravidae pre-eclampsia appears to be commonly, although not invariably, preceded by pregnancy-induced hypertension (Chesley 1978). Of 134 initially normotensive, nulliparous pregnant women who eventually became eclamptic, proteinuria developed after the earlier appearance of hypertension in 58 per cent. In about a third, hypertension and proteinuria were observed simultaneously—which, of course, does not necessarily mean that their onset was really simultaneous—and in only 8 per cent was proteinuria detected prior to hypertension.

The reported incidences of maternal and fetal complications of hypertensive disorders in pregnancy vary widely. Nevertheless, it is clear that these conditions constitute a common complication of pregnancy that may have devastating consequences for the mother and the baby (Chesley 1978; MacGillivray 1983). A vast number of medical and surgical regimens have therefore been tried, not only for the treatment, but also for the prevention of hypertensive disorders in pregnancy. Many of the so-called preventive measures used have been mild and probably harmless, but some have not been. As Zuspan and Ward (1964) put it, women with eclampsia have been 'blistered, bled, purged, packed, lavaged, irrigated, punctured, starved, sedated, anaesthetized, paralyzed, tranquillized, rendered hypotensive, drowned, been given diuretics, had mastectomies, been dehydrated, forcibly delivered, and neglected'.

Comparisons of the various strategies used in different countries reveal striking differences, in particular with regard to the use of hospital admission and the choice of drugs (Chamberlain *et al.* 1978; Lewis *et al.* 1980; Lindberg and Sandström 1981; Trudinger and Parik 1982). The role of diet and hospitalization for bed rest have already been considered in Chapters 18 and 39. In this chapter we have assessed the available evidence from randomized controlled trials of pharmacological approaches used either to prevent or to treat pregnancy-induced hypertension, pre-eclampsia, and eclampsia.

2 Prevention and treatment of pregnancy-induced hypertension and pre-eclampsia

Certain women appear to be at higher-than-average risk of developing pregnancy-induced hypertension. For example, women who are nulliparous are at twice the risk of parous women. Other factors that appear to be associated with increased risk include a family history of the condition, obesity (although this association may be due to the presence of chronically hypertensive multiparae among the obese women studied), excessive weight-gain in pregnancy, or specific deficiencies or excesses in nutrition. In principle, therefore, there may be a role for primary prevention, particularly in women at increased risk.

Moderate pregnancy-induced hypertension carries little risk to the mother or the fetus, other than the risks associated with development of severe hypertension, pre-eclampsia, and eclampsia. For this reason, the aim of pharmacologic treatment of moderate hypertensive disease in pregnancy has been to defer or prevent the development of severe hypertensive disease. Surveys in the United States, the United Kingdom, and Australia suggest that methyldopa is the most widely used drug in women with mild to moderate pregnancy-induced hypertension (Lewis *et al.* 1980; Trudinger and Parik 1982; Chamberlain *et al.* 1978), but beta-blockers, labetalol, and perhaps calcium channel blockers are rapidly being introduced into clinical practice. The modes of action of these drugs are summarized in Table 33.6. Although there are anecdotal reports in the literature on their use in women with mild to moderate hypertensive disease in pregnancy, there are few randomized controlled trials of sufficient size to allow reliable assessment of their effects on serious outcome measures (such as deterioration of the disease). Unfortunately, as will be seen, this is still the case even when overviews of all related randomized trials of a particular intervention are considered.

2.1 Diuretics

The rate of weight-gain in pregnancy reflects not only increase in tissue mass but also water retention. For this reason, excessive weight-gain has been used both to predict and to define pre-eclampsia (see Chapter 24). There is, however, no good evidence that excessive weight-gain due to water retention, or even frank oedema, defines a group of women at particular risk of developing pre-eclampsia (Robertson 1971; Friedman and Neff 1976). Nevertheless, many attempts have been made—and, indeed, are still being made by some obstetricians and midwives—to prevent retention of salt and water in pregnancy by prescribing diuretics or a rigidly sodium-free diet in the belief that this will prevent pre-eclampsia (Chesley 1978; MacGillivray 1983).

The effects of the prophylactic use of diuretics in normotensive pregnant women (with or without oedema or excessive weight-gain), and of their therapeutic use in moderate disease have been studied in 12 randomized trials (Collins *et al.* 1985a). Reliable data were available from 10 of these trials, involving nearly 7000 women and their babies, while in 2 other trials no reliable data were available (Finnerty and Bepko 1956; Zuspan *et al.* 1960). Significant evidence of prevention of 'pre-eclampsia' (defined wholly or partly by hypertension) was overwhelming (Table 33.2), even when oedema was not included as a diagnostic criterion. But, as the definitions of pre-eclampsia used depended heavily on increases in blood pressure, this evidence may simply reflect the well-known ability of diuretics to reduce blood pressure, rather than any improvement in outcome. When the data on proteinuric pre-eclampsia (Table 33.3), or on perinatal death (Table 33.2) are considered, there is no clear evidence of benefit, either because the numbers studied were too small, or because treatment was ineffective. Serious side-effects that had been attributed, in case reports, to diuretic treatment in pregnancy were not confirmed by these trials, which included nearly 7000 women and their babies. This

Table 33.2 Effect of diuretics in pregnancy for prevention/treatment of pre-eclampsia on any form of pre-eclampsia

Study	EXPT		CTRL		Odds ratio	Graph of odds ratios and confidence intervals
	n	(%)	*n*	(%)	(95% CI)	0.01 0.1 0.5 1 2 10 100
Weseley and Douglas (1962)	14/131	(10.69)	14/136	(10.29)	1.04 (0.48–2.28)	
Cuadros and Tatum (1964)	12/1011	(1.19)	35/760	(4.61)	0.27 (0.15–0.48)	
Menzies (1964)	14/57	(24.56)	24/48	(50.00)	0.34 (0.15–0.74)	
Campbell and MacGillivray (1975)	65/153	(42.48)	40/102	(39.22)	1.14 (0.69–1.90)	
Sibai *et al.* (1984)	1/10	(10.00)	2/10	(20.00)	0.47 (0.04–5.19)	
Flowers *et al.* (1962)	21/385	(5.45)	17/134	(12.69)	0.35 (0.16–0.73)	
Fallis *et al.* (1964)	6/38	(15.79)	18/40	(45.00)	0.26 (0.10–0.67)	
Landesman *et al.* (1965)	138/1370	(10.07)	175/1336	(13.10)	0.74 (0.59–0.94)	
Kraus *et al.* (1966)	15/506	(2.96)	20/524	(3.82)	0.77 (0.39–1.51)	
Tervila and Vartiainen (1971)	6/108	(5.56)	2/103	(1.94)	2.68 (0.65–10.98)	
Typical odds ratio (95% confidence interval)					0.66 (0.56–0.79)	

Table 33.2—*continued* Effect of diuretics in pregnancy for prevention/treatment of pre-eclampsia on severe hypertension/proteinuric pre-eclampsia

Study	EXPT		CTRL		Odds ratio	Graph of odds ratios and confidence intervals
	n	(%)	*n*	(%)	(95% CI)	0.01 0.1 0.5 1 2 10 100
Weseley and Douglas (1962)	3/131	(2.29)	2/136	(1.47)	1.56 (0.27–9.12)	
Cuadros and Tatum (1964)	1/1011	(0.10)	4/760	(0.53)	0.22 (0.04–1.29)	
Menzies (1964)	3/57	(5.26)	5/48	(10.42)	0.48 (0.11–2.04)	
Campbell and MacGillivray (1975)	19/153	(12.42)	15/102	(14.71)	0.82 (0.39–1.71)	
Sibai *et al.* (1984)	1/10	(10.00)	1/10	(10.00)	1.00 (0.06–17.25)	
Landesman *et al.* (1965)	20/1370	(1.46)	23/1336	(1.72)	0.85 (0.46–1.55)	
Tervila and Vartiainen (1971)	6/108	(5.56)	2/103	(1.94)	2.68 (0.65–10.98)	
Typical odds ratio (95% confidence interval)					0.85 (0.57–1.27)	

Effect of diuretics in pregnancy for prevention/treatment of pre-eclampsia on perinatal deaths

Study	EXPT *n*	(%)	CTRL *n*	(%)	Odds ratio (95% CI)	Graph
Weseley and Douglas (1962)	1/131	(0.76)	4/136	(2.94)	0.31 (0.05–1.80)	
Cuadros and Tatum (1964)	14/1011	(1.38)	13/760	(1.71)	0.81 (0.37–1.73)	
Menzies (1964)	3/57	(5.26)	2/48	(4.17)	1.27 (0.21–7.64)	
Campbell and MacGillivray (1975)	0/153	(0.00)	0/102	(0.00)	1.00 (1.00–1.00)	
Sibai *et al.* (1984)	0/10	(0.00)	0/10	(0.00)	1.00 (1.00–1.00)	
Flowers *et al.* (1962)	6/335	(1.79)	3/110	(2.73)	0.62 (0.14–2.88)	
Fallis *et al.* (1964)	1/34	(2.94)	3/40	(7.50)	0.41 (0.06–3.09)	
Landesman *et al.* (1965)	24/1370	(1.75)	19/1336	(1.42)	1.23 (0.68–2.26)	
Kraus *et al.* (1966)	14/506	(2.77)	16/524	(3.05)	0.90 (0.44–1.87)	
Tervila and Vartiainen (1971)	0/108	(0.00)	0/103	(0.00)	1.00 (1.00–1.00)	
Typical odds ratio (95% confidence interval)					0.91 (0.64–1.31)	

Table 33.2 —*continued* Effect of diuretics in pregnancy for prevention/treatment of pre-eclampsia on stillbirths

Study	EXPT		CTRL		Odds ratio	Graph of odds ratios and confidence intervals
	n	(%)	*n*	(%)	(95% CI)	0.01 0.1 0.5 1 2 10 100
Weseley and Douglas (1962)	1/131	(0.76)	2/136	(1.47)	0.53 (0.05–5.14)	
Cuadros and Tatum (1964)	6/1011	(0.59)	5/760	(0.66)	0.90 (0.27–2.98)	
Menzies (1964)	1/57	(1.75)	1/48	(2.08)	0.84 (0.05–13.75)	
Campbell and MacGillivray (1975)	0/153	(0.00)	0/102	(0.00)	1.00 (1.00–1.00)	
Sibai *et al.* (1984)	0/10	(0.00)	0/10	(0.00)	1.00 (1.00–1.00)	
Flowers *et al.* (1962)	3/335	(0.90)	2/110	(1.82)	0.44 (0.06–3.36)	
Fallis *et al.* (1964)	0/34	(0.00)	1/40	(2.50)	0.16 (0.00–8.03)	
Kraus *et al.* (1966)	6/506	(1.19)	9/524	(1.72)	0.69 (0.25–1.91)	
Tervila and Vartiainen (1971)	0/108	(0.00)	0/103	(0.00)	1.00 (1.00–1.00)	
Typical odds ratio (95% confidence interval)					0.68 (0.35–1.31)	

Effect of diuretics in pregnancy for prevention/treatment of pre-eclampsia on neonatal deaths

Study	EXPT *n*	(%)	CTRL *n*	(%)	Odds ratio (95% CI)	Graph
Weseley and Douglas (1962)	0/131	(0.00)	2/136	(1.47)	0.14 (0.01–2.24)	
Cuadros and Tatum (1964)	8/1011	(0.79)	8/760	(1.05)	0.75 (0.28–2.02)	
Menzies (1964)	2/57	(3.51)	1/48	(2.08)	1.66 (0.17–16.48)	
Campbell and MacGillivray (1975)	0/153	(0.00)	0/102	(0.00)	1.00 (1.00–1.00)	
Sibai *et al.* (1984)	0/10	(0.00)	0/10	(0.00)	1.00 (1.00–1.00)	
Flowers *et al.* (1962)	3/335	(0.90)	1/110	(0.91)	0.98 (0.10–9.62)	
Fallis *et al.* (1964)	1/34	(2.94)	2/40	(5.00)	0.59 (0.06–5.93)	
Kraus *et al.* (1966)	8/506	(1.58)	7/524	(1.34)	1.19 (0.43–3.29)	
Tervila and Vartiainen (1971)	0/108	(0.00)	0/103	(0.00)	1.00 (1.00–1.00)	
Typical odds ratio (95% confidence interval)					0.86 (0.47–1.59)	

suggests that the putative maternal and fetal risks of diuretic administration may have been overstated, perhaps due to selective case reporting.

Even collectively, these trials have been too small to provide reliable evidence of either the presence or the absence of any worthwhile effects of diuretic use on serious outcome measures, such as proteinuric pre-eclampsia or perinatal mortality. Reliable identification of subgroups of women among whom diuretics are effective (or among whom they are ineffective) is therefore not possible. So although separate overviews of trials in which diuretics were tested prophylactically (Table 33.3), and those in which diuretics were tested therapeutically (Table 33.4) are presented, these do not provide a reliable source of inference about any differences in the effects of diuretics in these different situations.

Table 33.3 Effect of diuretics in pregnancy for prevention of pre-eclampsia on any form of pre-eclampsia

Study	EXPT		CTRL		Odds ratio	Graph of odds ratios and confidence intervals
	n	(%)	*n*	(%)	(95% CI)	0.01 0.1 0.5 1 2 10 100
Cuadros and Tatum (1964)	12/1011	(1.19)	35/760	(4.61)	0.27 (0.15–0.48)	
Flowers *et al.* (1962)	21/385	(5.45)	17/134	(12.69)	0.35 (0.16–0.73)	
Fallis *et al.* (1964)	6/38	(15.79)	18/40	(45.00)	0.26 (0.10–0.67)	
Landesman *et al.* (1965)	138/1370	(10.07)	175/1336	(13.10)	0.74 (0.59–0.94)	
Kraus *et al.* (1966)	15/506	(2.96)	20/524	(3.82)	0.77 (0.39–1.51)	
Tervila and Vartiainen (1971)	6/108	(5.56)	2/103	(1.94)	2.68 (0.65–10.98)	
Typical odds ratio (95% confidence interval)					0.62 (0.51–0.75)	

Effect of diuretics in pregnancy for prevention of pre-eclampsia on severe hypertension/proteinuric pre-eclampsia

Study	EXPT *n*	(%)	CTRL *n*	(%)	Odds ratio (95% CI)	Graph
Cuadros and Tatum (1964)	1/1011	(0.10)	4/760	(0.53)	0.22 (0.04–1.29)	
Landesman *et al.* (1965)	20/1370	(1.46)	23/1336	(1.72)	0.85 (0.46–1.55)	
Tervila and Vartiainen (1971)	6/108	(5.56)	2/103	(1.94)	2.68 (0.65–10.98)	
Typical odds ratio (95% confidence interval)					0.88 (0.52–1.50)	

Effect of diuretics in pregnancy for prevention of pre-eclampsia on perinatal deaths

Study	EXPT *n*	(%)	CTRL *n*	(%)	Odds ratio (95% CI)	Graph
Cuadros and Tatum (1964)	14/1011	(1.38)	13/760	(1.71)	0.81 (0.37–1.73)	
Flowers *et al.* (1962)	6/335	(1.79)	3/110	(2.73)	0.62 (0.14–2.88)	
Fallis *et al.* (1964)	1/34	(2.94)	3/40	(7.50)	0.41 (0.06–3.09)	
Landesman *et al.* (1965)	24/1370	(1.75)	19/1336	(1.42)	1.23 (0.68–2.26)	
Kraus *et al.* (1966)	14/506	(2.77)	16/524	(3.05)	0.90 (0.44–1.87)	
Tervila and Vartiainen (1971)	0/108	(0.00)	0/103	(0.00)	1.00 (1.00–1.00)	
Typical odds ratio (95% confidence interval)					0.94 (0.65–1.38)	

2.2 Antithrombotic agents

Prostaglandins and thromboxane A_2 influence platelet–platelet and platelet–vessel wall interactions (Wallenburg 1987). Manipulation of prostaglandin and thromboxane synthesis has recently been pursued in attempts to prevent pregnancy-induced hypertensive disease in women thought to be at increased risk, either because of their past history or because of early signs or symptoms of pre-eclampsia in their current pregnancy. Changes in the coagulation system, with consumption of Factor VII (Redman *et al.* 1977), reduced circulating platelets (Redman *et al.* 1978), and increases in the levels of fibrin (or fibrinogen) degradation products, are well-documented in established pre-eclampsia (*Lancet* editorial 1986). The extent of the coagulopathy appears to be related to the severity of the pre-eclampsia, and although it has not yet been clearly established whether the associated intravascular coagulation is a primary or

Table 33.4 Effect of diuretics in pregnancy for treatment of pre-eclampsia on deterioration of pre-eclampsia

Study	EXPT		CTRL		Odds ratio	Graph of odds ratios and confidence intervals
	n	(%)	*n*	(%)	(95% CI)	0.01 0.1 0.5 1 2 10 100
Weseley and Douglas (1962)	14/131	(10.69)	14/136	(10.29)	1.04 (0.48–2.28)	
Menzies (1964)	14/57	(24.56)	24/48	(50.00)	0.34 (0.15–0.74)	
Campbell *et al.* (1975)	65/153	(42.48)	40/102	(39.22)	1.14 (0.69–1.90)	
Sibai *et al.* (1984)	1/10	(10.00)	2/10	(20.00)	0.47 (0.04–5.19)	
Typical odds ratio (95% confidence interval)					0.84 (0.58–1.22)	

Effect of diuretics in pregnancy for treatment of pre-eclampsia on severe hypertension/proteinuric pre-eclampsia

Study	EXPT *n*	(%)	CTRL *n*	(%)	Odds ratio (95% CI)	Graph
Weseley and Douglas (1962)	3/131	(2.3)	2/136	(1.5)	1.56 (027–9.12)	
Menzies (1964)	3/57	(5.26)	5/48	(10.42)	0.48 (0.11–2.04)	
Campbell *et al.* (1975)	19/153	(12.42)	15/102	(14.71)	0.82 (0.39–1.71)	
Sibai *et al.* (1984)	1/10	(10.00)	1/10	(10.00)	1.00 (0.06–17.25)	
Typical odds ratio (95% confidence interval)					0.81 (0.45–1.48)	

Effect of diuretics in pregnancy for treatment of pre-eclampsia on perinatal deaths

Study	EXPT *n*	(%)	CTRL *n*	(%)	Odds ratio (95% CI)	Graph
Weseley and Douglas (1962)	1/131	(0.76)	4/136	(2.94)	0.31 (0.05–1.80)	
Menzies (1964)	3/57	(5.26)	2/48	(4.17)	1.27 (0.21–7.64)	
Campbell and MacGillivray (1975)	0/153	(0.00)	0/102	(0.00)	1.00 (1.00–1.00)	
Sibai *et al.* (1984)	0/10	(0.00)	0/10	(0.00)	1.00 (1.00–1.00)	
Typical odds ratio (95% confidence interval)					0.62 (0.18–2.18)	

a secondary event, it may be an early feature of the disorder. Early activation of the clotting system may contribute directly to the later pathology of pre-eclampsia, by starting, or aggravating, the occlusive changes seen in the spiral arterioles ('acute atherosis'). The maternal syndrome of pre-eclampsia probably results from placental ischaemia, although definitive proof is still needed. The same spiral artery lesions are found in intrauterine growth retardation without pre-eclampsia (Sheppard and Bonnar 1976), suggesting that the two conditions may differ only with respect to the extent of the maternal response to the placental problem.

As a result, the use of anticoagulant (Howie *et al.* 1975) or antiplatelet (Beaufils *et al.* 1985; Wallenburg *et al.* 1986; Trudinger *et al.* 1988) agents has been considered for the prevention of pre-eclampsia and intrauterine growth retardation.

2.2.1 Anticoagulants

Because excessive thrombin action is thought to cause abnormalities in the maternal coagulation and fibrinolytic systems, women with pregnancy-induced hypertensive disorders have been treated with anticoagulants in an attempt to improve the clinical course of the disorder (Wallenburg 1987). Heparin, with or without dipyridamole, has been used in uncontrolled studies involving single cases or small series of patients (Page 1948; Maeck and Zilliacus 1948; Brain *et al.* 1967; Howie *et al.* 1975; Bonnar *et al.* 1975; Fairley *et al.* 1976). Heparin requires subcutaneous (or intravenous) administration, and its use in severe cases may be associated with dangerous side-effects (Howie *et al.* 1975). Warfarin has also been used prophylactically in an attempt to prevent recurrent pre-eclampsia in multiparae (Valentine and Baker 1977; Schramm 1979). But, as for heparin, these anecdotal reports did not provide any evidence of maternal or fetal benefit, while there was some suggestion of serious side-effects.

2.2.2 Antiplatelet agents

With the development of the pathophysiologic concept of selective, non-thrombin-mediated platelet activation in women with pregnancy-induced hypertensive disease, antiplatelet drugs have been considered for both prevention and treatment. Aspirin is a widely practicable antiplatelet agent which is thought to act by inhibiting the enzyme cyclo-oxygenase in the platelets, blocking the synthesis of the platelet-aggregating agent thromboxane A_2. It has been shown to prevent thrombotic occlusion of arteriovenous shunts (Lorenz *et al.* 1984) and coronary artery bypass grafts (Chesebro *et al.* 1982), and to reduce death and reinfarction in unstable angina and following myocardial infarction and cerebral ischaemic attacks (Antiplatelet Trialists' Collaboration 1988).

The first reports of aspirin use in pregnancy relate to relatively high doses (1.5–1.8 g per day) used to treat pre-eclampsia in two women (Goodlin *et al.* 1978; Jespersen 1980). Although platelet counts showed improvement, one of the two fetuses died after one week. In a later study, 5 thrombocytopenic women received 85 mg of aspirin per day in divided doses; platelet counts improved in every case, although no improvement of fetal condition was noted and there were 2 perinatal deaths (Goodlin 1983).

Recently, Beaufils and his colleagues (1985) reported an open randomized trial of antiplatelet prophylaxis in women at high risk of pre-eclampsia. In this study, marginally significant reductions in proteinuric pre-eclampsia, perinatal death, and severe intrauterine growth retardation were observed in the group allocated antiplatelet prophylaxis from 3 months' gestation until delivery. However, probably because of small numbers, the treatment groups were somewhat unbalanced with respect to certain entry prognostic variables, and allowance for this imbalance would further reduce the marginal statistical significance of the findings. The trial tested two drugs—150 mg aspirin and 300 mg dipyridamole daily—used in combination, despite the side-effects of dipyridamole (Persantine–Aspirin Reinfarction Study Research Group 1980), and the lack of evidence that dipyridamole enhances the clinical effect of aspirin (Antiplatelet Trialists' Collaboration 1988). Moreover, the dose of aspirin was more than that needed to inhibit platelet cyclo-oxygenase, so a smaller dose of aspirin might well have been as effective.

Even if it is not possible to reverse established pre-eclampsia, it may be that its progression (which is a consistent feature of the untreated disease) can be delayed. Since perinatal survival at the beginning of the 3rd trimester is known to improve rapidly with increasing maturity, a moderate delay in the onset of severe disease (for example, by one or two weeks) might be extremely important. Recently, Wallenburg and his colleagues (Wallenburg 1987; Wallenburg and Rotmans 1987) have reported the use of low-dose (60 mg/day) aspirin in women judged at 28 weeks' gestation to be at increased risk of pregnancy-induced hypertension or pre-eclampsia because of an increased pressor response to intravenous angiotensin II. This trial was placebo-controlled and tested the effects of aspirin alone. As with the trial by Beaufils and his colleagues (1985), the numbers were small and so, although promising (Table 33.5), the results must be regarded as far from conclusive. Several trials are now in progress, or are being planned, to determine more reliably any beneficial (or adverse) effects of low-dose aspirin in the prevention and treatment of pre-eclampsia. Until these studies have been completed it will remain unclear whether or not anti-platelet therapy should be adopted into routine clinical practice.

2.3 Antihypertensive agents

2.3.1 Methyldopa and clonidine

The most widely used antihypertensive agent in pregnancy is still methyldopa, although other agents, such as beta-blockers, are starting to be used more. The effect of methyldopa in pregnant women with hypertension has been studied in 4 randomized trials. In the largest of these (Redman *et al.* 1976; Mutch *et al.* 1977; Moar *et al.* 1978; Ounsted *et al.* 1980; Cockburn *et al.* 1982), 242 women with moderate hypertension developing in pregnancy (systolic blood pressure >140 mm Hg or diastolic blood pressure >90 mm Hg on two occasions before 28 weeks' gestation, or >150 mm Hg or >95 mm Hg, respectively, after 28 weeks and before 36 weeks) were randomly allocated to receive either methyldopa or routine care. Development of severe hypertension was significantly less common among women allocated methyldopa, but there was no evidence that the risk of proteinuric pre-eclampsia was reduced. A non-significant trend towards fewer stillbirths and neonatal deaths with methyldopa (1+0) compared with controls (3+2) was reinforced by the observation of fewer mid-pregnancy abortions in the methyldopa group (0 vs. 4), so that overall there was a statistically significant improvement in fetal outcome. Similar patterns were seen in the other, smaller trials (Leather *et al.* 1968; Arias and Zamora 1979; Welt *et al.* 1981), so that the overview of the trials provides clear evidence that methyldopa substantially reduces the risk of the development of severe hypertension (Table 37.7). However, as for diuretics, there is no significant

Table 33.5 Effect of antiplatelet therapy in pre-eclampsia/PIH on severe hypertension

Study	EXPT		CTRL		Odds ratio	Graph of odds ratios and confidence intervals
	n	(%)	*n*	(%)	(95% CI)	0.01 0.1 0.5 1 2 10 100
Wallenburg *et al.* (1986)	1/23	(4.35)	11/23	(47.83)	0.11 (0.03–0.40)	
Beaufils *et al.* (1985)	19/48	(39.58)	22/45	(48.89)	0.69 (0.30–1.55)	
Typical odds ratio (95% confidence interval)					0.41 (0.21–0.82)	

Effect of antiplatelet therapy in pre-eclampsia/PIH on proteinuria

Study	EXPT *n*	(%)	CTRL *n*	(%)	Odds ratio (95% CI)	Graph
Wallenburg *et al.* (1986)	0/23	(0.00)	8/23	(34.78)	0.09 (0.02–0.42)	
Beaufils *et al.* (1985)	0/48	(0.00)	6/45	(13.33)	0.11 (0.02–0.58)	
Typical odds ratio (95% confidence interval)					0.10 (0.03–0.31)	

Effect of antiplatelet therapy in pre-eclampsia/PIH on perinatal death

Study	EXPT *n*	(%)	CTRL *n*	(%)	Odds ratio (95% CI)	Graph
Wallenburg *et al.* (1986)	1/23	(4.35)	1/23	(4.35)	1.00 (0.06–16.50)	
Beaufils *et al.* (1985)	0/48	(0.00)	5/45	(11.11)	0.12 (0.02–0.69)	
Typical odds ratio (95% confidence interval)					0.22 (0.05–0.98)	

Table 33.6 Mode of action of various antihypertensive agents used in the treatment of hypertensive disorders in pregnancy*

Mode of action	Type of drug	Representative drugs
Central inhibition of sympathetic outflow; decrease in PVR.	α_2-adrenoceptor antagonists	Methyldopa, Clonidine
Depletion of norepinephrine stores in adrenergic neurons (brain and periphery); decrease in PVR	Adrenergic inhibitors	Reserpine, Guanethidine
Competitive inhibition of β-adrenergic activity; decrease in CO and various other hemodynamic effects, depending among others on presence or absence of Intrinsic Sympathomimetic Activity (ISA)	β-adrenoceptor antagonists β_1-selective	 Atenolol, Metroprolol Acebutolol,† Practolol
	$\beta_1 + \beta_2$	Propranolol, Pindolol,† Oxprenolo,† Timolol, Sotalol, Nadolol
Competitive inhibition of α-adrenergic activity; decrease in PVR	α_1-adrenoceptor antagonists	Prazosin, Ketanserin
Competitive inhibition of α− and β−adrenergic activity; decrease in PVR	$\alpha_1 + \beta_1 + \beta_2$-adrenoceptor antagonist	Labetalol
Direct relaxation of vascular smooth muscle; decrease in PVR	Direct vasodilators	Hydralazine, Minoxidil, Nitroprusside Diazoxide, Prostacyclin
Inhibition of influx of calcium-ions in vascular smooth muscle; decrease in PVR	Calcium antagonists	Nifedipine, Verapamil, Diltiazem
Inhibition of angiotensin II formation; decrease in PVR	Angiotensin-II converting enzyme inhibitors	Captopril Enalapril

* Most of the data derived from Kaplan (1986)
† These agents have Intrinsic Sympathomimetic Activity (ISA)
PVR = peripheral vascular resistance; CO = cardiac output

Table 33.7 Effect of methyldopa in pre-eclampsia/PIH on severe hypertension

Study	EXPT		CTRL		Odds ratio	Graph of odds ratios and confidence intervals
	n	(%)	*n*	(%)	(95% CI)	0.01 0.1 0.5 1 2 10 100
Welt *et al.* (1981)	0/7	(0.00)	1/7	(14.29)	0.14 (0.00–6.82)	
Redman *et al.* (1976)	2/117	(1.71)	16/125	(12.80)	0.20 (0.08–0.52)	
Arias and Zamora (1979)	2/29	(6.90)	10/29	(34.48)	0.19 (0.05–0.68)	
Typical odds ratio (95% confidence interval)					0.19 (0.09–0.41)	

Effect of methyldopa in pre-eclampsia/PIH on proteinuria

Study	EXPT *n*	(%)	CTRL *n*	(%)	Odds ratio (95% CI)	Graph
Weitz *et al.* (1987)	5/13	(38.46)	4/12	(33.33)	1.24 (0.25–6.14)	
Redman *et al.* (1976)	6/117	(5.13)	5/125	(4.00)	1.30 (0.39–4.34)	
Leather *et al.* (1968)	15/52	(28.85)	17/48	(35.42)	0.74 (0.32–1.71)	
Arias and Zamora (1979)	1/29	(3.45)	3/29	(10.34)	0.35 (0.05–2.61)	
Typical odds ratio (95% confidence interval)					0.86 (0.47–1.57)	

Effect of methyldopa in pre-eclampsia/PIH on perinatal death

Study	EXPT *n*	(%)	CTRL *n*	(%)	Odds ratio (95% CI)	Graph
Weitz *et al.* (1987)	0/13	(0.00)	0/12	(0.00)	1.00 (1.00–1.00)	
Redman *et al.* (1976)	1/117	(0.85)	5/125	(4.00)	0.27 (0.05–1.38)	
Leather *et al.* (1968)	6/52	(11.54)	6/48	(12.50)	0.91 (0.27–3.04)	
Arias and Zamora (1979)	0/29	(0.00)	1/29	(3.45)	0.14 (0.00–6.82)	
Typical odds ratio (95% confidence interval)					0.55 (0.21–1.40)	

effect on the incidence of proteinuria or perinatal death (Table 33.7).

Clonidine is similar to methyldopa in most ways, but it has a more rapid onset of action (about 30 minutes) compared with 4 hours for methyldopa (Kaplan 1986). Following a few case reports on the use of clonidine to treat moderate pregnancy-induced hypertension (Johnston and Aickin 1971; Parker *et al.* 1973), Horvath *et al.* (1985) reported a randomized, double-blind trial comparing methyldopa with clonidine. Of the 76 women with blood pressures in excess of 130/85 mm Hg, or with a rise of 30/15 mm Hg or more from previous stable values, 42 were allocated to oral methyldopa and 34 to oral clonidine until delivery. No differences were observed between groups with regard to maternal blood pressure control, development of proteinuria, incidence of fetal growth retardation, or neonatal condition, including neonatal blood pressures (Henderson-Smart *et al.* 1984).

2.3.2 Beta-blockers

Beta-blockers are known to reduce cardiac output, both by reducing heart rate and stroke volume (Kaplan 1986). The combined alpha- and beta-blocker labetalol lowers blood pressure by means of an alpha-adrenoceptor-mediated reduction of peripheral vascular resistance, but its beta-adrenoceptor blocking component also suppresses cardiac output (Kaplan 1986). A reduction in cardiac output may be an unfavourable haemodynamic effect where adequate perfusion of the maternal and uteroplacental circulation depends on maintaining the physiologically elevated cardiac output that occurs in pregnancy, particularly when the stroke volume is already reduced (for example, in severe pre-eclampsia; Wallenburg 1988). Reduction in cardiac output is much less pronounced with the class of beta-blockers (for example, oxprenolol) showing intrinsic sympathomimetic activity (Kaplan 1986), which may make these beta-blockers a more logical choice for treatment of hypertension in pregnancy. Two beta-blockers (atenolol and metoprolol) and one combined alpha- and beta-blocker (labetalol)—all without intrinsic sympathomimetic activity—have been studied in randomized, double-blind, placebo-controlled trials.

The study by Rubin *et al.* (1983a,b) indicated some advantage for the group of 60 women treated with atenolol. In the atenolol group only 2 women had to be withdrawn because of the development of severe hypertension, compared with 7 in the placebo group (and in 3 of these placebo group cases the babies required ventilation because of severe respiratory distress). Proteinuria following randomization was observed in 4 women in the atenolol group and 14 in the placebo group, while the number of hospital admissions appeared to be reduced by atenolol. No clinically important adverse effects were observed in the fetus or the neonate. Follow-up to 1 year of 55 children from each group did not identify any developmental differences between the atenolol and placebo-allocated groups (Reynolds *et al.* 1984), although any difference would have to be gross to be detectable in such a small study (Collins *et al.* 1985b).

In the randomized, double-blind, trial reported by Wichman *et al.* (1984), in which metoprolol was compared with placebo, 16 of 26 women in the metoprolol group and 19 of 26 allocated placebo developed severe hypertension; but no differences in the occurrence of proteinuria or perinatal mortality were observed.

Table 33.8 Effect of beta-blockers in pre-eclampsia/PIH on severe hypertension

Study	EXPT		CTRL		Odds ratio
	n	(%)	*n*	(%)	(95% CI)
Rubin *et al.* (1983)	2/60	(3.33)	7/60	(11.67)	0.30 (0.08–1.18)
Wichman *et al.* (1985)	16/26	(61.54)	19/26	(73.08)	0.60 (0.19–1.88)
Sibai *et al.* (1987)	5/92	(5.43)	14/94	(14.89)	0.36 (0.14–0.92)
Typical odds ratio (95% confidence interval)					0.41 (0.21–0.77)

Graph of odds ratios and confidence intervals: 0.01 0.1 0.5 1 2 10 100

Effect of beta-blockers in pre-eclampsia/PIH on proteinuria

Study	EXPT *n*	(%)	CTRL *n*	(%)	Odds ratio (95% CI)
Rubin *et al.* (1983)	4/60	(6.67)	14/60	(23.33)	0.27 (0.10–0.74)
Wichman *et al.* (1985)	11/26	(42.31)	11/26	(42.31)	1.00 (0.34–2.97)
Pickles *et al.* (unpub)	17/70	(24.29)	24/74	(32.43)	0.67 (0.33–1.38)
Sibai *et al.* (1987)	10/92	(10.87)	6/94	(6.38)	1.76 (0.63–4.90)
Typical odds ratio (95% confidence interval)					0.72 (0.46–1.15)

Effect of beta-blockers in pre-eclampsia/PIH on perinatal death

Study	EXPT *n*	(%)	CTRL *n*	(%)	Odds ratio (95% CI)
Rubin *et al.* (1983)	1/60	(1.67)	2/60	(3.33)	0.51 (0.05–4.97)
Wichman *et al.* (1984)	0/26	(0.00)	1/26	(3.85)	0.14 (0.00–6.82)
Pickles *et al.* (unpub)	0/70	(0.00)	0/74	(0.00)	1.00 (1.00–1.00)
Sibai *et al.* (1987)	1/100	(1.00)	0/100	(0.00)	7.39 (0.15–99.99)
Typical odds ratio (95% confidence interval)					0.67 (0.11–3.89)

Preliminary data have suggested that oral labetalol is effective in preventing a further increase in blood pressure in women with mild to moderate pregnancy-induced hypertension (Walker *et al.* 1982). In a trial conducted by Pickles and colleagues (1989), proteinuric pre-eclampsia was observed in 17 of 70 women allocated labetalol compared with 24 of 74 allocated placebo. No perinatal deaths were reported in either group.

In a further randomized trial of antihypertensive treatment in 161 women with mild to moderate hypertension in pregnancy, the combination of oral metoprolol and hydralazine was compared to routine care (Hogstedt *et al.* 1985). Hypertensive crises occurred significantly less frequently in the treated than in the control group, but this study did not provide any evidence that pre-eclampsia was prevented; and three of 82 treated women had a stillbirth compared with only 1 of 79 control patients.

Overviews of all available data from randomized trials of beta-blockers in women with early signs or symptoms of pre-eclampsia indicate that beta-blockers reduce the risk of severe hypertension developing (Table 33.8). Despite this, apart from the particularly promising results in one study (Rubin *et al.* 1983a) which are not supported by the available data from the other studies of beta-blockers, there is no evidence of any effect on the development of proteinuria (Table 33.8). Too few women have been studied overall for any reliable conclusions about the effects of beta-blockers on perinatal deaths, nor is there sufficient information to assess any serious adverse effects of these treatments on pregnancy outcome or infant development.

2.3.3 *Beta-blockers vs. methyldopa*

Five randomized trials provide data comparing the effects of beta-blockers (oxprenolol, atenolol, and labetalol) with methyldopa. Both beta-blockers and methyldopa have been shown to prevent the development of severe hypertension when compared with untreated controls. Direct randomized comparisons of these agents do not indicate any significantly greater effect on blood pressure control with beta-blockers than with methyldopa (Table 33.9). Similarly, the incidence of proteinuric pre-eclampsia appears to be similar in women allocated to beta-blockers and those allocated to

Table 33.9 Effect of beta-blockers vs. methyldopa in pre-eclampsia/PIH on severe hypertension

Study	EXPT		CTRL		Odds ratio	Graph of odds ratios and confidence intervals
	n	(%)	*n*	(%)	(95% CI)	0.01 0.1 0.5 1 2 10 100
Gallery *et al.* (1985)	46/97	(47.42)	30/89	(33.71)	1.76 (0.98–3.15)	
Fidler *et al.* (1983)	6/50	(12.00)	2/50	(4.00)	2.93 (0.70–12.35)	
Thorley (1984)	1/30	(3.33)	2/30	(6.67)	0.50 (0.05–5.02)	
Plouin *et al.* (1987)	12/91	(13.19)	22/85	(25.88)	0.44 (0.21–0.94)	
Redman *et al.* (1978)	20/39	(51.28)	15/35	(42.86)	1.40 (0.56–3.46)	
Typical odds ratio (95% confidence interval)					1.16 (0.79–1.72)	

Effect of beta-blockers vs methyldopa in pre-eclampsia/PIH on proteinuria

Study	EXPT *n*	(%)	CTRL *n*	(%)	Odds ratio (95% CI)	Graph
Gallery *et al.* (1985)	4/97	(4.12)	5/89	(5.62)	0.72 (0.19–2.76)	
Fidler *et al.* (1983)	5/50	(10.00)	5/50	(10.00)	1.00 (0.27–3.67)	
Thorley (1984)	5/30	(16.67)	3/30	(10.00)	1.76 (0.40–7.72)	
Plouin *et al.* (1987)	8/91	(8.79)	8/85	(9.41)	0.93 (0.33–2.59)	
Redman *et al.* (1978)	19/39	(48.72)	11/35	(31.43)	2.03 (0.81–5.11)	
Typical odds ratio (95% confidence interval)					1.25 (0.75–2.10)	

Table 33.9—*continued* Effect of beta-blockers vs. methyldopa in pre-eclampsia/PIH on perinatal death

Study	EXPT		CTRL		Odds ratio	Graph of odds ratios and confidence intervals
	n	(%)	*n*	(%)	(95% CI)	0.01 0.1 0.5 1 2 10 100
Gallery *et al.* (1985)	1/97	(1.03)	4/89	(4.49)	0.27 (0.05–1.58)	
Fidler *et al.* (1983)	0/50	(0.00)	0/50	(0.00)	1.00 (1.00–1.00)	
Thorley (1984)	0/30	(0.00)	0/30	(0.00)	1.00 (1.00–1.00)	
Plouin *et al.* (1987)	1/91	(1.10)	4/85	(4.71)	0.27 (0.05–1.61)	
Redman *et al.* (1978)	2/38	(5.26)	0/34	(0.00)	6.83 (0.42–99.99)	
Typical odds ratio (95% confidence interval)					0.46 (0.15–1.46)	

methyldopa. In only two of the trials were any perinatal deaths observed, and although there were slightly fewer in the beta-blocker groups of both trials, this difference is quite consistent with chance.

2.4 Summary

The small numbers of women studied in adequately controlled trials of antihypertensive medication for both the prevention and treatment of moderate hypertensive disease preclude definitive conclusions about their effects, even in overviews of all related trials. It seems likely that antihypertensive treatment prevents increases in blood pressure (Table 33.10), and for that reason *may* reduce the number of hospital admissions and emergency deliveries, but there is no clear evidence that antihypertensive treatment with any of the drugs available may defer or prevent the occurrence of proteinuric pre-eclampsia or associated problems such as fetal growth retardation and perinatal death (Table 33.10). Nor is there good evidence about the safety of such treatments, in particular, with respect to any developmental problems. At present there seems to be no reason to prefer any one of the tested beta-blockers, or to prefer labetalol to a pure beta-blocker, or indeed, to prefer beta-blockers to methyldopa.

3 Treatment of severe pre-eclampsia and eclampsia

Although treatment of hypertension does not strike at the basic disorder, it may still benefit the mother and fetus. One important objective in cases of severe hypertension in pregnancy is to reduce blood pressure in order to avoid hypertensive encephalopathy and cerebral haemorrhage. In severe hypertension, 'breakthrough' hyperperfusion and leakage of fluid through the blood–brain barrier may occur (Strandgaard *et al.* 1976). This occurs at mean arterial pressures of about 150 mm Hg or more in experimental animals (Goldby and Beilin 1972), but may be reached at lower blood pressure levels in previously normotensive individuals who suddenly become hypertensive (Kaplan 1986). For this reason, the aim in treating severely hypertensive pregnant women has been to keep the mean arterial blood pressure below 130–140 mm Hg (e.g. 170/110 mm Hg).

Severe disease in pregnancy-induced hypertension and pre-eclampsia are associated with a contracted circulating volume (Wallenburg 1988). Plasma volume expansion has, therefore, also been used for the treatment of patients with these conditions.

3.1 Antihypertensive agents

Surveys during the past decade indicate that hydralazine was the antihypertensive drug used most commonly in patients with severe pregnancy-induced hypertension and pre-eclampsia in the United States (Lewis *et al.* 1980), the United Kingdom (Chamberlain *et al.* 1978), Australia (Trudinger and Parik 1982), and Sweden (Lindberg and Sandström 1981), followed closely by diazoxide and, in the United Kingdom, by veratrum alkaloids. Methyldopa is also used in the treatment of severe hypertensive disease in pregnancy (Redman 1982), although it has the disadvantage of a relatively slow onset of action (about 4 hours), even when given intravenously (Kaplan 1986).

The primacy of hydralazine in the treatment of severe hypertensive disorders in pregnancy may be threatened by potent vasodilators (such as labetalol) that have been introduced more recently.

3.1.1 Hydralazine, labetalol, diazoxide, and methyldopa

The effects of the various drugs that are available for treating severe hypertension in pregnancy have been assessed in few adequately controlled randomized trials, involving only very small numbers of pregnant women. Three randomized studies have compared intravenous labetalol with intravenous hydralazine (Garden *et al.* 1982; Walker *et al.* 1983; Mabie *et al.* 1987). An overview of the results of these trials does not indicate any significant difference in the control of severe hypertension (Table 33.11), although it was suggested by one author that control was more simply and more consistently achieved with labetalol.

In another randomized trial, intravenous labetalol was compared with intravenous diazoxide (Michael 1986). Among 45 women treated with labetalol, 42 had a satisfactory and sustained reduction in blood pressure (diastolic blood pressure <85–90 mm Hg), none had a precipitous fall (<60/40) and 3 had no response, compared with 31, 8, and 6 women, respectively, among the 45 treated with diazoxide. In addition to the significantly better blood pressure control with labetalol, perinatal mortality was non-significantly better (0 vs. 3) (Table 33.12).

In another oral labetalol has been compared with oral methyldopa (Redman 1982) in 74 women with severe pregnancy-induced hypertension; in both groups delivery was delayed for an average of 5 weeks and there were no stillbirths in either group.

3.1.2 Other agents

There have been several recent reports of the treatment of moderate to severe pregnancy-induced hypertension with calcium channel blockers (Walters and Redman 1984; Allen *et al.* 1987; Constantine *et al.* 1987) and ketanserin, a specific serotonin receptor antagonist (Weiner *et al.* 1984; Hulme and Odendaal 1986; Voto *et al.* 1987). Intravenous infusions of prostacyclin have also been used to reduce blood pressure by producing vasodilatation (Goodlin 1980; Fidler *et al.* 1980; Belch *et al.* 1985; Jouppila *et al.* 1985). Prostacyclin infusions lower maternal blood pressure effectively, but can cause unpleasant side-effects (such as weakness, nausea, headaches, and bradycardia), and the blood pressure returns to its previously elevated levels as soon as the infusion is interrupted. In these few uncontrolled studies, no beneficial effects on fetal condition were apparent; moreover, prostacyclin infusion did not change placental or umbilical blood flow (Jouppila *et al.* 1985), and in two out of three patients reported by Fidler *et al.* (1980) fetal death occurred, perhaps as a result of a reduced placental perfusion.

3.1.3 Summary

The antihypertensive drugs discussed above all appear to be reasonably effective at reducing blood pressure and there is no good evidence that any one of them is better at doing so than any other. In clinical practice, therefore, the choice of drug should probably depend on the familiarity of an individual clinician with a particular drug, and on what is known about adverse maternal and fetal side-effects. In general, maternal side-effects are not different from those in the non-pregnant state, and are listed in pharmacology texts. All drugs used to treat hypertension in pregnancy cross the placenta (Broughton Pipkin 1986), and so may affect the fetus directly by means of their action within the fetal circulation, or indirectly, by their effect on utero-placental perfusion.

From what is known about direct and indirect adverse effects on fetus and neonate, hydralazine appears to be relatively safe. The use of labetalol in pregnancy has been found to be associated with marked fetal and neonatal alpha-adrenergic blockade, resulting in severe and long-lasting bradycardia, in particular after high doses (Garden *et al.* 1982; Woods and Malan 1983). The adverse effects of alpha-adrenergic blockade may, therefore, become clinically significant in the face of fetal and neonatal hypoxia (Woods and Malan 1983). Diazoxide may provoke a precipitous fall in maternal arterial pressure, leading to a reduction in uteroplacental perfusion, especially in severely pre-eclamptic women in whom placental blood flow is already compromised. In addition, hyperglycemia has been reported in the newborn after maternal treatment with diazoxide (Neuman *et al.* 1979).

There is as yet little clinical information on the fetal or neonatal effects of maternal use of calcium antagonists. Various problems have been observed in the neonatal period following their use in uncontrolled studies, but these effects could not be definitely attributed to maternal nifedipine ingestion (Allen *et al.* 1987; Constantine *et al.* 1987). As Broughton Pipkin (1986) points out, it should be borne in mind that both in chronically cannulated pregnant rhesus monkeys and in pregnant ewes the administration of nifedipine is associated with a degree of fetal hypoxemia and acidemia, and with a fall in arterial pressure. It is as yet unclear whether this must be considered a direct effect of the drug on fetal vasculature, or a consequence of its maternal haemodynamic effects.

Although nitroprusside has been used in these circumstances, it can lead to fetal cyanide toxicity (Naulty *et al.* 1981) and should therefore probably be avoided.

In summary, there are various drugs with different modes of action which, because they reduce maternal blood pressure effectively, may prevent the occurrence of acute hypertensive complications, such as encephalopathy or cerebral haemorrhage, in pregnant women with a severe hypertensive disorder. The few controlled trials available provide insufficient data with which to assess whether one drug is superior to another, either with regard to its antihypertensive effectiveness, or its potentially harmful or beneficial effects on fetal outcome. There is some evidence indicating that a precipitous fall in arterial blood pressure could jeopardize

Table 33.10 Effect of any antihypertensive therapy in pregnancy for the treatment of pre-eclampsia on severe hypertension

Treatment comparison and trial (date published)	Events/no. randomized (%) Anti-hypertensive	Control	Odds ratio (& 95% CI)	Graph of odds ratio (& 95% CI)	Odds reduction (± SE)
Diuretic vs. control (overview 4394)					
Wesley and Douglas (1962)	3/131 (2.29)	2/136 (1.47)	1.56 (0.27–9.12)		
Menzies (1964)	3/57 (5.26)	5/48 (10.42)	0.48 (0.11–2.04)		
Campbell and MacGillivray (1975)	19/153 (12.42)	15/102 (14.71)	0.82 (0.39–1.71)		
Sibai *et al.* (1984)	1/10 (10.00)	1/10 (10.00)	1.00 (0.06–17.25)		
All diuretic trials			0.81 (0.45–1.48)		
Methyldopa vs. control (overview 3997)					
Welt *et al.* (1981)	0/7 (0.00)	1/7 (14.29)	0.14 (0.00–6.82)		
Redham *et al.* (1976)	2/117 (1.71)	16/125 (12.80)	0.20 (0.08–0.52)		
Arias and Zamorsa (1979)	2/29 (6.90)	10/29 (34.48)	0.19 (0.05–0.68)		
All methyldopa trials			0.19 (0.09–0.41)		
β-blocker vs. control (overview 3998)					
Rubin *et al.* (1983a)	2/60 (3.33)	7/60 (11.67)	0.30 (0.08–1.18)		
Wichman *et al.* (1985)	16/26 (61.54)	19/26 (73.08)	0.60 (0.19–1.88)		
Sibai *et al.* (1987)	5/92 (5.43)	14/94 (14.89)	0.36 (0.14–0.92)		
All β-blocker trials			0.41 (0.21–0.77)		
ANY ANTIHYPERTENSIVE TRIAL			0.44 (0.30–0.65)		

Graph axis: 0.0, 0.5, 1.0, 1.5, 2.0 — Treated better | Treated worse

uteroplacental perfusion, and should therefore probably be avoided. Hydralazine is the oldest of the current generation of antihypertensive drugs, and appears still as effective and safe as other, more recently developed antihypertensive drugs.

3.2 Plasma volume expansion

Women with severe antepartum pre-eclampsia show haemoconcentration with a contracted circulating plasma volume (Wallenburg 1988). Over the past 25 years, several authors have recommended plasma volume expansion with non-crystalloid solutions such as dextran and salt poor albumin in attempts to correct intravascular volume and to improve the maternal systemic and uteroplacental circulation (Cloeren and Lippert 1972). Sehgal and Hitt (1980) studied the effect of plasma volume expansion with hyperosmolar solutions (dextran 40 and plasminate) in a randomized controlled trial and found that volume expansion was associated with significant improvements in haemoconcentration

Table 33.10 Effect of any antihypertensive therapy in pregnancy for the treatment of pre-eclampsia on perinatal death

Treatment comparison and trial (date published)	Events/no. randomized (%) andAnti-hypertensive	Control	Odds ratio (& 95% CI)	Graph of odds ratio (& 95% CI)	Odds reduction (± SE)
Diuretic vs. control (overview 4394)					
Weseley and Douglas (1962)	3/131 (0.76)	4/136 (2.94)	0.31 (0.05–1.80)		
Menzies (1964)	3/57 (5.26)	2/48 (4.17)	1.27 (0.21–7.64)		
Campbell and MacGillivray (1975)	0/153 (0.00)	0/102 (0.00)			
Sibai *et al.* (1984)	0/10 (0.00)	0/10 (0.00)			
All diuretic trials			(0.18–2.18)		
Methyldopa vs. control (overview 3997)					
Weitz *et al.* (1987)	0/13 (0.00)	1/12 (0.00)			
Redman *et al.* (1976)	1/117 (0.85)	5/125 (4.00)	0.27 (0.05–1.38)		
Leather *et al.* (1988)	6/52 (11.54)	6/48 (12.50)			
Arias and Zamosa (1979)	0/29 (0.00)	1/29 (3.45)	0.14 (0.00–6.82)		
All methyldopa trials			0.55 (0.21–1.40)		
β-blocker vs. control (overview 3998)					
Rubin *et al.* (1983*a*)	1/60 (1.67)	2/60 (3.33)	0.51 (0.05–4.97)		
Wichman *et al.* (1984)	0/26 (0.00)	1/26 (3.85)	0.14 (0.00–6.82)		
Pickles *et al.* (1989)	0/70 (0.00)	0/74 (0.00)			
Sibai *et al.* (1987)	1/100 (1.00)	0/100 (0.00)	7.39 (0.15–372.39)		
All β-blocker trials	2/256 (0.78)	3/260 (1.15)	0.67 (0.11–3.89)		
ANY ANTIHYPERTENSIVE TRIAL			0.59 (0.29–1.17)		

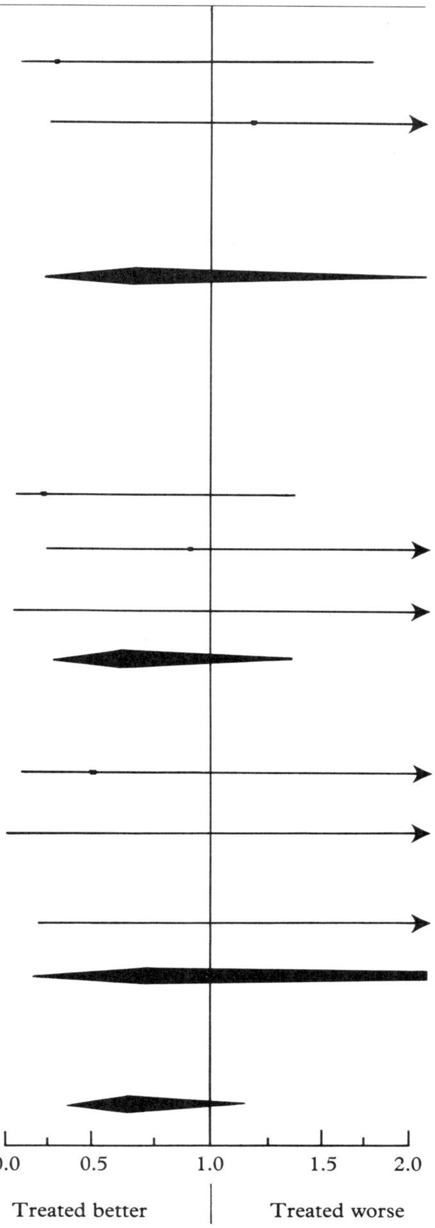

Graph axis: 0.0 0.5 1.0 1.5 2.0

Treated better | Treated worse

Table 33.11 Effect of labetalol vs. hydralazine in severe pregnancy-induced hypertension on severe hypertension as endpoint

Study	EXPT		CTRL		Odds ratio	Graph of odds ratios and confidence intervals
	n	(%)	*n*	(%)	(95% CI)	0.01 0.1 0.5 1 2 10 100
Walker *et al.* (1983)	4/11	(36.36)	5/11	(45.45)	0.70 (0.13–3.68)	
Mabie *et al.* (1987)	4/40	(10.00)	0/20	(0.00)	4.86 (0.57–41.03)	
Ashe *et al.* (1987)	1/10	(10.00)	2/10	(20.00)	0.47 (0.04–5.19)	
Typical odds ratio (95% confidence interval)					1.12 (0.36–3.54)	

Table 33.12 Effect of IV labetalol vs. IV diazoxide in severe pregnancy-induced hypertension on persistent severe hypertension

Study	EXPT		CTRL		Odds ratio	Graph of odds ratios and confidence intervals
	n	(%)	*n*	(%)	(95% CI)	0.01 0.1 0.5 1 2 10 100
Michael (1986)	3/45	(6.67)	6/45	(13.33)	0.48 (0.12–1.89)	
Typical odds ratio (95% confidence interval)					0.48 (0.12–1.89)	
Effect of IV labetalol vs. IV diazoxide in severe pregnancy-induced hypertension on perinatal death						
Michael (1986)	0/45	(0.00)	3/45	(6.67)	0.13 (0.01–1.28)	
Typical odds ratio (95% confidence interval)					0.13 (0.01–1.28)	

and output of urine, and a trend towards a lowering of mean arterial pressure.

In a recent uncontrolled study, Gallery and co-workers (1981; Gallery 1984) found that rapid replenishment of intravascular volume using a stable protein substitute decreased the arterial blood pressure for periods of 24 hours or more in pregnant women with generally moderate third trimester hypertension. Groenendijk *et al.* (1984) observed a trend towards reduced blood pressures following volume expansion in 10 pre-eclamptic women monitored using a Swan–Ganz catheter.

Although blood pressure was not restored to normal by volume expansion, these uncontrolled studies suggest that such treatment may be an effective adjunct to the administration of antihypertensive drugs and perhaps, by reducing the doses needed, might minimize the risks of any maternal and neonatal side-effects. It should be borne in mind, however, that intravascular volume expansion carries some risk of volume overload which may lead to pulmonary, and perhaps cerebral, oedema in pre-eclamptic women in whom colloid osmotic pressure is usually low (Benedetti and Carlson 1979). Volume expansion may be particularly dangerous after delivery, when central volumes and pressures tend to rise (Hankins *et al.* 1984), so that it should probably not be applied without monitoring pulmonary capillary wedge pressure (Wallenburg 1988).

Further studies are clearly needed to define the place of plasma volume expansion, with or without additional antihypertensive treatment, in the management of women with severe pregnancy-induced hypertension.

3.3 Anticonvulsant agents

Anticonvulsant and sedative drugs are widely used in the management of eclampsia, and in pregnant women with severe hypertensive disease and pre-eclampsia, in an attempt to prevent the occurrence of eclamptic seizures. In the United States, barbiturates are used in moderately severe pre-eclampsia, while parenteral magnesium sulphate is the treatment of choice in fulminating pre-eclampsia and eclampsia (Lewis *et al.* 1980). In contrast, magnesium sulphate is rarely used in Europe and Australia, the most frequent choice being diazepam, followed by barbiturates and chlormethiazole (Chamberlain *et al.* 1978; Trudinger and Parik

1982). In Sweden, many doctors still use 'lytic cocktails' consisting of hydralazine, chlorpromazine, and pethidine, in addition to diazepam and, sometimes, chlormethiazole (Lindberg and Sandström 1981). Since no adequately controlled clinical trials on the use of anticonvulsant drugs in pregnancy are available, the following review must be based on uncontrolled studies and anecdotal reports.

3.3.1 Magnesium sulphate

Only a small amount of magnesium appears to cross the blood–brain barrier after intravenous administration of magnesium sulphate (Thurnau *et al*. 1987) and it seems to act by pre-synaptic inhibition at the myoneural junction. Magnesium has little effect on blood pressure (Thiagarajah *et al.* 1985) and virtually no sedative effect.

The current popularity of magnesium sulphate in the United States reflects the management of eclampsia recommended by Pritchard and his colleagues (1984), based on their experience between 1955 and 1984 with 245 cases of eclampsia, including 83 cases occurring before delivery (Pritchard *et al.* 1984). A regimen of intravenous and intramuscular administration of magnesium sulphate, intravenous hydralazine, and delivery within 48 hours was associated with the death of only one mother, and only 8 of the 79 fetuses (10.1 per cent) who were alive when the diagnosis of eclampsia was made. Other reports generally support the efficacy of this treatment protocol, although the perinatal outcomes are not always as favourable (Harbert *et al.* 1968; Sibai *et al.* 1981).

Magnesium can attain life-threatening levels as a result of excessive dosage or diminished excretion (for example, due to renal failure). The single maternal death in Pritchard's series was caused by cardiorespiratory arrest due to an overdose, and three other women had magnesium-induced respiratory depression or arrest. Women receiving magnesium sulphate should therefore be closely monitored.

Magnesium readily crosses the placenta and high magnesium concentrations in cord blood have been shown to be associated with depression of the newborn (Lipsitz 1971). However, Stone and Pritchard (1970) found no clinical evidence of magnesium toxicity in the infants of mothers who had been treated with magnesium sulphate.

3.3.2 Diazepam

The benzodiazepines chlordiazepoxide and diazepam were introduced in the treatment of eclampsia and severe pre-eclampsia in the late 1960s as an alternative to the 'lytic cocktails' popular at that time (MacGillivray 1983). Diazepam acts by a direct depressant effect on the thalamus and hypothalamus. Following maternal intravenous administration it readily crosses the placenta to the fetus. It is very slowly metabolized and cleared in the neonate (Mandelli *et al.* 1975). Intravenous administration of diazepam in the mother may lead to loss of beat-to-beat variability in the fetal heart rate, and thus interfere with the clinical interpretation of the cardiotocogram (Scher *et al.* 1972). Given in high doses during labour, diazepam causes delayed onset of respiration, apnea, hypotonia, impaired metabolic response to cold, and poor sucking in the newborn infant (Cree *et al.* 1973). This well-documented neonatal depression may last several days because of the long plasma and clinical half-life of diazepam in the newborn.

3.3.3 Chlormethiazole

Following the first report by Duffus *et al.* (1969) of its use in Aberdeen, chlormethiazole has been widely used as a sedative and anticonvulsant in the treatment of severe pre-eclampsia and eclampsia. It acts rapidly following intravenous administration, and its effectiveness has been described in various reports of uncontrolled studies (Tischler 1973; Kristoffersen 1984; Johannesen 1984). Like the other anticonvulsants, chlormethiazole also crosses the placenta but, in contrast to diazepam, it is rapidly excreted by the fetus and the newborn (Tunstall *et al.* 1979).

3.3.4 Summary

The ideal anticonvulsant for use in severe pre-eclampsia and eclampsia is the one which is easiest to administer, is rapidly effective in arresting and preventing convulsions, has a wide safety limit for the mother, and is non-toxic and non-depressant to the baby (Campbell 1986). All the drugs discussed above appear to have a reliable and rapid anticonvulsant effect, but (as discussed) they differ with regard to their adverse effects on the fetus and neonate. The search for the ideal anticonvulsant to be used in severe pre-eclampsia and eclampsia continues (Slater *et al.* 1987).

4 Conclusions

4.1 Implications for current practice

Pharmacologic lowering of blood pressure constitutes a mainstay in the management of women with hypertensive disorders in pregnancy. There is some evidence from the overviews that antihypertensive treatment (diuretics, beta-blockers, methyldopa) of women with mild or moderate pregnancy-induced hypertensive disorders will prevent severe hypertension developing, but there is no evidence of an effect on the occurrence of proteinuric pre-eclampsia or perinatal mortality. This may be because there are no real beneficial effects on these more important outcome measures or perhaps more plausibly, given the marked effect on blood pressure, that the effects on severe pre-eclampsia and perinatal death could not be detected in the small trials published to date.

For the treatment of severe hypertensive disease, hydralazine appears to be effective in lowering blood pressure. Labetalol seem to be gaining in popularity, and although there is some evidence that it may produce a more controlled lowering of blood pressure than hydralazine or diazoxide, this requires further study.

The use of anticonvulsants is widespread, not only in the treatment of eclampsia but also in the management of pre-eclampsia to prevent seizures. The choice of drug appears to be determined by historical rather than by scientific data, and there is no reliable information as to how useful anticonvulsants really are in pre-eclampsia.

4.2 Implications for future research

The potential benefits of antiplatelet agents in both the prevention and treatment of pre-eclampsia deserve further investigation. Similarly, in view of the promising effects of beta-blockers and methyldopa on the development of severe hypertension (and in view of their widespread use by many doctors), there is an urgent need for further study in larger numbers of women.

The results of the small trials of plasma volume expansion conducted so far are also promising. Further study might help to determine whether this would be a practicable and effective way to reduce the need for (or dose of) antihypertensive therapy in severe pregnancy-induced hypertensive disorders.

In summary, at present, the treatment of hypertensive disorders in pregnancy appears to be largely based on clinical experience fed by anecdotal reports, rather than on reliable evidence from properly controlled trials of sufficient size. This does not seem appropriate given the large numbers of women who develop hypertensive disease in pregnancy and who are subsequently given the treatments discussed above. It might therefore be a prudent, rather than a disproportionate use of resources, to set up multicentre collaborative studies involving much larger numbers of women than have so far been studied in order to assess more reliably the effects of treatment on serious outcomes (such as proteinuric pre-eclampsia and perinatal mortality).

References

Allen J, Maigaard S, Forman A, Jacobsen P, Jespersen LT, Brogaard Hansen KP, Andersson KE (1987). Acute effects of nitrendipine in pregnancy-induced hypertension. Br J Obstet Gynaecol, 94: 222–226.

Antiplatelet Trialists' Collaboration (1988). Secondary prevention of vascular disease by prolonged antiplatelet therapy. Br Med J, 296: 320–331.

Arias F, Zamora J (1979). Antihypertensive treatment and pregnancy outcome in patients with mild chronic hypertension. Obstet Gynecol, 53: 489–494.

Ashe RG, Moodley J, Richards AM, Philpott RH (1987). Comparison of labetalol and dihydrallazine in hypertensive emergencies of pregnancy. S Afr Med J, 71: 354–356.

Beaufils M, Uzan S, Donsimoni R, Colau JC (1985). Prevention of pre-eclampsia by early antiplatelet therapy. Lancet, 1: 840–842.

Belch JJF, Thorburn J, Greer IA, Sarfo S, Prentice CRM (1985). Intravenous prostacyclin in the management of pregnancies complicated by severe hypertension. Clin Exp Hypertens, B4: 75–86.

Benedetti TJ, Carlson RW (1979). Studies of colloid osmotic pressure in pregnancy-induced hypertension. Am J Obstet Gynecol, 135: 308–311.

Bonnar J, Redman CWG, Sheppard BL (1975). Treatment of fetal growth retardation *in utero* with heparin and dipyridamole. Eur J Obstet Gynecol Reprod Biol, 5: 123–134.

Brain MC, Kuah KB, Dixon HG (1967). Heparin treatment of haemolysis and thrombocytopenia in pre-eclampsia. J Obstet Gynaecol Br Commnwlth, 74: 702–711.

Broughton Pipkin F (1986). The effects of maternal drug therapy on the fetus. In: Hypertension in Pregnancy. Sharp F, Symonds EM (eds). Ithaca, NY: Perinatology Press, pp 305–325.

Campbell DM, MacGillivray I (1975). The effect of a low calorie diet or a thiazide diuretic on the incidence of pre-eclampsia and on birthweight. Br J Obstet Gynaecol, 82: 572–577.

Campbell DM (1986). Clinical experiences and a review of chlormethiazole in the management of pre-eclampsia and eclampsia. Acta Psychiatr Scand (Suppl 329), 73: 175–181.

Chamberlain GVP, Lewis PJ, de Swiet M, Bulpitt CJ (1978). How obstetricians manage hypertension in pregnancy. Br Med J, 1:626–629.

Chesebro (1982) JH, Clements IP, Fuster V, Elveback LR, Smith HC, Bradsley WT, Frye RL, Holmes DR, Vlietstra RE, Pluth JR, Wallace RB, Puga FJ, Orszulak TA, Piehler JM, Schaff HV, Danielson GK (1982). A platelet inhibitor trial in coronary artery bypass operations. Benefit of perioperative dipyridamole and aspirin therapy on early postoperative vein graft patency. New Engl J Med, 307: 73–78.

Chesley LC (1978). Hypertensive Disorders in Pregnancy. New York: Appleton-Century-Crofts.

Cloeren SE, Lippert TH (1972). Effect of plasma expanders in toxemia of pregnancy. New Engl J Med, 287: 1356–1357.

Cockburn J, Moar VA, Ounsted MK, Redman CWG (1982). Final report of study on hypertension during pregnancy: The effects of specific treatment on the growth and development of the children. Lancet, 1: 647–649.

Collins R, Yusuf S, Peto R (1985a). Overview of randomised trials of diuretics in pregnancy. Br Med J, 290: 17–23.

Collins R, Chalmers I, Peto R (1985b). Antihypertensive treatment in pregnancy. Br Med J, 291: 1129.

Constantine G, Beevers DG, Reynolds AL, Luesley DM (1987). Nifedipine as a second line antihypertensive drug in pregnancy. Br J Obstet Gynaecol, 94: 1136–1142.

Cree JE, Meyer J, Hailey DM (1973). Diazepam in labour: its

metabolism and effect on the clinical condition and thermogenesis of the newborn. Br Med J, 4: 251–255.

Cuadros A, Tatum HJ (1964). The prophylactic and therapeutic use of bendroflumethiazide in pregnancy. Am J Obstet Gynecol, 89: 891–897.

Duffus GM, Tunstall ME, Condie RG, MacGillivray I (1969). Chlormethiazole in the prevention of eclampsia and the reduction of perinatal mortality. J Obstet Gynaecol Br Commnwlth, 76: 645–651.

Fairley KF, Addey FG, Ross IC, Kincaid-Smith P (1976). Heparin treatment in severe preeclampsia and glomerular nephritis in pregnancy. In: Hypertension in Pregnancy. Lindheimer MD, Katz AI, Zuspan FP (eds). New York: John Wiley, p 103.

Fallis NE, Plauche WC, Mosey LM, Langford HG (1964). Thiazide vs placebo in prophylaxis of toxemia of pregnancy in primigravid patients. Am J Obstet Gynecol, 88: 502–504.

Fidler J, Bennett MJ, de Swiet M, Ellis C, Lewis PJ (1980). Treatment of pregnancy hypertension with prostacyclin. Lancet, 2: 31–32.

Fidler J, Smith V, Fayers P, de Swiet M (1983). Randomised controlled comparative study of methyldopa and oxprenolol in treatment of hypertension in pregnancy. Br Med J, 286: 1927–1930.

Finnerty FA, Bepko FJ (1966). Lowering the perinatal mortality and the prematurity rate. The value of prophylactic diuretics in juveniles. JAMA, 195: 128–132.

Flowers CE, Grizzle JE, Easterling WE, Bonner OB (1962). Chlorthiazide as a prophylaxis against toxemia of pregnancy. Am J Obstet Gynecol, 84: 919–929.

Friedman EA, Neff RK (1976). Pregnancy outcome as related to hypertension, edema and proteinuria. In: Hypertension in Pregnancy. Lindheimer MD, Katz AI, Zuspan FP (eds). New York: John Wiley, pp 13–22.

Gallery EDM (1984). Volume homeostasis in normal and hypertensive human pregnancy. Seminars Nephrol, 4: 221–231.

Gallery EDM, Delprado W, Gyory AZ (1981). Antihypertensive effect of plasma volume expansion in pregnancy-associated hypertension. Austral NZ J Med, 11: 20–24.

Gallery EDM, Ross MR, Gyory AZ (1985). Antihypertensive treatment in pregnancy: analysis of different responses to oxprenolol and methyldopa. Br Med J, 291: 563–566.

Gant NF, Worley RJ (1980). Hypertension in Pregnancy. Concepts and management. New York: Appleton-Century-Crofts.

Garden A, Davey DA, Dommisse J (1982). Intravenous labetalol and intravenous dihydralazine in severe hypertension in pregnancy. Clin Exp Hypertens, B1: 371–383.

Goldby FS, Beilin LJ (1972). Relationship between arterial pressure and the permeability of arterioles to carbon particles in acute hypertension in the rat. Cardiovasc Res, 6: 384–390.

Goodlin RC (1980). Treatment of pregnancy hypertension with prostacyclin. Lancet, 2: 310.

Goodlin RC (1983). Correction of pregnancy-related thrombocytopenia with aspirin without improvement in fetal outcome. Am J Obstet Gynecol, 146: 862–864.

Goodlin RC, Haesslein HO, Fleming J (1978). Aspirin for the treatment of recurrent toxemia. Lancet, 2: 51.

Groenendijk R, Trimbos JBMJ, Wallenburg HCS (1984). Hemodynamic measurements in preeclampsia: preliminary observations. Am J Obstet Gynecol, 150: 232–236.

Hankins GDV, Wendel GD, Cunningham FG, Leveno KJ (1984). Longitudinal evaluation of hemodynamic changes in eclampsia. Am J Obstet Gynecol, 150: 506–512.

Harbert GM, Claiborne HA, McGaughey HS (1968). Convulsive toxemia. A report of 168 cases managed conservatively. Am J Obstet Gynecol, 10: 336–342.

Henderson-Smart DJ, Horvath JS, Phippard A, Korda A, Child A, Duggin GG, Hall BM, Storey B, Tiller DJ (1984). Effect of antihypertensive drugs on neonatal blood pressure. Clin Exp Pharmacol Physiol, 11: 351–354.

Hogstedt S, Lindberg S, Axelsson O, Lindmark G, Rane A, Sandström B, Lindberg BS (1985). A prospective controlled trial of metoprolol-hydralazine treatment in hypertension during pregnancy. Acta Obstet Gynecol Scand, 64: 505–510.

Horvath JS, Phippard A, Korda A, Henderson-Smart DJ, Child A, Tiller DJ (1985). Clonidine hydrochloride—A safe and effective antihypertensive agent in pregnancy. Obstet Gynecol, 66: 634–638.

Howie PW, Prentice CRM, Forbes CD (1975). Failure of heparin therapy to affect the clinical course of severe preeclampsia. Br J Obstet Gynaecol, 82: 711–717.

Hulme VA, Odendaal HJ (1986). Intrapartum treatment of preeclamptic hypertension by ketanserin. Am J Obstet Gynecol, 155: 260–263.

Jespersen J (1980). Disseminated intravascular coagulation in toxemia of pregnancy. Correction of the decreased platelet counts and raised levels of serum uric acid and fibrin(ogen) degradation products by aspirin. Thromb Res, 17: 743–746.

Johannesen P (1984). Eclampsia and severe cases of pre-eclampsia treated with chlormethiazole during a 10 year period. Scand J Clin Lab Invest, 44: 76–78.

Johnston CI, Aickin DR (1971). The control of high blood pressure during labour with clonidine ('Catapres'). Med J Austral, 2: 132–135.

Jouppila P, Kirkinen P, Koivula A, Ylikorkala O (1985). Failure of exogenous prostacyclin to change placental and fetal blood flow in preeclampsia. Am J Obstet Gynecol, 151: 661–665.

Kaplan NM (1986). Clinical Hypertension (4th edn). Baltimore: Williams & Wilkins, pp 180–272.

Kraus GW, Marchese JR, Yen SSC (1966). Prophylactic use of hydrochlorothiazide in pregnancy. JAMA, 198: 128–132.

Kristoffersen MB (1984). Chlormethiazole as the main therapeutic agent to pre-eclamptic/eclamptic patients. Scand J Clin Lab Invest, 44: 73–75.

Lancet (1986). Aspirin and pre-eclampsia (Editorial). Lancet, 1: 18–20.

Landesman R, Aguero O, Wilson K, La Russa R, Campbell W, Penaloza O (1965). The prophylactic use of chlorthalidone, a sulfonamide diuretic in pregnancy. J Obstet Gynaecol Br Commnwlth, 72: 1004–1010.

Leather HM, Humphreys DM, Baker P, Chadd MA (1968). A controlled trial of hypotensive agents in hypertension in pregnancy. Lancet, 2: 488–490.

Lewis PJ, Bulpitt CJ, Zuspan FP (1980). A comparison of current British and American practice in the management of hypertension in pregnancy. J Obstet Gynaecol, 1: 78–82.

Lindberg BS, Sandström B (1981). How Swedish obstetricians manage hypertension in pregnancy. Acta Obstet Gynecol Scand, 60: 327–331.

Lipsitz PJ (1971). The clinical and biochemical effects of excess magnesium in the newborn. Pediatrics, 47: 501–505.

Lorenz RL, Weber M, Kotzur J, Thiesen K, Schacky CV, Meister W (1984). Improved aortocoronary bypass patency by low-dose aspirin (100 mg daily). Lancet, 1: 1261–1264.

Mabie WC, Gonzalez AR, Sibai BM, Amon E (1987). A comparative trial of labetalol and hydralazine in the acute management of severe hypertension complicating pregnancy. Obstet Gynecol, 70: 328–333.

MacGillivray I (1983). Pre-eclampsia. The Hypertensive Disease of Pregnancy. London: W B Saunders Company Ltd.

Maeck JVS, Zilliacus H (1948). Heparin in the treatment of toxemia of pregnancy. Am J Obstet Gynecol, 55: 326–331.

Mandelli M, Morselli PL, Nordio S, Pandi G, Principi N, Sereni F, Tognoni G (1975). Placental transfer of diazepam and its disposition in the newborn. Clin Pharmacol Ther, 17: 564–572.

Menzies DN (1964). Controlled trial of chlorothiazide in treatment of early pre-eclampsia. Br Med J, 1: 739–742.

Michael CA (1986). Intravenous labetalol and intravenous diazoxide in severe hypertension complicating pregnancy. Austral NZ J Obstet Gynaecol, 26: 26–29.

Moar VA, Jefferies MA, Mutch LMM, Ounsted MK, Redman CWG (1978). Neonatal head circumference and the treatment of maternal hypertension. Br J Obstet Gynaecol, 85: 933–937.

Mutch LMM, Moar VA, Ounsted MK, Redman CWG (1977). Hypertension during pregnancy, with and without specific hypotensive treatment. II: The growth and development of the infant in the first year of life. Early Hum Dev, 1: 59–67.

Naulty J, Cefalo RC, Lewis PE (1981). Fetal toxicity of nitroprusside in the pregnant ewe. Am J Obstet Gynecol, 139: 708–711.

Neuman J, Weiss B, Rabello Y, Cabal L, Freedman RK (1979). Diazoxide for the acute control of severe hypertension complicating pregnancy: a pilot study. Obstet Gynecol, 53: 50–55.

Ounsted MK, Moar VA, Good FJ, Redman CWG (1980). Hypertension during pregnancy with and without specific treatment: The development of the children at the age of four years. Br J Obstet Gynaecol, 87: 19–24.

Page EW (1948). Use of heparin in preeclampsia. Am J Med, 4: 784.

Parker M, Le M, Coggins G (1973). The use of clonidine (catapres) in hypertensive and toxaemic syndromes of pregnancy. Austral NZ J Med, 3: 432.

Persantine–Aspirin Reinfarction Study Research Group (1980). Persantine and aspirin in coronary heart disease. Circulation, 62: 449-461.

Pickles CJ, Symonds EM, Broughton Pipkin F (1989). The fetal outcome in a randomized double-blind controlled trial of labetalol versus placebo in pregnancy-induced hypertension. Br J Obstet Gynaecol, 96: 38–43.

Plouin PE, Breart G, Maillard F, Papiernik E, Relier JP, Labetalol-Methyldopa Study Group (1987). Antihypertensive efficacy and perinatal safety of labetalol in the treatment of hypertension in pregnancy: a randomised comparison to methyldopa. Arch Mal Coeur, 80: 952–955.

Pritchard JA, Cunningham FG, Pritchard SA (1984). The Parkland Memorial Hospital protocol for treatment of eclampsia: evaluation of 245 cases. Am J Obstet Gynecol, 148: 951–960.

Redman CWG (1982). A controlled trial of the treatment of hypertension in pregnancy: Labetalol compared with methyldopa. In: The Investigation of Labetalol in the Management of Hypertension in Pregnancy. Riley AJ, Symonds EM (eds). International Congress Series No. 591. Amsterdam: Excerpta Medica, pp 101–110.

Redman CWG, Beilin LJ, Bonnar J, Ounsted MK (1976). Fetal outcome in trial of antihypertensive treatment in pregnancy. Lancet, 2: 753–756.

Redman CWG, Beilin LJ, Bonnar J (1977). Treatment of hypertension in pregnancy with methyl dopa: blood pressure control and side effects. Br J Obstet Gynaecol, 84: 419–426.

Redman CWG, Denson KWE, Beilin LJ, Bolton FG, Stirrat GM (1977). Factor-VIII consumption in pre-eclampsia. Lancet, 2: 1249–1252.

Reynolds B, Butters L, Evans J, Adams T, Rubin PC (1984). First year of life after the use of atenolol in pregnancy associated hypertension. Arch Dis Childhood, 59: 1061–1063.

Robertson EG (1971). The natural history of oedema during pregnancy. J Obstet Gynaecol Br Commnwlth, 78: 520–529.

Rubin PC, Butters L, Clark DM, Reynolds B, Sumner DJ, Steedman D, Low RA, Reid JL (1983a). Placebo-controlled trial of atenolol in treatment of pregnancy-associated hypertension. Lancet, 1: 431–434.

Rubin PC, Butters L, Reynolds B, Evans J, Sumner D, Low RA, Reid JL (1983b). Atenolol elimination in the neonate. Br J Clin Pharmacol, 16: 659–662.

Scher J, Hailey DM, Beard RW (1972). The effects of diazepam on the fetus. J Obstet Gynaecol Br Commnwlth, 79: 635–638.

Schramm M (1979). Prophylactic anticoagulation in the management of recurrent preeclampsia and fetal death. Austral NZ J Obstet Gynaecol, 19: 230–232.

Sehgal NN, Hitt JR (1980). Plasma volume expansion in the treatment of pre-eclampsia. Am J Obstet Gynecol, 138: 165–168.

Sheppard BL, Bonnar J (1981). An ultrastructural study of uteroplacental arteries in hypertensive and nomotensive pregnancy and fetal growth retardation. Br J Obstet Gynaecol 88: 695–705.

Sibai BM, McGubbin JH, Anderson GD, Lipshitz J, Dilts PV (1981). Eclampsia I. Observations from 67 recent cases. Obstet Gynecol, 58: 609–613.

Sibai BM, Grossman RA, Grossman HG (1984). Effects of diuretics on plasma volume in pregnancies with long-term hypertension. Am J Obstet Gynecol, 150: 831–835.

Sibai BM, Gonzalez AR, Mabie WC, Moretti M (1987). A comparison of labetalol plus hospitalization vs hospitalization alone in the management of preeclampsia remote from term. Obstet Gynecol, 70: 323–327.

Slater RM, Wilcox FL, Smith WD, Donnai P, Patrick J, Richardson T, Mawer GE, D'Souza SW, Anderton JM (1987). Phenytoin infusion in severe pre-eclampsia. Lancet, 1: 1417.

Stone SR, Pritchard JA (1970). Effect of maternally administered magnesium sulphate on the neonate. Obstet Gynecol, 35: 574–578.

Strandgaard S, MacKenzie ET, Jones JV (1976). Studies on the cerebral circulation of the baboon in acutely induced hypertension. Stroke, 7: 287–290.

Tervila L, Vartiainen E (1971). The effects and side effects of diuretics in the prophylaxis of toxaemia of pregnancy. Acta Obstet Gynecol Scand, 50: 351–356.

Thiagarajah S, Harbert GM Jr, Bourgeois FJ (1985). Magnesium sulfate and ritodrine hydrochloride: systemic and uterine hemodynamic effects. Am J Obstet Gynecol, 153: 666–674.

Thorley KJ (1984). Randomised trial of atenolol and methyl dopa in pregnancy related hypertension. Clin Exp Hypertens, B3: 168.

Thurnau GR, Kemp DB, Jarvis A (1987). Cerebrospinal fluid levels of magnesium in patients with preeclampsia after treatment with intravenous magnesium sulfate: a preliminary report. Am J Obstet Gynecol, 157: 1435–1438.

Tischler E (1973). Intravenous chlormethiazole in the management of severe pre-eclampsia. Austral NZ J Obstet Gynaecol, 13: 137–142.

Trudinger BJ, Parik I (1982). Attitudes to the management of hypertension in pregnancy: a survey of Australian fellows. Austral NZ J Obstet Gynaecol, 22: 191–197.

Trudinger B, Cook CM, Thompson R, Giles W, Connelly A (1988). Low-dose aspirin improves fetal weight in umbilical placental insufficiency. Am J Obstet Gynecol, 159: 681–685.

Tunstall ME, Campbell DM, Danson BM, Jostell KG (1979). Chlormethiazole treatment and breast feeding. Br J Obstet Gynaecol, 86: 793–798.

Valentine BH, Baker JL (1977). Treatment of recurrent pregnancy hypertension by prophylactic anticoagulation. Br J Obstet Gynaecol, 84: 309–311.

Voto LS, Zin C, Neira J, Lapidus AM, Margulies M (1987). Ketanserin versus α-methyldopa in the treatment of hypertension during pregnancy: a preliminary report. J Cardiovasc Pharmacol, 10 (Suppl 3): S101-S103.

Walker JJ, Belch JJF, Erwin L, McLaren M, Lang G, Forbes CD, Prentice CRM, Calder AA (1982). Labetalol and platelet function in pre-eclampsia. Lancet, 2: 279.

Walker JJ, Greer I, Calder AA (1983). Treatment of acute pregnancy-related hypertension: Labetalol and hydralazine compared. Postgrad Med J, 59 (Suppl 3): 168–170.

Wallenburg HCS (1987). Changes in the coagulation system and platelets in pregnancy-induced hypertension and pre-eclampsia. In: Hypertension in Pregnancy. Sharp F, Symonds EM (eds). Ithaca, NY: Perinatology Press, pp 227–248.

Wallenburg HCS (1988). Hemodynamics in hypertensive pregnancy. In: Hypertension in Pregnancy. Birkenhoger WH, Reid JL (eds). Handbook of Hypertension (Vol 10). Rubin PC (ed). Amsterdam: Elsevier, pp 66–102.

Wallenburg HCS, Rotmans N (1987). Prevention of recurrent idiopathic fetal growth retardation by low-dose aspirin and dipyridamole. Am J Obstet Gynecol, 157: 1230–1235.

Wallenburg HCS, Dekker GA, Makovitz JW, Rotmans P (1986). Low-dose aspirin prevents pregnancy-induced hypertension and pre-eclampsia in angiotensin-sensitive primigravidae. Lancet, 1: 1–3.

Walters BNJ, Redman CWG (1984). Treatment of severe pregnancy associated hypertension with the calcium antagonist nifedipine. Br J Obstet Gynaecol, 91: 330–336.

Weiner CP, Gelfan R, Socol ML (1984). Intrapartum treatment of preeclamptic hypertension by Ketanserin—a serotonin receptor antagonist. Am J Obstet Gynecol, 149: 576–578.

Weitz C, Khouzami V, Maxwell K, Johnson JWC (1987). Treatment of hypertension in pregnancy with methyldopa: a randomized double blind study. Int J Gynaecol Obstet, 25: 35–40.

Welt SI, Dorminy III JH, Jelovsek FR, Crenshaw MC, Gall SA (1981). The effect of prophylactic management and therapeutics on hypertensive disease in pregnancy: preliminary studies. Obstet Gynecol, 57: 557–564.

Weseley AC, Douglas GW (1962). Continuous use of chlorothiazide for prevention of toxemia of pregnancy. Obstet Gynecol, 19: 355–358.

Wichman K, Rydn G, Karlberg BE (1984). A placebo controlled trial of metoprolol in the treatment of hypertension in pregnancy. Scand J Clin Lab Invest, 169: 90–95.

Wichman K, Karlberg BE, Ryden G (1985). Metoprolol in the treatment of mild to moderate hypertension in pregnancy—effects on the mother. Clin Exp Hypertens, B4: 141–156.

Woods DL, Malan AF (1983). Side effects of labetalol in newborn infants. Br J Ostet Gynaecol, 90: 876.

Zuspan FP, Ward MC (1964). Treatment of eclampsia. South Med J, 57: 954–959.

Zuspan FP, Bell JD, Barnes AC (1960). Balance ward and double blind diuretic studies during pregnancy. Obstet Gynecol, 16: 543–49.

34 Infection in pregnancy

Elaine Wang and Fiona Smaill

1 Introduction

Infection has, in the past, been a major cause of both maternal and perinatal death. In most parts of the developed world today maternal deaths from infection are very rare. Nevertheless, maternal infection and colonization with pathogenic organisms continue to cause problems for both mothers and babies. As late as 1956 a randomized trial of antibiotics given to women in prolonged labour demonstrated a significant reduction in maternal morbidity and perinatal mortality in the group given the antibiotics (Smith *et al.* 1956). The prevalence of various forms of infection in pregnancy is higher in poorer women, and this fact may in part explain the greater frequency of adverse pregnancy outcomes among these women.

Organisms other than bacteria may lead to serious disease during pregnancy and the peripartum period. Such organisms include fungi, such as Candida species; viruses, such as herpes viruses; and protozoa, such as *Toxoplasma gondii*. In addition, a number of more fastidious organisms such as *Chlamydia trachomatis* and the genital mycoplasmas have now been linked with disease in pregnancy and childbirth.

Pregnant women are subject to the full range of acute and chronic infections to which non-pregnant people are also subject. Malaria, for example, is a major cause of maternal morbidity world-wide, and this has led the World Health Organization to recommend routine prophylaxis with chloroquine in endemic areas. Furthermore, routine antimalarial chemoprophylaxis has been shown in a randomized trial to reduce the incidence of low birthweight (Morley *et al.* 1964). In this chapter, however, we will focus on those infectious conditions which are of particular importance to those caring for pregnant women and their babies in developed countries.

The topics covered were chosen because of their particular importance in pregnancy.

2 Bacteriuria

Three to 8 per cent of pregnant women harbour significant numbers of bacteria in their urine, usually without exhibiting any symptoms. This asymptomatic bacteriuria may lead to complications such as acute cystitis and acute pyelonephritis, which are found in approximately 1 per cent of pregnancies (Little 1966; Harris and Gilstrap 1981; McFadyen *et al.* 1973; Kincaid-Smith and Bullen 1965; Whalley 1967; Dixon and Brant 1967; Harris 1979). Thus urinary tract infection is one of the most common medical complications of pregnancy. The prevalence of bacteriuria in pregnancy is higher in women of lower socioeconomic status. Parity and age play equivocal roles (Little 1966; McFadyen *et al.* 1973; Kass 1960; Williams *et al.* 1979). Fifteen to 45 per cent of untreated women with asymptomatic bacteriuria will develop symptomatic urinary tract infections (acute cystitis or pyelonephritis) (Table 34.1).

2.1 Screening for infection

The earliest studies on urinary tract infection by Kass (1960) defined infection as 100 million colony-forming units per litre or more in a clean catch urine, and these criteria are still widely accepted. Culture and colony count of a single voided specimen will detect 80 per cent of cases of asymptomatic infection, when compared to a catheterized specimen with 100 million colony-forming units per litre or more. The sensitivity of culture and colony count increases to 95 per cent if two consecutive specimens demonstrate the same organism (Kass 1960).

In patients with symptoms of urinary tract infection, the sensitivity of a single urine with 100 million colony-forming units per litre in predicting infection is 95 per cent. Colony counts of less than 100 million colony-forming units per litre are significant in non-pregnant women with symptoms of urinary tract infection (Stamm *et al.* 1980). The importance of these lower counts in pregnant women has not been evaluated.

False positive cultures and colony counts of clean catch voided urine will occur in between 85 per cent and 93 per cent of cases (Kass and Platt 1984). The specificity of the test depends on the care taken to minimize contamination when the specimen is collected. There is no information about sensitivity and specificity of culture and colony count in pregnancy.

The predictive value of a culture result depends on the prevalence of infection in the population studied (see Chapter 3.). With a prevalence of asymptomatic bacteriuria in pregnancy of 5 per cent, and assuming a specificity of 90 per cent for the test, the positive predictive value of a single urine culture is only 30 per cent.

Other more economical methods to screen for infection have been suggested. The predictive value of a positive history of previous urinary tract infection is not

Table 34.1 Effect of antibiotic vs. no treatment for asymptomatic bacteriuria in pregnancy on development of pyelonephritis

Study	EXPT		CTRL		Odds ratio
	n	(%)	*n*	(%)	(95% CI)
Elder *et al.* (1971)	4/133	(3.01)	27/147	(18.37)	0.21 (0.10–0.45)
Little (1966)	4/124	(3.23)	35/141	(24.82)	0.18 (0.09–0.36)
Kincaid-Smith and Bullen (1965)	2/61	(3.28)	20/55	(36.36)	0.12 (0.05–0.30)
Furness *et al.* (1975)	23/139	(16.55)	17/67	(25.37)	0.57 (0.27–1.19)
Gold *et al.* (1966)	0/35	(0.00)	4/30	(13.33)	0.10 (0.01–0.77)
Mulla (1960)	3/50	(6.00)	23/50	(46.00)	0.13 (0.05–0.31)
Williams *et al.* (1969)	5/85	(5.88)	18/78	(23.08)	0.24 (0.10–0.59)
Kass (1960)	0/42	(0.00)	20/48	(41.67)	0.09 (0.03–0.25)
Typical odds ratio (95% confidence interval)					0.20 (0.15–0.27)

Graph of odds ratios and confidence intervals: 0.01 0.1 0.5 1 2 10 100 better than that expected by chance (Little 1966; Chng and Hall 1982; Campos-Outcalt and Corta 1985). Semi-automated instruments to screen specimens for bacteriuria (Davis and Stager 1985), the detection of urinary nitrites (Campos-Outcalt and Corta 1985; Soisson *et al.* 1985), and microscopic analysis of a clean catch spun urine (Soisson *et al.* 1985) have been studied as alternatives. Although the sensitivity of semiautomated screens is 97 per cent, the specificity is low at 70 per cent (Davis and Stager 1985). The sensitivity of tests to detect urinary nitrites ranges from 45 per cent to 57 per cent (Campos-Outcalt and Corta 1985; Soisson *et al.* 1985), and the sensitivity of urinalysis for predicting infection is only 28 per cent (Soisson *et al.* 1985). These tests may have a role in identifying which urines should be cultured in the interests of cost-saving, but their sensitivity and specificity in pregnant women is not high enough to allow them to replace urine culture as an adequate screening test.

2.2 Treatment

Recognition and treatment of asymptomatic bacteriuria in pregnancy reduces the risk of pyelonephritis and at least its short term consequences to both mother and fetus. According to Kass and Platt (1984), screening for asymptomatic bacteriuria and treating the cases that are detected should prevent over 11 cases of pyelonephritis in every 1000 pregnancies screened. Acute pyelonephritis will not, however, be completely eradicated by treating all women with bacteriuria early in pregnancy. In one study, 34 per cent of patients hospitalized for acute pyelonephritis did not have significant bacteriuria demonstrated on their screening urine culture (Gilstrap *et al.* 1981a). Two further studies (Chng and Hall 1982; Lawson and Miller 1971) reported that 67 per cent and 80 per cent of women who developed acute urinary tract infection during pregnancy were negative on initial testing, but acute cystitis and acute pyelonephritis were not differentiated in these groups. That treatment of asymptomatic bacteriuria will, however, result in a substantially decreased risk of the development of pyelonephritis has been well demonstrated by all 8 of the published randomized controlled trials (Table 34.1).

The postulated relationship of asymptomatic bacteriuria in pregnancy with increased fetal mortality, preterm delivery, intrauterine growth retardation, and low birthweight infants is more tenuous. The associations are weak and controversial (Kass 1959; Kass 1960; Kincaid-Smith and Bullen 1965; Little 1966; Whalley 1967; Dixon and Brant 1967; Elder *et al.* 1971; Cunningham *et al.* 1973; Sever *et al.* 1979; Naeye 1979; Williams *et al.* 1979; Gilstrap *et al.* 1981b; McGrady *et al.* 1985). The earliest studies by Kass (1960) claimed that asymptomatic bacteriuria increased the risk of 'premature' delivery and neonatal death, and that these sequelae could be reduced by effective treatment. With the exception of a recently published trial assessing the effectiveness of antibiotic treatment of Group-B streptococcial bacteriuria (Thomsen *et al.* 1987) subsequent randomized controlled studies have not replicated the initial observations (Table 34.2).

The original approach to therapy for asymptomatic bacteriuria in pregnancy was continuous antibiotic therapy for the duration of pregnancy (Kass 1960; Kincaid-Smith and Bullen 1965). However, single-dose therapy for uncomplicated urinary tract infection in women who are not pregnant is well established (Souney and Polk 1982), and trials suggest that this is the case in pregnancy as well (Table 34.3). It has

Table 34.2 Effect of antibiotic vs. no treatment for asymptomatic bacteriuria in pregnancy on preterm delivery or low birthweight

Study	EXPT		CTRL		Odds ratio	Graph of odds ratios and confidence intervals
	n	(%)	*n*	(%)	(95% CI)	0.01 0.1 0.5 1 2 10 100
Elder *et al.* (1971)	17/133	(12.78)	16/145	(11.03)	1.18 (0.57–2.44)	
Little (1966)	10/124	(8.06)	13/141	(9.22)	0.86 (0.37–2.03)	
Kincaid-Smith and Bullen (1965)	9/61	(14.75)	12/56	(21.43)	0.64 (0.25–1.64)	
Furness *et al.* (1975)	24/118	(20.34)	10/52	(19.23)	1.07 (0.48–2.42)	
Gold *et al.* (1966)	2/35	(5.71)	0/30	(0.00)	6.60 (0.40–99.99)	
Kass (1960)	4/42	(9.52)	11/48	(22.92)	0.39 (0.13–1.16)	
Typical odds ratio (95% confidence interval)					0.89 (0.15–0.27)	

obvious advantages in terms of patient compliance, minimization of adverse effects, and financial savings. There have been attempts to compare other durations of therapy (Whalley and Cunningham 1977), but these have not yielded any useful guidelines for practice.

The available evidence from controlled trials suggests that where an isolate is known to be susceptible, sulphonamides, nitrofurantoin, ampicillin, and the first generation cephalosporins are equally effective in the treatment of asymptomatic bacteriuria (Harris *et al.* 1982; Pedler and Bint 1985; Brumfitt *et al.* 1979) (Table 34.4). Antibiotic treatment of bacteriuria in pregnancy has not been shown to reduce the risk of subsequent infection in the long term (Zinner and Kass 1971), but the only trial in which a follow-up was conducted is small.

2.3 Symptomatic urinary tract infection

Symptomatic lower urinary tract infection in pregnancy may respond to single dose treatment, but there is insufficient data (Masterton *et al.* 1985) for this treatment to be recommended.

Regular follow-up urine cultures must be obtained; failures, relapses, and recurrences treated appropriately; and when infection recurs, consideration given to continuous prophylactic therapy for the remainder of pregnancy. Nitrofurantoin 50 mg has been recommended (Bailey *et al.* 1986), but there have been no studies on its use in this situation. Recurrent infection during pregnancy may signify an underlying abnormality of the urinary tract and these women should be evaluated radiographically postpartum (Kincaid-Smith and Bullen 1965; Williams *et al.* 1979).

2.4 Pyelonephritis

Pyelonephritis is diagnosed clinically by the presence of fever, flank pain and dysuria, together with a positive urine culture. Patients should be hospitalized, and antibiotic therapy instituted parenterally after blood and urine cultures have been taken. Ampicillin, or a first generation cephalosporin, is appropriate initial treatment (Chow and Jewesson 1985) as infection is most likely to be due to *Escherichia coli*. Where there is concern about antibiotic resistance, or the patient is seriously ill, combination therapy with an aminoglycoside and ampicillin is appropriate. Careful monitoring of serum aminoglycoside levels throughout therapy is strongly recommended to minimize fetal exposure to the drug.

Patients with acute pyelonephritis are at risk of

Table 34.3 Effect of single dose vs. 5–7–day antibiotic for asymptomatic bacteriuria in pregnancy on persistent bacteriuria

Study	EXPT		CTRL		Odds ratio	Graph of odds ratios and confidence intervals
	n	(%)	*n*	(%)	(95% CI)	0.01 0.1 0.5 1 2 10 100
Bailey *et al.* (1983)	3/24	(12.50)	0/20	(0.00)	6.84 (0.67–70.12)	
Masterton *et al.* (1985)	6/52	(11.54)	3/38	(7.89)	1.49 (0.37–5.97)	
Bailey *et al.* (1986)	3/30	(10.00)	6/30	(20.00)	0.46 (0.11–1.89)	
Reeves (1975)	12/49	(24.49)	15/40	(37.50)	0.54 (0.22–1.34)	
Typical odds ratio (95% confidence interval)					0.79 (0.42–1.50)	

Table 34.4 Effect of broad spectrum penicillin vs. cephalosporin for asymptomatic bacteriuria in pregnancy on persistent bacteriuria

Study	EXPT		CTRL		Odds ratio	Graph of odds ratios and confidence intervals
	n	(%)	*n*	(%)	(95% CI)	0.01 0.1 0.5 1 2 10 100
Pedler and Bint (1985)	7/31	(22.58)	5/27	(18.52)	1.28 (0.36–4.51)	
Brumfitt *et al.* (1979)	2/23	(8.70)	2/22	(9.09)	0.95 (0.13–7.27)	
Harris *et al.* (1982)	7/24	(29.17)	9/20	(45.00)	0.51 (0.15–1.73)	
Typical odds ratio (95% confidence interval)					0.82 (0.37–1.83)	

relapse and recurrence of infection (Cunningham *et al.* 1973), but the only reported randomized trial of suppressive therapy for the remainder of pregnancy (Lenke *et al.* 1983) failed to detect any advantage over the alternative of close surveillance with cultures.

2.5 Conclusions

All pregnant women should be screened by culture and colony count of a clean catch urine. If this shows more than 100 million colony-forming units per litre, the diagnosis should be confirmed with a repeat culture, and appropriate antibiotic therapy instituted. Single-dose therapy should be tried initially, as this appears to be as effective as multi-dose regimens. This policy has been shown to reduce the risk of a serious disease, pyelonephritis.

Adequately controlled trials are still required to assess the relative values of different antimicrobial regimens for the treatment of asymptomatic bacteriuria.

3 Syphilis

Syphilis during pregnancy is particularly important because transmission of *Treponema pallidum* from mother to baby may result in the development of congenital syphilis, with tragic sequelae. The outcomes of such transmission may consist of preterm delivery (20 per cent), miscarriage or perinatal death (20 per cent), subclinical infection (20 per cent), or congenital infection with resulting handicap (40 per cent) (Stray-Pedersen 1983). Congenital syphilis can be largely prevented by treatment of the mother. Transmission to the fetus occurs particularly during the second trimester, although one report observed the organism in 2 of 5 conceptuses aborted during the first trimester (Harter and Benirschke 1976).

The incidence of maternal syphilis is relatively low. It has been estimated to be as high as two cases per 1000 pregnancies in one study from Australia (Bellingham 1973). However, studies from Norway and the United States estimate the rate to be one-tenth of that (Skarpaas and Loe 1980; Felman 1978). In England and Wales in 1979 there were 190 cases (0.3 per 1000) of primary or secondary syphilis, and 161 cases (0.27 per 1000) of early latent syphilis in some 600,000 women giving birth during that year (Williams 1985).

3.1 Diagnosis

Most women infected with *Treponema pallidum* are asymptomatic, and can only be identified by serological screening, such as at a premarital examination (Felman 1978) or prenatal examination (Skarpaas and Loe 1980). The vast majority of infections are diagnosed by the use of serologic tests. These consist of treponemal tests, which detect antibodies to *Treponema pallidum*, and non-treponemal tests, which detect antibodies to lipoidal antigens (Hart 1986). The main non-treponemal test is the Venereal Disease Research Laboratory (VDRL) test, and the usual treponemal tests are the fluorescent treponemal antibody absorption test (FTA-ABS) and the microhaemagglutination tests for syphilis (MHA-TP).

In the minority of patients who are suspected to have disease because of clinical findings, other diagnostic tests should include dark-field microscopic examination of a specimen taken from a lesion (Centers for Disease Control 1979), or fluorescent antibody staining of such a specimen (Daniels and Ferneyhough 1977). The sensitivity of these tests has been estimated to be between 74 and 95 per cent. This range may be due to differences in technical aspects of the performance of the test.

3.2 Screening during pregnancy

Although the wisdom of premarital screening has been questioned (Felman 1978), screening during pregnancy is still important because of the devastating effect of the disease on the baby. A programme of screening and treating those women found to be seropositive has been subjected to a detailed economic analysis (Stray-Pedersen 1983). Because of the major costs that result from a case of congenital syphilis, this analysis demonstrated the cost-effectiveness of such a programme despite the rarity of syphilis occurring in pregnancy. A similar analysis in the United Kingdom (Williams 1985) demonstrated a benefit to cost ratio of over 30 to 1 in economic terms for continuing a screening programme versus discontinuing it. Since transmission may occur later than the first trimester, serology should be repeated in women who are at increased risk of acquiring the infection (Bellingham 1973). These include the unmarried mother with a history of previous sexually transmitted infections.

In most countries, the VDRL continues to be cheaper to perform than treponemal serology, and an accepted procedure for screening is to perform the latter tests only when the VDRL is found to be positive (Hart 1986).

Treatment of mothers should consist of efficacious antibiotics, preferably a penicillin. Infants and sexual partners should be followed up, and treated if found to be infected. Sexual contact tracing usually involves close collaboration between the physician and public health officials.

3.3 Congenital syphilis

Diagnosis of congenital syphilis is difficult because the clinical presentation is variable and many patients are asymptomatic. Rathbun (1983) recommended that a complicated group of absolute, major, and minor criteria be accepted, including characteristic dental, mucosal, dermatologic, and bony findings, as well as cardiovascular, neurologic, and eye findings, in addition to laboratory tests.

Treatment has consisted of administration of penicillin by various routes and for different durations (Rathbun 1983). Treatment of infants is recommended when the adequacy of treatment of the mother is unknown, or if the mother received treatment for the first time during the pregnancy with a drug other than penicillin.

3.4 Conclusions

Screening programmes for the detection of asymptomatic syphilis should be continued despite the low incidence of maternal infection. Infected women should be promptly treated, preferably with penicillin. Appropriate follow-up of infants and sexual partners is essential.

The incidence of syphilis in pregnancy should be monitored as it may decrease to a point at which the screening policy is no longer cost-effective.

4 Gonorrhoea

Gonorrhoea is a serious infection in pregnancy, for both mother and baby. Maternal infection rates with *Neisseria gonorrhoeae* range from 1 to 5 per cent in different studies (Alexander 1984), although in one study based in an urban adolescent medicine clinic, the organism was recovered from at least one of three sites in 14.7 per cent of the sample (Chacko *et al.* 1982). However, this population was an urban, predominantly black, and younger group compared with pregnant women in general.

4.1 Maternal disease

Although the infection may be asymptomatic in the mother, pregnancy appears to increase the likelihood of both arthritis (Goobar and Clark 1964; Niles and Lowe 1966; Taylor *et al.* 1966) and systemic disease (Niles and Lowe 1966; Taylor *et al.* 1966; Davis 1945; Holmes *et al.* 1971). This dissemination may occur during the 2nd or 3rd trimesters (Goobar and Clark 1964; Niles and Lowe 1966; Taylor *et al.* 1966; Davis 1945; Holmes *et al.* 1971). Arthritis is the most frequent manifestation of disseminated disease, with either polyarticular or monoarticular involvement. The majority of patients have fever and shaking chills, and they may have a characteristic purpuric-petechial rash as well. Gonococci can be isolated from blood or petechial cultures in this form of infection (Holmes *et al.* 1971). It is quite possible, however, that at least some of the apparently increased incidence of disseminated disease observed during pregnancy results from better follow-up during this period (Hook and Holmes 1985).

Pregnant women may also present with any of the other symptoms of gonorrhoea associated with infections in the non-pregnant population. These include dysuria-sterile pyuria syndrome, cervicitis, proctitis, and conjunctivitis (Hook and Holmes 1985). Less commonly, acute bartholinitis, endometritis, and salpingitis may occur. Ascending infection during pregnancy may result in pelvic inflammatory disease other than salpingitis, including septic abortion after the 12th week of gestation.

In one study, septic abortion occurred in 13 (35 per cent) of 37 pregnant women hospitalized for symptomatic gonococcal infection (Sarrell and Pruett 1968). In that study, chorioamnionitis occurred after the 16th week in 8 cases (22 per cent). Chorioamnionitis may, in turn, lead to preterm labour (Russell 1979; Brunham *et al.* 1984). Edward and co-workers (1978) compared the outcomes of 19 women with gonococcal infection with 41 uninfected controls matched for age, parity, socioeconomic status, and date of delivery. They observed a significantly higher incidence of chorioamnionitis, preterm delivery, premature rupture of membranes, and delayed delivery after rupture of membranes in the infected group. In a non-randomized cohort comparison, prelabour rupture of membranes was observed in 6 (43 per cent) of 14 untreated women but only 4 (3 per cent) of 144 women who received treatment (Charles *et al.* 1970). Clearly, this dramatic difference must at least in part reflect selection bias.

4.2 Diagnosis

Culture remains the 'Gold Standard' for diagnosis of gonorrhoea in a woman. Although a Gram stain may effectively be used for diagnosing gonococcal urethritis in men (Jacobs and Kraus 1975; Barlow and Phillips 1978), or for diagnosing conjunctivitis, the Gram stain is not sensitive enough for specimens obtained from the female genital tract (Barlow and Phillips 1978).

Specimens for culture should be inoculated on a selective culture plate immediately, or sent in transport medium to reach the laboratory in the minimal time possible, since *Neisseria gonorrhoeae* are fairly fastidious organisms. The sensitivity of cultures is affected most by the quality of the specimen at the time of inoculation. Newer diagnostic techniques based on detection of gonococcal enzymes, antigens, DNA, or lipopolysaccharide have either not been found to be adequately sensitive or specific, or are no quicker than culture (Young *et al.* 1981; Aardoom *et al.* 1982; Stamm *et al.* 1984; Jaffe *et al.* 1982; Totten *et al.* 1983).

Screening for gonorrhoea during pregnancy is worthwhile because of the severe effects of infection on both the mother and her baby. It can be accomplished by obtaining specimens for culture at the first antenatal visit. In populations deemed 'at risk', either on demographic grounds, or because of a history of sexually transmitted disease (Holmes 1983), repeat cultures should be taken during the 3rd trimester.

Disseminated disease usually responds dramatically to the administration of penicillin (Holmes *et al.* 1971). The drug may be administered either as aqueous penicillin intravenously, or as intramuscular procaine penicillin, with an initial dose of 10 million units per day, reduced after clinical improvement has been observed, and then continued for 10 to 14 days. Oral treatment should consist of ampicillin or amoxycillin rather than phenoxymethyl penicillin, which has been associated with failures (Jaffe *et al.* 1982). If joint involvement has occurred, a longer duration of therapy is indicated. A repeat endocervical and rectal culture should be obtained as isolation of penicillin resistant gonococci is increasing (Totten *et al.* 1983; Rubin *et al.* 1983; Holmes 1983).

4.3 Neonatal disease

The most common gonococcal infection in neonates is conjunctivitis (Holmes *et al.* 1978). The clinical manifestations of ophthalmia neonatorum include conjunctival erythema, with ocular discharge and polymorphonuclear leukocytes in the Gram stain of the smear, occurring in an infant less than 30 days old (Sandstrom *et al.* 1982). Although gonococcal disease remains the most serious cause of ophthalmia neonatorum, other causes include chemical conjunctivitis from silver nitrate, which appears on the first day; infection with *Chlamydia trachomatis*, which occurs at 5 days to 2 weeks of age; infection with Herpes simplex, which occurs on day 2 to 3; and infection with other bacteria, occurring between 5 days and 3 weeks after birth. Gonococcal ophthalmia characteristically manifests itself early—at two to five days. However, indolent infections have occurred subsequently, and some infections have been asymptomatic (Brown *et al.* 1966; Mellin and Kent 1958; Armstrong *et al.* 1976; Valenton and Abendanio 1973; Podgore and Holmes 1981). Eyelid oedema, chemosis, and a progressively purulent exudate will develop. If left untreated, this infection may lead to permanent corneal damage and even perforation of the eye (Duke-Elder 1965).

4.4 Prevention

Obviously the ideal method of preventing neonatal ophthalmia is prevention or early treatment of maternal disease.

Crédé reported a reduction in incidence of ophthalmia neonatorum from 10 per cent to 0.3 per cent with the use of silver nitrate prophylaxis (Crédé 1881). Its success has been so dramatic that in 48 of 50 States in the United States prophylaxis for the prevention of gonococcal conjunctivitis is required by law (Smith and Halse 1955). A review of the literature revealed that open studies of tetracycline, erythromycin, and penicillin found that these agents were more effective than silver nitrate (Rothenberg 1979). This conclusion cannot be accepted uncritically because allocation to treatment agents was not randomized, and the groups may not have been comparable. Because of the declining incidence of gonococcal ophthalmia, the irritant effects of silver nitrate, and the recognition of the importance of chlamydia, regimens which are also active against the latter organism are now acceptable as alternatives (American Academy of Pediatrics, Committee on Drugs, Committee on Fetus and Newborn, Committee on Infectious Diseases 1980). In a randomized trial, the efficacy of erythromycin ointment over that of silver nitrate drops in preventing chlamydial conjunctivitis was confirmed (Hammerschlag *et al.* 1980). However, only 3 per cent of the study population was at risk for gonococcal ophthalmitis. None of these babies developed disease. No failures of treatment were observed in the retrospective studies of efficacy of penicillin antibiotics (Lewis 1946; Smith 1969; O'Brien and O'Connell 1972; Otiti 1975; Armstrong *et al.* 1976). These agents, however, are not recommended because of concern regarding sensitization of infants to penicillin.

4.4.1 Cost-effectiveness analysis

Rothenberg (1979) has proposed a model which may be used in deciding whether the adoption of a prophylactic programme is cost-effective. This model must include the cost of the prophylaxis which consists of: the cost of the prophylactic agent and its administration; the cost of follow-up of complications; the cost of treating cases; and the cost of missed cases and ensuing complications. Since treatment is recommended, the cost of screening would be common to all agents. The local situation with respect to incidence of maternal infection must be known and entered into the model in order to make the decision.

4.5 Conclusions

Screening by culture for gonorrhoea should be incorporated as a part of routine antenatal care because gonococcal infection can be seriously aggravated by pregnancy. Cultures should be repeated during pregnancy in high risk groups. Women found to be infected and their sexual partners should be promptly treated. Erythromycin ointment appears to be the most effective form of prophylaxis against neonatal ophthalmia.

There are a number of efficacious alternatives in the treatment of gonococcal infection in the mother and her infant. In most centres, this infection may still be effectively treated with penicillins. Since penicillinase-producing gonococci may become more widespread, however, the search for antibiotics that are safe for use in pregnancy must continue. As a number of different regimens are now available for prophylaxis of ophthalmia neonatorum, it is important to determine the most cost-effective one, particularly since a number of open studies suggest that the more expensive antibiotic ointments may be more effective and have fewer side-effects than silver nitrate drops (see also Chapter 75).

5 Rubella

Rubella is typically a mild childhood illness, associated with an erythematosus maculopapular rash and lymphadenopathy. Arthralgia and arthritis are common symptoms in adults, but up to 50 per cent of infections can be subclinical (Centers for Disease Control 1984). Maternal infection, occurring early in pregnancy, can lead to fetal death, low birthweight for gestational age, deafness, cataracts, jaundice, purpura, hepatosplenomegaly, congenital heart disease, and mental retardation. The objective of rubella vaccination programmes is to prevent fetal infection and the congenital rubella syndrome. The risk to the fetus of maternal infection at successive stages of pregnancy has been an area of controversy, recently addressed in a prospective study by Miller *et al.* (1982). Infants whose mothers had confirmed rubella at successive stages of pregnancy were followed for 2 years. No defects attributed to rubella were found in 63 children infected after 16 weeks, while all 9 infants infected before the 11th week had significant cardiac disease and deafness. Although fetal infection, as diagnosed by the presence of infant IgM antibody or persistence of IgG after the first year, occurred at all stages of pregnancy, the fetus appeared to be protected from damage after the 16th week of gestation.

5.1 Vaccination strategies

Rubella vaccine was first licensed in 1969. Two approaches to vaccination have been used—universal vaccination, and selective vaccination. In the United States, universal vaccination of young children to interrupt transmission has led to a significant decline in reported cases of rubella and the congenital rubella syndrome, but for a period in the late 1970s the majority of cases of reported rubella were in persons 15 years of age and older, and there had been little change in the proportion of this group who were seronegative from pre-vaccine years (Centers for Disease Control 1986; Dales and Chin 1982). A concerted effort over the last decade to vaccinate all susceptible adolescents and young adults has resulted in the lowest ever reported incidences of the congenital rubella syndrome and of rubella (Centers for Disease Control 1986). In 1985, the incidence of rubella in the United States was 0.25 cases per 100,000, down from 28 cases per 100,000 in 1969. Only 2 cases of the congenital rubella syndrome were reported in both 1984 and 1985, an incidence of 0.05 cases per 100,000 live births, but this figure is believed to be an underestimate of the actual total.

Selective immunization was adopted in the United Kingdom, and initially only girls aged 11–14 were vaccinated. The programme was later extended to include all seronegative women of childbearing age. Moderate epidemics continue to occur with a peak incidence of 16 cases per 100,000 during 1983 (Smithells *et al.* 1985). In the same year, 25 cases of the congenital rubella syndrome were registered in the United Kingdom, and the number of terminations of pregnancy for which rubella was given as the reason was 419 (Smithells *et al.* 1985; Office of Population Censuses and Surveys 1983). Vaccination acceptance was initially low, and has only recently reached 85 per cent (Dudgeon 1985). A rate of 100 per cent will be needed if congenital infection is to be eliminated.

5.2 Rubella serology testing and immunity

Haemagglutination-inhibition (HAI) antibody testing is the standard method of screening for the presence of rubella antibodies, but most laboratories now use alternative techniques which are generally simpler to perform and equally sensitive or more sensitive (Herrmann 1985). These include latex agglutination, fluorescence immunoassay, passive haemagglutination, haemolysis-in-gel, and enzyme immunoassay tests. It has been well established that the presence of rubella antibody, as detected by the haemagglutination-inhibition test, of greater than or equal to 1 in 8, correlates with clinical protection of the individual (Davis *et al.* 1971). The single radial haemolysis or haemolysis-in-gel test is widely used in Europe, and a level of 15 international units per millilitre is accepted as protective (Banatvala 1985).

Following an attack of rubella, life-long protection against disease usually develops. Reinfections can occur, but the majority of these are asymptomatic and detected only by a booster response in specific rubella antibody. Vaccination produces an overall lower antibody response than natural infection (Horstmann *et al.* 1985). Following vaccination, antibody as detected by haemagglutination-inhibition develops in more than 90 per cent of vaccinees (Robinson *et al.* 1982; Herrmann *et al.* 1982; Horstmann *et al.* 1985; O'Shea *et al.* 1982). These results, and clinical efficacy studies (Greaves *et al.* 1983; Stassburg *et al.* 1985), have shown that protection against infection can be expected in 95 per cent of vaccine recipients.

Those with undetectable antibody by haemagglutination-inhibition usually have antibody detected by a more sensitive assay (Horstmann *et al.* 1985) and typically have a booster response on revaccination (Robinson *et al.* 1982; Serdula *et al.* 1984; Balfour *et al.* 1981). The clinical significance of these low-level antibodies is uncertain, but it is generally believed that any detectable antibody titre specific for rubella should be considered protective (Centers for Disease Control 1984). Viraemia following virus challenge has been documented to occur rarely in this group (O'Shea *et al.* 1983). There has been debate about whether rubella reinfection that occurs during pregnancy can transmit the virus to the fetus. There have been case reports of maternal infection resulting in the birth of an infant with the congenital rubella syndrome (Eilard and Strannegard 1974), but this is a rare event and most studies of reinfection during pregnancy have not been associated with defects in the infant (Fogel *et al.* 1985; Morgan-Capner *et al.* 1985; Forsgren and Soren 1985).

5.3 Diagnosis of rubella in pregnancy

The diagnosis of rubella in a pregnant woman who has been exposed to or develops a rubella-like infection can frequently be difficult. The laboratory must be provided with a detailed history, as routine screening tests are inadequate and additional testing is required. A fourfold rise in IgG antibody confirms infection, but if the acute phase serum is drawn more than 7 days after the onset of rash, this may not be detected (Meyer *et al.* 1972). Rubella infection can also be confirmed by demonstrating rubella specific IgM antibody. False negative results can occur if the specimen is drawn too soon after the beginning of exposure (Enders 1985). Reinfection can also be accompanied by a low or moderate IgM antibody response, together with a significant and rapid rise in IgG antibody levels (Enders 1985). The pattern of antibody response to acute infection and reinfection will vary according to the test method used, and expert consultation may be required for interpretation of data.

Congenital rubella is confirmed serologically by the detection of rubella specific IgM antibody in a newborn infant's serum, or persistence of rubella IgG antibody for more than 3 months (Enders 1985). Virus isolation can be attempted from nasopharyngeal and urine specimens, as well as from involved tissues.

5.4 Safety of the vaccine

Pregnant women should not be given rubella vaccine, but if a pregnant woman is vaccinated unknowingly, or she becomes pregnant within 3 months after immunization, available data suggests that the risk of teratogenicity from live rubella vaccine is quite small. The Centers for Disease Control have maintained a register of susceptible women who received vaccine within 3 months before or after conception. None of the 144 infants whose mothers received the RA27/3 rubella vaccine were born with abnormalities consistent with the congenital rubella syndrome (Preblud and Williams 1985). As rubella vaccine virus has been isolated from fetal tissue following induced abortion, the risk is not zero. Based on these observations, the maximum theoretical risk for the occurrence of congenital rubella following vaccination is 2.6 per cent. Receipt of rubella vaccine in pregnancy is not ordinarily an indication for interruption of pregnancy (Preblud and Williams 1985).

Arthralgia and arthritis are well-recognized vaccine associated side-effects, occurring more frequently and tending to be more severe in susceptible women (Polk *et al.* 1982). There have been occasional reports of prolonged arthritis, neurological sequelae, and chronic rubella viraemia occurring following postpartum rubella immunization (Tingle *et al.* 1985), but no permanent joint destruction has been described.

5.5 Cost-effectiveness of rubella immunization

The most significant cost factors associated with rubella are related to the long term sequelae of congenital rubella and this has recently been estimated at US $30,000 per individual per year (Appell 1985). Analyses indicate that the costs of the congenital rubella syndrome outweigh that of vaccination several-fold, being true for vaccination of infants of both sexes, teenage girls, and postpartum women (Schoenbaum *et al.* 1976; White *et al.* 1985).

5.6 Conclusions

High immunization levels must be achieved and maintained, and all susceptible women of childbearing age should be identified and vaccinated. Routine screening of women not known to be immune, who do not have documented proof of rubella vaccination, should be performed in any health care setting and should be part of routine medical care. Where follow-up cannot be assured, rubella vaccination without prior serologic testing may be preferable (Centers for Disease Control 1984). Prenatal screening should be carried out on all pregnant women without documentation of immunity, and vaccination given following both delivery and abortion. It has been estimated that one-third to one-half of current cases of the congenital rubella syndrome could be prevented if postpartum vaccination programmes were fully implemented (Orenstein *et al.* 1984; Smithells *et al.* 1985).

Where maternal infection is diagnosed in the first 16 weeks of pregnancy, voluntary termination is recommended. Counselling regarding fetal risks can be difficult because of the often uncertain dates of gestation and exposure to infection. Routine use of immune serum globulin for post-exposure prophylaxis of rubella is not recommended (Schiff 1969), although it may have a role where maternal rubella occurs and termination of pregnancy is not an option.

Present strategies must be intensified and new methods developed to ensure a high uptake of rubella immunization. Continued surveillance is necessary to confirm that vaccine induced immunity will be lifelong. Further study is needed to assess the clinical significance of low-level antibody as detected by newer, more sensitive tests, and there is need for the establishment of a minimal acceptable antibody level that indicates immunity.

6 Candidiasis

Vaginal candidiasis causes an intensely irritating, pruritic vaginal discharge and is a frequent problem during pregnancy. The incidence in pregnant women has been estimated to be between 2 and 10 times higher than in non-pregnant women (Mead 1974; Gardner and Kaufman 1969). Colonization of the vagina has been observed in between 12 and 41 per cent of women in different studies (Gardner 1944; Plass *et al.* 1931). Some of these differences may be due to variation in culture techniques, patient populations, and definitions of infection. Suggested predisposing factors include antimicrobial usage and diabetes (Morton and Rashid 1977). The condition is more difficult to eradicate in pregnant women (Kimbell 1966).

Congenital candida infections affect infants of very low birthweight, and manifest themselves with pneumonia and skin infections (Dixon and Houston 1978; Whyte *et al.* 1982). These infections, however, are rare considering the high frequency of vaginal candidal carriage in pregnant women.

6.1 Diagnosis

The clinical diagnosis of vaginal candidiasis is neither specific nor sensitive (Oriel 1977). Typical symptoms include an irritating vaginal discharge and pruritus. Examination reveals reddened mucosa of the labia minora, introitus, and lower third of the vagina, with white patches and a thin discharge containing white flakes. Hurley and Morris (1964) noted that of 100 vaginal cultures that grew a candida species, 8 were from asymptomatic women without any abnormalities suggestive of candida; 49 were from patients with 'typical clinical manifestations'; and 43 were from patients with vaginitis that was not typical. Thus, diagnosis depends on recovery of candida on cultures.

Candidal colonization rates rise from less than 10 per cent of pregnant women in the 1st trimester to over 50 per cent in the 3rd trimester (Morton and Rashid 1977). The organism is usually soon cleared after delivery. In view of the low incidence of adverse effects on babies born to asymptomatic mothers, screening of pregnant women for candida is not indicated.

6.2 Treatment

Only one placebo-controlled trial of therapy for candidiasis (Ruiz-Velasco *et al.* 1978) has been reported. It showed that the incidence of candidiasis in both mothers and the infants to whom they subsequently gave birth was significantly reduced by the use of clotrimazole tablets and vulvar cream (Tables 34.5 and 34.6).

A variety of different agents, as well as different dosages and frequencies of administration, have been studied. A randomized comparison demonstrated the effectiveness of nystatin compared to hydrargaphen (Milne and Brown 1973), but most recent trials have compared nystatin with imidazole preparations (Table 34.7). These have shown imidazoles to be more effective than nystatin. There is no evidence that a 14-day course of antifungal therapy is any more effective in curing candidiasis than a 7-day course (Table 34.8), and at least some evidence to suggest that a 1–3-day course is sufficient (Table 34.9).

A new agent, butoconazole, has also been studied for the treatment of vaginal candidiasis. Both trials of this new agent, however, have been conducted in non-

Table 34.5 Effect of clotrimazole as antifungal therapy in pregnancy on bacteriologic cure of candida (mother)

Study	EXPT		CTRL		Odds ratio	Graph of odds ratios and confidence intervals
	n	(%)	*n*	(%)	(95% CI)	0.01 0.1 0.5 1 2 10 100
Ruiz-Velasco and Rosas-Arceo (1978)	6/50	(12.00)	27/50	(54.00)	0.15 (0.07–0.35)	
Typical odds ratio (95% confidence interval)					0.15 (0.07–0.35)	

Table 34.6 Effect of clotrimazole as antifungal therapy in pregnancy on infant colonization with candida

Study	EXPT		CTRL		Odds ratio	Graph of odds ratios and confidence intervals
	n	(%)	*n*	(%)	(95% CI)	0.01 0.1 0.5 1 2 10 100
Ruiz-Velasco and Rosas-Arceo (1978)	6/50	(12.00)	21/50	(42.00)	0.22 (0.09–0.53)	
Typical odds ratio (95% confidence interval)					0.22 (0.09–0.53)	

Table 34.7 Effect of imidazoles vs. nystatin as antifungal therapy in pregnancy on failure to control candidiasis

Study	EXPT *n*	EXPT (%)	CTRL *n*	CTRL (%)	Odds ratio (95% CI)	Graph of odds ratios and confidence intervals (0.01 0.1 0.5 1 2 10 100)
Tan *et al.* (1974)	1/13	(7.69)	13/19	(68.42)	0.09 (0.02–0.37)	
Higton (1973)	4/25	(16.00)	10/25	(40.00)	0.31 (0.09–1.06)	
Davis *et al.* (1974)	0/23	(0.00)	4/23	(17.39)	0.12 (0.02–0.89)	
McNellis *et al.* (1977)	48/291	(16.49)	114/244	(46.72)	0.24 (0.17–0.35)	
Typical odds ratio (95% confidence interval)					0.23 (0.16–0.32)	

Table 34.8 Effect of 7-day vs. 14-day course antifungal therapy in pregnancy on failure to control candidiasis

Study	EXPT *n*	EXPT (%)	CTRL *n*	CTRL (%)	Odds ratio (95% CI)	Graph of odds ratios and confidence intervals (0.01 0.1 0.5 1 2 10 100)
Eliot *et al.* (1979)	1/29	(3.45)	1/41	(2.44)	1.43 (0.08–24.35)	
Rubin *et al.* (1980)	11/32	(34.38)	19/35	(54.29)	0.45 (0.17–1.18)	
Pasquale *et al.* (1979)	0/14	(0.00)	1/10	(10.00)	0.09 (0.00–4.83)	
Typical odds ratio (95% confidence interval)					0.47 (0.19–1.13)	

Table 34.9 Effect of 1–3 day vs. 7–14 day course antifungal therapy in pregnancy on failure to control candidiasis

Study	EXPT *n*	EXPT (%)	CTRL *n*	CTRL (%)	Odds ratio (95% CI)	Graph of odds ratios and confidence intervals (0.01 0.1 0.5 1 2 10 100)
Pasquale *et al.* (1979)	13/25	(52.00)	1/24	(4.17)	9.93 (2.91–33.89)	
Bloch and Kretzel (1980)	11/55	(20.00)	8/54	(14.81)	1.43 (0.53–3.83)	
Typical odds ratio (95% confidence interval)					3.06 (1.42–6.59)	

pregnant women. In one study with a total of only 68 patients, no difference was observed in cure rate in the group receiving 3 days of butoconazole compared with 7 days of miconazole (Bradbeer *et al.* 1985). A multicentre study of 274 women comparing 3-day courses of butoconazole with clotrimazole revealed cure rates of 95 per cent and 91 per cent, respectively (Droegemueller *et al.* 1984).

6.3 Conclusions

The initial treatment of symptomatic vaginal candidiasis should consist of clotrimazole because it is more effective than nystatin. A 7-day course appears to be adequate. Repeat courses may be required, given the tendency of the infection to recur. No treatment is indicated in asymptomatic infection.

Results of studies conducted in non-pregnant women may not be generalizable to pregnant women. More definitive studies with adequate sample sizes are necessary to determine the efficacy of short courses of treatment, which are known to maximize compliance. Studies of methods to determine if there is a subgroup of women who are less likely to respond to short course therapy will also be important in clinical management. As new and more costly drugs become available, their cost-effectiveness must be examined (*Medical Letter* 1986).

7 *Trichomonas vaginalis*

The protozoan, *Trichomonas vaginalis*, is frequently isolated from vaginal secretions during pregnancy. While the incidence of colonization with the organism is 13 per cent to 23 per cent in women of childbearing age attending gynaecology clinics (Rein and Chapel 1975), higher rates are reported in selected groups. *Trichomonas vaginalis* infections have been found in up to 50 per cent of those attending clinics for sexually transmitted diseases (Spence *et al.* 1980; Fouts and Kraus 1980) and in 65 per cent of pregnant black women in South Africa (Hoosen *et al.* 1981). The organism was found in 32 of 868 antenatal patients (3.7 per cent) at the Royal Infirmary, Sheffield, United Kingdom (Bramley 1976), and in 286 of 473 women (60 per cent) attending the Dalhousie prenatal clinic in Halifax, Canada.

Infection with *T vaginalis* in pregnancy may cause severe symptomatic vaginitis in some women. In addition, it may have adverse effects on the course of pregnancy or on the newborn, although the role of the organism in these respects is highly uncertain. One randomized controlled trial reported no statistically significant difference in birthweight or gestational age at delivery when asymptomatic *T vaginalis* infection was either treated with a single dose of metronidazole, or left untreated (Ross and Van Middelkoop 1983). Unsubstantiated comments have, however, suggested that failure to treat severe trichomonal vaginitis leads to preterm delivery (Anonymous 1980), and case reports have implicated the organism as a cause of neonatal pneumonia (McLaren *et al.* 1983; Hiemstra *et al.* 1984). A study of 115 adolescent pregnancies reported an association between *T vaginalis* and low gestational age and birthweight (Hardy *et al.* 1984), but the high frequency of multiple sexually transmitted diseases in this group made it difficult to determine the specific significance of *T vaginalis* on fetal outcome. No significant difference in birthweight was found in a small cohort study comparing 115 women with persistent infection with *T vaginalis*, and 151 non-infected controls (Ross and Van Middelkoop 1983). As *T vaginalis* is often associated with other sexually transmitted organisms of significance in pregnancy, these should be specifically sought when *T vaginalis* has been identified.

Colonization of the neonate following vaginal delivery appears to be uncommon. *Trichomonas vaginalis* can be isolated from the vagina of female infants born to infected mothers in less than 1 per cent of cases (Al-Salihi *et al.* 1974; Bramley 1976). Clinical infection is rare, although the organism has been associated with vaginitis in the neonate (Al-Salihi *et al.* 1974). *Trichomonas vaginalis* can be isolated from the respiratory tract of infants (McLaren *et al.* 1983; Hiemstra *et al.* 1984), but there have been no prospective studies looking at the role of this organism in respiratory disease.

7.1 Diagnosis of infection

Trichomonas vaginalis infection cannot be readily diagnosed clinically (Spence *et al.* 1980; Fouts and Kraus 1980; McLellan *et al.* 1982). Up to 50 per cent of women with the organism are asymptomatic. Vaginal discharge is the most common complaint, but the classically described, green frothy discharge is found in only 12 per cent of women (Fouts and Kraus 1980).

Microscopic examination of a wet preparation of vaginal secretions is simple to perform and highly specific, but its sensitivity compared to culture may be as low as 50 per cent (Fouts and Kraus 1980). To maximize the sensitivity of a wet preparation, a drop of vaginal discharge diluted in saline should be examined under the microscope immediately. Cooling the secretions results in loss of the characteristic jerky motility of the organism. Culture is the best method to diagnose the disease, but the methodology is time-consuming and not generally available (Spence *et al.* 1980; Fouts and Kraus 1980). Selective media are inoculated with fresh vaginal secretions and examined daily for seven days.

Fixing and staining slides for the identification of *T vaginalis* frequently destroys the morphologic characteristics of trichomonads. Papanicolaou smears have been used to diagnose the disease, but the sensitivity of this method compared to culture is only 40 per cent (McLellan *et al.* 1982). Serologic tests for *T vaginalis* have been developed, but have not been found to be clinically useful (Mason 1979). A direct fluorescent antibody test for the detection of *T vaginalis* in vaginal secretions is available but, as yet, has not been clinically evaluated. No diagnostic test for *T vaginalis* has been evaluated specifically in pregnant women.

7.2 Treatment

Metronidazole is a highly effective treatment of infection with *T vaginalis* (Lossick 1982; Ross and van Middelkoop 1983). Both a single 2 g dose, and an extended 7-day regimen of 250 mg three times a day, are curative in more than 90 per cent of patients. The only available double-blinded randomized comparison of single and multiple dose regimens of metronidazole showed no statistically significant advantage of the multiple dose regimen (Thin *et al.* 1979). Because patient compliance is high with single-dose therapy, this regimen is preferred clinically. The sexual partner should be treated concomitantly with the patient (Lossick 1982).

Metronidazole readily crosses the placenta (Adamsons and Joelsson 1966). Although it has been found to be carcinogenic in rodents, and mutagenic for certain bacteria, there is no evidence of teratogenicity after its administration to pregnant women (Robinson and Mirchandani 1965; Peterson *et al.* 1966; Roe 1983). Most obstetricians, however, refrain from its use during the first trimester of pregnancy (Chow and Jewesson 1985).

Clotrimazole, an antifungal agent, has been shown to be effective *in vitro* against *T vaginalis* (Lossick 1982). It has promise as a local palliative treatment during pregnancy.

7.3 Conclusions

Based on currently available evidence, there is no reason to screen asymptomatic pregnant women for the presence of trichomonas. When symptoms are present, and local treatments do not give adequate relief, consideration should be given to a single 2 g dose of metronidazole to both the patient and her sexual partner. Although no teratogenic effects in humans have been demonstrated, they remain a possibility with the use of metronidazole, so its use should be avoided during the period of organogenesis.

Randomized trials of treatment for asymptomatic trichomoniasis in pregnancy may help to determine the role of *T vaginalis* in adverse outcomes of pregnancy and neonatal infection, as well as showing whether or not the treatment is effective. Prospective cohort studies should also be conducted, as it may be difficult to mount randomized trials large enough to demonstrate effects other than those of therapy on symptoms, or eradication of the organism. It is important that isolation procedures for other infectious agents be included in these studies since *T vaginalis* may simply be a marker of other sexually transmitted diseases.

If a wet preparation is accepted as the most readily available test, its low sensitivity compared to culture must be appreciated. There is a need for the development of more sensitive but easily performed diagnostic tests, and a need for controlled randomized studies to look at alternative treatment regimens, particularly local trichomonicidal agents such as clotrimazole.

8 Genital mycoplasmas

Genital mycoplasmas (*Mycoplasma hominis* and *Ureaplasma urealyticum*) have been postulated as causative agents of recurrent abortion, chorioamnionitis, preterm delivery, low birthweight, stillbirth, and postpartum fever. As these organisms are found in the vaginal secretions of between 35 and 93 per cent of pregnant women (Harrison *et al.* 1983; Taylor-Robinson and McCormack 1980; Harrison 1983; Hardy *et al.* 1984) it is important to determine whether or not they are, in fact, pathogenic.

The suggestion that genital mycoplasmas might be a cause of pregnancy wastage has largely been based on case-control studies, in which investigators obtained a higher rate of mycoplasma isolation from women who had the adverse outcomes in question than from pregnant women who did not have these abnormal outcomes (Driscoll *et al.* 1969; Kundsin and Driscoll 1970; Braun *et al.* 1971; McCormack *et al.* 1973; McCormack *et al.* 1975; Sompolisky *et al.* 1975; Shurin *et al.* 1975; Tafari *et al.* 1976; Wallace *et al.* 1978; Dische *et al.* 1979; Embree *et al.* 1980; Kass *et al.* 1981; Quinn *et al.* 1983a,b,c; Kundsin *et al.* 1984).

As is true of all such studies, other factors, both known and unknown, may have caused the adverse outcome, irrespective of the presence or absence of mycoplasma infection. For example, if such infections are simply markers for sexually transmitted disease in general, other organisms might be the actual causes. An increased prevalence of mycoplasma infection is associated with a number of factors associated with transmission of venereal diseases, including young age, non-white race, lower socioeconomic status, and greater sexual activity (Harrison *et al.* 1983). An additional and obvious flaw of these studies is the fact that the antimicrobial agents used are also effective against infections, other than mycoplasmas, which may be important in pregnancy loss (Taylor-Robinson and McCormack 1980). Hence, even if the treatments were effective, the role of mycoplasma infection as a cause of pregnancy loss would not be established.

In the light of these uncertainties, it is uncertain whether or not there is any value in screening for these organisms, or in treatment if they are isolated. Only one randomized trial examining the effects of treatment has been reported (Kass *et al.* 1981). Data was presented only for women who completed the full 6-week course of erythromycin or placebo. Unfortunately, there is no useful information to be gleaned from the published report of this trial. Initially, women were randomized to receive clindamycin, erythromycin, or placebo. No data were given for the 104 women who received clindamycin, as the drug was stated to have 'no therapeutic effect', as well as causing frequent gastrointestinal reactions. Less than half the women allocated to receive either erythromycin or placebo took the full 6-week course of treatment, and the compliance rate appears to have been lower in the women allocated to take erythromycin. The fact that data are presented only for compliers with the full 6-week course vitiates the purpose of randomization, and renders the comparisons as uninterpretable as the open, non-randomized comparisons of antibiotic administration

(Stray-Pedersen *et al.* 1978; Quinn *et al.* 1983a,b,c, 1985).

Conclusions

At the present time the role, if any, of mycoplasma colonization as a possible cause of adverse pregnancy outcome is unknown. Neither screening for the organisms nor treatment of colonized women are justified on the basis of present evidence.

In view of the high frequency of vaginal colonization with mycoplasmas, well-conducted randomized controlled trials should be carried out to assess the value, if any, of treating colonized women.

9 Toxoplasmosis

Maternal infection with the protozoan parasite *Toxoplasma gondii* acquired during pregnancy may result in congenital infection of the infant, sometimes with serious sequelae. Clinical manifestations of congenital toxoplasmosis, consisting of chorioretinitis, recurrent seizures, hydrocephalus, and intracranial calcifications, may be present at birth, or appear later (*Lancet* 1980). The vast majority of infections are asymptomatic in the mother, although lymphadenopathy may occur (Krick and Remington 1978).

The method of identifying asymptomatic infection is by observing a high antibody level to *T gondii* in the serum. Individuals can be infected only once, so a woman who is immune prior to pregnancy is not at risk of transmitting the organism to her infant.

Because infections are frequently asymptomatic, studies on congenital toxoplasmosis have relied on serological results to identify maternal infection. A definite maternal infection is defined by a seroconversion occurring during pregnancy. A probable infection is defined by a high antibody level with high specific IgM, indicating recent exposure.

Both the prevalence of seropositivity (indicative of past exposure), and the risk of acquisition during pregnancy, has been found to vary in different countries, and even in different regions within the same country (*Lancet* 1980; Vaage and Midtvedt 1975). This has been ascribed, at least in part, to different habits with respect to the handling and consumption of raw meat and the disposal of cat litter, both of which can be reservoirs of the organism (Desmonts and Couvreur 1974a,b). Congenital infections have usually been defined as recovery of the parasite from the placenta or cord blood, presence of antibody of the IgM class, and persistent elevation of antibodies in the baby 9 months after birth, since maternally derived antibody would have been lost by that time. The risk of acquisition of toxoplasmosis in the mother and the infant varies widely. In addition to true regional differences, the apparent risks may be confounded by the design of the study; by the timing of the first blood sampling; by serological assay methods which have different sensitivities; by different policies regarding interventions; and by the duration and assiduousness of the follow-up of infants. A study of the sequelae in infants with congenital toxoplasmosis (Wilson *et al.* 1980) demonstrates a major flaw which may so affect the results that it renders them uninterpretable: a substantial number of the patients who were examined for sequelae were actually referred to the study because of such sequelae. Nevertheless, there are undoubtedly real differences in the prevalence of toxoplasmosis, and these are reflected in the fact that routine screening for the condition is conducted in some countries (for example, in France, Belgium, and Luxembourg), but not in many others, such as the United Kingdom, or The Netherlands (Blondel 1986).

The risk of transmission of toxoplasmosis from mother to baby is also dependent on the time in the pregnancy that the maternal infection occurs (Desmonts and Couvreur 1974a,b). The frequency of infection rose from 17 per cent in infants whose mothers were infected during the 1st trimester, to 65 per cent in infants whose mothers acquired the infection in the 3rd trimester. Although the incidence of vertical transmission, based on serology, was highest in 3rd trimester infections, transmission during the 1st trimester is associated with more severe symptoms. Severe disease occurred in 14 per cent of 1st trimester transmissions versus 0 per cent of 3rd trimester transmissions (Desmonts and Couvreur 1974a,b). Some of the early infections may result in miscarriages. However, the high frequency of neonatal clinical disease after infections early in gestation has led French investigators to recommend therapeutic abortion, where feasible, and an antiprotozoan drug, spiromycin, when abortion is not possible (Desmonts and Couvreur 1974a,b).

A number of treatment protocols have been used. None of them have been evaluated in randomized clinical trials, either against placebo, or against each other. Because they have been shown to be efficacious in animal studies, the two main chemotherapeutic agents that have been studied are pyrimethamine-sulphonamide (and folinic acid), and spiramycin (Beattie 1984). Spiramycin has been prescribed more often during pregnancy because of the toxicity of pyrimethamine-sulpha, which may produce haematologic abnormalities in adults (Zighelboim *et al.* 1968) and has teratogenic potential (Wilson and Remington 1980).

In one study, women with a history of 'obstetric pathology' (defined as recurrent miscarriages or intra-uterine fetal death) were screened for evidence of previous toxoplasma infection (Zighelboim *et al.* 1968). Some patients with evidence of infection were treated with one of three treatment regimens effective against protozoans (spiramycin, tetracycline, and sulfamethoxypyridazine; pyrimethamine and sulfamethoxypyridazine; colimycin and pyrimethamine or spiramycin). Their progress was compared to that of a non-randomized control group that had not received treatment. No differences were found in the incidences of miscarriages or congenital malformations in the 81 treated patients compared with the 168 control patients.

Most other studies have examined the efficacy of antiprotozoan drugs in women who 'definitely' or 'probably' acquired the infection during their pregnancies. In a non-randomized cohort comparison, Desmonts and Couvreur observed a lower incidence of infection (measured by negative serology in the infants) in the treated group, although there was no difference in the frequency of clinical disease in a group treated with spiramycin compared with a control group (Desmonts and Couvreur 1974a,b).

Thalhammer and Heller-Szollosy (1979) screened 4310 pregnant women, and identified seroconversion in 19 and high titre in 18. All patients were treated and no disease developed in any of the infants. The authors concluded, however, that the low pick-up rate from such screening did not justify the expense of the programme. Desmonts and Couvreur (1974a,b) noted a lower incidence of congenital infection (demonstrated by serology) in infants born to mothers with toxoplasmosis who had been treated (24 per cent were seropositive compared with 56 per cent), but there was no difference in the incidence of clinical infection. Based on this model, screening would be cost-effective if the incidence of infection during pregnancy were at least 0.8 per cent, and treatment were at least 50 per cent effective.

Two detailed economic analyses on the subject of screening for toxoplasmosis have been published (Wilson and Remington 1980; Henderson *et al.* 1984). The former concluded that regionalized programmes for detection and treatment of toxoplasma infection during pregnancy may prove cost-effective in the United States (Wilson and Remington 1980). However, because of major uncertainties regarding risk of infection, the efficacy of treatment alternatives, and the details of the costs of implementing such a programme, their conclusion may not be valid. Using more satisfactory economic evaluation methodology, Henderson *et al.* (1984), in the United Kingdom, argued that the use of a health education programme would be more likely to be cost-effective than widespread toxoplasmosis screening. The education campaign would advise pregnant women against ingestion of raw or undercooked meat; to wash their hands after its preparation; to refrain from gardening, or to wear gloves when so engaged; and to have others clean the cat litter, or to do so only with rubber gloves. Hunter and co-workers (1983) also recommended that education of women was more appropriate than screening because of the low incidence of toxoplasmosis observed in their study (based in Birmingham, Alabama). Thus, universal screening of pregnant women cannot be recommended at this time.

Conclusions

The evidence of benefit from screening of pregnant women for toxoplasma antibodies is not sufficient to warrant this as a routine practice in countries where the prevalence of the disease during pregnancy is lower than 0.8 per cent. Women who have acquired toxoplasmosis during pregnancy should be treated with spiromycin. Therapeutic abortion should be offered to women who contract infection in the first trimester.

Much work is still necessary to determine the true frequency of infection and the sequelae of congenital toxoplasmosis. Neither spiromycin nor pyrimethamine-sulpha are very efficacious against this parasite and the latter agent is associated with a high frequency of side-effects in pregnant women. Trials are needed of new antiprotozoan drugs with potentially better efficacy and safety. Such studies will require prolonged follow-up as some of the sequelae of such infections may occur many years after birth.

10 *Chlamydia trachomatis*

Maternal infection with *Chlamydia trachomatis* is important primarily because of the potential adverse effects of infection on the newborn infant. The condition is often asymptomatic in the mother, and may not be detected clinically. Some infected women may have a mucopurulent cervicitis, salpingitis, or the urethral syndrome.

The prevalence of *C trachomatis* in pregnant women varies widely; estimates ranging from 2 per cent to 37 per cent have been reported (Alexander and Harrison 1983; Goh *et al.* 1982). Higher rates are found in young women, unmarried women, and black women, as well as women from lower socioeconomic groups and those attending inner-city antenatal clinics.

10.1 Neonatal infection

The newborn infant can acquire *C trachomatis* infection through contact with infected maternal genital secretions at birth. Inclusion conjunctivitis will develop in 18 to 50 per cent of infants born to infected mothers (Alexander and Harrison 1983), making *C trachomatis* the most common cause of neonatal conjunctivitis (Pierce *et al.* 1982). The estimated risk of an infant born to an infected mother developing chlamydial pneumonia ranges from 3 to 18 per cent (Alexander and Harrison 1983). Serologic evidence indicates that 67 per cent of infants exposed at birth to *C trachomatis* are infected before 6 months of age (Beem and Saxon 1982).

The role, if any, of *C trachomatis* as a cause of spontaneous abortion, preterm labour, and low birthweight has been less clearly defined (Harrison *et al.* 1983; Martin *et al.* 1982; Thompson *et al.* 1982).

10.2 Diagnosis

The diagnosis of maternal *C trachomatis* infection is made either by culture of the organism from an endocervical specimen, or by the identification of chlamydial antigens directly in endocervical smears. The detection of chlamydial antibodies has no role in routine diagnosis (Darougar 1985), and the sensitivity of cytological methods is poor (Geerling *et al.* 1985). Tissue culture is considered to be the 'Gold Standard' for diagnosis, but isolation rates may be influenced by laboratory experience in culture techniques, transport and storage of the specimen, and the time elapsed between sampling and inoculation (Darougar and Treharne 1982).

Commercial kits are available for the detection of chlamydial antigen using immunofluorescent staining or enzyme immunoassay (Centers for Disease Control 1985). Transport and storage of the specimen is uncomplicated, and processing rapid. Enzyme immunoassay is technically simple to perform, but immunofluorescent staining requires an experienced observer. The sensitivity of these tests compared to cell culture ranges from 70 per cent to 100 per cent (Stamm *et al.* 1984; Graber *et al.* 1985; Coudron *et al.* 1986; Chernesky *et al.* 1986; Forbes *et al.* 1986; Jones *et al.* 1984). Specificity is generally greater than 95 per cent. These figures should be interpreted cautiously, acknowledging the limitations of tissue culture as the 'Gold Standard'. Modification of antigen detection tests continues to occur, and published data may not reflect the current efficacy of commercial methods.

Only one study has looked at the use of these tests in pregnant women (Stamm *et al.* 1984). Results from screening 225 pregnant women, in whom the prevalence of infection was 13 per cent, gave the immunofluorescent staining test a sensitivity and specificity of 86 per cent and 99 per cent respectively. In this group, the predictive value for a positive test was 93 per cent and 98 per cent for a negative result.

If the prevalence of maternal infection exceeds 6 per cent, a cost–benefit analysis has shown that it is cost-effective to screen for chlamydia using cell-culture techniques, and treat those infected (Schachter and Grossman 1981). As less expensive diagnostic tests become available, screening may be justified at lower prevalence rates. The Centers for Disease Control recommend that pregnant women who satisfy the following criteria should have at least one prenatal culture: age less than 20 years, unmarried, history of other sexually transmitted disease, multiple sexual consorts, or partner with multiple consorts (Bell and Grayston 1986).

10.3 Treatment

There have been no randomized controlled trials to guide management of women found to be colonized with *C trachomatis* during pregnancy. Tetracycline is contraindicated (Klatersky-Genot 1970). Erythromycin is generally considered to be the drug of choice, but the optimal dose, duration, and timing of antibiotic therapy have not been established. In an open study, using as controls patients who refused therapy, Schachter *et al.* (1986) showed a significantly lower prevalence of chlamydial infection in infants born of infected mothers treated with erythromycin 250 mg (base) 4 times daily for 7 days at the 36th week of pregnancy. A 9 per cent overall failure rate was reported for the 107 women who completed a course of therapy, and an additional 3 per cent of the women could not tolerate the medication. Sexual partners were treated concurrently. McMillan *et al.* (1985), treating women with 500 mg erythromycin twice a day for 10 days, demonstrated a lower prevalence of disease in the newborn infants compared with that among infants born to mothers who, for unstated reasons, did not receive treatment. This comparison is likely to be biased and the final numbers available for follow-up (35 of 85, or 39 per cent) were small.

10.4 Conclusions

Women with a history or findings suggestive of chlamydial disease should have a firm diagnosis established, using either antigen detection methods or cell culture. If a diagnosis of chlamydial infection is made during pregnancy, the condition should be treated. Erythromycin is currently the antibiotic of choice.

Screening of all pregnant women for chlamydial infection, with appropriate treatment of those identified, may reduce neonatal transmission and infant disease. The value of routine screening will depend crucially on the prevalence of the condition in the population being screened. If the prevalence is less than 6 per cent, routine screening is probably not justified.

Further study is needed of newer diagnostic tests in screening pregnant women for *C trachomatis* infection. The natural history of *C trachomatis* infections in pregnancy is unknown, and the role of the organism in the adverse outcomes of pregnancy remains to be clarified. A well-designed placebo-controlled trial is required to clarify the usefulness of screening for and treating this condition. As erythromycin is not completely effective in eradicating infection, and because some women cannot tolerate the drug, trials of effective alternatives are needed.

11 Herpes simplex

Herpes simplex infection of the newborn, acquired from the mother, is a rare, but potentially very serious condition, occurring in between 1 in 2500 and 1 in 10,000 births (Sullivan-Bolyai *et al.* 1983; Arvin *et al.*

1982; Yeager *et al.* 1980). Its clinical presentation varies widely, from asymptomatic, through involvement of only the skin, to involvement of the eye or nervous system, or widespread dissemination (Whitley *et al.* 1980b; Yeager and Arvin 1984). With brain involvement or disseminated disease, Herpes simplex infection is fatal in 15 to 50 per cent of cases, and survivors are left with residua, despite antiviral therapy (Whitley *et al.* 1980b; Offit *et al.* 1982).

Whitley and co-workers described the course of disease in 56 babies diagnosed as having neonatal Herpes simplex infection (Whitley *et al.* 1980b). Forty-six per cent of these neonates were born preterm, with associated problems of respiratory distress syndrome, bacterial infection, and hyperglycaemia. Seventy per cent of the infants presented with only skin lesions, but nearly three-quarters of these disseminated. Twenty per cent of infants presented with central nervous system and visceral involvement. These data may vastly overestimate the severity of disease, as diagnostic suspicion bias may lead to investigation only of the more severely affected infants.

Vertical transmission is thought to be the route of infection, with a transmission from mother to baby of 50 per cent in primary herpes infections (Nahmias *et al.* 1971). However, the risk of transmission from a mother with a history of recurrent genital herpes who is shedding herpes virus at the time of delivery has been estimated in one prospective study to be no higher than 8 per cent (Prober *et al.* 1987).

11.1 Diagnosis

Thirty-six per cent of pregnant women diagnosed to have Herpes simplex infection on cytologic screening also have characteristic genital vesicles or ulcers (Nahmias *et al.* 1971). An additional 21 per cent have signs and symptoms such as non-specific cervical inflammation, dysuria, and pelvic pain. Thus, suggestive clinical findings are present in only half the women who show cytologic evidence of disease.

Vontver and co-workers (1979) found that cytologic smears lead to the diagnosis of Herpes simplex in only 43 per cent of lesions from which the virus could be cultured. Similarly, serology was of value only when paired sera of initial infections were available. Brown *et al.* (1979) have confirmed these observations, but noted the high specificity of these smears. Thus, only evidence from cultures or from electron microscopic examination of specimens are adequate to exclude the disease. The presence of characteristic cytological findings, however, allows the condition to be diagnosed with confidence.

11.2 Screening for viral shedding

A recently published study (Arvin *et al.* 1986) describes the natural history of Herpes simplex colonization in women. Four hundred and fourteen pregnant women with a history of recurrent genital herpes underwent regular sampling for herpes virus cultures during late pregnancy. Only one of 17 asymptomatic women with positive antepartum cultures had herpes virus recovered at the time of delivery, and this woman had a herpetic lesion at that time. Furthermore, none of the 5 asymptomatic mother–infant pairs who were shedding herpes virus at the time of delivery had positive antepartum cultures, despite repeated sampling during the 4 weeks prior to delivery—the most proximal previous culture being taken 1 to 10 days prior to delivery. Even the week prior to delivery asymptomatic excretors were not the same as the asymptomatic excretors at the time of delivery. Twenty per cent of women with lesions or a prodrome did shed herpes virus. Thus, clinical assessment remains the best criterion for diagnosing herpes virus shedding.

An economic analysis comparing a screening policy that included viral culture or cytology during the last 4 to 8 weeks of pregnancy versus using only a weekly history and physical examination (Binkin *et al.* 1984) found that the cost per case averted through screening would be approximately US $1.8 million.

11.3 Peripartum care of women with Herpes simplex infection

There have been no randomized trials to evaluate clinical policies for care of women with herpes in pregnancy, and the evidence on which recommended policy is based is weak indeed. The current recommendations of the Committee on Infectious Diseases for the American Academy of Pediatrics (1988) have been modified in the light of the results of recent cohort studies (Arvin *et al.* 1986; Prober 1987; Prober 1988). The previous recommendations for weekly cervical screening with viral cultures during the last five weeks of pregancy have been withdrawn. All women with lesions or a prodrome at the time of delivery should undergo sampling, and the sample should be examined with an electron microscope for herpes virus. If the results are not available at the time of delivery, it would be appropriate to assume that the woman has a herpes virus infection, and a caesarean section should be performed to deliver the baby, unless the membranes have been ruptured for longer than 4 to 6 hours.

Although vidarabine has been shown to be effective in treatment of Herpes simplex infections in a number of randomized trials (Whitley *et al.* 1980a; Whitley *et al.* 1977), it has limited use in genital herpes because it is an insoluble agent that requires a large fluid volume for intravenous administration. In addition, it is neurotoxic and myelotoxic (Hirsh and Schooley 1983). In some experimental models, it was found to be teratogenic, mutagenic, and carcinogenic (Hirsh and Schooley 1983). Another antiviral agent, acyclovir, has been found to reduce duration of viral shedding in genital herpes infections, with maximal effect on clinical symptoms in primary cases (Corey *et al.* 1982a; Bryson *et al.* 1983; Corey *et al.* 1982b; Fiddian *et al.* 1982; Reichmann *et al.* 1982). These published studies have all been conducted on non-pregnant individuals. No trials of either drug therapy or clinical management regimens have been reported in pregnant women.

11.4 Conclusions

Clinical assessment by history and physical examination, rather than repeated cultures, is the most effective approach to identifying women who are shedding virus at the time of delivery. Caesarean section should only be carried out if there is both clinical evidence of active disease, and the membranes are either intact, or have only recently (within 4 to 6 hours) ruptured. Even in these circumstances, unnecessary caesarean sections can be avoided if electron microscopy reveals no evidence of viral shedding.

Further studies are needed to develop practical and rapid methods of detecting Herpes simplex shedding at the time of delivery. A randomized trial of the efficacy of acyclovir (or any other antiviral agent) in reducing the risk of transmission to the baby, or the use of caesarean section, is required (Bryson *et al.* 1983).

12 Group B streptococcus

Group B streptococcus (*Streptococcus agalactiae*), with an incidence of 0.6 to 3.7 cases per 1000 live births (Baker 1977), has become the most frequent cause of overwhelming sepsis in neonates. The early, and most serious, form of infection is characterized by rapid onset of respiratory distress, sepsis, and shock. In this form, serotypes found in the maternal introital cultures are identical to those producing invasive disease in their infants, suggesting that transmission from mother to fetus is the most important route of spread (Anthony *et al.* 1979). The likelihood of disease, which occurs in 1 to 2 per cent of colonized babies, is directly related to the number of sites colonized and the density of colonization (Siegel and McCracken 1981). Infants with birthweights of less than 2500 g were observed by Boyer *et al.* (1983) to have a much higher overall attack rate, 7.9 per 1000 births vs. 1.9 per 1000 births of infants weighing 2500 g or more.

Attempts to prevent disease by antibiotics given to either all babies, or those considered to be at high risk, have proved disappointing. Three trials of antibiotics administered to the neonate with a view to reducing the incidence of group B streptococcal sepsis have been reported (Siegel *et al.* 1980, 1982; Pyati 1983; Gerard 1979). The available data suggest that infant sepsis with group B streptococcus can be reduced with antibiotic prophylaxis given to the baby (Table 34.10). Only 1 trial however (Pyati *et al.* 1983), reports data on deaths from group B streptococcus; there were 6 deaths in the antibiotic group and 8 in the control group (Table 34.11).

Based on the only trial for which this information has been made available (Siegel *et al.* 1980, 1982), antibiotic prophylaxis in the neonate was accompanied by an increase in sepsis with penicillin-resistant organisms (Table 34.12), and this resulted in a higher rate of deaths from infection in the neonates given antibiotics (Table 34.13). (Only total neonatal deaths, rather than total deaths from infection were reported for the trials by Pyati and Gerard; these were less frequent in the experimental group, but this difference was compatible with the play of chance (Table 34.14).)

Since attempts at prophylaxis after the baby has been delivered may be too late, attention has focused on studies of the effectiveness of antepartum and intrapartum antibiotics. An understanding of the natural history of group B streptococcal carriage is important for the interpretation of these studies. Sampling of the genital tract at any time between conception and delivery has revealed that between 5 and 25 per cent of

Table 34.10 Effect of prophylactic antibiotics for group B streptococcus in neonates on infant sepsis with group B streptococcus

Study	EXPT		CTRL		Odds ratio	Graph of odds ratios and confidence intervals
	n	(%)	*n*	(%)	(95% CI)	0.01 0.1 0.5 1 2 10 100
Pyati *et al.* (1983)	10/589	(1.70)	14/598	(2.34)	0.72 (0.32–1.62)	
Siegel *et al.* (1982)	10/16082	(0.06)	24/15976	(0.15)	0.44 (0.22–0.85)	
Gerard *et al.* (1979)	0/29	(0.00)	0/38	(0.00)	1.00 (1.00–1.00)	
Typical odds ratio (95% confidence interval)					0.54 (0.32–0.90)	

Table 34.11 Effect of prophylactic antibiotics for group B Streptococcus in neonates on neonatal deaths from group B Streptococcus

Study	EXPT		CTRL		Odds ratio	Graph of odds ratios and confidence intervals
	n	(%)	*n*	(%)	(95% CI)	0.01 0.1 0.5 1 2 10 100
Pyati *et al.* (1983)	6/589	(1.02)	8/598	(1.34)	0.76 (0.27–2.18)	
Typical odds ratio (95% confidence interval)					0.76 (0.27–2.18)	

Table 34.12 Effect of prophylactic antibiotics for group B Streptococcus in neonates on infant sepsis (penicillin resistant organisms)

Study	EXPT		CTRL		Odds ratio	Graph of odds ratios and confidence intervals
	n	(%)	*n*	(%)	(95% CI)	0.01 0.1 0.5 1 2 10 100
Siegel *et al.* (1982)	35/16082	(0.22)	26/15976	(0.16)	1.34 (0.81–2.21)	
Typical odds ratio (95% confidence interval)					1.34 (0.81–2.21)	

Table 34.13 Effect of prophylactic antibiotics for group B streptococcus in neonates on neonatal infectious deaths—all organisms

Study	EXPT		CTRL		Odds ratio	Graph of odds ratios and confidence intervals
	n	(%)	*n*	(%)	(95% CI)	0.01 0.1 0.5 1 2 10 100
Siegel *et al.* (1982)	18/16082	(0.11)	11/15976	(0.07)	1.61 (0.78–3.34)	
Typical odds ratio (95% confidence interval)					1.61 (0.78–3.34)	

pregnant women carry the organism. Three studies reported longitudinal follow-up of women found to be colonized (Anthony *et al.* 1978; Dillon *et al.* 1982; Hoogkamp-Korstanje *et al.* 1982). Anthony *et al.* (1978) reported on 382 women who had submitted four or more cultures in his protocol of 9 specimens. The overall carriage rate was 12 per cent. Over a third of the women in whom group B streptococci were recovered from initial cultures had lost these bacteria by the time of delivery. Approximately the same number who had initially been culture negative had acquired the organism by the time of delivery. Two other studies (Dillon *et al.* 1982; Hoogkamp-Korstanje *et al.* 1982) that employed anorectal specimens as well as vaginal specimens confirmed the lack of persistence of carriage.

Hall *et al.* (1976), in the only reported randomized trial of a course of antibiotics during pregnancy, found only a temporary eradication of group B streptococcal carriage, after a 7 day course of ampicillin administered during the 3rd trimester with no detectable effects on infant colonization (Table 34.15), or sepsis with group B streptococcus (Table 34.16). Merenstein and co-

Table 34.14 Effect of prophylactic antibiotics for group B streptococcus in neonates on all neonatal deaths

Study	EXPT		CTRL		Odds ratio	Graph of odds ratios and confidence intervals
	n	(%)	*n*	(%)	(95% CI)	0.01 0.1 0.5 1 2 10 100
Pyati *et al.* (1983)	49/589	(8.32)	64/598	(10.70)	0.76 (0.51–1.12)	
Gerard *et al.* (1979)	0/29	(0.00)	0/38	(0.00)	1.00 (1.00–1.00)	
Typical odds ratio (95% confidence interval)					0.76 (0.51–1.12)	

Table 34.15 Effect of antepartum antibiotics for group B streptococcus on infant colonization with group B streptococcus

Study	EXPT		CTRL		Odds ratio	Graph of odds ratios and confidence intervals
	n	(%)	*n*	(%)	(95% CI)	0.01 0.1 0.5 1 2 10 100
Hall *et al.* (1976)	6/25	(24.00)	10/33	(30.30)	0.73 (0.23–2.32)	
Typical odds ratio (95% confidence interval)					0.73 (0.23–2.32)	

Table 34.16 Effect of antepartum antibiotics for group B streptococcus on group B streptococcus sepsis

Study	EXPT		CTRL		Odds ratio	Graph of odds ratios and confidence intervals
	n	(%)	*n*	(%)	(95% CI)	0.01 0.1 0.5 1 2 10 100
Hall *et al.* (1976)	1/25	(4.00)	1/33	(3.03)	1.33 (0.08–22.41)	
Typical odds ratio (95% confidence interval)					1.33 (0.08–22.41)	

workers (1980), on the other hand, by treating women with either oral ampicillin or erythromycin from the 38th week of gestation right through to delivery, were able to reduce both maternal and infant colonization at delivery in these women significantly compared to a randomized no-treatment control group.

It thus appears that treatment during pregnancy, unless continued into labour, can have only a transient effect on the vaginal flora, and will not influence the rate of infant sepsis. It is quite likely, then, that screening during pregnancy and treatment of carriers may not eliminate the transmission of group B streptococcal disease (Anthony 1982).

Identification of carriage in the intrapartum period may be the ideal method of screening, as 58 per cent of infants born to mothers who are carriers during labour will be colonized with group B streptococcus, compared with only 12 per cent of infants born to culture negative mothers (Anthony *et al.* 1979).

Such screening would only be helpful if intrapartum antibiotics are efficacious in the prevention of transmission of infection from mother to baby. Five randomized controlled trials (Merenstein 1980; Easmon *et al.* 1983; Boyer *et al.* 1983; Lim *et al.* 1986 and Morales *et al.* 1986; Teres *et al.* 1987) have demonstrated a major reduction in group B streptococcus colonization in infants born to mothers treated with intrapartum antibiotics compared with infants of control mothers (Table 34.17). Even more importantly, infant sepsis with group B streptococcus was reduced in the treated groups in the 3 trials that reported sepsis rates (Table 34.18). The available data show a reduction in neonatal deaths from infection (Table 34.19). Boyer's study is perhaps the most interesting, as it demonstrates an effect of prophylaxis in a group of preterm infants—the subgroup most at risk for adverse sequelae.

As intrapartum prophylaxis of colonized pregnant women offers the possibility of reducing the incidence of infant sepsis, rapid methods for screening women in preterm labour are desirable. Lim and co-workers,

Table 34.17 Effect of intrapartum antibiotics for group B streptococcus on infant colonization with group B streptococcus

Study	EXPT		CTRL		Odds ratio	Graph of odds ratios and confidence intervals
	n	(%)	*n*	(%)	(95% CI)	0.01 0.1 0.5 1 2 10 100
Boyer and Gotoff (1986)	8/85	(9.41)	40/79	(50.63)	0.14 (0.07–0.27)	
Lim *et al.* (1986)	0/27	(0.00)	16/21	(76.19)	0.03 (0.01–0.12)	
Easmon *et al.* (1983)	1/38	(2.63)	22/49	(44.90)	0.12 (0.04–0.30)	
Merenstein *et al.* (1980)	0/20	(0.00)	8/24	(33.33)	0.11 (0.02–0.51)	
Typical odds ratio (95% confidence interval)					0.10 (0.07–0.15)	

Table 34.18 Effect of intrapartum antibiotics for group B streptococcus on infant sepsis with group B streptococcus

Study	EXPT		CTRL		Odds ratio	Graph of odds ratios and confidence intervals
	n	(%)	*n*	(%)	(95% CI)	0.01 0.1 0.5 1 2 10 100
Boyer and Gotoff (1986)	0/85	(0.00)	5/79	(6.33)	0.12 (0.02–0.70)	
Lim *et al.* (1986)	0/101	(0.00)	6/93	(6.45)	0.12 (0.02–0.60)	
Merenstein *et al.* (1980)	0/20	(0.00)	1/24	(4.17)	0.16 (0.00–8.19)	
Typical odds ratio (95% confidence interval)					0.12 (0.08–0.50)	

Table 34.19 Effect of intrapartum antibiotics for group B streptococcus on neonatal deaths from infection

Study	EXPT		CTRL		Odds ratio	Graph of odds ratios and confidence intervals
	n	(%)	*n*	(%)	(95% CI)	0.01 0.1 0.5 1 2 10 100
Boyer and Gotoff (1986)	0/85	(0.00)	2/79	(2.53)	0.12 (0.01–2.00)	
Lim *et al.* (1986)	0/101	(0.00)	0/93	(0.00)	1.00 (1.00–1.00)	
Merenstein *et al.* (1980)	0/20	(0.00)	0/24	(0.00)	1.00 (1.00–1.00)	
Typical odds ratio (95% confidence interval)					0.12 (0.01–2.00)	

using a modified broth culture and co-agglutination tests, were able to identify group B streptococcal colonized women relatively rapidly during the late 3rd trimester (Lim *et al.* 1986). By examining specimens after 5 and 20 hours of incubation, they differentiated lightly colonized from heavily colonized women. Expanding on their initial work with co-agglutination, these workers found a dose–response relationship between amount of colonization and time to identification. Heavily colonized women demonstrated a positive test within 5 hours, while others required 20 hours of incubation before their test became positive (Lim *et al.* 1987).

Reardon *et al.* (1984) examined the efficacy of a colorimetric method using a starch serum broth (Noble *et al.* 1983) in the identification of group B streptococci in the vaginal swabs obtained from 414 women. Group B streptococci are uniquely able to produce an orange carotenoid pigment under anaerobic conditions in broth culture. In this study, the colour change was 95 per cent sensitive and 99 per cent specific when compared to bacterial isolation. Noble's media required 12 hours for the colorimetric change to occur. A modified medium, with increased starch and serum content, only requires 6 hours, and has the potential advantage over co-agglutination of being interpretable by lay personnel (Wang *et al.* 1988). Other investigators have used direct examination of vaginal smears with Gram's stains and observed close to 100 per cent sensitivity and 67 per cent specificity (Holls *et al.* 1987; Feld *et al.* 1987). Latex particle agglutination tests, on the other hand, have a low sensitivity but high specificity, approximating 40 per cent and 99 per cent, respectively (Wald *et al.* 1987).

Conclusions

The efficacy of intrapartum administration of antibiotics in preventing neonatal sepsis with group B streptococcus has been clearly established. Antepartum or neonatal administration of antibiotics is relatively ineffective. For a pregnant woman in preterm labour, or a woman with either intrapartum fever or prolonged rupture of membranes, a vaginal sample should be obtained for rapid diagnosis, if this test is available. The woman should receive intrapartum intravenous ampicillin (or erythromycin if penicillin allergic) if either the test is positive or the result is unavailable.

The identification of the high risk patient remains a problem. Further studies using the new rapid diagnostic techniques should be tested in the labour and delivery suite so that results may be interpreted by the staff who are looking after patients. A cost–effectiveness evaluation incorporating such diagnostic techniques with chemoprophylaxis is required.

13 Acquired immunodeficiency syndrome

Acquired immunodeficiency syndrome has recently been identified as a major health problem, characterized by defects in the immune system, with attendant susceptibility to infections by opportunistic micro-organisms and specific tumours (Pinching and Jefferies 1985). As of May 1987, the total number of cases reported world-wide was 48,478 (LCDC 1987). This is an underestimate of the true number, because the last date of report for some countries was more than 6 months earlier, and diagnostic and reporting capabilities vary from country to country. Three-year survival after development of this disease is still practically nil, despite some promising chemotherapeutic agents, including interferon and azidothymidine (AZT).

Paediatric acquired immunodeficiency syndrome was first recognized in 1982 (MMWR 1982) and numerous case series have been reported since (Oleske *et al.* 1983; Rubinstein *et al.* 1983; Scott *et al.* 1984). The virus may be transmitted *in utero* and has been associated with a fetopathy, with characteristic dysmorphic features (Rubinstein and Bernstein 1986). The condition may present with recurrent bacterial infections and sepsis, persistent or recurrent thrush, and failure to thrive. Many of the infants are born preterm or small for gestational age, although this may be due to associated maternal risk factors. Later symptoms include lymphadenopathy, hepatosplenomegaly, chronic or recurrent diarrhoea, chronic pneumonitis, and salivary gland enlargement (Rubinstein and Bernstein 1986).

The aetiologic agent for this syndrome belongs to the retrovirus family and has been renamed human immunodeficiency virus-1 (HIV-1). Other names include lymphadenopathy associated virus (LAV) and human T lymphotrophic virus-III (HTLV-III) (Ziegler *et al.* 1985).

The organism in adults is usually transmitted sexually, but is also transmitted through blood and blood products, or by sharing needles. In paediatric cases, transmission may also occur from mother to infant, and this may occur *in utero* or peripartum (Rubinstein and Bernstein 1986), and through breast milk (Ziegler *et al.* 1985). Other studies have reported transmission rates from mother to baby of 50–65 per cent, the latter figure for women who had previously given birth to an affected infant (Scott *et al.* 1985a,b; Blanche *et al.* 1986).

Both asymptomatic and symptomatic women may transmit the infection to their infants. In one study, disease developed in mothers up to four years after the birth of the affected infant (Scott *et al.* 1985a,b). Thus, all women who belong to a risk group (see below) should be screened, not just those who are symptomatic. In addition, women who have had one affected infant may have subsequent infected infants (Scott *et al.* 1985a,b).

Screening should be offered to all women who belong to a high risk group for having a retroviral infection. Such women include:

(a) Those with evidence of HIV infection;

(b) Illicit intravenous drug users;

(c) Those born in countries with a high incidence of heterosexual transmission of acquired immunodeficiency syndrome;

(d) Those with a history of prostitution;

(e) Sex partners of illicit intravenous drug users, bisexual men, haemophiliacs, men born in countries with a high incidence of heterosexually transmitted acquired immunodeficiency syndrome.

There is no proven efficacious treatment for acquired immunodeficiency syndrome. Clinical trials are currently being conducted to study a number of drugs. Women who are found to carry the virus should be advised against pregnancy, or even to terminate pregnancy (Minkoff and Schwarz 1986).

More studies are needed to assess the risk of transmission of this disease from mother to baby. As newer agents are found to be efficacious in other populations, their use may be attempted in pregnant women and infants, although because of fetal risks, it may still be prudent to recommend abortion in infected women.

14 Conclusions

A review of the major infections which may complicate pregnancy and childbirth has been presented using data from studies which have been found to be methodologically sound. We have concentrated on infections in developed countries that are important either in terms of their incidence or associated morbidity.

Clear-cut recommendations can be made for the management of some specific infections, such as the treatment of vaginal candidiasis, and the inappropriateness of screening for this organism. As efficacious agents are identified, better forms of therapy, which may be less expensive or more convenient, must be tested through clinical trials, as illustrated in the studies on short course therapy for urinary tract infections. For many more situations, the basic information on which to make recommendations is simply not available. This includes the role of mycoplasmas in a number of postpartum complications, and the incidence of toxoplasma infection. Thus, for many situations, further therapeutic trials and economic analyses are necessary when developing management guidelines.

References

Section 1: Introduction

Morley D, Woodland M, Cuthbertson WFJ (1964). Controlled trial of pyrimethamine in pregnant women in an African village. Br Med J, 1: 667–668.

Smith JA, Jennison RF, Langley FA (1956). Perinatal infection and perinatal death. Clinical aspects. Lancet, 2: 903–906.

Section 2: Bacteriuria

Bailey RR, Bishop V, Peddie BA (1983). Comparison of a single dose with a 5-day course of co-trimoxazole for asymptomatic (covert) bacteriuria of pregnancy. Austral NZ J Obstet Gynaecol, 23: 139–141.

Bailey RR, Peddie BA, Bishop V (1986). Comparison of single dose with a five-day course of trimethoprim for asymptomatic (covert). bacteriuria of pregnancy. NZ Med J, 99: 501–503.

Brumfitt W, Franklin I, Hamilton-Miller J, Anderson F (1979). Comparison of pivmecillinam and cephadrine in bacteriuria in pregnancy and in acute urinary tract infection. Scand J Infect Dis, 11: 275–279.

Campos-Outcalt DE, Corta PJ (1985). Screening for asymptomatic bacteriuria in pregnancy. J Family Practice, 20: 589–591.

Chng PK, Hall MH (1982). Antenatal prediction of urinary tract infection in pregnancy. Br J Obstet Gynaecol, 89: 8–11.

Chow AW, Jewesson PJ (1985). Pharmacokinetics and safety of antimicrobial agents during pregnancy. Rev Infect Dis, 7: 287–313.

Cunningham FG, Morris GB, Mickal A (1973). Acute pyelonephritis of pregnancy: A clinical review. Obstet Gynecol, 42: 112–117.

Davis JR, Stager CE (1985). Detection of asymptomatic bacteriuria in obstetric patients with a semiautomated urine screen. Am J Obstet Gynecol, 151: 1069–1073.

Dixon HG, Brant HA (1967). The significance of bacteriuria in pregnancy. Lancet, 1: 19–20.

Elder HA, Santamarina BAG, Smith S, Kass EH (1971). The natural history of asymptomatic bacteriuria during pregnancy: The effect of tetracycline on the clinical course and the outcome of pregnancy. Am J Obstet Gynecol, 111: 441–462.

Furness ET, McDonald PJ, Beasley NV (1975). Urinary antiseptics in asymptomatic bacteriuria of pregnancy. NZ Med J, 81: 417–419.

Gilstrap LC, Cunningham FG, Whalley PJ (1981a). Acute pyelonephritis in pregnancy: An anterospective study. Obstet Gynecol, 57: 409–413.

Gilstrap LC, Leveno KJ, Cunningham FG, Whalley PJ, Roark ML (1981b). Renal infection and pregnancy outcome. Am J Obstet Gynecol, 141: 709–716.

Gold EM, Traub FB, Daichman I, Terris M (1966). Asymptomatic bacteriuria during pregnancy. Obstet Gynecol, 27: 206–209.

Harris RE (1979). The significance of eradication of bacteriuria during pregnancy. Obstet Gynecol, 53: 71–73.

Harris RE, Gilstrap LC (1974). Prevention of recurrent pyelonephritis during pregnancy. Obstet Gynecol, 44: 637–641.

Harris RE, Gilstrap LC (1981). Cystitis during pregnancy: A distinct clinical entity. Obstet Gynecol, 57: 578–580.

Harris RE, Gilstrap LC, Pretty A (1982). Single-dose antimicrobial therapy for asymptomatic bacteriuria during pregnancy. Obstet Gynecol, 59: 546–548.

Kass EH (1959). Bacteriuria and pyelonephritis of pregnancy. AMA Arch Intern Med, 105: 194–198.

Kass EH (1960). The role of asymptomatic bacteriuria in the pathogenesis of pyelonephritis. In: Biology of Pyelonephritis. Quinn EL, Kass EH (eds). Boston: Little, Brown, pp 399–412.

Kass EH, Platt R (1984). Urinary tract and genital mycoplasmal infection. In: Antenatal and Neonatal Screening. Wald NJ (ed). Oxford: Oxford University Press, pp 345–357.

Kincaid-Smith P, Bullen M (1965). Bacteriuria in pregnancy. Lancet, 1: 395–399.

Lawson DH, Miller AWF (1971). Screening for bacteriuria in pregnancy. Lancet, 1: 9–11.

Lenke RR, Van Dorsten JP, Schifrin BS (1983). Pyelonephritis in pregnancy: A prospective randomized trial to prevent recurrent disease evaluating suppressive therapy with nitrofurantoin and close surveillance. Am J Obstet Gynecol, 146: 953–957.

Little PJ (1966). The incidence of urinary tract infection in 5000 pregnant women. Lancet; 2: 925–928.

Masterton RG, Evans DC, Strike PW (1985). Single-dose amoxycillin in the treatment of bacteriuria of pregnancy and the puerperium—a controlled clinical trial. Br J Obstet Gynaecol, 92: 498–505.

McFadyen IR, Eykyn SJ, Gardner NHN, Vanier TM, Bennett AE, Mayo ME, Lloyd-Davies RW (1973). Bacteriuria in pregnancy. J Obstet Gynaecol Br Commnwlth, 80: 385–405.

McGrady GA, Daling JR, Peterson DR (1985). Maternal urinary tract infection and adverse fetal outcomes. Am J Epidemiol, 121: 377–381.

Mulla N (1960). Bacteriuria in pregnancy. Obstet Gynecol, 16: 89–92.

Naeye RL (1979). Causes of the excessive rates of perinatal mortality and prematurity in pregnancies complicated by maternal urinary tract infections. New Engl J Med, 300: 819–823.

Pedler SJ, Bint AJ (1985). Comparative study of amoxicillin-clavulanic acid and cephalexin in the treatment of bacteriuria during pregnancy. Antimicrob Agents Chemother, 27: 508–510.

Reeves DS (1975). Laboratory and clinical studies with sulfametopyrazine as a treatment for bacteriuria in pregnancy. J Antimicrob Chemother, 1: 171–186.

Sever JL, Ellenberg JH, Edmonds D (1979). Urinary tract infections during pregnancy: Maternal and pediatric findings. In: Infections of the Urinary Tract. Kass EH, Brumfitt W (eds). Chicago: University of Chicago Press, pp 19–21.

Soisson AP, Watson WJ, Benson WL, Read JA (1985). Value of a screening urinalysis in pregnancy. J Reprod Med, 30: 588–590.

Souney P, Polk BF (1982). Single-dose antimicrobial therapy for urinary tract infections in women. Rev Infect Dis, 4: 29–34.

Stamm WE, Wagner KF, Amsel R, Alexander ER, Turck M, Counts GW, Holmes KK (1980). Causes of the acute urethral syndrome in women. New Engl J Med, 303: 409–415.

Thomsen AC, Mørup L, Brogard-Hansen K (1987). Antibiotic elimination of Group-B streptrococci in urine in prevention of preterm labour. Lancet, 1: 591–593.

Whalley P (1967). Bacteriuria of pregnancy. Am J Obstet Gynecol, 97: 723–738.

Whalley PJ, Cunningham FG (1977). Short-term versus continuous antimicrobial therapy for asymptomatic bacteriuria in pregnancy. Obstet Gynecol, 49: 262–265.

Williams GL, Campbell H, Davies KJ (1969). Urinary concentrating ability in women with asymptomatic bacteriuria in pregnancy. Br Med J, 3: 212–215.

Williams JD, Reeves DS, Condie AP, Brumfitt W (1979). Significance of bacteriuria in pregnancy. In: Infections of the Urinary Tract. Kass EH, Brumfitt W (eds). Chicago: University of Chicago Press, pp 8–18.

Zinner SH, Kass EH (1971). Long term (10–14 years) follow up of bacteriuria of pregnancy. New Engl J Med, 285: 820–824.

Section 3: Syphilis

Bellingham FR (1973). Syphilis in pregnancy: Transplacental infection. Med J Austral, 2: 647–648.

Centers for Disease Control (1979). Criteria and techniques for the diagnosis of early syphilis. Atlanta: Department of Health, Education and Welfare Publication No. 98, p 386.

Daniels KC, Ferneyhough HS (1977). Specific direct fluorescent antibody detection of Treponema pallidum. Health Lab Sci, 14: 164–171.

Felman YM (1978). Should premarital syphilis serologies continue to be mandated by law? JAMA, 240: 459–460.

Hart G (1986). Syphilis tests in diagnostic and therapeutic decision making. Ann Intern Med, 104: 368–376.

Harter CA, Benirschke K (1976). Fetal syphilis in the first trimester. Am J Obstet Gynecol, 124: 705–711.

Rathbun KC (1983). Congenital syphilis: A proposal for improved surveillance, diagnosis, and treatment. Sex Transm Dis, 10: 93–99, 102–107.

Skarpaas T, Loe K (1980). Positive serologic syphilis reactions among pregnant women in Norway, 1964–1978. Tidsskr Nor Laegefor, 199: 1840–1843.

Stray-Pedersen B (1983). Economic evaluation of maternal screening to prevent congenital syphilis. Sex Transm Dis, 10: 167–172.

Williams K (1985). Screening for syphilis in pregnancy: An assessment of the costs and benefits. Community Medicine, 7: 37–42.

Section 4: Gonorrhoea

Aardoom HA, Hoop DD, Iserief SOA, Michel MF, Stolz E (1982). Detection of Neisseria gonorrhoea antigen by solid-phase enzyme immunoassay. Br J Vener Dis, 58: 359–362.

Alexander ER (1984). Maternal and infant sexually transmitted diseases. Urolog Clin North America, 11: 131–139.

American Academy of Pediatrics, Committee on Drugs, Committee on Fetus and Newborn, Committee on Infectious Diseases (1980). Prophylaxis and treatment of neonatal gonococcal infection. Pediatrics, 65: 1047–1048.

Armstrong JH, Zacharias F, Rein MF (1976). Ophthalmia neonatorum: A chart review. Pediatrics, 57: 884–892.

Barlow D, Phillips I (1978). Gonorrhea in women: Diagnostic, clinical, and laboratory aspects. Lancet, 1: 761–764.

Brown WM, Cowper HH, Hodgman JE (1966). Gonococcal ophthalmia among newborn infants at Los Angeles County General Hospital, 1957–1963. Public Health Rep, 81: 926–928.

Brunham RC, Holmes KK, Eschenback D (1984). Sexually Transmitted Diseases. New York: McGraw-Hill, pp 782–815.

Chacko MR, Phillips S, Jacobson MS (1982). Screening for

pharyngeal gonorrhoea in the urban teenager. Pediatrics, 70: 620–623.

Charles AG, Cohen S, Kass MB, Richman R (1970). Asymptomatic gonorrhea in prenatal patients. Am J Obstet Gynecol, 108: 595–599.

Crede CSF (1881). Die verhütung der augenent-sündung der Neugeborenen. Arch Gynäkol, 17: 50–53.

Davis CH (1945). Gonorrhoeal arthritis complicating pregnancy treated with penicillin. Am J Obstet Gynecol, 50: 215–218.

Duke-Elder S (1965). System of Ophthalmology. VIII. Disease of the Outer Eye. St Louis: Mosby, pp 115–127, 167–174.

Edward L, Barrada MI, Hamann AA, Hakanson EY (1978). Gonorrhea in pregnancy. Am J Obstet Gynecol, 132: 637–641.

Goobar JE, Clark GM (1964). Rheumatological manifestation of gonorrhoea. Arch Interamer Rheumatol, 7: 1–24.

Hammerschlag MR, Chandler JW, Alexander R, English M, Chiang WT, Koutsky L, Eschenbach DA, Smith JR (1980). Erythromycin ointment for ocular prophylaxis of neonatal chlamydial infection. JAMA, 244: 2291–2293.

Holmes KK (1983). Gonococcal infection. In: Infectious Diseases in the Fetus and Newborn. Remington JS, Klein JO (eds). Philadelphia: W B Saunders, pp 619–635.

Holmes KK, Counts GW, Beatty HN (1971). Disseminated gonococcal infection. Ann Intern Med, 74: 979–993.

Holmes KK, Buchanan TM, Adam JL, Eschenback DA (1978). Is serology useful in gonorrhea? A critical analysis of factors influencing serodiagnosis. In: Immunobiology of Neisseria Gonorrhoeae. Brooks GF, Gotslich EC, Holmes KK, Sawyer WD, Young FE (eds). Washington, DC: American Society for Microbiology, pp. 370–376.

Hook EW, Holmes KK (1985). Gonococcal infections. Ann Intern Med, 102: 229–243.

Jacobs NF, Kraus SF (1975). Gonococcal and nongonococcal urethritis in men: Clinical and laboratory differentiation. Ann Intern Med, 82: 7–12.

Jaffe HW, Kraus SJ, Edwards TA, Weinberger SS, Zubrzycki (1982). Diagnosis of gonorrhea using a genetic transformation test on mailed clinical specimens. J Infect Dis, 146: 275–279.

Lewis PM (1946). Penicillin in gonococcic conjunctivitis: Its use in 30 cases, compared with sulfonamides in 173 cases. Am J Ophthalmol, 29: 694–698.

Mellin GW, Kent MP (1958). Ophthalmia neonatorum: Is prophylaxis necessary? Pediatrics, 22: 1006–1015.

Niles JH, Lowe EW (1966). Gonococcal arthritis in pregnancy. Med Ann DC, 35: 69, 70, 74.

O'Brien NG, O'Connell E (1972). Gonococcal ophthalmia. J Irish Med J, 65: 370–371.

Otiti JML (1975). Ophthalmia neonatorum in Mbale Hospital, Uganda. E Afr Med J, 52: 644–647.

Podgore JK, Holmes KK (1981). Ocular gonococcal infection with minimal or no inflammatory response. JAMA, 246: 242–243.

Rothenberg (1979). Ophthalmia neonatorum due to Neisseria gonorrhoeae: Prevention and treatment. Sex Transm Dis, 6 (Suppl): 187–190.

Rubin GL, Peterson HB, Dorfman SF, Layde PM, Maze JM, Ory HW, Cates W (1983). Ectopic pregnancy in the United States. 1970 through 1978. JAMA, 249: 1725–729.

Russell P (1979). Inflammatory lesions of the human placenta: I. Clinical significance of acute chorioamnionitis. Am J Diagn Gynecol Obstet, 1: 127–132.

Sandström KI, Bell TA, Chandler JW, Wang, SP, Kuo C-C, Foy HM, Grayston JT, Cooney M, Smith AL, Holmes KK (1982). Diagnosis of neonatal purulent conjunctivitis caused by Chlamydia trachomatis and other organisms. In: Chlamydial Infections. Mardh PA, Holmes KK, Oriel JD, Piot P, Schachter J (eds). New York: Elsevier Biomedical, pp 217–220.

Sarrell PM, Pruett KA (1968). Symptomatic gonorrhea during pregnancy. Obstet Gynecol, 32: 670–673.

Smith CA, Halse L (1955). Ophthalmia neonatorum. Public Health Rep, 70: 462–470.

Smith JA (1969). Ophthalmia neonatorum in Glasgow. Scottish Med J, 14: 272–276.

Stamm WE, Cole B, Fennell C, Bonin P, Armstrong As, Herrmann JE, Holmes KK (1984). Antigen detection for the diagnosis of gonorrhea. J Clin Microbiol, 19: 399–403.

Taylor HA, Bradford SA, Patterson SP (1966). Gonococcal arthritis in pregnancy. Obstet Gynecol, 27: 766–782.

Totten PA, Holmes KK, Handsfield HH, Knapp JS, Perine PL, Falkowd S (1983). DNA hybridization technique for the detection of Neisseria gonorrhoeae in men with urethritis. J Infect Dis, 148: 462–471.

Valenton MJ, Abendanio R (1973). Gonorrheal conjunctivitis. Can J Ophthalmol, 8: 421–427.

Young H, Sarafian SK, McMillan A (1981). Reactivity of the limulus lysate assay with uterine cervical secretions: A preliminary evaluation. Br J Vener Dis, 57: 200–203.

Section 5: Rubella

Appell MW (1985). The multihandicapped child with congenital rubella: Impact on family and community. Rev Infect Dis, 7: S17-S21.

Balfour HH, Groth KE, Edelman CK, Amren DP, Best JM, Banatvala JE (1981). Rubella viraemia and antibody responses after rubella vaccination and reimmunization. Lancet, 1: 1078–1080.

Banatvala JE (1985). Rubella—continuing problems. Br J Obstet Gynaecol, 92: 193–196.

Centers for Disease Control (1984). Rubella prevention. Morbidity Mortality Weekly Review, 33: 301–318.

Centers for Disease Control (1986). Rubella and congenital rubella syndrome—United States, 1984–1985. Morbidity Mortality Weekly Review, 35: 129–135.

Dales LG, Chin J (1982). Public health implications of rubella antibody levels in California. Am J Public Health, 72: 167–172.

Davis WJ, Larson HE, Simsarian JP (1971). A study of rubella immunity and resistance to infection. JAMA, 215: 600–608.

Dudgeon JA (1985). Selective immunization: Protection of the individual. Rev Infect Dis, 7: S185-S190.

Eilard T, Strannegard O (1974). Rubella reinfection in pregnancy followed by transmission to the fetus. J Infect Dis, 129: 594–596.

Enders G (1985). Serologic test combinations for safe detection of rubella infections. Rev Infect Dis, 7: S113-S122.

Fogel A, Handsher R, Barnea B (1985). Subclinical rubella in pregnancy—occurrence and outcome. Israel J Med Science, 21: 133–138.

Forsgren M, Soren L (1985). Subclinical rubella reinfection in vaccinated women with rubella-specific IgM response during pregnancy and transmission of virus to the fetus. Scand J Infect Dis, 17: 337–341.

Greaves WL, Orenstein WA, Hinman AR, Nersesian WS (1983). Clinical efficacy of rubella vaccine. Pediatr Infect Dis, 2: 284–286.

Herrmann KL (1985). Available rubella serologic tests. Rev Infect Dis, 7: S108-S112.

Herrmann KL, Halstead SB, Wiebenga NH (1982). Rubella antibody persistence after immunization. JAMA, 247: 193–196.

Horstmann DM, Schluederberg A, Emmons JE, Evans BK, Randolph MR, Andiman WA (1985). Persistence of vaccine-induced immune responses to rubella—comparison with natural infection. Rev Infect Dis, 7: S80-S85.

Meyer HM, Parkman PD, Hopps HE (1972). The clinical application of laboratory diagnostic procedures for rubella and measles (rubeola). Am J Clin Path, 57: 803–812.

Miller E, Cradock-Watson JE, Pollock TM (1982). Consequences of confirmed maternal rubella at successive stages of pregnancy. Lancet, 2: 781–784.

Morgan-Capner P, Hodgson J, Hambling MH, Dulake C, Coleman TJ, Boswell PA, Watkins RP, Booth J, Stern H, Best JM, Banatrala JE (1985). Detection of rubella-specific IgM in subclinical rubella reinfection in pregnancy. Lancet, 1: 244–246.

Office of Population Censuses and Surveys (1983). Rubella associated terminations of pregnancy. Document No. AB 83/4.

Orenstein WA, Bart KJ, Hinman AR, Preblud SR, Greaves WL, Doster SW, Stetler HC, Sirotkin B (1984). The opportunity and obligation to eliminate rubella from the United States. JAMA, 251: 1988–1994.

O'Shea S, Best JM, Banatvala JE, Marshall WC, Dudgeon JA (1982). Rubella vaccination: Persistence of antibodies for up to 16 years. Br Med J, 285: 253–255.

O'Shea S, Best JM, Banatvala JE (1983). Viremia, virus excretion and antibody responses after challenge in volunteers with low levels of antibody to rubella virus. J Infect Dis, 148: 639–647.

Polk BF, Modlin JF, White JA, De Girolami PC (1982). A controlled comparison of joint reaction among women receiving one of two rubella vaccines. Am J Epidemiol, 115: 19–25.

Preblud SR, Williams NM (1985). Fetal risk associated with rubella vaccine: Implications for vaccination of susceptible women. Obstet Gynecol, 66: 121–123.

Robinson RG, Dudenhoeffer FE, Horoyd HJ, Baker LR, Bernstein DI, Cherry JD (1982). Rubella immunity in older children, teenagers and young adults: A comparison of immunity in those previously immunized with those unimmunized. J Pediatr, 101: 188–191.

Schiff GM (1969). Titered lots of immune globulin. Efficacy in the prevention of rubella. Am J Dis Child, 118: 322–327.

Schoenbaum SC, Hyde JN Jr, Bartoshesky L, Crampton K (1976). Benefit-cost analysis of rubella vaccination policy. New Engl J Med, 294: 306–310.

Serdula MK, Halstead SB, Wiebenga NH, Herrmann KL (1984). Serological response to rubella revaccination. JAMA, 251: 1974–1977.

Smithells RW, Sheppard S, Holzel H, Dickson A (1985). National congenital rubella surveillance programme 1 July 1971 – 30 June 1984. Br Med J, 291: 40–41.

Stassburg MA, Greenland S, Stephenson TG, Weiss BP, Auerbach D, Habel LA, Lieb LE (1985). Clinical effectiveness of rubella vaccine in a college population. Vaccine, 3: 109–111.

Tingle AJ, Chantler JK, Pot KH, Paty DW, Ford DK (1985). Post-partum rubella immunization: Association with development of prolonged arthritis, neurological sequelae and chronic rubella viremia. J Infect Dis, 152: 606–612.

White CC, Koplan JP, Orenstein WA (1985). Benefits, risks and costs of immunization for measles, mumps and rubella. Am J Public Health, 75: 739–744.

Section 6: Candidiasis

Bloch B, Kretzel A (1980). Econazole nitrate in the treatment of candidal vaginitis. S Afr Med J, 58: 314–316.

Bradbeer CS, Mayhew SR, Barlow D (1985). Butaconazole and miconazole in treating vaginal candidiasis. Genitourin Med, 61: 270–272.

Davis JE, Frudenfeld JH, Goddard JL (1974). Comparative evaluation of monistat and mycostatin in the treatment of vulvovaginal candidiasis. Obstet Gynecol, 44: 403–406.

Dixon BL, Houston CS (1978). Fatal neonatal pulmonary candidiasis. Radiology, 128: 132.

Droegemueller W, Adamson DG, Brown D, Cibley L, Fleury F, LePage ME, Henzl MR (1984). Three-day treatment with butaconazole nitrate for vulvovaginal candidiasis. Obstet Gynecol, 64: 530–534.

Eliott BW, Howat RCL, Mack AE (1979). A comparison between the effects of nystatin, clotrimazole, and miconazole on vaginal candidiasis. Br J Obstet Gynaecol, 86: 572–577.

Gardner HL (1944). Vaginal thrush. Texas State J Med, 40: 33–38.

Gardner HL, Kaufman RH (1969). Benign Diseases of the Vulva and Vagina. St Louis: Mosby, pp 149–167.

Higton BK (1973). A trial of clotrimazole and nystatin in vaginal candidiasis. J Obstet Gynaecol, 80: 992–995.

Hurley R, Morris ED (1964). The pathogenicity of candida species in the human vagina. J Obstet Gynaecol Br Commnwlth, 71: 692–695.

Kimbell NKB (1966). A new fungicidal cream in the treatment of vaginal candidiasis. J Obstet Gynaecol Br Commnwlth, 73: 319.

McNellis D, McLeod M, Lawson J, Pasquale SA (1977). Treatment of vulvovaginal candidiasis in pregnancy. A comparative study. Obstet Gynecol, 50: 674–678.

Mead PM (1974). Candida albicans. In: Infectious Diseases in Obstetrics and Gynecology. Monif GRF (ed). Hagerstown, MD: Harper & Row, p 242.

Medical Letter (1986). Butoconazole for vulvovaginal candidiasis. 28:68

Milne LFR, Brown ADG (1973). Comparison of nystatin ('Nystan') and hydrargaphen ('Penotrane') in the treatment of vaginal candidosis in pregnancy. Curr Med Res Opin, 1: 524–527.

Morton RS, Rashid S (1977). Candidal vaginitis. Natural history, predisposing factors and prevention. Proc R Soc Med, 70: Suppl 4: 3–6.

Oriel JD (1977). Clinical overview of candidal vaginitis. Proc R Soc Med, 70: Suppl 4: 7–9.

Pasquale SA, Lawson J, Sargent EC, Newdeck JP (1979). A dose response study with monistat cream. Obstet Gynecol, 53: 250–253.

Pigott PV (1972). An evaluation of a modified nystatin vaginal tablet in a multi-centre study. Curr Med Res Opin, 1: 159–165.

Plass ED, Hesseltine HC, Borts IH (1931). Monilia vulvovaginitis. Am J Obstet Gynecol, 21: 320–334.

Ruiz-Valasco V, Rosas-Arceo J (1978). Prophylactic clotrimazole treatment to prevent mycoses contamination of the newborn. Int J Gynaecol Obstet, 16: 70–71.

Rubin A, Russell JM, Mauff A (1980). Efficacy of econazole in the treatment of candidiasis and other vaginal discharges. S Afr Med J, 57: 407–408.

Tan CG, Milne LJR, Good CS, Loudon IDO (1974). A comparative trial of six day therapy with clotrimazole and nystatin in pregnant patients with vaginal candidiasis. Postgrad Med J, 50: July Suppl: 102–105.

Whyte RK, Hussain Z, deSa B (1982). Antenatal infections with candidal species. Arch Dis Childhood, 57: 528–535.

Section 7: Trichomonas

Adamsons K, Joelsson I (1966). The effects of pharmacologic agents upon the fetus and newborn. Am J Obstet Gynecol, 96: 437–460.

Al-Salihi FL, Curran JP, Wang JS (1974). Neonatal Trichomonas vaginalis: Report of three cases and review of the literature. Pediatrics, 53: 196–200.

Anonymous (1980). Management of normal pregnancy, labour and puerperium. Obstet Gynecol Surv, 35: 21–22.

Bramley M (1976). Study of female babies of women entering confinement with vaginal trichomoniasis. Br J Vener Dis, 52: 58–62.

Chow AW, Jewesson PJ (1985). Pharmacokinetics and safety of antimicrobial agents during pregnancy. Rev Infect Dis, 7: 287–313.

Fouts AC, Kraus SJ (1980). Trichomonas vaginalis: Reevaluation of its clinical presentation and laboratory diagnosis. J Infect Dis, 141: 137–143.

Hardy PH, Hardy JB, Nell EE, Graham DA, Spence MR, Rosenbaum RC (1984). Prevalence of six sexually transmitted disease agents among pregnant inner city adolescents and pregnancy outcome. Lancet, 2: 333–337.

Hiemstra I, Van Bel F, Berger HM (1984). Can Trichomonas vaginalis cause pneumonia in newborn babies? Br Med J (Clin Res), 289: 355–356.

Hoosen AA, Ross SM, Mulla MJ, Patel M (1981). The incidence of selected vaginal infections among pregnant urban blacks. S Afr Med J, 59: 827–829.

Lossick JG (1982). Treatment of Trichomonas vaginalis infections. Rev Infect Dis, 4 (Suppl): S801-S818.

Mason PR (1979). Serodiagnosis of Trichomonas vaginalis infection by the indirect immunofluorescent antibody test. J Clin Path, 32: 1211–1215.

McLaren LC, Davis LE, Healy GR, James CG (1983). Isolation of Trichomonas vaginalis from the respiratory tract of infants with respiratory disease. Pediatrics, 71: 888–890.

McLellan R, Spence MR, Brockman M, Raffel L, Smith JL (1982). The clinical diagnosis of trichomoniasis. Obstet Gynecol, 60: 30–34.

Peterson WF, Stauch JE, Ryder CD (1966). Metronidazole in pregnancy. Am J Obstet Gynecol, 94: 343–349.

Rein F, Chapel TA (1975). Trichomoniasis, candidiasis and the minor venereal diseases. Clin Obstet Gynecol, 18: 73–88.

Robinson SC, Mirchandani G (1965). Trichomonas vaginalis. Am J Obstet Gynecol, 93: 502–505.

Roe FJC (1983). Toxicologic evaluation of metronidazole with particular reference to carcinogenic, mutagenic and teratogenic potential. Surgery, 93: 158–164.

Ross SM, Van Middelkoop A (1983). Trichomonas infection in pregnancy—does it affect perinatal outcome? S Afr Med J, 63: 566–567.

Spence MR, Hollander DH, Smith J, McCaig L, Sewell D, Brockman M (1980). The clinical and laboratory diagnosis of Trichomonas vaginalis infection. Sex Transm Dis, 7: 168, 171.

Thin RN, Symonds MAE, Booker R, Cook S, Langlet F (1979). Double-blind comparison of a single dose and a five day course of metronidazole in the treatment of trichomoniasis. Br J Vener Dis, 55: 354–356.

Section 8: Genital mycoplasmas

Braun P, Lee YH, Klein JO, Marcy SM, Klein TA, Charles D, Levy P, Kass EH (1971). Birthweight and genital mycoplasmas in pregnancy. New Engl J Med, 284: 167–171.

Dische MR, Quinn PA, Czegledy-Nagy E, Sturgess JM (1979). Genital mycoplasma infection. Intrauterine infection: Pathologic study of the fetus and placenta. Am J Clin Pathol, 72: 167–174.

Driscoll SG, Knudsin RB, Horne HW, Scott JM (1969). Infections and first trimester losses: Possible role of mycoplasmas. Fertil Steril, 20: 1017–1019.

Embree JE, Krause VW, Embil JA, MacDonald S (1980). Placental infection with Mycoplasma hominis and Ureaplasma urealyticum: Clinical correlation. Obstet Gynecol, 56: 475–481.

Hardy PH, Hardy JB, Nell EE, Graham DA, Spence MR, Rosenbaum RC (1984). Prevalence of six sexually transmitted disease agents among pregnant inner-city adolescents and pregnancy outcome. Lancet, 2: 333–337.

Harrison HR (1983). Prospective studies of Mycoplasma hominis infection in pregnancy. Sex Transm Dis, 10: 311–317.

Harrison HR, Alexander ER, Weinstein L, Lewis M, Nash M, Sim DA (1983). Cervical Chlamydia trachomatis and mycoplasmal infection in pregnancy. JAMA, 250: 1721–1727.

Kass EH, McCormack WM, Lin JS, Rosner B, Munoz A (1981). Genital mycoplasmas as a cause of excess premature delivery. Trans Assoc Am Phys, 94: 261–266.

Kundsin RB, Driscoll SM (1970). Mycoplasmas and human reproductive failure. Surg Gynecol Obstet, 131: 89–92.

Kundsin RB, Driscoll SG, Monson RR, Yeh C, Biano SA, Cochran WD (1984). Association of Ureaplasma urealyticum in the placenta with perinatal morbidity and mortality. New Engl J Med, 310: 941–945.

McCormack WM, Lee YH, Lin JS, Rankin JS (1973). Genital mycoplasmas in postpartum fever. J Infect Dis, 127: 193–196.

McCormack WM, Rosner B, Lee YH, Rankin JS, Lin JS (1975). Isolation of genital mycoplasmas from blood obtained shortly after vaginal delivery. Lancet, 1: 596–599.

Quinn PA, Rubin S, Mocilla DM, Read SE, Chipman M (1983a). Serological evidence of Ureaplasma urealyticum infection in neonatal respiratory disease. Yale J Biol Med, 56: 565–572.

Quinn PA, Schewchuk AB, Shuber J, Lie KI, Ryan E, Sheu M, Chipman ML (1983b). Serologic evidence of Ureaplasma urealyticum infection in women with spontaneous pregnancy loss. Am J Obstet Gynecol, 145: 245–250.

Quinn PA, Shewchuk AM, Shuber J, Lie KI, Ryan E, Chipman LM, Nocilla DM (1983c). Efficacy of antibiotic therapy in preventing spontaneous pregnancy loss among couples colonized with genital mycoplasmas. Am J Obstet Gynecol, 145: 239–244.

Quinn PA, Butany J, Chipman M, Taylor J, Hannah W (1985). A prospective study of microbial infection in stillbirths and early neonatal death. Am J Obstet Gynecol, 151: 238–249.

Shurin PA, Alpert S, Rosner B, Driscoll SG, Lee YH, McCormack WM, Santamarina BAG, Kass EH (1975). Chorioamnionitis and colonization of the newborn infant with genital mycoplasmas. New Engl J Med, 293: 5–8.

Sompolisky D, Solomon F, Elkina L, Weintraub Z, Bukovsky I, Caspi E (1975). Infections with mycoplasma and bacteria in induced midtrimester abortion and fetal loss. Am J Obstet Gynecol, 121: 610–616.

Stray-Pedersen B, Eng J, Reikvam TM (1978). Uterine T-mycoplasma colonization in reproductive failure. Am J Obstet Gynecol, 130: 307–311.

Tafari N, Ross S, Naeye RL, Judge DM, Marboe C (1976). Mycoplasma T strains and perinatal death. Lancet, 1: 108–109.

Taylor-Robinson D, McCormack WM (1980). The genital mycoplasmas. New Engl J Med, 302: 1003–1010, 1063–1067.

Wallace RJ, Alpert S, Browne K, Lin JSL, McCormack WM (1978). Isolation of Mycoplasma hominis from blood cultures in patients with postpartum fever. Obstet Gynecol, 51: 181–185.

Section 9: Toxoplasmosis

Beattie CP (1984). Congenital toxoplasmosis. Br J Obstet Gynaecol, 91: 417–418.

Blondel B (1986). Antenatal care in the countries of the European Community over the last twenty years. In: Perinatal Care Delivery Systems. Kaminski M, Breart G, Buekens P, Huisjes HJ, McIlwaine G, Selbmann HK (eds). Oxford: Oxford University Press, pp 3–15.

Desmonts G, Couvreur J (1974a). Congenital toxoplasmosis. A prospective study of 378 pregnancies. New Engl J Med, 290: 1110–1116.

Desmonts G, Couvreur J (1974b). Toxoplasmosis in pregnancy and in transmission to the fetus. Bull NY Acad Med, 50: 146–159.

Henderson JP, Beattie CP, Hale EG, Wright T (1984). The evaluation of new services: Possibilities for preventing congenital toxoplasmosis. Int J Epidemiol, 13: 65–72.

Hunter K, Stagno S, Capps E, Smith RJ (1983). Prenatal screening of pregnant women for infections caused by cytomegalovirus, Epstein-Barr virus, herpes virus, rubella and Toxoplasma gondii. Am J Obstet Gynecol, 145: 269–273.

Koppe JG, Loewer-Sieger DH, De Roever-Bonnet H (1986). Results of a 20 year follow-up of congenital toxoplasmosis. Lancet, 1: 254–256.

Krick JA, Remington JS (1978). Current concepts in parasitology. Toxoplasmosis in the adult—an overview. New Engl J Med, 298: 550–553.

Lancet (1980). Congenital toxoplasmosis (Editorial). Lancet; 1: 578–579.

Thalhammer VO, Heller-Szollosy E (1979). Erfahrugen mit routinemabigem Toxoplasmose-screening der schwagen zwecks verhütung angeborener toxoplasmose. Eine prospektive untersuchung. Wien klin Wochenschr, 91: 20–25.

Vaage L, Midtvedt T (1975). Epidemiologic aspects of toxoplasmosis. II. The prevalence of positive toxoplasmin reactions in naval recruits from different parts of Norway. Scand J Infect Dis, 7: 218–221.

Wilson CB, Remington JS (1980). What can be done to prevent congenital toxoplasmosis? Am J Obstet Gynecol, 138: 357–363.

Wilson CB, Remington JS, Stagno S, Reynolds DW (1980). Development of adverse sequelae in children born with subclinical toxoplasmosis infection. Pediatrics, 66: 767–774.

Zighelboim I, Maekelt GA, Teppa P, Perera JR, de Teppa DG, Maniero P (1968). Reproductive wastage and toxoplasma antibodies. Am J Obstet Gynecol, 101: 839–843.

Section 10: Chlamydia

Alexander ER, Harrison HR (1983). Role of Chlamydia trachomatis in perinatal infection. Rev Infect Dis, 5: 713–719.

Beem MO, Saxon EM (1982). Chlamydia trachomatis infections of infants. In: Chlamydial Infections. Mardh PA, Holmes KK, Oriel JD, Piot P, Schachter J (eds). Amsterdam: Elsevier, pp 199–212.

Bell TA, Grayston JT (1986). Centers for Disease Control: Guidelines for prevention and control of Chlamydia trachomatis infections. Ann Intern Med, 104: 524–526.

Centers for Disease Control (1985). Chlamydia trachomatis infections. Morbidity Mortality Weekly Review, 34: 53S-74S.

Chernesky MA, Mahony JB, Stewart IO, Landis SJ, Seidleman W (1986). Chlamydia trachomatis in genital specimens by enzyme immunoassay, immunofluorescence and culture. J Infect Dis, 154: 141–148.

Coudron PE, Fedorko DP, Dawson MS, Kaplowitz LG, Brookman RR, Dalton HP, Davis BA (1986). Detection of Chlamydia trachomatis in genital specimens by the Microtrak TM direct specimen test. Am J Clin Path, 85: 89–92.

Darougar S (1985). The humoral immune response to chlamydial infection in humans. Rev Infect Dis, 7: 726–730.

Darougar S, Treharne JD (1982). Cell culture methods for the isolation of Chlamydia trachomatis—a review. In: Chlamydial Infections. Mardh PA, Holmes KK, Oriel JD, Piot P, Schachter J (eds). Amsterdam: Elsevier, pp 265–274.

Forbes BA, Bartholoma N, McMillan J, Roefara M, Weiner L, Welych L (1986). Evaluation of a monoclonal test to detect chlamydia in cervical and urethral specimens. J Clin Microbiol, 23: 1136–1137.

Geerling S, Nettum JA, Lindner LE, Miller SL, Dutton L, Wechter S (1985). Sensitivity and specificity of the Papanicolaou-stained cervical smear in the diagnosis of Chlamydia trachomatis infection. Acta Cytol, 29: 671–675.

Goh BT, Morgan-Capner P, Lim KS (1982). Chlamydial screening of pregnant women in a sexually transmitted diseases clinic. Br J Vener Dis, 58: 327–329.

Graber CD, Williamson O, Pike J, Valicenti J (1985). Detection of Chlamydia trachomatis infection in endocervical specimens using direct immunofluorescence. Obstet Gynecol, 66: 727–730.

Harrison HR, Alexander ER, Weinstein L, Lewis M, Nash M, Sim DA (1983). Cervical Chlamydia trachomatis and mycoplasma infections in pregnancy. JAMA, 250: 1721–1727.

Jones MF, Smith TF, Houglum AJ, Herrmann JE (1984). Detection of Chlamydia trachomatis in genital specimens by the Chlamydiazyme test. J Clin Microbiol, 20: 465–467.

Klatersky-Genot M (1970). Effects of tetracycline administered during pregnancy on the deciduous teeth. A double blind controlled study. Acta Stomatologica Belgica, 67: 107–124.

Martin DH, Koutsky L, Eschenback DA, Daling JR, Alexander ER, Benedetti JK, Holmes KK (1982). Prematurity and perinatal mortality in pregnancies complicated by maternal Chlamydia trachomatis infections. JAMA, 247: 1585–1588.

McMillan JA, Weiner LB, Lamberson HV, Hagen JH, Aubry RH, Abdul-Karim RW, Sunderji SG, Higgins AP (1985). Efficacy of maternal screening and therapy in the prevention of chlamydia infection of the newborn. Infection, 13: 263–266.

Pierce JM, Ward ME, Seal DV (1982). Ophthalmia neonatorum in the 1980's: Incidence, aetiology and treatment. Br J Ophthalmol, 66: 728–731.

Schachter J, Grossman M (1981). Chlamydial infections. Ann Rev Med, 3: 45–61.

Schachter J, Sweet RL, Grossman M, Landers D, Robbie M, Bishop E (1986). Experience with the routine use of erythromycin for chlamydial infections in pregnancy. New Engl J Med, 314: 276–279.

Stamm WE, Harrison HR, Alexander ER, Cles LD, Spence MR Quinn TC (1984). Diagnosis of Chlamydia trachomatis infections by direct immunofluorescence staining of genital secretions. Ann Intern Med, 101: 638–641.

Thompson S, Lopez B, Wong KH, Ramsey C, Thomas J, Reising G, Jenks B, Peacock W, Sanderson M, Goforth S, Zaidi A, Miller R, Klein L (1982). A prospective study of chlamydia and mycoplasma infections during pregnancy: Relation to pregnancy outcome and maternal morbidity. In: Chlamydial Infections. Mardh PA, Holmes KK, Oriel JD, Piot P, Schachter J (eds). Amsterdam: Elsevier, pp 155–158.

Section 11: Herpes simplex

Arvin AM, Yeager AS, Bruhn FW, Grossman M (1982). Neonatal Herpes simplex infection in the absence of mucocutaneous lesions. J Pediatr, 100: 715–721.

Arvin AM, Hensleigh PA, Prober CG, Au DS, Yasukawa LL, Witteck AE, Palumbo PE, Paryani SG, Yeager AS (1986). Failure of antepartum maternal cultures to predict the infant's risk of exposure to Herpes simplex at delivery. New Engl J Med, 315: 796–800.

Binkin NJ, Kaplan JP, Cates W (1984). Preventing neonatal herpes. The value of weekly viral cultures in pregnant women with recurrent genital herpes. JAMA, 251: 2816–2821.

Brown ST, Jaffe HW, Zaidi A, Filder R, Herrmann KL, Lylerla HC, Jove DF, Bodell JW (1979). Sensitivity and specificity of diagnostic tests for genital infection with herpes virus hominis. Sex Transm Dis, 6: 10–13.

Bryson Y, Dillon M, Lovett M, Acuna G, Taylor S, Cherry JD, Johnson L, Weismeir E, Growdon W, Creagh-Kirk T, Keeney R (1983). Treatment of first episodes of genital Herpes simplex virus infection with oral acyclovir. A randomized double-blind controlled trial in normal subjects. New Engl J Med, 308: 916–921.

Committee on Infectious Diseases (1988). Report 21st edition. Elk Grove Village, Illinois: American Academy of Pediatrics.

Corey L, Benedetti JK, Critchlow CW, Remington MR, Winter CA, Fahnlander AL, Smith K, Salter DL, Keeney RS, Davis LG, Hintz MA, Connor JG, Holmes KK (1982a). Double-blind controlled trial of topical acyclovir in genital Herpes simplex virus infections. Am J Med, 73 (1A): 326–334.

Corey L, Nahmias AJ, Guinan ME, Benedetti JK, Critchlow CW, Holmes KK (1982b). A trial of topical acyclovir in genital Herpes simplex virus infections. New Engl J Med, 306: 1313–1319.

Fiddian AP, Halsos AM, Kinge BR, Nilsen AE, Wikstrom K (1982). Oral acyclovir in the treatment of genital herpes. Preliminary report of a multicenter trial. Am J Med, 73 (1A): 335–337.

Hirsh MS, Schooley RT (1983). Treatment of herpes virus infections. New Engl J Med, 309: 963–970, 1034–1039.

Nahmias AJ, Josey WE, Naib ZM, Freeman MG, Hernandez RJ, Wheeler JH (1971). Perinatal risk associated with maternal genital Herpes simplex virus infection. Am J Obstet Gynecol, 110: 825–827.

Offit PA, Starr SE, Zolnick P, Plotkin S (1982). Acyclovir therapy in neonatal Herpes simplex virus infection. Pediatr Infect Dis, 1: 253–255.

Prober CG, Sullender WM, Yasukawa LL, Au DS, Yeager AS, Arvin AM (1987). Low risk of Herpes simplex virus infections in neonates exposed to the virus at the time of vaginal delivery to mothers with recurrent genital Herpes simplex virus infections. N Engl J Med, 316: 240–244.

Prober CG, Sullender WM, Yasukawa LL, Au DS, Arvin AM (1988). Use of routine viral cultures at delivery to identify infants exposed to herpes simplex infection. N Engl J Med, 318: 887–891.

Reichmann RC, Ginsberg M, Barrett-Connor E, Wyborny S, Connor JD, Redfield D, Savoia MC, Richman DD, Oxman MN, Dandliker PS, Badger G, Ashikaga T, Dolin R (1982). Controlled trial of oral acyclovir in the therapy of recurrent Herpes simplex genitalis. Am J Med, 73 (1A): 338–341.

Sullivan-Bolyai J, Hull HF, Wilson C, Corey L (1983). Neonatal Herpes simplex virus infection in King County, Washington: Increasing incidence and epidemiologic correlates. JAMA, 250: 3059–3062.

Vontver LA, Reeves WC, Rattray M, Corey L, Remington MA, Tolentino E, Schweid A, Holmes KK (1979). Clinical course and diagnosis of genital Herpes simplex virus infection and evaluation of topical surfactant therapy. Am J Obstet Gynecol, 133: 548–554.

Whitley RJ, Soon S, Dolin R, Galasso G, Chien LT, Alford CA, and the Collaborative Group (1977). Adenine arabinoside therapy of biopsy-proved Herpes simplex encephalitis: National Institute of Allergy and Infectious Diseases Collaborative Antiviral Study. New Engl J Med, 297: 289–294.

Whitley RJ, Nahmias AJ, Soong SJ, Galasso GG, Fleming CL, Alford CA (1980a). Vidarabine therapy of neonatal Herpes simplex virus infection. Pediatrics, 66: 495–501.

Whitley RJ, Nahmias AJ, Visintine AM, Fleming CL, Alford CA (1980b). The natural history of Herpes simplex virus infection of mother and newborn. Pediatrics, 66: 489–494.

Yeager AS, Arvin AM (1984). Reasons for the absence of a history of recurrent genital infections in mothers of neonates infected with Herpes simplex virus. Pediatrics, 73: 188–193.

Yeager AS, Arvin AM, Urbani LJ, Kemp JA III (1980). Relationship of antibody to outcome in neonatal Herpes simplex virus infections. Infect Immun, 29: 532–538.

Section 12: Group B streptococcus

Anthony BF (1982). Carriage of group B streptococci during pregnancy: A puzzler. J Infect Dis, 145: 789–793.

Anthony BF, Okada DM, Hobel CJ (1978). Epidemiology of group B streptococcus: Longitudinal observations during pregnancy. J Infect Dis, 137: 524–530.

Anthony, BF, Okada DM, Hobel CJ (1979). Epidemiology of the group B streptococcus: Maternal and nosocomial sources for infant acquisitions. J Pediatr, 95: 431–436.

Baker CJ (1977). Summary of the workshop on perinatal infections due to group B streptococcus. J Infect Dis, 136: 137–152.

Boyer KM, Gotoff SP (1986). Prevention of early-onset neonatal group B streptococcal disease with selective intrapartum chemoprophylaxis. New Engl J Med, 314: 1665–1669.

Boyer KM, Gadzala CA, Kelly PD, Gotoff SP (1983). Selective intrapartum chemoprophylaxis of neonatal group B streptococcal early onset disease. III. Interruption of mother-to-infant transmission. J Infect Dis, 148: 810–816.

Dillon HC, Gray E, Pass MA, Gray BM (1982). Anorectal and vaginal carriage of group B streptococci during pregnancy. J Infect Dis, 145: 794–799.

Easmon CSF, Hastings MJG, Deeley J, Bloxham B, Rivers RPA, Marwood R (1983). The effect of intrapartum chemoprophylaxis in the vertical transmission of group B streptococci. Br J Obstet Gynecol, 90: 633–635.

Feld SM, Harrigan JT (1987). Vaginal Gram stain as an immediate detector of group B streptococci in selected obstetric patients. Am J Obstet Gynecol, 156: 446–448.

Gerard P, Verghote-D'Hulst M, Bachy A, Duhaut G (1979). Group B streptococcal colonization of pregnant women and their neonates. Acta Paediatr Scand, 68: 819–823.

Hall RT, Barnes W, Krishnan L (1976). Antibiotic treatment of parturient women colonized with group B streptococci. Am J Obstet Gynecol, 124: 630–634.

Holls WM, Thomas J, Troyer V (1987). Cervical Gram stain for rapid detection of colonization with β-streptococcus. Obstet Gynecol, 69: 354–357.

Hoogkamp-Korstanje JAA, Gerards LJ, Cats BP (1982). Maternal carriage and neonatal acquisition of group B streptococci. J Infect Dis, 145: 800–803.

Lim DV, Morales WJ, Walsh AF, Katzanis D (1986). Reduction of morbidity and mortality rates for neonatal rates group B streptococcal disease through early diagnosis and chemoprophylaxis. J Clin Microbiol, 23: 489–492.

Lim DV, Morales WJ, Walsh AF (1987). Lim group B strep broth and coagglutination for rapid identification of group B streptococci in preterm pregnant women. J Clin Microbiol, 25: 452–452.

Merenstein GB, Todd WA, Brown G, Yost CC, Luzier T (1980). Group B beta-hemolytic streptococcus: Randomized controlled treatment study at term. Obstet Gynecol, 55: 315–318.

Morales WJ, Lim DV, Walsh AF (1986). Prevention of neonatal group B streptococcal sepsis by the use of a rapid screening test and selective intrapartum chemoprophylaxis. Am J Obstet Gynecol, 155: 979–983.

Noble MA, Bert J, West A (1983). Detection and identification of group B streptococci by use of pigment production. J Clin Microbiol, 36: 350–352.

Pyati SP, Pildes RS, Jacobs NM, Ramamurthy RS, Yeh TF, Raval DS, Lilien LD, Amma P, Metzger WI (1983). Penicillin in infants weighing two kilograms or less with early-onset group B streptococcal disease. New Engl J Med, 308: 1383–1389.

Reardon EP, Noble MA, Luther ER, Wort AJ, Bert J, Swift M (1984). Evaluation of rapid method for the detection of vaginal group B streptococci of women in labour. Am J Obstet Gynecol, 140: 575–578.

Siegel JD, McCracken GH (1981). Sepsis neonatorum. New Engl J Med, 304: 642–647.

Siegel JD, McCracken GH, Threlkeld N, Milvenan B, Rosenfield CR (1980). Single dose penicillin prophylaxis of neonatal group B streptococcal infections. A controlled trial in 18,738 newborn infants. New Engl J Med, 303: 769–775.

Siegel JD, McCracken GH, Threlkeld N, De Passe B, Rosenfield CR (1982). Single dose penicillin prophylaxis of neonatal group B streptococcal disease. Lancet, 1: 1426–1430.

Teres FO, Matorras R, Perea AG, Elorza MD (1987). Prevention of neonatal group B streptroccal spepsis. Ped Infect Dis J, 6: 874–876.

Wald ER, Dashefsky B, Green M, Harger J, Parise M, Korey C, Byers C (1987). Rapid detection of group B streptococci directly from vaginal swabs. J Clin Microbiol, 25: 573–574.

Wang E, Hammerberg O, Hunter D, Peng H, Richardson H (1988). Rapid detection of Group B streptococcal carriage in parturient women using a modified starch serum medium. Clin Invest Med, 11: 52–56.

Section 13: Acquired immunodeficiency syndrome

Blanche S, Dubois M, Ledeist F (1986). Prospective study on newborns of LAV seropositive mothers. International Conference on AIDS. Paris, France, June 1986.

Laboratory Centres for Disease Control (1987). Update:

'AIDS' in Canada. Laboratory Centres for Disease Control, May 4, 1987.

Minkoff HL, Schwarz RH (1986). AIDS: Time for obstetricians to get involved. Obstet Gynecol, 68: 267–268.

Morbidity Mortality Weekly Review (1982). Unexplained immunodeficiency and opportunistic infections in infants—New York, New Jersey, California. Morbidity Mortality Weekly Review, 31: 665–667.

Oleske J, Minnefor A, Cooper R, Thomas K, dela Cruz A, Ahdieh H, Guerrero I, Joshi VV, Desposito F (1983). Immune deficiency syndrome in children. JAMA, 249: 2345–2349.

Pinching AJ, Jefferies DJ (1985). AIDS and HTLV-III/LAV infection, consequences for obstetrics and perinatal medicine. Br J Obstet Gynecol, 92: 1211–1217.

Rubinstein A, Bernstein L (1986). The epidemiology of pediatric acquired immunodeficiency syndrome. Clin Immunol Immunopathol, 40: 115–121.

Rubinstein A, Sicklick M, Gupta A, Bernstein L, Klein N, Rubinstein E, Spigland I, Fruchter L, Litman N, Lee H, Hollander M (1983). Acquired immunodeficiency with reversed T_4/T_8 ratios in infants born to promiscuous and drug-addicted mothers. JAMA, 249: 2350–2356.

Scott GB, Buck BE, Leterman JG, Bloom FL, Parks WP (1984). Acquired immunodeficiency syndrome in infants. New Engl J Med, 310: 76–81.

Scott GB, Fischl MA, Klimas N, Fletcher MA, Dickinson GM, Levine RS, Parks WP (1985a). Mothers of infants with the acquired immunodeficiency syndrome. Evidence for both symptomatic and asymptomatic carriers. JAMA, 253: 363–366.

Scott GB, Fischl MA, Klimas N (1985b). Mothers of infants with the acquired immunodeficiency syndrome (AIDS): Outcome of subsequent pregnancies. International Conference on the Acquired Immunodeficiency Syndrome, Atlanta, Georgia, April 1985.

Ziegler JB, Cooper DA, Johnson RO, Gold J (1985). Postnatal transmission of AIDS-associated retrovirus from mother to infant. Lancet, 1: 896–897.

35 Rhesus isoimmunization

Jack Bennebroek Gravenhorst

1 Introduction

Isoimmunization against Rhesus antigens was once a major cause of perinatal mortality, neonatal morbidity, and long term disability and mental handicap. The condition is rarely seen today, now being responsible for less than 0.06 deaths per 1000 births in the United Kingdom in 1983 (Clarke *et al.* 1985). In The Netherlands the percentage of new Rh-immunizations went down from 3.5 in 1969 to 0.5 in 1986 (van Dijk 1988) and perinatal mortality from haemolytic disease was less than 0.05 per 1000 in 1983, 1984 and 1985 (Central Bureau of Statistics 1987). Although this reduction in the frequency of Rhesus (D) isoimmunization is sometimes credited entirely to the modern programmes of immunoprotection, it should not be forgotten that a large part of this reduction is the result of an increased proportion of one- and two-child families, in which the condition is unlikely to occur, and a decrease in the number of large families, in which it would be seen more frequently. The improved results in children who are born with the condition is at least in part explained by a general improvement in perinatal health, particularly of preterm infants. Nevertheless, the discovery, introduction, and utilization of anti-D gammaglobulin has been one of the major obstetrical achievements of the past quarter century.

2 History

In 1892 Ballantyne collected 65 cases of hydrops fetalis from the literature and noted, first, that the children were often preterm and anaemic, and second, that the condition occurred predominantly in multiparous women. Halban, in 1900, suggested isoimmunization as a possible cause for this condition, postulating antigen–antibody exchange across the placenta as the mechanism. The concept that fetal cells could cross the placental barrier and enter the mother's circulation was raised by Dienst in 1905, who suggested that a difference in blood groups between mother and child might be the cause of 'toxaemia'.

Little further progress in the understanding of the condition was achieved until the late 1930s. In 1938, Darrow came very close to the solution when she considered the destruction of red cells to be mediated by some form of immune reaction, and mentioned fetal haemoglobin as a possible antigen. A year later, Levine *et al.* (1939) reported a severe transfusion reaction in a woman who had received a transfusion of her husbands' blood, shortly after being delivered of a stillborn infant. The authors suggested that, as the woman had not been previously transfused, she might have been sensitized to an antigen in the fetus that had been inherited from the father.

From this time on progress was rapid. In 1940 Landsteiner and Wiener described the presence of the Rhesus antigen in 85 per cent of Caucasians. Shortly thereafter Wiener and Peters (1940) demonstrated that haemolytic transfusion reactions could occur when Rhesus positive blood was transfused to a Rhesus negative individual, and Levine *et al.* (1941) showed that isoimmunization against the Rhesus antigen was the predominant cause of haemolytic disease of the newborn. In 1946 Coombs and colleagues described the anti-human globulin test for the detection of incomplete antibodies. Solid evidence that maternal isoimmunization resulted from transplacental passage of fetal red blood cells was only obtained in 1954, when Chown demonstrated fetal haemoglobin in the maternal circulation.

Prior to the development of effective prophylaxis, treatment was directed either to the affected fetus or newborn. One of the early treatments of affected babies was simple transfusion, often with the blood of the father (Leonard 1945). That many of the infants so treated died is not surprising, as the father's blood almost certainly would have been Rhesus positive. After discovery of the Rhesus factor (Landsteiner and Wiener 1940), Rhesus negative blood was, of course, recommended for transfusion of the infant. Hart (1925) was the first to perform an exchange transfusion. His contribution was ignored, and it was another twenty years before the procedure was again attempted (Wiener and Peters 1940; Wiener *et al.* 1944), at first with little success. Randomized trials showing that exchange transfusion was an effective treatment for an affected newborn infant were carried out in the early 1950s (Mollison and Walker 1952; Armitage and Mollison 1953).

Elective preterm delivery of an affected fetus remained the cornerstone of treatment, but the timing of this intervention was problematical; too early delivery resulted in a baby too immature to survive, while waiting too long could result in intrauterine demise. Amniocentesis and spectrophotometric analysis of amniotic fluid was introduced by Bevis (1956), and later popularized by Liley (1961), as a means of evaluating the condition of the fetus, and hence helping to decide the best time for delivery. A therapeutic milestone was reached when Liley (1963) reported his success with intrauterine fetal transfusion, and described the technique of this procedure, thus adding a second useful approach to the care of an affected fetus.

Undoubtedly the major breakthrough was the almost simultaneous discovery and introduction of anti-D immunoprophylaxis by two independent groups of investigators, Clarke and co-workers in the United Kingdom (1963) and Freda *et al.* in the United States (1964). The effectiveness of anti-D immunoglobulin was demonstrated in a number of trials conducted in different countries. This form of prophylaxis has reduced the incidence of Rhesus (D) isoimmunization to such an extent that in many centres formerly rare forms of isoimmunization are now seen more often than isoimmunization due to Rhesus (D).

3 Prevention

Nine controlled trials of postpartum Rhesus (D) prophylaxis were carried out in the short time span from 1968 to 1971. The results of these trials, all of which compared the results of postpartum administration of anti-D gammaglobulin with those of either placebo-treated or unvaccinated controls, were clear-cut and unequivocal. The presence of Rhesus antibodies at 6 months postpartum was virtually eliminated. Only 6 instances of Rhesus sensitization occurred in the 2973 women who received anti-D gammaglobulin (0.2 per cent), compared to 186 such instances in the 2488 women in the control groups (7.5 per cent) (Table 35.1). The incidence of sensitization in a subsequent pregnancy was reported in 5 of these trials; it was 7 out of 438 treated women (1.2 per cent) compared with 41 out of 261 women in the control groups 15.7 per cent). (Table 35.2).

The question is not whether or not women at risk of Rhesus immunization should receive anti-D immunoglobulin, but which women should receive such prophylaxis, at what times and in what doses. This risk can occur in any situation in which Rhesus (D) positive cells enter the circulation of a Rhesus (D) negative woman, and it will vary with the amount of Rhesus (D) antigen to which she is exposed. The most common time for this to occur is at delivery of a Rhesus (D) positive baby, although there are many other instances in which a woman may be exposed to Rhesus (D) positive cells.

3.1 Routine use of prophylaxis

3.1.1 After delivery

From the randomized trials discussed above it appears that, without the administration of anti-D immunoglobulin, Rhesus (D) negative women who give birth to a Rhesus (D) positive baby, have a 7.5 per cent risk of developing Rhesus (D) antibodies within 6 months of delivery, and a much larger risk (17.5 per cent) of showing evidence of sensitization in a subsequent pregnancy.

ABO incompatibility, commonly believed to confer significant protection against the development of Rhesus (D) antibody formation (Nevanlinna and Vainio 1956; Bowman 1986), does not confer enough protection to warrant clinical consideration. In the 3 trials (Table 35.3) that looked specifically at the administration of anti-D immunoglobulin to women with ABO compatible babies, the same degree of protection was noted as that noted in all trials (Table 35.1).

Only one of the trials (Ascari *et al.* 1968) gave information on both ABO-compatible women treated within 72 hours of delivery and all Rhesus (D) negative women. In that trial the incidence of Rhesus immunization in untreated women was 51 out of 736 (6.9 per cent) overall compared with 32 out of 499 in the untreated women with ABO-compatible babies (6.4 per cent). It is clear that all Rhesus (D) negative women who give birth to a Rhesus (D) positive baby, or a baby whose Rhesus (D) status cannot be determined, should receive Rhesus (D) prophylaxis irrespective of their ABO status.

Table 35.1 Effect of anti-Rh-D prophlaxis postpartum (overall; irrespective of ABO status) on immunization after 6 months

Study	EXPT		CTRL		Odds ratio	Graph of odds ratios and confidence intervals
	n	(%)	*n*	(%)	(95% CI)	0.01 0.1 0.5 1 2 10 100
Stenchever *et al.* (1970)	1/26	(3.85)	2/28	(7.14)	0.54 (0.05–5.43)	
White *et al.* (1970)	0/160	(0.00)	3/153	(1.96)	0.13 (0.01–1.24)	
Clarke *et al.* (1971)	1/173	(0.58)	38/176	(21.59)	0.12 (0.06–0.24)	
Dudok De Wit *et al.* (1968)	3/333	(0.90)	17/329	(5.17)	0.23 (0.10–0.57)	
Woodrow *et al.* (1971)	0/153	(0.00)	13/362	(3.59)	0.23 (0.07–0.78)	
Robertson and Holmes (1969)	0/100	(0.00)	15/112	(13.39)	0.13 (0.05–0.38)	
Bishop and Krieger (1969)	0/95	(0.00)	11/92	(11.96)	0.12 (0.03–0.39)	
Ascari *et al.* (1968)	1/1081	(0.09)	51/736	(6.93)	0.09 (0.05–0.15)	
Chown *et al.* (1969)	0/852	(0.00)	36/500	(7.20)	0.06 (0.03–0.12)	
Typical odds ratio (95% confidence interval)					0.11 (0.08–0.15)	

Table 35.2 Effect of anti-Rh-D prophylaxis postpartum (overall; irrespective of ABO status) on immunization on subsequent pregnancy

Study	EXPT		CTRL		Odds ratio	Graph of odds ratios and confidence intervals
	n	(%)	*n*	(%)	(95% CI)	0.01 0.1 0.5 1 2 10 100
White *et al.* (1970)	0/13	(0.00)	1/8	(12.50)	0.07 (0.00–4.10)	
Clarke *et al.* (1971)	2/88	(2.27)	20/45	(44.44)	0.05 (0.02–0.13)	
Woodrow *et al.* (1971)	3/128	(2.34)	13/127	(10.24)	0.26 (0.10–0.72)	
Ascari *et al.* (1968)	1/81	(1.23)	7/63	(11.11)	0.15 (0.04–0.65)	
Chown *et al.* (1969)	1/28	(3.57)	0/18	(0.00)	5.17 (0.09–99.99)	
Typical odds ratio (95% confidence interval)					0.13 (0.07–0.23)	

It is reasonably well established that 20 microgram of anti-D immunoglobulin will neutralize the antigenicity of 1 ml of Rhesus (D) positive red cells or 2 ml of whole blood (Pollack *et al.* 1971b). Hence, the usually administered dose of 300 microgram is sufficient to protect against a feto-maternal bleed of 30 ml. Since a fetomaternal transfusion of more than 30 ml occurs in approximately 0.6 per cent of deliveries (Zipursky 1977), reducing the standard dose administered will either increase the risk of having administered too little, or will require routine screening for feto-maternal transfusions that are larger than compensated for by the amount of anti-D immunoglobulin used.

The relative cost-effectiveness of a small dose of anti-D immunoglobulin coupled with screening for the amount of feto-maternal transfusion vs. routine administration of a higher dose will depend on local circumstances and the relative costs of anti-D immunoglobulin and of laboratory screening.

The trials in which doses of less than 200 microgram

Table 35.3 Effect of anti-Rh-D prophylaxis postpartum <72 hours in ABO-compatible cases on immunization after 6 months

Study	EXPT		CTRL		Odds ratio	Graph of odds ratios and confidence intervals
	n	(%)	*n*	(%)	(95% CI)	0.01 0.1 0.5 1 2 10 100
Stenchever *et al.* (1970)	1/26	(3.85)	2/28	(7.14)	0.54 (0.05–5.43)	
White *et al.* (1970)	0/160	(0.00)	3/153	(1.96)	0.13 (0.01–1.24)	
Ascari *et al.* (1968)	1/781	(0.13)	32/499	(6.41)	0.08 (0.04–0.17)	
Typical odds ratio (95% confidence interval)					0.10 (0.05–0.19)	

Table 35.4 Effect of <200μg anti-Rh-D postpartum vs. higher doses on immunization at 6 months

Study	EXPT		CTRL		Odds ratio	Graph of odds ratios and confidence intervals
	n	(%)	*n*	(%)	(95% CI)	0.01 0.1 0.5 1 2 10 100
Medical Research Council (1974)	1/459	(0.22)	9/1341	(0.67)	0.44 (0.11–1.83)	
Chown *et al.* (1969)	0/858	(0.00)	0/358	(0.00)	1.00 (1.00–1.00)	
Godel *et al.* (1968)	0/53	(0.00)	0/65	(0.00)	1.00 (1.00–1.00)	
Typical odds ratio (95% confidence interval)					0.44 (0.11–1.83)	

Table 35.5 Effect of <301μg anti-Rh-D postpartum vs. higher doses on immunization at 6 months

Study	EXPT		CTRL		Odds ratio	Graph of odds ratios and confidence intervals
	n	(%)	*n*	(%)	(95% CI)	0.01 0.1 0.5 1 2 10 100
Ascari *et al.* (1968)	0/300	(0.00)	1/781	(0.13)	0.25 (0.00–19.95)	
Chown *et al.* (1969)	0/852	(0.00)	0/364	(0.00)	1.00 (1.00–1.00)	
Godel *et al.* (1968)	0/53	(0.00)	0/65	(0.00)	1.00 (1.00–1.00)	
Typical odds ratio (95% confidence interval)					0.25 (0.00–19.95)	

were compared with 200 microgram or more (Table 35.4), and trials using 300 microgram or less with those using more than 300 microgram (Table 35.5) showed no statistically significant differences in the incidence of Rhesus immunization at 6 months. The small number of isoimmunizations (none in 2 of the 3 trials) are not sufficient to show a true difference, even if such a difference did exist.

The best time to administer the anti-D immunoglobulin would be as soon as possible after delivery, but immediate administration is not practical in view of the time required to determine the blood group of the baby. From the trials that have been conducted, it would appear that an interval of up to 72 hours is compatible with effective prophylaxis. Samson and Mollison (1975) have demonstrated that 100 microgram anti-D immunoglobulin intramuscularly 13 days after an intravenous injection of 1 ml of Rhesus (D) positive cells still appears to have some suppressive effect on Rhesus immunization. The conclusion to be drawn from this observation is that anti-D immunoglobulin is better given late than not at all.

3.1.2 During pregnancy

Reporting on the McMaster Rhesus conference, Davey and Zipursky (1979) summarized the results of 11 studies, in which 262 of a total of 30,155 women (0.87 per cent; range: 0.3 to 5.65 per cent) already had Rhesus (D) antibodies during their first pregnancy. Most immunizations took place after 28 weeks of gestation.

This had been the rationale for proposing the antenatal administration of anti-D immunoglobulin as first suggested and tested by Zipursky and Israels (1967). Large scale collaborative studies were carried out subsequently in a number of centres, sometimes with contemporary and sometimes with historical controls (Bowman and Pollock 1978; Bartsch and Hermann 1979; Zipursky and Blajchman 1979; Davey 1979). Doses of 200 to 300 microgram of anti-D immunoglobulin were given at 34 or 28 weeks or at both 28 and 34 weeks, and a further dose was administered after delivery to all women giving birth to a Rhesus (D) positive child. Controls received the anti-D immunoglobulin only after delivery. Separate series of primigravidae and multigravidae were studied. The results of these studies have suggested that antenatal administration of anti-D immunoglobulin is an effective means of further reducing the incidence of Rhesus immunization. Although the passive antibodies given to the mother are also transferred to the fetus, these small amounts have never been shown to have any adverse effects.

Recently, Huchet *et al.* (1987) reported a randomized controlled trial conducted in 23 maternity units in Paris, France, in which 1969 Rhesus negative nulliparous women were assigned to either a treatment group receiving 100 microgram of anti-D immunoglobulin at 28 weeks of gestation and again at 34 weeks of gestation, or to a control group on the basis of an even or odd year of birth. Both treated and control women received a standard dose of 100 microgram anti-D immunoglobulin after delivery if the baby was Rh positive. There were 6 instances of immunization during pregnancy in the control group as compared to only one in the treatment group (Table 35.6). Of the women who were reviewed at 2 to 12 months after the birth of a Rhesus positive infant, 7 showed evidence of immunization in the control group as compared to only one in the treatment group. When women with a Rhesus positive baby, who had not only been nulliparae but also primigravidae at randomization, were considered, 4 of 360 in the control group and none of 362 in the treatment group were immunized (Table 35.6).

The evidence suggests that an antenatal anti-D immunoglobulin programme could reduce the remaining incidence of Rhesus immunization from 0.6 to 0.06 per cent (Davey 1979). Some state that the additional cost of an antenatal programme is small in comparison to the cost of antenatal diagnosis, treatment, and hospitalization of the mother, combined with the cost of intensive care and treatment of the child suffering from haemolytic disease, and the cost of treating long term handicaps (Bowman 1985; Wible-Kant and Beer 1983; Lim *et al.* 1982). Others point out that limiting the number of pregnancies in women who are already immunized, and ensuring the administration of anti-D immunoglobulin to every eligible woman after delivery or abortion would be a far more cost-effective way to reduce the incidence of haemolytic disease in communities in which this is not already practised (Davey 1979; Tovey 1980; Bennebroek Gravenhorst and Woodfield 1985).

3.2 Special circumstances

3.2.1 After delivery

Large feto-maternal haemorrhages of more than 30 ml can occur after even an uneventful delivery in about 0.5 per cent of deliveries (Zipursky 1977). For this reason, counts of fetal cells in maternal blood have become routine after delivery in some centres, although the high cost of this precludes universal use. After traumatic deliveries and with manual removal of the placenta the risk of a large feto-maternal haemorrhage is increased. With caesarean section, in addition to the usual route of feto-maternal transfusion, passage of fetal blood from the umbilical cord spilled into the peritoneal cavity can also take place (Hindeman 1966). Fetal cell counts in these circumstances allow the determination of whether or not the dose of anti-D immunoglobulin given has been sufficient, and whether an additional dose of anti-D immunoglobulin is required. The same will apply when an unexpectedly anaemic infant is born, since this may have been due to a large feto-maternal bleed.

3.2.2 Early pregnancy loss

Placental trauma associated with either spontaneous or induced abortion can cause feto-maternal bleeding (Matthews and Matthews 1969; Bennebroek Gravenhorst *et al.* 1986). The incidence of feto-maternal bleeding in spontaneous abortion was estimated at about 6 to 7 per cent during the first trimester of pregnancy (Goldman and Eckerling 1972). In the second trimester, incidences of 20 per cent and more have been reported (Queenan *et al.* 1971; Matthews and Matthews 1969; Voigt and Britt 1969). Bennebroek Gravenhorst *et al.* (1986) reported the presence of feto-maternal transfusion in 40 per cent of abortions performed by aspirotomy between 12 and 18 weeks of gestation. The fetal red cell counts in maternal blood indicated that the amount transfused was more than 1 ml in 6.8 per cent of the cases.

Table 35.6 Effect of anti-Rh-D in pregnancy on positive Kleihauer at 32–35 weeks

Study	EXPT		CTRL		Odds ratio	Graph of odds ratios and confidence intervals
	n	(%)	*n*	(%)	(95% CI)	0.01 0.1 0.5 1 2 10 100
Huchet *et al.* (1987)	39/927	(4.21)	67/957	(7.00)	0.59 (0.40–0.87)	
Typical odds ratio (95% confidence interval)					0.59 (0.40–0.87)	

Effect of anti-Rh-D in pregnancy on positive Kleihauer at delivery in pregnancy with a Rh+ fetus

Study	EXPT *n*	(%)	CTRL *n*	(%)	Odds ratio (95% CI)
Huchet *et al.* (1987)	73/599	(12.19)	119/590	(20.17)	0.55 (0.41–0.76)
Typical odds ratio (95% confidence interval)					0.55 (0.41–0.76)

Effect of anti-Rh-D in pregnancy in Kleihauer > 1/10,000 in pregnancy with a Rh+ fetus

Study	EXPT *n*	(%)	CTRL *n*	(%)	Odds ratio (95% CI)
Huchet *et al.* (1987)	31/599	(5.18)	32/590	(5.42)	0.95 (0.57–1.58)
Typical odds ratio (95% confidence interval)					0.95 (0.57–1.58)

Effect of anti-Rh-D in pregnancy on immunization in pregnancy

Study	EXPT *n*	(%)	CTRL *n*	(%)	Odds ratio (95% CI)
Huchet *et al.* (1987)	1/927	(0.11)	6/955	(0.63)	0.25 (0.06–1.08)
Typical odds ratio (95% confidence interval)					0.25 (0.06–1.08)

Effect of anti-Rh-D in pregnancy on immunization in pregnancy with a Rh+ fetus

Study	EXPT *n*	(%)	CTRL *n*	(%)	Odds ratio (95% CI)
Huchet *et al.* (1987)	1/599	(0.17)	6/590	(1.02)	0.23 (0.05–1.03)
Typical odds ratio (95% confidence interval)					0.23 (0.05–1.03)

Effect of anti-Rh-D in pregnancy on immunization at 2–12 months—primiparae

Study	EXPT *n*	(%)	CTRL *n*	(%)	Odds ratio (95% CI)
Huchet *et al.* (1987)	1/472	(0.21)	7/468	(1.50)	0.22 (0.05–0.88)
Typical odds ratio (95% confidence interval)					0.22 (0.05–0.88)

Effect of anti-Rh-D in pregnancy on immunization at 2–12 months—primigravidae

Study	EXPT *n*	(%)	CTRL *n*	(%)	Odds ratio (95% CI)
Huchet *et al.* (1987)	0/362	(0.00)	4/360	(1.11)	0.13 (0.02–0.95)
Typical odds ratio (95% confidence interval)					0.13 (0.02–0.95)

Effect of anti-Rh-D in pregnancy on neonatal jaundice

Study	EXPT *n*	(%)	CTRL *n*	(%)	Odds ratio (95% CI)
Huchet *et al.* (1987)	1/927	(0.11)	4/955	(0.42)	0.31 (0.05–1.79)
Typical odds ratio (95% confidence interval)					0.31 (0.05–1.79)

Retrospective studies have shown that without protection 3 to 4 per cent of Rhesus (D) negative women are immunized by an early abortion in the first pregnancy (Freda *et al.* 1970; Queenan *et al.* 1971; Goldman and Eckerling 1972). With late abortion an incidence of immunization of 8 to 9 per cent has been reported (Freda *et al.* 1970; Goldman and Eckerling 1972). Siminowitz (1979) reported immunization rates in the next pregnancy of 3.6 per cent in Rhesus (D) negative women after unprotected abortion (11 out of 300 women) as compared to 0.4 per cent (13 out of 3080) women when 50 microgram of anti-D immunoglobulin was given after the abortion. Similar findings were reported by other investigators (Kiss and Szoke 1974; Hensleigh *et al.* 1977; Keith and Bozorgi 1977). From these studies it would appear that up to 13 weeks of pregnancy a dose of 50 to 75 micrograms is sufficient to ensure adequate protection. In the second trimester the standard postpartum dose of 200 to 300 microgram is recommended.

Katz and Marcus (1972) have pointed out that in ruptured ectopic pregnancies fetal blood may be resorbed from the maternal peritoneal cavity and enter the maternal circulation. They found that 9 out of 38 women with ruptured tubal pregnancies between 6 and 10 weeks of gestation had a significant number of fetal erythrocytes in their circulation, suggesting that anti-D immunoglobulin should be administered to all Rhesus (D) women in these circumstances.

3.2.3 Events in pregnancy

Abdominal trauma, placenta praevia, placental abruption, or any form of uterine bleeding may on occasion cause feto-maternal transfusion (Turchetti *et al.* 1965; Renaer *et al.* 1976). This may sometimes be suspected on the basis of the findings at cardiotocography performed for these indications. Even without any obvious cause feto-maternal transfusion may occur. In a series of 5001 pregnancies, Van de Putte *et al.* (1972) found 6 feto-maternal transfusions that were large enough to account for 4 perinatal deaths and 2 cases of severe neonatal anaemia. Unexplained fetal or intrapartum death, or the birth of a pale, distressed child should alert the obstetrician to the possibility of a feto-maternal transfusion.

3.2.4 Interventions in pregnancy

Feto-maternal haemorrhage has been documented as a consequence of chorion villus sampling (Mariona *et al.* 1986; Brambati *et al.* 1986); amniocentesis (Blajchman *et al.* 1974; Lachman *et al.* 1977; Goldstein and Pezzlo 1978; Schmidt *et al.* 1980; Lele *et al.* 1982; Mennuti *et al.* 1980; Thomsen *et al.* 1983; Hill *et al.* 1980; Chard *et al.* 1976); placentocentesis (Fairweather *et al.* 1980); and fetoscopy (Fairweather *et al.* 1980).

In chorion villus sampling, to the present day, the only evidence for such bleeding consists of an elevation of the maternal serum alpha-fetoprotein concentration after the procedure (Brambatti *et al.* 1986). It should be realized that this does not necessarily mean that red cells have entered the maternal circulation. The elevation may be due to maternal uptake of placental cell protein. Nevertheless, it is generally recommended that 50 to 75 microgram of anti-D immunoglobulin should be administered to Rhesus (D) negative women after chorion villus sampling.

Amniocentesis in early and late pregnancy is also associated with an increased risk of feto-maternal transfusion. In early pregnancy most of the evidence is based on the increase in serum alpha-fetoprotein concentrations generally observed after the procedure. Again, this does not necessarily equate with passage of fetal red blood cells. A number of investigators have reported a reduction in the frequency of feto-maternal transfusion when ultrasound was used to guide the amniocentesis (Schmidt *et al.* 1980; Mennuti *et al.* 1983). In the 3rd trimester the frequency of feto-maternal transfusion associated with amniocentesis is certainly not negligible (Harrison and Campbell 1975; Platt *et al.* 1978). In genetic amniocentesis a dose of 50 to 75 microgram anti-D immunoglobulin is probably sufficient. Later in pregnancy a dose of 200 to 300 microgram is more appropriate, as this dose will also afford protection against Rhesus immunization for the remainder of the pregnancy.

Several authors (Vos 1967; Pollock 1968; Hochhuli 1977; Gjode *et al.* 1980; Stine *et al.* 1985) have described feto-maternal transfusion after external cephalic version (see Chapter 42). A standard dose of anti-D immunoglobulin is probably required.

3.2.5 Non-pregnancy related

The administration of anti-D immunoglobulin after transfusion with Rhesus (D) positive blood has been shown to provide effective prophylaxis (Roszner *et al.* 1975; Bowman 1976; Keith *et al.* 1976). Ennker *et al.* (1979) reviewed 80 cases in which anti-D immunoglobulin was used after mismatched transfusions. The volume of blood transfused ranged from 10 ml to 1250 ml of whole blood.

The optimal dose of anti-D immunoglobulin was determined by Pollack *et al.* (1971b), who found no failures of prophylaxis when a dose of 20 microgram anti-D immunoglobulin per millilitre of transfused blood was used. As intramuscular injection of anti-D immunoglobulin is very painful, the anti-D immunoglobulin should be administered intravenously. To prevent serious side-effects the infusion should be administered slowly (25 ml per hour). For this purpose it is best to use anti-D immunoglobulin prepared by ion-exchange chromatography at a dilution of 1000–2500 microgram in 100 ml containing 2 per cent (w/v) human albumin. Larger amounts, if required, should be administered over several days (Ennker *et al.* 1979).

4 Screening and diagnosis

All women should have routine determination of their Rhesus (D) status in early pregnancy. Women who are Rhesus (D) negative should be further screened for the presence of antibodies, as the Rhesus (D) antigens are the main cause of isoimmunization in the absence of Rhesus (D) prophylaxis. The other Rhesus antigens are far less immunogenic, but occasionally can cause serious clinical problems. Anti-Kell, anti-Kidd, anti-Duffy, and some of the more rare antigens can also cause haemolytic disease in the fetus and newborn (Weinstein 1982). For this reason, many centres screen all pregnant women for Rhesus and other blood group antibodies (Bowell *et al.* 1986).

The presence of antibodies indicates that the fetus may become affected if it carries the antigen to which the antibodies were formed. The presence of antibodies does not tell whether or not the fetus does carry the antigen. It is therefore helpful to determine whether the woman's partner is homozygous or heterozygous for the antigen. If the father is homozygous, the fetus will carry the antigen; if the father is heterozygous, there is a 50 per cent risk that it will. Zygosity of the Rhesus (D) antigen cannot be determined with certainty, but it can be estimated with a probability ranging between 80 and 96 per cent (Race 1954).

On occasion, knowledge of the blood type of the fetus at an early stage of gestation can be of help in the management of pregnancy in women with severe Rhesus immunization and a heterozygous partner. It is possible to obtain fetal red cells by chorion villus sampling as early as 8 to 11 weeks of gestation (Kanhai *et al.* 1987). Using sensitive immunofluorescence techniques it is possible to detect one fetal Rhesus (D) positive red cell among 4000 maternal Rhesus (D) negative erythrocytes (Gemke *et al.* 1986). Knowledge of the blood type of the fetus makes it possible to avoid the use of invasive diagnostic procedures later in pregnancy if the fetus proves to be Rhesus (D) negative, and permits the offer of a termination to a woman with a history of severe Rhesus (D) haemolytic disease in previously affected pregnancies if the fetus is Rhesus (D) positive (Kanhai *et al.* 1987).

The presence and level of an antibody titre does not always predict the presence or severity of disease, although in a first affected pregnancy there is a reasonable correlation between the antibody titre and the severity of disease (Bowman 1984).

The major prognostic determinant of the severity of disease is the past obstetric history. Bowman (1978, 1984) showed that the severity of the disease in previous pregnancies, in combination with serial antibody titres, will give a reasonably accurate assessment of the severity of the haemolytic disease in the current pregnancy about 62 per cent of the time, but not, however, with sufficient precision to determine the optimal time for intervention. For this, amniocentesis and spectrophotometric analysis of haemoglobin degradation products (bilirubin) in the amniotic fluid are required. This must be repeated at regular intervals, depending upon the level and change in the level of amniotic fluid bilirubin.

The timing of intervention will depend primarily on this level (Liley 1961), although hydropic changes and hepatomegaly found on ultrasound (Buscaglia *et al.* 1986; Vintzileos *et al.* 1986), as well as more or less typical features on antenatal cardiotocography (Mondanlou *et al.* 1977; Visser 1982; Katz *et al.* 1983), may help to determine whether and when intervention is necessary.

5 Treatment

Preterm delivery was formerly the only method of antenatal management available. A multicentre factorial design randomized trial was planned in 1948, and the results were reported by Mollison and Walker in 1952 and by Armitage and Mollison in 1953. The practice of preterm induction between 35 and 37 weeks of gestation was 'associated with a reduced incidence of stillbirth but this was outweighed by the increased incidence of neonatal deaths; hence the total death rate in the "induced group" was higher than in the group allowed to go to spontaneous delivery' (Mollison and Walker 1952). The total death rate in the induced group was 28 out of 77 (36 per cent), while that in the spontaneous group was 26 out of 108 (24 per cent). Interesting as these trial reports were at the time, they do not, of course, apply to current care.

Pre-emptive delivery before the fetus is too severely affected to be effectively treated by postnatal therapy remains the mainstay of treatment. When, however, the pregnancy cannot be carried to a stage of fetal maturity that would allow delivery of an infant who can be successfully treated by the currently available methods of intensive neonatal care, intrauterine transfusion is the treatment of choice.

The introduction of intrauterine transfusion by Liley in 1963 has dramatically changed the outlook for the very preterm fetus with haemolytic disease. Refinements in technique, and especially the use of modern ultrasound equipment, have facilitated the procedure and improved the results (Clewell *et al.* 1981; Frigoletto *et al.* 1981; Larkin *et al.* 1982; Bennebroek Gravenhorst and Woudenberg 1982; Buscaglia *et al.* 1986).

In its original design, intrauterine transfusion was based on the fact that red cells can be absorbed from the fetal peritoneal cavity and enter the fetal circulation (Mellish and Wolman 1958; Taylor *et al.* 1966). By infusing Rhesus (D) negative packed cells into the fetal peritoneal cavity, fetal anaemia can be corrected and delivery may be postponed to a more advanced stage in pregnancy. The procedure can be started as early as 21 to 22 weeks of gestation and can be repeated if necessary. More recently, techniques of intravascular fetal transfusions have been described (Rodeck *et al.* 1984; Hobbins *et al.* 1985; Grannum *et al.* 1986a,b; de Crespigny *et al.* 1985; Berkowitz *et al.* 1986; Nicolaides *et al.* 1986). The advantages of these methods have not been evaluated against intraperitoneal transfusions, but the latter also have not been tested in controlled trials.

In early published series, overall survival rates were 28 to 62 per cent (Whitfield *et al.* 1972; Bowman *et al.* 1969; Robertson *et al.* 1976). In more recent studies, a perinatal survival rate of 69 to 92 per cent has been reported (Bowman and Manning 1983; Berkowitz and Hobbins 1981; Clewell *et al.* 1981; Larkin *et al.* 1982; Harman *et al.* 1983; Scott *et al.* 1984). The two major factors in determining survival are the presence or absence of hydrops and the likelihood of fetal trauma. With hydropic infants mortality rates range between 25 and 75 per cent (Bowman and Manning 1983; Larkin *et al.* 1982; Bennebroek Gravenhorst and Woudenberg 1982; Scott et al. 1984).

The risk of traumatic death has decreased considerably since the use of real time ultrasound. The current fetal mortality risk per procedure is estimated at 2 to 3 per cent with intraperitoneal transfusions (Bennebroek Gravenhorst and Woudenberg 1982; Scott *et al.* 1984). A close approximation of the direct mortality risk for intravascular transfusion is not yet possible.

Maternal morbidity occurs in 1 to 2 per cent of the cases. Infection, hepatitis, and placental abruption have all been reported (Mandelbaum and Brough 1967; Bowman 1978; Larkin *et al.* 1982).

In follow-up studies of 450 infants surviving after intrauterine transfusion, 78 per cent appeared normal, 17.1 per cent had minor and 5.1 per cent severe neurological damage (Hardyment *et al.* 1979). Ellis (1980) and Ruys (1982) reported 15 per cent abnormalities after intrauterine transfusion. White *et al.* (1978) reported that if the transfused infants are compared with controls matched for gestational age, birthweight, and mode of delivery, no statistically significant differences were found.

Other treatments that have been used include plasmapheresis from early pregnancy onward (Angela *et al.* 1980); immune suppression with promethazine (Gusdon 1981; Charles and Blumenthal 1982); and desensitization by oral administration of Rhesus (D) red blood cells (Bierme *et al.* 1979). The claimed benefits of the latter two methods have not been found by other investigators (Stenchever 1978; Caudle and Scott 1982; Gold *et al.* 1983). Corticosteroids do lower the bilirubin concentration of amniotic fluid but do not have a beneficial influence on the clinical situation and may mislead the clinician (Navot *et al.* 1982).

Plasmapheresis in which large volumes of plasma are removed and replaced with donor plasma is used in some centres as a method of management of haemolytic disease in severely immunized women with at least two prior stillbirths and a probable Rhesus (D) homozygous partner (Clarke *et al.* 1970; Graham-Pole *et al.* 1974; Fraser *et al.* 1976; Pepperell and Cooper 1978).

In our centre we have treated 27 mothers with weekly small volume plasmapheresis (600 ml) starting at an early stage of pregnancy. Four mothers gave birth to a Rhesus (D) negative infant. Of the remaining 23 Rhesus (D) positive infants 15 (65 per cent) survived. Intrauterine transfusion was carried out in only 4 of these pregnancies (Bennebroek Gravenhorst and Kanhai 1986). These results suggest that small volume plasmapheresis may be as effective as the more demanding large volume plasmapheresis that are usually recommended.

6 Conclusions

Haemolytic disease of the fetus and newborn, while by no means the frequent problem that it once was, remains a problem that requires constant vigilance and attention to prophylactic care. Although effective prophylaxis is available it must be properly used. Situations in which Rhesus immunization does occur have become sufficiently rare and its treatment is sufficiently complex to warrant regionalization of care for these women and babies.

References

Angela E, Robinson E, Tovey LAD (1980). Intensive plasma exchange in the management of severe Rh disease. Br J Haematol, 45: 621–631.

Armitage P, Mollison PL (1953). Further analysis of controlled trials of treatment of haemolytic disease of the newborn. J Obstet Gynaecol Br Empire, 60: 605–620.

Ascari WG, Allen AE, Baker WJ, Pollack W (1968). Rho(D) immune globulin (human) evaluation in women at risk of Rh immunization. JAMA, 205: 1–4.

Ballantyne JW (1892). The Diseases and Deformations of the Foetus. Edinburgh: Oliver & Boyd.

Bartsch FR, Hermann M (1979). Proceedings of the McMaster Rh Conference. Vox Sang, 36: 50–64.

Bennebroek Gravenhorst J, Kanhai HHH (1986). Rhesus-antagonisme. Ned Tijdschr Geneeskd, 130: 1220–1224.

Bennebroek Gravenhorst J, Van Woudenberg J (1982). Intrauterine fetal transfusion in severe RH isoimmunization. In: Paediatrics and Blood Transfusion. Smit Sibinga CTH, Forfar JO (eds). The Hague/Boston/London: Martinus Nijhof, pp 171–175.

Bennebroek Gravenhorst J, Woodfield DG (1985). Isoimmunization in pregnancy: diagnosis, treatment and prevention.

In: Supportive Therapy in Haematology. Das PC, Smit Sibinga CT, Halie MR (eds). Boston: Martinus Nijhoff, pp 129–137.

Bennebroek Gravenhorst J, Beintema-Dubbeldam A, van Lith DAF, Beekhuizen W (1986). Elevation of maternal alpha-fetoprotein serum levels in relation to fetomaternal haemorrhage after second trimester pregnancy termination by aspirotomy. Br J Obstet Gynaecol, 93: 1302–1304.

Berkowitz RL, Hobbins JC (1981). Intrauterine transfusion utilizing ultrasound. Obstet Gynecol, 57: 33–36.

Berkowitz RL, Chitkara U, Goldberg JD, Wilkins I, Chervenak FA, Lynch L (1986a). Intrauterine intravascular transfusions for severe red blood cell isoimmunization: Ultrasound-guided percutaneous approach. Am J Obstet Gynecol, 155: 574–581.

Berkowitz RL, Chitkara U, Goldberg JD, Wilkins I, Chevernak FA (1986b). Intrauterine transfusion in utero: the percutaneous approach. Am J Obstet Gynecol, 154: 622–623.

Bevis DCA (1956). Blood pigments in haemolytic disease of the newborn. J Obstet Gynaecol Br Empire, 63: 68–75.

Bierme SJ, Blanc M, Abbal M, Fournie A (1979). Oral Rh treatment for severely immunised mothers. Lancet, i: 604–605.

Bishop GJ, Krieger VI (1969). One millilitre injections of Rho(D) immune globulin in prevention of Rh immunization. A further report on the clinical trial. Med J Austral, 2: 171–174.

Blajchman MA, Maudsley RF, Uchida I, Zipursky A (1974). Diagnostic amniocentesis and fetal-maternal bleeding. Lancet, i: 993–994.

Bowell PJ, Allen DL, Entwistle CC (1986). Bloodgroup antibody screening tests during pregnancy. Br J Obstet Gynaecol, 93: 1038–1043.

Bowman H (1976). Effectiveness of prophylactic Rh immuno suppression after transfusion with D-positive blood. Am J Obstet Gynecol, 124: 80–84.

Bowman JM (1978). The management of Rh-isoimmunization. Obstet Gynecol, 52: 1–16.

Bowman JM (1984). Rhesus haemolytic disease. In: Antenatal and Neonatal Screening. Wald NJ (ed). Oxford: Oxford University Press, pp 314–344.

Bowman JM (1985). Controversies in Rh prophylaxis. Who needs Rh immunoglobulin and when should it be given? Am J Obstet Gynecol, 151: 289–294.

Bowman JM (1986). Feto-maternal ABO incompatibility and erythroblastosis fetalis. Vox Sang, 50: 104–106.

Bowman JM, Manning FA (1983). Intrauterine fetal transfusions: Winnipeg 1982. Obstet Gynecol, 61: 203–209.

Bowman JM, Pollock JM (1978). Antenatal prophylaxis of Rh isoimmunization: 28 weeks-gestation service program. Can Med Assoc J, 118: 627–630.

Bowman JM, Friesen RF, Bowman WD, McInnis A, Barnes P, Grewar D (1969). Fetal transfusion in severe Rh isoimmunization. JAMA, 207: 1101–1106.

Brambatti B, Guercilena S, Bonacchi I, Oldrini A, Lanzani A, Piceni L (1986). Feto-maternal transfusion after chorionic villus sampling: clinical implications. Human Reproduction 1: 37–40.

Buscaglia M, Ferrazzi E, Zuliani G, Caccamo ML, Pardi G (1986). Ultrasound contributions to the management of the severely isoimmunized fetus. J Perinat Med, 14: 51–58.

Caudle MR, Scott JR (1982). The potential role of immunosuppression plasmapheresis and desensitization as treatment modalities for Rh immunization. Clin Obstet Gynecol, 25: 313–319.

Central Bureau of Statistics (1987). Unpublished data from the Netherlands' Central Bureau of Statistics.

Chard T, Kitau MJ, Ledward R, Coltart T, Embury S, Seller MJ (1976). Elevated levels of maternal plasma alpha-fetoprotein after amniocentesis. Br J Obstet Gynaecol, 83: 33–34.

Charles AG, Blumenthal LS (1982). Promethazine Hydrochloride therapy in severely Rh-sensitized pregnancies. Obstet Gynecol, 60: 627–630.

Chown B (1954). Anaemia from bleeding of the fetus into the maternal circulation. Lancet, i: 1213–1215.

Chown B, Duff AM, James J, Nation E, Ellement M, Buchanan DI, Beck P, Martin JK, Godel JC, McHugh M, Jarosch JM, De Veber II, Holland C, Cunningham TA, MacLachlan TB, Blum E, Bryans FE, Stout TD, Decker J, Bowman JM, Lewis M, Peddie LJ, Kaita H, Anderson C, Van Dyk C (1969). Prevention of Primary Rh Immunization: First report of the Western Canadian Trial, 1966–1968. Can Med Assoc J, 100: 1021–1024.

Clarke CA, Donohoe WTA, McConnell RB, Woodrow JC, Finn R, Krevans JR, Kulke W, Lehane D, Sheppard PM (1963). Further experimental studies on the prevention of Rh haemolytic disease. Br Med J, i: 979–984.

Clarke CA, Bradley J, Elson CJ, Donohoe WTA (1970). Intensive plasmapheresis as a therapeutic measure in Rhesus immunized women. Lancet, i: 793–799.

Clarke CA, Donohoe WTA, Finn R, Lehane D, McConnell RB, Sheppard PM, Towers SH, Woodrow JC, Bowley CC, Tovey LAD, Bias WM, Krevans JR (Medical Research Council Working Party) (1971). Prevention of Rh-haemolytic disease: final results of the 'high risk' clinical trial. Br Med J, 2: 607–609.

Clarke CA, Mollison PL, Whitfield AGW (1985). Death from rhesus haemolytic disease in England and Wales in 1982 and 1983. Br Med J, 291: 17–19.

Clewell WH, Dunne MG, Johnson ML, Bowes WA (1981). Fetal transfusion with real-time ultrasound guidance. Obstet Gynecol, 57: 516–520.

Coombs RRA, Mourant AE, Race RR (1946). A new test for the detection of weak and 'incomplete' Rh agglutinins. Br J Exp Path, 26: 255–266.

Darrow RR (1938). Icterus gravis (Erythroblastosis) neonatorum. An examination of etiologic considerations. Arch Path, 25: 378–417.

Davey M (1979). The prevention of Rhesus-isoimmunization. Clin Obstet Gynaecol, 6: 509–530.

Davey MG, Zipursky A (1979). Proceedings of the McMaster Rh Conference. Vox Sang, 36: 50–64.

de Crespigny CH, Robinson HP, Quinn M, Doyle L, Ross E, Gauchi M (1985). Ultrasound-guided fetal blood transfusion for severe rhesus isoimmunization. Obstet Gynecol, 66: 529–532.

Dienst A (1905). Das Eklampsiegift, vorlaufige Mitteilung. Zbl Gynäkol 29: 353–364.

Dudok de Wit C, Borst-Eilers E, Weerdt CHM, Kloosterman GJ (1968). Prevention of RH immunization. A controlled trial with a comparatively low dose of anti-D immunoglobulin. Br Med J, 4: 477–479.

Ellis MI (1980). Follow-up study of survivors after intrauterine transfusion. Dev Med Child Neurol, 22: 48–54.

Ennker J, Maas DHN, Schneider J (1979). Immunoprophylactic anti Rh(D) treatment after mismatched transfusions. Eur J Obstet Gynecol Reprod Biol, 9: 117–124.

Fairweather DVI, Ward RHT, Modell B (1980). Obstetric aspects of midtrimester fetal bloodsampling by needling or fetoscopy. Br J Obstet Gynecol, 87: 87–99.

Fraser ID, Bennet MO, Bothamley JE, Airth GR (1976). Intensive antenatal plasmapheresis in severe rhesus isoimmunization. Lancet, i: 6–9.

Freda VJ, Gorman JG, Pollack W (1964). Successful prevention of experimental RH sensitization in man with an anti-RH gamma2-globin antibody preparation: A preliminary report. Transfusion, 4: 26–32.

Freda VJ, Gorman JG, Galen RS, Treacy N (1970). The threat of Rh immunization from abortion. Lancet, ii: 147–148.

Frigoletto FD, Umanski I, Birnholz J, Acker D, Easterday CL, Harris GBC, Griscom NT (1981). Intrauterine fetal transfusion in 365 fetuses during fifteen years. Am J Obstet Gynecol, 139: 781–788.

Gemke RJBJ, Kanhai HHH, Overbeeke MA, Maas CJ, Bennebroek Gravenhorst J, Bernini LF, Engelfriet CP, Veer MB (1986). ABO and Rhesus phenotyping of fetal erythrocytes in the first trimester of pregnancy. Br J Haematol, 64: 689–697.

Gjode P, Rasmussen Th, Jorgensen J (1980). Fetomaternal bleeding during attempts at external version. Br J Obstet Gynaecol, 87: 571–573.

Godel JC, Buchanan DI, Jarosch JM, McHugh M (1968). Significance of Rh-sensitization during pregnancy: its relation to a preventive programme. Br Med J, 4: 479–482.

Gold WR, Queenan JT, Woody J, Sacher RA (1983). Oral desensitization in Rh disease. Am J Obstet Gynecol, 146: 980–981.

Goldman JA, Eckerling B (1972). Prevention of Rh immunization after abortion with anti-Rho(D)-immuno globulin. Obstet Gynecol, 40: 366–370.

Goldstein AI, Pezzlo F (1978). Fetal-maternal hemorrhage after amniocentesis. Incidence, degree and ramification. Int J Gynaecol Obstet, 16: 187–189.

Graham-Pole J, Barr W, Willoughby MLN (1974). Continuous-flow exchange-plasmapheresis in severe Rhesus isoimmunization. Lancet, i: 1051.

Grannum PA, Copel JA, Plaxe SC, Scioscia AL, Hobbins JC (1986). In utero exchange transfusion by direct intravascular injection in severe erythroblastosis fetalis. New Engl J Med, 314: 1431–1434.

Gusdon JP (1981). The treatment of erythroblastosis with promethazine. J Reprod Med, 26: 454–458.

Halban J (1900). Agglutinationsversuche mit mutterlichen und kindlichen Blute. Wien klin Wochenschr, 24: 545–548.

Hardyment AF, Salvador HS, Towell ME, Carpenter CW, Jan JE, Tingle AJ (1979). Follow-up of intrauterine transfused surviving children. Am J Obstet Gynecol, 133: 235–241.

Harman CR, Manning FA, Bowman JM, Lange IR (1983). Severe Rh disease—poor outcome is not inevitable. Am J Obstet Gynecol, 145: 823–829.

Harrison R, Campbell S, Craft I (1975). Risk of feto-maternal haemorrhage resulting from amniocentesis with or without ultrasound placental localization. Obstet Gynecol, 46: 389–391.

Hart AP (1925). Familial icterus gravis of the newborn and its treatment. Can Med Assoc J, 15: 1008.

Hensleigh PA, Dixon LW, Hall E, Kitay DZ, Jackson JE (1977). Reduced dose of Rh(D) immuno globulin following induced first trimester abortion. Am J Obstet Gynecol, 129: 413–416.

Hill LM, Platt LD, Kellogg B (1980). Rh sensitization after genetic amniocentesis. Obstet Gynecol, 56: 459–461.

Hindeman P (1966). Untersuchungen über die transperitoneale Spateinschwemmung fetaler Erythrocyten in den mutterlichen Kreislauf. Bibl Gynäkol, 38: 23–29.

Hobbins JC, Grannum PA, Romero R, Reece EA, Mahoney MJ (1985) Percutaneous umbilical blood sampling. Am J Obstet Gynecol, 152: 1–6.

Hochhuli E (1977). Kritik zur auszere Wendung in Terminnahe bei Beckenendlage. Z Geburtsh Perinatol, 181: 325–328.

Huchet J, Dallemagne S, Huchet Cl, Brossard Y, Larsen M, Parnet-Mathieu F (1987). Application anté-partum du traitement préventif d'immunisation Rhésus D chez les femmes Rhésus négatif. J Gynécol Obstét Biol Réprod, 16: 101–111.

Kanhai HHH, Bennebroek Gravenhorst J, Gemke RJ, Overbeeke MA, Bernini LF, Beverstock GC (1987). Fetal blood group determination in first trimester pregnancy for the management of severe immunization. Am J Obstet Gynecol, 156: 120–123.

Katz J, Marcus RG (1972). The risk of Rh isoimmunisation in ruptured tubal pregnancy. Br Med J, 3: 667–669.

Katz M, Meizner I, Shani N, Insler V (1983). Clinical significance of sinusoidal fetal heart rate pattern. Br J Obstet Gynaecol, 90: 832–836.

Keith L, Bozorgi N (1977). Small dose anti-Rh therapy after first trimester abortion. Int J Gynaecol Obstet, 15: 235–237.

Keith L, Berger GS, Pollack W (1976). The transfusion of Rh positive blood into Rh negative women. Am J Obstet Gynecol, 125: 502–505.

Kiss D, Szoke B (1974). Prevention der Rh-isoimmunisation in verbindung mit Spontan Abortus und Schwangerschaftsunterbrechungen. Zbl Gynäkol, 96: 389–401.

Lachman E, Hingley SM, Bates G, Ward AM, Stewart CR, Duncan LB (1977). Detection and measurement of fetomaternal haemorrhage: serum alpha-protein and Kleihauer technique. Br Med J, 1: 1377–1379.

Landsteiner K, Wiener AS (1940). An agglutinable factor in human blood recognized by immune sera for Rhesus blood. Proc Soc Exp Biol Med, 43: 223.

Larkin RM, Knochel JQ, Lee TG (1982). Intrauterine transfusions: new techniques and results. Clin Obstet Gynecol, 25: 303–312.

Lele AS, Carmody PJ, Hurd ME, O'Leary JA (1982). Fetomaternal bleeding following diagnostic amniocentesis. Obstet Gynecol, 60: 60–64.

Leonard MF (1945). Haemolytic disease of the newborn (erythroblastosis foetalis). Clinical analysis of fifty-five cases with special reference to pathogenesis, prognosis and therapy. J Pediatr, 27: 249-255.

Levine PH, Newark NJ, Stetson RE (1939). An unusual case of intra-group agglutination. JAMA, 113: 126–127.

Levine Ph, Katzin EM, Burnham L (1941). Isoimmunization

in pregnancy. Its possible bearing on the etiology of erythroblastosis foetalis. JAMA, 116: 825–827.

Liley AW (1961). Liquor amnii analysis in management of pregnancy complicated by rhesus sensitization. Am J Obstet Gynecol, 82: 1359–1370.

Liley AW (1963). Intrauterine transfusion of foetus in haemolytic disease. Br Med J, 2: 1107–1109.

Lim OW, Fleisher AA, Ziel HK (1982). Reduction of rho(D)-sensitization: a cost–effective analysis. Obstet Gynecol, 59: 477–480.

Mandelbaum B, Brough J (1967). Hepatitis following multiple intrauterine transfusions. Obstet Gynecol, 30: 188–191.

Mariona FG, Syner FN, Koppitich F (1986). Chorionic villi sampling changes maternal serum alpha-fetoprotein. Prenat Diagn, 6: 69–73.

Matthews CD, Matthews AEB (1969). Transplacental haemorrhage in spontaneous and induced abortion. Lancet, i: 694–695.

Medical Research Council (1974). Controlled trial of various anti-D dosages in suppression of Rh sensitization following pregnancy. Br Med J, 2: 75–80.

Mellish P, Wolman IJ (1958). Intraperitoneal blood transfusion. Am J Med Sci, 235: 717–725.

Mennuti MT, Brummond W, Crombleholm WR, Schwarz RH, Arvan DH (1980). Fetal-maternal bleeding associated with genetic amniocentesis. Obstet Gynecol, 55: 48–54.

Mennuti T, Digaetano A, McDonnell A, Cohen AW, Liston RM (1983) Fetal-maternal bleeding associated with genetic amniocentesis: Real-time versus static ultrasound. Obstet Gynecol, 62: 26–30.

Mollison PL, Walker W (1952). Controlled trials of the treatment of haemolytic disease of the newborn. Lancet, i: 429–433.

Mondanlou HD, Freeman RK, Ortitz O, Hinkes P, Pillsbury G (1977). Sinusoidal fetal heart rate pattern and severe fetal anemia. Obstet Gynecol, 49: 537–541.

Navot D, Rozen E, Sadovski E (1982). Effect of dexamethasone on amniotic fluid absorbance in Rh-sensitized pregnancies. Br J Obstet Gynaecol, 89: 456–458.

Nevanlinna HR, Vainio T (1956). The influence of mother-child ABO incompatibility on Rh immunization. Vox Sang, 1: 26–36.

Nicolaides KH, Soothill PW, Rodeck CH, Clewell W (1986). Rh disease: Fetal blood transfusion by cordocentesis. Fetal Therapy 1: 185–192.

Pepperell RJ, Cooper IA (1978). Intensive antenatal plasmapheresis in severe Rhesus isoimmunization. Austral NZ J Obstet Gynaecol, 18: 121–126.

Platt LD, Manning FA, Lemay M (1978). Real-time B-scan-directed amniocentesis. Am J Obstet Gynecol, 130: 700–703.

Pollack W, Ascari WQ, Crispen JF, O'Connor RR, Ho TY (1971a). Studies on Rh prophylaxis II. Rh immune prophylaxis after transfusion with Rh-positive blood. Transfusion, 11: 340–344.

Pollack W, Ascari WQ, Kochesky RR, O'Connor RR, Ho TY, Tripodi D (1971b). Studies on Rh prophylaxis I. Relationship between doses of anti-Rh and size of antigenic stimulus. Transfusion, 11: 333–339.

Pollock A (1968). Transplacental haemorrhage after external cephalic version. Lancet, i: 612.

Queenan JT, Kubarych SF, Shah S, Holland B (1971). Role of induced abortion in rhesus immunization. Lancet, i: 815–817.

Race RR (1954). Cited by Mollison PL (1979). Bloodtransfusion in Clinical Medicine (6th edn). Oxford: Blackwell Scientific Publications, p 297.

Renaer M, Van de Putte I, Vermylen C (1976). Massive feto-maternal haemorrhage as a cause of perinatal mortality and morbidity. Eur J Obstet Gynecol Reprod Biol, 3: 125–140.

Robertson EG, Brown A, Ellis MI, Walker W (1976). Intrauterine transfusion in the management of severe rhesus isoimmunization. Br J Obstet Gynaecol, 83: 694–697.

Robertson JG, Holmes CM (1969). A clinical trial of anti-Rho(D) immunoglobulin in the prevention of Rho(D) immunization. J Obstet Gynaecol Br Commnwlth, 76: 252–259.

Rodeck CH, Nicolaides H, Warsof LS, Fysh J, Gamsu HR, Kemp JR (1984). The management of severe isoimmunization by fetoscopic intravascular transfusions. Am J Obstet Gynecol, 150: 769–774.

Roszner P, Kaufmann HM, Moeller HG, Kruger D (1975). Die immunprophylaktische behandlung von Rh-fehltransfusionen. Zbl Gynäkol, 97: 1507–1517.

Ruys JH (1982). Development of infants surviving intrauterine transfusions. In: Paediatrics and Bloodtransfusion. Smit Sibinga CTH, Forfar JO (eds). The Hague/Boston/London: Martinus Nijhoff, pp 177–183.

Samson D, Mollison PL (1975). Effect on primary Rh immunisation of delayed administration of anti Rh. Immunology, 28: 349–357.

Schmidt W, Gabelmann J, Garoff L, Kubli K (1980). Feto-Maternelle Transfusionen nach amniocentese in der Fruhschwangerschaft, eine Auswertung von 1000 Fallen. Z Geburtsh Perinatol, 184: 359–365.

Scott JR, Kochenour NK, Larkin R, Scott M (1984). Changes in the management of severely Rh-immunized patients. Am J Obstet Gynecol, 149: 336–341.

Simonovitz I (1979). Proceedings of the McMaster Rh Conference. Vox Sang, 36: 50–64.

Stenchever MA (1978). Promethazine hydrochloride: Use in patients with Rh isoimmunization. Am J Obstet Gynecol, 130: 665–668.

Stenchever MA, Davies IJ, Weisman R, Gross S (1970). Rho(D)immunoglobulin: a double blind clinical trial. Am J Obstet Gynecol, 106: 316–317.

Stine LE, Phelan JP, Do RW, Eglinton GS, Dorsten JP van, Schifrin BS (1985). Update on external version performed at term. Obstet Gynecol, 65: 642–646.

Taylor WW, Scott DE, Pritchard JA (1966). Fate of compatible adult erythrocytes in the fetal peritoneal cavity. Obstet Gynecol, 28: 175–181.

Thomson SG, Isager-Sally L, Lange AP, Saurbrey N, Gronvall S, Schioler V (1983). Elevated maternal serum alphafetoprotein caused by midtrimester amniocentesis: A prognostic factor. Obstet Gynecol, 62: 297–300.

Tovey GH (1980). Should anti-D immunoglobulin be given antenatally? Lancet, 2: 466–468.

Turchetti G, Palagi R, Lattanzi, E (1965). Anaemia in the newborn due to transplacental fetal haemorrhage. Obstet Gynecol, 26: 698–701.

van Dijk BA (1988). Incidentie van immunisatie tegen het rhesus (D) en andere erythrocyten bloedgroepantigenen. Paper presented at the Symposium of the Central Laboratory of the Netherlands Red Cross Blood Transfusion service. 28 January 1988.

Van de Putte I, Renaer M, Vermeylen C (1972). Counting fetal erythrocytes as a diagnostic aid in perinatal death and morbidity. Am J Obstet Gynecol, 114: 850–856.

Vintzileos AM, Campbell WA, Storlazzi E, Mirochnick MH, Escoto DT, Nochimson DJ (1986). Fetal liver ultrasound measurements in isoimmunized pregnancies. Obstet Gynecol, 68: 162–167.

Visser GHA (1982). Antepartum sinusoidal and decelerative heart rate patterns in Rh disease. Am J Obstet Gynecol, 143: 538–544.

Voigt C, Britt RP (1969). Feto-maternal haemorrhage in therapeutic abortion. Br Med J, 4: 395–396.

Vos GH (1967). The effect of external version on antenatal immunization by the Rh factor. Vox Sang, 12: 390–396.

Weinstein L (1982). Irregular antibodies causing haemolytic disease of the newborn: a continuing problem. Clin Obstet Gynecol, 25: 321–332.

White CA, Visscher RD, Visscher HC, Wade ME (1970). Rho(D) immune prophylaxis: a double-blind cooperative study. Obstet Gynecol, 36: 341–346.

White CA, Goplerud CP, Kisker CT, Stehbens JA, Kitchell M, Taylor JC (1978). Intrauterine fetal transfusion, 1965–1976, with an assessment of the surviving children. Am J Obstet Gynecol, 130: 933–939.

Whitfield CR, Thompson W, Armstrong MJ, Reid McC (1972). Intrauterine fetal transfusion for severe rhesus haemolytic disease. J Obstet Gynaecol Br Commnwlth, 79: 931–940.

Wible-Kant J, Beer AE (1983). Antepartum Rh immune globulin. Clin Perinatol, 10: 343–355.

Wiener AS, Peters HR (1940). Hemolytic reactions following transfusions of blood of the homologous group, with three cases in which the same agglutinogen was responsible. Ann Intern Med, 13: 2306–2322.

Wiener AS, Wexler IB, Gamrin E (1944). Haemolytic disease of the foetus and the newborn infant with special reference to transfusion therapy and the use of biological test for detecting Rh sensitivity. Am J Dis Child, 68: 317–323.

Woodrow JC, Clarke CA, McConnell RB, Towers SH, Donohoe WTA (1971). Prevention of Rh-haemolytical disease: results of the Liverpool 'low-risk' clinical trial. Br Med J, 2: 610–612.

Zipursky A (1977). Rh hemolytic disease of the newborn—the disease eradicated by immunology. Clin Obstet Gynecol, 20: 759–772.

Zipursky A, Blajchman M (1979). Proceedings of the McMaster Rh Conference. Vox Sang, 36: 50–64.

Zipursky A, Israels LG (1967). The pathogenesis and prevention of Rh immunization. Can Med Assoc J 97: 1245–1257.

36 Diabetes in pregnancy

David J. S. Hunter

1 Introduction

Perinatal mortality in pregnancy complicated by diabetes has dropped tenfold in the last four decades compared with a fourfold to fivefold drop overall (Macfarlane and Mugford 1984). In a review of data on pregnant diabetic women from 26 teaching hospitals in the 1940s, Peel and Oakley (1949) found that the perinatal mortality was 40 per cent, whereas at the present time perinatal mortality rates are reported that are not significantly different from those of the population at large (Oloffson *et al.* 1984; Tevaarwerk *et al.* 1981). We have reached the stage where success must be measured by parameters other than perinatal mortality alone (Oloffson *et al.* 1984).

The precise reasons for this remarkable change are not immediately apparent. A number of factors may all have played a part. These would include, among others: increasing acceptance by physicians of the importance of tight control of diabetes; the introduction of programmes to achieve this control; the development of home glucose monitoring to facilitate such programmes; gradual trends towards prolongation of pregnancy; and advances in neonatal care. This chapter will review the components of care that have evolved in managing pregnancy complicated by diabetes, and will try to define the relative importance of each.

2 Definition and classification

Before proceeding further, it would be appropriate to review the current definition of diabetes. Diabetes is a disturbance of multiple metabolic pathways, rather than of glucose metabolism alone, although the effects on carbohydrate metabolism are the most apparent. The World Health Organization Expert Committee on Diabetes Mellitus (1980) defined the diagnostic criteria of diabetes as a random venous plasma glucose level greater than 11 mmol/l (200 mg/dl) or a fasting value of greater than 8 mmol/l (140 mg/dl), in the presence of symptoms of diabetes (polyuria, polydypsia, ketoacidosis).

Normal plasma glucose values were defined by this committee as less than 8 mmol/l on a random sample, and less than 6 mmol/l fasting. Values between the normal and those of diabetes are 'equivocal', and evaluation with a glucose challenge is recommended (75 g taken orally after an overnight fast). Venous plasma values over 11 mmol/l, 2 hours post challenge are diagnostic of diabetes, and values between 8 and 11 mmol/l are termed 'impaired glucose tolerance'.

To establish the diagnosis of diabetes in the absence of symptoms of diabetes, at least one additional abnormal glucose value is required, such as a 1 hour post challenge glucose value greater than 11 mmol/l or an elevated 2 hour or fasting glucose value on a repeat occasion.

Although there is general consensus on the impact of overt diabetes in pregnancy, the significance and appropriate management of lesser degrees of hyperglycaemia is widely debated (see Chapter 25).

The subclassification of patients with established

diabetes preceding pregnancy (White 1949), which relates perinatal mortality to duration of diabetes or presence of microvascular damage, is still widely used. Although a review of 1196 pregnancies from several centres prior to 1977 showed a significantly higher perinatal mortality in White Class D as compared to Class B diabetics (Gabbe 1978), a review of 1043 pregnancies reported since that time, including the McMaster series, fails to show such a relationship (Table 36.1). Pedersen *et al.* (1974) added the occurrence of pyelonephritis, ketoacidosis, pre-eclampsia, and inadequate antenatal care as prognostically bad signs in diabetic women. While these factors can all adversely influence perinatal morbidity, it is unlikely that they would predict significant differences in the perinatal mortality rate. These classifications therefore, although indicating increased risk of morbidity, do not quantify that risk, and are probably of most value when used to compare series of pregnant diabetics between centres.

Table 36.1 Perinatal mortality and White's classification derived from reports since 1977 (data from Gabbe *et al.* 1977a; Kitzmiller *et al.* 1978; Adashi *et al.* 1979; Coustan *et al.* 1980; Jovanovic *et al.* 1981; Kitzmiller *et al.* 1981; Ylinen *et al.* 1981; Jovanovic and Jovanovic 1984; and the unpublished McMaster series, 1987)

		Perinatal mortality	
White's class	No. of cases	No.	Per 1000
B	465	13	27.9
C	257	7	27.2
D, R & F	321	10	31.2
R/F*	96	6	62.5
Total	1139	36	31.6

* Obtained from reports that separately identify class R/F

3 Care for diabetic pregnancy

3.1 Prepregnancy counselling and assessment

Increasingly, diabetic patients wish to discuss the prospects and implications of pregnancy prior to conception. At this time, the topics of major importance to be discussed are the risks to the fetus and neonate, including the likelihood of miscarriage and risk of congenital anomaly, and the risk to the mother, particularly the significance of diabetic retinopathy and nephropathy in those women so affected. This is an opportune time to discuss the general management of diabetes in pregnancy, the importance of tight control just before and during pregnancy in order to reduce the risks, and the need for accurate estimation of the date of conception.

Despite the acknowledged risk of aberrant fetal growth and the (occasional) need for elective delivery for which accurate information on the duration of pregnancy is mandatory, some diabetic women still present with uncertain dates. This can easily be prevented by instructing diabetic women to maintain routinely a permanent record of their menstrual periods, and to seek advice whenever these are unduly delayed. Similarly, women with irregular cycles can be requested to keep a basal body temperature chart in order to record the onset of pregnancy accurately.

Since diabetes is a chronic and progressive disease, the advice may need to include a discussion of the fact that postponement of pregnancy until a later age may eventually worsen the prognosis for the pregnancy.

While preconception clinics may fulfil an important role, it must be emphasized that the provision of adequate preconceptional care and advice does not depend on the establishment or provision of such specialized clinics. It is far more important that all those involved in the care of young diabetic women be critically aware of the importance of pregnancy, both emotionally and biologically. Not infrequently information is given too late, for fear that undue emphasis on the risks and dangers may create unwarranted anxiety. There is ample evidence, however, that for the majority of women full information will lessen rather than augment anxiety (see Chapter 8). Moreover, involving women in their care from the very beginning of pregnancy is likely to increase compliance with the measures that are considered to be of real importance for improving outcomes.

3.1.1 Risk of congenital anomalies

Diabetes is associated with an increased incidence of congenital anomalies (Mills 1982). Precise estimation of the risk is difficult because of the lack of consensus in defining major and minor anomalies, and a bias towards increased diagnosis and reporting of anomalies in infants of diabetic mothers.

Molsted-Pedersen *et al.* (1964) reported a congenital anomaly rate of 6.4 per cent in 853 infants of diabetic mothers compared with 2.1 per cent in 1212 infants of non-diabetic controls (relative risk: 3.0). The incidence of major anomalies was 5.2 per cent and 1.2 per cent respectively. Strict comparison cannot be made, however, as the control group was collected over a 6 months' period, and the diabetic series was spread over 37 years.

From the Collaborative Perinatal Project, Chung and Myrianthopoulos (1975) reported a major malformation rate in 499 infants of diabetic mothers of 17.6 per cent as compared to 8.4 per cent in 47,408 infants of non-diabetic mothers (relative risk: 2.1). Although this was a prospective study and provided concurrent controls, the definition of major anomaly included torticollis (5 cases); inguinal hernia (12 cases); contracture of hip (4 cases); metatarsus adductus (7 cases); cavernous haemangioma (4 cases); cardiac enlargement (9 cases); and hypospadias (7 cases), which together contributed 50 of the 88 so-called major anomalies reported. Furthermore, the study was institutionally rather than population based with the potential, therefore, of selection bias.

Kucera (1971) reviewed the world literature between 1945 and 1965, which consisted of 47 papers that described 340 anomalies in 7111 infants of diabetic mothers (4.8 per cent). A control series was derived from World Health Organization data along with his own series from Czechoslovakia. A total of 7124 anomalies were described among 431,764 infants of non-diabetic mothers (1.7 per cent). The incidence of some of the anomalies reported are listed in Table 36.2. It can be seen that cardiac anomalies are the most frequent, occurring over four times as often in the children of diabetic as in those of non-diabetic women. Vertebral anomalies, although not as common as cardiac anomalies, occur 50 times more frequently in children of diabetic than in children of non-diabetic women (Table 36.2).

Table 36.2 The number, incidence, and relative risk of selected anomalies in diabetics and non-diabetics (from Kucera 1971)

Anomally	Diabetics		Non-diabetics		Relative risk
	No.	Rate per 1000	No.	Rate per 1000	
Anencephaly	21	3.0	407	0.9	3.3
Spina bifida	14	2.0	636	1.4	1.4
Neural tube defect	33	4.6	1043	2.4	1.9
Cardiac	71	10.0	1007	2.3	4.3
Caudal regression	5	0.7	2	0.004	175
All vertebral	11	1.5	12	0.03	50
Cleft palate	6	0.8	313	0.7	1.1
Total anomalies	340	47.9	7124	16.5	2.9
Total patients	7101		431,764		

Grix (1982) found that 14 of 32 malformed infants of diabetic mothers born in southern California between 1973 and 1980 had multiple malformations; 12 of these 14 also had vertebral defects, hemivertebra being the most common.

Infants of diabetic mothers are at increased risk of neural tube defects. Milunski *et al.* (1982) reported 8 neural tube defects in a series of 411 diabetics, a rate 19 times the frequency found in non-diabetics. However, 7 of the 8 were anencephalics and Kucera's data (1971) also suggest the increased incidence lies more with anencephaly than with spina bifida. It is unclear at present whether diabetic women would derive added benefit over the general population from screening with serum alpha-fetoprotein as suggested by Milunsky *et al.* (1982). First, the increased risk of neural tube defects relates mainly to anencephaly which readily could be diagnosed by ultrasound. Second, alpha-fetoprotein levels in diabetics may be 60 per cent less than those in non-diabetics at the same gestational age (Wald *et al.* 1979). Reference values for serum alpha-fetoprotein based on a total population of pregnant women may therefore be entirely inadequate to estimate the risk of neural tube defects in a diabetic pregnancy.

The reason for the threefold increase of congenital anomalies in diabetes is not clear. It is unlikely for insulin to be responsible, since this hormone does not cross the placenta and since, at the time of embryogenesis, the fetus does not produce insulin (Like and Orci 1972). In animals there is evidence to incriminate excessive glucose and/or the broad metabolic derangement of diabetes as a cause of malformations. Sadler (1980) found that whole embryo cultures of mice exposed to diabetic levels of glucose had a high frequency of neural tube defects (exencephaly), and Baker *et al.* (1980) found that uncontrolled diabetes in the rat produced lumbosacral malformations analogous to those occurring in the offspring of diabetic women. Control of diabetes during the period of organ differentiation significantly reduced the number of lumbosacral defects compared to those occurring in the litters of the uncontrolled animals (Baker *et al.* 1980).

There are indications that in human pregnancies as well, the incidence of congenital anomalies can be reduced by controlling diabetes prior to, or during the early weeks of pregnancy. Miller *et al.* (1981) and Ylinen *et al.* (1984) have shown a significant correlation between elevated haemoglobin A_1 levels in the 1st trimester of pregnancy and an increased incidence of congenital malformations. Women with normal haemoglobin A_1 levels had an incidence of anomalies similar to the population at large. Fuhrmann *et al.* (1984) admitted 56 women to a prepregnancy clinic to achieve good control of diabetes and compared them to 144 women who did not join the clinic until the 8th week of pregnancy. Only 1 of the 56 women had a baby with malformations (cardiac), whereas 9 of the 144 women who joined the clinic after the 8th week had an infant with congenital anomalies; 3 of these were fatal, 3 were severe and 3 minor.

Although there are clear difficulties involved, and anxieties generated when trying to establish tight control before or during the early weeks of pregnancy (Steele *et al.* 1982), congenital anomalies are now the leading cause of perinatal mortality in diabetics (Cousins 1983). In view of the serious possibility that tight early control of the diabetes will reduce the risk, there is a pressing need to encourage preconceptional care for diabetic women. Obviously, such care would need to be based on adequate collaboration with and between diabetologist and obstetrician.

3.1.2 Other risks to fetus and neonate

3.1.2.1 Risk of miscarriage The difficulty in establishing the risk of miscarriage for diabetic women is threefold. First, the background incidence of spontaneous abortion is very difficult to obtain. Second, the definition of abortion varies from loss of pregnancy before the 20th to loss before the 28th week. Third, any reported incidence in a group of diabetic women from a clinical or personal series may suffer from the error of selection bias. A recent retrospective analysis of 164 pregnancies in 78 insulin-dependent diabetic women between 1956 and 1975 showed 17.1 per cent spontaneous abortions, compared to a background incidence of abortion of 8.8 per cent during that time period (Sutherland and Pritchard 1986). Despite the fact that this study was population based (the city of Aberdeen), the background incidence of spontaneous abortion is low, when compared to other series. Kalter (1987) reviewed over 50 articles published between 1950 and 1986 and noted the incidence of spontaneous abortion in diabetic women to be 10.0 ± 0.3 per cent. He concluded that the incidence of spontaneous abortion in diabetic women was not greater than that in the population at large.

3.1.2.2 Risk of preterm delivery The risk of preterm delivery in diabetic women relates mainly to the widespread policy of elective delivery before term. Although there is an increasing tendency to allow diabetic women to enter into labour spontaneously and to try to reduce the incidence of elective preterm induction or caesarean section, this change in approach to management is not as yet universally implemented.

3.1.2.3 Risks associated with aberrant fetal growth There is still an increased incidence of macrosomia even with the best diabetic control currently available. The real risk accompanying an excessively large baby is that of birth trauma, discussed below. Intrauterine growth retardation is not typically associated with diabetes unless the diabetes is complicated by microvascular disease, in particular nephropathy. Women with vascular complications of diabetes will need particularly careful counselling for reasons explained below.

3.1.2.4 Long term outcome for the infant In view of the severe metabolic disturbance of the fetal milieu, it is not surprising that there has been interest in the long term neurological development of infants of diabetic mothers. Churchill *et al.* (1969) studied the relationship between maternal ketosis and subsequent neurological development of the infant. The mean intelligence quotient at 4 years of age was 94.4 in 33 infants whose mothers had shown acetonuria greater than 1+ within 24 hours before birth, compared to a mean value of 103 (p = 0.001) in 33 matched non-diabetic controls. Stehbens *et al.* (1977) found a correlation between a lower intelligence quotient of children at 5 years of age and the presence of acetonuria in pregnancy (defined as a positive dipstick for acetone during 6-hourly urine tests while in hospital). They also noted a similar correlation of low intelligence quotient with low birthweight, but because of the small sample size in their study, they were unable to differentiate the relative importance of these two factors. There are inadequate data to assess the impact of acetonuria separately from the impact of low birthweight on intellectual development in childhood.

Cummins and Norrish (1980) found a normal intelligence quotient distribution in 51 infants of diabetic mothers delivered between 1964 and 1972. The mean intelligence quotient of 13 children whose mothers experienced hypoglycaemia during pregnancy reported by Churchill *et al.* (1969) was 105 and not significantly different from the control group.

Kitzmiller *et al.* (1981) reviewed 18 of 24 infants born to mothers with diabetic nephropathy, at a mean infant age of 20 ± 7.6 months. The mean gestational age at the time of delivery was 35.1 ± 2.3 weeks. Three infants had a head circumference below the 3rd percentile; one of these had multiple other anomalies including caudal regression, and the other two were small for gestational age. Only one of the 18 infants had a low Denver Developmental Screening Test Index. This child had been born at 33 weeks and had suffered from respiratory distress syndrome.

Finally, it is reassuring for the woman to learn that the risk of her children developing juvenile onset diabetes is in the order of 2 per cent or less (Zanona 1976).

3.1.3 Maternal risks

3.1.3.1 Risks associated with nephropathy Nephropathy without significant hypertension and a normal serum creatinine is associated with a good fetal outcome. The prognosis worsens in the presence of hypertension or impaired renal function (Kitzmiller *et al.* 1981).

Davison *et al.* (1985) presents an encouraging picture from a review of 29 studies, published since 1950, involving 1902 pregnancies in 1311 women with pre-existing renal disease. A steady decrease in perinatal mortality over the three decades was found despite an increasing rate of preterm birth. They attribute the improvement to intensive obstetric care and a greater reliance on the judicious and deliberate use of preterm delivery made possible by the increased skills in neonatology. Neither Davison *et al.* (1985) nor Kitzmiller *et al.* (1981) could therefore support the previously held opinion that underlying renal disease is an indication for termination of pregnancy (Pedersen 1977a,b).

However, Davison *et al.* (1985) recommended that pregnancy was best restricted to women whose preconceptional serum creatinine levels are less than 175 μmol/l (2 mg/100 ml) and whose diastolic blood pressure is 90 mm Hg or less. They cautioned that renal disease that does not cause symptoms, or disrupt homeostasis in non-pregnant individuals, can certainly jeopardize pregnancy performance in some women. They also cautioned that, although the majority of women with renal disease do not experience deterioration during pregnancy, some women do suffer significant deterioration of renal function that does not improve after delivery.

3.1.3.2 Risks associated with retinopathy There is also concern about the effect of pregnancy on women with proliferative retinopathy. Two recent studies (Johnston 1980; Moloney and Drury 1982) have compared retinal changes in diabetic women throughout pregnancy with a control group. Despite the fact that in one of these studies (Moloney and Drury 1982), the pregnant group tended to start with more severe retinopathy than the controls, pregnancy still appeared to be associated with a deterioration in both background and proliferative retinopathy. The background changes regressed after delivery but there was no regression in neovascularization. However, only 4 women in their series had proliferative retinopathy. Johnston (1980) compared 30 pregnant women who had proliferative retinopathy with 27 controls matched for age and duration of disease, who had never been pregnant. He noted that with intensive laser treatment throughout pregnancy, visual acuity was maintained so that no difference existed at completion of pregnancy between a control group and the pregnant group. He also observed that a similar number of women became blind in the control group (2) as compared to the pregnant group; and, most important of all, that the visual acuity was the same in those whose pregnancies were interrupted as in those that went to term.

Price *et al.* (1984) followed 13 women with retinopathy, including 5 who had proliferative retinopathy by serial ophthalmological examinations during pregnancy and afterwards. They found no evidence of progression during pregnancy. Cassar *et al.* (1978) found retinopathy present in 12 of 67 diabetic patients. Nine of these had minimal retinopathy and none of these worsened during pregnancy. Of 4 with proliferative retinopathy, 1 showed regression and 2 showed advance, but normal vision was preserved by photocoagulation.

Perinatal mortality rates in patients with retinopathy would appear to be low, but morbidity is high; in particular preterm birth, low birthweight, and pre-eclampsia (Price *et al.* 1984; Reece *et al.* 1986). There would seem to be little evidence, therefore, that the presence of proliferative retinopathy should still be considered an absolute contraindication to pregnancy as suggested, for example, by White (1971). Optimal outcome, both ophthalmological and perinatal, will depend on skilled supervision from the two disciplines.

3.1.4 Methods of control of blood glucose

Blood glucose levels can now be monitored effectively and controlled by the woman at home using either chemstrips or a glucometer (Peacock *et al.* 1979; Stubbs *et al.* 1980; Schneider *et al.* 1980; Varner 1983), combined with readily available skilled support, predominantly through telephone contact.

The aim is to establish normal levels of blood glucose both fasting, and before and after meals. There is variation in what is considered normal in this context. Noting that plasma glucose values rarely exceed 120 mg/dl (6.6 mmol/l) in normal pregnancy, Gabbe (1985) suggests that ideal control is reflected by a fasting level of <90 mg/dl (5.0 mmol/l), <120 mg/dl (6.6 mmol/l) 2 hours after a meal, and <105 mg/dl (5.8 mmol/l) before a meal. Adequate control is assessed either by calculating mean blood glucose levels at these times, or from the level of glycosylated haemoglobin. Insulin is administered usually before breakfast and supper, either as a short-acting insulin alone or in combination with a medium-acting insulin. Occasionally a third or even fourth injection is required.

Much interest has been generated in the continuous subcutaneous infusion of insulin with a pump, and there is no question that for certain women with variable insulin requirements, this provides an acceptable alternative (Potter *et al.* 1980). Pumps, however, are expensive and the women need to be reliable and capable of mastering the complexities of the programme (Raskin 1982). Although nocturnal hypoglycaemia remains a serious concern (Zinman 1982), the risks of hyperglycaemia from pump failure have been minimized by incorporating alarm systems into the design.

Whether the pump in fact achieves better control than conventional methods is debatable. Kitzmiller *et al.* (1985) followed 21 women managed with continuous subcutaneous infusion of insulin through the first 10 weeks of pregnancy, and subsequently by conventional intermittent injections. They noted that the tight control achieved with continuous subcutaneous infusion was also achieved with conventional therapy and concluded that a randomized trial is required to establish the place, if any, of continuous subcutaneous infusion.

Two randomized crossover trials (Schiffrin and Belmonte 1982; Reeves *et al.* 1982) also concluded that equal control was achieved with a conventional intensive regime of injections as with the pump. Since then, 4 such trials have been reported. Three of these (Botta *et al.* 1986; Carta *et al.* 1986; Coustan *et al.* 1986) looked predominantly at metabolic control and all 3 concluded that control could be achieved equally well with conventional insulin therapy as with continuous subcutaneous infusion. The fourth (Laatikainen *et al.* 1987) studied the influence on diabetic retinopathy and noted a worsening of retinopathy in 8 of 22 women allocated to continuous subcutaneous infusion compared with 2 of 18 allocated to conventional insulin therapy. These results should be interpreted with caution, however, since there were more women with pre-existent retinopathy in the group allocated to continuous infusion than in the control group (13 of 22 vs. 6 of 18), and since worsening of retinopathy occurred nearly as frequently in the women who declined continuous infusion and were therefore treated in the conventional manner as in those who actually did receive continuous insulin infusion (3 of 9 vs. 5 of 13).

In those trials that provide data, no effects were noted on the incidence of caesarean section (Botta *et al.* 1986; Carta *et al.* 1986; Coustan *et al.* 1986), preterm birth (Carta *et al.* 1986), congenital malformations (Carta *et al.* 1986; Coustan *et al.* 1986), perinatal mortality (Botta *et al.* 1986; Carta *et al.* 1986; Coustan *et al.* 1986), or neonatal hypoglycaemia (Coustan *et al.* 1986).

The early promise, therefore, of easily and safely obtained tight control has not been realized, at least not above that achieved with conventional treatment, and the clinical application of these devices remains limited to a select group of women. It is likely that the secret to good control lies not so much with the method of insulin administration, but with the obsessiveness with which blood glucose levels are measured and adjustments in insulin therapy made.

3.2 Care in pregnancy

3.2.1 General care

The first few weeks of pregnancy are a period of readjustment and many women require re-education about their diabetes and its control. Rotation of insulin injection sites, the interaction of diet and exercise, and the dietary requirements of pregnancy may be unfamiliar to many women. Specialist care in and for pregnancy needs to start as early as possible. Gestational age, when doubtful, will need to be estimated precisely as soon as possible by pregnancy tests and/or early ultrasound. Hypoglycaemia can be troublesome at this stage and control may be difficult to achieve because of poor motivation, nausea, and vomiting, or changes in the hormonal milieu. Considerable education is needed to resist over-treatment of impending hypoglycaemic reactions. Glucose or sugar should be avoided; milk or a light snack, which can be repeated if necessary, are more appropriate. All diabetic women should be provided with glucagon for emergency situations.

In addition to routine prenatal assessment, obstetric care at this time should include assessment of renal function in women who have hypertension or proteinuria, and retinoscopy, particularly in diabetics who have had their condition for more than 10 years. Urine cultures should be repeated regularly in those with nephropathy. Detailed ultrasound at approximately 18 weeks (possibly with serum alpha-fetoprotein measurement) is recommended for reasons to be given.

A diabetic woman without nephropathy or retinopathy, and with no other complications of pregnancy, usually experiences an uneventful 2nd trimester. The educational and readjustment processes are hopefully complete as far as possible, and, unless there is a risk of compromised fetal growth or early pre-eclampsia, little need exists for intensive obstetric supervision at this time. Women with hypertension may need to be followed closely and, if necessary, treated with hypotensive drugs. Serial uric acid estimations and assessment of renal function can be particularly useful in following these pregnancies. In the absence of superimposed pre-eclampsia or raised creatinine from impaired renal function, the uric acid level should not increase by more than 30 μmol/l per week or increase above 350 μmol/l (Redman *et al.* 1976; Dunlop and Davison 1977). Increases above this level or rate tend to indicate the development of superimposed pre-eclampsia with its additional influence on perinatal outcome.

As so much emphasis is placed on the control of diabetes in the last trimester, the evidence that is available to associate tight control with improved perinatal outcome will be reviewed later in this chapter.

3.2.2 Timing of delivery

Pre-empting pregnancy has long been one of the classical management strategies applied in diabetic pregnancy. The rationale for early delivery was based on the observation that the neonatal death rate fell below the rising stillbirth rate at and after 36 weeks of gestation (Peel and Oakley 1949; Hagbard 1956). As a result, Peel Peel and Oakley (1949) recommended that delivery should take place in the 36th week of pregnancy; a recommendation that was widely accepted at the time. The perinatal mortality rate of diabetics delivered in their hospital (King's College Hospital, London) before and after this practice was introduced is shown in Table 36.3. As noted later by Peel (1972), this did not improve the perinatal mortality rate, and this might have been recognized earlier had the policy been evaluated by a controlled trial at the outset. Nevertheless, the concern

Table 36.3 Perinatal mortality in King's College Hospital, London before and after the policy of routine delivery at 36 weeks started before 1950 (Peel and Oakley 1949; Brudenell 1975)

Years	No. births	Stillbirths		First week deaths		Perinatal mortality per 1000
		No.	Per 1000	No.	Per 1000	
1942–49	141	16	11.3	20	16.0	25.5
1951–55	132	20	15.2	22	19.6	31.8
1956–60	186	13	7.0	17	9.8	16.1
1961–65	213	13	6.1	11	5.5	11.3
1966–70	176	7	4.0	8	4.7	8.5

that the intrauterine death rate rises dramatically after 36 weeks still exists (Duhring 1977). It is likely, however, that this concern is based on inaccurate recollection of the original reports.

Peel and Oakley (1949) (Fig. 36.1), showed a fluctuating percentage of stillbirths from 36 to 40 weeks' gestation, and Hagbard (1956) showed a modest rise in the stillbirth rate from 35 to 38 weeks, but after that the rate was not significantly higher.

Despite the fact that the extent of risk of intrauterine death after 37 weeks is not known precisely, many women are now being allowed to continue pregnancy to 38 or more weeks of gestation. Of the last 171 diabetic women delivered at McMaster since 1979, 103 (60 per cent) were delivered after 37 weeks' gestation. This rate can be compared to the 50 per cent rate reported by Coustan *et al.* (1980), the 35 per cent rate reported by Kitzmiller *et al.* (1978), and the 84 per cent rate reported by Drury (1984). Both Murphy *et al.* (1984) and Jovanovic *et al.* (1981) report a mean gestational age at delivery of 39 weeks for uncomplicated diabetics. These 6 series include 430 women delivered after the 37th week of pregnancy with only 1 intrauterine death (a rate of 2.3 per 1000). There would seem little reason to terminate an otherwise uncomplicated pregnancy in a diabetic woman before term, or even before the expected date of delivery.

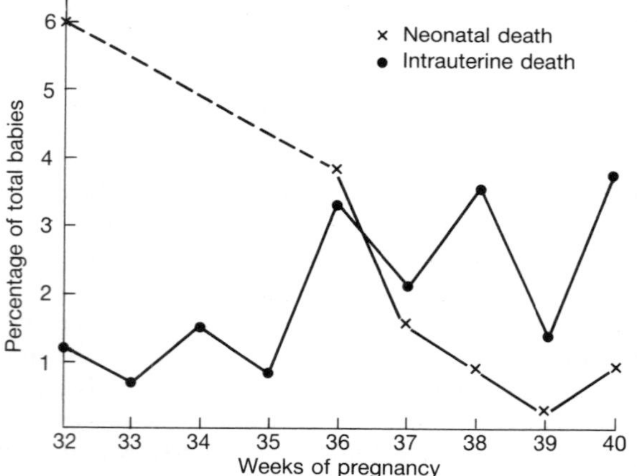

Fig. 36.1 Facsimile of the graph presented by Peel and Oakley (1949) on the relationship btween perinatal mortality and gestational age in diabetic pregnancies

3.2.3 Pulmonary maturity assessment

Assessment of pulmonary maturity has until recently been a prerequisite for planned delivery of the diabetic woman. Although there has been concern about the reliability of the lecithin/sphingomyelin ratio in women with diabetes (Robert *et al.* 1976), there is increasing evidence to suggest that in well-controlled diabetics, the lecithin/sphingomyelin ratio reflects the same degree of pulmonary surfactant production, and therefore the same risk of hyaline membrane disease, as in non-diabetics (Jovanovic *et al.* 1981; Gabbe *et al.* 1981; Dudley and Black 1985; Landon *et al.* 1986). The much publicized shortcomings of this test may have related to a variety of factors. In part they may have been due to the inherent deficiencies of the test itself, or to its frequent use between 36 and 37 weeks' gestation, when the prevalence of respiratory distress is lower than it is earlier in pregnancy. Also, diabetic mothers are frequently delivered by elective caesarean section, which predisposes the neonate to the wet lung syndrome and/or transient tachypnea of the newborn (Cohen and Carson 1985). Finally, the infants of poorly controlled diabetic mothers may have a disturbance in the development of pulmonary maturity, possibly mediated through decreased prolactin levels (Saltzman *et al.* 1986), or through direct interference in the synthesis of phosphatidyl choline by high fetal insulin levels (Carlson *et al.* 1984), or by impaired structural development (B R Bhavnani *et al.*, personal communication, 1987). Although pulmonary development in the fetus of diabetic mothers is intriguing, the problem will become less important as delivery is delayed to a later gestational age and as elective caesarean section is used less frequently.

3.3 Care for labour and delivery

Although most people would agree with Freinkel *et al.* (1985) that caesarean section in diabetics, as in all women, should only be performed for obstetric indications, no one would appear to have put their expressed conservatism into practice as completely as Stronge *et al.* (1986) from Dublin (who still reported a caesarean section rate of 20 per cent). Murphy *et al.* (1984) allowed more women to labour between 1979 and 1982 than between 1973 and 1978, but their caesarean section rate remained unchanged (42.8 per cent and 48.8 per cent) during the two periods. Kitzmiller *et al.* (1978) reported a caesarean section rate of 72.3 per cent in 147 diabetic women, and the rate in McMaster has remained unchanged at approximately 60 per cent since 1979, nearly three times the overall caesarean rate in the hospital. The caesarean section rate in diabetics is probably no more than an exaggerated reflection of the use of caesarean section in general, probably with a proportionally large input of elective and of repeat operations.

As blood glucose levels can be controlled confidently throughout labour with a glucose infusion with insulin added (West and Lowy 1977; Caplan *et al.* 1982), the residual danger of vaginal delivery in these women appears to be that of birth trauma, particularly brachial plexus injury secondary to shoulder dystocia and macrosomia. Acker *et al.* (1985) reported that 12.5 per cent of vaginally delivered neonates who weighed more than 4000 g experienced shoulder dystocia. As this complication was not predictable from the labour pattern and 85 per cent delivered the head spontaneously, they recommended that caesarean section be used to avoid birth trauma (fracture and brachial palsy) in the presence of suspected macrosomia. However, as only 12.7 per cent of infants weighing over 4000 g with shoulder dystocia had birth trauma (possibly a high incidence in itself), 200 caesarean sections would be required in women with macrosomic infants to prevent 3 cases of birth trauma. As approximately 10 per cent of women at more than 37 weeks' gestation will have an infant weighing more than 4000 g (Thomson *et al.* 1968), this recommendation, if adopted, would cause a large increase in the already high caesarean section rate.

It is probably enough at this stage merely to advise caution in managing the labour and delivery of a diabetic woman with a suspected large infant.

3.4 Care after birth

All insulin therapy should cease with delivery of the placenta and thereafter insulin requirements should be recalibrated according to blood glucose levels. Although hypoglycaemia affects from 10 to 50 per cent of the neonates (Tevaarwerk *et al.* 1981), Coustan *et al.* (1980) found that only 1 of 76 infants of diabetic mothers required intravenous therapy for 24 hours; the remainder had transient hypoglycaemia responding to oral feeding. Hypoglycaemia can occur in some infants within the first hour of life (Farquhar 1954); consequently, early feeding should be instituted and blood glucose levels should be measured half-hourly for the first 2 hours of life. Routine separation of the newborn from the mother into a neonatal intensive care unit is inappropriate. Skilled assessment of the infant at birth, exclusion of serious anomalies, and careful observation over the first 12 to 24 hours of life is the ideal management for these infants. Intensive care should be reserved for infants with specific problems.

Family planning is an important consideration. There is no contraindication to the use of low dose oral contraceptives, particularly in young (less than 35), non-obese, non-hypertensive, non-smoking diabetics (Health and Welfare Canada 1985). The development of headaches or hypertension is an indication to change to alternative methods. The intrauterine device has until recently been a reasonable alternative, but adverse publicity, along with concern over its effectiveness in diabetics (Gosden *et al.* 1982), is making it a less acceptable alternative. Barrier methods, of course, also make a reasonable alternative if contraceptive failure would not pose serious problems. For all women, the risk of pregnancy has to be carefully weighed against the risk of the proposed method of contraception.

In general, sterilization if required is better not performed at the time of caesarean section if this can be avoided, in view of the increased risk that the newborn may have still undiagnosed cardiac anomalies. It is well known that an unsuccessful outcome of pregnancy is a strong determinant of the wish for subsequent reversal of sterilization. If necessary, the procedure can easily be performed by laparoscopy within the next few months.

Women with nephropathy or retinopathy should be counselled carefully about limiting family size.

4 Control of diabetes and outcome

4.1 Congenital malformations

Miller *et al.* (1981) and Ylinen *et al.* (1984) have shown a significant correlation between elevated glycosylated haemoglobin levels (indicative of episodes of hyperglycaemia) in the 1st trimester of pregnancy and an increased incidence of congenital malformations, while diabetic women with normal levels of glycosylated haemoglobin had not more congenital anomalies in their offspring than did non-diabetic women. Fuhrmann *et al.* (1984) compared 56 women admitted to a prepregnancy clinic with 144 women who did not join the clinic for tight control until after the 8th week of pregnancy. Of the 56 women controlled early in pregnancy only one had an infant with a malformation (of the heart), whereas 9 of the 144 women who joined the clinic after the 8th week had infants with congenital malformations; of these, three were fatal, three severe and three minor.

4.2 Perinatal mortality

The most convincing evidence linking maternal blood glucose level to perinatal mortality is the non-random cohort study of Karlsson and Kjellmer (1972) obtained between 1961 and 1970. Of 38 women whose mean blood glucose from 32 weeks' gestation to delivery exceeded 150 mg/dl (8.3 mmol/l), 9 (23.6 per cent) had a perinatal loss as compared to two of 52 women (3.8 per cent) whose mean blood glucose was below 100 mg/

dl (5.5 mmol/l) (p = 0.002). Of the 77 women whose mean blood glucose was in the intermediate range, 12 (15.6 per cent) had a perinatal loss (p = 0.003).

Jovanovic and Peterson (1980) reviewed 11 series published between 1922 and 1979 in which blood glucose values were reported. They showed a linear relationship between the mean maternal blood glucose and perinatal mortality with zero perinatal mortality predicted when mean blood glucose was 83 mg/dl (4.6 mmol/l). This tends to support the hypothesis of a significant correlation, but it must be kept in mind that methods for measurement of blood glucose have changed since the early studies, and some of the later studies have included women with gestational diabetes.

Although there now seems to be general agreement that tight control of diabetes reduces perinatal mortality, the true contribution of tight control to decreased perinatal mortality cannot be separated from that made by the total programme of care. A proper study to explore whether tight control actually does improve outcome would now be difficult to mount, since many would probably consider it as unethical to 'deny' diabetic women the apparently obvious benefits of tight control.

4.3 Perinatal morbidity

Several studies have related good control to low perinatal morbidity (Kitzmiller *et al.* 1978; Coustan *et al.* 1980). Jovanovic *et al.* (1981) found that the infants of 52 women with established diabetes, who agreed to a programme of strict control and completed pregnancy with normal glycosylated haemoglobin levels, had the same incidence of neonatal complications (hypoglycaemia, hyperbilirubinaemia, respiratory distress) as 52 matched controls. Landon (1986) found that newborns of 43 diabetic women with mean blood glucose levels less than 110 mg/dl (6.1 mmol/l) had significantly less hypoglycaemia and respiratory distress than those of 32 diabetics with mean blood glucose values greater than 110 mg/ml. Although there was no significant difference in the incidence of hyperbilirubinaemia in Landon's series, Ylinen *et al.* (1981) found this incidence to be higher when glycosylated haemoglobin levels were elevated in the 3rd trimester. Tevaarwerk *et al.* (1981) reported a higher incidence of these neonatal complications in their series of 110 well-controlled diabetics than in the population at large, but the incidence was much lower than that generally reported in infants of diabetic mothers.

The incidence of macrosomia has been used as a measure of glycaemic control, but there is increasing evidence that despite good control approximately 30 per cent of the women will have an infant with a birthweight greater than the 90th percentile for gestational age. (Coustan *et al.* 1980; Kitzmiller *et al.* 1978; Miller 1983).

In the McMaster series, the incidence of a birthweight more than the 90th percentile for gestational age is also 30 per cent, and 18 per cent of the babies weigh more than the 95th percentile for gestational age. Furthermore, there is no relationship between the birthweight percentile and glycosylated haemoglobin measured in the last 4 weeks prior to delivery (Fig. 36.2). Similarly, Karlsson and Kjellmer (1972) found no association between birthweight and the mean blood glucose levels from 32 weeks' gestation onwards. The lack of correlation between glycosylated haemoglobin and birthweight is puzzling and has been noted by other authors (Miller 1983; Fadel *et al.* 1981; Yatscoff *et al.* 1985a). It also appears that glycosylated serum protein levels fail to correlate with birthweight (Yatscoff *et al.* 1985b).

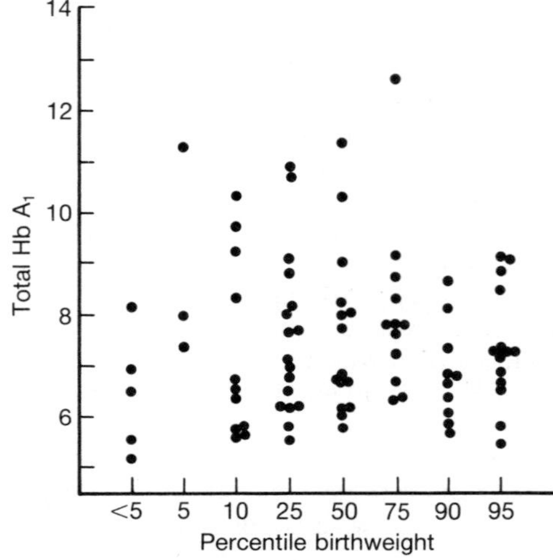

Fig. 36.2 Relationship between glycosylated haemoglobin and birthweight (date from McMaster University)

In trying to examine birthweight associations four points need to be emphasized. First, by definition, 10 per cent of newborn infants will weigh more than the 90th centile of weight for gestational age. Second, even minor elevations of blood glucose appear to be associated with a 20 per cent incidence of macrosomia (Coustan *et al.* 1984, Gabbe *et al.* 1977a,b). Third, even in well-controlled diabetics, the availability of glucose exceeds that in non-diabetics (Persson and Turnell 1975; Gillmer *et al.* 1975). It is possible, therefore, that a fetus with a strong growth potential may achieve an excessive size in the presence of minor excesses (or even normal levels) of maternal blood glucose. Fourth, it is possible that a wide range of glucose values are associated with normal glycosylated haemoglobin levels (Langer and Mazze 1986).

It is interesting that fetal insulin production, as reflected in C-peptide levels in amniotic fluid, is increased even in well-controlled diabetics (Tyden *et al.* 1984). Furthermore, although increased levels of C-peptide (particularly in response to an arginine infusion) are associated with macrosomia and neonatal hypoglycaemia (Fallucca *et al.* 1985), the association with hypoglycaemia is stronger than with macrosomia, suggesting again that factors other than glucose and insulin play a role in the production of fetal macrosomia.

In clinical terms, the ideal endpoint or combination of endpoints against which to measure the appropriate degree of control have not been defined. Euglycaemia may be ideal, but is unattainable in most women. A normal glycosylated haemoglobin might be achieved in most women, but this may not reflect euglycaemia. Although glycosylated protein levels do not reflect minor degrees of hyperglycaemia (Yatscoff *et al.* 1985b), they correlate with mean blood glucose values over the proceeding 7 days (Morris *et al.* 1985). This could allow more frequent reappraisal of diabetic control with the possible benefit of a rapid feedback and continued adjustment of insulin dosages where indicated.

An important consideration as pregnancy moves into the last trimester, is the assessment of fetal well-being and timing of delivery. Fetal assessment is discussed in detail elsewhere in this book (see Chapters 27, 28, 29, and 30). Jovanovic and Jovanovic (1984) and Murphy *et al.* (1984) rely heavily on the woman's perception of fetal activity to indicate fetal well-being, using non-stress cardiotocography only when fetal compromise is suspected. This would appear to be a rational approach in need of further careful evaluation.

4.4 Evidence from randomized trial

Despite the importance of the subject to date the benefits and drawbacks of tight control of diabetes in pregnancy have been assessed in only one randomized trial (Farrag 1987; Tables 36.4 and 36.5). In this trial 60 women were randomly allocated to one of three groups: very tight control (aiming to keep blood sugar levels below 5.6 mmol/l), tight control (blood sugar levels between 5.6 and 6.7 mmol/l), and moderate control (blood sugar levels between 6.7 and 8.9 mmol/l).

The data shown in Table 36.4 indicate that very tight control is associated with a high incidence of episodes of hypoglycaemia in early pregnancy in particular and confers no benefits in the other pregnancy outcomes studied compared to keeping blood sugar levels below 6.7 mmol/l. On the other hand, a policy that allows

Table 36.4 Effect of very tight vs. tight control of diabetes in pregnancy on hypoglycaemia in first half of pregnancy

Study	EXPT		CTRL		Odds ratio	Graph of odds ratios and confidence intervals
	n	(%)	*n*	(%)	(95% CI)	0.01 0.1 0.5 1 2 10 100
Farrag (1987)	7/16	(43.75)	0/29	(0.00)	25.96 (4.91–99.99)	
Typical odds ratio (95% confidence interval)					25.96 (4.91–99.99)	

Effect of very tight vs. tight control of diabetes in pregnancy on pre-eclampsia

Study	EXPT *n*	(%)	CTRL *n*	(%)	Odds ratio (95% CI)	Graph
Farrag (1987)	1/16	(6.25)	0/29	(0.00)	16.65 (0.28–99.99)	
Typical odds ratio (95% confidence interval)					16.65 (0.28–99.99)	

Effect of very tight vs. tight control of diabetes in pregnancy on transient hypertension

Study	EXPT *n*	(%)	CTRL *n*	(%)	Odds ratio (95% CI)	Graph
Farrag (1987)	0/16	(0.00)	1/29	(3.45)	0.21 (0.00–12.72)	
Typical odds ratio (95% confidence interval)					0.21 (0.00–12.72)	

Effect of very tight vs. tight control of diabetes in pregnancy on urinary tract infection

Study	EXPT *n*	(%)	CTRL *n*	(%)	Odds ratio (95% CI)	Graph
Farrag (1987)	0/16	(0.00)	0/29	(0.00)	1.00 (1.00–1.00)	
Typical odds ratio (95% confidence interval)					1.00 (1.00–1.00)	

Table 36.4 — *continued* Effect of very tight vs. tight control of diabetes in pregnancy on caesarean section

Study	EXPT n	(%)	CTRL n	(%)	Odds ratio (95% CI)	Graph of odds ratios and confidence intervals
Farrag (1987)	2/16	(12.50)	3/29	(10.34)	1.24 (0.18–8.45)	
Typical odds ratio (95% confidence interval)					1.24 (0.18–8.45)	

Effect of very tight vs. tight control of diabetes in pregnancy on birthweight >90th centile

Study	EXPT n	(%)	CTRL n	(%)	Odds ratio (95% CI)	Graph of odds ratios and confidence intervals
Farrag (1987)	0/16	(0.00)	0/29	(0.00)	1.00 (1.00–1.00)	
Typical odds ratio (95% confidence interval)					1.00 (1.00–1.00)	

Effect of very tight vs. tight control of diabetes in pregnancy on preterm labour

Study	EXPT n	(%)	CTRL n	(%)	Odds ratio (95% CI)	Graph of odds ratios and confidence intervals
Farrag (1987)	1/16	(6.25)	0/29	(0.00)	16.65 (0.28–99.99)	
Typical odds ratio (95% confidence interval)					16.65 (0.28–99.99)	

Effect of very tight vs. tight control of diabetes in pregnancy on perinatal mortality

Study	EXPT n	(%)	CTRL n	(%)	Odds ratio (95% CI)	Graph of odds ratios and confidence intervals
Farrag (1987)	0/16	(0.00)	0/29	(0.00)	1.00 (1.00–1.00)	
Typical odds ratio (95% confidence interval)					1.00 (1.00–1.00)	

Effect of very tight vs. tight control of diabetes in pregnancy on respiratory distress syndrome

Study	EXPT n	(%)	CTRL n	(%)	Odds ratio (95% CI)	Graph of odds ratios and confidence intervals
Farrag (1987)	1/16	(6.25)	2/29	(6.90)	0.90 (0.08–10.16)	
Typical odds ratio (95% confidence interval)					0.90 (0.08–10.16)	

Graph scale: 0.01, 0.1, 0.5, 1, 2, 10, 100

Table 36.5 Effect of tight vs. moderate control of diabetes in pregnancy on hypoglycaemia in first half of pregnancy

Study	EXPT n	(%)	CTRL n	(%)	Odds ratio (95% CI)	Graph of odds ratios and confidence intervals
Farrag (1987)	0/29	(0.00)	0/15	(0.00)	1.00 (1.00–1.00)	
Typical odds ratio (95% confidence interval)					1.00 (1.00–1.00)	

Effect of tight vs. moderate control of diabetes in pregnancy on pre-eclampsia

Study	EXPT n	(%)	CTRL n	(%)	Odds ratio (95% CI)	Graph of odds ratios and confidence intervals
Farrag (1987)	0/29	(0.00)	3/15	(20.00)	0.05 (0.00–0.53)	
Typical odds ratio (95% confidence interval)					0.05 (0.00–0.53)	

Graph scale: 0.01, 0.1, 0.5, 1, 2, 10, 100

Table 36.5 — *continued* Effect of tight vs. moderate control of diabetes in pregnancy on transient hypertemsion

Study	EXPT *n*	EXPT (%)	CTRL *n*	CTRL (%)	Odds ratio (95% CI)	Graph of odds ratios and confidence intervals (0.01 0.1 0.5 1 2 10 100)
Farrag (1987)	1/29	(3.45)	2/15	(13.33)	0.22 (0.02–2.52)	
Typical odds ratio (95% confidence interval)					0.22 (0.02–2.52)	

Effect of tight vs. moderate control of diabetes in pregnancy on urinary tract infection

Study	EXPT *n*	EXPT (%)	CTRL *n*	CTRL (%)	Odds ratio (95% CI)	Graph
Farrag (1987)	0/29	(0.00)	2/15	(13.33)	0.05 (0.00–0.96)	
Typical odds ratio (95% confidence interval)					0.05 (0.00–0.96)	

Effect of tight vs. moderate control of diabetes in pregnancy on caesarean section

Study	EXPT *n*	EXPT (%)	CTRL *n*	CTRL (%)	Odds ratio (95% CI)	Graph
Farrag (1987)	3/29	(10.34)	6/15	(40.00)	0.17 (0.04–0.78)	
Typical odds ratio (95% confidence interval)					0.17 (0.04–0.78)	

Effect of tight vs. moderate control of diabetes in pregnancy on birthweight >90th centile

Study	EXPT *n*	EXPT (%)	CTRL *n*	CTRL (%)	Odds ratio (95% CI)	Graph
Farrag (1987)	0/29	(0.00)	13/15	(86.67)	0.02 (0.00–0.07)	
Typical odds ratio (95% confidence interval)					0.02 (0.00–0.07)	

Effect of tight vs. moderate control of diabetes in pregnancy on preterm labour

Study	EXPT *n*	EXPT (%)	CTRL *n*	CTRL (%)	Odds ratio (95% CI)	Graph
Farrag (1987)	0/29	(0.00)	2/15	(13.33)	0.05 (0.00–0.96)	
Typical odds ratio (95% confidence interval)					0.05 (0.00–0.96)	

Effect of tight vs. moderate control of diabetes in pregnancy on perinatal mortality

Study	EXPT *n*	EXPT (%)	CTRL *n*	CTRL (%)	Odds ratio (95% CI)	Graph
Farrag (1987)	0/29	(0.00)	2/15	(13.33)	0.05 (0.00–0.96)	
Typical odds ratio (95% confidence interval)					0.05 (0.00–0.96)	

Effect of tight vs. moderate control of diabetes in pregnancy on respiratory distress syndrome

Study	EXPT *n*	EXPT (%)	CTRL *n*	CTRL (%)	Odds ratio (95% CI)	Graph
Farrag (1987)	2/29	(6.90)	6/15	(40.00)	0.11 (0.02–0.56)	
Typical odds ratio (95% confidence interval)					0.11 (0.02–0.56)	

blood sugar levels to rise up to 8.9 mmol/l is associated with a higher incidence of caesarean section, birthweight above the 90th centile of weight for gestation, and a trend towards an increase in urinary tract infection, hypertension, preterm labour, respiratory distress syndrome, and perinatal mortality (Table 36.5). This evidence confirms the conclusion from observational studies that keeping blood sugars within a well-controlled range is better than either too strict or too lenient a regimen.

5 Conclusions

Currently, there is considerable evidence to suggest that pregnancy in diabetic women may be managed with fewer obstetric interventions than are usually practised. While there is no question that, overall, specialized care and collaboration of and between various disciplines will achieve the best results, access to this can be difficult for geographical reasons, scarcity of resources, and reluctance to either refer or be referred. As suggested by Connell *et al.* (1985), however, good perinatal outcome does not have to be the sole prerogative of tertiary care centres. Focusing attention on those women with specific complications of diabetes and/or pregnancy will allow the majority of diabetic women to be treated as normal pregnant women, with the one major exception of careful control of blood glucose levels.

Prolongation of pregnancy, associated with a decreased need to assess pulmonary maturity and the judicious use of caesarean section, may further reduce both neonatal and maternal morbidity and may allow pregnant women with diabetes to feel more like their non-diabetic counterparts.

Much has been achieved in improving the care for and outcome of pregnancies in diabetic women without resort to randomized clinical trials. This has undoubtedly and to a large extent been successful. Yet, it has also resulted in a blurring of the contributions made by the various components of care and in doubts about the validity of some claims as to their effectiveness. Similarly, the policies of early and preterm delivery that were used in the past, without the support of well-designed studies, resulted in an unnecessarily high morbidity. The legacy of this lingers on as a reminder of the need for well-designed trials to assess the value both of current treatments and of suggestions for their improvement.

In the meantime, better survey data on the diabetic population are still needed, as data that refer only to those women who attend tertiary care centres can be seriously misleading. Survey data may still allow deficiencies in the total system of care to be identified, thus leading to further improvements in the care that is available to these women.

One can only admire the fortitude with which diabetic women cope with their disease, and the way in which they rise to the added challenge of pregnancy and parenthood. Their doctors should continue to strive to define a programme of care that is the least disruptive and best tailored to meet the circumstances of each individual woman. It is equally important that we avoid manoeuvres and interventions that are, at best, of unproven benefit and socially disruptive, and, at worst, liable to do more harm than good. We should also be extremely careful before advising women against pregnancy. To deny a diabetic woman the chance of reproduction can be seen as the ultimate affirmation of the hopelessness of her disease.

References

Acker DB, Sachs BP, Friedman EA (1985). Risk factors for shoulder dystocia. Obstet Gynecol, 66: 762–768.

Adashi EY, Pinto H, Tyson JE (1979). Impact of maternal euglycemia on fetal outcome in diabetic pregnancy. Am J Obstet Gynecol, 133: 268–274.

Baker S, Eglar JM, Klein SH, Goldman AS (1980). Meticulous control of diabetes during organogenesis prevents congenital lumbosacral defects in rats. Diabetes, 30: 955–959.

Botta RM, Sinagra D, Angelico MC, Bompiani GD (1986). Confronto fra terapia insulinica tradizionale ottimizzata e con microinfusore in gravide affette da diabete mellito di tipo I. Minerva Med, 77: 657–661.

Brudenell M (1975). Care of the clinical diabetic woman in pregnancy and labour. In: Carbohydrate Metabolism in Pregnancy and the Newborn. Sutherland HW, Stowers JM (eds). London: Churchill Livingstone, p 222.

Caplan RH, Pagliara AS, Beguin EA, Smiley CA, Bina-Frymark M, Goettl KA, Hartigan JM, Tankersley JC, Peck TM (1982). Constant intravenous insulin infusion during labour and delivery in diabetes mellitus. Diabetes Care, 5: 6–10.

Carlson KS, Smith BT, Post M (1984). Insulin acts on the fibroblast to inhibit glucocorticoid stimulation of lung maturity. J Appl Physiol, 57: 1577–1579.

Carta Q, Meriggi E, Trossarelli GF, Catella G, Dal Molin V, Menato G, Gagliardi L, Massobrio M, Vitelli A (1986). Continuous subcutaneous insulin infusion versus intensive conventional insulin therapy in Type I and Type II diabetic pregnancy. Diabetes Metab, 12: 121–129.

Cassar J, Kohner EM, Hamilton AM, Gordon H, Joplin GF (1978). Diabetic retinopathy and pregnancy. Diabetologia, 15: 105–111.

Chung CS, Myrianthopoulos NC (1975). Factors affecting risks of congenital malformations. II Effect of maternal diabetes. Birth Defects, 11: No. 10, pp 1–38.

Churchill JA, Berendes HW, Nemore J (1969). Neuropsychological deficits in children of diabetic mothers. Am J Obstet Gynecol, 105: 257–258.

Cohen M, Carson BS (1985). Respiratory morbidity benefit of awaiting onset of labor after elective cesarean section. Obstet Gynecol, 65: 818–823.

Connell FA, Fadheim C, Emanuel I (1985). Diabetes in pregnancy: A population based study of incidence, referral for care and perinatal mortality. Am J Obstet Gynecol, 151: 598–603.

Cousins L (1983). Congenital anomalies among infants of diabetic mothers. Am J Obstet Gynecol, 147: 333–338.

Coustan DR, Imarah J (1984). Prophylactic insulin treatment of gestational diabetes reduces the incidence of macrosomia operative delivery and birth trauma. Am J Obstet Gynecol, 150: 836–842.

Coustan DR, Berkowitz RL, Hobbins JC (1980). Tight metabolic control of overt diabetes in pregnancy. Am J Med, 68: 845–852.

Coustan DR, Reece EA, Sherwin RS, Rudolf MCJ, Bates SE, Sockin SM, Holford T, Tamborlane WV (1986). A randomized clinical trial of the insulin pump vs intensive conventional therapy in diabetic pregnancies. JAMA, 255: 631–636.

Cummins M, Norrish M (1980). Follow-up of children of diabetic mothers. Arch Dis Child, 55: 259–264.

Davison JM, Katz Al, Linheimer MD (1985). Kidney disease and pregnancy: Obstetric outcome and long term renal prognosis. Clin Perinatol, 12: 497–519.

Drury MI (1984). Diabetes in pregnancy—Matthews Duncan revisited. Irish J Med Sci, 153: 144–151.

Dudley DKL, Black DM (1985). Reliability of lecithin/sphyngomyelin ratios in diabetic pregnancy. Obstet Gynecol, 66: 521–524.

Duhring JL (1977). Discussion on: A modern approach to management of pregnant diabetics. Am J Obstet Gynecol, 128: 614.

Dunlop W, Davison JM (1977). The effect of normal pregnancy upon the renal handling of uric acid. Br J Obstet Gynaecol, 84: 13–21.

Fadel HE, Reynolds A, Stallings M, Abraham EC (1981). Minor (glycosylated) hemoglobins in cord blood of infants of diabetic mothers. Am J Obstet Gynecol, 139: 397–402.

Fallucca F, Gargulo P, Troili F, Zicari D, Pimpinalla G, Maldonato A, Maggi E, Gerlin G, Pachi A (1985). Amniotic fluid insulin C-peptide concentrations and fetal morbidity in infants of diabetic mothers. Am J Obstet Gynecol, 153: 534–540.

Farquhar JW (1954). Control of the blood sugar level in the neonatal period. Arch Dis Child, 29: 519–529.

Farrag OAM (1987). Prospective study of 3 metabolic regimens in pregnant diabetics. Austral NZ J Obstet Gynaecol, 27: 6–9.

Freinkel N, Dooley SL, Metzger BE (1985). Care of the pregnant woman with insulin dependent diabetes. New Engl J Med, 313: 96–101.

Fuhrmann K, Reiher H, Semmler K, Glockner E (1984). The effect of intensified conventional insulin therapy before and during pregnancy on malformation rate in offspring of diabetic mothers. Exp Clin Endocrinol, 83: 173–177.

Gabbe SG (1978). Application of scientific rationale to the management of the pregnant diabetic. Seminars Perinatol, 2: 361–371.

Gabbe (1985). Management of diabetes mellitus in pregnancy. Am J Obstet Gynecol, 153: 824–828.

Gabbe SG, Mestman JH, Freeman RK, Goebelsmann UT, Lowensohn RI, Nochimson D, Cetrulo C, Quilligan EJ (1977a). Management and outcome of pregnancy in diabetes mellitus, Classes B to R. Am J Obstet Gynecol, 129: 723–732.

Gabbe SG, Mestman JH, Freeman RK, Anderson GV, Lowensohn RI (1977b). Management and outcome of Class A diabetes mellitus. Am J Obstet Gynecol, 127: 465–469.

Gabbe SG, Lowensohn RI, Mestman JH, Freeman RK, Goebelsmann U (1981). Lecithin/sphyngemyelin ratio in diabetic pregnancy. Obstet Gynecol, 66: 521–524.

Gillmer MDG, Beard RW, Brooke FM, Oakley NW (1975). Carbohydrate metabolism in pregnancy, Part I—Diurnal plasma glucose profile in normal and diabetic women. Br Med J, 3: 399–402.

Gosden C, Ross A, Steel J, Springbett A (1982). Intrauterine contraceptive devices in diabetic women. Lancet, i: 530–534.

Grix A (1982). Malformations in infants of diabetic mothers. Am J Med Genet, 13: 131–137.

Hagbard L (1956). Pregnancy and diabetes mellitus—A clinical study. Acta Obstet Gynecol Scand, 35: (Suppl) 1.

Health and Welfare Canada (1985). Guidelines for the direction for use of estrogen progestogen combination oral contraceptives. Report on Oral Contraceptives.

Johnston GP (1980). Pregnancy and diabetic retinopathy. Am J Opthalmol, 90: 519–524.

Jovanovic R, Jovanovic L (1984). Obstetric management when normoglycemia is maintained in diabetic pregnant women with vascular compromise. Am J Obstet Gynecol, 149: 617–623.

Jovanovic L, Peterson CM (1980). Management of the pregnant diabetic woman. Diabetes Care, 3: 63–68.

Jovanovic L, Druzin M, Peterson CM (1981). Effect of euglycemia on the outcome of pregnancy in insulin-dependent diabetic women as compared to normal controls. Am J Med Genet, 71: 921–927.

Kalter H (1987). Diabetes and spontaneous, abortion: An historical review. Am J Obstet Gynecol, 156: 1243–1253.

Karlsson K, Kjellmer I (1972). The outcome of diabetic pregnancies in relation to the mothers' blood sugar level. Am J Obstet Gynecol, 112: 213–220.

Kitzmiller JL, Cloherty JP, Younger MD, Tabatabaii A, Rothchild SB, Sosenko I, Epstein MF, Singh S, Neff RK (1978). Diabetic pregnancy and perinatal morbidity. Am J Obstet Gynecol, 131: 560–580.

Kitzmiller JL, Brown ER, Phillipe M, Stark AR, Acker D, Kaldany A, Singh S, Hare JW (1981). Diabetic nephropathy and perinatal outcome. Am J Obstet Gynecol, 141: 741–751.

Kitzmiller JL, Younger MD, Hare JW, Phillippe M, Vignati L, Fargnoli B, Grause A (1985). Continuous subcutaneous insulin therapy during early pregnancy. Obstet Gynecol, 66: 606–611.

Kucera J (1971). Rate and type of congenital anomalies amongst offspring of diabetic women. J Reprod Med, 7: 61–70.

Laatikainen L, Teramo K, Hieta-Heikurainen H, Koivisto V, Pelkonen R (1987). A controlled study of the influence of continuous subcutaneous insulin infusion treatment on diabetic retinopathy during pregnancy. Acta Med Scand, 221: 367–376.

Landon MB, Piana RP, Main EK, Mennuti MT, Gabbe SG (1986). Glycemic control does reduce neonatal morbidity in diabetic pregnancies, Sixth Annual Meeting, The Society of Perinatal Obstetricians, Abstract 171.

Langer O, Mazze R (1986). The relationship between verified self monitored blood glucose and HBA1, for pregnant and nonpregnant diabetics, Sixth Annual Meeting, The Society of Perinatal Obstetricians, Abstract 37.

Like A, Orci L (1972). Embryogenesis of the human pancreatic islets A light and electron microscopic study. Diabetes, 21: 511–534.

Macfarlane A, Mugford M (1984). Birth Counts. Statistics of Pregnancy and Childbirth. London: Her Majesty's Stationery Office, p 10.

Miller JM (1983). A reappraisal of 'tight control' in diabetic pregnancies. Am J Obstet Gynecol, 147: 158–162.

Miller E, Hare JW, Cloherty JP, Dunn PJ, Gleason RE, Soeldner JS, Kitzmiller JK (1981). Elevated maternal hemoglobin A1c in early pregnancy and major congenital anomalies in infants of diabetic mothers. New Engl J Med, 304: 1331–1334.

Mills JL (1982). Malformations in infants of diabetic mothers. Teratology, 25: 385–394.

Milunsky A, Alpert E, Kitzmiller JL, Younger MD, Neff RK (1982). Prenatal diagnosis of neural tube defects. VIII The importance of serum alpha-fetoprotein screening in diabetic pregnant women. Am J Obstet Gynecol, 142: 1030–1032.

Moloney JBM, Drury MI (1982). The effect of pregnancy on the natural course of diabetic retinopathy. Am J Opthalmol, 93: 745–756.

Molsted-Pedersen L, Tygstrup I, Pedersen J (1964). Congenital malformations in newborn infants of diabetic women. Lancet, i: 1124–1126.

Morris MA, Grandis AS, Litton J (1985). The correlations of glycosylated serum protein and glycosylated hemoglobulin concentrations with blood glucose in diabetic pregnancy. Am J Obstet Gynecol, 153: 257–260.

Murphy J, Peters J, Morris P, Hayes TM, Pearson JF (1984). Conservative management of pregnancy in diabetic women. Br Med J, 288: 1203–1205.

Oloffson P, Liedholm H, Sartor G, Sjöberg U, Svenningsen NW, Ursing D (1984). Diabetes and pregnancy. A 21-year Swedish material. Acta Obstet Gynecol Scand (Suppl), 122: 3–62.

Peacock L, Hunter JC, Walford S, Allison SP, Davison J, Clarke P, Symonds EM, Tattersall RB (1979). Self monitoring of blood glucose in diabetic pregnancy. Br Med J, 2: 1333–1336.

Pedersen J (1977a). The Pregnant Diabetic and Her Newborn. Copenhagen: Munksgaard, p 194.

Pedersen J (1977b). The Pregnant Diabetic and Her Newborn (2nd edn). Baltimore: Williams & Wilkins, p 9.

Pedersen J, Molsted-Pedersen L, Andersen B (1974). Assessors of fetal perinatal mortality in diabetic pregnancy. Diabetes, 23: 302–305.

Peel J (1972). A historical review of diabetes and pregnancy. J Obstet Gynaecol Br Commnwlth, 79: 385–395.

Peel J, Oakley W (1949). The management of pregnancy in diabetics. In: Transactions of the 12th British Congress of Obstetrics and Gynaecology. London: Royal College of Obstetricians and Gynaecologists, p 161.

Persson B, Turnell NO (1975). Metabolic control in diabetic pregnancy. Am J Obstet Gynecol, 122: 737–745.

Potter JM, Reckless JPD, Cullen DR (1980). Subcutaneous continuous insulin infusion and control of blood glucose concentration in diabetics in third trimester of pregnancy. Br Med J, 280: 1099–1101.

Price JH, Hadden DR, Archer DB, Harley J McDG (1984). Diabetic retinopathy in pregnancy. Br J Obstet Gynaecol, 91: 11–17.

Raskin P (1982). Treatment of Type I diabetes with portable insulin infusion devices. Diabetes Care, 5 (Suppl 1): 48–52.

Redman CWG, Beilin LJ, Bonnar J, Wilkinson RH (1976). Plasma urate measurements in predicting fetal death in hypertensive pregnancy. Lancet, i: 1370–1373.

Reece EA, Lockwood CJ, Tuck ST, Hobbins JC (1986). Pregnancy outcome and severe diabetic retinopathy, Sixth Annual Meeting, The Society of Perinatal Obstetricians, Abstract 40.

Reeves ML, Seigler DE, Ryan EA, Skyler JD (1982). Glycemic control in insulin dependent diabetes mellitus comparing outpatient intensified conventional therapy with continuous subcutaneous of insulin infusion. Am J Med, 72: 673–680.

Robert MF, Nett RK, Hubbell JP, Taeusch HW, Avery ME (1976). Association between maternal diabetes and the respiratory distress syndrome in the newborn. New Engl J Med, 294: 357–360.

Sadler TW (1980). Effects of maternal diabetes on early embryogenesis. The teratogenic potential of diabetic serum. Teratology, 21: 339–347.

Saltzman DH, Barbieri RL, Frigoletto FD (1986). Decreased fetal cord prolactin concentration in diabetic pregnancy. Am J Obstet Gynecol, 154: 1035–1038.

Schiffrin A and Bellmonte MN (1982). Comparison between continuous subcutaneous insulin infusion and multiple injections of insulin. Diabetes, 31: 255–264.

Schneider JM, Curet LB, Olson RW, Shay G (1980). Ambulatory care of the pregnant diabetic. Obstet Gynecol, 56: 144–149.

Steele JM, Johnstone FD, Smith AF, Duncan LJP (1982). Five years experience of a 'prepregnancy' clinic for insulin dependent diabetics. Br Med J, 285: 353–356.

Stehbens JA, Baker GL, Kitchell M (1977). Outcome at ages 1, 3, and 5 years of children born to diabetic women. Am J Obstet Gynecol, 127: 408–413.

Stronge JM, Foley ME, Drury MI (1986). Diabetes mellitus and pregnancy. New Engl J Med, 314: 58–59.

Stubbs SM, Brudenell JM, Pyke DA, Watkins PJ, Stubbs WA, Aberti KGMM (1980). Management of the pregnant diabetic: Home or hospital with or without glucose meters. Lancet, i: 1122–1124.

Sutherland HW, and Pritchard CW (1986). Increased incidence of spontaneous abortion in pregnancies complicated by maternal diabetes mellitus. Am J Obstet Gynecol, 155: 135–138.

Tevaarwerk GJM, Harding PGR, Milne KJ, Jaco NT, Rodger NW, Hurst C (1981). Pregnancy in diabetic women: Outcome with a program aimed at normoglycemia before meals. Can Med Assoc J, 125: 435–440.

Thomson AM, Billewicz WZ, Hytten FE (1968). The assessment of fetal growth. J Obstet Gynaecol Br Commnwlth, 75: 903–916.

Tyden O, Berne C, Eriksson UJ, Hansson U, Stangenberg M, Person B (1984). Amniotic fluid C-peptide and phosphatidyl glycerol in diabetic pregnancy. J Perinat Med, 12: 69–73.

Varner MW (1983). Efficacy of home glucose monitoring in diabetic pregnancy. Am J Med, 75: 592–596.

Wald NJ, Cuckle HS, Boreham J, Stirrat GM, Turnbull AC (1979). Maternal serum alpha-fetoprotein and diabetes mellitus. Br J Obstet Gynaecol, 86: 101–105.

West TET, Lowy C (1977). Control of blood glucose during labour in diabetic women with combined glucose and low-dose insulin infusion. Br Med J, 1: 1252–1254.

White P (1971). Pregnancy and diabetics. In: Joslins Diabetes Mellitus. Marble A, White P, Bradley RF, Krall LP (eds). Philadelphia: Lea & Febiger, pp 581–598.

White P (1949). Pregnancy complicating diabetes. Am J Med, 7: 609–616.

World Health Organization (1980). Expert Committee on Diabetes Mellitus, WHO Tech Report, 646: 1–79.

Yatscoff RW, Mehta A, Dean H (1985a). Cord blood glycosylated hemoglobin: Correlation with maternal glycosylated hemoglobin and birthweight. Am J Obstet Gynecol, 152: 861–866.

Yatscoff RW, Mehta A, Dean H (1985b). Maternal and cord blood glycated albumin and total serum: Correlation with maternal glycemic control and birthweight. Am J Obstet Gynecol, 153: 783–788.

Ylinen K, Raivio K, Teramo K (1981). HbA1 predicts the perinatal outcome in insulin-dependent diabetic pregnancies. Br J Obstet Gynaecol, 88: 961–967.

Ylinen K, Aula P, Stenman U-H, Kesaniemi-Koukkanen T, Teramok K (1984). Risk of minor and major fetal malformations in diabetics with high hemoglobin A1c values in early pregnancy. Br Med J, 289: 345–346.

Zinman B (1982). Insulin infusion pumps: Therapeutic implications (Editorial). Clin Invest Med, 5: 91.

Zanona J (1976). Considerations on genetic counselling In: Diabetes and Other Endocrine Disorders during Pregnancy and in the Newborn. New MI, Fiser RH (eds)., New York: Alan R. Liss, pp 1–12.

37 Bleeding during the latter half of pregnancy

Robert Fraser and Robert Watson

1 Introduction

Although, in the Western world at least, bleeding in the second half of pregnancy is no longer a common cause of maternal death, it continues to be a major cause of perinatal mortality, and of both maternal and infant morbidity. Not all of these adverse outcomes are due to the bleeding itself; some of them are caused by the underlying pathology, or by our efforts to deal with it.

The frequency of bleeding in the second half of pregnancy in the total population is difficult to assess. There are no widely accepted criteria for the diagnosis. Ascertainment rates depend in part on the quality and availability of antenatal care. The low incidences reported from some centres may only mean that some episodes of bleeding, perhaps judged to be trivial by the sufferers, did not come to the attention of clinicians and thus are not reported at all. The high incidence reported in some hospital series is biased by the fact that women with bleeding are more likely than women without complications to be sent to a referral centre. Two community studies (Paintin 1962; Roberts 1970) respectively reported rates of 3 per cent and 4.8 per cent of all births.

In most series approximately half the women who present with bleeding in the second half of pregnancy are eventually found to have either placental abruption or placenta praevia. No firm diagnosis can be made in the other half, and they are considered to have haemorrhage of uncertain or indeterminate origin (Watson 1982). In a small proportion of women who bleed, the bleeding arises from lower genital tract. This is rarely serious as far as the pregnancy is concerned.

2 Placental abruption

2.1 Introduction

Placental abruption, or retroplacental haemorrhage, is a major contributor to perinatal mortality amongst normally formed fetuses. Although maternal mortality is fortunately now rare, maternal morbidity in the forms of haemorrhage, shock, disseminated intravascular coagulation, and renal failure is sufficiently frequent to justify concerned and intensive treatment of those affected (Table 37.1).

The condition presents diagnostic difficulties that result in poor comparability between published series. The pathological diagnosis is made retrospectively on examination of the placenta, by the finding of adherent retroplacental clot, crater formation and placental infarction, but as many as 4.5 per cent of placentae may show such changes (Fox 1978). Although the clinical diagnosis is made in between 0.5–1.5 per cent of births in most series, there is no vaginal bleeding before delivery in 20–35 per cent of cases. Placental abruption

Table 37.1 Collected series of placental abruptions: incidence, maternal mortality and morbidity, perinatal mortality

			Maternal complication rate amongst mothers with placental abruption			PNMR amongst babies delivered after abruption	Distribution of perinatal deaths related to admission and delivery		
Author, year, and country of origin	Years surveyed	Incidence (%)	Maternal deaths (%)	Maternal renal failure (%)	Maternal coagulation defect (%)	PNMR (per 1000 births)	IUFD before admission (% of PN deaths)	IUFD after admission (% of PN deaths)	NND (% of PN deaths)
Page *et al.* (1954) USA	1930–50	225/41,412 (0.54)	4/225 (1.7)	4/225 (1.7)	13/225 (5.7)	101/225 (448)	—	—	—
Douglas *et al.* (1955) USA	1932–54	398/71,826 (0.55)	5/398 (1.3)			138/398 (347)	83/138 (60)	32/138 (23)	23/138 (17)
Porter (1960) USA	1950–58	283/54,286 (0.52)	5/283 (1.8)	11/283 (3.9)	12/283 (4.2)	—	188/285 (87)	—	—
Paintin (1962) UK	1949–58	223/30,383 (0.73)	—	0	—	51/223 (228)	—	—	—
Hibbard (1966) UK	1952–64	506/43,620 (1.16)	1/506 (0.2)	6/506 (1.2)	42/206† (20.0)	295/510 (507)	148/259 (57)	47/259 (18)	64/259 (25)
de Valera (1968) Eire	1956–66	1394/51,401 (2.70)	2/1394 (0.1)	—	—	—	—	—	—
Roberts (1970) UK	1965–68	283/13,656 (2.07)	—	—	—	43/283 (152)	—	—	—
Golditch and Boyce (1970) USA	1960–68	130/26,743 (0.48)	0/130 (0.0)	—	6/130 (4.6)	39/130 (300)	15/39 (38)	4/39 (10)	20/39 (52)
Lunan (1973) UK	1966–70	379/29,456 (1.30)	1/379 (0.3)	1/379 (0.3)	17/379 (4.5)	146/384 (380)	78/146 (53)	35/146 (24)	33/146 (23)
Blair (1973) UK	1965–69	189/23,465 (0.81)	1/189 (0.5)	3/189 (1.5)	21/189 (11.1)	106/189 (550)	55/106 (53)	29/106 (27)	21/106 (20)
Knab (1978) USA	1963–77	434/35,133 (1.24)	—	—	—	122/388‡ (317)	31/122 (25)	27/122 (22)	64/122 (53)
Paterson (1979) UK	1968–75	193/35,217 (0.55)	0/193 (0.00)	0/193 (0.0)	1/193 (0.5)	68/196 (346)	49/68 (72)	5/68 (7)	14/68 (21)
Green-Thompson (1982) South Africa	1981	157/23,323 (0.67)	—	—	—	—	—	—	—
Caffrey (1983) Nigeria	1977	64/10,747 (0.60)	—	—	—	49/64 (765)	—	—	—
Bansal (1985) Kenya	1983	18/23,084 (0.07)	—	—	—	18/21 (857)	—	—	—
Okonofua (1985) Nigeria	1982–83	98/6,637 (1.47)	—	—	—	66/98 (673)	51/66 (77)	7/66 (11)	8/66 (12)

— Information not abstracted from publication
† Only 206 women had coagulation studies performed
‡ Analysis of cases for one hospital only

may enter into the differential diagnosis of almost any pregnant woman with abdominal or back pain. In one prospective series with a live fetus at presentation (Hurd *et al.* 1983) the clinical diagnosis was made with confidence, but in error, in 10 per cent of cases, and only diagnosed *after* delivery in 38 per cent.

Placental abruption was at one time a major cause of maternal death. Maternal mortality directly attributed to placental abruption has now become a rarity in developed countries (Table 37.1). In the latest maternal mortality report for England and Wales, a rate of 1.04 deaths from placental abruption per million maternities was recorded, during the years 1979–81 (Department of Health and Social Security 1986). In one series of 22 maternal deaths attributed to placental abruption between 1950 and 1968 reported from Dublin (de Valera 1968), 15 were due to renal failure and 7 to haemorrhagic shock, usually in women with a coagulation defect.

Postpartum haemorrhage is twice as common in

women with abruption as in the unselected hospital population (Hibbard and Jeffcoate 1966). Emergency hysterectomy has occasionally been required (Pritchard and Brekken 1967).

Even in modern series a perinatal mortality rate in cases of abruption of less than 300 per 1000 is rarely recorded. In the developing world the rate continues to exceed 500 per 1000 (Table 37.1). In modern series fetal death before admission to hospital commonly contributes 50 per cent or more of the perinatal losses (Blair 1973; Paterson 1979; Hurd *et al.* 1983). Neonatal deaths are principally attributed to the complications of delivery too early in pregnancy. Amongst surviving infants, rates of respiratory distress, patent ductus arteriosus, low Apgar scores, and anaemia are more common than in unselected hospital series (Hurd *et al.* 1983).

2.2 Aetiology and possible scope for prevention

It is rare to identify an aetiological factor in placental abruption. There is an association with increasing age and parity, although it has been suggested that this is an effect of parity, independent of age (Hibbard and Jeffcoate 1966). Some cases have followed abdominal trauma, others followed sudden reduction in uterine volume, typically seen at spontaneous or artificial membrane rupture in cases of polyhydramnios. Occasional cases have a temporal relationship to attempts at external cephalic version (see Chapter 31). In a recently reported randomized controlled trial two women in 310 had abruption within 6 hours of the attempt at version. There were no abruptions in the 330 controls (Kasule *et al.* 1985). This whole series had a relatively low incidence of placental abruption.

There is no evidence of a relationship to diagnostic amniocentesis performed in early pregnancy (Tabor *et al.* 1986).

The relationship of pregnancy induced hypertension to the aetiology of placental abruption remains controversial. Data from the Collaborative Perinatal Project confirm a higher rate of intrapartum hypertension in women with abruption, but no significant excess of hypertension was recorded in the antenatal period before the abruption occurred (Naeye *et al.* 1977). A recent study found no excess of pre-eclampsia or pregnancy induced hypertension in women with abruption (Paterson 1979).

The suggestion that maternal folic acid deficiency may have an aetiological role in abruption (Hibbard and Jeffcoate 1966) has not been confirmed (see Chapter 19). In one hospital series relating to women with a high rate of dietary folate deficiency, supplementation during the prepregnancy period and during pregnancy itself had no detectable prophylactic effect on recurrent placental abruption (de Valera 1968). In another series the introduction of routine folate supplementation had no detectable effect on the incidence of abruption (Golditch and Boyce 1970). A large prospective study found no association between a low serum folate level and abruption in either the index pregnancy or previous pregnancies, and in a placebo controlled randomized study of folic acid supplementation in pregnancy the abruption rate was 1.0 per cent in the supplemented group and 0.8 per cent in the placebo group (Hall 1972).

The pathological changes typical of abruption—decidual necrosis at the margin of the placenta, and large placental infarcts—are more common in cigarette smokers. According to Naeye *et al.* (1977) the frequency of decidual necrosis increases with the number of cigarettes smoked, and may follow nicotine-induced arteriolar spasm. Naeye (1980) also claimed that placental abruption is one and a half times more frequent in smokers than non-smokers, and giving up smoking in pregnancy may be associated with a protective effect. Controlled trials on smoking withdrawal in pregnancy (see Chapter 16) have not been large enough to determine whether or not this is true. Placental abruption is associated with pre-existing intrauterine growth retardation (Hibbard and Jeffcoate 1966), but these data have not been analysed for any independent effect of maternal smoking.

The probable importance of maternal factors in the aetiology of placental abruption is emphasized by the recurrence rate in subsequent pregnancies, which is reported as being between 5.6 per cent and 17.3 per cent (Paterson 1979; Hibbard and Jeffcoate 1966).

2.3 Pathological findings

The lesions most commonly found are increased prevalence of thrombosed arteries and necrosis of the decidua basalis—particularly at the periphery of the placenta. Infarcts and fibrosis of the terminal villi are common in the placental parenchyma (Naeye *et al.* 1977).

Blood escaping under the necrotic decidua takes one or several of the following courses. It may (1) dissect under the membranes, and remain concealed, or reach the cervix and become revealed vaginal bleeding (antepartum haemorrhage); (2) rupture the membranes and enter the amniotic fluid; (3) dissect under the placenta increasing the area of separation; or (4) infiltrate the myometrium producing the typical purple discoloration known as the 'Couvelaire Uterus' (Egley and Cefalo 1985).

2.4 Clinical findings

Various attempts have been made to classify the severity of placental abruption using the clinical findings, estimated blood loss, or extent of placental infarction. Two typical schemes are shown in Table 37.2.

Table 37.2 Classifications of severity of placental abruption

Clinical findings (Page 1954)	Pathological and clinical findings (Knabb 1978)
Grade 0 Unrecognized before delivery	*Mild* *Clot covers <1/6th placental surface* Blood losses <400 ml No symptoms
Grade 1 External bleeding only or mild uterine hypertonus No maternal shock	*Moderate* Clot >1/6th <2/3rds surface Blood loss 400–1000 ml Increased uterine tone and tenderness
Grade 2 Uterine hypertonus Uterine tenderness Possible external bleeding	*Severe* Clot >2/3rds surface. Blood loss >1000 ml Tense painful uterus
Grade 3 Maternal shock and/or coagulation defect Uterine hypertonus Intrauterine fetal death	

The recently published study of Hurd and colleagues (1983) provides a valuable insight into the clinical spectrum of this disease, because their analysis included those cases which were not suspected before delivery. These are the cases graded as 0 by Page (Table 37.2). Because of the unique nature of the Hurd and colleagues' study it will be quoted extensively. There were 59 cases of placental abruption, 50 with a live fetus on admission, and 9 in which fetal death had occurred. A further 3 cases were clinically diagnosed in the antenatal period as having abruption, but this diagnosis could not be confirmed on inspection of the placenta.

Amongst the 50 women with a live fetus, 39 (78 per cent) had vaginal bleeding. In 13 cases an initial diagnosis of idiopathic preterm labour was made. This association between occult abruption and the onset of preterm labour is well recognized. Whether the presence of extravasated blood in the myometrium triggers uterine activity, or a fetal response to a hostile uterine environment initiates labour, is unresolved.

Fetal distress, diagnosed as repeated late fetal heart rate decelerations, severe variable decelerations, or sustained bradycardia, was common after admission in the group clinically diagnosed as abruption. Thirty-three women had backache or uterine tenderness. The conjunction of backache with a posteriorly placed placenta is suspicious. The differential diagnosis of such complaints includes, pyelonephritis; red degeneration in a fibroid, the onset of labour, and orthopaedic problems such as lumbar or sacroiliac strain.

High frequency contractions (more than 5 in 10 minutes) were noted in 17 per cent of the series of Hurd *et al.* (1983). Sustained uterine hypertonus was diagnosed in a similar proportion. These figures seem low when compared with those reported in retrospective series because of the inclusion of the grade 0 cases. Uterine hypertonus is a very common physical sign in the more severe grades of abruption, particularly when the fetus has died *in utero* (Pritchard and Brekken 1967).

Ultrasound examination of the uterus and contents, when available, has an important role in the differential diagnosis of antepartum haemorrhage. Most important is its ability to localize the placenta. A low-lying placenta brings placenta praevia into the differential diagnosis, while a posterior placenta might make the diagnosis of abruption more likely in a woman with back pain. The diagnosis of retroplacental haematoma by ultrasound is not always straightforward. In Hurd and colleagues' series, although all the women had ultrasound examination, only 1 retroplacental haematoma was recognized. The difficulty arises from the similar ultrasound appearances associated with fresh retroplacental bleeding, organized haematomata, placental infarction, and non-pathological areas of sonolucency representing endometrial venules, normal decidua basalis, or normal subplacental myometrium (Jouppila and Kirkinen 1982).

In Hurd and colleagues study, 11 of the 50 women with live fetuses on admission were found to have a 'marginal abruption' (covering less than 5 per cent of placental surface area), and these were evenly distributed between the asymptomatic and symptomatic cases. The mean area of placenta affected was 40 per cent, but all but one of the women with a dead fetus on admission had more than 50 per cent of the surface area affected.

Abruption may occur at any stage of gestation. In one series of 193 cases there were 34 cases (18 per cent) before 32 weeks, 77 cases (40 per cent) between 34 and 37 weeks, and 82 cases (42 per cent) after 37 weeks (Paterson 1979). In this series it was considered that the abruption took place after the woman had become established in labour in 42 cases (22 per cent).

In severe abruption (Page's Grade 3) there may be heavy vaginal bleeding, or evidence of increasing abdominal girth if the blood is retained within the uterus. The woman is usually in severe pain, and may be shocked as a result of hypovolaemia. Absence of clotting may be obvious in the vaginal blood loss. Other signs of clotting defect might be bleeding from the gums, or venepuncture sites, or haematuria.

The rate of coagulation defects reported in different series of placental abruption varies for at least two reasons: first, the defect may be less common in recent years because of improved care, particularly in the matter of volume replacement; second, the criteria on which the diagnosis is made varies between clinical and laboratory measurements. These have been classified by Letsky (1985) (Table 37.3). Some series include cases of Letsky's Stage 2, others only Stage 3. In a series of 141 cases of severe abruption in which the fetus was dead, severe hypofibrinogenaemia (Stage 3) was present in 38 per cent (Pritchard and Brekken 1967). Green-Thompson (1982) in South Africa records a similar incidence of 35 per cent where the fetus is dead, but points out the rarity of a significant coagulation defect with a live fetus.

In the shocked hypovolaemic woman with heavy vaginal bleeding it may be impossible to exclude placenta praevia on clinical grounds. A deeply engaged presenting part might suggest abruption, but usually the uterus is too tense for this sign to be elicited.

Table 37.3 Spectrum of severity of disseminated intravascular coagulation (after Letsky 1985)

Severity of DIC		*In vitro* findings
Stage 1	Low grade compensated	Raised fibrin degradation products Increased soluble fibrin complexes
Stage 2	Uncompensated, but no haemostatic failure	As above, and in addition, Fibrinogen level falls Platelet count falls Reduced factors V and VIII
Stage 3	Rampant, with haemostatic failure	Very low platelet counts Very low fibrinogen levels High fibrin degradation products levels

Stage 2 is common after mild or moderate abruption. Stage 3 is more often seen after severe abruption.

2.5 Treatment

In suspected mild abruption the symptoms may resolve, and if there has been bleeding this may cease, with the fetal condition apparently satisfactory. It may be impossible to confirm the diagnosis, and care should be as for the women with antepartum haemorrhage of uncertain origin. It would seem likely that the conditions are present for further and possibly more serious placental separation, but no evidence exists to show this is a significant risk. The common pre-existence of fetal growth retardation (Hibbard and Jeffcoate 1966), further complicated by a reduced area for placental perfusion due to the abruption, would suggest that fetal monitoring should be instituted (see Chapters 3 and 28).

In moderate and severe abruption, maternal resuscitation and analgesia are priorities. The amount of blood loss may not be obvious—some may have been lost before admission, and large volumes of blood may be retained in the uterus. Clinical signs of hypovolaemia may be masked by increased peripheral resistance. Cerebral and cardiac perfusion may be preserved, and renal blood flow jeopardized (Muldoon 1969). This will become manifest by oliguria.

Using historical controls, Muldoon suggested that the insertion of a central venous pressure monitor allowed a more accurate assessment of under (and over) transfusion. He showed that those monitored by central venous pressure had a greater amount of blood transfused, a lower rate of oliguria in the first 24 hours post-abruption, and a lower rate of puerperal anaemia (Muldoon 1969). Cannulation of subclavian and jugular veins are rightly considered tasks for those with special experience. If such expertise is not available, basilic vein catheterization in the upper arm should be within the capabilities of all doctors supervising women with abruption. A satisfactory 'blind' placement can be obtained in 85 per cent of cases (Ryan 1977).

The use of whole blood has become traditional in volume replacement in these women. It is likely, however, that a crystalloid infusion to precede the blood would be beneficial (Moss 1972). Letsky recommends fresh frozen plasma at the rate of 1 unit for every 4–6 units of bank red cells transfused, to replenish labile clotting factors, which are not present in the stored blood (Letsky 1985).

Plasma substitutes such as plasma protein, dextran, gelatin, and starch may produce adverse reactions, and dextran in particular can interfere with platelet function *in vivo* and cross-matching *in vitro*. Letsky considers polygeline (Haemaccel) to be the best available colloid pending the availability of red cells for transfusion. In one randomized study of patients undergoing aortic surgery, colloid infusions had no detectable benefits over crystalloids, when physiological endpoints were used to monitor fluid replacement (Virgilio 1979).

No systematic attempts have been made to study alternatives to blood transfusion in this condition, although at least one Jehovah's Witness who refused blood and blood products despite severe haemorrhage and disseminated intravascular coagulation associated with eclampsia has survived (Reid *et al.* 1986).

A clotting defect should be sought, although defects of clinical significance are rare when there is a live fetus (Green-Thompson 1982). Recognition of a clotting defect depends on a high index of suspicion, and serial studies of coagulation factors. A prolongation of the bedside clotting time may be significant, but the usefulness of this test has been questioned, as false positives may cause unnecessary panic (Letsky 1985). The laboratory tests which suggest that disseminated intravascular coagulation is developing are progressive falls in the platelet count and fibrinogen titre, prolongation of the thrombin time and partial thromboplastin time, and elevation of urinary or plasma fibrin degradation products (Letsky 1985) (Table 37.3).

The process of disseminated intravascular coagulation usually starts to resolve after delivery (Sher 1977). Maintaining circulating volume assists the clearance of fibrin degradation products from the plasma (Letsky 1985).

The use of blood and blood products in this condition has been discussed by Letsky. She points out that fresh blood is rarely available, because of the requirement to screen it for infections, and recommends the use of bank blood or red cell concentrates, with fresh frozen plasma, the latter providing all coagulation factors apart from platelets. Freeze-dried plasma is easier to store and handle, but is deficient in Factors V and VIII. There is a suggestion that concentrated fibrinogen should not be used as it may 'feed the fire', and encourage further disseminated intravascular coagulation. The same criticism could be levelled at frozen or dried plasma presumably, and earlier authors have claimed that fibrinogen has been used to good effect when surgery is indicated, or in the arrest of bleeding from a flaccid postpartum uterus, and in a case of multiple lower genital tract lacerations (Pritchard and Brekken 1967). Platelet transfusions may have a place if the above manoeuvres fail to achieve haemostasis, but the same theoretical objection to their use exists (Letsky 1985).

Heparin therapy has the ability to break the 'vicious cycle' of disseminated intravascular coagulation, but most authorities consider its use inappropriate in situations where the circulation is not intact, and this obviously includes abruption. The contrary objection to antifibrinolytic drugs exists, in that they might prevent the removal of microvascular thrombi in vital organs such as brain or kidney (Letsky 1985). Their possible use in uterine inertia is discussed below. The restoration of circulating volume, and emptying of the uterus are the cornerstones of treatment. Specific replacement of coagulation factors should be done under laboratory control.

Analgesia, when required, is best administered as narcotics (morphine/pethidine intramuscularly or intravenously) supplemented by self-administered nitrous oxide/oxygen mixtures (see Chapter 57). Most anaesthetists are reluctant to offer epidural analgesia to women with a placental abruption for two reasons: first, because epidural haemorrhage may develop in the woman with an undiagnosed clotting defect; and second, because of the unpredictable extent of peripheral blood pooling, which may result in hypotension in a woman already having difficulty maintaining perfusion of vital organs.

2.6 Delivery

When the fetus is alive, a decision about delivery in its interest should be made in the light of its considered maturity, and the past experience of the obstetricians and paediatricians concerned. The best mode of delivery is a matter of debate. Only one controlled trial comparing vaginal delivery with caesarean section in cases of abruption after 36 weeks' gestation has been reported (Okonofua and Olatunbosun 1985). It showed a perinatal loss of 12/23 (52 per cent) in those delivered vaginally vs. 3/18 (16 per cent) in those delivered by emergency caesarean section. Interpretation of this pioneering trial is rather difficult. Allocation to delivery groups was alternate rather than randomized, 2 women who refused caesarean section were placed in the vaginal delivery group, 2 who were originally allocated to vaginal delivery, but eventually delivered by caesarean section for failure to progress, were not analysed. Preterm labourers were excluded. This trial was undertaken in a centre, Ife, Nigeria, where electronic fetal heart rate monitoring was *not* available. One can only speculate as to whether or not similar results would be found in units with more sophisticated technology, and trials in such centres are obviously required.

In the early series reviewed in Fig. 37.1, policy was directed towards vaginal delivery at all reasonable costs. This was because the newborn prognosis was so poor (especially for preterm infants), and if the mother recovered from a potentially serious operation she was left with a scarred uterus (Porter 1960; Hibbard and Jeffcoate 1966). Indeed, in Porter's paper a point at issue was whether *maternal* mortality could have been reduced by caesarean section.

A change of policy towards early caesarean section in the fetal interest developed after the publications of three later series (Golditch and Boyce 1970; Lunan 1973; Knab 1978). Improvements in resuscitation and anaesthetic techniques were also being reported (Phillips and Evans 1970), and improved survival of the preterm newborn has been generally achieved. Based on their retrospective analyses these authors noted that a number of normally formed infants were lost in the hours between diagnosis and delivery (see Table 37.1). Golditch and Boyce (1970) suggested that if the fetal heart was present on admission, caesarean section should be performed as soon as maternal blood replacement had started. Lunan (1973) noted that of the 35 fetal deaths occurring after admission, 14 came without warning. He hypothesized that these were due to extension of the placental separation, and that they might have been saved by earlier emergency caesarean section. In his series, as in the other two discussed here, continuous fetal heart rate monitoring was *not* available. Because of uterine tenderness, tenseness, and the interference with heart sound transmission when the abruption has taken place under an anterior placenta, auscultation of the fetal heart cannot be relied on to detect fetal distress or even to confirm the presence of a live fetus. Although not available at the time that these studies were undertaken, a hand-held Doppler or ultrasound visualization of the fetal heart can be very useful in those circumstances today. Knab (1978) noted that most of the post-admission fetal deaths occurred in fetuses delivered more than 2 hours after admission. In view of this he made an elegant case for a randomized controlled trial of intention to deliver vaginally, or abdominally in cases where vaginal delivery was not imminent. It is ironic that later reviewers have used Knab's data when suggesting that such a trial may be unethical (Green-Thompson 1982).

Current practice appears to favour early resort to caesarean section where the fetus is judged viable, but Hurd's study included an attempt to deliver vaginally, using continuous electronic fetal heart rate monitoring, and synthetic oxytocin infusions, in the absence of contraindications (Hurd *et al.* 1983). Of his 31 women with a live fetus diagnosed before delivery as having abruption, 16 were delivered by caesarean section for the following indications: fetal distress 9, uterine hypertonus 2, disseminated intramuscular coagulation and unfavourable cervix 1, preterm breech 3, transverse lie 1. Of the 15 women delivered vaginally, 7 had no evidence of fetal distress, 3 had irregular fetal heart rate patterns but normal fetal scalp blood pH, and 5 had fetal distress in late labour when vaginal delivery was a more reasonable option than caesarean section. One of these babies was lost before delivery, but this was ascribed to poor attention by the staff, who were not available when the fetal heart rate pattern of distress developed. This study suggests that a 50 per cent reduction in caesarean section rate might be possible without a significant effect on the perinatal mortality rate. Such a reduction would seem to be in the maternal interest.

Analysis of the delivery modes in the grade 0 abruption patients in Hurd's study is also of interest (Hurd *et al.* 1983). Fifteen of the 19 women gave birth vaginally to healthy infants, and 4 were delivered by emergency caesarean section (1 for transverse lie, 2 preterm breech presentations, and only 1 for fetal distress).

In severe abruption, where there is a dead fetus, most authorities favour vaginal delivery except where there is an obvious obstetric indication for caesarean section, such as transverse lie. In most published series a handful of cases are reported where uterine contractions could not be stimulated, or the clinical shock associated with haemorrhage has been uncontrollable, and in such rare cases caesarean section has been undertaken. These are also the cases in which coagulation defects are most common, and maternal risks are considerable (Pritchard and Brekken 1967).

When there is no satisfactory response to oxytocin, prostaglandins may be administered to attempt to stimulate contractions. An aetiological factor in uterine inertia may be a direct inhibitory effect of high concentrations of fibrin degradation products on myometrial activity (Basu 1969). One small uncontrolled trial of Aprotinin (Trasylol) in this situation has been reported (Sher 1977). The drug-induced inhibition of fibrinolysis was postulated to reduce the levels of fibrin degradation products, thus removing the blocking effect on the myometrial contractility. No controlled trial of this interesting therapeutic approach has been undertaken, and others have suggested that antifibrinolytic drugs are contraindicated in disseminated intravascular coagulation, because of the risk of thrombosis in the small vessels of kidney and/or brain (Letsky 1985).

When caesarean section in a woman with disseminated intravascular coagulation is judged to be inevitable, it should be undertaken after close consultation with anaesthetic and haematological colleagues. Volume replacement and transfusions of whole blood, frozen plasma, and specific coagulation factors should be given before and during the surgical procedure.

2.7 Conclusions

A well-equipped hospital should be able to provide adequate emergency treatment for the mother, and will usually be able to safely deliver a fetus that is alive on admission. Survival of such liveborn infants will depend on the quality of neonatal care. Advances in the management of this condition will come if some means of predicting abruption should be developed. Further information about aetiology is required before prevention of the disorder can be contemplated.

3 Placenta praevia

3.1 Introduction

Placenta praevia is defined as a placenta which is situated wholly or partially in the lower uterine segment.

The overall prevalence of placenta praevia, calculated from various series reported in the literature over the past 20 years is 0.55 per cent, ranging from 0.29 per cent (Green-Thompson 1982) to 1.24 per cent (de Valera 1968). Variations in the reported prevalence of placenta praevia among studies are due to differences in definition, the duration of pregnancy at the time that diagnosis is made, and sociomedical characteristics of the population studied (Brenner *et al.* 1978). There is also wide variation in the relative frequency of the different types or degrees of placenta praevia reported in the literature, in particular the proportion of major degrees of placenta praevia, which range from 25 per cent (Brenner *et al.* 1978) to 53 per cent (Macafee *et al.* 1962) with most authors reporting a frequency of around 40 to 45 per cent (Pedowitz 1965; Hibbard 1966; Cotton *et al.* 1980; Silver *et al.* 1984). These differences are of more than academic interest, as it is generally accepted that there is an increasing incidence of mortality and morbidity to mother and fetus as the placenta becomes more centrally placed (Beischer and Mackay 1986). Classifications of placenta praevia are displayed more fully in Table 37.4.

Placenta praevia is seldom responsible for maternal death in recently reported series. The major cause of both mortality and morbidity is haemorrhage; prevention and effective treatment of haemorrhage has reduced the gravity of the condition. There were no maternal deaths in 583 cases of placenta praevia at the Royal Maternity Hospital, Belfast during the years 1963 to 1977 (Myerscough 1982). The Report on Confidential Enquiries into Maternal Deaths in England and Wales 1979–1981 records only three deaths associated with placenta praevia in 1,942,859 total births. Two of the deaths were associated with placenta praevia/accreta. One woman who died was allowed home despite vaginal bleeding late in the 2nd trimester and an ultrasound examination which confirmed placenta praevia.

With modern care a perinatal mortality rate of 50–60 per 1000 is now attainable (Gordon 1969; Myerscough 1982; MacDonald 1984; Silver *et al.* 1984), and for surviving infants long term physical growth and psychomotor development is generally normal (Naeye 1978).

3.2 Aetiology and possible scope for prevention

Placenta praevia results from implantation of the fertilized ovum low in the cavity of the uterus, the actual implantation site being in the isthmus or in the immediate neighbourhood of the isthmus (Myerscough 1982). The exact reasons for this occurrence are not known. A large placental surface area may be the explanation in multiple pregnancy or in the extremely rare condition of placenta membranacea, but the placenta in placenta praevia of singleton pregnancies is not larger than normal (Green-Thompson 1982). Advanced age and parity is associated with the development of placenta praevia, although the relative importance of these two factors is disputed. Eastman and Hellman (1964) found age to be a more important factor, whereas Pedowitz (1965), Nelson and Huston (1971), Naeye (1978), and Clark *et al.* (1985) find increasing parity to have a more significant effect. Maternal age is the most important risk factor in cases of recurrent placenta praevia (Gorodeski *et al.* 1981).

Table 37.4 Classification of placenta praevia

British	Degree 1	The greater part of the placenta is attached to the active contractile portion of the uterus or upper segment and only the lower margin of its dips into the lower segment.
	Degree 2	The margin of the placenta reaches down to the internal os.
	Degree 3	The placenta completely covers the internal os when closed, but does not entirely do so when the os is well dilated.
	Degree 4	The centre of the placenta corresponds, or very nearly corresponds, with the internal os.
American	Marginal	The margin of the placenta extends to, but does not encroach upon the cervical os.
	Partial	The placenta covers a portion of the cervical os.
	Total	The placenta covers the os entirely.
Ultrasound	Low Lying	
	Partial	
	Complete/Total	

Deficient endometrium may be an aetiological factor, and in theory, any event damaging the endometrial lining of the uterus could result in decidual deficiency. Thus, possible predisposing factors would include uterine scars, previous uterine adhesions, endometritis, curettage, manual removal of the placenta, submucous leiomyoma, multiparity, and adenomyosis (Breen *et al.* 1977). Women with one or more previous miscarriages have been reported to be at increased risk of placenta praevia (Record and McKeown 1956; Brenner *et al.* 1978), and there appears to be an increased risk following dilatation and curettage and evacuation of retained products of conception (Rose and Chapman 1986). Barret *et al.* (1981) found that the risk of placenta praevia was six times greater for women with a history of induced 1st trimester abortion than for women without such a history, but other studies have been unable to show any association between legal abortion and placenta praevia (Harlap and Davis 1975; Schoenbaum *et al.* 1980; Madore *et al.* 1981; Grimes and Techman 1984). The lack of association with termination of pregnancy may be related to the method of suction curettage in contrast to sharp curettage (Rose and Chapman 1986).

Bender (1954) first suggested the relationship between previous caesarean section scars and the subsequent development of placenta praevia. Singh *et al.* (1981) reported a 3.9 per cent incidence of placenta praevia among women with previous caesarean section, while Clark *et al.* (1985) demonstrated an almost linear increase in placenta praevia with the number of previous caesarean sections, rising to 10 per cent in women who had four or more previous caesareans.

MacGillvray *et al.* (1986) have shown an increased rate of male to female sex at birth among women with placenta praevia. An increase in the sex ratio at birth is associated with insemination early or late in the menstrual cycle (Harlap 1979). MacGillvray *et al.* (1986)

have postulated that such early or late insemination may result in delayed development and implantation of the blastocyst, and that this may be a predisposing factor in placenta praevia.

3.3 Pathological findings

The placenta is often irregular in shape and variable in thickness, and frequently the cord has a marginal or vellamentous insertion (Percival 1980; Clayton *et al.* 1985). Myerscough (1982) states that 'every variety of malformation of the placenta (bipartita, succenturata, membranacea, fenestrata, and accreta) together with abnormalities in the insertion of the cord and the distribution of the umbilical vessels are more common and that such irregularities of the placenta and cord affect the well-being of the fetus and interfere with its growth and development.'

Placenta membranacea, while quoted in most standard textbooks as a cause of placenta praevia, is in fact an extremely rare placental anomaly, with only a handful of cases having been reported world-wide (Fox 1978).

There is an association between placenta praevia and placenta accreta (Kistner *et al.* 1952; Read *et al.* 1980) and a strong association between placenta praevia/accreta and prior multiple caesarean sections (Clark *et al.* 1985).

Vellamentous insertion of the cord is associated with multiple pregnancy, placenta praevia, and bipartite placenta (Carp *et al.* 1979). There is a risk of damage to the exposed and unprotected fetal vessels with resultant serious and often fatal fetal haemorrhage. Bleeding from vasa praevia is, however, an extremely rare clinical condition, for despite the obvious danger of fetal blood loss from damaged vellamentous vessels it has been estimated that this accident occurs in only 2 per cent of velamentous cords (Quek and Tan 1972). The fetus is at greater risk from compression of the vellamentous vessels against the wall of the pelvis during delivery; fetal distress under such circumstances is common and fetal death by no means rare (Fox 1978).

Naeye (1978), using material from the Collaborative Perinatal Project, found that the placentae in fatal cases of placenta praevia were growth-retarded, with an increased frequency of necrosis of the decidua basalis and thrombi at the placental margin. He also showed an increased frequency of villous hyperplasia in the placentae and excessive erythropoiesis in the liver and other fetal organs, in fatal cases. He attributed the decidual necrosis and marginal thrombi to premature separation of the placentae from the uterine wall, and the villous hyperplasia and excessive fetal erythropoiesis, as a response to fetal haemorrhage. The women with placental villous hyperplasia had a history of recurrent maternal vaginal bleeding often starting in the 2nd trimester of pregnancy. Microscopic abnormalities were no more frequent in the placentae of the placenta praevia survivors than in the placentae of survivors who did not have placenta praevia.

3.4 Clinical findings

3.4.1 Vaginal bleeding

Vaginal bleeding associated with placenta praevia is due to separation of the placenta from its attachment in the lower segment. The bleeding is usually painless, bright red, and variable in amount. The degree of bleeding is proportional to the extent of the separation, but the first haemorrhage is seldom severe. A history of warning haemorrhage or of recurrent slight vaginal bleeding is commonly obtained from women who are later found to have placenta praevia (Myerscough 1982), although in approximately one in six cases there is no warning haemorrhage before the onset of labour (Macafee 1962; Morgan 1965).

It is generally believed that the blood loss is maternal and comes mainly from the uterine wall from which the placenta has been detached, and only to a very slight extent from the separated portion of the placenta. Although it is widely recognized that in the rare condition of vasa praevia the blood loss is fetal, it may well be that in a proportion of cases of placenta praevia the vaginal bleeding may also contain blood of fetal origin. The work of Naeye (1978) suggests that there is fetal bleeding, which results in fetal anaemia and compensatory erythropoiesis in the fetus and villous hyperplasia in the placenta, preceding fetal death in cases of placenta praevia. McShane *et al.* (1985) have shown a statistically significant direct correlation between fetal anaemia requiring neonatal transfusion and the degree of antenatal maternal blood loss. Cotton *et al.* (1980) recorded an 18.7 per cent incidence of anaemia in the neonates and emphasized the need to always determine whether any fetal component is present in 3rd trimester blood loss. This possibility may be tested by examining the blood from the vaginal haemorrhage for the presence of fetal red cells. A number of tests are available, all of which depend upon sodium hydroxide haemolysing maternal cells and leaving fetal cells intact. The method of Gelsthorpe (1960) is simple and effective. Two to three drops of blood are added to a small test-tube half-filled with a 1 per cent aqueous solution of sodium hydroxide. The test-tube is shaken and allowed to stand for 90 seconds. A brown-green solution indicates maternal blood cells which have undergone haemolysis, whereas a red solution identifies fetal cells.

Placenta praevia may cause vaginal bleeding from as early as 16 weeks' gestation up to the delivery of the fetus at term, but bleeding is more likely to occur after 32 weeks' gestation. Gabert (1971) reported that in approximately 80 per cent of cases the initial bleed occurred after 31 weeks' gestation. Onset of bleeding before 20 weeks' gestation is associated with a very poor fetal prognosis (McShane *et al.* 1985), and some have shown that the earlier in pregnancy the initial haemorrhage occurs the greater is the incidence of prematurity (Pedowitz 1965; Crenshaw *et al.* 1973; Silver *et al.* 1984).

It is generally accepted that there is an increasing incidence of mortality and morbidity to mother and fetus as the placenta becomes more centrally placed (Beischer and Mackay 1986). Pedowitz (1965) states that 'fetal salvage obtained with expectant therapy is directly related to the incidence of total placenta praevia, and this accounts for the varying degrees of success reported by different investigators'. Review of the literature, however, shows conflicting evidence on this subject. Some authors have shown a higher fetal mortality and morbidity in major degrees compared to minor degrees of placenta praevia (Pedowitz 1965; Crenshaw *et al.* 1973), but neither Hibbard (1969) nor Cotton *et al.* (1980) could find any evidence of increased fetal mortality with total placental praeviae. Pedowitz (1965) and Crenshaw *et al.* (1973) reported that the initial bleeding occurred earlier, and that there was a greater incidence of recurrent bleeding in total placenta praevia. Hibbard (1969), however, states that in his series the type of praevia bore no relationship to the total blood loss, number of bleeding episodes, or fetal outcome, although the majority of women bleeding into hypovolaemic shock were classified as having a total praevia. Cotton *et al.* (1980) found that the degree of praevia was not related to mortality, overall fetal or maternal morbidity, gestational age at delivery, birthweight, initial presentation of bleeding, estimated blood loss prior to delivery, or indication for termination of pregnancy. They did show a statistically significant increase in total estimated blood loss and number of units transfused when the total praevias were compared to the marginal forms, but this was only demonstrated by the statistically dubious technique of excluding the intermediate partial praevias from the calculations.

3.4.2 Asymptomatic placenta praevia

All placentae praeviae are asymptomatic prior to the first onset of bleeding (Green-Thompson 1982). With the introduction of routine ultrasound scanning in the early 2nd trimester approximately 5–6 per cent of placentae are found to be low-lying (Rizos *et al.* 1979; Gillieson *et al.* 1982). Low-lying placenta, where the lower edge approaches the internal os as defined by ultrasound in early pregnancy, may be thought of as an earlier stage of placenta praevia, but studies have shown the condition to be an anatomical variant of a normally placed placenta (King 1973; Wexler and Gottesfeld 1977; Chapman *et al.* 1979). Over 90 per cent of cases of asymptomatic placenta praevia diagnosed by ultrasound in the early 2nd trimester remain asymptomatic and become normally situated subsequently (Rizos *et al.* 1979; Chapman *et al.* 1979; Ruparelia and Chapman 1985). The mechanism whereby the placenta 'migrates' (King 1973) away from the cervix and lower uterine segment with advancing gestational age has not been fully elucidated. The various theories involve either changes in the architecture of the lower uterine segment with advancing gestation or 'dynamic placentation' in which microscopic placental separations and reattachments occur throughout the 2nd and 3rd trimesters. The fraction of uterine wall covered by the placenta diminishes from one-half at 16 weeks' gestation to one-quarter to one-third at term (Rizos *et al.* 1979). To some extent the phenomenon of placental migration may be an artefact due to technical inexperience with ultrasonography or to inadequate bladder distension preventing satisfactory outlining of the cervix and lower uterus (Chapman *et al.* 1979).

Most authors have recommended routine rescanning later in the pregnancy for women in whom a low-lying placenta has been found. Kurjak and Barsic (1977) scanned their patients every 2–3 weeks, while King (1973) and Rizos *et al.* (1979) performed a repeat scan every 4–8 weeks. Comeau *et al.* (1983) found the overall risk of placenta praevia in the 3rd trimester to be 5.6 per cent if the placenta covered any of the cervix early in gestation. However, when placenta praevia was found to persist after 30 weeks' gestation, the risk for clinically significant bleeding at delivery was 28.8 per cent. On the basis of these findings they recommended that women with low or cervical placental implantation found early in gestation should be rescanned between 30 and 32 weeks gestation. Ruparelia and Chapman (1985) specifically addressed themselves to the value of follow-up ultrasound in a prospective study of 100 women found to have an asymptomatic low-lying placenta diagnosed by ultrasound before 20 weeks' gestation. All women with early low-lying placenta were rescanned at 32 and 36 weeks to check on placental position. On rescanning at 32 weeks, 94 women (94 per cent) had a placenta in a normal position. In the remaining 6 women a persistent low-lying placenta was detected on rescan at 36 weeks. Four of these women in whom the low-lying placenta was anteriorly positioned delivered vaginally, while only 2 of the original 100 women with low-lying placenta had placenta praevia requiring caesarean section. Antepartum haemorrhage occurred only in these 2 women, in both of whom the placenta was in a low-lying posterior position. Thus both Comeau *et al.* (1983) and Ruparelia and Chapman (1985) have shown that approximately 6 per cent of women diagnosed as having a low-lying placenta in the early 2nd trimester will have a persisting placenta praevia at 30–32 weeks. Of this small number, however, approximately one-third to one-quarter will have significant bleeding.

It would seem appropriate therefore that any asymptomatic women being found to have a low-lying placenta on ultrasound after 32 weeks should be managed as a symptomatic placenta praevia by expectant conservative management.

3.4.3 Signs

The patient's general condition depends mainly on the extent of placental separation and resultant blood loss, but may also be influenced by the woman's previous clinical state. An anaemic women who bleeds will present in a worse clinical state (Green-Thompson 1982) than a woman who was healthy prior to the onset of bleeding. On abdominal examination the uterus is soft and not tender, and fetal parts are readily palpable. The fetal heart is usually heard.

Painless vaginal bleeding in the absence of labour is the most common presentation. Cotton *et al.* (1980) report that bleeding in the absence of labour occurred in 70.6 per cent of their patients. An additional 20.6 per cent had evidence of uterine activity as well as clinically significant bleeding, and in 11 per cent there was premature rupture of the membranes. Although it is well recognized that a small proportion of women with placenta praevia do not bleed until the onset of labour, this constitutes *less* than 2 per cent of cases of placenta praevia (Cotton *et al.* 1980).

Some form of fetal malpresentation (transverse, oblique or unstable lie, and breech presentation) is common. Pedowitz (1965) recorded transverse lie in 13.5 per cent and Crenshaw *et al.* (1973) and Cotton *et al.* (1980) found a fetal malpresentation in approximately one-third of all cases. In cephalic presentation, the presenting part is invariably high and is often displaced slightly from the midline (Myerscough 1982). Although an abnormally high presenting part may alert the clinician, this may not be pertinent in those populations where engagement occurs late in labour (Green-Thompson 1982). There are conflicting reports in the literature concerning the effect of placenta praevia on fetal growth. Varma (1973), Naeye (1978) and Neri *et al.* (1980) have all shown an increased incidence of fetal growth retardation, particularly associated with those cases where there has been repeated episodes of vaginal bleeding. Naeye (1978) showed that surviving infants were growth-retarded at birth, their head circumferences being less retarded than their body weights, a pattern characteristic of late fetal undernutrition. However, for the survivors the long term consequences were few with normal long term physical growth and psychomotor development and only a small excess of neurological abnormalities.

Other workers, however, have been unable to show any increased incidence of growth retardation in placenta praevia (Gabert 1971; Brenner *et al.* 1978; Nicolaides *et al.* 1982; Silver *et al.* 1984). Chapman *et al.* (1979) found a significant association between low-lying placentae diagnosed by ultrasound before 24 weeks' gestation and small-for-dates infants, whereas Ruparelia and Chapman (1985) found no increased incidence of growth retardation in 100 women diagnosed as having a low-lying placenta on ultrasound before 20 weeks' gestation. The contribution of placental growth and location to fetal development requires further study (Comeau *et al.* 1983).

3.5 Treatment

Initial care for a woman with bleeding in the second half of pregnancy is the same, irrespective of the suspected cause of bleeding. Arrangements should be made for her immediate transfer by ambulance to a fully equipped maternity hospital. If she is shocked, the first priority is resuscitation by volume replacement. If a woman with placenta praevia is moribund, caesarean section should be undertaken at the same time as resuscitation is proceeding. After the necessary emergency care has been given, the subsequent management depends on the following factors:

1. Whether the fetus is dead, alive but distressed, or alive and not distressed.
2. Whether the bleeding is continuing.
3. Whether the woman is in labour.
4. The estimated gestation.

If the fetus is alive and vaginal bleeding is present on admission to hospital, a sample of vaginal blood should be collected as soon as possible and tested for the presence of fetal haemoglobin.

A digital examination is absolutely contraindicated when there is any possibility of placenta praevia, except in theatre when termination of pregnancy is forced by bleeding or labour, or when the pregnancy has reached an adequate gestation for safe termination. The really dangerous haemorrhage is often the one that has been provoked by ill-advised obstetric interference, such as digital examination of the cervical canal at or very shortly after the time of the warning haemorrhage. Although it is widely appreciated that vaginal examination may provoke separation of the placenta with massive haemorrhage, it is sometimes not realized that a rectal examination is even more dangerous, as it is virtually certain that the placenta will not be detected by the examining finger before it is separated and serious bleeding provoked (Scott 1981).

If bleeding is less severe or has stopped, confirmation of the diagnosis by ultrasound should be performed at the earliest opportunity. The early and accurate diagnosis of placenta praevia is imperative to spare those women with a normally implanted placenta the economic, emotional, and social expense of conservative care with possibly long term hospitalization (Crenshaw *et al.* 1973). Ultrasound localization, if available, is the method of choice, being accurate, non-invasive and, as far as is known, safe (Donald and Abdulla 1968; Robinson and Garret 197O; Bowie *et al.* 1978). Bowie *et al.* (1978) reported 1 false negative in 13 cases of proven placenta praevia and 19 false positive diagnosis in 151 women who did not have placenta praevia. Vaginal examination of the woman in theatre may be the only diagnostic method available in some circumstances (Green-Thompson 1982).

There is no agreement in the literature with regard to the benefits or hazards of early speculum examination. Hibbard (1969) and Crenshaw *et al.* (1973) reported that a gentle speculum examination of the vagina and cervix to rule out local causes of bleeding was not associated with additional maternal haemorrhage, whereas Brenner *et al.* (1978) consider it unwise to examine women with prematurity and vaginal bleeding with a speculum until the absence of placenta praevia is confirmed by ultrasound or other means. Scott (1981) specifically stresses that a speculum examination is not recommended initially, while Myerscough (1982) points out that local causes of antepartum haemorrhage are seldom associated with more than a moderate degree of bleeding or blood stained discharge. Neither approach has been subjected to a clinical trial.

The primary object of expectant conservative management, first introduced in 1945 by Macafee (1945) in Britain and Johnson *et al.* (1945) in the United States of America, is to reduce the number of premature births by allowing the pregnancy to continue until the baby has grown to a size and age that will give a reasonable chance of survival. Figures from the Royal Maternity Hospital, Belfast covering the years 1932 to 1977 show a progressive decline in fetal death rate from placenta praevia from over 50 per cent to less than 5 per cent (Myerscough 1982).

The Macafee regimen requires that from the time of the initial diagnosis of placenta praevia until delivery the woman must remain in a fully equipped and staffed maternity hospital, because of the risks to both mother and fetus from further major haemorrhage. In the United States of America many workers have adopted a policy of permitting selected women to return home as part of expectant management (Hibbard 1969; Cotton *et al.* 1980; Silver *et al.* 1984). Cotton *et al.* (1980) reported that the vast majority of women sent home required readmission to hospital for significant maternal bleeding, but there were no maternal deaths and no significant difference in perinatal outcome compared to those women kept in hospital. An interesting comparison of home versus hospital expectant management has been reported (D'Angelo and Irwin 1984). On the basis of a retrospective analysis of different unit policies these workers suggested that retention of the mother in hospital until delivery was justified on the grounds of reduced neonatal mortality and morbidity and cost of treatment. There were no maternal deaths in the women allowed home. Observational studies from areas with no facilities for antenatal admission are of interest. In one United States series of 355 maternities where no obstetric or midwifery supervision was sought, there was 1 antepartum death from placenta praevia (Kaunitz *et al.* 1984).

With every episode of bleeding, the Rhesus negative woman should have a Kleihauer test performed for the presence of fetal cells, and be given prophylactic immune anti-D if fetal cells are present.

Preterm birth continues to be a major problem even when expectant management is used. Brenner *et al.* (1978) found that about 40 per cent of women with placenta praevia had rupture of the membranes, spontaneous labour, haemorrhage, or other problems that resulted in delivery before 37 weeks' gestation. The limitations of expectant management are elegantly illustrated by Brenner's cumulative delivery rate graph (Brenner *et al.* 1978) (Fig 37.1).

During the period of expectant management maternal and fetal well-being should be monitored. The mother should not be allowed to become anaemic, and her haemoglobin should be maintained at a normal level by haematinics (see Chapter 19), or if necessary by transfusion. Most authors recommend fetal monitoring by biophysical or biochemical tests (see Chapters 28, 29 and 30).

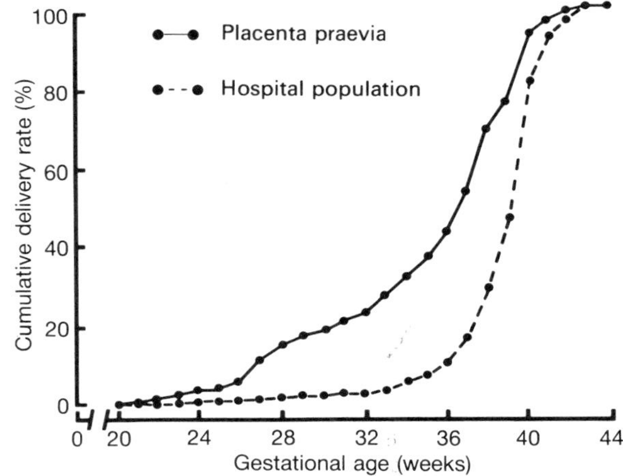

Fig. 37.1 Cumulative delivery rate by gestational age in women with placenta praevia (from Brenner *et al.* (1978)

3.6 Elective delivery

The case made in 1945 for delaying delivery until 37 weeks on the grounds that fetal outcome is improved by awaiting maturity (Macafee 1945) has come to be generally accepted during the ensuing years (Myerscough 1982). The benefits of added fetal maturity are considered to outweigh the risk to both mother and fetus associated with a further severe maternal haemorrhage that might occur during expectant therapy. Over the past several years, however, obstetric practice and neonatal care have undergone fundamental changes, and some clinicians have suggested that an 'aggressive' policy may improve fetal outcome. They have advocated the use of tocolysis to inhibit preterm labour, repeated blood transfusions when needed to maintain a satisfactory maternal condition, and elective preterm delivery after 34 weeks when amniocentesis has confirmed fetal pulmonary maturity (Cotton *et al.* 1980; Neri *et al.* 1980; Silver *et al.* 1984). No controlled trials to evaluate this approach have been carried out.

With improved ultrasound diagnosis many authorities suggest elective caesarean section without prior digital confirmation (Scott 1981; Myerscough 1982; Beischer and Mackay 1986). This approach has considerable merit since digital examination may cause serious haemorrhage. McShane *et al.* (1985) performed caesarean section in stable patients without digital examination, and the diagnosis of placenta praevia was confirmed in all cases. Digital examination in theatre certainly has a place, especially where ultrasound is not available, when the ultrasound appearances are equivocal, or the clinical signs of placenta praevia are not confirmed by ultrasound. If digital examination is indicated, it should be carried out in theatre with the staff scrubbed and prepared for immediate caesarean section should catastrophic haemorrhage be provoked. Digital exploration in theatre without anaesthesia seems to us unwise, as it adds the risk of the need for a crash induction of anaesthesia to an already potentially dangerous situation. The practice is advocated by some because it avoids the risk of an unnecessary anaesthetic being administered to a woman who does not have placenta praevia.

There is no place for epidural anaesthesia in a woman who is actively bleeding, as further lowering of the blood pressure brought about by epidural anaesthesia may tip the balance against the fetus. Anaesthetic opinion is, however, divided on the wisdom of using epidural anaesthesia in stable patients for digital examination in theatre, or for elective caesarean section without prior digital exploration. Moir (1980) considers that placenta praevia is an absolute contraindication to epidural anaesthesia because of the problems of volume replacement in a vasodilated patient, but Crawford (1985) has claimed that epidural is safe in experienced hands.

There is almost no indication for vaginal delivery in the care of women with even marginal placenta praevia whose babies have attained a viable age (Crenshaw *et al.* 1973). Nesbitt (1962) found that fetal salvage in placenta praevia was lowest in hospitals with a low caesarean section rate. Over the years many workers have reported an improvement in fetal survival when babies of viable age are delivered abdominally (Grant 1955; Pedowitz 1965; Macafee 1962; Nelson and Huston 1971). The fetal hazards of vaginal delivery include profuse maternal haemorrhage, malpresentation, cord accidents, placental separation, fetal haemorrhage, and dystocia resulting from a posterior placental implantation (Stallworthy 1951). If the fetus is previable, malformed, or dead, vaginal delivery may be appropriate (Myerscough 1982).

If at digital examination in theatre at 37–38 weeks no placenta praevia is found, the accepted treatment is to terminate the pregnancy by amniotomy in the belief that an alternative cause of antepartum haemorrhage may be associated with compromised placental function (Walker *et al.* 1976). Willocks (1971) has challenged this policy. In a retrospective review of 307 such cases at the Queen Mothers Hospital, Glasgow, he was unable to demonstrate a single fetal loss which could have been avoided by routine induction of labour following digital exploration which excluded placenta praevia. Furthermore, of the 148 women allowed to await a spontaneous onset of labour, the caesarean section rate was 5.4 per cent, compared to 12.5 per cent in the 105 women whose labours were induced.

Caesarean section for placenta praevia can be daunting even for the most experienced surgeon, and should never be delegated to an unsupervised junior colleague (Department of Health and Social Security (1986), Report on the Confidential Enquiry into Maternal Deaths in England and Wales 1979–1981). For the experienced operator the lower segment transverse incision is recommended (Myerscough 1982). A vertical lower segment (de Lee incision) or a classical upper segment incision may occasionally be indicated when the lower segment has failed to form or where the placenta is anterior or complete, but the classical incision with its consequent long term disadvantages is rarely justified (Scott 1981) (see Chapters 70 and 72). If a low transverse incision is employed, large uterine vessels will be cut, and should a low transverse incision tear during extraction of the fetus, haemorrhage may be overwhelming (Morgan 1965). With a lower segment incision the placenta, if anterior, will present at once. Myerscough (1982) advises against cutting or tearing through the organ with a view to delivering the baby through it, as this may result in fetal blood loss which may prove fatal for the baby. Whenever possible the operator should reach around the placenta, carefully separating it off until the membranes are reached. The umbilical cord should be clamped immediately following delivery to reduce the danger of fetal blood loss via the placenta.

Postpartum haemorrhage is more common in placenta praevia (Williamson and Greeley 1945). Separation of the placenta is often irregular, and the contractile effect of the muscle of the lower segment is inefficient. The operator should proceed as expeditiously as possible with placental removal and closure of the uterine incision. Often haemostasis can be secured with one continuous atraumatic suture (Scott 1981). Failing the direct control of bleeding with accurate suturing and oxytocics, packing of the uterus is possible, but this is difficult since the uterine scar might be disrupted, if performed vaginally after caesarean section, or the pack may be accidentally sutured into the uterine wound if done at the time of caesarean section (Green-Thompson 1982). Caesarean hysterectomy may be necessary in some circumstances to save the mother's life, but should be performed before she is in extremis (Scott 1981). Aortic compression can be a life-saving method of temporarily controlling torrential haemorrhage following delivery until hysterectomy, or internal iliac ligation can be performed (Department of Health and Social Security (1986); Report on Confidential Enquiries into Maternal Deaths in England and Wales 1979–1981).

Placenta accreta is not infrequently present in association with placenta praevia. Morgan (1965) reported an incidence of 2.6 per cent in her series of 536 cases of placenta praevia. All obstetricians should, however, be aware of the strong association between placenta accreta and placenta praevia in women with prior caesarean section. The reported incidence of prior caesarean section in women with placenta praevia/accreta is from 43 per cent to 60 per cent (Kistner *et al.* 1952; Read *et al.* 1980; Clark *et al.* 1985). Clark *et al.* (1985) found the risk of placenta accreta to be 5 per cent in women with placenta praevia and no previous caesarean section, rising to 67 per cent in women with four prior caesarean sections. McHattie (1972) reported an overall 42 per cent maternal mortality rate among women with placenta praevia accreta who did not undergo hysterectomy, and concluded that total hysterectomy is the treatment of choice. However, if the woman is young, of low parity, and bleeding is not severe an attempt should be made to conserve the uterus. Clark *et al.* (1985) reported that 28 per cent of women with placenta praevia/accreta were managed conservatively without hysterectomy. Such management included curettage, local excision, and repair or oversewing of the implantation site. Myerscough (1982) advises that on occasions it may be prudent to leave the adherent portion of the placenta *in situ*, supported if necessary by a uterine pack, and quotes two such recorded cases (Torbet and Tsoutsoplides 1968).

Haemorrhage due to coagulation disorders is rare in placenta praevia. Hibbard (1969) reported only one instance of clotting deficiency in his series of 475 cases of placenta praevia. Crenshaw *et al.* (1973) reported one case of haemorrhage in association with a coagulation defect in a woman who had an intrauterine death 5 days prior to the bleeding.

4 Bleeding of uncertain origin

4.1 Introduction

In both clinical presentation and retrospective classification, haemorrhage of undetermined or uncertain origin is the most common type of antepartum haemorrhage. Although in some cases the cause of bleeding later becomes clear, in the majority no cause can be demonstrated. The importance of this subgroup lies in its frequency, the clinical problems it presents in diagnosis and management, and the associated high fetal loss, which is often greater than in proven placenta praevia (Table 37.5).

Table 37.5 Antepartum haemorrhage of uncertain origin: frequency and perinatal mortality

Author	Percentage of all APH	Perinatal mortality (%)
Paintin (1962)	60.8	7.6
Butler and Bonham (1963)	72.0	9.1
Macafee and Harley (1963)	41.1	15.7
Roberts (1970)	48.2	5.6
Willocks (1971)	61.9	14.2
Watson (1982)	74.3	3.5

Haemorrhage of uncertain origin is a collective clinical category, and must include minor but unrecognized cases of all specific types of antepartum haemorrhage—placenta praevia, localized abruption, marginal haemorrhage, cervical and vaginal lesions, and excessive show. Despite this heterogeneity, the condition is epidemiologically distinct from both placental abruption and placenta praevia in terms of age, parity, social class, and gestation at delivery (Paintin 1962).

4.2 Aetiology and pathological findings

Some authors, notably Scott (1960, 1981) have reported that the commonest source of bleeding in this category of antepartum haemorrhage is from the edge of a normally situated placenta—marginal haemorrhage. It does not have the same inherent tendency to extension as does placental abruption, as it occurs from the edge of the chorionic plate. The haemorrhage extends onto the maternal surface of the placenta but does not indent the basal plate, a feature which distinguishes the lesion from true retroplacental clot (Fox 1978).

A cervical or vaginal cause of bleeding is unlikely to pose any threat to the fetus, and inclusion of such cases in the haemorrhage of uncertain origin category would lessen the incidence of related perinatal mortality, which is principally due to prematurity. In this context it is of interest to note that Macafee and Harley (1963), who recorded a low incidence of haemorrhage of undetermined origin, reported a high perinatal mortality, whereas Watson (1982) with a high incidence of uncertain haemorrhage found a much lower perinatal mortality rate. These differences in perinatal mortality are probably also influenced by improvements in neonatal care of the preterm infant which have occurred since the 1960s.

4.3 Clinical findings

The clinical presentation of bleeding of unknown origin is painless antepartum haemorrhage without the signs associated with placenta praevia. In the majority of cases the blood loss is not of an extent to cause serious concern, and usually settles spontaneously (Scott 1981). The most serious threat to the fetus is preterm labour and delivery. In approximately 60 per cent of cases the bleeding occurs before 37 weeks' gestation, and in this group 15 per cent will deliver preterm within 10 days of the initial haemorrhage (Watson 1982). An increased incidence of preterm labour is well recognized in both placenta praevia and placental abruption, but it is less well appreciated that haemorrhage of uncertain origin precedes preterm labour in many instances (Schnoeneck 1955). In those cases where there is a circumvallate placenta there may also be drainage of fluid per vaginum (hydrorrhoea gravidarum) due to serum extruding from the annular clot (Naftolin *et al.* 1973)

4.4 Care

The management of painless antepartum haemorrhage depends, among other factors, primarily upon the gestation of the fetus at the time of the initial bleed. A policy of expectant treatment is appropriate in the preterm period, whereas intervention is generally considered more suitable in those infants who are mature at the time of the initial haemorrhage. An ultrasound examination for placental localization should be performed as soon as possible, and if placenta praevia is diagnosed or cannot be excluded, then management should follow the plan already discussed for placenta praevia. When the placenta is clearly defined in the upper segment the woman should be allowed home after a period of rest and observation in hospital provided that she has no recurrence of bleeding (Willocks 1971; Donald 1974). The risk to the fetus in such cases is preterm delivery, and the great majority of perinatal deaths are due to preterm delivery occurring within 7 to 10 days of the initial haemorrhage (Roberts 1970; Watson 1982). No randomized prospective trial has been performed to assess the risks of discharging such women home, but a retrospective survey has not suggested any advantage in retaining them in hospital if they remain undelivered for 10 days (Watson 1982). After the bleeding has settled, and before discharge from hospital, both a speculum examination to exclude a local cause for the bleeding, and a digital examination to exclude advanced cervical dilatation should be performed.

If a policy of expectant management is adopted, fetal well-being should be monitored. It is generally recommended that induction of labour should be performed at 38 weeks' when the fetus is mature. This policy is based on the belief that the placenta may have to some extent been damaged by the haemorrhage and its functional reserve reduced (Walker *et al.* 1976; Scott 1981). While it is accepted that in cases of haemorrhage of uncertain origin the fetus is at risk (Murdoch and Foulkes 1952), most of the evidence suggests that little of the risk is due to placental insufficiency, and that the real danger to the fetus is from preterm birth (Roberts 1970; Willocks 1971). Routine induction of labour at 38 weeks should not be performed, and women should be allowed to go into spontaneous labour. Willocks (1971), in a review of 307 cases of haemorrhage of uncertain origin, awaited spontaneous labour in 148 women with no fetal losses.

5 Bleeding due to local causes

The reported incidence of antepartum haemorrhages due to local causes varies widely in different series. Paintin (1962) reported only 8 cases of local bleeding in 910 cases of antepartum haemorrhage, while Roberts (1970) found that lower genital tract causes accounted for 9 per cent of all cases of antepartum haemorrhage using the Cardiff Births Survey. Green-Thompson (1982) considers local causes to be an important group, and reported that local causes were responsible for the bleeding in 35 per cent of a series of women attending the antepartum haemorrhage clinic at King Edward VIII Hospital, Durban.

The local causes of bleeding include trichomoniasis, cervical ectropion, varicosities of vulva and introitus, cervical polyps, and cervical neoplasia. They pose no direct threat to the pregnancy *per se*, but require appropriate care in diagnosis and treatment. They will not be further discussed in this chapter.

6 Conclusions

Bleeding in the second half of pregnancy constitutes a possibly life-threatening condition. All professionals who care for women during pregnancy and childbirth must be aware of the causes, pathogenesis, and prognosis of such bleeding, and have a clear plan in mind for its differential diagnosis and management.

Improvements in neonatal care mean that the age in gestation at which delivery in the interests of the fetus becomes justified must be kept under review.

References

Bansal YP (1985). A profile of intra-partum and post-partum aspects of ante-partum haemorrhage from Pumwani Maternity Hospital, Nairobi. East Afr Med J, 62: 807–812.

Barrett JM, Boehm FH, Killam AP (1981). Induced abortion : A risk factor for placenta praevia. Am J Obstet Gynecol, 141: 769–772.

Basu HK (1969). Fibrinolysis and abruptio placentae. J Obstet Gynaecol Br Commnwlth, 76: 481–496.

Beischer NA, Mackay EV (1986). Obstetrics and The Newborn. London: Baillière Tindall.

Beischer NA, Reid S, Brown JB, Macafee CAJ (1970). The value of urinary oestriol estimations in patients with antepartum haemorrhage. Austral NZ J Obstet Gynaecol, 10: 191–204.

Bender S (1954). Placenta previa and previous lower segment cesarean section. Surg Gynecol Obstet, 98: 625–628.

Blair RG (1973). Abruption of the placenta : A review of 189 cases occurring between 1965 and 1969. J Obstet Gynaecol Br Commnwlth, 80: 242–245.

Bowie JA, Rochester D, Cedkin AV, Cooke WT, Krunzmann A (1978). Accuracy of placental localization by ultrasound. Radiology, 128: 177–180.

Breen JL, Neubecker R, Gregori CA, Franklin JE (1977). Placenta accreta, increta and percreta. A survey of 40 cases. Obstet Gynecol, 49: 43–47.

Brenner WE, Edelman DA, Hendricks CH (1978). Characteristics of patients with placenta praevia and results of 'expectant management'. Am J Obstet Gynecol, 132: 180–189.

Butler NR, Bonham DG (1963). The First Report of the 1958 British Perinatal Mortality Survey. Edinburgh/London: E and S Livingstone.

Caffrey KT (1983). Antepartum haemorrhage, a profile from an urban hospital, Kadiena, Nigeria. East Afr Med J, 60: 801–804.

Carp HJA, Mashiach S, Serr DM (1979). Vasa previa : A major complication and its management. Obstet Gynecol, 53: 273–275.

Chapman MG, Furness ET, Jones WR, Sheat JH (1979). Significance of the ultrasound location of placenta site in early pregnancy. Br J Obstet Gynaecol, 86: 846–848.

Clark SL, Koonings PP, Phelan JP (1985). Placenta praevia/accreta and prior Cesarean section. Obstet Gynecol, 66: 89–92.

Clayton SG, Lewis TLT, Pinker GD (1985). Obstetrics by Ten Teachers (14th edn). London: Edward Arnold.

Comeau J, Shaw L, Marcell CC, Lavery JP (1983). Early placenta previa and delivery outcome. Obstet Gynecol, 61: 577–580.

Cotton DB, Read JA, Paul RH, Quilligan EJ (1980). The conservative aggressive management of placenta praevia. Am J Obstet Gynecol, 137: 687–695.

Crawford JS (1985). Principles and Practices of Obstetric Anaesthesia (15th edn). Oxford: Blackwell Scientific Publications.

Crenshaw C, Darnell Jones DE, Parker RT (1973). Placenta previa : A survey of twenty years experience with improved perinatal survival by expectant therapy and cesarean delivery. Obstet Gynecol Surv, 28: 461–470.

D'Angelo LJ, Irwin LF (1984). Conservative management of placenta previa : a cost benefit analysis. Am J Obstet Gynecol, 149: 320–323.

Department of Health and Social Security (1986). Report on Health and Social Subjects 29. Report on Confidential Enquiries into Maternal Deaths in England and Wales 1979–81. London: Her Majesty's Stationery Office.

de Valera E (1968). Abruptio Placentae. Am J Obstet Gynecol, 100: 599–606.

Donald I (1974). Antepartum haemorrhage. In: Practical Obstetric Problems (5th edn). London: Lloyd-Luke (Medical Books), pp 363–428.

Donald I, Abdulla UJ (1968). Placentography by sonar. J Obstet Gynaecol Br Commnwlth, 75: 1993–2006.

Douglas RG, Buchman MI, MacDonald FA (1955). Premature Separation of the normally implanted placenta. J Obstet Gynaecol Br Empire, 62: 710-736.

Eastman JN, Hellman LM (1964). Williams Obstetrics (13th edn). New York: Appleton-Century-Crofts.

Egley C, Cefalo RC (1985). Abruptio Placentae. In: Progress in Obstetrics and Gynaecology 5. Edinburgh: Churchill Livingstone, pp 108–120.

Fox H (1978). Pathology of the Placenta. London: W B Saunders.

Gabert HA (1971). Placenta previa and fetal growth. Obstet Gynecol, 38: 403–406.

Gelsthorpe K (1960). A rapid method of differentiating foetal from maternal blood. Vox Sang, 5, No.2: 172–175.

Gillieson MS, Winter-Muram HT, Muran D (1982). Low-lying placenta. Radiology, 144: 577–580.

Golditch IA, Boyce NE (1970). Management of Abruptio Placentae. JAMA, 212: 288–293.

Gordon H (1969). Modern Trends in Obstetrics, Vol.4. London: Butterworths, p 257.

Gorodeski IG, Bahari CM, Schachter A, Neri A (1981). Recurrent placenta praevia. Eur J Obstet Gynaecol Reprod Biol, 12: 7–11.

Grant FG (1955). Placenta praevia: review of 200 cases. J Obstet Gynaecol Br Empire, 62: 497–503.

Green-Thompson RW (1982). Antepartum haemorrhage. Clin Obstet Gynaecol, 9: 479–515.

Grimes DA, Techman T (1984). Legal abortion and placenta previa. Am J Obstet Gynecol, 149: 501–504.

Hall MH (1972). Folic acid deficiency and abruptio placentae. J Obstet Gynaecol Br Commnwlth, 79: 222–225.

Harlap S (1979). Gender of infants conceived on different days of the menstrual cycle. New Engl J Med, 300: 1445–1448.

Harlap S, Davies AM (1975). Late sequelae of induced abortion: complications and outcome of pregnancy and labour. Am J Epidemiol, 102: 217–224.

Hibbard LT (1969). Placenta praevia. Am J Obstet Gynecol, 104: 172–184.

Hibbard BM, Jeffcoate TNA (1966). Abruptio Placentae. Obstet. Gynecol, 27: 155–167.

Hurd WH, Miodovnik M, Hertzberg V, Lavin JP (1983). Selective management of Abruptio Placentae: a prospective study. Obstet Gynecol, 61: 467–473.

Johnson HW, Williamson JC, Greeley AV (1945). The conservative management of some varieties of placenta praevia. Am J Obstet Gynecol, 50: 398–406.

Jouppila P, Kirkinen P (1982). Problems associated with the

ultrasonic diagnosis of abruptio placentae. Int J Gynaecol Obstet, 21: 5–11.

Kasule J, Chimbira THK, Brown I McL (1985). Controlled trial of external cephalic version. Br J Obstet Gynaecol, 92: 14–18.

Kaunitz AM, Spence C, Danielson TS, Rochat RW, Grimes DA (1984). Perinatal and maternal mortality in a religious group avoiding obstetric care. Am J Obstet Gynecol, 150: 826–831.

King DL (1973). Placental migration demonstrated by ultrasonography. Radiology, 109: 167–170.

Kistner RW, Hertig AT, Reid DE (1952). Simultaneously occurring placenta previa and placenta accreta. Surg Gynecol Obstet, 94: 141–151.

Knab DR (1978). Abruptio Placentae : An assessment of the time and method of delivery. Obstet Gynecol, 52: 625–629.

Kurjak A, Barsic B (1977). Changes of placental site diagnosed by repeated ultrasonic examination. Acta Obstet Gynecol Scand, 56: 161–165.

Letsky EA (1985). Coagulation Problems During Pregnancy. Edinburgh: Churchill Livingstone.

Lunan CB (1973). The management of abruptio placentae. J Obstet Gynaecol Br Commnwlth, 80: 120–124.

Macafee CHG (1945). Placenta praevia—study of 174 cases. J Obstet Gynaecol Br Empire, 52: 313–324.

Macafee CHG (1962). Placenta praevia. Postgrad Med J, 38: 254–256.

Macafee CHG, Harley JMG (1963). Antepartum haemorrhage. In: British Obstetric Practice, Obstetrics, (3rd edn). Claye A (ed). London: Heinemann.

Macafee CHG, Millar WG, Hartley G (1962). Maternal and foetal mortality in placenta praevia. J Obstet Gynaecol Br Commnwlth. 69: 203–212.

MacDonald D (1984). Discussion following paper by D'Angelo LJ, Irwin LF. Conservative management of placenta praevia : A cost benefit analysis. Am J Obstet Gynecol, 149: 323.

MacGillivray I, Davey D, Isaacs S (1986). Placenta praevia and sex ratio at birth. Br Med J, 292: 371–372.

Madore C, Hawes WE, Many F, Hexter AC (1981). A study on the effects of induced abortion on subsequent pregnancy outcome. Am J Obstet Gynecol, 139: 516–521.

McHattie TJ (1972). Placenta previa accreta. Obstet Gynecol, 40: 795–798.

McShane PM, Heye PS, Epstein MF (1985). Maternal and perinatal mortality resulting from placenta previa. Obstet Gynecol, 65: 176–182.

Moir DD (1980). Obstetric anaesthesia and analgesia (2nd edn). London: Baillière Tindall.

Morgan J (1965). Placenta praevia : report on a series of 538 cases (1938–1962). J Obstet Gynaecol Br Commnwlth, 72: 700–705.

Moss G (1972). An argument in favour of electrolyte solutions for early resuscitation. Surg Clin N America, 52: 3–17.

Muldoon MJ (1969). The use of central venous pressure monitoring in abruptio placentae. J Obstet Gynaecol Br Commnwlth, 76: 225–228.

Murdoch JD, Foulkes JF (1952). Antepartum haemorrhage. J Obstet Gynaecol Br Empire, 59: 786–794.

Myerscough PR (1982). Munro Kerr's Operative Obstetrics. 10th edn. London: Baillière Tindall.

Naeye RL (1978). Placenta praevia. Predisposing factors and effects on the fetus and surviving infants. Obstet Gynecol, 52: 521–525.

Naeye RL (1980). Abruptio placentae and placenta praevia : Frequency, perinatal mortality and cigarette smoking. Obstet Gynecol, 55: 701–704.

Naeye RL, Harknes WL, Utts J (1977). Abruptio placentae and perinatal death : a prospective study. Am J Obstet Gynecol, 128: 701–704.

Naftolin F, Khudr G, Benirschke K, Hutchinson DL (1973). The syndrome of chronic abruptio placentae, hydrorrhea and circumvallate placenta. Am J Obstet Gynecol, 116: 347–350.

Nelson HB, Huston JE (1971). Placenta praevia, a possible solution to the associated high fetal mortality rate. J Reprod Med, 7: 188–194.

Neri A, Gorodesky I, Bahary C, Ovadia Y (1980). Impact of placenta previa on intrauterine fetal growth. Israel J Med Sci, 16: 429–432.

Nesbitt REL, Yankauer A, Schlesinger ER, Allaway NC (1962). Investigation of perinatal mortality rates associated with placenta previa in upstate New York 1942–1958. New Engl J Med, 267: 381–386.

Nicolaides KH, Faratian B, Symonds EM (1982). Effect of low implantation of the placenta on maternal blood pressure and placental function. Br J Obstet Gynaecol, 89: 806–810.

Okonofua FE, Olatunbosun OA (1985). Caesarean versus vaginal delivery in abruptio placentae associated with live fetuses. Int J Gynaecol Obstet, 23: 471–474.

Page EW, King EB, Merril JA (1954). Abruptio Placentae : dangers of delay in delivery. Obstet Gynecol, 3: 385–393.

Paintin DB (1962). The epidemiology of ante-partum haemorrhage : A study of all births in a community. J Obstet Gynaecol Br Commnwlth, 69: 614–623.

Paterson MEL (1979). The aetiology and outcome of abruptio placentae. Acta Obstet Gynecol Scand, 58: 31–35.

Pedowitz P (1965). Placenta praevia. An evaluation of expectant management and the factors responsible for fetal wastage. Am J Obstet Gynecol, 93: 16–25.

Percival R (1980). Holland and Brews Manual of Obstetrics 14th edn. Edinburgh: Churchill Livingstone.

Phillips JM, Evans JA (1970). Acute anaesthetic and obstetric management of patients with severe abruptio placentae. Anaesth Analgesia, 49: 998–1004.

Porter J (1960). Conservative treatment of abruptio placentae: a study of 283 cases. Obstet Gynecol 15: 696–697.

Pritchard JA, Brekken AL (1967). Clinical and laboratory studies on severe abruptio placentae. Am J Obstet Gynecol, 97: 681–695.

Quek SP, Tan KL (1972). Vasa praevia. Austral NZ J Obstet Gynaecol, 12: 206–209.

Read JA, Cotton DB, Miller FC (1980). Placenta accreta. Changing clinical aspects and outcome. Obstet Gynecol, 56: 31–34.

Record RG, McKeown T (1956). Investigation of foetal mortality associated with placenta praevia. Br J Prev Social Med, 10: 25–31.

Reid MF, Nohr K, Birks RJS (1986). Eclampsia and haemorrhage in a Jehovah's Witness. Anaesthesia, 41: 324–325.

Rizos N, Doran TA, Miskin M, Benzie RJ, Ford JA (1979).

Natural history of placenta previa ascertained by diagnostic ultrasound. Am J Obstet Gynecol, 133: 287–291.

Roberts G (1970). Unclassified antepartum haemorrhage. Incidence and perinatal mortality in a community. J Obstet Gynaecol Br Commnwlth. 77: 492–495.

Robertson JG (1970). Placenta Praevia. Practitioner, 204: 383–392.

Robinson AK, Garret WJ (1970). Ultrasonic visualization of the placenta. Med J Austral, 2: 1062–1064.

Rose GL, Chapman MG (1986). Aetiological factors in placenta praevia—a case controlled study. Br J Obstet Gynaecol, 93: 586–588.

Ruparelia BA, Chapman MG (1985). Early low-lying placentae—ultrasonic assessment, progress and outcome. Eur J Obstet Gynaecol Reprod Biol, 20: 209–213.

Ryan DW (1977). An evaluation of basilic vein catheterization. Resuscitation, 5: 163–168.

Schnoeneck FJ (1955). Obstetric causes of premature labour. Obstet Gynecol, 6: 444–446.

Schoenbaum SC, Monson RR, Stubblefield PG, Darney PD, Ryan KJ (1980). Outcome and delivery following an induced or spontaneous abortion. Am J Obstet Gynecol, 136: 19–24.

Scott JS (1960). Placenta extrachorialis (placenta marginata and placenta circumvallata). J Obstet Gynaecol Br Empire, 67: 904–918.

Scott JS (1981). Antepartum haemorrhage. In: Integrated Obstetrics and Gynaecology for postgraduates (3rd edn). Dewhurst J (ed). Oxford: Blackwell Scientific Publications pp 248–258.

Sher G (1977). Pathogenesis and management of uterine inertia complicating abruptio placentae with consumption coagulopathy. Am J Obstet Gynecol, 129: 164–170.

Silver R, Depp R, Sabbagha RE, Dooley SL, Sokol ML, Tamura RK (1984). Placenta praevia : Aggressive expectant management. Am J Obstet Gynecol, 150: 15–22.

Singh PM, Rodrigues C, Gupta AN (1981). Placenta previa and previous Cesarean section. Acta Obstet Gynecol Scand, 292: 371–372.

Stallworthy J (1951). Dangerous placenta (Joseph Price oration) Am J Obstet Gynecol, 61: 720–737.

Tabor A, Madsen M, Obel EB, Philip J, Bang J, Norgaard-Pedersen B (1986). Randomized controlled trial of genetic amniocentesis in 4606 low risk women. Lancet, i: 1287–1292.

Torbet TE, Tsoutsoplides GC (1968). Placenta praevia accreta : conservative management. J Obstet Gynaecol Br Commnwlth. 75: 737–740.

Varma TR (1973). Fetal growth and placental function in patients with placenta praevia. J Obstet Gynecol Br Commnwlth, 80: 311–315.

Virgilio RJ (1979). Crystalloid vs. Colloid resuscitation: is one better? Surgery, 85: 129–139.

Walker J, MacGillivray I, Macnaughton MC (1976). Combined Textbook of Obstetrics and Gynaecology. (9th edn). Edinburgh: Churchill Livingstone.

Watson R (1982). Antepartum haemorrhage of uncertain origin. Br J Clin Practice, 36: 222–226.

Wexler P, Gottesfeld KR (1977). Second trimester placenta previa. An apparently normal presentation. Obstet Gynecol, 50: 706–709.

Williamson HC, Greeley AV (1945). Management of placenta previa: 12 year study. Am J Obstet Gynecol, 50: 398–406.

Willocks J (1971). Antepartum haemorrhage of uncertain origin. J Obstet Gynaecol Br Commnwlth, 78: 987–991.

38 Hormone administration for the maintenance of pregnancy

Peter A. Goldstein, Henry S. Sacks, and Thomas C. Chalmers

1 Introduction

Over the last fifty years, hormones have been given to pregnant women in attempts to prevent miscarriage, fetal death, preterm delivery, and other adverse outcomes of pregnancy. As early as 1929, Allen and Corner established that in rabbits, an extract of the corpus luteum was needed to maintain progestational proliferation of the endometrium during pregnancy after ovariectomy (Allen and Corner 1929). In the mid-1930s, researchers began to suspect a link between hormonal and placental abnormalities and complications of pregnancy. In 1935, Smith and Smith examined the origin of abnormal levels of serum and urine 'prolan' and 'estrin' in women with late pregnancy toxaemia and eclampsia (Smith and Smith 1935). They found that the placentae of the toxaemic and eclamptic patients showed a marked excess of 'prolan' but a low level of 'estrin' when compared to pregnant women without these conditions. They argued that their 'results would certainly favour the conclusion that the high level of prolan found in cases of late pregnancy toxemia, as well as the tendency towards low levels of estrin, originate in a placental abnormality' (pp 179–180). Smith and Smith (1939) went on to report an increased incidence of elevated levels of an 'anterior pituitary-like hormone' in women whose pregnancies were complicated by pre-eclampsia, eclampsia, and 'premature delivery'. A few years later, White and Hunt (1943) found that 'accidents characteristic of diabetic pregnancies . . . appear(ed) to be related to an imbalance of the pregnancy hormones, oestrogen, progesterone and chorionic gonadotropin'.

White and Hunt's (1943) study of 125 pregnant diabetic women showed that 77 of them had demonstrable hormonal imbalances, while 7 were considered to have had an imbalance, judged by their histories and clinical signs. The hormonal imbalances included elevated levels of human chorionic gonadotropin (hCG), depressed levels of oestrogen, and decreased levels of pregnanediol excretion. The investigators went on to assert that 'accidents, toxemia, prematurity, and fetal death' could be 'predicted by an increase in chorionic gonadotropin and a decrease in pregnanediol excretion,' and that these complications could be prevented by 'continuous substitutional estrogen and progesterone therapy'.

Oestrogen, progesterone, and hCG are all needed to maintain an environment that is compatible with fetal development (Siiteri *et al.* 1977; Fainstat and Bhat 1983; Jones 1983; Rothchild 1983; Friberg 1985; Madenes 1985). The basic assumption in the early studies in which the relationship between steroid hormones and failed pregnancies was examined was that the uterine environment became inhospitable to the developing fetus due to a failure of hCG to stimulate oestrogen and progesterone secretion. Thus, it was believed that any prophylactic measures that aimed to prevent the loss of the fetus due to premature delivery, miscarriage, or stillbirth would require the recreation of the normal hormonal environment. Based on animal models, Smith and Smith (1944), Pencharz (1940), and Smith (1948) argued that the synthetic oestrogen, diethylstilboestrol (DES), was the therapeutic agent of choice. It was thought that diethylstilboestrol would cause an increase in placental progesterone secretion because of its stimulatory effects on hCG secretion without responding to negative inhibition by progesterone (Smith and Smith 1944).

The conclusion that deficiencies of endogenous hormone secretion call for replacement therapy is a classic example of the danger of applying pathophysiologic reasoning to therapeutic action without first testing the hypothesis by means of adequately designed trials.

2 Oestrogens

Diethylstilboestrol was administered to pregnant women on a wide scale over a period of over 30 years. Although the drug is no longer administered prophylactically to pregnant women, the history of its introduction to, and withdrawal from, clinical practice is relevant in any assessment of the use of other hormones (like progestagens and hCG) which are still used prophylactically in pregnancy.

Between 1950 and 1954, the conclusions reached in at least six clinical studies strongly endorsed the use of diethylstilboestrol (Smith and Smith 1954; Gitman and Koplowitz 1950; Davis and Fugo 1950; Ross 1953; Pena 1954; White *et al.* 1953). None of these studies included controls randomly assigned to conventional treatment, and none employed double-blinding. Five other contemporary studies, however, employed concurrent controls and in three of these neither the patients nor the investigators were aware of the experimental group assignment (Crowder *et al.* 1950; Robinson and Shettles 1952; Ferguson 1953; Dieckmann *et al.* 1953; Medical Research Council 1955): these studies did not observe the positive effects of diethylstilboestrol previously reported.

Smith and Smith (1949) was excluded from the present study for two reasons. First, there was evidence that this study was not truly randomized; they state that 'as far as was possible, alternate primigravidous women . . . were treated', but 387 women were in the treated group and 555 were in the control, and there was no mention of withdrawals. Second, there were internal inconsistencies which made accurate determinations of pregnancy outcomes impossible.

Data derived from all trials deemed to be reasonably well controlled are presented in Tables 38.1–38.5. The frequency of miscarriage, stillbirth, neonatal death, all of these outcomes combined, and 'premature' delivery

Table 38.1 Effect of diethylstilboestrol in pregnancy on miscarriage

Study	EXPT		CTRL		Odds ratio	Graph of odds ratios and confidence intervals
	n	(%)	*n*	(%)	(95% CI)	0.01 0.1 0.5 1 2 10 100
Dieckmann *et al.* (1953)	34/840	(4.05)	17/806	(2.11)	1.91 (1.09–3.33)	
Medical Research Council (1955)	6/76	(7.89)	6/71	(8.45)	0.93 (0.29–3.02)	
Berle and Behnke (1977)	55/134	(41.04)	52/131	(39.69)	1.06 (0.65–1.73)	
Robinson and Shettles (1952)	6/51	(11.76)	10/42	(23.81)	0.43 (0.15–1.27)	
Ferguson (1953)	6/190	(3.16)	5/203	(2.46)	1.29 (0.39–4.27)	
Crowder *et al.* (1950)	31/63	(49.21)	16/37	(43.24)	1.27 (0.56–2.85)	
Typical odds ratio (95% confidence interval)					1.20 (0.89–1.62)	

Table 38.2 Effect of diethylstilboestrol in pregnancy on stillbirth

Study	EXPT		CTRL		Odds ratio	Graph of odds ratios and confidence intervals
	n	(%)	*n*	(%)	(95% CI)	0.01 0.1 0.5 1 2 10 100
Dieckmann *et al.* (1953)	7/840	(0.83)	8/806	(0.99)	0.84 (0.30–2.32)	
Medical Research Council (1955)	9/76	(11.84)	7/71	(9.86)	1.23 (0.44–3.45)	
Ferguson (1953)	3/190	(1.58)	4/190	(2.11)	0.75 (0.17–3.33)	
Crowder *et al.* (1950)	0/63	(0.00)	0/37	(0.00)	1.00 (1.00–1.00)	
Typical odds ratio (95% confidence interval)					0.95 (0.50–1.83)	

Table 38.3 Effect of diethylstilboestrol in pregnancy on neonatal death

Study	EXPT		CTRL		Odds ratio	Graph of odds ratios and confidence intervals
	n	(%)	*n*	(%)	(95% CI)	0.01 0.1 0.5 1 2 10 100
Dieckmann *et al.* (1953)	16/840	(1.90)	4/806	(0.50)	3.23 (1.34–7.80)	
Medical Research Council (1955)	8/76	(10.53)	10/71	(14.08)	0.72 (0.27–1.92)	
Ferguson (1953)	4/190	(2.11)	7/203	(3.45)	0.61 (0.18–2.02)	
Typical odds ratio (95% confidence interval)					1.31 (0.74–2.34)	

Table 38.4 Effect of diethylstilboestrol in pregnancy on miscarriage, stillbirth, or neonatal death

Study	EXPT		CTRL		Odds ratio	Graph of odds ratios and confidence intervals
	n	(%)	*n*	(%)	(95% CI)	0.01 0.1 0.5 1 2 10 100
Dieckmann *et al.* (1953)	57/840	(6.79)	29/806	(3.60)	1.90 (1.23–2.94)	
Medical Research Council (1955)	23/76	(30.26)	23/71	(32.39)	0.91 (0.45–1.82)	
Ferguson (1953)	13/190	(6.84)	16/203	(7.88)	0.86 (0.40–1.83)	
Typical odds ratio (95% confidence interval)					1.38 (0.99–1.92)	

Table 38.5 Effect of diethylstilboestrol in pregnancy on 'prematurity' (<2500 g or <38 weeks' gestation)

Study	EXPT		CTRL		Odds ratio	Graph of odds ratios and confidence intervals
	n	(%)	*n*	(%)	(95% CI)	0.01 0.1 0.5 1 2 10 100
Swyer and Daley (1954)	11/227	(4.85)	12/233	(5.15)	0.94 (0.41–2.17)	
Dieckmann *et al.* (1953)	59/840	(7.02)	36/806	(4.47)	1.60 (1.06–2.42)	
Ferguson (1953)	35/190	(18.42)	26/203	(12.81)	1.53 (0.89–2.64)	
Typical odds ratio (95% confidence interval)					1.47 (1.08–2.00)	

(less than 38 weeks' gestation or birthweight less than 2500 g) in women given diethylstilboestrol is compared with that among untreated control women. These data show that no protective effect of diethylstilboestrol was demonstrable. Furthermore, as was pointed out in a reanalysis of one of these trials 25 years later (Brackbill and Berendes 1978), the data in one of the published reports (Dieckmann *et al.* 1953) actually showed an *increased* incidence of miscarriages, 'premature' deliveries and neonatal deaths associated with the drug that was statistically significant.

Although claims that diethylstilboestrol was an effective prophylactic against poor pregnancy outcome were challenged by the results of these adequately designed trials, the use of the drug in pregnancy continued into the 1970s. The first inkling that something might have gone wrong came in 1970 when Herbst and Scully reported 7 cases of vaginal adenocarcinoma (a very rare cancer in women less than 50 years old) within a 2 year period in young women whose mothers had received diethylstilboestrol while pregnant with them (Herbst and Scully 1970). The following year, Herbst and others found a strong positive correlation between maternal stilboestrol therapy and tumour appearance in young women (Herbst *et al.* 1971). Later that year, a similar observation was made in a second study (Greenwald *et al.* 1971). Within 6 months of publication of the first paper describing these possible adverse effects, the Food and Drug Administration issued a bulletin stating that the use of diethylstilboestrol was contraindicated in pregnancy (FDA 1971). Subsequent analyses of observational data suggested that the risk of developing vaginal adenocarcinoma after exposure to diethylstilboestrol *in utero* lay between 1.4 and 14 per 10,000 female fetuses exposed (Herbst 1979).

These rare malignancies were not the only adverse effects of the drug, however. The least biased estimates of the effects of diethylstilboestrol exposure on more common adverse outcomes have been derived from the follow-up, of women and fetuses entered into 3 of the original randomized trials. The 25-year follow-up of the randomized trial conducted by Dieckmann in Chicago (Bibbo *et al.* 1977) confirmed that a large proportion of exposed daughters had vaginal adenosis (67 per cent compared with 4 per cent in controls) and circumferential ridges of the vagina and cervix (40 per cent compared with none in the controls). Exposed daughters also had a higher incidence of irregular menstrual cycles and had fewer pregnancies (Senekjian *et al.* 1988). Comparison of the outcome of pregnancies in daughters who had been exposed as fetuses to diethylstilboestrol with that of daughters whose mothers had been given a placebo revealed a significantly greater incidence of 'premature' live births, perinatal deaths, spontaneous abortions, and ectopic pregnancies in the diethylstilboestrol-exposed group (Herbst *et al.* 1980).

Adverse effects of diethylstilboestrol exposure on the reproductive tract were not confined to the female offspring. Diethylstilboestrol-exposed sons were found to have an increased incidence of epididymal cysts, hypotrophic testes, and capsular induration of the testes (Bibbo *et al.* 1977). Semen analysis revealed that they also tended to have a relatively low ejaculate volume and impaired sperm motility.

The results of the 27-year follow-up (Beral and Colwell 1981) of cases entered into the British Medical Research Council's trial was in several respects complementary to the Chicago trial follow-up. In addition, of the men exposed as fetuses to diethylstilboestrol, half as many were married, or living as married, as among the non-exposed men (34 per cent and 62 per cent respectively). Follow-up of adults who as fetuses were entered into the other British trial of diethylstilboestrol (Swyer and Law 1954) revealed an unexpected but dramatic excess of psychiatric problems among those exposed to diethylstilboestrol *in utero* (Vessey *et al.* 1983).

Long term follow-up of the mothers entered into both the Chicago and Medical Research Council trials (Bibbo *et al.* 1978; Beral and Colwell 1980) indicated that they may have been put at increased risk of breast cancer by exposure to diethylstilboestrol during pregnancy. This risk appears to have been supported by the findings in a larger, non-randomized cohort study (Greenberg *et al.* 1984).

A non-randomized cohort study commissioned by the National Cancer Institute to study the incidence and natural history of genital tract anomalies and cancer in offspring exposed *in utero* to synthetic estrogens—the DESAD Project (Sestili 1977)—has generated data based on larger samples which support many of the observations made in the follow-up studies based on randomized cohorts. Children of women who received diethylstilboestrol have impaired fertility (Barnes *et al.* 1980), increased incidence of structural anomalies of the cervix, vagina, uterus, and ovaries (Jeffries *et al.* 1984; Kaufman *et al.* 1977), increased incidence of cervical and vaginal dysplasia and carcinoma *in situ* (Kaufman *et al.* 1981; Robboy *et al.* 1984), and an increased incidence of vaginal epithelial changes (O'Brien *et al.* 1979; Robboy *et al.* 1979). There is some evidence that the extent of the vaginal epithelial changes decreases with the passage of time (Noller *et al.* 1983).

Despite the existence of a vast body of literature describing the failures of diethylstilboestrol, a recently published non-randomized study, employing historical controls, asserted that: 'Diethylstilboestrol was efficacious in improving pregnancy outcome when initiated in the early stages of high-risk pregnancies' (Horne 1985).

3 Progestagens

The use of progestagens in attempts to maintain pregnancy began at the time that prophylactic oestrogens were introduced into clinical practice. In contrast to oestrogens, however, the use of progestagens during pregnancy continues. The proportion of progestagens that are prescribed as prophylactics in pregnancy ranges from 3 to 25 per cent in different countries (Tognoni *et al.* 1980). A recent survey in England revealed that 1 in 6 general practitioners uses progestagens in this way (Everett *et al.*, in press). In the light of the tragic consequences of ignoring the results of controlled trials of diethylstilboestrol, one might hope that the prophylactic use of progestagens in pregnancy is based on strong evidence that these drugs are more likely to do good than harm.

We have identified 20 reports of controlled trials in which a progestagen has been compared with either a placebo or no treatment during pregnancy (Turner *et al.* 1966; Swyer and Daley 1953; Johnson *et al.* 1975; Yemini *et al.* 1985; Goldzieher 1964; Govaerts-Videtzky *et al.* 1965; Shearman and Garrett 1963;

Hauth *et al.* 1983; Fuchs and Stakemann 1960; Erny *et al.* 1986; Klopper and MacNaughton 1965; LeVine 1964; Brenner and Hendricks 1962; Hartikainen-Sorri *et al.* 1980; Moller and Fuchs 1965; Tognoni *et al.* 1980; Sondergaard *et al.* 1985; Dalton 1962; Papiernik-Berkhauser 1970; Souka *et al.* 1980). In addition we identified two trials in which the effects of a combination of a progestagen and an oestrogen was assessed (Medical Research Council 1955; Berle and Behnke 1977).

Of these 22 controlled trials, 4 had to be excluded from our analysis, 3 because insufficient endpoint data were provided (Turner *et al.* 1966; Erny *et al.* 1986; Moller and Fuchs 1965), and 1 because the treatment code had not been broken at the time of the report (Govaerts-Videtzky *et al.* 1965). The identity of the treatment groups was not revealed in the first report of another of the trials (Shearman and Garrett 1963), but it was made available in a subsequent publication (Shearman 1968).

Full details of the methods we have used to minimize bias in our analyses of the 18 trials that remained for analysis have been published elsewhere (Goldstein *et al*, in press). One of the studies examined twin pregnancies (Hartikainen-Sorri *et al.* 1980) and, as some of these pregnancies ended with different outcomes for the two babies, all pregnancies in that particular study were considered to have had two individual outcomes. Analysis with or without including the 2 trials in which an oestrogen was administered concomitantly with a progestogen (Medical Research Council 1955; Berle and Behnke 1977), made no difference to the conclusions. Therefore they have been included in the results presented here.

Table 38.6 Effect of progestogens in pregnancy on miscarriage

Study	EXPT		CTRL		Odds ratio	Graph of odds ratios and confidence intervals
	n	(%)	*n*	(%)	(95% CI)	0.01 0.1 0.5 1 2 10 100
Shearman (1968)	5/27	(18.52)	5/23	(21.74)	0.82 (0.21–3.25)	
Hartikainen-Sorri *et al.* (1980)	0/78	(0.00)	0/76	(0.00)	1.00 (1.00–1.00)	
Sondergaard *et al.* (1985)	17/23	(73.91)	17/19	(89.47)	0.37 (0.08–1.72)	
Hauth *et al.* (1983)	0/80	(0.00)	0/88	(0.00)	1.00 (1.00–1.00)	
Dalton (1969)	0/76	(0.00)	0/74	(0.00)	1.00 (1.00–1.00)	
Yemini *et al.* (1985)	8/39	(20.51)	3/40	(7.50)	2.92 (0.82–10.36)	
Le Vine (1964)	3/15	(20.00)	7/14	(50.00)	0.28 (0.06–1.25)	
Klopper and MacNaughton (1965)	8/18	(44.44)	5/15	(33.33)	1.57 (0.39–6.25)	
Goldzieher (1964)	5/23	(21.74)	5/31	(16.13)	1.44 (0.36–5.70)	
Johnson *et al.* (1975)	0/18	(0.00)	4/25	(16.00)	0.16 (0.02–1.23)	
Medical Research Council (1955)	6/76	(7.89)	6/71	(8.45)	0.93 (0.29–3.02)	
Brenner and Hendricks (1962)	0/97	(0.00)	0/98	(0.00)	1.00 (1.00–1.00)	
Berle and Behnke (1977)	55/134	(41.04)	52/131	(39.69)	1.06 (0.65–1.73)	
Tognoni *et al.* (1980)	26/71	(36.62)	22/68	(32.35)	1.21 (0.60–2.42)	
Souka *et al.* (1980)	17/25	(68.00)	14/25	(56.00)	1.65 (0.53–5.10)	
Swyer and Daley (1953)	11/60	(18.33)	13/53	(24.53)	0.69 (0.28–1.70)	
Typical odds ratio (95% confidence interval)					1.01 (0.76–1.34)	

Table 38.7 Effect of progestogens in pregnancy on stillbirth

Study	EXPT		CTRL		Odds ratio	Graph of odds ratios and confidence intervals
	n	(%)	*n*	(%)	(95% CI)	0.01 0.1 0.5 1 2 10 100
Hartikainen-Sorri *et al.* (1980)	1/78	(1.28)	1/76	(1.32)	0.97 (0.06–15.72)	
Hauth *et al.* (1983)	1/80	(1.25)	3/88	(3.41)	0.40 (0.05–2.88)	
Dalton (1969)	1/62	(1.61)	3/66	(4.55)	0.38 (0.05–2.78)	
Yemini *et al.* (1985)	0/39	(0.00)	0/40	(0.00)	1.00 (1.00–1.00)	
Le Vine (1964)	0/15	(0.00)	0/14	(0.00)	1.00 (1.00–1.00)	
Klopper and MacNaughton (1965)	0/18	(0.00)	0/15	(0.00)	1.00 (1.00–1.00)	
Goldzieher (1964)	0/23	(0.00)	0/31	(0.00)	1.00 (1.00–1.00)	
Fuchs and Stakemann (1960)	0/63	(0.00)	2/63	(3.17)	0.13 (0.01–2.15)	
Johnson *et al.* (1975)	0/18	(0.00)	1/25	(4.00)	0.18 (0.00–9.52)	
Medical Research Council (1955)	9/76	(11.84)	7/71	(9.86)	1.23 (0.44–3.45)	
Brenner and Hendricks (1962)	0/97	(0.00)	1/98	(1.02)	0.14 (0.00–6.89)	
Tognoni *et al.* (1980)	0/71	(0.00)	0/68	(0.00)	1.00 (1.00–1.00)	
Swyer and Daley (1953)	0/60	(0.00)	0/53	(0.00)	1.00 (1.00–1.00)	
Typical odds ratio (95% confidence interval)					0.65 (0.31–1.36)	

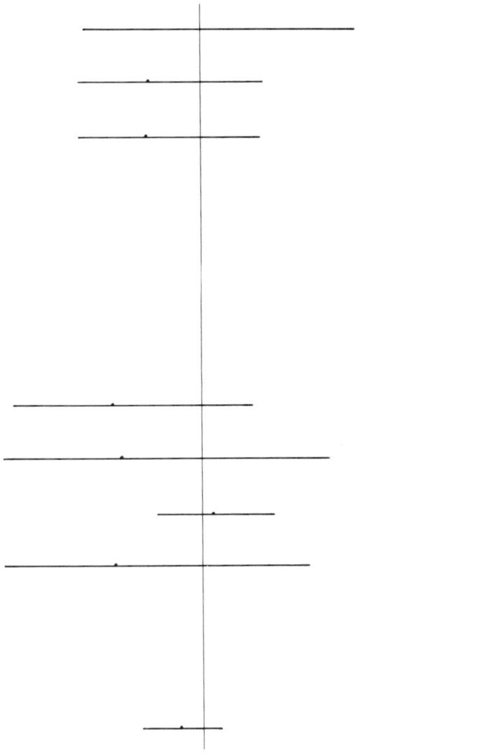

Table 38.8 Effect of progestogens in pregnancy on neonatal death

Study	EXPT		CTRL		Odds ratio	Graph of odds ratios and confidence intervals
	n	(%)	*n*	(%)	(95% CI)	0.01 0.1 0.5 1 2 10 100
Hartikainen-Sorri *et al.* (1980)	3/78	(3.85)	1/76	(1.32)	2.70 (0.37–19.56)	
Hauth *et al.* (1983)	2/80	(2.50)	0/88	(0.00)	8.27 (0.51–99.99)	
Yemini *et al.* (1985)	0/39	(0.00)	0/40	(0.00)	1.00 (1.00–1.00)	
Le Vine (1964)	1/15	(6.67)	0/14	(0.00)	6.91 (0.14–99.99)	
Johnson *et al.* (1975)	0/18	(0.00)	2/25	(8.00)	0.17 (0.01–2.95)	
Medical Research Council (1955)	8/76	(10.53)	10/71	(14.08)	0.72 (0.27–1.92)	
Brenner and Hendricks (1962)	1/97	(1.03)	0/98	(0.00)	7.47 (0.15–99.99)	
Swyer and Daley (1953)	1/60	(1.67)	0/53	(0.00)	6.58 (0.13–99.99)	
Typical odds ratio (95% confidence interval)					1.22 (0.57–2.61)	

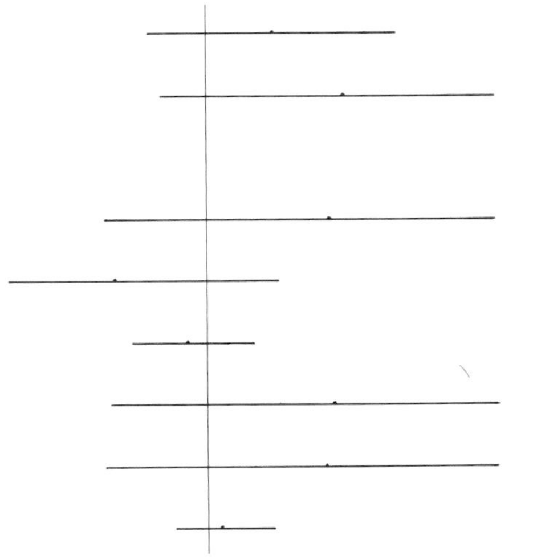

There is no evidence from the available data that progestagens reduce the risk of miscarriage (Table 38.6), stillbirth (Table 38.7), neonatal death (Table 38.8) or the combined risk of these three adverse outcomes of pregnancy (Table 38.9). There is some suggestion (Table 38.10) that these drugs may reduce the risk of 'prematurity', variously defined as delivery prior to 38 weeks' gestation and/or low birthweight (<2500 g). Of the 4 placebo-controlled studies in which data on duration of gestation were available, 2 suggested a lengthening of gestation (Johnson *et al.* 1975; Yemini *et al.* 1985), whereas the 2 others suggested a reduction in gestational duration with progesterone treatment (Brenner and Hendricks 1962; LeVine 1964).

The rationale for administering progesterone in early pregnancy to women with a history of recurrent miscarriage (three or more spontaneous abortions) is that, since the corpus luteum is the principal source of progesterone during the early stages of pregnancy, luteal defects might lead, through decreased progesterone production, to recurrent miscarriage. Using the 3 trials from which data relating to this particular category of women could be obtained (although not data providing biochemical confirmation of the diagnosis) (Swyer and Daley 1953; Goldzieher 1964; LeVine 1969), Daya (1988) conducted a meta-analysis which tested and sustained the hypothesis that administration of progesterone reduces the risk of miscarriage in these circumstances (Odds ratio 0.342, 95 per cent Confidence interval 0.147–0.796). Although these data are suggestive of a protective effect of progesterone, we agree with Daya (1988) that they should not be used as a basis for giving the drug except within the context of larger, better trials which include follow-up at least until the end of the neonatal period.

In those studies that have mentioned it, no significant side-effects were observed in either mother or child following therapy (7 of the studies failed to mention side-effects at all). One study (Hartikainen-Sorri *et al.* 1980), however, reported that treated (progesterone) infants had just over twice the incidence of respiratory problems as that among control infants.

Only one of the trials (Dalton 1962) has been the subject of a long term follow-up study, and there are conflicting interpretations of the findings (Dalton 1976; Lynch *et al.* 1978; Lynch and Mychalkiw 1978). Dalton (1976) reported that children whose mothers had received progesterone for toxaemia during pregnancy showed greater academic achievement at 9 to 10 years of age than did normal or toxaemic controls. Reappraisals of Dalton's study populations failed to demonstrate the reported increase in academic achievement (Lynch *et al.* 1978; Lynch and Mychalkiw 1978). The results of the follow-up studies are confounded, however, by the comingling of uncontrolled and controlled data.

Although the other progestagen follow-up studies have been largely anecdotal and uncontrolled, there have been suggestions that fetal exposure to the drug may increase the risk of oesophageal atresia (Lammer and Cordero 1986), cardiac, neurological, neural tube and other major malformations (Nora *et al.* 1978), and female masculinization (Wilkins *et al.* 1958; Wilkins 1960) and 'tomboyishness' in girls (Ehrhardt and Money 1967). Other studies, however, have failed to detect these adverse effects (Varma and Morsman 1982;

Table 38.9 Effect of progestogens in pregnancy on miscarriage, stillbirth, or neonatal death

Study	EXPT		CTRL		Odds ratio	Graph of odds ratios and confidence intervals
	n	(%)	*n*	(%)	(95% CI)	0.01 0.1 0.5 1 2 10 100
Hartikainen-Sorri *et al.* (1980)	4/78	(5.13)	2/76	(2.63)	1.94 (0.38–9.87)	
Hauth *et al.* (1983)	3/80	(3.75)	3/88	(3.41)	1.10 (0.22–5.61)	
Yemini *et al.* (1985)	8/39	(20.51)	3/40	(7.50)	2.92 (0.82–10.36)	
Le Vine (1964)	4/15	(26.67)	7/14	(50.00)	0.38 (0.09–1.68)	
Johnson *et al.* (1975)	0/18	(0.00)	7/25	(28.00)	0.13 (0.03–0.68)	
Brenner and Hendricks (1962)	1/97	(1.03)	1/98	(1.02)	1.01 (0.06–16.27)	
Swyer and Daley (1953)	12/60	(20.00)	13/53	(24.53)	0.77 (0.32–1.87)	
Typical odds ratio (95% confidence interval)					0.85 (0.50–1.44)	

Table 38.10 Effect of progestogens in pregnancy on 'prematurity' (<2500 g or <38 weeks' gestation)

Study	EXPT		CTRL		Odds ratio	Graph of odds ratios and confidence intervals
	n	(%)	*n*	(%)	(95% CI)	0.01 0.1 0.5 1 2 10 100
Hartikainen-Sorri *et al.* (1980)	24/78	(30.77)	18/76	(23.68)	1.43 (0.70–2.89)	
Sondergaard *et al.* (1985)	0/23	(0.00)	0/19	(0.00)	1.00 (1.00–1.00)	
Papiernik (1970)	2/50	(4.00)	9/49	(18.37)	0.24 (0.07–0.82)	
Hauth *et al.* (1983)	6/80	(7.50)	8/88	(9.09)	0.81 (0.27–2.42)	
Yemini *et al.* (1985)	5/39	(12.82)	14/40	(35.00)	0.30 (0.11–0.84)	
Le Vine (1964)	3/15	(20.00)	3/14	(21.43)	0.92 (0.16–5.38)	
Goldzieher (1964)	0/23	(0.00)	0/31	(0.00)	1.00 (1.00–1.00)	
Fuchs and Stakemann (1960)	35/63	(55.56)	33/63	(52.38)	1.14 (0.56–2.28)	
Johnson *et al.* (1975)	0/18	(0.00)	9/25	(36.00)	0.12 (0.03–0.52)	
Swyer and Daley (1953)	1/60	(1.67)	1/53	(1.89)	0.88 (0.05–14.36)	
Typical odds ratio (95% confidence interval)					0.73 (0.51–1.06)	

Uher *et al.* 1965; Kester *et al.* 1980) and so the safety of progestagens remains an open question.

4 Human chorionic gonadotrophin

Two controlled trials (Svigos 1982; Harrison 1985) have assessed whether human chorionic gonadotrophin reduces the risk of miscarriage in women with a past history of repeated early pregnancy loss (Table 38.11). The first of these (Svigos 1982) reported simply the frequency of 'continuing pregnancies' in the two groups; attempts to contact the author to clarify the meaning of this term failed, but we have assumed that the numbers of 'non-continuing pregnancies' were the numbers of miscarriages. Data from both trials suggest that prophylactic administration of human chorionic gonadotrophin is effective in reducing the risk of miscarriage in women with a past history of repeated early pregnancy loss. In the only trial that presented complete data on pregnancy outcome (Harrison 1985), three times as many treated pregnancies ended with a live birth than did control pregnancies. This statistically significant difference ($X^2 = 4.95, p < 0.05$) reflected the reduced risk of miscarriage (Odds ratio = 0.056, 95 per cent Confidence interval = 0.0094–0.36). Although these results are statistically significant, they must be interpreted with caution due to the small number (n = 20) of patients in the study. Nevertheless, they are

Table 38.11 Effect of human chorionic gonadotrophin in early pregnancy on miscarriage

Study	EXPT		CTRL		Odds ratio	Graph of odds ratios and confidence intervals
	n	(%)	*n*	(%)	(95% CI)	0.01 0.1 0.5 1 2 10 100
Harrison (1985)	0/10	(0.00)	7/10	(70.00)	0.05 (0.01–0.32)	
Svigos (1982)	1/17	(5.88)	9/15	(60.00)	0.09 (0.02–0.38)	
Typical odds ratio (95% confidence interval)					0.07 (0.02–0.22)	

encouraging and strongly suggest that the study should be replicated on larger samples of participants. To date, there has been no reported follow-up study of infants or children whose mothers were given human chorionic gonadotrophin during pregnancy and such follow-up studies should certainly be conducted in the context of further well-controlled trials.

5 Conclusions

Of the treatments examined, oestrogens have been shown to be both ineffective and, more tragically, harmful. There has never been any scientific basis for prescribing oestrogens in pregnancy. The diethylstilboestrol tragedy could very well have been avoided, either by conducting, from introduction of the drug, a large, well-designed randomized controlled trial, or by conducting a meta-analysis of the small, properly controlled trials reported prior to 1953.

The same standards of evidence should be applied to both progestagens and hCG. In spite of the fact that progestagens continue to be prescribed on a wide scale, there is no good evidence that they are either effective or safe. If they are to be prescribed at all, they should only be prescribed within the context of further trials designed to address the many uncertainties about their effects in the short and longer term. Ultrasound examination during the 1st trimester of pregnancy has made it clear that a significant proportion of the women who have received progestagens in the past have been carrying non-viable pregnancies. Any future trials mounted to assess the effects of progestagen administration in early pregnancy should involve only those pregnancies in which ultrasonography has confirmed that the fetus is alive. On the other hand, there is some evidence that progesterone may be of benefit in very early pregnancy, before fetal viability can be demonstrated, to compensate for luteal phase deficiency. This hypothesis can only be substantiated by conducting appropriately designed trials, such as that currently being run at McMaster University (Daya 1988).

The two small trials of human chorionic gonadotrophin suggest that it may reduce the risk of miscarriage in women who have a history of repeated early pregnancy loss. Here again, future trials should involve only those pregnancies in which ultrasonography has shown the fetus to be alive.

In the present state of knowledge, hormone administration of any type in pregnancy should be used only within controlled clinical trials until the ratio of benefits to hazards has been established more clearly.

References

Allen WM, Corner GM (1929). Physiology of the corpus luteum. III. Normal growth and implantation of embryos after very early ablation of the ovaries, under the influence of extracts from the corpus luteum. Am J Physiol, 88: 340–346.

Barnes AB, Colton T, Gunderson J, Noller KL, Tilley BC, Strama T, Townsend DE, Hatab P, O'Brien PC (1980). Fertility and outcome of pregnancy in women exposed *in utero* to diethylstilbestrol. New Engl J Med, 302: 609–613.

Beral V, Colwell L (1980). Randomized trial of high doses of stilboestrol and ethisterone in pregnancy: long-term follow-up mothers. Br Med J, 281: 1098–1101.

Beral V, Colwell L (1981). Randomized trial of high doses of stilboestrol and ethisterone therapy in pregnancy: long-term follow-up of the children. J Epidemiol Community Health, 35: 155–160.

Berle P, Behnke, K (1977). Ueber behandlungserfolge der drohenden fehlgeburt. Geburtsh Frauenheilkd, 37: 139–142.

Bibbo M, Gill WB, Azizi F, Blough R, Fang VS, Rosenfield RL, Schumacher GFB, Sleeper K, Sonek MG, Wied GL (1977). Follow-up study of male and female offspring of DES-exposed mothers. Obstet Gynecol, 49:1–8.

Bibbo M, Haenszel WM, Wied GL, Hubby M, Herbst AL (1978). A twenty five year follow-up study of women exposed to diethylstilbestrol during pregnancy. New Engl J Med, 298: 763–767.

Brackbill Y, Berendes HW (1978). Dangers of diethylstilboestrol: Review of a 1953 paper. Lancet, 2: 520.

Brenner WE, Hendricks CH (1962). Effect of medroxyprogesterone acetate upon the duration and characteristics of human gestation and labor. Am J Obstet Gynecol, 83: 1094–1098.

Crowder RE, Bills ES, Broadbent JS (1950). The management of threatened abortion: a study of 100 cases. Am J Obstet Gynecol, 60: 896–899.

Dalton K (1969). Controlled trials in the prophylactic value of progesterone in the treatment of pre-eclamptic toxaemia. J Obstet Gynaecol Br Commnwlth, 69: 463–468.

Dalton K (1976). Prenatal progestrone and educational attainments. Br J Psychiat, 129: 438–442.

Davis ME, Fugo NW (1950). Steroids in the treatment of early pregnancy complications. JAMA, 142: 778–785.

Daya S, (in press). Efficacy of progesterone support for pregnancy in women with recurrent miscarriage: a meta-analysis of controlled trials. Br J Obstet Gynaecol.

Dieckmann WJ, Davis ME, Rynkiewicz LM, Pottinger RE (1953). Does the administration of diethylstilboestrol during pregnancy have therapeutic value? Am J Obstet Gynecol, 66: 1062–1075.

Ehrhardt AA, Money J (1967). Progestin-induced hermaphroditism: IQ and psychosexual identity in a study of ten girls. J Sex Res, 3: 83–100.

Erny R, Pigne A, Prouvost C, Gamerre M, Malet C, Serment

H, Barrat J (1986). The effects of oral administration of progesterone for premature labor. Am J Obstet Gynecol, 154: 525–529.

Everett CB, Ashurst H, Chalmers I (1987). Reported management of threatened miscarriages by general practitioners in Wessex. Br Med J, 295: 583–586.

Fainstat T, Bhat N. (1983). Recurrent abortion and progesterone therapy. In: Progesterone and Progestins. Wayne Bardin C, Milgram E, Mauvais-Jarvis P (eds). New York: Raven Press, pp 259–276.

FDA Drug Bulletin (1971). Diethylstilbestrol contraindicated in pregnancy. US Dept of Health, Education, and Welfare.

Ferguson JH (1953). Effect of stilboestrol on pregnancy compared to the effect of a placebo. Am J Obstet Gynecol, 65: 592–601.

Friberg J. (1985). Pregnancy endocrinology. In: Principles of Medical Therapy in Pregnancy. Gleicher N (ed). New York and London: Plenum Medical Book Co, pp 145–151.

Fuchs F, Stakemann G (1960). Treatment of threatened premature labor with large doses of progesterone. Am J Obstet Gynecol, 79: 172–176.

Gitman L, Koplowitz A (1950). Use of diethylstilbestrol in complications of pregnancy. NY State J Med, 50: 2823–2824.

Goldstein PA, Berrier J, Rosen S, Sacks HS, Chalmers TC (in press). A meta-analysis of randomized control trials of progestational agents in pregnancy. Br J Obstet Gynaecol.

Goldzieher JW (1964). Double-blind trial of a progestin in habitual abortion. JAMA, 188: 651–654.

Govaerts-Videtzky M, Martin L, Hubinont PO (1965). A double-blind study of progestogen treatment in spontaneous abortion. J Obstet Gynaecol Br Commnwlth, 72: 1034.

Greenberg ER, Barnes AB, Resseguie L, Barrett JA, Burnside S, Lanza LL, Neff RK, Stevens M, Young RH, Colton T (1984). Breast cancer in mothers given diethylstilbestrol in pregnancy. New Engl J Med, 311: 1393–1398

Greenwald P, Barlow JJ, Nasca PC, Burnett WS (1971). Vaginal cancer after maternal treatment with synthetic estrogens. New Engl J Med, 285: 390–392.

Harrison RF (1985). Treatment of habitual abortion with human chorionic gonadotrophin: results of open and placebo-controlled studies. Eur J Obstet Gynecol Reprod Biol, 20: 159–168.

Hartikainen-Sorri AL, Kauppila A, Tuimala R (1980). Inefficacy of 17-*alpha*-hydroxyprogestone caproate in the prevention of prematurity in twin pregnancy. Obstet Gynecol, 56: 692–695.

Hauth JC, Gilstrap III LC, Brekken AL, Hauth JM (1983). The effect of 17-*alpha*-hydroxyprogesterone caproate on pregnancy outcome in an active-duty military population. Am J Obstet Gynecol, 146: 187–190.

Herbst AL (1979) DES-associated clear cell adenocarcinoma of the vagina and cervix. Obstet Gynecol Surv, 34: 844

Herbst AL, Scully RE (1970). Adenocarcinoma of the vagina in adolescence: A report of 7 cases including 6 clear-cell carcinomas (so called mesonephromas). Cancer, 25: 745–757.

Herbst AL, Hubby MM, Blough RR, Azizi F (1980). A comparison of pregnancy experience in DES-exposed and DES-unexposed daughters. J Reprod Med, 24: 62–69

Herbst AL, Ulfelder H, Poskanzer DC (1971). Adenocarcinoma of the vagina: Association of maternal stilbestrol therapy with tumor appearance in young women. N Engl J Med, 284: 878–881.

Horne HW (1985). Evidence of improved pregnancy outcome with diethylstilbestrol (DES) treatment of women with previous pregnancy failures: A retrospective analysis. J Chron Dis, 38: 873–880.

Jeffries JA, Robboy SJ, O'Brien PC, Bergstralh EJ, Labarthe DR, Barnes AB, Noller KL, Hatab PA, Kaufman RH, Townsend DE (1984). Structural anomalies of the cervix and vagina in women enrolled in the Diethylstilbestrol Adenosis (DESAD) Project. Am J Obstet Gynecol, 148: 59–66.

Johnson JWC, Austin KL, Jones GS, Davis GH, King TM (1975). Efficacy of 17-*alpha*-hydroxyprogesterone caproate in the prevention of premature labor. N Engl J Med, 293: 675–680.

Jones GS. (1983). The historic review of the clinical use of progesterone and progestins. In: Progesterone and Progestins Wayne Bardin C, Milgram E, Mauvais-Jarvis P (eds), New York: Raven Press, pp 189–202.

Kaufman RH, Binder GL, Gray PM, Adam E (1977). Upper genital tract changes associated with exposure *in utero* to diethylstilbestrol. Am J Obstet Gynecol, 128: 51–59.

Kaufman RH, Korhonen MO, Strama T, Adam E, Kaplan A (1981). Development of clear cell adenocarcinoma in DES-exposed offspring under observation. Obstet Gynecol, 59: 68S–72S.

Kester P, Green R, Finch SJ, Williams K (1980). Prenatal 'female hormone' administration and pyschosexual development in human males. Psychoneuroendocrinology, 5: 269–285.

Klopper A, MacNaughton M (1965). Hormones in recurrent abortion. J Obstet Gynaecol Br Commnwlth, 72: 1022–1028.

Lammer EJ, Cordero JF (1986). Exogenous sex hormone exposure and the risk for major malformations. JAMA, 255: 3128–3132.

Le Vine L (1964). Habitual abortion—A controlled study of progestational therapy. West J Surg Obst Gynecol, 72: 30–36.

Lynch A, Mychalkiw W, Hutt SJ (1978). Prenatal progesterone I. Its effect on development and on intellectual and academic achievement. Early Hum Dev, 2/4: 305–322.

Lynch A, Mychalkiw W (1978). Prenatal progesterone II. Its role in the treatment of pre-eclamptic toxaemia and its effect on the offspring's intelligence: a reappraisal. Early Hum Dev, 2/4: 323–339.

Madenes AE (1985). Endocrinology of the placenta. In: Principle of Medical Therapy in Pregnancy. Gleicher N (ed). New York and London: Plenum Medical Book Co. pp 152–162.

Medical Research Council (1955). The use of hormones (diethylstilbestrol, estrogen, ethisterone, corpus luteum hormone) in the management of pregnancy in diabetics. Report to the Medical Research Council by their conference on diabetes and pregnancy. Lancet, 2: 833–836.

Moller KJA, Fuchs F (1965). Double-blind controlled trial of 6-methyl, 17-acetoprogesteron i threatened abortion. J Obstet Gynaecol Br Commnwlth, 72: 1042–1044.

Noller KL, Townsend DE, Kaufman RH, Barnes AB, Robboy SJ, Fish CR, Jeffries JA, Bergstralh EJ, O'Brien PC, McGorray SP, Scully R (1983). Maturation of vaginal and cervical epithelium in women exposed *in uterus* to diethylstilbestrol (DESAD-Project). Am J Obstet Gynecol, 146: 279–285.

Nora JJ, Nora AH, Blu J, Ingram J, Fountain A, Peterson M, Lortscher RH, Kimberling WD (1978). Exogenous progestagen and estrogen implicated in birth defects. JAMA, 240: 837–843.

O'Brien PC, Noller KL, Robboy SJ, Barnes AB, Kaufman RH, Tilley BC, Townsend DE (1979). Vaginal epithelial changes in young women enrolled in the National Cooperative Diethylstilbestrol Adenosis (DESAD) Project. Obstet Gynecol, 53: 300–308.

Papiernik-Berkhauer E (1970). Etude en double aveugle d'un médicament prévenant la survenue prématurée de l'accouchement chez femmes 'à risque élève' d'accouchement prématuré. In: Edition Schering, Serie IV, fiche 3, pp 65–68.

Pena EF (1954). Prevention of abortion. Am J Surg, 87: 95–96.

Pencharz RI (1940). Effect of estrogens and androgen alone and in combination with chorionic gonadotropin on ovary of hypophysectomized rat. Science, 91: 554.

Robboy SJ, Kaufman RH, Prat J, Welch WR, Gaffey T, Scully RE, Richart R, Fenoglio CM, Virate R, Tilley BC (1979). Pathologic findings in young women enrolled in the National Cooperative Diethylstilbestrol Adenosis Project. Obstet Gynecol, 53: 309–317.

Robboy SJ, Noller KL, O'Brien P, Kaufman RH, Townsend D, Barnes AB, Gundersen J, Lawrence WD, Bergstrahl E, McGorray S, Tilley BC, Anton J, Chazen G (1984). Increased incidence of cervical and vaginal dysplasia in 3980 diethylstilbestrol-exposed young women. JAMA, 252: 2979–2983.

Robinson D, Shettles LB (1952). Use of diethylstilboestrol in threatened abortion. Am J Obstet Gynecol, 63: 1330–1333.

Ross JW (1953). Further report on the use of diethylstilbestrol in the treatment of threatened abortion. J Nat Med Assoc, 45: 223.

Rothchild I. (1983). Role of progesterone in initiating and maintaining pregnancy. In: Progesterone and Progestins. Wayne Bardin C, Milgram E, Mauvais-Jarvis P (eds). New York: Raven Press, pp 219–229.

Senekjian EK, Potkul RK, Frey K, Herbst AL (1988). Infertility among daughters either exposed or not exposed to diethylstilbestrol. Am J Obstet Gynecol, 158: 493–498.

Sestili MA (1977). Genital tract anomalies and cancer in females exposed *in utero* to diethylstilbestrol: Brief report on the DESAD project. Public Health Reports, 92: 481–484.

Shearman RP (1968). Hormonal treatment of habitual abortion. In: Progress in infertility. Kistner RW (ed). London: J and A Churchill, pp 767–777.

Shearman RP, Garrett WJ (1963). Double-blind study of effect of 17-hydroxyprogesterone caproate on abortion rate. Br Med J, 1: 292–295.

Siiteri PK, Febres F, Clemens LE, Chang, RJ, Gondos, B, Stites, D (1977). Progesterone and maintenance of pregnancy: Is progesterone nature's immunosuppressant? Ann NY Acad Sci, 286: 384–397.

Smith GV, Smith OW (1935). Evidence for the placental origin of the excessive prolan of late pregnancy toxemia and eclampsia. Surg Gynecol Obstet, 61: 175–183.

Smith GV, Smith OW (1939). The anterior pituitary-like hormone in late pregnancy toxemia. Am J Obstet Gynecol, 38: 618–624.

Smith GV, Smith OW (1954). Prophylactic hormone therapy. Relation to complications of pregnancy. Obstet Gynecol, 4: 129–141.

Smith OW (1948). Diethylstilbestrol in the prevention and treatment of complications of pregnancy. Am J Obstet Gynecol, 56: 821–834.

Smith OW, Smith GVS (1944). Pituitary stimulating property of stilbestrol as compared with that of estrone. Proc Soc Exp Biol Med, 57:198–200.

Smith OW, Smith GVS (1949). The influence of diethlylstilbestrol on the progress and outcome of pregnancy as based on a comparison of treated with untreated primigravidas. Am J Obstet Gynecol 58: 994–1009.

Sondergaard F, Ottesen B, Detlefsen GU, Schierup L, Pederson SC, Lebech PE (1985). Traitment par la progesterone des menaces d'accouchement prématuré avec taux bas de progesterone plasmatique. Contraception-fertilité-sexualité, 3: 1227–1231.

Souka AR, Osman M, Sibaie F, Einen MA (1980). Therapeutic value of indomethacin in threatened abortion. Prostaglandins, 19: 457–460.

Svigos J (1982). Preliminary experience with the use of human chorionic gonadotrophin therapy in women with repeated abortion. Clin Reprod Fertil, 1: 131–135.

Swyer GIM, Daley D (1953). Progesterone implantation in habitual abortion. Br Med J, 1: 1073–1077.

Swyer GIM, Law RG (1954). An evaluation of the prophylactic ante-natal use of stilboestrol: preliminary report. J Endocrinol, 10: 6–7.

Tognoni G, Ferrario L, Inzalaco M, Crosignani PG (1980). Progestagens in threatened abortion. Lancet, 2: 1242–1243.

Turner, SJ, Mizock, GB, Feldman, GL (1966). Prolonged gynecologic and endocrine manifestations subsequent to administration of medroxyprogesterone acetate during pregnancy. Am J Obstet Gynecol, 95: 222–227.

Uher J, Jirasek JE, Cernoch A (1965). On the activity of 16-methylen-6-dehydro-17-alpha-acetoxyprogesterone (MDAP) on the human foetus. Gynaecologia, 159: 377–383.

Varma TR, Morsman J (1982). Evaluation of the use of Proluton-Depot (hydroxyprogesterone hexanoate) in early pregnancy. Int J Gynaecol Obstet, 20: 13–17.

Vessey MP, Fairweather DVI, Norman-Smith B, Buckley J (1983). A randomized double-blind controlled trial of the value of stilboestrol therapy in pregnancy: long-term follow-up of mothers and their offspring. Br J Obstet Gynaecol, 90: 1007–1017.

White P, Hunt H (1943). Pregnancy complicating diabetes. J Clin Endocrinol, 3: 500–511.

White P, Koshy P, Duckers J (1953). The management of pregnancy complicating diabetes and of children of diabetic mothers. Med Clin N America, 37: 1481–1496.

Wilkins L (1960). Masculinization of female fetus due to use of orally given progestins. JAMA, 172: 118–122.

Wilkins L, Jones HW, Holman GH, Stempfel RS (1958). Masculinization of the female fetus associated with administration of oral and intramuscular progestins during gestation: Non-adrenal female pseudohermaphrodism. J Clin Endocrinol Metab, 18: 559–585.

Yemini M, Borenstein R, Dreazen E, Apelman Z, Mogilner BM, Kessler I, Lancet M (1985). Prevention of premature labor by 17-*alpha*-hydroxyprogesterone caproate. Am J Obstet Gynecol, 151: 574–577.

39 Bed rest and hospitalization during pregnancy

Caroline Crowther and Iain Chalmers

1 Introduction

Bed rest is a relatively common prescription for women whose pregnancies are complicated by one or more of a wide variety of conditions. These include bleeding, multiple pregnancy, pre-eclampsia, fetal growth retardation, and threatened preterm delivery. Women with such pregnancy complications may be advised to rest in bed at home; alternatively they may be admitted to hospital, both to facilitate bed rest and to permit closer investigation and surveillance of their pregnancies.

The extent to which women are advised to rest in bed at home or to come into hospital for rest varies considerably, but such advice is very common in some places. The information available suggests that most British general practitioners advise women with bleeding in early pregnancy to rest in bed at home (Everett *et al.* 1987). As far as hospitalization during pregnancy is concerned, between 20 and 25 per cent of women giving birth in England and Wales will have spent more than five days in hospital during pregnancy (Office of Population Censuses and Surveys 1984). This pattern of obstetric practice is not surprising. In 1959, a report published by the Ministry of Health (Ministry of Health 1959) recommended that, over and above the beds needed for lying-in, hospitals should make provision for some 20 to 25 per cent of women to be admitted during pregnancy. A subsequent report (Department of Health and Social Security 1970) recommended that the proportion of maternity beds available for antenatal care should be at least 25 per cent, so that 'the resources of modern medicine can be available to all mothers and babies'. Despite the far-reaching implications of these recommendations, no evidence was produced in the reports to show that any benefit could be expected from implementing these proposals. This is regrettable. Hospitalization during pregnancy not infrequently results in financial and social costs for pregnant women and their families. A number of studies have made it clear that antenatal hospitalization is often a disruptive and stressful experience (Rosen 1975; White and Ritchie 1984; Berardi 1985; Ford 1987; Curry MA, unpublished observations). In addition, adoption of these policies has involved substantial costs to the health services (Acker *et al.* 1986). Routine hospitalization for uncomplicated twin pregnancy has been estimated to have cost the British National Health Service about £2.5 million per 1000 pregnancies so managed in 1985 (Saunders *et al.* 1985). The available evidence suggests that these costs are comparable in France (Papiernik 1983; Tresmontant *et al.* 1983), but substantially higher in the United States (Powers and Miller 1979).

In this chapter we review the rather scanty evidence which is available about the effects of bed rest and hospitalization on the outcome of pregnancies complicated by either early bleeding, multiple pregnancy or pre-eclampsia. The role of bed rest and hospitalization in the care of women with bleeding in late pregnancy and those who threaten to deliver preterm has been reviewed in other chapters (see Chapters 37 and 44).

2 Threatened miscarriage

Bleeding in early pregnancy has prompted advice to rest in bed since at least the time of Hippocrates (cited in Diddle *et al.* 1953). A majority of 20 current textbooks of obstetrics recently reviewed by Everett (Everett *et al.* 1987) recommended prescription of bed rest for threatened miscarriage (although a number noted that the effectiveness of the policy has not been established). Current medical practice reflects this consensus. A recent survey of the management of threatened miscarriage by general practitioners working in the Wessex Region of England (Everett *et al.* 1987), for example, showed that the vast majority prescribe bed rest in these circumstances, even though only a small minority thought it was mandatory and a third admitted that they thought it was usually ineffective. Nearly three-quarters of the general practitioners surveyed expressed a concern, however, that if they did not recommend bed rest they might be held responsible for a subsequent miscarriage.

The only reported attempt to undertake any form of controlled evaluation of the effectiveness of bed rest in the management of threatened miscarriage was made over 30 years ago (Diddle *et al.* 1953). Three groups of women booked to deliver in three different hospitals were given three different kinds of advice if bleeding started in early pregnancy. Of the women who, in one hospital, were prescribed immediate hospitalization for bed rest, 59 per cent (70/119) went on to miscarry, compared with 81 per cent (987/1214) of those attending the second hospital, who were advised to rest as much as possible in bed at home. However, women booked to deliver at the third hospital were instructed to continue leading their lives as normally as possible and only 54 per cent (64/119) of these went on to miscarry. The results of this study thus give no support to the view that a policy of advising bed rest reduces the risk of miscarriage after bleeding occurs in early pregnancy.

Bed rest is sometimes advised for many days if spotting or bleeding is persistent, and this may cause considerable difficulty at home (Romito 1989). Yet, in a substantial proportion of these pregnancies, the fetus is already dead, so no amount of bed rest is likely to be of help in this respect. The presence of a non-viable pregnancy can now be demonstrated either by low serum levels of the beta-subunit of human chorionic gonadotrophin in very early pregnancies, or by ultrasonography thereafter. Because there is currently no valid basis for advising women with threatened miscarriages one way or the other with regard to bed rest, the preferences of individual women should probably dominate both in deciding the extent of diagnostic activity, and whether or not to rest in bed. There is obviously scope for conducting randomized trials to assess the value of bed rest in pregnancies in which fetal viability has been confirmed so, that decisions can be based on better information than is currently available.

3 Multiple pregnancy

3.1 Routine hospitalization of women with twin pregnancies

Prolonged bed rest in twin pregnancy aimed at increasing the duration of gestation, improving fetal growth, and decreasing perinatal mortality has been advocated for half a century (Hirst 1938), although there is still no concensus as to the optimum time when this should be started or discontinued (Powers and Miller 1979), nor whether rest should be in hospital or at home (Mueller-Heubach 1984; Hays and Smeltzer 1986). More than 30 years ago, Russell (1952) observed that there were fewer perinatal deaths and that babies had a higher average birthweight among twins born to women of higher social classes compared to those in the lower social classes. He believed that these differences were explained because, compared with working-class women, middle-class women had had better nutrition during childhood and had better physiques, better diets during their pregnancies, and more leisure, and consequently more rest during their pregnancies. Russell suggested that if 'the great wastage of child life associated with twin pregnancy' was to be significantly reduced then 'the most important measure likely to bring this about is a general improvement in the physical and social conditions of the lower income groups'. Because this involved long-term social policies, he suggested that, as an interim measure, 'consideration might be given to admitting to hospital all twin mothers at the 30th week in order by diet and rest to tide them over the danger period'.

These and similar recommendations (Brown and Dixon 1963; Barter *et al.* 1965) were reinforced by the results of studies using either historical controls (Laursen 1973; Persson *et al.* 1979) or non-randomized concurrent controls (usually women who could not or would not comply with the recommendation of hospitalization) (Jeffrey *et al.* 1974; Komaromy and Lampé 1977; Misenheimer and Kaltreider 1978; Kappel *et al.* 1985). In several countries it became common practice to admit women with a multiple pregnancy to hospital for rest for varying periods between 29 and 36 weeks of gestation, and this policy continues to be widespread. The Scottish Twin Study (Patel *et al.* 1983), for example, showed that 40 per cent of women with a twin pregnancy were admitted towards the end of the 2nd trimester and the beginning of the 3rd trimester for the sole indication of bed rest. This was the commonest single reason for antenatal hospital admission of women with multiple pregnancies. A recent survey in the Northern Regional Health Authority in England revealed similar patterns of practice there (Lowry and Stafford 1985). A Canadian survey has shown that one in three women with twin pregnancies is hospitalized for rest prophylactically (Zilbert and Gray 1980). Papiernik and his colleagues (Papiernik 1983; Tresmontant *et al.* 1983) reported that 80 per cent of women in a French series were offered hospital admission during pregnancy.

The cost and possible benefits of bed rest for twin pregnancy were reviewed by Powers and Miller in 1979. They focused accurately on the core of the problem: 'answering the question of the efficacy of bed rest is becoming increasingly important. Already in the reported English literature a minimum of 88 women years of bed rest has been expended on healthy mothers solely to prolong their twin pregnancies and still its efficacy is unproved' (Powers and Miller 1979).

The first reported attempt to make a controlled evaluation of the policy was published by Weekes and his colleagues in 1977. They took advantage of a 'natural experiment' by comparing the outcomes of twin pregnancies managed by three obstetric teams that had different policies. Sixty women cared for by one of the teams were hospitalized routinely for rest; one of the other teams inserted a cervical suture in the 37 women under their care; and 36 women were cared for by a third team that used neither of these active approaches. Although it should be noted that the sample studied was not large, there were no statistically significant differences between the outcomes in the three groups in respect of mean gestational age at delivery, the incidence of preterm delivery, or mean birthweight.

In a comparable non-randomized cohort study, O'Connor and colleagues (1981) compared pregnancy outcome in 101 women with twin pregnancies who were cared for in a centre where outpatient management was the rule, with 137 women cared for by specialists working in another centre in which hospital admission for bed rest between 30 and 36 weeks' gestation was advocated routinely. No advantage of hospitalization could be detected.

Only recently has the policy of routine hospitalization of women with twin pregnancies for bed rest been evaluated in controlled trials (Hartikainen-Sorri and Jouppila 1984; Saunders *et al.* 1985; Crowther *et al.*, in press (a)). In Oulu, Finland, Hartikainen-Sorri and Jouppila (1984) allocated 78 women (on the basis of their birth date) either to be hospitalized routinely for bed rest starting at the beginning of the 30th week of pregnancy, or to specialized out-patient antenatal care and admission only if complications arose. The randomized trial conducted by Saunders and his colleagues (1985) in Harare, Zimbabwe, compared a policy of routine admission to hospital at 32 weeks' gestation with a policy of selective admission (at a mean gestational age of 37 weeks) for complications, or for labour. A further randomized trial in Harare (Crowther *et al.*, in press (a)) compared a policy of routine hospitalization beginning between 28 and 30 weeks with selective admission (at a mean gestational age of 35 weeks) only when complications developed.

There is some suggestion from the data derived from these three controlled trials that one beneficial result of routine hospitalization may be a decreased risk of developing hypertension (Table 39.1). These observations should be regarded with caution because it will

Table 39.1 Effect of hospitalization for bed rest in twin pregnancy on development of hypertension

Study	EXPT		CTRL		Odds ratio	Graph of odds ratios and confidence intervals
	n	(%)	*n*	(%)	(95% CI)	0.01 0.1 0.5 1 2 10 100
Saunders *et al.* (1985)	4/105	(3.81)	5/107	(4.67)	0.81 (0.21–3.07)	
Crowther (in press (a))	3/58	(5.17)	9/60	(15.00)	0.34 (0.10–1.13)	
Hartikainen-Sorri and Jouppila	3/32	(9.38)	9/45	(20.00)	0.45 (0.13–1.56)	
Typical odds ratio (95% confidence interval)					0.48 (0.24–1.00)	

Table 39.2 Effect of hospitalization for bed rest in twin pregnancy on low birthweight

Study	EXPT		CTRL		Odds ratio	Graph of odds ratios and confidence intervals
	n	(%)	*n*	(%)	(95% CI)	0.01 0.1 0.5 1 2 10 100
Saunders *et al.* (1985)	76/210	(36.19)	92/214	(42.99)	0.75 (0.51–1.11)	
Crowther (in press (a))	68/116	(58.62)	77/120	(64.17)	0.79 (0.47–1.34)	
Hartikainen-Sorri and Jouppila	22/64	(34.38)	27/90	(30.00)	1.22 (0.62–2.43)	
Typical odds ratio (95% confidence interval)					0.83 (0.63–1.10)	

have been difficult both to standardize assessments of blood pressure and to blind observers to the experimental group of the participants. The assessment of birthweight is less subject to these problems of observer bias, however, and the data also suggest the possibility that a reduced incidence of low birthweight may result from routine hospitalization (Table 39.2). All of the differences observed are compatible with chance variation, however, and in other respects, the available data provide no support for the policy of routine hospitalization of women with twin pregnancies. Indeed they suggest it may have adverse effects: the risk of (spontaneous) preterm birth appears to have been *increased* by routine hospitalization (Table 39.3), an observation reflected in an increased incidence of very low births weight (Table 39.4). Neither do the data on infant morbidity and mortality provide any support for the policy: no differences were detected in the incidence of depressed Apgar score (Table 39.5), admission to the special care nursery (Table 39.6), or perinatal mortality (Table 39.7).

Of the three trials of routine hospitalization in twin

Table 39.3 Effect of hospitalization for bed rest in twin pregnancy on preterm delivery

Study	EXPT		CTRL		Odds ratio	Graph of odds ratios and confidence intervals
	n	(%)	*n*	(%)	(95% CI)	0.01 0.1 0.5 1 2 10 100
Saunders *et al.* (1985)	64/210	(30.48)	40/214	(18.69)	1.89 (1.21–2.94)	
Crowther (in press (a))	72/116	(62.07)	80/120	(66.67)	0.82 (0.48–1.39)	
Hartikainen-Sorri and Jouppila	22/64	(34.38)	22/90	(24.44)	1.62 (0.80–3.29)	
Typical odds ratio (95% confidence interval)					1.39 (1.02–1.89)	

Table 39.4 Effect of hospitalization for bed rest in twin pregnancy on very low birthweight

Study	EXPT		CTRL		Odds ratio	Graph of odds ratios and confidence intervals
	n	(%)	*n*	(%)	(95% CI)	0.01 0.1 0.5 1 2 10 100
Saunders *et al.* (1985)	4/210	(1.90)	1/214	(0.47)	3.42 (0.59–19.93)	
Crowther (in press (a))	1/116	(0.86)	2/120	(1.67)	0.53 (0.05–5.13)	
Hartikainen-Sorri and Jouppila	4/64	(6.25)	2/90	(2.22)	2.91 (0.56–15.17)	
Typical odds ratio (95% confidence interval)					2.12 (0.73–6.16)	

Table 39.5 Effect of hospitalization for bed rest in twin pregnancy on Apgar score <7 at 1 minute

Study	EXPT		CTRL		Odds ratio	Graph of odds ratios and confidence intervals
	n	(%)	*n*	(%)	(95% CI)	0.01 0.1 0.5 1 2 10 100
Crowther (in press (a))	22/116	(18.97)	36/120	(30.00)	0.55 (0.31–1.00)	
Saunders *et al.* (1985)	24/210	(11.43)	21/214	(9.81)	1.19 (0.64–2.20)	
Hartikainen-Sorri and Jouppila	10/64	(15.63)	10/90	(11.11)	1.49 (0.57–3.85)	
Typical odds ratio (95% confidence interval)					0.88 (0.60–1.31)	

Table 39.6 Effect of hospitalization for bed rest in twin pregnancy on admission to special care nursery

Study	EXPT		CTRL		Odds ratio	Graph of odds ratios and confidence intervals
	n	(%)	*n*	(%)	(95% CI)	0.01 0.1 0.5 1 2 10 100
Crowther (in press (a))	42/116	(36.21)	41/120	(34.17)	1.09 (0.64–1.86)	
Typical odds ratio (95% confidence interval)					1.09 (0.64–1.86)	

Table 39.7 Effect of hospitalization for bed rest in twin pregnancy on perinatal death

Study	EXPT		CTRL		Odds ratio	Graph of odds ratios and confidence intervals
	n	(%)	*n*	(%)	(95% CI)	0.01 0.1 0.5 1 2 10 100
Saunders *et al.* (1985)	8/210	(3.81)	5/214	(2.34)	1.64 (0.54–4.94)	
Crowther (in press (a))	4/112	(3.57)	12/120	(10.00)	0.37 (0.13–1.02)	
Hartikainen-Sorri and Jouppila	3/64	(4.69)	0/90	(0.00)	11.45 (1.14–99.99)	
Typical odds ratio (95% confidence interval)					0.95 (0.47–1.93)	

pregnancy, the one with the most encouraging results is the trial in which women were admitted earliest (at an average of 29 weeks) in pregnancy (Crowther *et al.*, in press (a)). The incidence of hypertension, preterm delivery, low birthweight, very low birthweight, depressed Apgar score, and perinatal mortality were all reduced, although the majority of these apparent effects are very easily ascribable to chance variation. Furthermore, the possibility that the policy may have adverse effects should not be dismissed lightly. The results of the trial in Oulu, Finland, prompted the abandonment of routine hospital admission there.

3.2 Routine hospitalization of women with multiple pregnancies at greater than average risk of adverse outcome

Some obstetricians have suggested applying the policy of hospitalization for bed rest in multiple pregnancy only to those women deemed to be at higher than average risk of complications (MacGillivray 1975; Houlton *et al.* 1982). Sometimes this advice has been prompted by evidence suggesting adverse effects of routine hospitalization (Van der Pol *et al.* 1982; Hartikainen-Sorri 1986). Although this more conservative advice is more likely to be justified than recommendations that a diagnosis of twin pregnancy, of itself, is sufficient reason for hospitalization, there is remarkably little good evidence to support hospitalization even of those women with multiple pregnancies that are at above average risk of adverse outcome. Only two such selective policies have been evaluated in randomized trials. The first of these (Crowther *et al.* 1989) involved women with twin pregnancies deemed by cervical scoring (Neilson *et al.* 1988) to be at increased risk of preterm delivery. Among 70 women hospitalized between 28 and 34 weeks' gestation, 51 (72.9 per cent) delivered preterm (<37 weeks) compared to 55 (79.7 per cent) of 69 women in the control group. This difference is not statistically significant, but again, it suggests that a modest beneficial effect of routine hospitalization relatively early in pregnancy may await discovery.

In the only other randomized evaluation of hospitalization for women with multiple pregnancies at above average risk (Crowther *et al.*, in press (b)), 19 women with triplet pregnancies were randomly allocated to hospitalization from 26 weeks' gestation onwards, or to a selectively admitted control group (who were admitted at a mean gestational age of 33 weeks' gestation). Again, although the comparisons between the hospitalized and control groups tended to suggest beneficial effects of routine hospitalization, the differences observed could easily reflect the play of chance, and they do not provide a basis for widespread adoption of the policy.

4 Hypertension

4.1 Non-proteinuric hypertension

The policy of hospitalization for bed rest in pregnancy complicated by hypertension was introduced by Hamlin (1952) as part of a management plan which aimed to reduce the incidence of pre-eclampsia and abolish eclampsia. The plan also involved increased vigilance in antenatal care and a high protein, high vitamin, and low carbohydrate diet. Introduction of this policy was associated with a fall in the rate of serious complications associated with pre-eclampsia (Hamlin 1952) and so it became adopted by others (Dawson 1953).

The first serious challenge to the idea that hospitalization was an effective component of the Hamlin approach came in a report published by Mathews and his colleagues in 1971. Using the same study design (historical controls) as that used to support the introduction of the policy a quarter of a century earlier, they observed a decrease in the incidence of eclampsia and perinatal mortality when the policy of hospitalization for bed rest in women with non-proteinuric hypertension was abandoned in favour of ambulatory management at home with a self-monitoring plan.

Mathews went on to address the hypothesis arising from his earlier observations in a randomized trial (Mathews 1977). Women with a diastolic blood pressure of between 90 and 109 mm Hg (unaccompanied by proteinuria), and a singleton pregnancy of at least 28 weeks' duration, were randomly allocated to one of four groups: bed rest in hospital with barbiturate sedation; bed rest in hospital without sedation; normal activity at home with sedation; and normal activity at home without sedation. Women allocated to the two domiciliary policies were told to go about their activities as normally as possible and were given written instructions emphasizing the importance of symptoms and of testing their urine for protein with 'Albustix' every day. More recently, a second randomized trial to evaluate the effects of hospitalization for rest in women with non-proteinuric hypertension has been completed (Crowther *et al.*, in press (c)). The characteristics of the women recruited were similar to those in Mathews' trial, but no barbiturate sedatives were used. Taken together, the data provided by these trials provide the only well-controlled evaluation of the policy of hospitalization for non-proteinuric hypertension. Unfortunately, no clear picture concerning the value of the policy emerges. One of the trials suggests that hospitalization may have a beneficial effect on the evolution of pre-eclampsia, while the other tends to suggest the opposite (Table 39.8 and Table 39.9). There are also contrasting patterns of preterm delivery in the two trials (Table 39.10). The best estimate of the effect of the policy on the risk of perinatal mortality is very imprecise due to the small number of perinatal deaths in the two studies (Table 39.11).

4.2 Proteinuric hypertension

When proteinuria develops in addition to hypertension in pregnancy, the risks for both mother and fetus are substantially increased (see Chapter 33). Admission to hospital is considered necessary for thorough evaluation and increased surveillance to detect any deteri-

Table 39.8 Effect of hospitalization for non-proteinuric hypertension in pregnancy on diastolic BP >109 mm Hg

Study	EXPT		CTRL		Odds ratio	Graph of odds ratios and confidence intervals
	n	(%)	*n*	(%)	(95% CI)	0.01 0.1 0.5 1 2 10 100
Crowther (in press (c))	25/110	(22.73)	42/108	(38.89)	0.47 (0.26–0.83)	
Mathews (1977)	15/71	(21.13)	6/64	(9.38)	2.43 (0.96–6.15)	
Typical odds ratio (95% confidence interval)					0.74 (0.45–1.21)	

Table 39.9 Effect of hospitalization for non-proteinuric hypertension in pregnancy on development of proteinuria

Study	EXPT		CTRL		Odds ratio	Graph of odds ratios and confidence intervals
	n	(%)	*n*	(%)	(95% CI)	0.01 0.1 0.5 1 2 10 100
Crowther (in press (c))	18/110	(16.36)	27/108	(25.00)	0.59 (0.31–1.14)	
Mathews (1977)	5/71	(7.04)	3/64	(4.69)	1.52 (0.37–6.33)	
Typical odds ratio (95% confidence interval)					0.70 (0.38–1.26)	

Table 39.10 Effect of hospitalization for non-proteinuric hypertension in pregnancy on preterm delivery

Study	EXPT		CTRL		Odds ratio	Graph of odds ratios and confidence intervals
	n	(%)	*n*	(%)	(95% CI)	0.01 0.1 0.5 1 2 10 100
Crowther (in press (c))	13/110	(11.82)	24/108	(22.22)	0.48 (0.24–0.97)	
Mathews (1977)	2/71	(2.82)	1/64	(1.56)	1.77 (0.18–17.40)	
Typical odds ratio (95% confidence interval)					0.54 (0.27–1.05)	

Table 39.11 Effect of hospitalization for non-proteinuric hypertension in pregnancy on perinatal death (excluding lethal congenital malformations)

Study	EXPT		CTRL		Odds ratio	Graph of odds ratios and confidence intervals
	n	(%)	*n*	(%)	(95% CI)	0.01 0.1 0.5 1 2 10 100
Crowther (in press (c))	2/110	(1.82)	1/108	(0.93)	1.92 (0.20–18.69)	
Mathews (1977)	2/71	(2.82)	1/64	(1.56)	1.77 (0.18–17.40)	
Typical odds ratio (95% confidence interval)					1.85 (0.37–9.25)	

Table 39.12 Effect of strict bed rest for proteinuric hypertension in pregnancy on perinatal death

Study	EXPT		CTRL		Odds ratio	Graph of odds ratios and confidence intervals
	n	(%)	*n*	(%)	(95% CI)	0.01 0.1 0.5 1 2 10 100
Crowther (in press (d))	11/53	(20.75)	8/52	(15.38)	1.43 (0.53–3.85)	
Mathews *et al.* (1982)	2/20	(10.00)	4/20	(20.00)	0.47 (0.08–2.58)	
Typical odds ratio (95% confidence interval)					1.08 (0.46–2.55)	

oration in maternal or fetal condition as soon as possible. Whether the hospitalization should be linked with strict rest in bed, however, is less clear.

In addition to their research on non-albuminuric hypertension, Mathews and his colleagues (1980, 1982) have also reported the results of a randomized controlled trial to assess the value of strict bed rest for women hospitalized because of albuminuric hypertension. Forty women with a diastolic blood pressure of at least 90 mm Hg and more than a trace of proteinuria, were randomly allocated to either complete bed rest, or ambulation as desired. Three women in each group were excluded from the analysis for a variety of reasons.

A number of intermediate outcomes were examined. Although daily increases in serum placental lactogen levels were greater in the rested group, the differences were not statistically significant. There was no evidence of improved renal function in the rested group. Five patients in each group had both hyperuricaemia and grossly small for gestational age fetuses on clinical examination. All 5 patients confined to bed developed the premonitory symptoms of eclampsia (increasing headache, visual disturbances, epigastric pain, and vomiting), compared to only one of those allocated to ambulation. The development of these symptoms led to 'emergency' caesarean section in all but one woman, who gave birth to a very growth-retarded, immature fetus.

Crowther (in press (d)) has recently replicated Mathews' trial. One hundred and five women with a diastolic blood pressure between 90 and 109 mm Hg, more than a trace of proteinuria, and a singleton pregnancy of at least 28 weeks' gestation, were randomly allocated to strict bed rest or ambulation as desired. Although there was an increase in the incidence of diastolic blood pressure greater than 109 mm Hg in the group of women confined to bed, this group was less likely than controls to experience a worsening of their proteinuria. Neither of these differences was statistically significant, however. The trial did not detect any effect of the policy on the incidence of preterm delivery, low birthweight, depressed Apgar score, or admission to the special care nursery.

Using all of the data derived from the two trials provides little in the way of clues concerning the effect of the policy on the risk of perinatal mortality (Table 39.12).

5 Conclusions

5.1 Implications for current practice

As we noted at the beginning of this chapter, hospitalization during pregnancy is costly and disruptive for many families. It is surprising, therefore, that its use has been the subject of such a small amount of well-controlled research (Lancet editorial 1981). There are circumstances in which discussion with individual women who have one of the conditions we have reviewed will make it clear that a prescription for rest, either at home or in hospital, would be welcome. As there is no strong evidence that this is likely to have harmful effects, such women's views should be taken into account in deciding which form of care is appropriate. By the same token, however, women with either bleeding in early pregnancy, uncomplicated multiple pregnancy, or non-albuminuric hypertension should not be coerced into resting in bed at home or in hospital, against their better judgement. There is currently no good evidence to support such recommendations.

5.2 Implications for future research

None of the foregoing should be taken to mean that the available evidence is satisfactory. Controlled evaluation of these policies is a very recent phenomenon and further research of this kind should help to clarify whether some, as yet unidentified benefits of hospitalization for rest outweigh its undoubted costs.

The currently available evidence from controlled trials, and the fact that the neonatal morbidity and mortality associated with twin pregnancy is particularly high among babies delivered prior to 32 weeks' gestation, suggest that rest from relatively early in pregnancy may be the most appropriate policy to assess. The current Australian multicentre trial of routine hospitalization of women with multiple pregnancies from 26 to 30 weeks' gestation (MacLennan A, personal communication), and the detailed plans that have been drawn up for such a trial in Canada (Young 1986), represent the kind of further research that will provide a more rational basis for assessing whether the substantial costs associated with implementing such a policy are likely to be outweighed by a reduction in neonatal mortality and morbidity. In places in which either the resources required to implement such a costly policy could not be made available, or scepticism about the value of hospitalization is particularly strong, trials restricted to women at higher than average risk of delivering preterm may be more appropriate. Similar considerations apply in respect of hospitalization for non-albuminuric hypertension. In the current climate of financial retrenchment, the evaluation of policies of antenatal hospitalization in such trials should by now have become as easy as their unvalidated introduction seems to have been during the era of economic expansion.

References

Acker D, Sapir J, Sachs B, Friedman E (1986). Diagnostic related groups and the obstetrician: Antepartum admission. Am J Obstet Gynecol, 155: 780–783.

Barter RH, Hsu I, Erkenbeck RV, Pugsley LQ (1965). The prevention of prematurity in multiple pregnancy. Am J Obstet Gynecol, 91: 787–791.

Berardi JC (1985). Mécanisme en jeu dans la prévention communautaire de la prématurité: Etude d'une population d'immigrés maghrebines. Paper presented at Symposium on the Prevention of Preterm Birth, 19–22 May, 1985, Evian, France.

Brown EJ, Dixon HG (1963). Twin pregnancy. Br J Obstet Gynaecol, 70: 251–257.

Crowther CA, Neilson JP, Verkuyl DAA, Bannerman C, Ashurst HM (1989). Preterm labour in twin pregnancies: can it be prevented by hospital admission? Br J Obstet Gynaecol, 96: 850–853.

Crowther CA, Verkuyl DAA, Bannerman C, Neilson JP, Ashurst HM (in press (a)). The effects of hospitalization for bed rest on fetal growth, neonatal morbidity, and length of gestation in twin pregnancy. Br J Obstet Gynaecol.

Crowther CA, Verkuyl DAA, Ashworth F, Bannerman C, Ashurst HM (in press (b)). The effects of hospitalization for bed rest on duration of pregnancy, fetal growth, and neonatal morbidity in triplet pregnancies.

Crowther CA, Boumeester A, Ashurst H (in press (c)). Home management versus hospitalisation for women with non-proteinuric hypertension in pregnancy.

Crowther CA, Boumeester A, Ashurst H (in press (d)). Strict bed rest versus ambulation as desired in women with proteinuric hypertension in pregnancy.

Dawson B (1953). The prevention of eclampsia—an Australian experiment. J Obstet Gynaecol Br Commnwlth, 60: 80–84.

Department of Health and Social Security, Central Health Services Council Standing Midwifery and Maternity Advisory Committee (Chairman: Sir J Peel) (1970). Domiciliary Midwifery and Maternity Bed Needs. London: Her Majesty's Stationery Office.

Diddle AW, O'Connor KA, Jack R, Pearce RL (1953). Evaluation of bed rest in threatened abortion. Obstet Gynecol, 2: 63–67.

Everett, CB, Ashurst, H, Chalmers I (1987). Reported management of threatened miscarriage by general practitioners in Wessex. Br Med J, 295: 583–586.

Ford M (1987). Perceived Stress, Social Support and Adaptive Responses in Antepartum Hospitalized Women. Thesis submitted for the Master of Science in Nursing, University of Toronto.

Hamlin RMJ (1952). The prevention of eclampsia and pre-eclampsia. Lancet, 1: 64–68.

Hartikainen-Sorri AL (1986). Is routine hospitalisation of twin pregnancy necessary? Acta Genet Med Gemellol, 34: 189–192.

Hartikainen-Sorri AL, Jouppila P (1984). Is routine hospitalisation needed in the antenatal care of twin pregnancy? J Perinat Med, 12: 31–34.

Hays PM, Smeltzer JS (1986). Multiple gestation. Clin Obstet Gynecol, 29: 264–285.

Hirst JC (1938). Maternal and fetal expectations with multiple pregnancy. Am J Obstet Gynecol, 37: 634–643.

Houlton MCC, Marivate M, Philpott RHP (1982). Factors associated with preterm labour and changes in the cervix before labour in twin pregnancy. Br J Obstet Gynaecol, 89: 190–194.

Jeffrey RL, Bowes WA, Delaney JJ (1974). Role of bed rest in twin gestation. Obstet Gynecol, 43: 822–826.

Kappel B, Hansen KB, Moller J, Faaborg-Andersen J (1985). Bed rest in twin pregnancy. Acta Genet Med Gemellol, 34: 67–71.

Komaromy B, Lampe L (1977). The value of bed rest in twin pregnancies. Int J Gynaecol Obstet, 15: 262–266.

Lancet (1981). Bed rest in obstetrics (Editorial). Lancet, i: 137–138.

Laursen B (1973). Twin pregnancy. Acta Obstet Gynecol Scand, 52: 367–371.

Lowry MF, Stafford JM (unpublished report) (1985). Northern Region Twin Study, 1984.

MacGillivray I (1975). Management of multiple pregnancy. In: Human Multiple Reproduction. MacGillivray I, Nylander PPS, Corney G (eds). London: W B Saunders, pp 124–135.

Mathews DD (1977). A randomised controlled trial of bed rest and sedation or normal activity and non-sedation in the management of non-albuminuric hypertension in late pregnancy. Br J Obstet Gynaecol, 84: 108–114.

Mathews DD, Patel IR, Sengupta SM (1971). Outpatient management of toxaemia. J Obstet Gynaecol Br Commnwlth, 78: 610–619.

Mathews DD, Agarwal V, Shuttleworth TP (1980). The effect of rest and ambulation on plasma urea and urate levels in pregnant women with proteinuric hypertension. Br J Obstet Gynaecol, 87: 1095–1098.

Mathews DD, Agarwal V, Shuttleworth TP (1982). A randomised controlled trial of complete bed rest versus ambulation in the management of proteinuric hypertension during pregnancy. Br J Obstet Gynaecol, 89: 128–131.

Ministry of Health (1959). Report of the Maternity Services Committee (Chairman: the Earl of Cranbrook). London: Her Majesty's Stationery Office.

Misenheimer HR, Kaltreider DF (1978). Effects of decreased prenatal activity in patients with twin pregnancy. Obstet Gynecol, 51: 692–694.

Mueller-Heubach E (1984). Complications of multiple gestation. Clin Obstet Gynecol, 27: 1003–1013.

Neilson JP, Verkuyl DAA, Crowther CA, Bannerman C (1988). Preterm labor in twin pregnancies: prediction by cervical assessment. Obstet Gynecol, 72: 719–723.

O'Connor MC, Arias E, Royston JP, Dalrymple IJ (1981). The merits of special antenatal care for twin pregnancies. Br J Obstet Gynaecol, 88: 222–230.

Office of Population Censuses and Surveys (1984). Hospital In-patient Enquiry: Maternity Statistics 1979 to 1981. OPCS Monitor MB4 84/1.

Papiernik E (1983). Social cost of twin births. Acta Genet Med Gemellol, 32: 105–111.

Patel N, Barrie W, Campbell D, Howat R, Melrose E, Redford D, McIlwaine G, Smalls M (1983). Scottish Twin Study. Glasgow: Greater Glasgow Health Board and Departments of Child Health and Obstetrics, University of Glasgow.

Persson PH, Grennert L, Gensser G, Kullander S (1979). On improved outcome of twin pregnancies. Acta Obstet Gynecol Scand, 58: 3–7.

Powers WF, Miller TC (1979). Bed rest in twin pregnancy: Identification of a critical period and its cost implications. Am J Obstet Gynecol, 134: 23–29.

Romito P (1989). Women's paid and unpaid work during pregnancy. Working and Occasional Paper No 10, London: Thomas Coram Research Unit.

Rosen EL (1975). Concerns of an obstetric patient experiencing long-term hospitalisation. J Obstet Gynecol Neonatal Nurs , 4: 15–19.

Russell JK (1952). Maternal and foetal hazards associated with twin pregnancy. J Obstet Gynaecol Br Empire, 59: 208–213.

Saunders MC, Dick JS, Brown I McL, McPherson K, Chalmers I (1985). The effects of hospital admission for bedrest on the duration of twin pregnancy: A randomised trial. Lancet, 2: 793–795.

Tresmontant R, Heluin G, Papiernik E (1983). Cost of care and prevention of preterm births in twin pregnancies. Acta Genet Med Gemellol, 32: 99–103.

Van der Pol JG, Bleker OP, Treffers PE (1982). Clinical bedrest in twin pregnancies. Eur J Obstet Gynecol Reprod Biol, 14: 75–80.

Weekes ARL, Menzies DN, DeBoer CH (1977). The relative efficacy of bed rest, cervical suture and no treatment in the management of twin pregnancy. Br J Obstet Gynaecol, 84: 161–164.

White M, Ritchie J (1984). Psychological stressors in antepartum hospitalisation: Reports of pregnant women. Matern Child Nurs J, 13: 47–56.

Young DC (1986). A Multicenter Randomized Controlled Trial of Prophylactic Hospital Admission of Twin Pregnancies in Prevention of Preterm Birth at Gestations less than 32 Completed Weeks. MSc thesis, McMaster University.

Zilbert AW, Gray JH (1980). Atlantic Provinces Twin Study 1977–1978. Nova Scotia Medical Bulletin 153.

40 Cervical cerclage to prolong pregnancy

Adrian Grant

1 Introduction

'In 1658, Cole and Culpepper wrote in the *Practice of Physick* that "the second fault in women which hindered conception is when the seed is not retained or the orifice of the womb is so slack that it cannot rightly contract itself to keep in the seed; which is chiefly caused by abortion, or hard labor and childbirth, whereby the fibers of the womb are broken in pieces one from another and they, and the inner orifice of the womb overmuch slackened." In an issue of the *Lancet* published 1865, Gream mentioned the term "cervical incompetence".' (cited by Harger 1983).

In normal pregnancy the uterine cervix is thought to act as a sphincter. A congenital or traumatically-acquired weakness of the cervix, or the unusual physiological circumstance of multiple pregnancy, are factors which may render the cervix incapable of performing this function. Belief in such 'incompetence' of the cervix is the basis for performing the operation of cervical cerclage.

1.1 Diagnosis of cervical incompetence

There is no truly diagnostic test for cervical incompetence. Currently, the decision to insert a cervical suture is most commonly based on past obstetric history and, to a lesser extent, clinical assessment of the cervix during pregnancy by vaginal examination. McDonald (1980) describes the features from previous pregnancies which he feels are most suggestive of cervical incompetence as: 'the history of one or more mid-trimester abortions, with early rupture of the membranes, usually before the onset of labour. There is absence of significant haemorrhage. The labours are short and relatively pain-free: the fetus is born alive. Repeated middle term miscarriages at the same time of gestation are significant.' The diagnosis of cervical incompetence may be made on the basis of a single vaginal examination or serial clinical assessments of the cervix which suggest dilatation. Other symptoms, such as mucous vaginal discharge, lower abdominal discomfort and a bearing down sensation, or signs, such as visualization of the membranes bulging through the cervix, either are very uncommon or may appear too late to be helpful in prevention of miscarriage. Ultrasound visualization of the cervix in early pregnancy (Brook *et al.* 1981, Jackson *et al.* 1984) may allow a more objective assessment of the cervical dilatation but its usefulness is controversial (Witter 1984). Other methods to assess the cervical compliance and resistance between pregnancies with intracervical balloons (Neuman *et al.* 1980) or graduated dilators (Anthony *et al.* 1982), like ultrasound visualization, still require appropriate evaluation.

1.2 Techniques of cervical cerclage

A variety of surgical techniques and suture materials have been used to treat cervical incompetence, but there are basically two main variants of cervical cerclage. In the type of operation associated with Shirodkar's name, a circular incision is made around the cervix at the level of the internal os; the vagina and bladder are dissected away; and an encircling suture of fascia lata strip or mersilene tape is placed in the region of the internal os and lower uterine segment. The suture is subsequently buried in the cervix to reduce the risk of sepsis (Shirodkar 1960). This may make it difficult to divide later in pregnancy, and Shirodkar advocated elective caesarean section for delivery, especially for those women in whom there was a possibility of further pregnancies. To circumvent this problem others subsequently modified his operation (Green-Armytage and Browne 1957) by tying the knot superficially. This made it relatively easy to remove the suture, either electively at 38 weeks' gestation, or, if labour began, earlier than this.

A number of techniques have been developed which do not require dissecting the bladder from the uterus. The most commonly employed variant is that associated with the name of McDonald (1957). A purse string suture of heavy silk, mersilene tape, or nylon is placed as high as possible around the cervix to approximate to the level of the internal os, but without dissecting back the bladder. About five bites are made into the exocervix; the knot is tied superficially and usually anteriorly with the ends left long to facilitate subsequent division.

A third variant has been recommended for patients with very short or amputated cervices. A transabdominal (Benson and Durfee 1965) or vaginal (Ritter 1978) approach is used to place an encircling suture above the cardinal and uterosacral ligaments. This approach is only very rarely used because it is more difficult, carries a higher morbidity rate and requires at least one, if not two, intra-abdominal operations.

1.3 Variations in the use of cervical cerclage

There is considerable variation in the frequency with which cervical cerclage is performed. For example, in France the insertion rate is about 30 per 1000 births (Rumeau-Rouquette *et al.* 1984), whereas the rate in Scotland in 1976 was 5 per 1000 (Cole 1982). A survey conducted in Britain in 1979 revealed that an average of about eight sutures are inserted for every 1000 births, but rates reported by individual obstetricians varied from 0 per 1000 to 80 per 1000 births managed (MRC Working Party on Preterm Labour 1979). In part, this wide variation reflects the difficulties in making a definite diagnosis of cervical incompetence; but it is also an expression of the lack of satisfactory evidence concerning the efficacy of cervical cerclage and the fact that the operation may also entail hazards.

1.4 Complications of cervical cerclage

Table 40.1 lists documented complications of cerclage (Harger 1980; Lipshitz 1975; Kuhn and Pepperell 1977; Aarnoudse and Huisjes 1979; Heinemann *et al.* 1977; Charles and Edwards 1981; Loos *et al.* 1985; Lindberg 1979; Robboy 1973; Bates and Cropley 1977; Berchuck and Sokol 1984; Page 1958; Dunn *et al.* 1959; Department of Health and Social Security 1982). Reported rates are low but variable, probably reflecting in part the experience of the operator and the variant of operation used, and in part the completeness or incompleteness of the reporting.

Table 40.1 Complications of cervical cerclage (see text for references)

cervical laceration
premature rupture of membranes
stimulation of myometrial activity
sepsis
endotoxic shock
cervical dystocia
cervical stenosis
vesico-vaginal fistula
uterine rupture
complications of anaesthesia
maternal death

2 Observational studies to evaluate cervical cerclage

Most published articles on cervical cerclage are reports of case series. The common practice of comparing the outcome in a current pregnancy treated by cerclage with the performance in previous pregnancies is clearly inappropriate. Yet, despite this, studies of this type are still being reported (for example, Wright 1987). Data for Norway and Aberdeen (Bakketeig *et al.* 1979; Carr-Hill and Hall 1985) linking information relating to successive pregnancies in the same woman suggest (Table 40.2) that although the risk of another preterm delivery increases between three- and fourfold after one preterm delivery, there is still an 85 per cent chance of a subsequent pregnancy going to term. After 2 preterm deliveries, this chance decreases to 70 per cent (Table 40.2) equivalent to about an eightfold increase in risk compared with the risk of preterm delivery following 2 term pregnancies. Most case series of cervical cerclage report 'success' rates at about this level, although some suggest somewhat higher delivery rates at term.

Two reports (Keirse *et al.* 1978; Rush 1979) have compared patients with prespecified past obstetric histories (e.g. previous 2nd-trimester abortion or preterm delivery) who were treated with cerclage, with other

Table 40.2 Risk of recurrent preterm* delivery (data from Bakketeig *et al.*1979 in Norway, and Carr-Hill and Hall 1985 in Aberdeen)

First birth	Second birth	Per cent preterm* delivery in the subsequent pregnancy	
		Norway	Aberdeen
preterm*		14	15
>36 weeks		4	5
preterm	preterm	28	32
preterm	>36 weeks	6	12
>36 weeks	preterm	9	23
>36 weeks	>36 weeks	3	4

* preterm defined as 16–36 weeks in Norway and 21–36 weeks in Aberdeen

patients with a similar past history who were managed without suture over the same time-period. Neither study suggested any benefit from cerclage, but it is impossible to know in such 'observational' studies what factors determined which patients were treated with cerclage and which were not, and the results must therefore be interpreted with caution.

Weekes and colleagues (1977) profited from variations in the way that individual obstetricians in Liverpool managed twin pregnancy. One group of patients received prophylactic cerclage, another group routine bed rest, and a third group neither. Differences in either the characteristics of patients referred to particular specialists or in other respects of management could have biased the comparison, and the numbers are inadequate for firm conclusions. Nevertheless, this study gives no support to the suggestion that there is prolongation of twin pregnancies after prophylactic cerclage.

One other non-randomized cohort study (Sinha *et al.* 1979) has addressed the role of cervical cerclage in twin pregnancy. Eighty-eight women with a twin pregnancy seen in one hospital had cervical suture electively inserted and these were compared with 76 women with twin pregnancy cared for in another hospital where cervical cerclage was not used. The incidence of spontaneous onset of labour before 36 weeks was higher in the cervical suture group (24/88) than in the women without suture (6/76). More than half of the women who had a suture inserted sustained cervical damage.

The undoubted problems of selection bias which beset these observational studies are most satisfactorily overcome by random treatment allocation (Bergsjø 1980; Chalmers 1984).

3 Randomized controlled trials of cervical cerclage

3.1 Description of the trials

Four randomized controlled trials of cerclage have been published to date (Dor *et al.* 1982; Rush *et al.* 1984; Lazar *et al.* 1984; Forster *et al.* 1986) and interim results of a fifth (the MRC/RCOG Cervical Cerclage Trial—Macnaughton 1981; Grant 1981–85) have recently been published (MRC/RCOG Working Party on Cervical Cerclage 1988). The designs of these studies are summarized in Table 40.3.

The first was conducted by Dor and his colleagues (1982) in Israel. 342 women attending the infertility clinic who conceived following induction of ovulation were closely monitored by ultrasound. The 50 cases of twin pregnancy were recruited to the trial in the 13th week and 25 were randomly allocated to cerclage with a McDonald suture using double silk stitches, the remaining 25 acting as controls.

The study conducted by Rush in South Africa (1984) involved 194 women with singleton pregnancies with a high risk (30 per cent) of having a late miscarriage or a preterm delivery. The women were randomly allocated either to have a McDonald-type suture of monofilament Nylon inserted, or to be managed without a suture. All but two of the women received the treatment to which they had been allocated (Table 40.3).

The third trial was conducted by Lazar and his colleagues (1984) in France and was mounted in the context of existing high rates of cervical cerclage. A 'historical' comparison had been performed (Lazar *et al.* 1979) which suggested that the rate of preterm delivery was halved by cerclage when two groups of women at 'moderate' risk were compared in two successive time periods when the rates of cerclage were 5 per cent and 18 per cent respectively. The extent to which this change could be attributed to cerclage was uncertain and there was worry about possible adverse effects of the operation. A weighted scoring system was used to assess the eligibility of potential subjects, the aim being to exclude from the trial women at high risk (who would be managed with cerclage) and women at low risk (who would be managed conservatively). (Details of this are given in the report of the trial.) However, as judged by its eventual preterm delivery rate (6 per cent) the trial population was, in fact, at relatively very low risk. The trial design was 'pragmatic' (Schwartz *et al.* 1980), that is, compared two management policies—90 per cent of those allocated to cerclage had a cervical suture inserted and 11 per cent of the control group were also managed with cerclage (Table 40.3). The sealed envelope method of random allocation was definitely violated in one of the four clinical centres, with more women, especially those at higher risk, being allocated cerclage. Despite the selection bias which thus operated in this centre the investigators chose to include the data from this centre because secondary analyses conducted after excluding these cases did not make any difference to the conclusions reached after analysing the data from all four centres.

Table 40.3 Randomized controlled trials of cervical cerclage—Study design

	Dor *et al.* 1982	Rush *et al.* 1984	Lazar *et al.* 1984	Forster *et al.* 1986	MRC/RCOG 1988
Total no. subjects	50 (100 fetuses)	194	506	242	905
Eligibility criteria	Twin pregnancies	2–4 previous pregnancies of < 37 weeks—at least one between 14 & 36 weeks	'moderate risk' as judged by scoring system	Not stated	obstetricians uncertain about advisability of cerclage
Management of experimental group	McDonald suture used in all cases (100%)	McDonald suture inserted in 95 out of the 96 cases (99%)	McDonald suture inserted in 242 of the 268 cases (90%)	cerclage (technique not stated) inserted in all 112 cases (100%)	suture (method not prescribed) inserted in 417 of 454 cases (92%)
Management of control group	suture withheld in all cases (100%)	suture withheld in 97 of the 98 cases (99%)	suture withheld in 212 of the 238 cases (89%)	Stutz pessary; use of cerclage not stated	suture withheld in 418 of 451 cases (93%)
Source of participants	infertility clinic (induction of ovulation) Tel-Aviv, Israel	reproductive failure clinic, Groote Schuur Hospital, Cape Town, South Africa	four maternity units in France	one maternity unit in German Federal Republic	130 obstetricians in nine countries
Time of entry	13th week	15–21 weeks	10–28 weeks	Not stated but probably very variable	95% before 20 weeks
Method of allocation	'random'	random numbers, sealed envelopes	random numbers, envelopes	first letter of surname	telephone randomization

The report of a fourth trial was published in 1986. Förster and his colleagues in the German Democratic Republic compared cerclage with Stutz pessary for both prophylactic and therapeutic indications. The original intention was to include a third group managed with bed rest and without cerclage or pessary but in the first 8 patients in this group 'further opening of the cervical os and shortening of the cervix' was judged to make it necessary to treat them all with cerclage or pessary. It is not stated what eligibility criteria were used nor is it clear from the published report at what gestational age treatment was started, but it is implied in the discussion that some cases were treated before 18 weeks and some as late as after 32 weeks. The choice of treatment was based on the first letter of the patient's surname, a method of allocation which is notoriously prone to selection bias because the allocation is known before eligibility has been decided. The 16 per cent difference in the sizes of the two trial groups could be due to chance only, but could also be a reflection of such selection bias. Because Stutz pessaries were used in the control group and because of the worries about selection bias this study will be considered separately from the other four trials in the review which follows later.

At the time of writing, the MRC/RCOG Cervical Cerclage Trial is still recruiting cases. Interim analyses of completed case records up to the end of 1986 have recently been published (MRC/RCOG Working Party on Cervical Cerclage 1988). The entry criterion—obstetricians' uncertainty as to the advisability of cerclage—was intentionally loose. The current wide variation in the clinical use of the procedure is reflected in differences in the types of cases for which particular obstetricians are uncertain about whether to perform the operation. It was argued that all cases which would meet rigid entry criteria would be entered into a trial with open criteria by those obstetricians whose uncertainty happened to coincide with the rigid criteria; the bonus would be the entry of other types of cases for which other obstetricians were uncertain about the advisability of cerclage. In practice, three-quarters of the women entered have had one or more 2nd-trimester miscarriages or preterm deliveries, a further 10 per cent have had a history of possible past cervical damage (for example, cone biopsy or cervical amputation); in the remaining 15 per cent of cases cerclage was considered on the basis of other indications such as previous termination of pregnancy and/or, previous 1st-trimester miscarriage. The trial groups are well balanced in respect of these various indications. The design of the trial was pragmatic. It was recognized that the clinical situation might change as pregnancy progressed and the aim was to compare two *policies* in the form of recommended management at trial entry. In fact (Table 40.3)

92 per cent of those allocated to cerclage received a suture (of those who did not, for 5 per cent it was the patient's wishes and 3 per cent miscarried before the stitch could be inserted), and of those allocated to the control group 7 per cent had cerclage (5 per cent because the cervix was judged to be opening and 2 per cent because the patient decided after entry that she would like a suture).

More than one hundred obstetricians (from nine countries) have contributed cases to this trial. Although randomization within specialist was not performed, cerclage and control cases are evenly distributed for each participating obstetrician. Most cases (95 per cent) were entered before 20 completed weeks of gestation; the latest gestation at entry was 29 weeks. Cases were entered and randomized by telephone. Most obstetricians used the telephone randomization service provided by the Clinical Trial Service Unit in Oxford but other randomization centres were established in Italy, Zimbabwe, and Hungary.

3.2 The effects of cervical cerclage on the subsequent management of pregnancy

In all 3 trials for which data are available, the use of cerclage was associated with more intensive antenatal management as judged by admission to hospital (Table 40.4) and the use of oral tocolytics (Table 40.5). In the French trial, this was partially, though not completely, explained by the finding that more women in the cerclage group (22 per cent) reported 'uterine pains' than in the control (18 per cent).

In the same 3 trials induction of labour was more common in the cerclage group (Table 40.6). However, if in the French trial the data from the centre where the randomization was breached are excluded, this trial no longer shows a statistically significant difference in the rate of induction.

All four trials (for which data are available) had higher caesarean section rates in the cerclage groups and the 95 per cent confidence interval for the typical odds ratio derived from these data only just includes unity (Table 40.7). In the MRC/RCOG trial the overall difference reflected a difference in emergency caesareans.

3.3 The effects of cervical cerclage on pregnancy outcome

The aim of the operation of cervical cerclage is to

Table 40.4 Effect of cervical cerclage (all trials) on additional admissions to hospital

Study	EXPT *n*	EXPT (%)	CTRL *n*	CTRL (%)	Odds ratio (95% CI)	Graph of odds ratios and confidence intervals (0.01 0.1 0.5 1 2 10 100)
MRC/RCOG (1988)	135/454	(29.74)	114/451	(25.28)	1.25 (0.93–1.67)	
Rush *et al.* (1984)	30/96	(31.25)	19/98	(19.39)	1.87 (0.98–3.57)	
Lazar *et al.* (1984)	85/268	(31.72)	41/238	(17.23)	2.17 (1.45–3.24)	
Typical odds ratio (95% confidence interval)					1.55 (1.24–1.93)	

Table 40.5 Effect of cervical cerclage (all trials) on administration of oral tocolytics

Study	EXPT *n*	EXPT (%)	CTRL *n*	CTRL (%)	Odds ratio (95% CI)	Graph of odds ratios and confidence intervals (0.01 0.1 0.5 1 2 10 100)
MRC/RCOG (1988)	113/454	(24.89)	107/451	(23.73)	1.07 (0.79–1.44)	
Rush *et al.* (1984)	12/96	(12.50)	8/98	(8.16)	1.59 (0.63–4.01)	
Lazar *et al.* (1984)	127/268	(47.39)	73/238	(30.67)	2.01 (1.41–2.87)	
Typical odds ratio (95% confidence interval)					1.40 (1.12–1.75)	

Table 40.6 Effect of cervical cerclage (all trials) on induction of labour

Study	EXPT		CTRL		Odds ratio	Graph of odds ratios and confidence intervals
	n	(%)	*n*	(%)	(95% CI)	0.01 0.1 0.5 1 2 10 100
MRC/RCOG (1988)	85/454	(18.72)	69/451	(15.30)	1.27 (0.90–1.80)	
Rush *et al.* (1984)	9/96	(9.38)	8/98	(8.16)	1.16 (0.43–3.14)	
Lazar *et al.* (1984)	49/268	(18.28)	39/238	(16.39)	1.14 (0.72–1.81)	
Typical odds ratio (95% confidence interval)					1.22 (0.93–1.59)	

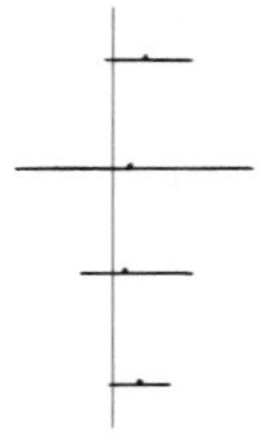

Table 40.7 Effect of cervical cerclage (all trials) on caesarean section

Study	EXPT		CTRL		Odds ratio	Graph of odds ratios and confidence intervals
	n	(%)	*n*	(%)	(95% CI)	0.01 0.1 0.5 1 2 10 100
MRC/RCOG (1988)	68/454	(14.98)	56/451	(12.42)	1.24 (0.85–1.81)	
Rush *et al.* (1984)	19/96	(19.79)	18/98	(18.37)	1.10 (0.54–2.24)	
Dor *et al.* (1982)	9/25	(36.00)	7/25	(28.00)	1.43 (0.44–4.65)	
Lazar *et al.* (1984)	33/268	(12.31)	22/238	(9.24)	1.37 (0.78–2.40)	
Typical odds ratio (95% confidence interval)					1.26 (0.95–1.66)	

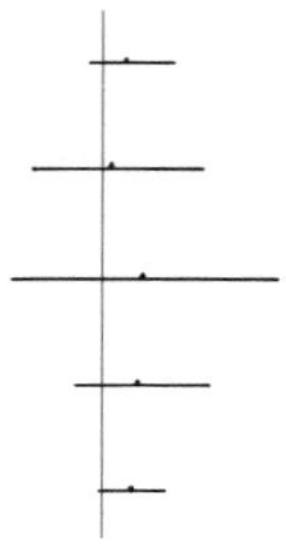

prolong pregnancy and thereby reduce fetal and neonatal mortality and morbidity. There is no other obvious mechanism whereby a beneficial effect of cerclage could be mediated and prolongation of pregnancy by cerclage was the main hypothesis addressed in all four trials. Advances in neonatal care have meant that the traditional definition of early delivery before 37 completed weeks (preterm delivery) is less clinically meaningful than a cut-off earlier in pregnancy. Most obstetricians would agree that a shift in the time of delivery from before to after 32 weeks would be clinically important, whereas a shift from 33 weeks to 37 weeks while desirable, would be less important.

The trials are not consistent in the direction of differences observed between the cerclage and control groups. The three smaller trials show a tendency towards shorter gestation and higher mortality in the cerclage groups (Tables 40.8, 40.9 and 40.10).

As discussed earlier there are worries about selection bias distorting the results of the French trial (Lazar *et al.* 1984). But the major limitation of this trial is the very low risk of the trial population as judged by overall rates of preterm delivery of 6 per cent and delivery before 33 weeks of 1 per cent; rates which are similar to those in the general population. Cervical cerclage is an unusual intervention in that plausibly it may precipitate miscarriage or preterm delivery—the very things that its use aims to prevent. The balance between possible prevention of early delivery, and early delivery precipitated by the procedure, is likely to change with the risk level of those treated. At levels of risk as low as those observed in the French trial any possible beneficial effect could be overwhelmed by any adverse effect caused by the procedure.

The small Israeli trial (Dor *et al.* 1982) was limited to twin pregnancies which were otherwise at no special risk of early delivery. For this reason the trial is not directly comparable to the other trials and together with the 24 twin pregnancies in the interim analysis of the MRC/RCOG trial it will be considered later in a separate section on twin pregnancies.

The South African trial (Rush *et al.* 1984) included singleton pregnancies at quite high risk of preterm delivery (33 per cent) and of delivery before 33 weeks (11 per cent). Rates of early delivery were higher in the cerclage group (Tables 40.8 and 40.9) but the confidence intervals are very wide (delivery prior to 33 weeks: odds ratio = 1.26; 95 per cent confidence

Table 40.8 Effect of cervical cerclage (all trials) on delivery <33 weeks' gestation

Study	EXPT		CTRL		Odds ratio	Graph of odds ratios and confidence intervals
	n	(%)	*n*	(%)	(95% CI)	0.01 0.1 0.5 1 2 10 100
MRC/RCOG (1988)	59/454	(13.00)	82/451	(18.18)	0.67 (0.47–0.97)	
Rush *et al.* (1984)	12/96	(12.50)	10/98	(10.20)	1.26 (0.52–3.04)	
Dor *et al.* (1982)	6/25	(24.00)	5/25	(20.00)	1.26 (0.33–4.73)	
Lazar *et al.* (1984)	4/268	(1.49)	1/238	(0.42)	2.99 (0.51–17.41)	
Typical odds ratio (95% confidence interval)					0.79 (0.58–1.09)	

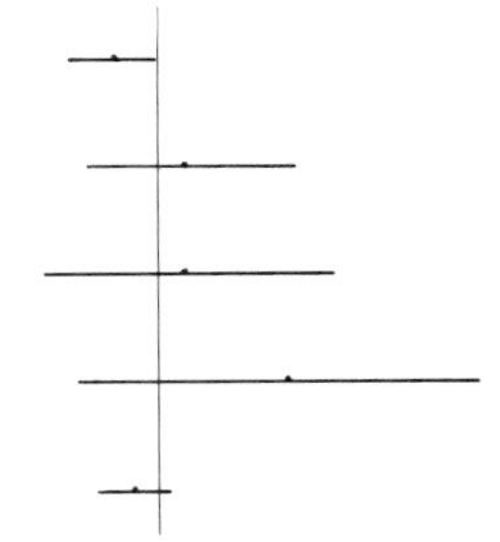

Table 40.9 Effect of cervical cerclage (all trials) on delivery <37 weeks' gestation

Study	EXPT		CTRL		Odds ratio	Graph of odds ratios and confidence intervals
	n	(%)	*n*	(%)	(95% CI)	0.01 0.1 0.5 1 2 10 100
MRC/RCOG (1988)	124/454	(27.31)	146/451	(32.37)	0.79 (0.59–1.04)	
Rush *et al.* (1984)	33/96	(34.38)	31/98	(31.63)	1.13 (0.62–2.06)	
Dor *et al.* (1982)	13/25	(52.00)	14/25	(56.00)	0.85 (0.28–2.57)	
Lazar *et al.* (1984)	18/268	(6.72)	13/238	(5.46)	1.24 (0.60–2.57)	
Typical odds ratio (95% confidence interval)					0.88 (0.69–1.11)	

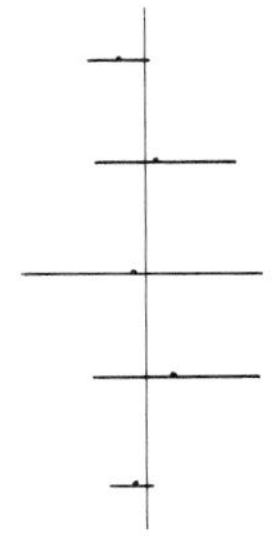

Table 40.10 Effect of cervical cerclage (all trials) on miscarriage, stillbirth, or neonatal death

Study	EXPT		CTRL		Odds ratio	Graph of odds ratios and confidence intervals
	n	(%)	*n*	(%)	(95% CI)	0.01 0.1 0.5 1 2 10 100
MRC/RCOG (1988)	37/454	(8.15)	54/451	(11.97)	0.66 (0.43–1.01)	
Rush *et al.* (1984)	9/96	(9.38)	9/98	(9.18)	1.02 (0.39–2.69)	
Dor *et al.* (1982)	7/25	(28.00)	6/25	(24.00)	1.23 (0.35–4.28)	
Lazar *et al.* (1984)	2/268	(0.75)	1/238	(0.42)	1.74 (0.18–16.84)	
Typical odds ratio (95% confidence interval)					0.76 (0.52–1.10)	

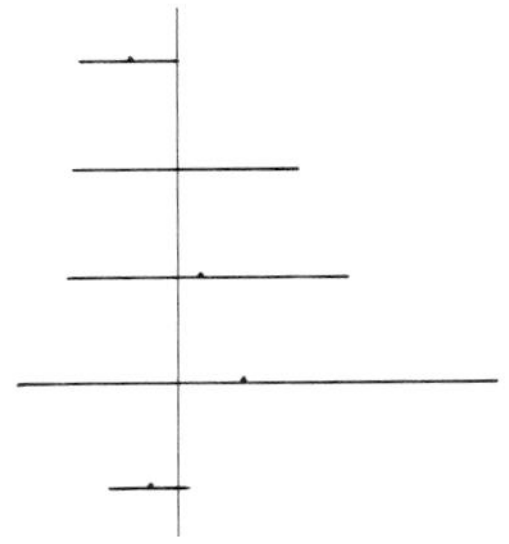

interval 0.52–3.04). So these results are compatible with a major benefit or a major adverse effect of the procedure on gestational age. The mortality rate (9 per cent) was the same in the 2 trial groups (Table 40.10).

Substantially the largest amount of data is provided by the interim results of the MRC/RCOG trial and these tend to suggest a beneficial effect of cerclage. The difference between the 2 trial groups in deliveries before 33 weeks, 13.0 per cent vs. 18.2 per cent (Table 40.8) is just statistically significant at the 5 per cent level (odds ratio = 0.67; 95 per cent confidence interval 0.47–0.97). Another way of putting these results is that an estimated 20 women must have cervical sutures inserted to prevent one delivery before 33 weeks, but the number of women requiring sutures to achieve this effect may be as few as 10 or as many as 100. The number of deliveries between 33 and 36 weeks is the same in the 2 trial groups, so the 5 per cent difference between the groups persists for the incidence of preterm birth (27 per cent vs. 32 per cent) but gives a smaller relative reduction (odds ratio = 0.79; 95 per cent confidence interval 0.59–1.04, Table 40.9). The mortality difference is in the same direction and similar order of magnitude (odds ratio = 0.66; 95 per cent confidence interval 0.43–1.01, Table 40.10) and reflects both a lower rate of miscarriage or stillbirth and (particularly) a lower rate of neonatal death.

3.4 Cervical cerclage for specific indications

The relatively broad entry criteria of the MRC/RCOG trial has led to the recruitment of women considered to be at risk of 'cervical incompetence' for a variety of reasons. The usefulness of cervical cerclage is likely to depend on the indications for the operation. Possible differential effects of cervical cerclage have been investigated in secondary analyses of the MRC/RCOG data stratified by possible indications for cerclage, such as past obstetric history of 2nd-trimester miscarriage or preterm delivery, or previous surgery to the cervix, or

Table 40.11 Effect of prophylactic cervical cerclage after previous 2nd-trimester miscarriage and/or preterm delivery on delivery <33 weeks' gestation

Study	EXPT *n*	EXPT (%)	CTRL *n*	CTRL (%)	Odds ratio (95% CI)	Graph of odds ratios and confidence intervals (0.01 0.1 0.5 1 2 10 100)
MRC/RCOG (1988)	43/325	(13.23)	61/305	(20.00)	0.61 (0.40–0.93)	
Rush *et al.* (1984)	12/96	(12.50)	10/98	(10.20)	1.26 (0.52–3.04)	
Typical odds ratio (95% confidence interval)					0.70 (0.48–1.02)	

Effect of prophylactic cervical cerclage after previous 2nd-trimester miscarriage and/or preterm delivery on delivery <37 weeks' gestation

Study	EXPT *n*	EXPT (%)	CTRL *n*	CTRL (%)	Odds ratio (95% CI)	Graph of odds ratios and confidence intervals
MRC/RCOG (1988)	88/325	(27.08)	105/305	(34.43)	0.71 (0.50–0.99)	
Rush *et al.* (1984)	33/96	(34.38)	31/98	(31.63)	1.13 (0.62–2.06)	
Typical odds ratio (95% confidence interval)					0.79 (0.59–1.07)	

Effect of prophylactic cervical cerclage after previous 2nd-trimester miscarriage and/or preterm delivery on miscarriage, stillbirth, or neonatal death

Study	EXPT *n*	EXPT (%)	CTRL *n*	CTRL (%)	Odds ratio (95% CI)	Graph of odds ratios and confidence intervals (0.01 0.1 0.5 1 2 10 100)
MRC/RCOG (1988)	25/325	(7.69)	41/305	(13.44)	0.54 (0.33–0.90)	
Rush *et al.* (1984)	9/87	(10.34)	9/89	(10.11)	1.03 (0.39–2.71)	
Typical odds ratio (95% confidence interval)					0.62 (0.40–0.98)	

multiple pregnancy. Three of the strata generated in this way are broadly similar to women recruited to the other 3 trials.

3.4.1 Cervical cerclage after previous 2nd trimester miscarriage and/or preterm delivery

Six hundred and thirty women (70 per cent) in the MRC/RCOG interim analysis had singleton pregnancies and a past history of one or more 2nd-trimester miscarriage or preterm delivery (but no history of surgery to the cervix). These characteristics are similar to the entry criteria of the South African trial (Rush *et al.* 1984). Table 40.11 is an 'overview' of the outcome in these two trials in respect of delivery before 33 weeks, preterm delivery and fetal or neonatal death. As discussed earlier, the South African trial, if anything, suggested a small adverse effect of cerclage but with wide confidence intervals. In contrast the stratified analysis of the MRC/RCOG data suggests a large beneficial effect of the operation with estimates of the odds ratios of 0.61, 0.71, and 0.54, in respect of these three outcomes. In fact this analysis revealed that most of the differences observed in the primary analyses were in women with a past history of 2nd-trimester miscarriage or preterm delivery. Furthermore, the more early deliveries in the past the greater the apparent benefit. The MRC/RCOG trial provides 80 per cent of the data in Table 40.11 so the 'typical odds ratios' are from 0.6–0.8 with confidence intervals between about 0.4 and 1.1. To put these results in another way, the estimate is that the insertion of about 18 cervical sutures will prevent 1 delivery before 33 weeks but this statement cannot be made with great confidence.

3.4.2 Previous surgery to the cervix as an indication for cervical cerclage

Only 96 cases in the MRC/RCOG interim analysis had a past history of cone biopsy or cervical amputation. The odds ratios for the main measures of outcome were all near unity, but with such wide confidence intervals these analyses are of little practical usefulness. Far larger numbers are required.

Table 40.12 Effect of prophylactic cervical cerclage in twin pregnancy on delivery <33 weeks' gestation

Study	EXPT n	EXPT (%)	CTRL n	CTRL (%)	Odds ratio (95% CI)	Graph of odds ratios and confidence intervals (0.01 0.1 0.5 1 2 10 100)
MRC/RCOG (1988)	1/10	(10.00)	4/14	(28.57)	0.34 (0.05–2.40)	
Dor *et al.* (1982)	6/25	(24.00)	5/25	(20.00)	1.26 (0.33–4.73)	
Typical odds ratio (95% confidence interval)					0.83 (0.28–2.49)	

Effect of prophylactic cervical cerclage in twin pregnancy on delivery <37 week's gestation

Study	EXPT n	EXPT (%)	CTRL n	CTRL (%)	Odds ratio (95% CI)	Graph
MRC/RCOG (1988)	6/10	(60.00)	7/14	(50.00)	1.47 (0.30–7.25)	
Dor *et al.* (1982)	13/25	(52.00)	14/25	(56.00)	0.85 (0.28–2.57)	
Typical odds ratio (95% confidence interval)					1.02 (0.41–2.52)	

Effect of prophylactic cervical cerclage in twin pregnancy on miscarriage, stillbirth, or neonatal death

Study	EXPT n	EXPT (%)	CTRL n	CTRL (%)	Odds ratio (95% CI)	Graph
MRC/RCOG (1988)	1/10	(10.00)	1/14	(7.14)	1.43 (0.08–25.35)	
Dor *et al.* (1982)	7/25	(28.00)	6/25	(24.00)	1.23 (0.35–4.28)	
Typical odds ratio (95% confidence interval)					1.26 (0.40–3.96)	

3.4.3 Twin pregnancy as an indication for cervical cerclage

The 50 cases in the Israeli trial (Dor *et al.* 1982) were all twin pregnancies and there were 24 twin pregnancies in the interim analysis of the MRC/RCOG trial. The outcome in respect of the three principal measures of outcome for these 74 cases is summarized in Table 40.12; the data are too sparse to allow any conclusions. In the Dor study, 14 of the 50 fetuses in the cerclage group did not survive the early neonatal period as opposed to 11 of the 50 in the control group. The timing of these losses was generally similar in the two groups. In the sutured group three women aborted in the 14th, 16th, and 17th weeks while in the non-sutured group two women aborted at 15 and 16 weeks. This demonstrates how difficult it is to judge whether in an individual case the insertion of a cervical suture actually caused an abortion. Three women in each group subsequently delivered prior to 33 completed weeks. The extra miscarriage in the sutured group is largely responsible for the difference in mortality: 39 (78 per cent) survived the neonatal period in the control group compared with 36 (72 per cent) in the cerclage group.

3.4.4 Cervical cerclage for other reasons in women at moderate or low risk of early delivery

One hundred and fifty-five women (17 per cent) included in the interim analysis of the MRC/RCOG trial had neither a previous 2nd-trimester miscarriage, nor preterm delivery, nor previous surgery to the cervix nor twin pregnancy. Many had histories of previous 1st-trimester miscarriages. This stratum seems most similar to the French trial and the outcome of these two groups is summarized in Table 40.13. Again the data are too few to be useful clinically, the confidence intervals of the typical odds ratios being very wide.

3.5 Cervical cerclage vs. Stutz pessary

The East German trial conducted by Förster and his colleagues (1986) compared cervical cerclage with Stutz pessary. As discussed earlier, there are major worries about selection bias. There were fewer deliveries before 33 weeks and before 37 weeks, and fewer fetal or neonatal deaths in the cerclage group, but the trial is too small to be clinically useful and the confidence intervals of the odds ratios are very wide (Table 40.14).

Table 40.13 Effect of prophylactic cervical cerclage for moderate risk of early delivery on delivery <33 weeks' gestation

Study	EXPT *n*	EXPT (%)	CTRL *n*	CTRL (%)	Odds ratio (95% CI)	Graph of odds ratios and confidence intervals (0.01 0.1 0.5 1 2 10 100)
MRC/RCOG (1988)	6/73	(8.22)	7/82	(8.54)	0.96 (0.31–2.98)	
Lazar *et al.* (1984)	4/268	(1.49)	1/238	(0.42)	2.99 (0.51–17.41)	
Typical odds ratio (95% confidence interval)					1.34 (0.52–3.47)	

Effect of prophylactic cervical cerclage for moderate risk of early delivery on delivery <37 weeks' gestation

Study	EXPT *n*	EXPT (%)	CTRL *n*	CTRL (%)	Odds ratio (95% CI)	Graph
MRC/RCOG (1988)	14/73	(19.18)	19/82	(23.17)	0.79 (0.37–1.70)	
Lazar *et al.* (1984)	18/268	(6.72)	13/238	(5.46)	1.24 (0.60–2.57)	
Typical odds ratio (95% confidence interval)					1.00 (0.59–1.70)	

Effect of prophylactic cervical cerclage for moderate risk of early delivery on miscarriage, stillbirth, or neonatal death

Study	EXPT *n*	EXPT (%)	CTRL *n*	CTRL (%)	Odds ratio (95% CI)	Graph
MRC/RCOG (1988)	3/73	(4.11)	5/82	(6.10)	0.67 (0.16–2.77)	
Lazar *et al.* (1984)	2/268	(0.75)	1/238	(0.42)	1.74 (0.18–16.84)	
Typical odds ratio (95% confidence interval)					0.87 (0.26–2.92)	

Table 40.14 Effect of Stutz pessary vs. cervical cerclage on delivery <33 weeks' gestation

Study	EXPT		CTRL		Odds ratio	Graph of odds ratios and confidence intervals
	n	(%)	*n*	(%)	(95% CI)	0.01 0.1 0.5 1 2 10 100
Förster *et al.* (1986)	7/130	(5.38)	10/112	(8.93)	0.58 (0.22–1.56)	
Typical odds ratio (95% confidence interval)					0.58 (0.22–1.56)	

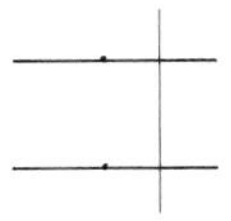

Effect of Stutz pessary vs. cervical cerclage on delivery <37 weeks' gestation

Study	EXPT		CTRL		Odds ratio	Graph of odds ratios and confidence intervals
Förster *et al.* (1986)	26/130	(20.00)	26/112	(23.21)	0.83 (0.45–1.53)	
Typical odds ratio (95% confidence interval)					0.83 (0.45–1.53)	

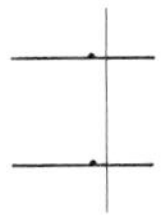

Effect of Stutz pessary vs. cervical cerclage on miscarriage, stillbirth, or neonatal death

Study	EXPT		CTRL		Odds ratio	Graph of odds ratios and confidence intervals
Förster *et al.* (1986)	5/130	(3.85)	6/112	(5.36)	0.71 (0.21–2.37)	
Typical odds ratio (95% confidence interval)					0.71 (0.21–2.37)	

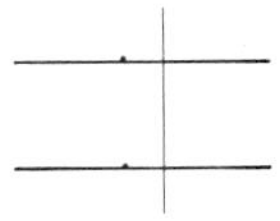

Table 40.15 Effect of cervical cerclage (all trials) on pre-labour rupture of membranes

Study	EXPT		CTRL		Odds ratio	Graph of odds ratios and confidence intervals
	n	(%)	*n*	(%)	(95% CI)	0.01 0.1 0.5 1 2 10 100
Rush *et al.* (1984)	18/96	(18.75)	12/98	(12.24)	1.64 (0.75–3.57)	
Dor *et al.* (1982)	2/25	(8.00)	3/25	(12.00)	0.65 (0.10–4.03)	
Typical odds ratio (95% confidence interval)					1.42 (0.70–2.91)	

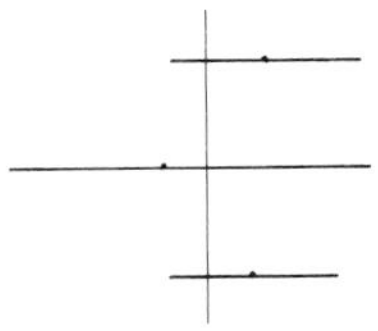

Table 40.16 Effect of cervical cerclage (all trials) on puerperal pyrexia

Study	EXPT		CTRL		Odds ratio	Graph of odds ratios and confidence intervals
	n	(%)	*n*	(%)	(95% CI)	0.01 0.1 0.5 1 2 10 100
MRC/RCOG (1988)	16/276	(5.80)	8/266	(3.01)	1.93 (0.85–4.37)	
Rush *et al.* (1984)	10/96	(10.42)	3/98	(3.06)	3.22 (1.05–9.91)	
Typical odds ratio (95% confidence interval)					2.31 (1.19–4.47)	

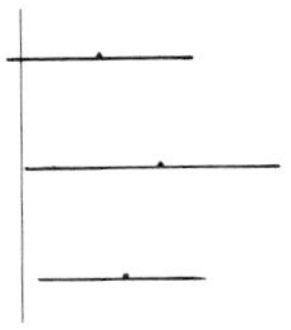

3.6 Evidence from the randomized trials of possible adverse effects of cervical cerclage

A wide variety of possible adverse effects of cervical cerclage were reported in the interim analysis of the MRC/RCOG trial. It was impossible to ascribe many of them to the operation with any confidence. Cervical trauma and difficulties in removing the stitch were each reported in six of the 450 cases with cerclage. Prelabour rupture of the membranes was associated with cervical cerclage in the South African trial (Rush *et al.* 1984) but this difference was not observed in the Israeli trial (Table 40.15). Puerperal pyrexia was reported more frequently in the cerclage group of both the MRC/RCOG trial and the South African trial (Table 40.16). This is consistent with the observational studies mentioned earlier and appears to be a real effect of the operation.

4 Conclusions

4.1 Implications for current practice

The operation of cervical cerclage may undoubtedly have adverse effects. These may be the, albeit uncommon, types of morbidity listed in Table 40.1, or increased medical intervention, for example admission to hospital and (probably) induction of labour and caesarean section. These events must be taken into account when considering the use of the operation.

The aim of the operation is to prolong pregnancy and thereby improve fetal and neonatal outcome. The 'classical' history of cervical incompetence is spontaneous miscarriage in the middle of pregnancy. The beneficial effect of cervical cerclage (if it has any) is therefore most likely to be a shift in the time of delivery of the (few) cases with true 'cervical incompetence' from the 2nd trimester to a time in gestation at which survival of the baby is more likely. On the basis of the evidence currently available the use of the operation in cases characterized by previous 2nd-trimester miscarriage or preterm delivery can be estimated to prevent 1 delivery before 33 weeks, about every 20 times it is used. This estimate is not very secure, however, and the true effect may be somewhat less or greater than this. Nevertheless, the suggestion of increasing effectiveness with increasing numbers of early deliveries in the past from the MRC/RCOG trial would seem to support the existence of the condition of 'cervical incompetence'. (Given that individual British gynaecologists only use the operation on average about 6 times each year, and would thus expect to see a difference of one less preterm delivery every 4 years, it is not surprising that clinical impressions have led to such a wide variation in the use of the operation.)

The evidence for the use of the operation in other circumstances, such as following cervical surgery, or in twin pregnancies, show no suggestion of benefit unlike when the decision is based on past obstetric history of 2nd-trimester miscarriage or preterm delivery. The data are, however, too sparse to reach any firm conclusion on this.

Unlike many clinical treatments cervical cerclage has the 'paradoxical' potential to both prevent and *cause* early delivery. The balance between these two effects is likely to depend on the inherent risk of early delivery in the cases treated. Taking this consideration and the other recognized adverse effects of the operation into account it seems sensible to limit the use of the operation to cases with a high likelihood of benefit. Current evidence suggests that increasing numbers of previous 2nd-trimester abortions or preterm deliveries constitute the firmest basis for making this decision. There is currently no good evidence to support the use of cervical cerclage on the basis of previous surgery to the cervix, multiple pregnancy, or other indications.

4.2 Implications for future research

The 1850 cases entered into the 5 randomized controlled trials reviewed in this chapter provide a less than adequate basis for clinical decisions about the use of cervical cerclage. A further 200 women have joined the MRC/RCOG trial but ideally far larger numbers are required, particularly for the important analyses of subgroups. The future of the MRC/RCOG trial is uncertain but at the time of writing it seems likely that recruitment will end soon, partly because the rate of recruitment has fallen and partly for financial reasons.

Prophylactic cervical cerclage looks most promising when based on a past history of previous 2nd-trimester miscarriage and, or preterm delivery. These are known, however, to have a variety of causes (Haxton and Bell 1983), not many of which could be altered by cervical cerclage. Better discrimination between those women who might benefit from cerclage and those who could not is urgently needed. This might be on the basis of a 'classical history of incompetence' for example, or by improved clinical methods of diagnosis. This research would probably be most satisfactorily performed in centres where cervical cerclage is used very little.

There is still controversy about the most appropriate technique to use for cervical cerclage. The Shirodkar approach is claimed to be more effective than the McDonald technique but it is more invasive and almost certainly associated with more side-effects. No formal randomized comparison has been made, but there is scope within the MRC/RCOG trial to compare the relative effects of the two techniques on outcome.

Cervical cerclage remains inadequately evaluated. The shame is that more randomized studies have not been conducted. Nevertheless, the trials which have been mounted are beginning to provide good evidence about the balance between the benefits and hazards. They provide a template for future research into the effectiveness of the procedure.

References

Aarnoudse JG, Huisjes HJ (1979). Complications of cerclage. Acta Obstet Gynecol Scand, 58: 255–257.

Anthony GS, Calder AA, Macnaughton MC (1982). Cervical resistance in patients with previous spontaneous mid-trimester abortion. Br J Obstet Gynaecol, 89: 1046–1049.

Bakketeig LS, Hoffman HJ, Harley EE (1979). The tendency to repeat gestational age and birthweight in successive births. Am J Obstet Gynecol, 135: 1086–1103.

Bates JL, Cropley T (1977). Complication of cervical cerclage. Lancet, ii: 1035.

Benson RC, Durfee R (1965). Transabdominal cervico-uterine cerclage during pregnancy for the treatment of cervical incompetence. Obstet Gynecol, 25: 145–155.

Berchuck A, Sokol RJ (1984). Cervicovaginal fistula formation: a new complication of Shirodkar cerclage. Am J Perinatol, i: 263–265.

Bergsjø P (1980). Aggressive cervical cerclage (letter). Am J Obstet Gynecol, 149: 240–241.

Brook I, Feingold M, Schwartz A, Zakut H (1981). Ultrasonography in the diagnosis of cervical incompetence in pregnancy—a new diagnostic approach. Br J Obstet Gynaecol, 88: 640–643.

Carr-Hill RA, Hall MH (1985). The repetition of spontaneous preterm labour. Br J Obstet Gynaecol, 92: 921–928.

Chalmers I (1984). Confronting Cochrane's challenge to obstetrics. Br J Obstet Gynaecol, 91:721–723.

Charles D, Edwards WR (1981). Infectious complications of cervical cerclage. Am J Obstet Gynecol, 141: 1065–1071.

Cole SK (1982). Cervical suture in Scotland: strengths and weaknesses in the use of routine clinical summaries. Br J Obstet Gynaecol, 89: 528–535.

Department of Health and Social Security (1982). Report on Confidential Enquiries into Maternal Deaths in England and Wales 1976–1978. Report on Health and Social Subjects No. 26, London: Her Majesty's Stationery Office.

Dor J, Shalev J, Mashiach G, Blankstein J, Serr DM (1982). Elective cervical suture of twin pregnancies diagnosed ultrasonically in the first trimester following induced ovulation. Gynaecol Obstet Invest, 13: 55–60.

Dunn LJ, Robinson JC, Steer CM (1959). Maternal death following suture of incompetent cervix during pregnancy. Am J Obstet Gynecol, 78: 335–339.

Förster Von F, During R, Schwarzlos G (1986). Treatment of cervical incompetence—cerclage or pessary? Zbl Gynäkol, 108: 230–237.

Grant A (ed) (1981–85) MRC/RCOG Randomized Cervical Cerclage Trial Newsletters 1–10. Oxford: National Perinatal Epidemiology Unit.

Green-Armytage VB, Browne JCM (1957). Habitual abortion due to insufficiency of the internal cervical os. Br Med J, 2: 128–131.

Harger JH (1980). Comparison of success and morbidity in cervical cerclage procedures. Obstet Gynecol, 56: 543–548.

Harger JH (1983). Cervical cerclage: patient selection, morbidity, and success rates. Clinics Perinatol, 10: 321–341.

Haxton MJ, Bell J (1983). Fetal anatomical abnormalities and other associated factors in middle-trimester abortion and their relevance to patient counselling. Br J Obstet Gynaecol, 90: 501–506.

Heinemann M-H, Tang C-K, Kramer EE (1977). Placental bacteremia and maternal sepsis complicating Shirodkar procedure. Am J Obstet Gynecol, 128: 226–228.

Jackson G, Pendleton HJ, Nichol B, Wittmann BK (1984). Diagnostic ultrasound in the assessment of patients with incompetent cervix. Br J Obstet Gynaecol, 91: 232–236.

Keirse MJN, Rush RW, Anderson ABM, Turnbull AC (1978). Risk of pre-term delivery in patients with previous pre-term delivery and/or abortion. Br J Obstet Gynaecol, 85: 81–85.

Kuhn RJP, Pepperell RJ (1977). Cervical ligation: a review of 242 pregnancies. Austral NZ J Obstet Gynaecol, 17: 79–83.

Lazar P, Servent R, Dreyfus J, Gueguen S, Papiernik E (1979). Comparison of two successive policies of cervical cerclage for the prevention of preterm birth. Eur J Obstet Gynaecol Reprod Biol, 9: 307–312.

Lazar P, Gueguen S, Dreyfus J, Renaud R, Pontonnier G, Papiernik E (1984). Multicentred controlled trial of cervical cerclage in women at moderate risk of preterm delivery. Br J Obstet Gynaecol, 91: 731–735.

Lindberg BS (1979). Maternal sepsis, uterine rupture and coagulopathy complicating cervical cerclage. Acta Obstet Gynecol Scand, 58: 317–319.

Lipshitz J (1975). Cerclage in the treatment of incompetent cervix. S Afr Med J, 99: (Obstetrics and Gynaecology Suppl): 2013–2015.

Loos W, Fischbach F, Graeff H (1985). Bacterial contamination of the cervix and complications during pregnancy after cerclage. Geburtshilfe Frauenheilk, 45: 646–650.

Macnaughton MC (1981). MRC/RCOG Cervical Cerclage Trial. Lancet, i: 1320.

McDonald IA (1957). Suture of the cervix for inevitable miscarriage. J Obstet Gynaecol Br Empire. 64: 346–350.

McDonald IA (1980). Cervical cerclage. Clin Obstet Gynaecol, 7: 461–479.

MRC/RCOG Working Party on Cervical Cerclage (1988). Interim report of the Medical Research Council/Royal College of Obstretricians and Gynaecologist multicentre randomised trial of cervical cerclage. Br J Obstet Gynaecol, 95: 437–445.

MRC Working Party on Preterm Labour (1979). Unpublished results of questionnaire.

Neuman MR, Merkatz IR, Selim MA, Zador IE, Roux JF (1980). Continuous monitoring of the cervical dilatation during labour and the measurement of cervical compliance in the human. In: Dilatation of the Uterine Cervix. Naftolin F, Stubblefield PG (eds). New York: Raven Press.

Page, EM (1958). Incompetent internal os of the cervix causing late abortion and premature labour. Technique for surgical repair. Obstet Gynecol, 12: 509–515.

Ritter HA (1978). Surgical closure of the incompetent cervix: 15 years' experience. Int J Gynecol Obstet, 16: 194–196.
Robboy MS (1973). The management of cervical incompetence. UCLA experience with cerclage procedures. Obstet Gynecol, 41: 108–112.
Rumeau-Rouquette C, du Mazaubrun C, Rabarison Y (1984). Naître en France; 10 ans d'évolution 1972–1981. INSERM, Paris, pp 70–71.
Rush RW (1979). Incidence of pre-term delivery in patients with previous pre-term delivery and/or abortion. S Afr Med J, 56: 1085–1087.
Rush RW, Isaacs S, McPherson K, Jones L, Chalmers I, Grant A. (1984). A randomized controlled trial of cervical cerclage in women at high risk of preterm delivery. Br J Obstet Gynaecol, 91: 724–730.
Schwartz D, Flamant R, Lellouch J (1980). Clinical Trials. London: Academic Press.
Shirodkar VN (1960). Habitual abortion in the second trimester. In: Contributions to Obstetrics and Gynaecology. Shirodkar VN (ed). Edinburgh: Livingstone.
Sinha DP, Nandakumar VC, Brough AK, Beebeejaun MS (1979). Relative cervical incompetence in twin pregnancy: assessment and efficacy of cervical suture. Acta Genet Med Gemellol, 28: 327–331.
Weekes ARL, Menzies DN, De Boer CH (1977). The relative efficacy of bed rest, cervical suture and no treatment in the management of twin pregnancy. Br J Obstet Gynaecol, 84: 161–164.
Witter FR (1984) Negative sonographic findings followed by rapid cervical dilatation due to cervical incompetence. Obstet Gynecol, 64: 136–137.
Wright EA (1987). Fetal salvage with cervical cerclage. Int J Gynaecol Obstet, 25: 13–16.

41 Abdominal decompression during pregnancy

G. Justus Hofmeyr

1 Introduction

Regular antenatal assessment of symptomless women has become the norm in developed countries. Among the more compelling justifications for this costly exercise is the need to detect impaired fetal growth and hypertension. Suboptimal maternal blood flow to the placenta is thought to be an important feature of both these conditions, yet there are no well-validated methods to increase the uteroplacental circulation. The concept that repeated brief decompression of the abdominal region may increase the flow of blood to the placenta has over the years intrigued a number of enthusiasts, but has not found acceptance in mainstream obstetric practice.

The principle of abdominal decompression was conceived in 1954 as an alternative method to curarization for relieving the resistance of the abdominal wall musculature to the forward movement of the contracting uterus during the first stage of labour (Heyns 1959). The first suit designed to decompress the entire abdominal circumference came into use in 1957, following experiments with a bucket-type suction apparatus applied to the anterior abdominal wall. The observation of unanticipated additional effects of the procedure such as the relief of the pain of labour, curtailment of the duration of labour, and improved fetal oxygenation prompted further investigation of the effects of abdominal decompression on physiological parameters and on clinical outcome in normal and abnormal pregnancies. The enthusiastic use of abdominal decompression in various centres during the 1960s and early 1970s has waned in recent years, although sporadic reports of its use continue to appear.

2 Technique

The apparatus consists of an airtight plastic suit worn over a rigid frame, or spacer, which encircles the woman's abdomen (Fig. 41.1). She is able to reduce the pressure within the spacer in accordance with her level of tolerance, usually to between −50 and −100 mm Hg, by progressively occluding (with her thumb) the vent in an exhaust tube connected to a high-flow vacuum pump. This is maintained for about 15 seconds in the minute over half an hour, 3 times daily to 3 times weekly during the antenatal period, or during labour to coincide with each uterine contraction. Considerable interference with breathing may be experienced, and dizziness and syncope may occur, presumably because of reduced cardiac return (Blecher 1967).

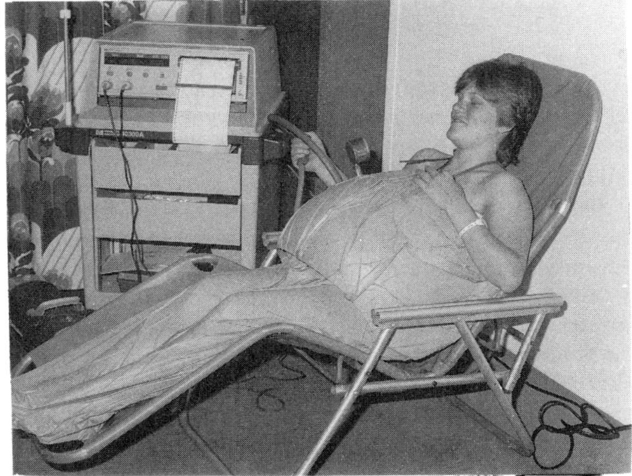

Fig. 41.1 Abdominal decompression equipment.

3 Physiological effects

On the whole, the few physiological studies of abdominal decompression have been poorly controlled and documented. The available data suggest that the technique may reduce intrauterine pressure (Heyns *et al.* 1962), increase maternal placental blood flow (Blecher 1968; Coxon and Haggith 1971) and increase fetal movements and fetal heart rate accelerations and oscillatory frequency (Pavelka and Salzer 1981). One recently reported study (Stange and Vaclavinkova 1983) found that abdominal decompression was associated with an increase in maternal cutaneous blood flow and a slight decrease in transcutaneous pO_2. The latter was thought by the investigators to be an artefact. No change was observed in either the baseline level or variability of the fetal heart rate.

It is obviously important to assess whether abdominal decompression can cause the physiological changes through which its possible clinical effects are likely to be mediated. The advent of blood velocity measurement with ultrasound using the Doppler effect (see Chapter 27) offers an opportunity to assess more rigorously whether or not abdominal decompression affects uteroplacental blood flow.

4 Prophylactic use in normal pregnancies

4.1 Short term effects

Information is available from two controlled trials about the effects of using abdominal decompression prophylactically in normal pregnancies. Coxon *et al.* (1973) compared the effects of high (−70 mm Hg) with low (−20 mm Hg) level abdominal decompression in healthy nulliparous women. The prospective randomized study of Liddicoat (1968) was mounted to assess the effects of the technique on child development (see below). No perinatal data other than the mortality rate were analysed, but the original hospital notes of a proportion (256/329) of the women who participated in this study have been traced, and it is now possible to report on some perinatal details (Hofmeyr and Metrikin, unpublished data).

Only the trial of Coxon *et al.* (1973) provides information about the effect of abdominal decompression on the incidence of pre-eclampsia. The rate of admission to hospital for pre-eclampsia was similar in the two groups, although the mean duration of hospital stay was significantly shorter in the high decompression group (5.0 vs. 10.6 days). None of the available data suggest that prophylactic abdominal decompression affects duration of gestation (Table 41.1) or birth weight (Table 41.2). In the only trial in which it was reported (Coxon *et al.* 1973) mean (SEM) placental weight was actually statistically significantly lower in the high decompression group (627 vs. 653 g, $p < 0.05$). The available data give no support to suggestions based on poorly controlled observations that prophylactic abdominal decompression has a beneficial effect on the condition of the infant at birth. The incidence of depressed Apgar score (Table 41.3) is similar whether or not decompression is used. If anything, the perinatal mortality rate appears to be increased by prophylactic decompression (Table 41.4) although this may reflect a chance excess of deaths from causes unlikely to be influenced by the intervention.

Table 41.1 Mean (SEM) duration of gestation (weeks) of initially normal pregnancies with and without abdominal decompression

	Decompression	Control
Hofmeyr and Metrikin (unpub)	39.2 (0.2)	39.2 (0.2)
Coxon *et al.* (1973)	40.2 (0.09)	4.01 (0.09)

Table 41.2 Mean (SEM) birthweight (g) of babies born to women with initially normal pregnancies with and without abdominal decompression

	Decompression	Control
Coxon *et al.* (1973)	3250 (30)	3310 (30)
Hofmeyr and Metrikin (unpub)	3220 (44)	3223 (48)

4.2 Effect on child development

It was because Heyns (1962) had reported a higher developmental quotient in children whose mothers had received antenatal decompression than children in a non-randomized control group, that Liddicoat (1968) mounted her carefully controlled trial of the effects of abdominal decompression on child development. Of 37 multiparous and 348 nulliparous women with uncomplicated pregnancies who agreed to accept either management protocol, 331 underwent intelligence testing and then 329 were allocated by randomized numbers (administered by an independent person) to receive antenatal decompression or routine physiotherapy classes. The drop-out rate reached 45 per cent by 9 months and 56 per cent by 3 years of age, but the groups remained comparable in terms of maternal intelligence scores. Although the developmental scores (assessed blind to allocation) were very slightly higher in the study group at 28 days and at 3 years of age, the differences were not statistically significant.

Liddicoat (1968) observed that the mothers who had received abdominal decompression (who had also been

Table 41.3 Effect of prophylactic abdominal decompression in pregnancy on Apgar score <4 at 1 minute

Study	EXPT *n*	EXPT (%)	CTRL *n*	CTRL (%)	Odds ratio (95% CI)	Graph of odds ratios and confidence intervals (0.01 0.1 0.5 1 2 10 100)
Hofmeyr and Metrikin (unpub)	3/121	(2.48)	3/121	(2.48)	1.00 (0.20–5.04)	
Typical odds ratio (95% confidence interval)					1.00 (0.20–5.04)	

Table 41.4 Effect of prophylactic abdominal decompression in pregnancy on perinatal mortality

Study	EXPT *n*	EXPT (%)	CTRL *n*	CTRL (%)	Odds ratio (95% CI)	Graph of odds ratios and confidence intervals (0.01 0.1 0.5 1 2 10 100)
Liddicoat (1968)	6/141	(4.26)	3/157	(1.91)	2.22 (0.59–8.37)	
Coxon *et al.* (1973)	3/200	(1.50)	1/211	(0.47)	2.89 (0.40–20.70)	
Typical odds ratio (95% confidence interval)					2.41 (0.80–7.25)	

exposed to reports in the news media that abdominal decompression produced developmentally exceptional children) frequently gave manifestly unrealistic accounts of their children's abilities. At 3 years of age, 11 children were untestable. Of the 5 untestable children in the decompression group, 4 were untestable on account of uncontrollable temper tantrums and extreme irritability. The 6 control children who were untestable were so on account of shy, overdependent, nervous behaviour and obstinate refusal. Among the children tested, 14/89 children in the decompression group were noted to be undisciplined or aggressive compared with only 2/90 in the control group ($p = 0.0013$, Fisher's exact probability test) (Liddicoat 1967, unpublished data). It is at least possible that these differences in behaviour patterns between the groups resulted from a difference in parental expectations. The expectation of parents that, as a result of certain childbirth practices, a child has above average intelligence may influence their child rearing practices and family dynamics.

5 Abdominal decompression for treatment of the compromised fetus

In contrast to the lack of evidence that prophylactic abdominal decompression in normal pregnancies has any beneficial effects, there is some evidence that the technique may have a place in the management of pregnancies in which the risk of fetal compromise is increased. Three relevant trials have been reported. The article co-authored by Blecher and Heyns (1967) presented the results of comparisons between abdominal decompression and drug therapy in two separate study populations of women, all of whom had either pre-eclampsia, essential hypertension or chronic nephritis. Allocation to decompression or drug treatment was not at random but by strict alternation. Additional data have been abstracted from an unpublished doctoral thesis (Blecher 1967) for incorporation in the tables which follow.

In the second of the three relevant controlled trials, MacRae *et al.* (1971) randomly allocated 28 women with clinical evidence of impaired fetal growth and low urinary oestriol levels to receive abdominal decompression. In the third trial, Varma and Curzen (1973) alternately allocated 140 patients with certain gestational age and ultrasound measurement of the biparietal diameter below the 10th percentile, to receive abdominal decompression or to act as controls. Unfortunately, the alternate selection of patients was compromised by the exchange of 7 pairs of patients because of non-acceptance of the decompression procedure. Reference to a more detailed unpublished report of this trial (Varma 1975) has made it clear that it is not possible to reanalyse the data by allocated treatment to achieve an unbiased comparison, but the data have been included in the analysis presented below because of the high level of compliance (90 per cent) with the allocated treatment.

In the trial reported by Blecher and Heyns (1967), abdominal decompression appeared to have a beneficial effect on the progression of pre-eclampsia (Table 41.5).

Table 41.5 Effect of abdominal decompression for treatment of fetal compromise on unchanged or worsening pre-eclampsia

Study	EXPT		CTRL		Odds ratio	Graph of odds ratios and confidence intervals
	n	(%)	*n*	(%)	(95% CI)	0.01 0.1 0.5 1 2 10 100
Blecher (1967)	8/42	(19.05)	20/38	(52.63)	0.23 (0.09–0.58)	
Typical odds ratio (95% confidence interval)					0.23 (0.09–0.58)	

In both of the other controlled trials (MacRae *et al.* 1971; Varma and Curzen 1973) abdominal decompression appeared to be associated with a significantly greater increase in levels of urinary oestriol, although only Varma and Curzen actually presented data (1.68 (1.21) vs. 0.91 (0.74) mg per week (mean (SD)). In addition, Varma and Curzen (1973) found that abdominal decompression was associated with statistically significantly faster weekly growth in the fetal biparietal diameter (2.08 (0.36) vs. 1.49 (0.71) mm per week (mean (SD)). These differences between experimental and control groups in the Varma and Curzen trial were reflected in somewhat less use of induction of labour for 'placental insufficiency' in the decompression group (Table 41.6). Varma and Curzen also reported less fetal distress during labour in the group who had received decompression (Table 41.7).

Observer bias and possibly reporting bias may account for some or all of the putative effects of abdominal decompression noted above. The assessment of birthweight is less subject to large observer biases and data are available from all three trials. Abdominal decompression was associated with a substantial reduction in the incidence of low birthweight in two of the three trials (Table 41.8) and an increase in mean birthweight (2800(591) g vs. 2296(364) g) and placental weight in the third (MacRae *et al.* 1971). The available data suggest a reduction in the incidence of both depressed Apgar score (Table 41.9) and perinatal mortality (Table 41.10).

The studies reviewed above are thus suggestive of a beneficial effect of abdominal decompression on fetuses with impaired growth, but their methodological shortcomings limit their conclusiveness. Unfortunately, studies which are methodologically less sound continue to appear (Pavelka and Salzer 1981).

6 The effect of abdominal decompression during labour

Only one controlled trial has examined the effects of abdominal decompression used in labour. Matthews and Loeffler (1968) randomly allocated 20 healthy nulliparous women in early labour to receive abdominal decompression or to act as controls. Fetal scalp blood

Table 41.6 Effect of abdominal decompression for treatment of fetal compromise on induction for placental insufficiency

Study	EXPT		CTRL		Odds ratio	Graph of odds ratios and confidence intervals
	n	(%)	*n*	(%)	(95% CI)	0.01 0.1 0.5 1 2 10 100
Varma and Curzen (1973)	20/70	(28.57)	27/70	(38.57)	0.64 (0.32–1.29)	
Typical odds ratio (95% confidence interval)					0.64 (0.32–1.29)	

Table 41.7 Effect of abdominal decompression for treatment of fetal compromise on fetal distress in labour

Study	EXPT		CTRL		Odds ratio	Graph of odds ratios and confidence intervals
	n	(%)	*n*	(%)	(95% CI)	0.01 0.1 0.5 1 2 10 100
Varma and Curzen (1973)	10/70	(14.29)	27/70	(38.57)	0.29 (0.14–0.61)	
Typical odds ratio (95% confidence interval)					0.29 (0.14–0.61)	

Table 41.8 Effect of abdominal decompression for treatment of fetal compromise on low birthweight

Study	EXPT		CTRL		Odds ratio	Graph of odds ratios and confidence intervals
	n	(%)	*n*	(%)	(95% CI)	0.01 0.1 0.5 1 2 10 100
Varma and Curzen (1973)	18/70	(25.71)	58/70	(82.86)	0.10 (0.05–0.20)	
Blecher (1967)	40/84	(47.62)	55/80	(68.75)	0.42 (0.23–0.78)	
Typical odds ratio (95% confidence interval)					0.22 (0.14–0.34)	

Table 41.9 Effect of abdominal decompression for treatment of fetal compromise on Apgar score <6 at 1 minute

Study	EXPT		CTRL		Odds ratio	Graph of odds ratios and confidence intervals
	n	(%)	*n*	(%)	(95% CI)	0.01 0.1 0.5 1 2 10 100
Varma and Curzen (1973)	7/70	(10.00)	27/70	(38.57)	0.21 (0.10–0.46)	
Typical odds ratio (95% confidence interval)					0.21 (0.10–0.46)	

Table 41.10 Effect of abdominal decompression for treatment of fetal compromise on perinatal mortality

Study	EXPT		CTRL		Odds ratio	Graph of odds ratios and confidence intervals
	n	(%)	*n*	(%)	(95% CI)	0.01 0.1 0.5 1 2 10 100
Blecher (1967)	10/84	(11.90)	24/87	(27.59)	0.38 (0.18–0.79)	
MacRae *et al.* (1971)	1/28	(3.57)	2/28	(7.14)	0.50 (0.05–5.02)	
Varma and Curzen (1973)	2/70	(2.86)	8/70	(11.43)	0.28 (0.08–1.00)	
Typical odds ratio (95% confidence interval)					0.36 (0.19–0.67)	

Table 41.11 Effects of intrapartum abdominal decompression on changes in fetal scalp blood indices (Matthews and Loeffler 1968)

Parameter	Experimental	Control	Sig
Difference in blood–gas values after 20 minutes	$n = 10$	$n = 10$	p
pH (Mean (SEM))	+0.05 (0.03)	+0.01 (0.02)	NS
CO_2 mm Hg (Mean (SEM))	−9.1 (4.4)	−3.9 (1.9)	NS
BD mEq/1 (Mean (SEM))	−0.9 (1.5)	+0.8 (0.9)	NS
O_2 saturation % (Mean (SEM))	−0.86 (3.3)	−2.78 (4.1)	NS

gas indices tended to be better in the decompression groups, but the differences are easily ascribable to chance (Table 41.11). No information is available on other outcomes, including pain (Matthews, personal communication).

7 Conclusions

The notion that prophylactic abdominal decompression improves perinatal outcome and child development has provided a salutary lesson concerning the danger of drawing conclusions from poorly controlled clinical trials. There is some evidence that abdominal decompression may be of value in certain abnormal states of pregnancy but the studies reported to date are not of sufficient methodological quality to support the use of abdominal decompression except within the context of further, methodologically sound, controlled trials. Nevertheless, there are so few options for managing the compromised fetus other than elective delivery that it is important to subject abdominal decompression to further evaluation.

The advent of Doppler blood flow measurement offers an opportunity to assess the effect of abdominal decompression on uteroplacental and fetal blood flow. Future research should perhaps include the effects on blood flow and, more importantly, the clinical effects of abdominal decompression in conditions such as pre-eclampsia and impaired fetal growth. The role of the technique in the relief of labour pain, the augmentation of labour, and for the management of acute fetal distress should also be investigated further.

References

Blecher JA (1967). Aspects of the Physiology of Abdominal Decompression and Its Usage in the Toxaemias of Pregnancy and in Foetal Distress in Labour. MD thesis, University of the Witwatersrand, South Africa. 1: 12–22.

Blecher JA (1968). The volume of the maternal placental circulation before and after abdominal decompression. S Afr J Med Sci, 33: 43–48.

Blecher JA, Heyns OS (1967). Abdominal decompression in the treatment of the toxaemias of pregnancy. Lancet, 2: 621–625.

Coxon A, Fairweather DVI, Smyth CN, Frankenberg J, Vessey M (1973). A randomised double blind clinical trial of abdominal decompression for the prevention of pre-eclampsia. J Obstet Gynaecol Br Commnwlth, 80: 1081–1085.

Coxon A, Haggith JW (1971). The effects of abdominal decompression on vascular haemodynamics in pregnancy and labour. J Obstet Gynaecol Br Commnwlth, 78: 49–54.

Heyns OS (1959). Abdominal decompression in the first stage of labour. J Obstet Gynaecol Br Commnwlth, 66: 220–228.

Heyns OS (1962). Use of abdominal decompression in pregnancy and labour to improve foetal oxygenation. Dev Med Child Neurol, 4: 473–482.

Heyns OS, Samson NS, Graham JAC (1962). Influence of abdominal decompression on intra amniotic pressure and fetal oxygenation. Lancet, 1: 289–292.

Liddicoat R (1968). The effects of maternal antenatal decompression treatment on infant mental development. S Afr Med J, 42: 203–211.

MacRae DJ, Mohamedally SM, Willmot MP (1971). Clinical and endocrinological aspects of dysmaturity and the use of intermittent abdominal decompression in pregnancy. J Obstet Gynaecol Br Commnwlth, 78: 636–641.

Matthews DP, Loeffler FE (1968). The effect of abdominal decompression on fetal oxygenation during pregnancy and early labour. J Obstet Gynaecol Br Commnwlth, 75: 268–270.

Pavelka R, Salzer H (1981). Abdominal decompression. An approach towards treating placental insufficiency. Gynecol Obstet Invest, 12: 317-324.

Stange L, Vaclavinkova V (1983). Maternal blood flow and pO_2 changes during abdominal decompression treatment of poor intrauterine fetal growth. Int J Gynaecol Obstet, 21: 419–421.

Varma TR (1975). An Investigation into the Effect of Abdominal Decompression on Fetal Growth and Placental Function. PhD thesis, University of London.

Varma TR, Curzen P (1973). The effects of abdominal decompression on pregnancy complicated by the small-for-dates fetus. J Obstet Gynaecol Br Commnwlth, 80: 1086–1094.

42 Breech presentation and abnormal lie in late pregnancy

G. Justus Hofmeyr

1 Breech presentation

Breech presentation is sometimes associated with maternal or fetal abnormalities, but often it is simply an error of orientation that places a healthy mother and a healthy baby at risk of either a complicated vaginal delivery or caesarean section. Given the mobility of the fetus within the uterine cavity and the extreme variability of its position in early pregnancy, it is perhaps surprising that at the time of delivery the rate of breech presentation is as low as 3 to 4 per cent, and for singleton babies weighing more than 2500 g, 2.6 to 3 per cent (Kauppila 1975). The probability of breech presentation is to some extent increased by nulliparity (Westgren *et al.* 1985), previous breech birth (Tompkins 1946), uterine anomaly, contracted pelvis (Ranney 1973), use of anticonvulsant drugs (Robertson 1984), placenta praevia, cornual placenta (Stevenson 1950; Fianu and Vaclavinkova 1978), decreased or increased volume of amniotic fluid, curtailed gestation, fetal anomaly or fetal death, multiple pregnancy, extended fetal legs (Tompkins 1946), short umbilical cord (Soernes and Bakke 1986), decreased fetal activity (Moessinger *et al.* 1982), and impaired fetal growth (Westgren *et al.* 1985).

One may infer from these associations that the preponderance of cephalic presentations is the result of the active accommodation of the appropriately proportioned fetus to the appropriately shaped uterine cavity (Stevenson 1951). It is presumed that the vigorous fetus whose flexed legs occupy the narrower lower uterine pole is more likely to change position by kicking itself around than the fetus whose legs occupy the roomier upper uterine pole. This tendency is reduced when the breadth of space in the upper segment is encroached upon, and when engagement of the presenting part in the pelvic brim is prevented. Diminished amniotic fluid reduces the fetus's freedom to alter position, while excessive amniotic fluid reduces the effect of spacial factors, the fetus being positioned more randomly.

1.1 Risks of breech presentation

Breech presentation *per se* poses risk to the mother in that it increases the likelihood of caesarean section, and to the fetus because of the hazards of breech delivery. The likelihood of either of these consequences depends upon the obstetric situation and the policy of the institution towards breech delivery.

The rate of caesarean section for breech presentation has increased in recent years (see Chapter 69). National figures vary from, for example, 45 per cent for Norway (1983), 54 per cent for Canada (1980–81), 76 per cent for the United States (1983), and England and Wales (1980), to 93 per cent for Sweden (1981) (Notzon *et al.* 1987). There is also a variation among institutions (Green *et al.* 1982). The risk to the mother of the immediate and long term complications of caesarean section is thus a serious consideration (Collea *et al.* 1980) (see Chapters 69 and 70).

The increased risk, if any, to the baby from vaginal breech delivery is difficult to determine. Various estimates of the perinatal mortality attributable to breech presentation have varied from 0 to 35 per 1000 (Kauppila 1975). Rovinksy *et al.* (1973) have estimated the fetal risk in breech presentation, corrected for abnormalities which may have caused the malpresentation, to be four times that for cephalic presentation.

1.2 Diagnosis of breech presentation

Routine antenatal examination in late pregnancy should include assessment of the fetal presentation. Because the presentation is subject to spontaneous change, even in established labour at term, such assessment is valid only for the time at which it is made. It is a worthwhile routine to recheck the presentation immediately before performing caesarean section for supposed malpresentation.

Breech presentation may be suspected when there is a history of subcostal discomfort, or of fetal kicking felt in the lower uterus. Abdominal examination of the lower portion of the uterus reveals a fetal pole which lacks the firmness and spherical outline of the fetal head, and the recess between the head and shoulders. This finding should be confirmed by pelvic examination to exclude a deeply engaged fetal head, as fetal shoulders may be clinically indistinguishable from the breech. The head may be identified in the upper uterine segment by means of ballottement; because of the flexibility of the fetal neck, the movement of the head through the amniotic fluid has the characteristics of a free spherical structure. Movement of the breech, which must be accompanied by movement of the entire trunk, gives a characteristic impression of inertia. If doubt exists, findings may be confirmed with ultrasound.

1.3 Spontaneous cephalic version

Spontaneous changes of fetal polarity occur with decreasing frequency during the 3rd trimester of pregnancy, and more frequently from the breech to the vertex presentation than the reverse. The incidence of breech presentation at 29 to 32 weeks' gestation has been reported to be 14 per cent (Hughey 1985), and incidences reported at 32 weeks' range from 16 per cent (Scheer and Nubar 1976) and 15 per cent (Sorenson *et al.* 1979) to 6.7 per cent (Westgren *et al.* 1985). Westgren *et al.* (1985) found the likelihood of spontaneous cephalic version after 32 weeks' gestation to be 57 per cent and after 36 weeks 25 per cent. This was least for multiparae with a history of previous breech birth, intermediate for nulliparae and greatest for multiparae without a previous breech birth. Spontaneous version was less likely in pregnancies with extended fetal legs and short umbilical cord and was unrelated to placental position. Gottlicher and Madjaric (1985) found that spontaneous cephalic version occurred in 16 per cent of nulliparae and 58 per cent of multiparae after 33 weeks' gestation.

1.4 Promoting spontaneous cephalic version

A great variety of techniques has been used to promote correction of breech presentation. A midwifery technique claimed to be effective is to ask the mother to lie supine, hips slightly elevated and hips and knees flexed, and to gently roll through 180 degrees from side to side for 10 minutes, repeating this three times a day (S Lees, personal communication). Traditional midwives in Gazankulu, South Africa, attempt to correct abnormal presentations during labour by manually shaking the uterus while the mother is in the knee–elbow position on the floor (M Price, personal communication). Fomicheva (1979) reported an 87 per cent success rate using a 'complex of physical exercises' at 34–35 weeks' gestation, and even laser acupuncture has been used to promote external cephalic version (DiExng 1985).

Use of the knee–chest position by Elkins (1982) was associated with spontaneous version and normal vaginal birth in 65 of 71 women with ultrasound-confirmed breech presentation after 37 weeks' gestation. The woman is instructed to kneel with hips flexed slightly more than 90 degrees but thighs not pressing against the abdomen, and head, shoulders, and upper chest flat on the mattress. This is done for 15 minutes every 2 hours of waking for 5 days. Hofmeyr (1983) observed that during a study in which 60 women with breech presentation were enrolled, spontaneous cephalic version occurred in 5 women shortly after ultrasound examination and before enrolment in the study. It was usual for these women to turn over onto their hands and knees before alighting from the sonar examination couch. It was suggested that displacement of the presenting breech by the distended bladder requested for ultrasound examination may have contributed to the versions, and that this principle merited further investigation. Chenia and Crowther (1987) incorporated this suggestion as a modification of Elkins's procedure in a prospective randomized study. Seventy-six black African women with breech presentation beyond 37 weeks' gestation were allocated by randomized sealed envelope to practise the knee–chest procedure for 15 minutes prior to getting up in the morning (preferably with a full bladder), at midday and in the evening for 7 days, or to serve as controls. The small and statistically insignificant therapeutic gain of 8.6 per cent is consistent, at the 95 per cent confidence level, with anything between a true gain of 30 per cent and a negative effect of 13 per cent (normal approximation of the binomial distribution). The effectiveness, if any, of the knee–chest position is yet to be confirmed by controlled investigation.

In a randomized trial, Bung *et al.* (1987) studied the efficacy of a maternal positioning exercise—raising of the pelvis, abduction of the thighs, and relaxed abdominal breathing—for the purpose of promoting spontaneous version of the fetus from breech to vertex. The baby delivered as a breech in 9/30 (30 per cent) in the exercise group, compared to 14/31 (45 per cent) in the untreated control group. The participants reported that the exercises, which they practised for between 10 minutes and 60 minutes a day, were relaxing and comfortable.

2 External cephalic version

The wide variation of opinion on the usefulness of external cephalic version was succinctly summarized by MacArthur (1964) who wrote: 'There are those who enthusiastically recommend it, those who violently oppose it, and still others who express a rather elegant distaste for it.'

2.1 Factors influencing the decision to attempt external cephalic version

The decision whether or not to attempt external cephalic version will be influenced by the relative utility to mother and baby of having a cephalic presentation at the time of birth, the likelihood of spontaneous conversion to a cephalic presentation, the risks to the mother and baby of external cephalic version, and the effectiveness of version in achieving a cephalic presentation at the time of birth. The very existence of a breech presentation may be an indication of fetal compromise associated with an inappropriate volume of amniotic fluid or fetal lethargy, and conversion to a cephalic presentation will not greatly reduce that risk.

Successful performance of external cephalic version is a satisfying event. Immediate 'success' rates, however, are irrelevant. The important question is whether or not external cephalic version is more likely than expectant management to be followed by cephalic presentation at the onset of labour.

Before the use of tocolytic drugs, external cephalic version was almost always attempted before 36 weeks' gestation, because the procedure was rarely found to be successful after that gestational period. By the mid 1970s, reports of a fetal mortality rate in the region of 1 per cent (Bradley-Watson 1975), and the increasing popularity of caesarean section for breech delivery (Lyons and Papsin 1978) resulted in declining use of the procedure.

In 1975 Saling and Müller-Holve reported that external cephalic version could be achieved in the majority of cases after 37 weeks' gestation, provided that the uterus was relaxed with betamimetic agents. There are fundamental differences between external cephalic version attempted before term and at term, and it is essential that these two approaches be considered separately.

Delay of external cephalic version attempts until term allows time for spontaneous version to take place in a maximal number of cases, and also allows time for any complications that may contraindicate attempts at external cephalic version, or that may require delivery by caesarean section, to become apparent. Examples of such conditions would include, among others, poor fetal growth, pre-eclampsia, or antepartum haemorrhage. Thus, by waiting until term, fewer unnecessary attempts at external cephalic version are required.

External cephalic version before term is usually carried out without adjuvant medication, although it is at times facilitated by sedation or anaesthesia. At term, betamimetic agents are frequently used to relax the uterus. Fetal bradycardia following external cephalic version before term has been managed by reversion to the breech presentation, while complications at term can be managed by prompt abdominal delivery of the mature infant. The fetal mortality rate associated with external cephalic version at term has been reported to be lower than that before term (Müller-Holve 1979). Following successful external cephalic version at term, fewer reversions to the breech presentation occur. The major disadvantage of delaying external cephalic version till term is that the opportunity to attempt external cephalic version may be missed in women whose membranes rupture or whose labour commences before term. Indeed, it has been suggested that the latter complication may be promoted by the persistent breech presentation (Rannay 1973).

2.2 External cephalic version before term

The effectiveness of external cephalic version before term remains controversial. Although non-randomized studies suggest that it may reduce the incidence of breech delivery (Table 42.1), three randomized controlled trials of external cephalic version before term have failed to demonstrate any effect of the procedure on the incidence of breech birth, caesarean section rates and perinatal outcome (Tables 42.2, 42.3, 42.4, 45.5).

2.3 External cephalic version at term

Studies of external cephalic version at term show more consistency. The results of non-randomized studies of external cephalic version at term are shown in Table 42.6. The effect on the incidence of breech birth, compared with a preceding period of time when external cephalic version was not attempted, is very similar to that found in the non-randomized studies of external cephalic version before term, i.e. a reduction in the incidence of breech delivery to about 1.5 per cent. This was achieved by attempting external cephalic version in 2.2 per cent of the obstetric population, as compared to 5.7 per cent in the studies with complete data for external cephalic version before term (Table 42.1).

Three randomized trials of external cephalic version at term have been published (Tables 42.7, 42.8, 42.9). All three showed that the external cephalic version significantly reduces the incidence of breech presentation at birth (Table 42.7). Factors found in various studies to influence the success rate of external cephalic

Table 42.1 External cephalic version before term. Success rate, incidence of breech delivery with and without ECV policy, and fetal mortality related to ECV attempts

Authors	ECV attempts (patients)	Vertex at birth	Breech birth >2500 g	Breech birth 'control' period or unit	Fetal deaths
Ryder (1943)	214	198 (92.5%)	–	–	0
Beischer and Townsend (1960)	356	–	173/ 5605 (3.1%)	61/ 1430 (4.3%)	2
MacArthur (1964)	617	582 (94.5%)	35/ 2078 (1.2%)	47/ 1381 (3.4%)	0
Thornhill (1965)	78	66 (84.6%)	–	–	0
Friedlander (1966)	706	692* (98.0%)	–	–	0
Ellis (1968)	314	258 (82.2%)	–	–	3
Bock (1969)	296	240 (81.1%)	124/ 6058 (2.05%)	136/ 4316 (3.15%)	1
Bradley-Watson (1975)	866	806 (93%)	– (2.5%)	–	8
Ylikarkala and Hartikainen-Sorri (1977)	491	374 (76.2%)	±545/18,783 (2.9%)	±688/15,279 (4.5%)	0
Total†	4177	3745 (90%)	877/33,424 (2.62%)	932/22,406 (4.16%)	16 (0.4%)

* Immediate ECV success only
† Excluding incomplete data

Table 42.2 Effect of external cephalic version before term on non-cephalic births

Study	EXPT		CTRL		Odds ratio	Graph of odds ratios and confidence intervals
	n	(%)	n	(%)	(95% CI)	0.01 0.1 0.5 1 2 10 100
Mensink and Huisjes (1980)	20/50	(40.00)	20/52	(38.46)	1.07 (0.48–2.35)	
Kasule *et al.* (1985)	162/310	(52.26)	168/330	(50.91)	1.06 (0.77–1.44)	
Brosset (1956)	15/74	(20.27)	16/73	(21.92)	0.91 (0.41–2.00)	
Typical odds ratio (95% confidence interval)					1.04 (0.79–1.36)	

Table 42.3 Effect of external cephalic version before term on caesarean section

Study	EXPT		CTRL		Odds ratio	Graph of odds ratios and confidence intervals
	n	(%)	n	(%)	(95% CI)	0.01 0.1 0.5 1 2 10 100
Mensink and Huisjes (1980)	7/50	(14.00)	4/52	(7.69)	1.91 (0.55–6.65)	
Kasule *et al.* (1985)	51/310	(16.45)	52/330	(15.76)	1.05 (0.69–1.60)	
Typical odds ratio (95% confidence interval)					1.12 (0.75–1.67)	

Table 42.4 Effect of external cephalic version before term on Apgar score <7 at 1 minute

Study	EXPT		CTRL		Odds ratio	Graph of odds ratios and confidence intervals
	n	(%)	*n*	(%)	(95% CI)	0.01 0.1 0.5 1 2 10 100
Mensink and Huisjes (1980)	6/50	(12.00)	10/52	(19.23)	0.58 (0.20–1.68)	
Kasule *et al.* (1985)	11/310	(3.55)	12/330	(3.64)	0.97 (0.42–2.24)	
Typical odds ratio (95% confidence interval)					0.80 (0.42–1.54)	

Table 42.5 Effect of external cephalic version before term on perinatal mortality

Study	EXPT		CTRL		Odds ratio	Graph of odds ratios and confidence intervals
	n	(%)	*n*	(%)	(95% CI)	0.01 0.1 0.5 1 2 10 100
Mensink and Huisjes (1980)	1/50	(2.00)	3/52	(5.77)	0.37 (0.05–2.72)	
Kasule *et al.* (1985)	8/310	(2.58)	5/330	(1.52)	1.71 (0.57–5.12)	
Typical odds ratio (95% confidence interval)					1.20 (0.46–3.13)	

Table 42.6 Reported influence of a policy of external cephalic version at term on the overall incidence of breech birth

Authors	Successful ECV	Breech birth rate	
		without ECV	with ECV
Saling and Müller-Holve (1975)	43/ 57 (75%)	88/ 2291 (3.8%)	28/ 1702 (1.6%)
Fall and Nillson (1979)	37/ 53 (70%)	– (2.8%)	41/ 2492 (1.6%)
Morrison *et al.* (1986)	207/304 (68%)	589/12,942 (4.6%)	366/13,221 (2.8%)
Rabinovici *et al.* (1986)	39/ 58 (67%)	119/ 3447 (3.5%)	133/ 4494 (2.5%)
Total*	326/472 (69%)	796/18,680 (4.3%)	535/19,417 (2.8%)

* Excluding incomplete data

Table 42.7 Effect of external cephalic version at term on non-cephalic births

Study	EXPT		CTRL		Odds ratio	Graph of odds ratios and confidence intervals
	n	(%)	*n*	(%)	(95% CI)	0.01 0.1 0.5 1 2 10 100
Van Dorsten *et al.* (1981)	8/25	(32.00)	19/23	(82.61)	0.13 (0.04–0.41)	
Hofmeyr (1983)	1/30	(3.33)	20/30	(66.67)	0.06 (0.02–0.19)	
Brocks *et al.* (1984)	17/31	(54.84)	29/34	(85.29)	0.23 (0.08–0.68)	
Typical odds ratio (95% confidence interval)					0.13 (0.07–0.23)	

Table 42.8 Effect of external cephalic version at term on caesarean section

Study	EXPT *n*	EXPT (%)	CTRL *n*	CTRL (%)	Odds ratio (95% CI)	Graph of odds ratios and confidence intervals (0.01 0.1 0.5 1 2 10 100)
Van Dorsten *et al.* (1981)	7/25	(28.00)	17/23	(73.91)	0.17 (0.05–0.51)	
Hofmeyr (1983)	6/30	(20.00)	13/30	(43.33)	0.35 (0.12–1.02)	
Brocks *et al.* (1984)	7/31	(22.58)	12/34	(35.29)	0.55 (0.19–1.58)	
Typical odds ratio (95% confidence interval)					0.32 (0.17–0.60)	

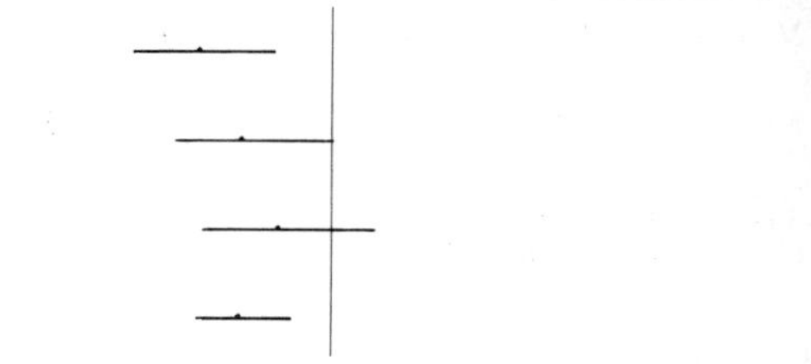

Table 42.9 Effect of external cephalic version at term on Apgar score <7 at 1 minute

Study	EXPT *n*	EXPT (%)	CTRL *n*	CTRL (%)	Odds ratio (95% CI)	Graph of odds ratios and confidence intervals (0.01 0.1 0.5 1 2 10 100)
Van Dorsten *et al.* (1981)	9/25	(36.00)	7/23	(30.43)	1.28 (0.39–4.20)	
Hofmeyr (1983)	3/30	(10.00)	5/30	(16.67)	0.57 (0.13–2.48)	
Typical odds ratio (95% confidence interval)					0.93 (0.37–2.34)	

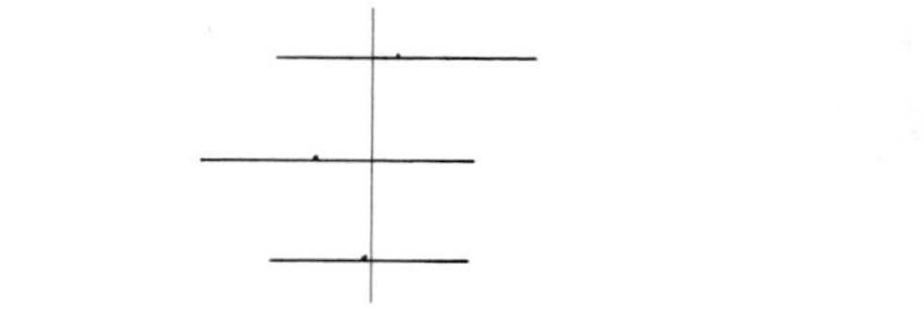

version at term are shown in Table 42.10. In general, these factors have a similar effect on the probability of spontaneous version (Hofmeyr *et al.* 1986). The fact that increasing gestational age and extended fetal legs seem to have less effect on the success of external cephalic version at term than that reported for external cephalic version before term may be related to the use of betamimetics to relax the uterus in the term studies.

Pooling of the data from these randomized trials indicates that in carefully selected patients the incidence of cephalic birth may be increased from about 22 per cent to 70 per cent, and the rate of caesarean section reduced from 42 per cent to 20 per cent (Table 42.8).

One trial (Robertson *et al.* 1987) has compared the effectiveness of external cephalic version with and without ritodrine tocolysis. The results were virtually identical: 5/30 (17 per cent) of the babies in the tocolysis group remained as a breech, compared to 6/28 (21 per cent) in the control group; 8/30 (27 per cent) women in the tocolysis group had caesarean sections, compared to 5/28 (18 per cent) in the control group. No differences in neonatal outcome were noted.

2.4 External cephalic version during labour

External cephalic version during labour is worthy of consideration as an extension of the trend towards version later in pregnancy (Hofmeyr 1983). In theory, this approach has several advantages. Maximum time would be allowed for spontaneous version to take place and for possible contraindications to external cephalic version to appear, thus limiting the number of attempts of versions that would be necessary. The risks of external cephalic version may be reduced further by performing the procedure in the labour ward, with continuous subsequent monitoring of the fetal condition until delivery. In cases assessed as unsuitable for vaginal breech birth, the external cephalic version may be attempted in the operating theatre, and in the event of failure followed immediately by caesarean section. A further advantage is that in Rh negative women, Anti-D gammaglobulin can be administered after delivery, and the unnecessary use in the 40 per cent of these women who will have Rh negative babies can be avoided. Disadvantages of the approach would include the inconvenience of version as an emergency rather than as an elective procedure, and the increased risk that the membranes may rupture spontaneously before external cephalic version can be attempted.

Earlier reports have included occasional references to attempted external cephalic versions during labour. Friedlander (1966) was successful in 3 out of 5 attempts, and Saling and Müller-Holve (1975) in 3 out of 6 attempts during labour, while Ranney (1973) referred to 2 successful cases. Ferguson and Dyson (1985) reported a series of 15 attempted external cephalic

Table 42.10 Factors associated with a decreased success rate for external cephalic version at term

Authors	Increased gestation	Nulli-parity	Extended legs	Anterior placenta	Lateral/ cornual placenta	Caucasian patient	Decreased liquor, lower birthweight
Saling and Müller-Holve (1975)	No	No	trend				
Fianu and Václavinková (1979)					Yes		
Van Dorsten *et al.* (1981)	No	trend					
Pluta *et al.* (1981)		Yes					
Kirkinen and Ylöstalo (1982)	No	No		Yes	No		Yes
Stine *et al.* (1985)	No	No	No				
Dyson *et al.* (1986)		Yes					
Hofmeyr *et al.* (1986)		trend	No		Yes	Yes	
Morrison *et al.* (1986)	Yes			No			
Rabinovici *et al.* (1986)	No	Yes		Yes			
Brocks *et al.* (1984)		Yes		Yes			

versions during labour in women considered unsuitable for vaginal breech delivery and who had intact membranes. External cephalic version was successful in 11 (73 per cent) and caesarean section avoided in 10 of these women. Attempts at external cephalic version after spontaneous rupture of the membranes were 'uniformly unsuccessful'.

Because of the disadvantages mentioned, it is unlikely that external cephalic version during labour will become a first-line approach for breech presentation. However, when breech presentation is encountered during labour prior to rupture of the membranes, the limited data available to date suggest that external cephalic version with tocolysis is a reasonable procedure to consider.

2.5 The risk of attempted external cephalic version

The risk of attempted external cephalic version to the mother is exceedingly small. It consists of the possibility of adverse effects from any of the drugs used to facilitate version and the hazards of placental abruption, a rare but recognized complication of external cephalic version. In 1969, Alexander and Newton reported a case of acute renal failure following attempted external cephalic version. Placental abruption was suspected but not proven, and the patient recovered completely. No cases of serious maternal complications have been reported since that time.

The small but real risks of external cephalic version to the fetus are related to its gestational age, and to the methods employed. External cephalic version performed before term has been associated with a fetal mortality of up to 1 per cent (Bradley-Watson 1975). Müller-Holve (1979) found that the complication rate was greater when external cephalic version was attempted before 37 weeks' gestation; when general anaesthesia or a state close to general anaesthesia was induced; and when the placenta was situated anteriorly.

A review of the literature has revealed four reports of fetal death associated with external cephalic version at term (Table 42.11), and none when nitrous oxide and general anaesthesia were not used (Table 42.12). It may be that the mature fetus is better able to withstand the procedure, but the introduction of ultrasonography and cardiotocography to exclude fetal compromise may also

Table 42.11 Fetal mortality in reported series of external cephalic version at term using nitrous oxide or general anaesthesia

Authors	No. of patients	Successful ECV	Cephalic at birth	Fetal deaths
Saling and Müller-Holve (1975)	57	43 (75%)	40/54 (74%)	0
Berg and Kunze (1977)	10	7 (70%)	7 (70%)	1
Müller-Holve (1979)*	407	252 (62%)	–	3
Pluta *et al.* (1981)	508	268 (53%)	268 (53%)	0
Total	982	570 (58%)	315/572 (55%)	4 (0.4%)

* Abstracted from literature review

Table 42.12 Fetal mortality in reported series of external cephalic version at term without nitrous oxide or general anaesthesia

Authors	No. of patients	Successful ECV	Cephalic at birth	Fetal deaths
Müller-Holve (1979)	30	21 (70%)	–	0
Fall and Nillson (1979)	53	37 (70%)	38 (72%)	0
Fianu and Václavinková (1979)	74	48 (65%)	41 (55%)	0
Brocks *et al.* (1984)	74	30 (41%)	34 (46%)	0
Stine *et al.* (1985)*	148	108 (73%)	95/142 (67%)	0
Dyson *et al.* (1986)	158	122 (77%)	122 (77%)	0
Hofmeyr *et al.* (1986)*	80	62 (78%)	62 (78%)	0
Morrisen *et al.* (1986)	304	207 (68%)	201 (66%)	0
Rabinovici *et al.* (1986)	58	39 (67%)	40 (69%)	0
Total	979	674 (69%)	633/943 (67%)	0

* Cases from earlier randomized trials included

be responsible for the improved fetal outcome when external cephalic version is performed at term. Cardiotocographic recordings following attempted external cephalic version revealed baseline bradycardia lasting for 1 to 12 minutes in 9 per cent of cases, and a statistically significant reduction in fetal activity and fetal heart rate reactivity and variability compared with measurements made prior to external cephalic version (Hofmeyr and Sonnendecker 1983). Phelan *et al.* (1984) found bradycardia in 8 per cent and other abnormalities in 11 per cent of cardiotocograph recordings following an attempted external cephalic version. Decreased fetal heart rate variability was more common after than before attempted external cephalic version. All changes were temporary, however, and perinatal outcome was not worse in the group with fetal heart rate changes. The persistence of fetal heart rate and activity changes for some time after attempted external cephalic version suggests that these changes may result from a disturbance of oxygenation. For this reason, a limitation of the period of continuous pressure on the uterus to 5 minutes has been recommended (Hofmeyr 1983). Attempted external cephalic version has not resulted in changes in circulating blood levels of human placental lactogen and free estriol (Dudenhausen *et al.* 1981).

Isolated cases of fetal compromise as a result of attempted external cephalic version have been reported. A case of feto-maternal haemorrhage estimated to be in excess of 25 ml and presenting with maternal haemoglobinuria has been reported following external cephalic version under general anaesthesia at 35 weeks' gestation (Pollock 1968). Luyet *et al.* (1976) reported a case of massive feto-maternal bleeding and fetal death after external cephalic version. Gjøde *et al.* (1980) reported feto-maternal bleeding of 0.1 to 1.5 ml in 28 per cent of 50 women following attempted external cephalic version after 30 weeks' gestation (median gestation 37 weeks), and recommended routine administration of anti-D serum to Rh-negative women undergoing attempted external cephalic version (see Chapter 35).

Developmental screening at 2 to 5 years of 116 children subjected to attempted external cephalic version failed to demonstrate any additional risk for cerebral motor disturbances (Kouam 1985).

Compound presentation, often involving the vertex and feet, may follow successful external cephalic version, particularly when performed at term. Ang (1978) reported 2 such cases discovered at caesarean section performed for other reasons, and found reports of 12 cases in a review of the literature. I have encountered 1 such case, in which vaginal delivery followed spontaneous resolution of the foot and vertex presentation. Ang (1978), however, recommends delivery by caesarean section in such situations. Friedlander (1966) has suggested that the risk of compound presentation may be reduced by performing external cephalic version in the direction of a backward somersault when the fetal legs are extended. He argues that any obstruction encountered by the feet will tend to cause flexion of the legs.

Chapman *et al.* (1978) have reported one case of fetal spinal cord transection thought to be the result of inadvertent extension of the fetal neck during a failed attempt at external cephalic version at 36 weeks' gestation. Saling and Müller-Holve (1975) recommended the use of a backward somersault technique in which the primary manoeuvre is pressure against the fetal forehead. When a backward somersault is used, the primary pressure should be against the breech, which causes flexion rather than extension of the fetal spine.

Thus, attempted external cephalic version must be recognized as an invasive procedure that involves some risk to the fetus. Provided that fetal well-being is confirmed and monitored, and provided that appropriate precautions are observed, the risk to the mature fetus appears to be very small.

3 Oblique and transverse lie

Breech presentation is an error of polarity in which the forces necessary to maintain a longitudinal lie of the fetus are intact. Oblique and transverse lies are the result of an entirely different situation, in that the fetus fails to adopt a longitudinal lie. Abnormal lie is associated with multiparity, abdominal laxity, uterine and fetal anomalies, shortening of the longitudinal axis of the uterus by fundal or low-lying placenta (Stevenson 1949), and conditions which prevent the engagement of the presenting part such as pelvic tumour and small pelvic inlet. Clinical diagnostic features include the appearance of an unusually wide uterine outline and the absence of a palpable fetal pole symmetrically above or in the pelvic brim. Abnormal lie, particularly oblique lie, may be transitory and related to maternal position. Oblique lie is frequently erroneously diagnosed during ultrasound examination because of displacement of the presenting part by the over-distended maternal bladder.

When non-longitudinal lie is encountered after 32 weeks' gestation, underlying abnormalities should be sought. Further management options include antepartum attempts at external version, version at term followed by induction of labour, or expectant management with or without intrapartum attempted version if the abnormal lie persists.

The role of external version in the management of oblique and transverse lie has not been assessed in a randomized trial. A number of descriptive case series have been reported (Stevenson 1949; Hibbard and Schumann 1973; Ranney 1973). With expectant management most cases of abnormal lie will revert to the longitudinal lie by the time of delivery. The persistence rate of transverse lies has been found to be only 12 per cent (Fried 1984), 16 per cent (Hughey 1985) and in transverse lies documented after 37 weeks' gestation, 17 per cent (Phelan *et al.* 1986). Given the high spontaneous version rate and the unstable nature of the non-longitudinal lie with a high probability of reversion following external cephalic version (Phelan *et al.* 1986), there does not appear to be a strong case for external version prior to labour or planned delivery.

The risk of delaying intervention until the onset of labour is that cord prolapse or strong labour may occur prior to the woman's arrival at hospital. Phelan *et al.* (1986) followed the progress of 29 women with transverse lie after 37 weeks' gestation. Although only 5 (17 per cent) transverse lies persisted in labour, 13 women underwent caesarean section (45 per cent) and major complications included 2 cases of cord prolapse, one spontaneous rupture of the uterus in a grand multipara, and one neonatal death. These authors recommended that once fetal lung maturity is assured, external version should be attempted in the delivery area, presumably (though not stated) followed by induction of labour. While oxytocin is being administered, the longitudinal lie is maintained by gentle lateral pressure on the uterus until such time as it is felt to be stable, or can be made so by amniotomy. This is similar to the technique of 'stabilizing induction' reported by Edwards and Nicholson (1969). For failed version or unfavourable obstetric situations, such as fetal macrosomia without a favourable obstetric history, Phelan *et al.* (1986) recommend elective caesarean section.

Care of the woman with a transverse or oblique lie encountered during labour is more straightforward, as the choice lies between caesarean section and external version. Phelan *et al.* (1985) undertook a prospective uncontrolled study of external version for transverse lie in labour. Prerequisites were normal ultrasound and cardiotocographic assessment, and absence of contraindications to external version. Of 69 cases encountered (0.4 per cent of the obstetric population), 12 were enrolled in the study. Ritodrine was infused at 100 to 350 micrograms per minute. If cephalic presentation was obtained, the betamimetic infusion was stopped and the fetal position maintained until uterine tone returned. Provided the cervix was sufficiently dilated, the membranes were ruptured and internal fetal heart monitoring was commenced. Nine fetuses were converted to a cephalic presentation and 1 to breech. There were 6 normal vaginal deliveries. In addition to this 50 per cent reduction in the caesarean section rate, the need for midline uterine incisions in caesarean sections for transverse lie was reduced. There were no fetal or maternal complications associated with the procedure, though larger studies are needed to evaluate potential risks.

In the absence of controlled trials, the timing of intervention in pregnancies complicated by non-longitudinal lie must remain a matter of clinical judgement. The advantage of gaining fetal maturity, allowing time for spontaneous version to take place and allowing labour to begin spontaneously must be weighed against the risk of membrane rupture or cord prolapse before the version can be attempted. Once labour has begun or the decision has been made to terminate the pregnancy, the small reported experience indicates that attempted version in selected cases with immediate recourse to caesarean section if necessary, is a reasonable option. Further evaluation of its place in modern obstetrics is required.

4 Conclusions

The history of external cephalic version before term

provides a salutary example of the tendency for invasive obstetric procedures with impressive immediate results to become routine practice without proper evaluation. To date, the efficacy of external cephalic version before term is in serious doubt.

External cephalic version for breech presentation at term substantially reduces the incidence of breech birth and caesarean section. Appropriate selection and surveillance is important to ensure an acceptably low complication rate.

Further research is needed to evaluate the effectiveness of postural management of breech presentation and to determine the place and optimal timing of external version attempts for non longitudinal lie.

References

Alexander L, Newton J (1969). Acute renal failure after attempted external cephalic version. J Obstet Gynaecol Br Commnwlth, 76: 711–712.

Ang LT (1978). Compound presentation following external version. Austral NZ J Obstet Gynaecol, 18: 213–214.

Beischer NA, Townsend L (1960). External cephalic version in breech presentation. J Obstet Gynaecol Br Commnwlth, 67: 668–671.

Berg D, Kunze U (1977). Critical remarks on external cephalic version under tocolysis. Report on a case of antepartum fetal death. J Perinat Med, 5: 32–38.

Bock JE (1969). The influence of prophylactic external cephalic version on the incidence of breech delivery. Acta Obstet Gynecol Scand, 48: 215–221.

Bradley-Watson PJ (1975). The decreasing value of external cephalic version in modern obstetric practice. Am J Obstet Gynecol, 123: 237–240.

Brocks V, Philipsen T, Secher NJ (1984). A randomized trial of external cephalic version with tocolysis in late pregnancy. Br J Obstet Gynaecol, 91: 653–656.

Brosset A (1956). The value of prophylactic external version in cases of breech presentation. Acta Obstet Gynecol Scand, 35: 55–562.

Bung P, Huch R, Huch A (1987). Ist die indische wendung eine erfolgreiche Methode zur senkung der Beckenendlagefrequenz? Geburtsh Frauenheilk, 47: 202–205.

Chapman GP, Weller RD, Normand ILS, Gibbens D (1978). Spinal cord transection *in utero*. Br Med J, 2: 398.

Chenia F, Crowther C (1987). Does advice to assume the knee–chest position reduce the incidence of breech presentation at delivery? A randomized clinical trial. Birth, 14: 75–78.

Collea JV, Chein C, Quilligan EJ (1980). The randomised management of term frank breech presentation: a study of 208 cases. Am J Obstet Gynecol, 137: 235–243.

DiExng AH (1985). Observation of the conversion rate of breech presentation by laser acupuncture. Chung Hua Fu Chan Ko Tsa Chih, 20: 326–329 (Chi).

Dudenhausen JW, Pluta M, Forsterling R, Gesche J, Saling E (1981). Humanes plazentares Laktogen und unkonjugiertes Ostriol im mutterlich Blut vor und nach auserer wendung des Kindes aus Beckenendlage in schadellage in Terminnale. Geburtsh Frauenheilk, 41: 407–409.

Dyson DC, Ferguson JE, Hensleigh P (1986). Antepartum external cephalic version under tocolysis. Obstet Gynecol, 67: 63–68.

Edwards RL, Nicholson HO (1969). The management of the unstable lie in late pregnancy. J Obstet Gynaecol Br Commnwlth, 76: 713–718.

Elkins VH (1982). In: Effectiveness and Satisfaction in Antenatal Care. Enkin M, Chalmers I (eds). London: Spastics International Medical Publishers, p 216.

Ellis R (1968). External cephalic version under anaesthesia. J Obstet Gynaecol Br Commnwlth, 75: 865–870.

Fall O, Nilsson BA (1979). External cephalic version in breech presentation under tocolysis. Obstet Gynecol, 53: 712–715.

Ferguson JE, Dyson DC (1985). Intrapartum external cephalic version. Am J Obstet Gynecol, 152: 297–298.

Fianu S, Vaclavinkova V (1978). The site of placental attachment as a factor in the aetiology of breech presentation. Acta Obstet Gynecol Scand, 57: 371–372.

Fianu S, Vaclavinkova V (1979). External cephalic version in the management of breech presentation with special reference to the placental localisation. Acta Obstet Gynecol Scand, 58: 209–201.

Fomicheva VV (1979). Correction of pelvic presentation of the fetus by a complex of physical exercises (English abstract). Vopr Okhr Materin Det, 24: 73–76.

Fried AW, Cloutier M, Woodring JH, Shier RW (1984). Sonography of the transverse fetal lie. Am J Radiol, 142: 421–423.

Friedlander D (1966). External cephalic version in the management of breech presentation. Am J Obstet Gynecol, 95: 906–913.

Gjøde R, Rasmussen TB, Jorgensen J (1980). Fetomaternal bleeding during attempts at external version. Br J Obstet Gynaecol, 87: 571–573.

Gottlicher S, Madjaric J (1985). The position of the human foetus during pregnancy and the probability of a spontaneous change to vertex presentation in primiparae and multiparae. Geburtsh Frauenheilk, 45: 534–538.

Green JE, McLean F, Smith LP, Usher R (1982). Has an increased caesarean section rate for term breech delivery reduced the incidence of birth asphyxia, trauma and death? Am J Obstet Gynecol, 142: 643–648.

Hibbard LT, Schumann WR (1973). Prophylactic external cephalic version in an obstetric practice. Am J Obstet Gynecol, 116: 511–516.

Hofmeyr GJ (1983). Effect of external cephalic version in late pregnancy on breech presentation and caesarean section rate: a controlled trial. Br J Obstet Gynaecol, 90: 392–399.

Hofmeyr GJ, Sonnendecker EWW (1983). Cardiotocographic changes after external cephalic version. Br J Obstet Gynaecol, 90: 914–918.

Hofmeyr GJ, Sadan O, Myer IG, Galal KC, Simko G (1986). External cephalic version and spontaneous version rates: ethnic and other determinants. Br J Obstet Gynaecol, 93: 13–16.

Hughey MJ (1985). Fetal position during pregnancy. Am J Obstet Gynecol, 153: 885–886.

Kasule J, Chimbira THK, Brown IMcL (1985). Controlled trial of external cephalic version. Br J Obstet Gynaecol, 92: 14–18.

Kauppila O (1975). The perinatal mortality in breech deliveries and observations on affecting factors, a retrospective study of 2227 cases. Acta Obstet Gynecol Scand (Suppl), 39: 1–79.

Kirkinen P, Ylostalo P (1982). Ultrasonic examination before, external version of breech presentation. Gynecol Obstet Invest, 13: 90–97.

Kouam L (1985). Child development after abdominal version of the fetus from breech presentation to vertex presentation near term. Geburtsh Frauenheilk, 45: 83–90.

Luyet F, Schmid J, Maroni E, Duc G (1976). Massive fetomaternal transfusion during external cephalic version with fatal outcome. Arch Gynaekol, 221: 273–275.

Lyons ER, Papsin FR (1978). Caesarean section in the management of breech presentation. Am J Obstet Gynecol, 130: 558–561.

MacArthur JL (1964). Reduction of the hazards of breech presentation by external cephalic version. Am J Obstet Gynecol, 88: 302–306.

Mensink WFA, Huisjes HJ (1980). Is external version useful in breech presentation? (English abstract). Ned Tijdschr Geneeskd, 124: 1828–1831.

Morrison JC, Myatt RE, Martin JN, Meeks GR, Martin RW, Bacovaz ET, Wiser WL (1986). External cephalic version of the breech presentation under tocolysis. Am J Obstet Gynecol, 154: 900–903.

Moessinger AC, Blaus WA, Marone PA, Polsen DC (1982). Umbilical cord length as an index of fetal activity: experimental study and clinical implications. Pediatr Res, 16: 109-112.

Müller-Holve W (1979). Causes of complications in external cephalic versions (English abstract). Geburtsh Frauenheilk, 39: 635–641.

Notzon FC, Placek PJ, Taftel SS (1987). Comparisons of national cesarean section rates. New Engl J Med, 316: 386–389.

Phelan JP, Stine LE, Mueller E, McCart D, Yeh S (1984). Observations of fetal heart rate characteristics related to external cephalic version and tocolysis. Am J Obstet Gynecol, 149: 658–661.

Phelan JP, Stine LE, Edwards NB, Clark SL, Horenstein J (1985). The role of external version in the intrapartum management of the transverse lie presentation. Am J Obstet Gynecol, 151: 724–726.

Phelan JP, Boucher M, Mueller E, McCart D, Horenstein J, Clark SL (1986). The nonlaboring transverse lie: A management dilemma. J Reprod Med, 31: 184–186.

Pluta M, Schmidt S, Giffei JM, Saling E (1981). Die ausere wendung des Feten aus Beckenendlage schadellage in Terminnale unter Tokolyse. Z Geburtsh Perinat, 1985: 207–215.

Pollock A (1968). Transplacental haemorrhage after external cephalic version. Lancet, (i): 612.

Rabinovici J, Barkai G, Shaler J, Serr DM, Mashiach S (1986). Impact of a protocol for external cephalic version under tocolysis at term. Israel J Med Sci, 22: 34–40.

Ranney B (1973). The gentle art of external cephalic version. Am J Obstet Gynecol, 116: 239–248.

Robertson AW, Kopelman JN, Read JA, Duff P, Magelssen DJ, Dashow EE (1987). External cephalic version at term: is a tocolytic necessary? Obstet Gynecol, 70: 896–899.

Robertson IS (1984). Breech presentation associated with anticonvulsant drugs. J Obstet Gynecol, 4: 174–177.

Ryder GH (1943). Breech presentation treated by cephalic versions in the consecutive deliveries of 1700 women. Am J Obstet Gynecol, 45: 1004–1025.

Rovinsky JJ, Miller JA, Kaplan S (1973). Management of breech presentation at term. Am J Obstet Gynecol, 115: 497–513.

Saling E, Müller-Holve W (1975). External cephalic version under tocolysis. J Perinat Med, 3: 115–122.

Scheer K, Nubar J (1976). Variation of fetal presentation with gestational age. Am J Obstet Gynecol, 125: 269–270.

Soernes T, Bakke T (1986). The length of human umbilical cord in vertex and breech presentations. Am J Obstet Gynecol, 154: 1086–1087.

Sorenson T, Hasch E, Lange AP (1979). Fetal presentation during pregnancy. Lancet, ii: 477.

Stevenson CS (1949). Transverse or oblique presentation of the fetus in the last ten weeks of pregnancy: its causes, general nature and treatment. Am J Obstet Gynecol, 58: 432–446.

Stevenson CS (1950). The principal cause of breech presentation in single term pregnancies. Am J Obstet Gynecol, 60: 41–53.

Stevenson CS (1951). Certain concepts in the handling of breech and transverse presentations in late pregnancy. Am J Obstet Gynecol, 62: 488–505.

Stine CE, Phelan JP, Wallace R, Eglinton GS, van Dorsten JP, Schifrin BS (1985). Update on external cephalic version performed at term. Obstet Gynecol, 65: 642–646.

Thornhill PE (1965). Changes in fetal polarity near term—spontaneous and external version. Am J Obstet Gynecol, 93: 306–308.

Tompkins P (1946). An inquiry into the cause of breech presentation. Am J Obstet Gynecol, 51: 595–602.

Van Dorsten JP, Schifrin BS, Wallace RL (1981). Randomized control trial of external cephalic version with tocolysis in late pregnancy. Am J Obstet Gynecol, 141: 417–424.

Westgren M, Edvall H, Nordstrom E, Svalenius E (1985). Spontaneous cephalic version of breech presentation in the last trimester. Br J Obstet Gynaecol, 92: 19–22.

Ylikorkala O, Hartikainen-Sorri A (1977). Value of external version in fetal malpresentation in combination with the use of ultrasound. Acta Obstet Gynecol Scand, 56: 63-67.

Appendix 42.1 Technique of external cephalic version at term

Absolute contraindications

1. Multiple pregnancy
2. Antepartum haemorrhage
3. Placenta praevia
4. Caesarean section necessary irrespective of the presentation
5. Ruptured membranes
6. Severe fetal anomaly

Relative contraindications

1. Previous caesarean section
2. Hypertension
3. Impaired fetal growth
4. Obesity

Prerequisites

1. Recent ultrasound examination, or clinical assessment of adequate amniotic fluid volume and fetal growth (e.g. symphysis fundus measurement at least 30 cm).
2. Normal cardiotocography, or history of a consistent fetal movement pattern.
3. Informed consent.

Procedure (Fig. 42.1)

1. Position the mother on her side on a narrow examination couch, her back supported at about 45 degrees against the wall with a cushion. For a forward somersault the fetal back should be uppermost, for a backward somersault towards the couch. Preferably attempt a backward somersault first.
2. Apply (talcum) powder to the abdomen.

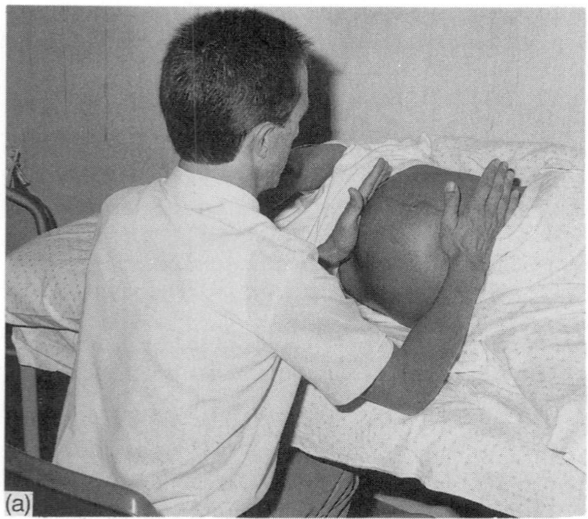
(a)

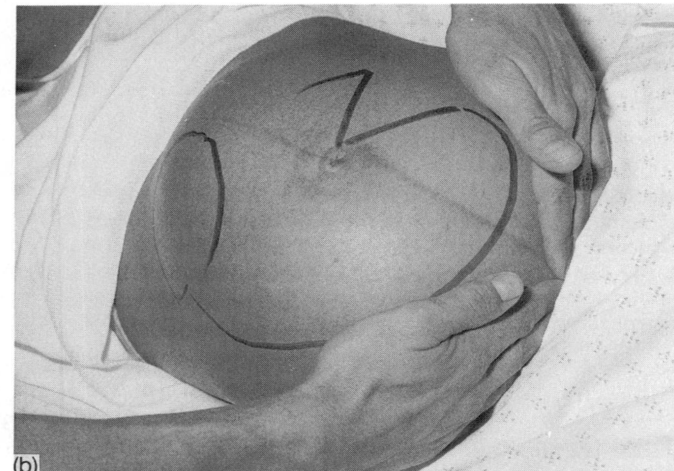
(b)

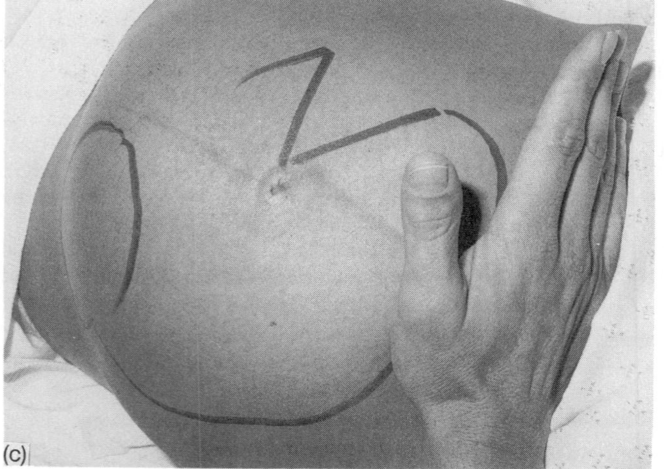
(c)

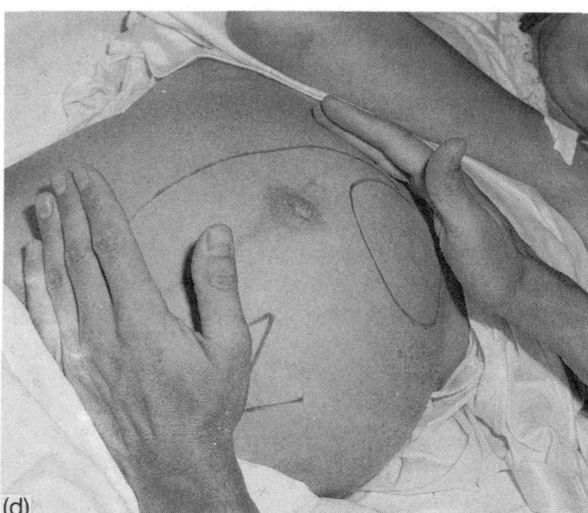
(d)

Fig. 42.1 Use of the semi-lateral position for ECV (Hofmeyr 1983).

3. Administer a tocolytic agent, e.g. hexoprenaline sulphate (Ipradol), 5 μg intravenous infusion over 20 sec, and provided maternal pulse remains below 120/min, a further 5 μg over 20 sec. Others have used intravenous infusions for 15 min before and during the procedure, of terbutaline sulphate (Bricanyl) 5 μg/min or ritodrine hydrochloride (Yutopar) 100 μg/min; terbutaline sulphate 250 μg intravenous infusion over 1–2 min; Fenoterol (Partusisten) 5 μg/min intravenous infusion 20 to 50 μg; isoxuprine 10 mg intramuscular injection: or salbutamol (Ventolin) infusion in increasing dosage up to 20 μg/min.
4. At all times steady and patiently persistent pressure is more effective than jerky or prodding movements.
5. If the breech is engaged or not easily mobilized, lift it from the pelvis by gently and slowly insinuating four fingertips of each hand between the breech and the pubic bones (Fig 42.1b). Rarely, disengagement of the breech *per vaginam* may be necessary.
6. Sit alongside the woman on a kitchen-type chair, elbow resting on the couch, and gently move the breech upwards towards the iliac fossa and then the upper flank, using the hypothenar edge of the palm (Fig 42.1c). This movement alone may result in version.
7. If necessary, use the other hand to guide the head towards the flank nearest the couch, then into the pelvis.
8. If unsuccessful, reposition the mother with her head at the opposite end of the couch, and attempt version in the opposite direction (Fig 42.1d).
9. If the head becomes inaccessible behind the costal margin, begin by guiding the head toward the flank in the direction of a forward somersault, then lift the breech and continue as above.
10. If unsuccessful, a similar technique may be attempted with the operator standing and the woman in only 15 degrees lateral tilt.
11. Auscultate the fetal heart every 2 min during the procedure, maintaining the fetal position while doing so. If bradycardia occurs, stop the procedure until the fetal heart rate has returned to normal.
12. Limit the duration of continuous pressure to 5 min per attempt. Allow at least 3 min rest between attempts.
13. After version maintain the longitudinal lie by gentle lateral pressure on each side of the uterus until it is felt to be stable.
14. Continue observation until repeat cardiotocography is normal or until fetal movements are felt and the heart rate is normal.
15. If persistent fetal distress is suspected, consider abdominal delivery.

43 Prelabour rupture of the membranes preterm

Marc J. N. C. Keirse, Arne Ohlsson, Pieter E. Treffers, and Humphrey H. H. Kanhai

'Premature rupture of the membranes is such a common and important event in obstetrics that it is surprising to find a tremendous divergence of opinion concerning its proper management'

Mead 1980

1 Introduction

Prelabour rupture of the membranes in the preterm period poses one of the most important therapeutic dilemmas in current obstetric practice. The incidence of the condition in the general population of pregnant women is only about 1 per cent (Kanhai 1981; Gibbs and Blanco 1982). However, if elective preterm deliveries, fetal death before labour, and twin pregnancies are excluded, then the incidence among women ultimately delivering either preterm (less than 37 weeks) or very preterm (less than 32 weeks; see Chapter 74) ranges between 40 and 60 per cent (Kanhai 1981; White *et al.* 1986; Verloove-Vanhorick and Verwey 1987; Van Kamp *et al.* 1989).

The divergence of opinion as to what constitutes the best care for these women was recently emphasized by the results of a questionnaire conducted among members of the Society of Perinatal Obstetricians in the United States and Canada (Capeless and Mead 1987). Ninety-seven per cent of these obstetricians reported that they would recommend 'expectant management' for women admitted with prelabour rupture of the membranes before 32 weeks of gestation; but opinions on the content of 'expectant management' varied enormously. The highest level of agreement reached related to an initial ultrasound examination; 245 of 261 respondents (94 per cent) said they would use it. All other issues relating to diagnostic follow-up and treatment provided a wide disparity of views, on occasions even among members of the same departments. Such disparity of views as to what constitutes the best form of care for women with preterm prelabour rupture of the membranes is not confined to North America, as surveys in Australia (Trudinger and Boshell 1987) and Europe (Keirse 1984, and unpublished data) have demonstrated.

2 Defining the problem

2.1 Prelabour rupture

Prelabour rupture of the membranes is often referred to as 'premature' rupture of the membranes. There is general consensus that this term should only be applied to situations in which it is clear that the membranes did not rupture at or after the onset of labour. There is less consensus on how long the interval (usually named the latent period; see Chapter 64) between rupture of the membranes and the onset of uterine contractions should be in order to substantiate the judgment that rupture of the membranes did not coincide with the onset of labour. Naturally, the longer the interval that is required, the stricter the definition will be and the fewer the number of women that will be considered to have prelabour rupture of the membranes. There are, however, no international recommendations or agreements as to how long the interval should be. This undoubtedly hinders epidemiological studies and comparisons of data from different centres, but it has virtually no direct consequences in considering what type of care is appropriate.

In this and the related Chapter on prelabour rupture of membranes at term (see Chapter 64) we have deliberately used the term 'prelabour' rather than 'premature', partly because of the ambiguity of the word 'premature' (see Chapter 74), and partly to avoid the confusion created by the use of different latent periods to define the condition. In essence, this chapter deals only with spontaneous rupture of the membranes preterm that does not coincide with or follow the onset of clinically detectable uterine contractions. This does not imply that the latent period between membrane rupture and the onset of uterine contractions is unimportant; nor does it imply ignorance of the fact that no pregnant uterus can ever be defined as entirely quiescent during pregnancy.

2.2 Preterm gestation

By international agreement preterm is now defined as a gestational age of less than 37 weeks, i.e. less than 259 days (FIGO News 1976; World Health Organization 1977; see also Chapter 74). This is not to say that the nature and the quantity of the risk associated with prelabour rupture of the membranes remains the same throughout the period of gestation defined as being preterm. On the contrary, general awareness that there are very different risks from early to late preterm gestations has already led to the introduction of new terms: for example, 'very preterm' to denote a gestational age of less than 32 weeks (see Chapter 74).

With regard to prelabour rupture of the membranes, preterm gestations can be divided into three broad categories, which represent different levels of anticipated fetal 'maturity' and may therefore require different forms of care. Prelabour rupture of the membranes may thus occur at a gestational age at which the infant has no chances of intact survival when brought into the outside world. It may occur at gestational ages at which the infant's chances of intact survival are nearly identical to those that apply at term. In between these two categories, there is a range of gestational ages at which the chances of survival will depend very much on the type of care that is given pre- and postnatally. For obvious reasons, the dividing lines between these three categories of gestational ages, important as they may be for the provision of care, cannot be sharply defined.

At the extreme lower end of the preterm gestational age range, all chances of improving perinatal outcome will depend entirely on the possibilities for maintaining an ongoing pregnancy. Any measures to achieve that end are likely to confer more benefit than harm to the infant, although the same does not necessarily apply to the mother. At the very other end of the preterm gestational age range, care policies should differ little, if at all, from those that apply after rupture of the membranes at term (see Chapter 64). At these gestational ages, the available evidence suggests that most active interventions and interferences with the spontaneous evolution of events should be considered to be potentially more harmful than beneficial. It is the category of gestational ages in between these two ends of the spectrum, roughly between 26 and 34 weeks, that present the greatest challenges for care.

2.3 Associated risks

By far the most common consequence of prelabour rupture of the membranes is preterm delivery. Irrespective of whether there is recognizable uterine contractility or not on admission, nearly all women with prelabour rupture of the membranes in the preterm period will, sooner or later, deliver preterm. Irrespective of how early in gestation they are, the majority of them will do so within a week (Taylor and Garite 1984; Beydoun and Yasin 1986; Kragt and Keirse 1989). The likelihood that delivery will be delayed for a week or longer is much greater at very early gestational ages than later in pregnancy, ranging from about 40 per cent when the membranes rupture before 24 weeks to less than 20 per cent if they rupture after 34 weeks (see also Chapter 64). Nevertheless, at all gestational ages delays of more than a week will be achieved by less than half of the women.

Prelabour rupture of the membranes may be associated with a variety of maternal, fetal, and obstetrical problems that are more common in women delivering preterm than in women delivering at term (see Chapter 74). It is often not appreciated that in about half of the women who deliver preterm after spontaneous preterm labour associated with pre-existent pathology in mother or fetus, the ultimate delivery process does not start with uterine contractions, but with prelabour rupture of the membranes (Kanhai 1981; Van Kamp *et al.* 1989). A careful assessment of the fetal and maternal condition is therefore required before any assessment of the risks of prelabour rupture of the membranes can be made, and certainly before any care options are put into practice.

The infant's ultimate chances of survival relate far more to gestational age at delivery than to gestational age at rupture of the membranes (Taylor and Garite

1984; Beydoun and Yasin 1986). This is because the degree of maturity of various organ systems, most notably the brain and the lungs, is the main determinant of mortality and morbidity. Infectious morbidity, mostly due to ascending intrauterine infection, is the second most important hazard for the baby. This risk too appears to be larger at lower gestational ages, possibly because of the relative immaturity of antibacterial defence mechanisms, but possibly also because of changes in the bacteriostatic properties of amniotic fluid with advancing gestational age (Naeye and Ross 1982).

The consequences of prelabour rupture of the membranes preterm are not limited to these two main risks of immaturity and infection. They also include increased risks of pulmonary hypoplasia and various deformities associated with persistent oligohydramnios (Nimrod *et al.* 1984; Taylor and Garite 1984; Thibeault *et al.* 1985; Bhutani *et al.* 1986); placental abruption (Breese 1961; Nelson *et al.* 1986; Vintzileos *et al.* 1987b); umbilical cord complications, either immediately or when labour supervenes (Fayez *et al.* 1978; Moberg *et al.* 1984); and mechanical difficulties, if caesarean section becomes necessary, of delivering a baby from a uterus that contains little, if any amniotic fluid and has a poorly developed lower segment (see Chapters 70 and 74).

3 Diagnosis

3.1 Ruptured membranes

The diagnosis of rupture of the membranes is in many instances obvious from the sudden gush of clear amniotic fluid from the vagina and its continued dribbling thereafter. If the rupture has occurred recently, it will often be possible to collect some fluid by sitting the woman on a suitable receptacle. Alternatively, it may be possible to obtain a sample from a pool of amniotic fluid in the posterior fornix on speculum examination. If, on the other hand, the rupture has occurred some hours previously and most fluid has escaped from the vagina, it may be difficult or impossible to establish or confirm the diagnosis with any degree of confidence. In these circumstances, much depends on taking a careful history from the woman. Information can be obtained as to when and how the gush of fluid occurred; whether anything like it has ever happened before (this should differentiate membrane rupture from the minor degrees of urinary incontinence that are sometimes present in late pregnancy; see Chapter 79); approximately how much fluid was lost (expressed in terms of spoonfuls, cupfuls or other familiar measures of volume); what the colour was like; whether it smelled of anything; and whether there was anything else remarkable. The latter question may elicit a comment on the presence of white or greasy particles, an answer that will be more reliable if it is not prompted by the wording of the question.

More rarely in early than in late gestation, and seldom before 32 weeks, vernix particles may be seen trapped in the pubic hair. Since there can be no doubt as to their origin, the diagnosis should be clear when this sign is present. If fluid is available, differentiation between amniotic fluid and urine, or vaginal secretions, is essential. Kragt and Keirse (1989) found that 20 per cent of women with preterm gestations who came to a labour and delivery unit with a primary complaint of 'aqueous discharge' did not have ruptured membranes.

On the whole, differentiation between amniotic fluid and urine is straightforward. If there are difficulties, most of them can be resolved by asking the woman to produce a sample of urine for comparison. Amniotic fluid contains protein while urine usually does not; this may readily allow differentiation with any one of the dip sticks that are commonly used to test urine at antenatal visits. Amniotic fluid, when put on a glass slide and allowed to dry, will assume a typical fern-like pattern when viewed under the microscope; urine will show no such pattern. The pH of urine will usually be acidic; that of amniotic fluid will be higher, at 7.1 to 7.3. Vernix particles or meconium, if present, are of course diagnostic for amniotic fluid and are never present in urine. Other tests, such as creatinine or uric acid determinations, all of which show much higher levels in urine than in amniotic fluid, are rarely, if ever needed.

Several tests have been developed for the specific purpose of differentiating liquor amnii, not only from urine, but also from various vaginal secretions and fluids (Friedman and McElin 1969; Smith 1976; Iannetta 1984; Rochelson *et al.* 1987). Some of the tests that have been advocated for the diagnosis of ruptured membranes are of little use in preterm gestations, because the contents of amniotic fluid change with gestational age. For instance, the nile blue test is likely to give false negative results below 36 weeks of gestation: the percentage of orange staining anucleate cells, on which the test depends, is only 10 per cent at 36 weeks and less than 1 per cent at 32 weeks (Brosens and Gordon 1965). Other tests, such as the recently introduced colorimetric alpha-fetoprotein monoclonal antibody test (Rochelson *et al.* 1987), have been designed especially for preterm gestations, but have not yet been adequately evaluated.

Among the various tests, the nitrazine test is probably the most widely used. Nitrazine paper changes colour from yellow-green to dark blue at a pH of 6.5 or more (Smith 1976), while the vaginal pH in pregnancy is usually between 4.5 and 6.0. Although nitrazine paper turns dark blue when exposed to the alkaline pH of amniotic fluid, it also does so on exposure to tap water, antiseptic solutions, cervical mucus, semen, blood, and even urine if the latter is alkaline (Friedman and McElin 1969; Smith 1976). This is why most people insist on using an additional test, usually microscopic observation of ferning, to limit the number of false positive results, which are in the order of about 15 per cent (Friedman and McElin 1969; Smith 1976; Rochelson *et al.* 1987). Although false positive and false negative results occur with all of these tests, the fern test is less likely to produce false positive results; unfortunately it has a higher rate of false negatives (Friedman and McElin 1969; Smith 1976), also when examined specifically at preterm gestations (Rochelson *et al.* 1987).

The invasive technique of transabdominal injection of dyes such as Evans blue, methylene blue, indigo carmine or sodium fluorescein into the amniotic cavity in order to watch for their subsequent appearance from the vagina (Atlay and Sutherst 1970; Smith 1976) cannot be justified.

Ultrasound, on the other hand, can be helpful in confirming the diagnosis. Although oligohydramnios due to rupture of the membranes does not differ from that due to other causes (such as severe fetal growth retardation or renal agenesis), the combination of a history of sudden release of liquor with ultrasound characteristics of oligohydramnios is unlikely to lead to an erroneous diagnosis.

Making the correct diagnosis in suspected prelabour rupture of the membranes is usually straightforward. High (hindwater) leaks may cause confusion, as may a long interval between membrane rupture and admission for care. Delay in presentation at hospital is likely only in those women who, for one reason or another, have had inadequate antenatal education and poor access to care. Usually these will be those with poor socioeconomic status, who unfortunately also appear to be at higher risk not only of prelabour rupture of the membranes (Reid 1970; Johnson *et al.* 1981; Perkins 1982), but also of infectious complications when prelabour rupture of the membranes occurs (Naeye and Blanc 1970; Naeye and Ross 1982; Perkins 1982). The development of more sophisticated tests for the diagnosis of prolonged ruptured membranes is not the most sensible approach to the problems faced by the women who are at increased risk of this problem. The provision of improved antenatal care more generally for such women should be seen as a more important challenge.

Regrettably, there is a dearth of information as to whether high (hindwater) rupture of the membranes should be considered as a clinically distinct entity from low rupture. This lack of information relates both to how these two types of rupture can be identified, and to whether or not these two types of rupture warrant different forms of care. In the absence of such data, the only practical proposition for care is to ignore such subdivisions and to concentrate on clinical signs that are known to correlate with outcome.

3.2 Vaginal examination

There are several statements in the literature that vaginal examination either introduces or increases the risk of intrauterine infection. No controlled comparisons have been conducted to substantiate or refute the belief that 'once an examination has been performed, the clock of infection starts to tick'.

Opinion in general is divided along two lines. The first, and most widely propagated opinion, holds that a careful, sterile speculum or digital examination should be carried out in all women with prelabour rupture of the membranes. The second, advocates that all vaginal examinations, whether by gloved fingers or by speculum, should be avoided unless women are in active labour. These two policies have not been evaluated in unbiased comparisons.

There has been only one controlled trial that purported to investigate the use of vaginal examination after prelabour rupture of the membranes. It was conducted by Munson and her colleagues (1985), but the authors did not state how they 'randomly selected' women 'from the outpatient clinics and labor admitting rooms' to have vaginal examinations. They reported that women were entered 'regardless of the presence of labor, rupture of the membranes, or maternal illness'. The only outcome that was addressed related to whether speculum examination could provide the same information on cervical effacement and dilatation as a digital examination. Munson *et al.* (1985) concluded that 'speculum examination should be adequate for most patients with ruptured membranes'. Unfortunately, they provided no information on the clinical consequences of the alternative policies, nor on how to identify women not belonging to the category of 'most patients'.

There is no reason to perform vaginal examinations unless they provide information that cannot be obtained by less invasive procedures, and unless that information is likely to be useful in determining the further pattern of care. This does not necessarily rule out the potential value of a single, careful vaginal examination to establish whether the membranes are ruptured or not, to determine fetal position, and to rule out complications (such as presentation or actual prolapse of the umbilical cord). On the negative side, are observational data that the risk of infection is higher when such examinations are performed (Schutte *et al.* 1983a), but from these data it is impossible to ascertain whether the risk of infection causally relates to the vaginal examination itself, to the prior risk of infection before the examination, or to whatever is done as a consequence of the examination.

In the absence of controlled comparisons, which seem to be urgently required, one can only speculate about the differential effects of any one of four possible diagnostic policies. These policies are: digital vaginal examination alone, speculum examination alone, both digital and speculum examination, and neither of these examinations. Evaluation of these policies would have to include positive and negative predictive values of the procedures (see Chapter 3) in confirming the ruptured membranes; the additional diagnoses that can be made and their utility in determining further patterns of care. It should also entail the risks and benefits to mother and baby; the likelihood of introducing infection; and the degree of maternal discomfort experienced.

The question of whether digital or speculum examination is better is only secondary to the more important question of whether it is better to avoid the introduction of any foreign objects, whether it be gloved fingers or a speculum. There is probably little benefit to be derived from performing both examinations instead of only one of them. On balance, the information that can be obtained by speculum examination, which may include visualization of amniotic fluid 'pooling' in the posterior fornix, collection of some of that fluid for nitrazine test, microscopic examination for ferning, or phosphatidylglycerol determination, and the collection of material for culture or screening for group B streptococci (see Chapter 34), would seem to be superior to that obtained by digital examination. On the other hand, speculum examination is likely to be more unpleasant for the mother than digital examination. Speculum examination is also unlikely to provide much useful information if the membranes have been ruptured for some time because the likelihood of observing amniotic fluid decreases rapidly within hours after rupture of the membranes.

3.3 Assessing the risk of infection

Any woman with prelabour rupture of the membranes should be assessed for signs of intrauterine infection. These include fever, maternal and fetal tachycardia, and leucocytosis. If either one of these is accompanied by a tender uterus and foul smelling liquor, there will be no doubt about the diagnosis. However, uterine tenderness and fetid discharge are late signs of intrauterine infection. Very different frequencies are thus reported for these symptoms (Koh *et al.* 1979; Gibbs *et al.* 1980; Ferguson *et al.* 1985). In a retrospective study of 171 women with a clinical diagnosis of acute chorioamnionitis, Gibbs and his colleagues (1980) found that foul-smelling amniotic fluid was present in 22 per cent of cases and uterine tenderness in 13 per cent of cases. The main issue, however, is not how to recognize fulminant intrauterine infection, but how to detect it in its incipient stages. The earliest clinical signs of intra-amniotic infection are thought to be fetal tachycardia and a slight elevation of maternal temperature (Gibbs 1977), but both signs are rather nonspecific. A few years ago, there were hopes that the estimation of C-reactive protein in the maternal circulation might be reasonably reliable as an early sign of intrauterine infection (Evans *et al.* 1980; Farb *et al.* 1983; Hawrylyshyn *et al.* 1983; Romem and Artal 1984). These hopes have not materialized; nor has the value (if any) of using C-reactive protein estimation ever been assessed in controlled comparisons.

Although intrauterine infection may on occasions precede rupture of the membranes (Naeye and Peters 1980; Guzick and Winn 1985), the main risk is infection ascending from the vagina into the uterine cavity. Information on the presence of pathogens may therefore be useful, particularly about those organisms that are the main bacteria responsible for the majority of fetal infections, such as the group B *streptococci*, *Escherichia coli*, and *Bacteroides*. The demonstration of vaginal colonization with one type of bacterium or another does not necessarily mean, however, that intrauterine infection will occur, nor that, if it does occur, it will be caused by these bacteria (see Chapter 34). Whether information on colonization is helpful in guiding the subsequent pattern of care is not known. What is known, is that intrapartum antibiotic treatment of mothers carrying group B streptococci in the vagina reduces the incidence of neonatal sepsis and neonatal death from infection (see Chapter 34). In some populations, colonization with these bacteria is found in up to 20 per cent of women with prelabour rupture of the membranes (Iams *et al.* 1985). In populations with a high prevalence of group B streptococci carriership, therefore, it would seem well worthwhile obtaining information on colonization in order to institute appropriate treatment before delivery (see Chapter 34). In view of the frequency with which clinical or subclinical infection ultimately develops after prelabour rupture of the membranes preterm, screening for these and other pathogens is probably beneficial in most, if not all populations.

In the past there have been several diagnostic protocols involving the use of amniocentesis, both for fetal lung maturity studies, and for identifying fetuses at risk of developing infectious morbidity (Garite *et al.* 1979, 1981; Cotton *et al.* 1984a; Schmidt *et al.* 1984; Iams *et al.* 1985; Feinstein *et al.* 1986). If bacteria are present in the amniotic fluid, it would seem logical and appropriate to remove the fetus from the infected environment in order to decrease infectious morbidity and mortality. Fetal infection most commonly results from swallowing or aspirating infected amniotic fluid and, irrespective of whether antibiotic treatment adequately reaches the fetus, it will be near impossible to adequately sterilize the uterine cavity. Fetal infection can also arise as a result of haematogenous spread through infected fetal vessels of the chorionic plate and umbilical cord, resulting in primary fetal septicaemia before bacteria are discovered in the amniotic fluid.

The problems associated with the use of amniocentesis have been the failure to obtain amniotic fluid in a significant proportion of cases; the invasiveness and risks associated with the diagnostic procedure itself; and, most importantly, the lack of a strong correlation between the results of diagnostic tests applied to the liquor and the development of fetal infection. Bacteria are not found in all women with clinical signs of intra-amniotic infection, nor are they always absent in women without signs of infection (Listwa *et al.* 1976; Larsen *et al.* 1976; Gibbs 1977; Gonik and Cotton 1985; Feinstein *et al.* 1986). Some have suggested that the presence of white blood cells in the amniotic fluid, rather than bacteria, is a better predictor of infectious morbidity (Larsen *et al.* 1974, 1976), but this has not been confirmed by others (Listwa *et al.* 1976; Gibbs 1977; Gonik and Cotton 1985) and the utility of the approach has never been demonstrated.

There has been only one controlled trial to assess the value of amniocentesis for fetal maturity tests and detection of intrauterine infection by Gram stain and culture after prelabour rupture of the membranes preterm (Cotton *et al.* 1984b). Of 64 eligible women between 24 and 36 weeks of gestation, 17 (26 per cent) were excluded because amniocentesis was not considered to be feasible because of lack of liquor or because of the position of the umbilical cord. In two of the 25 women (8 per cent) then randomized to the amniocentesis group, amniocentesis failed. The resulting overall 'failure rate' of 34 per cent is comparable with other controlled (Garite *et al.* 1981; Iams *et al.* 1985) and uncontrolled studies in which failure rates of amniocentesis have been reported to be in the range of 30 to 50 per cent (Garite *et al.* 1979; Cotton *et al.* 1984a).

The protocol of the controlled trial reported by Cotton and his colleagues (1984a) envisaged effecting delivery when pulmonary maturity or bacteria in the amniotic fluid were identified, and repeating the amniocentesis after 48 hours and then at weekly intervals if neither pulmonary maturity nor bacteria were identified. The use of amniocentesis did not, however, reduce the proportion of women receiving tocolytic agents (59 vs. 71 per cent) or corticosteroids (18 vs. 17 per cent). Nor was there a statistically significant reduction in the number of women delivered because of clinical amnionitis (8 vs. 13 per cent), or in the number of perinatal deaths (one infant from each group died, both from fulminant early neonatal sepsis). The only statistically significant differences observed were in the frequency of fetal distress, as judged from cardiotocographic tracings, and in the average number of days that the infants remained in hospital after the mother had been discharged. Both these outcomes were more favourable (lower) in the amniocentesis group, but both may have been influenced by knowledge of the group assignment. On the whole, there is thus inadequate evidence to judge whether the use of amniocentesis in women with prelabour rupture of the membranes confers more benefit than harm to mother and baby.

Vintzileos and his colleagues (Feinstein *et al.* 1986; Vintzileos *et al.* 1985a,b, 1986a,b,c,d, 1987a) reported on a number of measures, including amniocentesis, non-stress cardiotocography, and biophysical profiles, for prediction or early recognition of intrauterine infection in women with prelabour rupture of the membranes preterm. In due course, all of these procedures were stated to be 'useful' in selecting 'candidates for fetal infection and therefore in need for prompt delivery'. Their series of papers on the subject (referred to above) either had no controls or only historical controls, and dealt with women from 25 weeks of gestation onwards without signs of labour, infection, bleeding, or fetal distress.

Comparison of the many reports of these authors indicates higher positive and negative predictive values both for non-stress cardiotocography and biophysical profile than for amniocentesis as a means to detect intrauterine infection. Unfortunately, comparison of these reports also reveals such glaring biases, that the data must be regarded as inadequate for guiding clinical practice. For example, comparison of 3 papers which reported on 'consecutive series' of 73 women (Vintzileos *et al.* 1985a, 1987a; Feinstein *et al.* 1986), with another report on 'all women' admitted for prelabour rupture of the membranes in a 23 months' period (Vintzileos *et al.* 1986a), reveals that two series of 73 admissions were collected (Feinstein *et al.* 1986) over a period of time during which a maximum number of 127 women were admitted in total (Vintzileos *et al.* 1986a). Although the authors believed 'that the similarity between the historic and study groups permitted a meaningful clinical comparison' (Vintzileos *et al.* 1987a), it is clear that, even without such discrepancies, historical controls are entirely inadequate to judge the utility of these procedures (see Chapter 1).

Goldstein *et al.* (1988) recently reported that all of 17 women with prelabour rupture of the membranes before 33 weeks of gestation in whom at least one episode of gross fetal body movement and/or fetal breathing movements lasting more than 30 seconds was observed had negative amniotic fluid cultures at amniocentesis (95 per cent confidence interval of positive culture: 0–16 per cent). On the other hand, all of the 13 women in whom fetal breathing movements were absent and in whom the duration of total fetal body movements was confined to 50 seconds or less, had positive amniotic fluid cultures (95 per cent confidence interval: 79–100 per cent).

It would thus appear from these data and from those of Vintzileos and his colleagues (discussed above) that fetal behaviour may change markedly when intra-amniotic infection develops. These changes in fetal behaviour may prove to be as reliable for the detection of intrauterine infection as the more invasive technique of amniocentesis. Whether the use of these parameters will prove valuable in determining the most appropriate pattern of care, however, cannot be determined by the type of studies that have been conducted thus far. For this, it will be necessary to demonstrate, in controlled comparisons, that the information obtained by these tests and the clinical action that is based on it improve perinatal outcome beyond that observed when these tests are not used.

3.4 Assessing the risk of fetal immaturity

Assessing the risk of fetal immaturity largely depends on a careful assessment of gestational age and on ascertainment of any such assessments made earlier in pregnancy (see also Chapter 74). On the basis of gestational age alone, there will usually be little difficulty in identifying fetuses who are profoundly immature. Nor will there be much difficulty in identifying some fetuses who have attained a level of maturity that, at least for the practical purpose of providing care, differs little from that which would be attained at term. In between these two categories, and most typically between 26 and 34 weeks of gestation, weighing the risk of relative immaturity is considerably more difficult.

More specific information on the degree of maturity than can be implied from fetal age is limited to organ systems that can be tested, and to inferences that can be drawn from the test results. Information on fetal pulmonary maturity, even when sought by the same means (i.e. amniocentesis) as information on infection, takes on a different level of importance than the information on intrauterine infection. There is no good reason to strive actively for early delivery merely because pulmonary maturity appears to be adequate, yet several clinical protocols have implied that consequence of the demonstration of adequate fetal lung maturity (Garite *et al.* 1981; Iams *et al.* 1985). The fact that an adequate level of pulmonary maturity decreases mortality and morbidity from respiratory disorders, does not necessarily mean that all other causes of mortality and morbidity associated with preterm birth, most notably intraventricular haemorrhage, will be prevented (see Chapter 74).

The main gain that can be obtained from demonstrating pulmonary maturity, whether this is based on analysis of amniotic fluid obtained vaginally or by amniocentesis, is that measures to promote pulmonary maturity, such as corticosteroid administration, may then be regarded as superfluous. It is not that delivery will thenceforth be without hazards for the infant, or that the main or only risk for the infant now becomes infection rather than preterm birth.

The only controlled trial on amniocentesis for examining fetal pulmonary maturity after prelabour rupture of the membranes is that of Cotton *et al.* (1984b), which was discussed above. When amniotic fluid for investigation of fetal pulmonary maturity is collected from the vagina, there is wide consensus that determination of phosphatidylglycerol is the test to be used, because this compound is virtually absent from any body fluids other than lung surfactant (Stedman *et al.* 1981). As for amniocentesis, however, the utility of this approach in the care for women with prelabour rupture of the membranes has not been assessed.

4 Care of the woman with prelabour rupture of the membranes preterm

Alternative care options for women with prelabour rupture of the membranes are often presented as 'conservative (or expectant) management' versus 'aggressive (or active) management'. Unfortunately, these jargon descriptions are of little help. No single approach is ever entirely 'conservative'. Protocols described as 'conservative' often refer to absence of drug treatment with corticosteroids or tocolytic agents (Varner and Galask 1981; Graham *et al.* 1982; Beydoun and Yasin 1986), but sometimes they mean exactly the opposite (Andreyko *et al.* 1984). They may include a variety of procedures, such as routine speculum examination (Varner and Galask 1981; Beydoun and Yasin 1986), attempts to obtain amniotic fluid by amniocentesis (Barrett and Boehm 1982; Ismail *et al.* 1985), or caesarean section if the infant presents by the breech (Graham *et al.* 1982). Some or all of these approaches would be considered as 'aggressive' by others. Approaches that are described as 'aggressive' may imply little more than the administration of corticosteroids and tocolytics, which is labelled as 'conservative management' by others (Andreyko *et al.* 1984). They may also, as they often do at term, imply attempts to induce labour or effect delivery in an attempt to prevent intrauterine infection (Garite *et al.* 1981; Iams *et al.* 1985; Nelson *et al.* 1985).

This is not to suggest that there is no justification for deciding, in a particular case, whether the primary objective should be to effect delivery, or alternatively, to prolong pregnancy. Rather, it suggests that the labels 'aggressive' and 'conservative' are too heterogeneous to be applied to that decision, and to the other aspects of care for these women.

Preterm delivery is *the* main consequence of prelabour rupture of the membranes preterm. Where adequate facilities for intensive perinatal and neonatal care are lacking, the most effective form of care, therefore, is referral to a centre where such facilities are readily available (see Chapter 74). It is possible, of course, that leakage will stop and that amniotic fluid will accumulate again. This, however, is the exception rather than the rule (Beydoun and Yasin 1986). It must be infinitely better for both mother and baby to be referred back to the original caregivers because the problem apparently solved itself, than to be referred at the last minute when fetal compromise or preterm delivery have become inevitable.

If there are no detectable uterine contractions following prelabour rupture of the membranes preterm, and there is no evidence of infection, then it is the concern that infection may supervene (and, to a lesser extent, that pulmonary hypoplasia may develop as a result of prolonged oligohydramnios) that dominate in considering what kind of care is appropriate. These concerns have led some clinicians to try to seal the membranes (Baumgarten and Moser 1986) or to occlude the cervix with a catheter specially designed for that purpose (Ogita *et al.* 1984) in attempts to reduce these risks. No controlled data are available to assess the merits, if any, of these approaches. Measures directed more specifically at decreasing the risk of ascending infection have also included continuous infusion of an antiseptic solution (polyvinylpyrrolidine iodine) through a catheter introduced deep into the vagina (Saling 1979). Again, no controlled evaluations of the assumed benefits of this approach have been reported, and the method certainly has the disadvantage that women must remain bedbound and attached to the end of a catheter for it to be administered.

Four approaches have been evaluated in controlled comparisons of alternative forms of care for women whose membranes ruptured preterm and in whom there is no evidence of either uterine contractions or infection. These comparisons have dealt with the prophylactic use of antibiotics; the prophylactic use of tocolytic drugs; the use of corticosteroids to promote fetal pulmonary maturity; and induction of labour in women with or without evidence suggestive of adequate fetal lung maturity. Some of the controlled comparisons have evaluated combinations of these interventions.

4.1 Prophylactic antibiotics

Four controlled trials have been reported on the use of prophylactic antibiotics after prelabour rupture of the membranes and before the onset of labour. Two of these studies were conducted more than 20 years ago (Lebherz *et al.* 1963; Brelje *et al.* 1966) and they included women at variable gestational ages, so that it is not clear how many of them were preterm. These studies also dealt with antibiotics that would nowadays not be used. The two more recent studies (Dunlop *et al.* 1986; Amon *et al.* 1988) included fewer women than the older studies, but all women were at less than 35 weeks of gestation. One of the recent studies (Dunlop *et al.* 1986) used a factorial design, testing the use of oral ritodrine as well as that of antibiotic prophylaxis. The four studies show considerable heterogeneity and they are not entirely beyond suspicion of selection bias, either at or after treatment allocation.

Lebherz *et al.* (1963) reported on 1896 women (out of an unstated number) with prelabour rupture of the membranes who had been treated in a double-blind fashion twice daily with 150 mg demethyltetracycline or placebo. It is not known how many of these women were preterm, but 359 (19 per cent) of their 1912 infants weighed less than 2500 g and 27 (1.4 per cent) weighed less than 1000 g at birth. Brelje *et al.* (1966) conducted a double-blind study in which a vaginal suppository containing either 6 mg nitrofurazone or placebo was inserted every 6 hours until delivery in women whose membranes had been ruptured for at least 6 hours and who had a normal temperature and were not in labour. The number of women entered into the trial is not entirely clear. The authors report cultures at entry for 376 women, but data on infection and infant outcome are reported for only 367 women. These 367 include 109 women whose number of cultures were stated to be so incomplete 'as to make them useless for analysis', and 258 women who had enough cultures to be included in the analyses. Only 85 of the 258 women (33 per cent) for whom this outcome is reported delivered a 'premature' infant. In 1966 this is likely to have related to a birthweight below 2500 g rather than to preterm gestation (see Chapter 74). Dunlop *et al.* (1986) randomized 48 women with prelabour rupture of the membranes between 26 and 34 weeks of gestation into 4 groups. All women were treated with dexamethasone. Half of them received 250–500 mg cephalexin every 6 hours, and half received no antibiotics; half of the women in both groups received oral ritodrine and half did not. Lastly, Amon *et al.* (1988) randomly allocated 43 women to receive ampicillin and 39 to receive no antibiotic prophylaxis; their method of randomization is not described and the use of corticosteroids or tocolytic drugs was at the discretion of the attending physician.

Overall, the results of the trials show no reduction in the incidence of intrauterine infection as manifested by signs of maternal infection before delivery (Table 43.1) or by evidence of neonatal infection after birth (Table 43.2). The typical odds ratio for maternal infection before delivery, which usually related to amnionitis or chorioamnionitis, was 1.17 with a 95 per cent confidence interval of 0.72 to 1.88 (Table 43.1). The typical odds ratio for neonatal infection was 1.03 (confidence interval: 0.52–2.03; Table 43.2). Data on neonatal pneumonia, a more reliable indicator of intrauterine infection than other neonatal infections, were available in two reports, both of which also provided data on neonatal sepsis. Neither of these two outcomes occurred less frequently with than without antibiotic prophylaxis (Table 43.3). Consequently, the number of deaths that could be attributed to infection across the four trials was nearly identical in the groups with and without antibiotic prophylaxis. The typical odds ratio was 1.11, with a 95 per cent confidence interval of 0.45 to 2.73 (Table 43.4). Also the total number of fetal and neonatal deaths, excluding infants with lethal malformations, showed no difference between the two groups (Table 43.5). The typical odds ratio for this outcome was 0.76 with a confidence interval of 0.50 to 1.17 (Table 43.5). This is the more remarkable since in one of the trials, reported some 25 years ago, there had been 18 infants weighing less than 1000 g at birth in the control group as compared with only 9 in the antibiotic group (Lebherz *et al.* 1963). Seventeen of the 39 deaths in the control group as compared with only 6 of the 27 deaths in the antibiotic group had been among these infants (Lebherz *et al.* 1963).

The only statistically significant difference observed was in the incidence of infectious morbidity in the mother postpartum. This was significantly lower in women who had received antibiotic prophylaxis (Table 43.6), with an odds ratio of 0.58 (confidence interval: 0.43–0.80). It is not clear, however, whether a similar reduction in the incidence of infectious morbidity might have been achieved with antibiotic treatment starting at, instead of before delivery.

4.2 Prophylactic oral tocolytics

Only two studies have addressed the question of whether the administration of tocolytic drugs might improve outcome in women not in labour after prelabour rupture of the membranes preterm (between 25 and 34 weeks of gestation) (Levy *et al.* 1985; Dunlop *et al.* 1986). Both studies were small (comprising respectively 41 and 48 women); neither was double-blind; nor can one be confident from the reports that either was free of selection bias at the time of allocation. In both studies, the tocolytic treatment used was oral ritodrine. In one of the two studies (Dunlop *et al.* 1986), women in the two groups were also randomly allocated to receive either prophylactic antibiotics or no antibiotics, which resulted in 4 groups of 12 women each. All of the women in this trial also received dexamethasone to promote fetal lung maturity. In the other trial (Levy *et al.* 1985), none of these additional treatments were used or studied.

The incidence of delivery within 48 hours was lower in women receiving ritodrine prophylaxis, but only one of the two trials provided this information (Table 43.7).

Table 43.1 Effect of prophylactic antibiotics for prelabour rupture of the membranes on maternal infection before delivery

Study	EXPT		CTRL		Odds ratio	Graph of odds ratios and confidence intervals
	n	(%)	*n*	(%)	(95% CI)	0.01 0.1 0.5 1 2 10 100
Brelje *et al.* (1966)	35/193	(18.13)	28/174	(16.09)	1.15 (0.67–1.99)	
Dunlop *et al.* (1986)	3/24	(12.50)	4/24	(16.67)	0.72 (0.15–3.52)	
Amon *et al.* (1988)	7/43	(16.28)	4/39	(10.26)	1.67 (0.47–5.91)	
Typical odds ratio (95% confidence interval)					1.17 (0.72–1.88)	

Table 43.2 Effect of prophylactic antibiotics for prelabour rupture of the membranes on neonatal infection

Study	EXPT		CTRL		Odds ratio	Graph of odds ratios and confidence intervals
	n	(%)	*n*	(%)	(95% CI)	0.01 0.1 0.5 1 2 10 100
Brelje *et al.* (1966)	14/193	(7.25)	16/174	(9.20)	0.77 (0.37–1.63)	
Dunlop *et al.* (1986)	5/24	(20.83)	1/24	(4.17)	4.45 (0.82–24.17)	
Typical odds ratio (95% confidence interval)					1.03 (0.52–2.03)	

Table 43.3 Effect of prophylactic antibiotics for prelabour rupture of the membranes on neonatal pneumonia

Study	EXPT		CTRL		Odds ratio	Graph of odds ratios and confidence intervals
	n	(%)	*n*	(%)	(95% CI)	0.01 0.1 0.5 1 2 10 100
Brelje *et al.* (1966)	3/193	(1.55)	4/174	(2.30)	0.67 (0.15–3.00)	
Amon *et al.* (1988)	4/43	(9.30)	2/39	(5.13)	1.84 (0.35–9.60)	
Typical odds ratio (95% confidence interval)					1.06 (0.35–3.21)	

Effect of prophylactic antibiotics for prelabour rupture of the membranes on neonatal sepsis

Study	EXPT		CTRL		Odds ratio	Graph of odds ratios and confidence intervals
Brelje *et al.* (1966)	1/193	(0.52)	1/174	(0.57)	0.90 (0.06–14.52)	
Amon *et al.* (1988)	1/43	(2.33)	6/39	(15.38)	0.19 (0.04–0.90)	
Typical odds ratio (95% confidence interval)					0.28 (0.07–1.06)	

Table 43.4 Effect of prophylactic antibiotics for prelabour rupture of the membranes on perinatal death due to infection

Study	EXPT		CTRL		Odds ratio	Graph of odds ratios and confidence intervals
	n	(%)	*n*	(%)	(95% CI)	0.01 0.1 0.5 1 2 10 100
Brelje *et al.* (1966)	1/193	(0.52)	0/174	(0.00)	6.70 (0.13–99.99)	
Lebherz *et al.* (1963)	7/950	(0.74)	8/962	(0.83)	0.89 (0.32–2.45)	
Dunlop *et al.* (1986)	1/24	(4.17)	0/24	(0.00)	7.39 (0.15–99.99)	
Amon *et al.* (1988)	1/43	(2.33)	1/39	(2.56)	0.91 (0.06–14.78)	
Typical odds ratio (95% confidence interval)					1.11 (0.45–2.73)	

Table 43.5 Effect of prophylactic antibiotics for prelabour rupture of the membranes on fetal and neonatal death (excluding malformations)

Study	EXPT		CTRL		Odds ratio	Graph of odds ratios and confidence intervals
	n	(%)	*n*	(%)	(95% CI)	0.01 0.1 0.5 1 2 10 100
Lebherz *et al.* (1963)	27/945	(2.86)	39/960	(4.06)	0.70 (0.43–1.14)	
Brelje *et al.* (1966)	5/193	(2.59)	3/174	(1.72)	1.50 (0.37–6.09)	
Dunlop *et al.* (1986)	4/24	(16.67)	1/24	(4.17)	3.71 (0.59–23.21)	
Amon *et al.* (1988)	2/43	(4.65)	6/39	(15.38)	0.30 (0.07–1.28)	
Typical odds ratio (95% confidence interval)					0.76 (0.50–1.17)	

Table 43.6 Effect of prophylactic antibiotics for prelabour rupture of the membranes on infectious morbidity postpartum

Study	EXPT		CTRL		Odds ratio	Graph of odds ratios and confidence intervals
	n	(%)	*n*	(%)	(95% CI)	0.01 0.1 0.5 1 2 10 100
Lebherz *et al.* (1963)	33/941	(3.51)	70/955	(7.33)	0.48 (0.32–0.71)	
Brelje *et al.* (1966)	19/193	(9.84)	17/174	(9.77)	1.01 (0.51–2.01)	
Dunlop *et al.* (1986)	3/24	(12.50)	8/24	(33.33)	0.32 (0.08–1.19)	
Amon *et al.* (1988)	5/43	(11.63)	3/39	(7.69)	1.56 (0.36–6.64)	
Typical odds ratio (95% confidence interval)					0.58 (0.42–0.80)	

Table 43.7 Effect of prophylactic betamimetics after prelabour rupture of the membranes on delivery within 48 hours

Study	EXPT		CTRL		Odds ratio	Graph of odds ratios and confidence intervals
	n	(%)	*n*	(%)	(95% CI)	0.01 0.1 0.5 1 2 10 100
Levy and Warsof (1985)	2/21	(9.52)	9/21	(42.86)	0.19 (0.05–0.72)	
Typical odds ratio (95% confidence interval)					0.19 (0.05–0.72)	
Effect of prophylactic betamimetics after prelabour rupture of the membranes on delivery within 10 days						
Levy and Warsof (1985)	17/21	(80.95)	20/21	(95.24)	0.26 (0.04–1.67)	
Dunlop *et al.* (1986)	17/24	(70.83)	17/24	(70.83)	1.00 (0.29–3.43)	
Typical odds ratio (95% confidence interval)					0.66 (0.24–1.85)	

The incidence of delivery within 10 days was not detectably different between the two groups (Table 43.7). One of the trials, which also studied antibiotic prophylaxis in a factorial design, provided no information on infection according to whether women had received ritodrine or not (Dunlop *et al.* 1986). Only one trial thus allowed assessment of the incidence of infection in mother and baby by allocation to tocolytic prophylaxis (Levy *et al.* 1985). The 95 per cent confidence intervals for both maternal infection (defined as induction for suspected chorioamnionitis) and neonatal infection (defined as positive blood, urine, or cerebrospinal cultures in the infant) are too wide for any meaningful conclusions to be drawn (Table 43.8). The number of women was also too small to assess the influence of tocolytic prophylaxis on perinatal mortality, available for both trials, or on respiratory distress, available for only one trial (Table 43.9).

These data, and data from other placebo-controlled trials on the prophylactic use of oral betamimetic drugs in women without ruptured membranes discussed elsewhere (see Chapter 44), offer no support for suggestions that prophylactic tocolysis before the onset of uterine contractions is worthwhile in women with prelabour rupture of the membranes.

4.3 Corticosteroid administration

For many years, there has been considerable discussion as to whether or not rupture of the membranes enhances fetal pulmonary maturity (Gillebrand 1967; Chiswick and Burnard 1973; Yoon and Harper 1973; Jones *et al.* 1975; Mead 1980; Wennergren *et al.* 1986; Coustan 1987). Inherent in this discussion has been not only the question as to whether prelabour rupture of the membranes offers the infant some protection against the development of respiratory distress syndrome, but also whether that protection might be of a sufficient degree to override any beneficial effect of

Table 43.8 Effect of prophylactic betamimetics after prelabour rupture of the membranes on maternal infection

Study	EXPT		CTRL		Odds ratio	Graph of odds ratios and confidence intervals
	n	(%)	*n*	(%)	(95% CI)	0.01 0.1 0.5 1 2 10 100
Levy and Warsof (1985)	3/21	(14.29)	1/21	(4.76)	2.94 (0.38–22.53)	
Typical odds ratio (95% confidence interval)					2.94 (0.38–22.53)	
Effect of prophylactic betamimetics after prelabour rupture of the membranes on neonatal infection						
Levy and Warsof (1985)	0/21	(0.00)	0/21	(0.00)	1.00 (1.00–1.00)	
Typical odds ratio (95% confidence interval)					1.00 (1.00–1.00)	

Table 43.9 Effect of prophylactic betamimetics after prelabour rupture of the membranes on perinatal mortality (excluding malformations)

Study	EXPT		CTRL		Odds ratio	Graph of odds ratios and confidence intervals
	n	(%)	*n*	(%)	(95% CI)	0.01 0.1 0.5 1 2 10 100
Dunlop *et al.* (1986)	3/24	(12.50)	1/24	(4.17)	2.91 (0.38–22.06)	
Levy and Warsof (1985)	0/21	(0.00)	1/21	(4.76)	0.14 (0.00–6.82)	
Typical odds ratio (95% confidence interval)					1.52 (0.25–9.22)	
Effect of prophylactic betamimetics after prelabour rupture of the membranes on respiratory distress syndrome						
Dunlop *et al.* (1986)	8/24	(33.33)	7/24	(29.17)	1.21 (0.36–4.05)	
Typical odds ratio (95% confidence interval)					1.21 (0.36–4.05)	

the administration of corticosteroids on pulmonary maturity. Because corticosteroids are known to have immunosuppressive effects, there has also been concern that administering them to women with prelabour rupture of the membranes might increase susceptibility to intrauterine infection and mask early signs of infection, thereby causing a delay in its diagnosis (Beck and Johnson 1980).

As discussed by Crowley (see Chapter 45), there is no evidence from the randomized controlled trials that either of these mechanisms has resulted in an increased incidence of perinatal infections in women with prolonged rupture of the membranes. Her analysis, however, concentrated on the presence of ruptured membranes rather than on whether rupture of the membranes had occurred before labour. To clarify the effects of corticosteroid administration, she also excluded controlled comparisons in which corticosteroid administration was part of a wider 'management protocol' that was being evaluated against an alternative policy.

There is justified concern that corticosteroids are more likely both to be superfluous and to be hazardous in women with prelabour rupture of the membranes. We therefore searched for all controlled comparisons in which women with prelabour rupture of the membranes were allocated either to receive or not to receive corticosteroids, irrespective of whether or not allocation to corticosteroid treatment was part of a larger 'package of care'. Seven trials were found (Block *et al.* 1977; Collaborative Group on Antenatal Steroid Therapy 1981; Garite *et al.* 1981; Schmidt *et al.* 1984; Iams *et al.* 1985; Nelson *et al.* 1985; Morales *et al.* 1986). A further trial (Simpson and Harbert 1985), in which the method of randomization was not described, was excluded because 'on rare occasions patients were assigned to betamethasone at the discretion of one of the attending physicians' (Simpson and Harbert 1985). Only 3 of the 7 trials dealt exclusively with women who were not in labour at the time of admission to the study (Iams *et al.* 1985; Nelson *et al.* 1985; Morales *et al.* 1986). Separate analysis of these trials provided no evidence that the effects of corticosteroid administration differed from those observed in the trials that also incorporated women with uterine contractions after prelabour rupture of the membranes. Moreover, in all three of these trials some of the women received tocolytic drug treatment in addition to corticosteroids, indicating that some uterine contractility was likely to have been present either at or shortly after entry into the trial. All controlled comparisons involving women with prelabour rupture of the membranes have therefore been considered together, irrespective of whether or not there was evidence of labour at the time of randomization.

Four of the trials (Block *et al.* 1977; Collaborative Group on Antenatal Steroid Therapy 1981; Schmidt *et al.* 1984; Morales *et al.* 1986) were included in the chapter by Crowley (Chapter 45). In the other three trials (Garite *et al.* 1981; Iams *et al.* 1985; Nelson *et al.* 1985), allocation to corticosteroid administration always implied the use of two further interventions. Women assigned to the corticosteroid group received tocolytic agents (ethanol, magnesium sulphate, or betamimetics) when necessary to delay delivery for at least 24 hours. In two of the trials (Garite *et al.* 1981; Iams *et al.* 1985), women allocated to the control group received no tocolysis; in the other trial (Nelson *et al.* 1985) there were two control groups, one with and one without tocolytic treatment. In all three trials, allocation to corticosteroid administration also implied that delivery was instituted 48 to 72 hours after the start of corticosteroid administration. This was not done in the women assigned to the control group, except in the study reported by Nelson *et al.* (1985), in which delivery was effected in one, but not in the other of the two control groups. For the overviews presented in Tables 43.10 and 43.11, control data for the study of Nelson *et al.* (1985) have been limited to the one group which, except for corticosteroid administration, received identical care to the women given corticosteroids.

The data from all 7 trials, shown in Tables 43.10 and 43.11, further substantiate the conclusions reached by Crowley (see Chapter 45). Irrespective of any effects that prelabour rupture of the membranes itself may have on fetal pulmonary maturity, the incidence of respiratory distress syndrome was reduced by corticosteroid administration. The typical odds ratio derived from the 7 trials was 0.55 with a 95 per cent confidence interval of 0.40 to 0.75, which is statistically highly significant (Table 43.10). The incidence of neonatal infection, albeit available for only 5 of these trials, was not statistically significantly higher in the corticosteroid-treated group than in the control group. The typical odds of 1.61 (confidence interval 0.87–2.98) and the odds of the individual trials (Table 43.11) suggest that corticosteroid administration may be more likely to increase than to decrease the incidence of neonatal infection. Yet, that effect, which remains unproven at present, has probably less influence than the benefit derived in terms of a lower incidence of respiratory distress.

If corticosteroid treatment in women at imminent risk of preterm delivery should be different for those

Table 43.10 Effect of corticosteroids after prelabour rupture of the membranes on respiratory distress syndrome

Study	EXPT		CTRL		Odds ratio	Graph of odds ratios and confidence intervals
	n	(%)	*n*	(%)	(95% CI)	0.01 0.1 0.5 1 2 10 100
Block *et al.* (1977)	3/25	(12.00)	5/26	(19.23)	0.59 (0.13–2.61)	
Morales *et al.* (1986)	30/121	(24.79)	63/124	(50.81)	0.33 (0.20–0.56)	
Collaborative Group (1981)	15/153	(9.80)	17/135	(12.59)	0.75 (0.36–1.57)	
Nelson *et al.* (1985)	10/22	(45.45)	11/22	(50.00)	0.84 (0.26–2.70)	
Schmidt *et al.* (1984)	7/24	(29.17)	6/17	(35.29)	0.76 (0.20–2.84)	
Garite *et al.* (1981)	14/80	(17.50)	17/79	(21.52)	0.78 (0.35–1.70)	
Iams *et al.* (1985)	10/38	(26.32)	12/35	(34.29)	0.69 (0.25–1.86)	
Typical odds ratio (95% confidence interval)					0.55 (0.40–0.75)	

Table 43.11 Effect of corticosteroids after prelabour rupture of the membranes on neonatal infection

Study	EXPT		CTRL		Odds ratio	Graph of odds ratios and confidence intervals
	n	(%)	*n*	(%)	(95% CI)	0.01 0.1 0.5 1 2 10 100
Morales *et al.* (1986)	11/121	(9.09)	11/124	(8.87)	1.03 (0.43–2.46)	
Nelson *et al.* (1985)	5/22	(22.73)	0/22	(0.00)	9.07 (1.44–57.16)	
Schmidt *et al.* (1984)	4/24	(16.67)	3/17	(17.65)	0.93 (0.18–4.78)	
Garite *et al.* (1981)	4/80	(5.00)	0/79	(0.00)	7.58 (1.05–54.87)	
Iams *et al.* (1985)	4/38	(10.53)	3/35	(8.57)	1.25 (0.27–5.88)	
Typical odds ratio (95% confidence interval)					1.61 (0.87–2.98)	

with and those without prelabour rupture of the membranes, then the difference should probably be dictated by only two factors. The first is the likelihood that fetal pulmonary maturity is sufficient to forego corticosteroid-induced enhancement. The second is the likelihood that delivery will be delayed for a sufficiently long time to ensure spontaneous maturation. After prelabour rupture of the membranes, adequate pulmonary maturity can sometimes be implied from the presence of vernix in the leaking amniotic fluid, or assured from other tests, such as phosphatidylglycerol determination in the collected fluid. In centres where such tests are practised, it is logical to forego corticosteroid administration when pulmonary maturity is judged to be adequate. The problem is, however, that the test results will often not be available in time to institute corticosteroid treatment when it is necessary. The second factor, the likelihood that delivery will be delayed for a sufficiently long time to ensure further spontaneous maturation between admission and delivery, is considerably less frequent with than *without* ruptured membranes (Kragt and Keirse 1989).

We also conducted a separate analysis of the 3 trials (Garite *et al.* 1981; Iams *et al.* 1985; Nelson *et al.* 1985) that compared corticosteroid administration followed by active measures to effect delivery with an expectant policy that included neither corticosteroid administration nor active measures to effect delivery. The pooled data (Table 43.12) showed no statistically significant difference in the incidence of respiratory distress syndrome between the two policies. In two of the trials (Garite *et al.* 1981; Iams *et al.* 1985), but not in the third (Nelson *et al.* 1985), there were fewer cases of respiratory distress syndrome in the group with the corticosteroid and active delivery policy than in the group without the active delivery policy (Table 43.12).

On balance, the evidence does not plead for a more restrictive use of corticosteroids in women with ruptured membranes, than in women without ruptured membranes. On the contrary, women admitted with the primary complaint of preterm uterine contractions are less likely to deliver within 48 hours than those admitted with a primary complaint of prelabour rupture of the membranes (Kragt and Keirse 1989). It could thus be argued that prelabour rupture of the membranes should provide a stronger incentive for the use of corticosteroids than the mere presence of preterm uterine contractility. Whether the theoretical possibility of

Table 43.12 Effect of corticosteroids after prelabour rupture of the membranes on respiratory distress syndrome with induction of labour

Study	EXPT		CTRL		Odds ratio	Graph of odds ratios and confidence intervals
	n	(%)	*n*	(%)	(95% CI)	0.01 0.1 0.5 1 2 10 100
Nelson *et al.* (1985)	10/22	(45.45)	8/24	(33.33)	1.65 (0.51–5.31)	
Garite *et al.* (1981)	14/80	(17.50)	17/79	(21.52)	0.78 (0.35–1.70)	
Iams *et al.* (1985)	10/38	(26.32)	12/35	(34.29)	0.69 (0.25–1.86)	
Typical odds ratio (95% confidence interval)					0.88 (0.51–1.52)	

an increased risk of perinatal infections should lead to concomitant antibiotic treatment cannot be assessed from the data that are currently available. However, this is certainly worth considering and definitely worth investigating in further controlled comparisons.

4.4 Induction of labour

Two controlled comparisons have been reported in which women were assigned either to an 'active' policy intended to effect delivery, or to a control policy in which no such measures were taken (Nelson *et al.* 1985; Spinnato *et al.* 1987). Other controlled comparisons in which a policy of effecting delivery was preceded by corticosteroid treatment have been discussed earlier in this chapter (see Table 43.12).

One of the two available studies (Nelson *et al.* 1985) has also been referred to above because corticosteroid treatment was given to one of the groups. In the two remaining groups (neither of which received corticosteroids), delivery was either instituted between 24 and 48 hours after prelabour rupture of the membranes, or women were observed without active measures to effect delivery or arrest labour when it occurred. The gestational ages at entry ranged from 28 to 34 weeks, with a mean of 32 weeks in both trial groups. The women in whom delivery was to be instituted between 24 and 48 hours received betamimetic drug treatment if labour occurred within the first 24 hours, presumably to make the group comparable to the one receiving corticosteroids, and this occurred in 7 of 22 women. Women in the actively treated group had a mean (SD) latency period of 95 (130) hours as compared with 33 (16) hours in those with expectant care.

In the other study (Spinnato *et al.* 1987), women were entered if they had prelabour rupture of the membranes between 25 and 36 weeks of gestation, and if analysis of amniotic fluid (obtained either transvaginally or transabdominally) indicated adequate pulmonary maturity. Women who were in labour at the time of admission were allowed to deliver; the remainder were randomized by sealed envelopes either to be delivered promptly (by induction of labour if there was a vertex presentation and by caesarean section for all other presentations), or to receive expectant care. Of 114 women enrolled in the study, 15 were subsequently excluded; of the remaining women, 52 had been in labour and did not qualify for randomization. This left only 47 who had been assigned to one or other of the two policies. The number of women excluded between randomization and analysis is not given, but all 15 excluded women may have been in that category, although 7 of the exclusions were stated to have been due to preterm labour (Spinnato *et al.* 1987). The mean (SD) interval between prelabour rupture of the membranes and delivery averaged 18 (12) hours in the group with the active policy, and 121 (195) hours in the group with expectant care.

Taken together, the results of these two trials do not suggest any protective effect of the more active policy in respect of either maternal sepsis (Table 43.13) or infant outcome measures, such as neonatal infection, neonatal sepsis, respiratory distress syndrome, intracranial haemorrhage, and perinatal death not due to congenital malformations (Table 43.14). On the whole the tendency is for most outcomes to be less favourable in the group with the active policy, and this also applies when criteria such as mechanical ventilation for more than 24 hours, or oxygen therapy for more than 3 days, are considered (Table 43.14). Neither of the two trials showed a statistically significant influence of the alternative policies on the duration of neonatal hospitalization. In the trial of Nelson *et al.* (1985) the mean (SD) duration of neonatal hospitalization was 25 (21) days in the actively treated group as compared with 20 (9) days

Table 43.13 Effect of induction of delivery after prelabour rupture of membranes preterm on maternal sepsis

Study	EXPT		CTRL		Odds ratio	Graph of odds ratios and confidence intervals
	n	(%)	*n*	(%)	(95% CI)	0.01 0.1 0.5 1 2 10 100
Nelson *et al.* (1985)	4/22	(18.18)	3/24	(12.50)	1.54 (0.31–7.57)	
Typical odds ratio (95% confidence interval)					1.54 (0.31–7.57)	

Effect of induction of delivery after prelabour rupture of membranes preterm on caesarean section

Study	EXPT		CTRL		Odds ratio	
Nelson *et al.* (1985)	6/22	(27.27)	4/24	(16.67)	1.84 (0.46–7.37)	
Spinnato *et al.* (1987)	4/26	(15.38)	3/21	(14.29)	1.09 (0.22–5.38)	
Typical odds ratio (95% confidence interval)					1.47 (0.52–4.19)	

Table 43.14 Effect of induction of delivery after prelabour rupture of membranes preterm on neonatal infection

Study	EXPT		CTRL		Odds ratio	Graph of odds ratios and confidence intervals
	n	(%)	*n*	(%)	(95% CI)	0.01 0.1 0.5 1 2 10 100
Spinnato *et al.* (1987)	6/26	(23.08)	3/21	(14.29)	1.74 (0.41–7.40)	
Typical odds ratio (95% confidence interval)					1.74 (0.41–7.40)	

Effect of induction of delivery after prelabour rupture of membranes preterm on neonatal sepsis

Study	EXPT		CTRL		Odds ratio	Graph of odds ratios and confidence intervals
	n	(%)	*n*	(%)	(95% CI)	0.01 0.1 0.5 1 2 10 100
Nelson *et al.* (1985)	0/22	(0.00)	1/24	(4.17)	0.15 (0.00–7.44)	
Spinnato *et al.* (1987)	6/26	(23.08)	2/21	(9.52)	2.56 (0.56–11.62)	
Typical odds ratio (95% confidence interval)					1.77 (0.43–7.25)	

Effect of induction of delivery after prelabour rupture of membranes preterm on respiratory distress syndrome

Study	EXPT		CTRL		Odds ratio	Graph of odds ratios and confidence intervals
	n	(%)	*n*	(%)	(95% CI)	0.01 0.1 0.5 1 2 10 100
Nelson *et al.* (1985)	11/22	(50.00)	8/24	(33.33)	1.96 (0.61–6.26)	
Spinnato *et al.* (1987)	2/26	(7.69)	0/21	(0.00)	6.35 (0.38–99.99)	
Typical odds ratio (95% confidence interval)					2.32 (0.79–6.80)	

Effect of induction of delivery after prelabour rupture of membranes preterm on intracranial haemorrhage

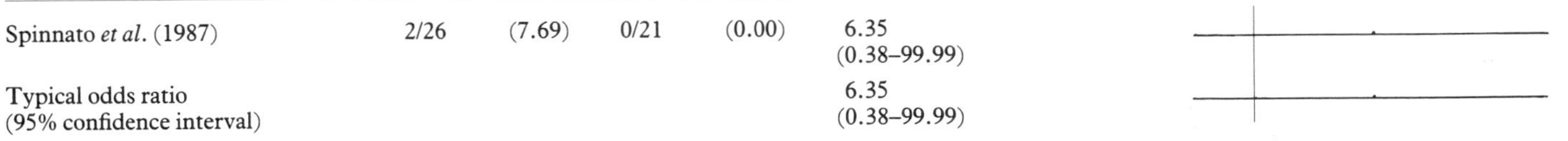

Study	EXPT		CTRL		Odds ratio	Graph of odds ratios and confidence intervals
Spinnato *et al.* (1987)	2/26	(7.69)	0/21	(0.00)	6.35 (0.38–99.99)	
Typical odds ratio (95% confidence interval)					6.35 (0.38–99.99)	

Effect of induction of delivery after prelabour rupture of membranes preterm on perinatal death (excluding malformations)

Study	EXPT		CTRL		Odds ratio	Graph of odds ratios and confidence intervals
	n	(%)	*n*	(%)	(95% CI)	0.01 0.1 0.5 1 2 10 100
Nelson *et al.* (1985)	1/22	(4.55)	0/24	(0.00)	8.09 (0.16–99.99)	
Spinnato *et al.* (1987)	2/26	(7.69)	2/21	(9.52)	0.79 (0.10–6.10)	
Typical odds ratio (95% confidence interval)					1.30 (0.21–7.94)	

Effect of induction of delivery after prelabour rupture of membranes preterm on mechanical ventilation >24 hours

Study	EXPT		CTRL		Odds ratio	Graph of odds ratios and confidence intervals
	n	(%)	*n*	(%)	(95% CI)	0.01 0.1 0.5 1 2 10 100
Spinnato *et al.* (1987)	2/26	(7.69)	0/21	(0.00)	6.35 (0.38–99.99)	
Typical odds ratio (95% confidence interval)					6.35 (0.38–99.99)	

Effect of induction of delivery after prelabour rupture of membranes preterm on oxygen therapy >3 days

Study	EXPT		CTRL		Odds ratio	Graph of odds ratios and confidence intervals
	n	(%)	*n*	(%)	(95% CI)	0.01 0.1 0.5 1 2 10 100
Spinnato *et al.* (1987)	7/25	(28.00)	5/21	(23.81)	1.24 (0.33–4.57)	
Typical odds ratio (95% confidence interval)					1.24 (0.33–4.57)	

in the expectant group. In the study of Spinnato *et al.* (1987) the mean was 13 days in the active group and 17 days in the expectant group. These two small trials therefore provide no evidence for any beneficial effect of measures to bring about labour or delivery after prelabour rupture of the membranes preterm. If anything, the available evidence would seem to suggest that such policies may cause more harm than benefit (see also Chapter 64).

4.5 Surveillance

The majority of women will experience labour within hours or a few days after rupture of the membranes. At that time, major reassessment is necessary and special attention should be devoted to signs of infection or cord complications, irrespective of whether these were considered to be absent before the start of uterine contractions. In some women, however, labour will be delayed much longer. Among these women will be some in whom the diagnosis of ruptured membranes was made erroneously and others in whom the rupture did not occur at the lower pole of the amniotic sac but higher up in the uterus.

Provided that mother and fetus are well at the initial assessments, the main preoccupations in the first few days after rupture of the membranes obviously centre on detecting the onset of infection and the onset of uterine contractions. Regular assessments of maternal temperature, other vital signs, uterine contractility, and fetal heart rate are therefore mandatory. It is not clear whether regular determinations of leucocyte counts add anything to this surveillance, particularly as some of these determinations will of necessity be performed and interpreted by on-duty personnel, whose admiration for technology and laboratory results may on occasions exceed their common sense. Variation in leucocyte counts can be quite large, particularly when the influences of labour or corticosteroid administration are added.

Other elements of surveillance are guided by the other complications which are known to occur more frequently after prelabour rupture of the membranes. These are primarily related to compression or prolapse of the umbilical cord, placental abruption, and the development of fetal deformities and lung hypoplasia.

Prolapse of the umbilical cord is a well-recognized complication of prelabour rupture of the membranes. It may occur either at the time of membrane rupture or later. There are many cases reported in the literature of mothers and babies in whom the umbilical cord prolapses when labour eventually supervenes several days or weeks after rupture of the membranes. Any change in an apparently stable situation, such as a resuming loss of liquor or the onset of uterine contractions, should alert the caregiver to this possibility. Cardiotocography and a careful ultrasound examination may be useful in these circumstances.

Compression of the umbilical cord may occur due to the loss of the protective effect of amniotic fluid (Gabbe *et al.* 1976; Moberg *et al.* 1984), which reduces local increases in pressure by distributing them more evenly. The risk of local increases in pressure escalates with the onset of uterine contractions and the resulting increases in intrauterine pressure. The incidence of severe decelerations of the fetal heart rate appears to be directly related to the degree of oligohydramnios (Moberg *et al.* 1984; Vintzileos *et al.* 1985b). Careful monitoring of the fetal heart rate is therefore essential, especially as soon as labour-like uterine activity occurs.

Although the association is not universally recognized, there are several reports of placental abruption occurring some time after prelabour rupture of the membranes. In a study of some 45,000 deliveries, Breese (1961) reported an incidence of placental abruption of 7.4 per cent among women with prelabour rupture of the membranes preterm (preterm at that time being defined as an infant birthweight of 500 to 2500 g), as compared with an incidence of only 2.0 per cent in all women giving birth to infants of 500 g or more. More recent studies have estimated the absolute risk of developing placental abruption some time after prelabour rupture of the membranes to be in the order of 4 (Nelson *et al.* 1986) to 6 (Vintzileos *et al.* 1987b) per cent, with the highest risk being observed in women who have severe oligohydramnios. The nature of the association between prelabour rupture of the membranes and placental abruption is not known. Unfortunately, this lack of understanding of the aetiology provides no clues for specific preventive measures. The appearance of any blood loss in a woman with ruptured membranes should be considered as a serious warning sign, however, and should be dealt with appropriately (see Chapter 37).

Prolonged rupture of the membranes with oligohydramnios for several weeks may lead to the development of fetal deformities that appear to result from this lack of liquor. Among these are pulmonary hypoplasia, which is the most dreaded of these complications, as well as a spectrum of fetal postural and compression abnormalities (Nimrod *et al.* 1984; Thibeault *et al.* 1985; Fox and Moessinger 1985; Bhutani *et al.* 1986). The development of fetal pulmonary hypoplasia has been ascribed to a number of factors, such as fetal constraint, thoracic and abdominal compression that reduces the space available for lung growth, decreased fetal breathing movements, and excessive loss of lung fluid interfering with intrauterine lung expansion (Wigglesworth *et al.* 1981; Wigglesworth and Desai 1982; Hislop *et al.* 1984; Tabor *et al.* 1986; Bhutani *et al.* 1986). The incidence of fetal pulmonary hypoplasia after prelabour rupture of the membranes is hard to estimate. This is because, first, there is a wide gradation in the severity of the condition, and second, the risk of developing it appears to depend on the severity and duration of the oligohydramnios as well as on the gestational age at which rupture of the membranes occurs (Wigglesworth and Desai 1982; Thibeault *et al.* 1985; Beydoun and Yasin 1986; Bhutani *et al.* 1986). The risk appears to be large when the amniotic fluid leak occurs in the first half of the 2nd trimester and results in virtual absence of amniotic fluid for several weeks (Wigglesworth and Desai 1982; Taylor and Garite 1984; Bhutani *et al.* 1986).

It would appear that pulmonary hypoplasia becomes the rule rather than the exception when oligohydramnios has been severe enough and of long enough duration to cause positional deformities (Thibeault *et al.* 1985). It has been suggested that the presence of fetal breathing movements may indicate that lung growth is preserved, and conversely that consistent absence of these movements correlates strongly with the presence or subsequent development of pulmonary hypoplasia (Blott *et al.* 1987). These conclusions were based on observations made in only 11 women. Others, also reporting on a small number of investigations, found that fetuses with oligohydramnios and lung hypoplasia exhibited breathing movements for a higher portion of the time and at higher rates than fetuses with oligohydramnios and normal lung development (Fox and Moessinger 1985). More data are thus needed before reliable conclusions can be drawn with regard to the risk of pulmonary hypoplasia and its prediction.

In the surveillance of women with prelabour rupture of the membranes, much prognostic relevance may be attached to the reaccumulation of amniotic fluid. Although its prognostic significance is hard to quantify, renewed accumulation of amniotic fluid is likely to defer intrauterine infection; to prevent cord complications; to lower the risk of placental abruption; to reduce the increased risk of pulmonary hypoplasia; and, possibly as a consequence of all of these, to decrease the likelihood of preterm delivery (Gonik *et al.* 1985; Thibeault *et al.* 1985; Vintzileos *et al.* 1985b; Beydoun and Yasin 1986; Vintzileos *et al.* 1987b). Some quantitative assessment of the amount of amniotic fluid or the dimensions of intrauterine amniotic fluid pools by ultrasound may therefore be a useful criterion in surveillance after prelabour rupture of the membranes. Although such assessments have not been shown to actually improve outcome, they are likely to identify a group of women and babies for whom prelabour rupture of the membranes poses less of a threat than is normally anticipated. For some of these women it may imply that they can return home with a reasonable degree of safety, although this too has never been assessed in controlled comparisons.

5 Care after the onset of labour

Stimulation of intrauterine prostaglandin synthesis is thought to be the main mechanism by which rupture of the membranes eventually leads to uterine contractions (Mitchell *et al.* 1977; Keirse 1979). This stimulation of prostaglandin synthesis is probably due to disruption of the continuity between fetal membranes and decidua over a rather large area of the uterus (Keirse *et al.* 1983). It has also been shown *in vitro* that bacterial products can stimulate prostaglandin synthesis in the fetal membranes (Bejar *et al.* 1981; Lamont *et al.* 1985;

Bennett *et al.* 1987). Intrauterine infection, as is well known from clinical observations (Romero *et al.* 1988), may therefore be an even more powerful stimulus for enhancing prostaglandin synthesis and the ensuing uterine contractility than rupture of the membranes by itself. The clinical consequences of this are that the question should always be raised as to whether the onset of uterine contractions is not the result of intrauterine infection.

5.1 With signs of intrauterine infection

If labour is considered to be secondary to intrauterine infection, it should be allowed to proceed to delivery as swiftly as possible in the interests of both mother and fetus, irrespective of the latter's degree of maturity. The other main option that needs to be envisaged is whether the woman should be referred to a centre with better facilities for perinatal and neonatal care. When this is the case, it should also lead to a careful scrutiny of possible inadequacies in the institution's referral policies that had prevented referral before the development of intrauterine infection. Decisions about the method of delivery and whether caesarean section will be necessary, should differ little from that for other preterm deliveries (see Chapter 74), except for the fact that significant maternal morbidity is likely to be a certainty rather than a theoretical risk when caesarean section is required.

The issue as to whether antibiotics should be administered at once in these circumstances has not been addressed by controlled studies. However, clinical common sense, as well as extrapolation of data from controlled trials on the intrapartum use of antibiotics for group B haemolytic streptococci (see Chapter 34), provide enough evidence to justify antibiotic treatment when clinical signs of intrauterine infection are present. Arguments against intrapartum antibiotic treatment are, first, that it might induce bacterial resistance or superinfection with resistant bacteria in the infant and, second, that it may interfere with establishing a diagnosis of infection in the neonate. The fear that bacterial resistance may develop is not entirely unjustified, but it is based mainly on theoretical considerations that need to be substantiated by solid evidence before they can justify withholding effective treatment from both mother and fetus. Arguments that intrapartum antibiotic treatment may interfere with the diagnosis of infection in the neonate should not be overemphasized. A diagnosis of infection, and even sepsis, in the preterm infant is often difficult to make with confidence. Most infants with infections acquired before birth receive treatment well before bacteriological evidence of infection is available. In many infants who are treated on the basis of clinical symptoms there is never any solid bacteriological confirmation of clinically diagnosed infection. It is therefore impossible to justify withholding treatment before birth, merely to demonstrate that treatment given after birth is really necessary. Studies that have compared intrapartum with immediate postpartum antibiotic treatment for intra-amniotic infection (Sperling *et al.* 1987; Gilstrap *et al.* 1988) tend to support the use of antibiotic treatment as soon as a clinical diagnosis of intrauterine infection is reached. Although the comparisons reported in these studies were not derived from controlled trials and are, therefore, prone to bias, they suggest that the incidence of neonatal sepsis may be lower in infants whose mothers received antibiotics before delivery (Sperling *et al.* 1987; Gilstrap *et al.* 1988). Moreover, data from controlled comparisons in women harbouring group B streptococci have convincingly demonstrated a lower incidence of neonatal infection and death from infection after intrapartum antibiotic treatment (see Chapter 34).

5.2 With or without suggestive evidence of fetal maturity

When there is suggestive evidence, on the basis of either gestational age or fetal lung maturity tests, that fetal pulmonary maturity is adequate, preterm labour should probably be allowed to proceed to preterm delivery. Considerations, such as the anticipated duration of neonatal hospitalization, infant–mother separation, and the costs of neonatal care, should take second place to considerations that the risk of infection, if not already present, is likely to be increased if other care options are chosen.

When there is no evidence to indicate that the fetal lungs are mature enough, corticosteroids should be administered. Current evidence, discussed above (Tables 43.10 and 43.11), suggests that the benefits of this approach are likely to outweigh its theoretical hazards. This probably applies irrespective of whether or not delivery is likely to be delayed sufficiently long for the treatment to have its maximal effect. From the available evidence (see Chapter 45) it appears that a short interval between corticosteroid administration and delivery is better than no interval at all. At the same time, if the interval between corticosteroid administration and delivery is relatively short, the fear that intrauterine infection may be enhanced or masked becomes less worrisome.

There are also situations in which the fetus is so immature as to have no chances of withstanding extrauterine life successfully. Any attempts to prolong pregnancy in these circumstances should not only consider what might and can be gained in terms of infant outcome, but should heavily weigh both the maternal risks and the opinion of the parents.

5.3 Intravenous tocolytics

As discussed elsewhere (see Chapter 44), there is no

evidence that tocolytic agents, *per se*, improve perinatal outcome. Improvement in outcome can be derived from using the time that is gained before delivery to institute measures that are known to be effective in improving outcome for the preterm infant. There is also a slight possibility that some prolongation of the interval until delivery might be beneficial (Schutte *et al.* 1983b).

Three controlled trials have been reported on the use of tocolytic drugs versus no tocolysis in preterm labour following prelabour rupture of the membranes (Christensen *et al.* 1980; Garite *et al.* 1987; Weiner *et al.* 1988). One of these (Weiner *et al.* 1988), which reported on what was described as 'aggressive tocolysis for premature labor associated with premature rupture of the membranes', could not be interpreted reliably. The word 'premature' apparently had a different meaning from what is commonly understood by 'premature rupture of the membranes', for 21 per cent of the women had uterine contractions (and 8 per cent had 'regular contractions') before rupture of the membranes. In addition, the authors excluded from their analysis as many as 31 per cent of the women randomized to either one of the two policies (Weiner *et al.* 1988; see also Chapter 44). Data from the other two trials have been combined in Table 43.15.

Christensen *et al.* (1980) allocated 14 women to intravenous ritodrine followed by oral maintenance treatment and 16 women to placebo in a double-blind fashion. Women were between 28 and 36 weeks of gestation, and had no signs of intrauterine infection. Only urogenital carriers of group B streptococci or *E coli* were treated with antibiotics (ampicillin) during labour. Corticosteroids were apparently not administered in either group, although exact information on this aspect is not available in their report. Garite and his colleagues (1987) conducted a study in which 79 women admitted with prelabour rupture of the membranes were randomized to an intent either to treat or not to treat women with a tocolytic agent, if and when uterine contractions started before 31 weeks of gestation. Only 5 of the 79 women had regular contractions on admission, although some degree of contractility was present in 30 of them (38 per cent). None of the women received corticosteroids or antibiotics. The drug treatment, which was actually given to 23 of the 39 women randomized to the 'intention to treat' group, consisted of intravenous ritodrine followed by oral maintenance until the end of the 31st week. The remaining 16 women (41 per cent), who had been scheduled to receive ritodrine, did not receive the drug either because they had developed chorioamnionitis, or because they had gone beyond 31 weeks of gestation, or because the cervix was too dilated at the time that treatment was due to begin.

The combined data of the two trials (Christensen *et al.* 1980; Garite *et al.* 1987) show no statistically significant delay of delivery with betamimetic drug treatment (Table 43.15), and only one of the two trials shows a small delay of 24 hours to be more frequent in treated than in untreated women (Table 43.15). None of the other outcomes reported, whether they related to infant mortality and morbidity, or infectious morbidity in the mother, indicated that tocolytic treatment in any way influenced the outcome for mother or baby (Table 43.15). In the absence of further data on the effects of betamimetic drugs in preterm labour after prelabour rupture of the membranes, it can only be concluded that there is no evidence to consider their effects as being distinctly different from those in other preterm labours discussed elsewhere (see Chapter 44).

A trial of indomethacin to arrest preterm labour after rupture of the membranes was reported by Gamissans and his colleagues (Gamissans *et al.* 1982; Gamissans and Balasch 1984). It is not clear, however, how often the membranes ruptured before as opposed to after the onset of labour, and all women in both the indomethacin and the placebo group also received ritodrine to arrest labour (see Chapter 44). There were no statistically significant differences in any of the outcome measures, which included delay of delivery, recurrence of preterm labour, preterm delivery, infant birthweight, mortality, and respiratory morbidity (Gamissans and Balasch 1984). Delay of delivery for more than 10 days was achieved in 22 of 38 women (58 per cent) treated with ritodrine and indomethacin, compared with 20 of 36 women (55 per cent) who received only ritodrine.

The totality of the evidence available is too weak to indicate whether preterm labour which starts with uterine contractions should be considered to be different from that which follows rupture of the membranes. In the absence of evidence to the contrary, the answers to questions on the effects of tocolysis should be the same irrespective of whether preterm labour is preceded by rupture of the membranes.

5.4 Amnioinfusion

Decelerations of the fetal heart rate during preterm labour occur more frequently if the membranes have ruptured before the onset of labour. Many of the abnormal fetal heart rate patterns are suggestive of umbilical cord compression, and may well be due to the loss of the protective effect of amniotic fluid (Moberg *et al.* 1984). Gabbe and his colleagues (1976) showed in chronic experiments in the Rhesus monkey that removal of amniotic fluid produced variable deceleration patterns in the fetal heart rate, and that the frequency of these decelerations could be markedly reduced by infusion of normal saline to replace the volume lost. Later, Miyazaki and Taylor (1983) observed that variable

Table 43.15 Effect of tocolytic treatment during preterm labour after prelabour rupture of the membranes on delivery <24 hours

Study	EXPT *n*	EXPT (%)	CTRL *n*	CTRL (%)	Odds ratio (95% CI)	Graph of odds ratios and confidence intervals (0.01, 0.1, 0.5, 1, 2, 10, 100)
Christensen *et al.* (1980)	0/14	(0.00)	6/16	(37.50)	0.10 (0.02–0.60)	
Garite *et al.* (1987)	4/39	(10.26)	4/40	(10.00)	1.03 (0.24–4.40)	
Typical odds ratio (95% confidence interval)					0.41 (0.13–1.25)	

Effect of tocolytic treatment during preterm labour after prelabour rupture of the membranes on delivery <48 hours

Study	EXPT *n*	EXPT (%)	CTRL *n*	CTRL (%)	Odds ratio (95% CI)
Christensen *et al.* (1980)	7/14	(50.00)	9/16	(56.25)	0.78 (0.19–3.22)
Garite *et al.* (1987)	9/39	(23.08)	10/40	(25.00)	0.90 (0.32–2.51)
Typical odds ratio (95% confidence interval)					0.86 (0.37–1.97)

Effect of tocolytic treatment during preterm labour after prelabour rupture of the membranes on delivery <1 week

Study	EXPT *n*	EXPT (%)	CTRL *n*	CTRL (%)	Odds ratio (95% CI)
Christensen *et al.* (1980)	11/14	(78.57)	15/16	(93.75)	0.28 (0.04–2.24)
Garite *et al.* (1987)	27/39	(69.23)	27/40	(67.50)	1.08 (0.42–2.78)
Typical odds ratio (95% confidence interval)					0.86 (0.36–2.03)

Effect of tocolytic treatment during preterm labour after prelabour rupture of the membranes on delivery <32 weeks

Study	EXPT *n*	EXPT (%)	CTRL *n*	CTRL (%)	Odds ratio (95% CI)
Garite *et al.* (1987)	31/39	(79.49)	34/40	(85.00)	0.69 (0.22–2.17)
Typical odds ratio (95% confidence interval)					0.69 (0.22–2.17)

Effect of tocolytic treatment during preterm labour after prelabour rupture of the membranes on perinatal death (excluding malformations)

Study	EXPT *n*	EXPT (%)	CTRL *n*	CTRL (%)	Odds ratio (95% CI)
Christensen *et al.* (1980)	1/14	(7.14)	0/16	(0.00)	8.52 (0.17–99.99)
Garite *et al.* (1987)	5/39	(12.82)	2/40	(5.00)	2.60 (0.56–12.16)
Typical odds ratio (95% confidence interval)					3.05 (0.73–12.81)

Effect of tocolytic treatment during preterm labour after prelabour rupture of membranes on respiratory distress syndrome

Study	EXPT *n*	EXPT (%)	CTRL *n*	CTRL (%)	Odds ratio (95% CI)
Christensen *et al.* (1980)	2/14	(14.29)	1/16	(6.25)	2.37 (0.23–24.88)
Garite *et al.* (1987)	20/39	(51.28)	23/40	(57.50)	0.78 (0.32–1.88)
Typical odds ratio (95% confidence interval)					0.89 (0.39–2.04)

Effect of tocolytic treatment during preterm labour after prelabour rupture of the membranes on neonatal sepsis

Study	EXPT		CTRL		Odds ratio	Graph of odds ratios and confidence intervals
	n	(%)	*n*	(%)	(95% CI)	0.01 0.1 0.5 1 2 10 100
Garite *et al.* (1987)	1/39	(2.56)	2/40	(5.00)	0.52 (0.05–5.13)	
Typical odds ratio (95% confidence interval)					0.52 (0.05–5.13)	

Effect of tocolytic treatment during preterm labour after prelabour rupture of the membranes on severe intraventricular haemorrhage

Study	EXPT *n*	(%)	CTRL *n*	(%)	Odds ratio (95% CI)	Graph
Garite *et al.* (1987)	3/39	(7.69)	2/40	(5.00)	1.57 (0.26–9.47)	
Typical odds ratio (95% confidence interval)					1.57 (0.26–9.47)	

Effect of tocolytic treatment during preterm labour after prelabour rupture of the membranes on chorioamnionitis

Study	EXPT *n*	(%)	CTRL *n*	(%)	Odds ratio (95% CI)	Graph
Christensen *et al.* (1980)	1/14	(7.14)	1/16	(6.25)	1.15 (0.07–19.41)	
Garite *et al.* (1987)	14/39	(35.90)	7/40	(17.50)	2.54 (0.94–6.84)	
Typical odds ratio (95% confidence interval)					2.33 (0.91–5.93)	

Effect of tocolytic treatment during preterm labour after prelabour rupture of the membranes on endomyometritis postpartum

Study	EXPT *n*	(%)	CTRL *n*	(%)	Odds ratio (95% CI)	Graph
Christensen *et al.* (1980)	1/14	(7.14)	1/16	(6.25)	1.15 (0.07–19.41)	
Garite *et al.* (1987)	10/39	(25.64)	6/40	(15.00)	1.92 (0.64–5.70)	
Typical odds ratio (95% confidence interval)					1.79 (0.65–4.96)	

decelerations in fetal heart rate during human labour often disappeared when saline was infused into the intrauterine cavity through a transcervical intrauterine pressure catheter. Although these decelerations are not always indicative of fetal hypoxaemia and acidosis, they certainly result in a higher need for fetal scalp blood sampling and often lead to an increased caesarean section rate (Moberg *et al.* 1984). Reducing the incidence of such decelerations may therefore be beneficial, not only in lowering the incidence of fetal hypoxia, but also in reducing the need for other interventions such as scalp blood sampling of a preterm fetus and caesarean section in a possibly infected environment.

Only one controlled trial has addressed the relative merits and hazards of using amnioinfusion during labour in women with prelabour rupture of the membranes preterm (Nageotte *et al.* 1985). The authors assigned 66 women 'in a random fashion' (details of how this was achieved are not given) to receive amnioinfusion during labour, or to a control group who would not receive amnioinfusion. Five women were excluded, apparently all before labour, either because of antepartum fetal distress or because a non-vertex presentation was diagnosed at some time between 'random' allocation and implementation of the policy. Twenty-nine women received an amnioinfusion of normal saline at 37°C through an intrauterine pressure catheter inserted through the cervix. The saline was delivered at a rate of 10 ml per minute in the first hour and 3 ml per minute thereafter. The 32 women in the control group also had an intrauterine pressure catheter inserted for monitoring purposes. Gestational ages at delivery ranged from 26 to 35 weeks.

The authors reported a statistically significant reduction in the number of mild, moderate, and severe variable decelerations per hour in the infused group as compared with the control group. The number of women who experienced such decelerations is not reported, but 7 women in the control group underwent caesarean section because of fetal distress compared with only one in the amnioinfusion group. The mean (SD) number of decelerations per hour was reduced from 18.0 (6.0) in the control group to 7.2 (7.0) in the group receiving amnioinfusion. Umbilical blood pH values at birth were statistically significantly higher in the infused group than in the control group, with mean (SD) arterial pH values of respectively 7.34 (0.05) and 7.23 (0.08). As shown in Table 43.16, the procedure did not produce a detectable increase in the incidence of endometritis postpartum; 3 of the 4 cases of endometritis occurred in women who had undergone caesarean section. Although the only outcomes that were influenced to a statistically significant extent were the mean number of decelerations and the average umbilical pH (which may or may not explain the difference in caesarean section rates), this study warrants replication.

Limiting further controlled trials to women with prelabour rupture of the membranes who already show some evidence of fetal heart decelerations may be advantageous in two respects. First, the women and babies entered into such a study would be less likely to experience harm for no potential benefit than those without fetal heart rate decelerations. Second, firm conclusions on the beneficial effects, if any, of this approach may be more readily reached when there is a higher prevalence of the adverse outcomes, such as fetal hypoxia and caesarean section, which one is trying to prevent.

6 Conclusions

6.1 Implications for current practice

Prelabour rupture of the membranes preterm precedes nearly half of all preterm deliveries. It adds its own specific problems to those of preterm labour and preterm delivery considered more generally (see Chapters 44 and 74). The number of recommendations for current practice that can be adequately substantiated is considerably smaller than the number of opinions about what does or does not constitute adequate care for these women and their babies. This applies both to the specialized diagnostic tests and to the various treatments that are applied in these circumstances.

Any woman with a history suggestive of prelabour rupture of the membranes in the preterm period should be assessed as soon as possible. Attention should be directed to whether the membranes are indeed ruptured; to a careful review of the menstrual history and assessment of gestational age; to possible signs of incipient or established infection; to signs of fetal distress due to cord compression or prolapse; and to signs of uterine contractions.

For the woman who is not in labour, is not infected, and shows no evidence of fetal distress or other fetal or maternal pathology, continuation of the pregnancy is more likely to be beneficial than harmful. The limited evidence that is available suggests that measures to effect delivery do more harm than good. In view of the frequency with which preterm delivery will follow

Table 43.16 Effect of amnioinfusion for prelabour rupture of the membranes on caesarean section

Study	EXPT		CTRL		Odds ratio	Graph of odds ratios and confidence intervals
	n	(%)	*n*	(%)	(95% CI)	0.01 0.1 0.5 1 2 10 100
Nageotte *et al.* (1985)	2/29	(6.90)	7/32	(21.88)	0.31 (0.08–1.26)	
Typical odds ratio (95% confidence interval)					0.31 (0.08–1.26)	

Effect of amnioinfusion for prelabour rupture of the membranes on neonatal death

Study	EXPT *n*	(%)	CTRL *n*	(%)	Odds ratio (95% CI)	Graph
Nageotte *et al.* (1985)	1/29	(3.45)	2/32	(6.25)	0.55 (0.06–5.56)	
Typical odds ratio (95% confidence interval)					0.55 (0.06–5.56)	

Effect of amnioinfusion for prelabour rupture of the membranes on endometritis

Study	EXPT *n*	(%)	CTRL *n*	(%)	Odds ratio (95% CI)	Graph
Nageotte *et al.* (1985)	1/29	(3.45)	3/32	(9.38)	0.39 (0.05–2.89)	
Typical odds ratio (95% confidence interval)					0.39 (0.05–2.89)	

prelabour rupture of the membranes, corticosteroids should be administered if pulmonary maturity is likely to be inadequate. Whether corticosteroid treatment should be combined routinely with antibiotic treatment cannot be determined on the basis of the available evidence. On balance, combining antibiotics with corticosteroids is likely to do more good than harm and such a policy is certainly worth investigating in a controlled manner.

In populations with a high prevalence of group B streptococci carriers, either screening for the organism or antibiotic treatment should be adopted. In all other populations, an initial culture should be part of the care provided after prelabour rupture of the membranes preterm. Since the main risk is ascending infection, there is no justification for amniocentesis in order to obtain culture data directly from within the uterus.

An important consideration in respect of all the specific elements of care mentioned above is that, despite the initial lack of uterine contractions, nearly all women with prelabour rupture of the membranes preterm will eventually deliver preterm, and the majority of them will do so within a week of rupturing their membranes. There is no evidence, however, that the prophylactic use of oral betamimetic agents before uterine contractions begin is of any value in preventing the onset of labour.

By contrast with uncomplicated prelabour rupture of the membranes preterm, antibiotic treatment should be started and delivery effected if there are signs of intrauterine infection. These objectives should be pursued with adequately intensive surveillance, and the presence of a skilled neonatologist at birth.

Except for the special circumstances mentioned above, there is little evidence that the onset of preterm labour after rupture of the membranes requires forms of care that are distinctly different from those normally required in preterm labour. Due consideration should be given, however, to the possibility that the initiation of labour may have resulted from intrauterine infection, and that it may entail an increased risk of cord prolapse.

6.2 Implications for future research

Considering the magnitude of the problem and the wealth of literature on the subject, it is surprising how few controlled comparisons are available to guide the important choices that need to be made in the care for women with prelabour rupture of the membranes preterm. There are a number of issues that would appear to merit priority among clinical investigators.

First, there is a need to assess whether or not the prognosis of hindwater rupture is comparable to that associated with forewater rupture because it is plausible that the former may be a more benign condition. Investigations aimed at distinguishing these two forms of prelabour rupture of the membranes preterm are likely to be worthwhile.

Second, the relative merits and hazards of the various diagnostic elements in this condition, including vaginal examination (digital or speculum), should be assessed not only in terms of their predictive properties and consequences for determining the pattern of subsequent care, but also in terms of the maternal discomfort they entail. The same applies to the many measures, such as ultrasound assessment of liquor volume and fetal breathing and other movements, that are used both for initial diagnosis and in subsequent surveillance.

Third, a formal, randomized comparison of elective versus selective use of antibiotics in women with prelabour rupture of the membranes preterm, irrespective of whether or not uterine contractions are present, would seem to be high on the list of priorities. At a lower level of priority could be randomized comparisons of elective versus selective use of antibiotics instituted either at the onset of labour, or after delivery.

Lastly, further controlled trials are required to assess whether amnioinfusion has a role in the management of labour when oligohydramnios has resulted from prelabour rupture of the membranes, either in all women, or in those in whom there is suggestive evidence of umbilical cord compression.

References

Amon E, Lewis SV, Sibai BM, Villar MA, Arheart KL (1988). Ampicillin prophylaxis in preterm premature rupture of membranes: A prospective randomized study. Am J Obstet Gynecol, 159: 539–543.

Andreyko JL, Chen CP, Shennan AT, Milligan JE (1984). Results of conservative management of premature rupture of the membranes. Am J Obstet Gynecol, 148: 600–604.

Atlay RD, Sutherst JR (1970). Premature rupture of the fetal membranes confirmed by intra-amniotic injection of dye (Evans blue T-1824). Am J Obstet Gynecol, 108: 993–994.

Barrett JM, Boehm FH (1982). Comparison of aggressive and conservative management of premature rupture of fetal membranes. Am J Obstet Gynecol, 144: 12–16.

Baumgarten K, Moser S (1986). Technique of fibrin adhesion for premature rupture of membranes during pregnancy. J Perinat Med, 14: 43–49.

Beck JC, Johnson JWC (1980). Maternal administration of glucocorticoids. Clin Obstet Gynecol, 23: 93–113.

Bejar R, Curbelo V, Davis C, Gluck L (1981). Premature labor. II: Bacterial sources of phospholipase. Obstet Gynecol, 57: 479–482.

Bennett PR, Rose MP, Myatt L, Elder MG (1987). Preterm labor: Stimulation of arachidonic metabolism in human amnion cells by bacterial products. Am J Obstet Gynecol, 156: 649–655.

Beydoun SN, Yasin SY (1986). Premature rupture of the membranes before 28 weeks: Conservative management. Am J Obstet Gynecol, 155: 471–479.

Bhutani VK, Abbasi S, Weiner S (1986). Neonatal pulmonary manifestations due to prolonged amniotic leak. Am J Perinatol, 3: 225–230.

Block MF, Kling OR, Crosby WM (1977). Antenatal glucocorticoid therapy for the prevention of respiratory distress syndrome in the premature infant. Obstet Gynecol, 50: 186–190.

Blott M, Greenough A, Nicolaides KH, Moscoso G, Gibb D, Campbell S (1987). Fetal breathing movements as predictor of favourable pregnancy outcome after oligohydramnios due to membrane rupture in second trimester. Lancet, 2: 129–131.

Breese MW (1961). Spontaneous premature rupture of the membranes. Am J Obstet Gynecol, 81: 1086–1093.

Brelje MC, Kaltreider DF, Kassir L (1966). The use of vaginal antibiotics in premature rupture of the membranes. Am J Obstet Gynecol, 94: 889–897.

Brosens I, Gordon H (1965). The cytological diagnosis of ruptured membranes using nile blue sulphate staining. J Obstet Gynaecol Br Commnwlth, 72: 342–346.

Capeless E, Mead PB (1987). Management of preterm rupture of membranes: Lack of a national consensus. Am J Obstet Gynecol, 157: 11–12.

Chiswick ML, Burnard E (1973). Respiratory distress syndrome. Lancet, 1: 1060–1062.

Christensen KK, Ingemarsson I, Leideman T, Solum H, Svenningsen N (1980). Effect of ritodrine on labor after premature rupture of the membranes. Obstet Gynecol, 55: 187–190.

Collaborative Group on Antenatal Steroid Therapy (1981). Effect of antenatal dexamethasone administration on the prevention of respiratory distress syndrome. Am J Obstet Gynecol, 141: 276–287.

Cotton DB, Hill LM, Strassner HT, Platt LD, Ledger WJ (1984a). Use of amniocentesis in preterm gestation with ruptured membranes. Obstet Gynecol, 63: 38–43.

Cotton DB, Gonik B, Bottoms SF (1984b). Conservative versus aggressive management of preterm rupture of membranes. A randomized trial of amniocentesis. Am J Perinatol, 1: 322–324.

Coustan DR (1987). Clinical aspects of antenatal enhancement of pulmonary maturity. Clin Perinatol, 14: 697–711.

Dunlop PDM, Crowley PA, Lamont RF, Hawkins DF (1986). Preterm ruptured membranes, no contractions. J Obstet Gynaecol, 7: 92–96.

Evans MI, Haij SN, Devoe LD, Angerman NS, Moawad AH (1980). C-reactive protein as a predictor of infectious morbidity with premature rupture of the membranes. Am J Obstet Gynecol, 138: 648–652.

Farb HF, Arnesen M. Geistler P, Knox GE (1983). C-reactive protein with premature rupture of membranes and premature labor. Obstet Gynecol, 62: 49–51.

Fayez JA, Hasan AA, Jonas HS, Miller GL (1978). Management of premature rupture of the membranes. Obstet Gynecol, 52: 17–21.

FIGO News (1976). Lists of gynecologic and obstetrical terms and definitions. Int J Gynaecol Obstet, 14: 570–576.

Feinstein SJ, Vintzileos AM, Lodeiro JG, Campbell WA, Weinbaum PJ, Nochimson DJ (1986). Amniocentesis with premature rupture of the membranes. Obstet Gynecol, 68: 147–152.

Ferguson MG, Rhodes PG, Morrison JC, Puckett CM (1985). Clinical amniotic fluid infection and its effect on the neonate. Am J Obstet Gynecol, 151: 1058–1061.

Fox HE, Moessinger AC (1985). Fetal breathing movements and lung hypoplasia: Preliminary human observations. Am J Obstet Gynecol, 151: 531–533.

Friedman ML, McElin TW (1969). Diagnosis of ruptured fetal membranes. Clinical study and review of literature. Am J Obstet Gynecol, 104: 544–550.

Gabbe SG, Ettinger BB, Freeman RK, Martin CB (1976). Umbilical cord compression associated with amniotomy: Laboratory observations. Am J Obstet Gynecol, 126: 353–355.

Gamissans O, Cararach V, Serra J (1982). The role of prostaglandin-inhibitors, beta-adrenergic drugs and glucocorticoids in the management of threatened preterm labor. In: Beta-mimetic Drugs in Obstetrics and Perinatology. Jung H, Lamberti G (eds). Stuttgart: Georg Thieme, pp 71–84.

Gamissans O, Balasch J (1984). Prostaglandin synthetase inhibitors in the treatment of preterm labor. In: Preterm Birth: Causes, Prevention and Management. Fuchs F, Stubblefield PG (eds). New York: Macmillan, pp 223–248.

Garite TJ, Freeman RK, Linzey EM, Braly PS, (1979). The use of amniocentesis in patients with premature rupture of membranes. Obstet Gynecol, 54: 226–230.

Garite TJ, Freeman RK, Linzey EM, Braly PS, Dorchester WL (1981). Prospective randomized study of corticosteroids in the management of premature rupture of the membranes and the premature gestation. Am J Obstet Gynecol, 141: 508–515.

Garite TJ, Keegan KA, Freeman RK, Nageotte MP (1987). A randomized trial of ritodrine tocolysis versus expectant management in patients with premature rupture of membranes at 25 to 30 weeks of gestation. Am J Obstet Gynecol, 157: 388–393.

Gibbs RS (1977). Diagnosis of intra-amniotic infection. Seminars Perinatol, 1: 71–77.

Gibbs RS, Blanco JD (1982). Premature rupture of the membranes. Obstet Gynecol, 60: 671–679.

Gibbs RS, Castillo MS, Rodgers PJ (1980). Management of acute chorioamnionitis. Am J Obstet Gynecol, 136: 709–713.

Gillebrand PN (1967). Premature rupture of the membranes and prematurity. J Obstet Gynaecol Br Commnwlth, 74: 678–683.

Gilstrap LC, Leveno KJ, Cox SM, Burris JS, Mashburn M, Rosenfeld CR (1988). Intrapartum treatment of acute chorioamnionitis: Impact on neonatal sepsis. Am J Obstet Gynecol, 159: 579–583.

Goldstein I, Romero R, Merrill S, Wan M, O'Connor TZ, Mazor M, Hobbins JC (1988). Fetal body and breathing movements as predictors of intraamniotic infection in preterm premature rupture of membranes. Am J Obstet Gynecol, 159: 363–368.

Gonik B, Cotton DB (1985). The use of amniocentesis in preterm premature rupture of membranes. Am J Perinatol, 2: 21–24.

Gonik B, Bottoms SF, Cotton DB (1985). Amniotic fluid volume as a risk factor in preterm premature rupture of the membranes. Obstet Gynecol, 65: 456–459.

Graham L, Gilstrap LC, Hauth JC, Kodack-Garza S (1982). Conservative management of patients with premature rupture of fetal membranes. Obstet Gynecol, 59: 607–610.

Guzick DS, Winn K (1985). The association of chorioamnionitis with preterm delivery. Obstet Gynecol, 65: 11–16.

Hawrylyshyn P, Bernstein P, Milligan JE, Soldin S, Pollard A, Papsin FR (1983). Premature rupture of membranes: The role of C-reactive protein in the prediction of chorioamnionitis. Am J Obstet Gynecol, 147: 240–246.

Hislop A, Fairweather DVI, Blackwell RJ, Howard S (1984). The effect of amniocentesis and drainage of amniotic fluid on lung development in Macaca fascicularis. Br J Obstet Gynaecol, 91: 835–842.

Iams JD, Talbert ML, Barrows H, Sachs L (1985). Management of preterm prematurely ruptured membranes: A prospective randomized comparison of observation vs use of steroids and timed delivery. Am J Obstet Gynecol, 151: 32–38.

Iannetta O (1984). A new simple test for detecting rupture of the fetal membranes. Obstet Gynecol, 63: 575–576.

Ismail MA, Zinaman MJ, Lowensohn RI, Moaward AH (1985). The significance of C-reactive protein levels in women with premature rupture of membranes. Am J Obstet Gynecol, 151: 541–544.

Johnson JW, Daikoku NH, Niebyl JR, Johnson TRB, Khouzami VA, Witter RF (1981). Premature rupture of membranes and prolonged latency. Obstet Gynecol, 57: 547–556.

Jones MD, Burd LT, Bowes WA, Battaglia FC, Lubchenko LO (1975). Failure of association of premature rupture of the membranes with respiratory-distress syndrome. New Engl J Med, 292: 1253–1257.

Kanhai HHH (1981). Achtergronden en Konsekwenties van Vroeggeboorte. Leiden University: MD thesis.

Keirse MJNC (1979). Epidemiology of pre-term labour. In: Human Parturition. Keirse MJNC, Anderson ABM, Bennebroek Gravenhorst J (eds). The Hague: Leiden University Press, pp 219–234.

Keirse MJNC (1984). A survey of tocolytic drug treatment in preterm labour. Br J Obstet Gynaecol, 91: 424–430.

Keirse MJNC, Thiery M, Parewijck W, Mitchell MD (1983). Chronic stimulation of uterine prostaglandin synthesis during cervical ripening before the onset of labor. Prostaglandins, 25: 671–682.

Koh KS, Chan FH, Monfared AH, Ledger WJ, Paul RH (1979). The changing perinatal and maternal outcome in chorioamnionitis. Obstet Gynecol, 53: 730–734.

Kragt H, Keirse MJNC (1989). How accurate is a woman's diagnosis of threatened preterm delivery? (submitted for publication).

Lamont RF, Rose MP, Elder MG (1985). Effect of bacterial products on prostaglandin E production by amnion cells. Lancet, 2: 1331–1333.

Larsen JW, Goldkrand JW, Hanson TM, Miller CK (1974). Intrauterine infection on an obstetric service. Obstet Gynecol, 43: 838–843.

Larsen JW, Weis KR, Lenihan JP, Crumrine M, Heggers JP (1976). Significance of neutrophils and bacteria in the amniotic fluid of patients in labor. Obstet Gynecol, 47: 143–147.

Lebherz TB, Hellman LP, Madding R, Anctil A, Arje SL (1963). Double-blind study of premature rupture of the membranes. Am J Obstet Gynecol, 87: 218–225.

Levy DL, Warsof SL (1985). Oral ritodrine and preterm premature rupture of membranes. Obstet Gynecol, 66: 621–623.

Listwa HM, Dobek AS, Cartpenter J, Gibbs RS (1976). The predictability of intrauterine infection by analysis of amniotic fluid. Obstet Gynecol, 48: 31–34.

Mead FB (1980). Management of the patient with premature rupture of the membranes. Clin Perinatol, 7: 243–255.

Mitchell MD, Keirse MJNC, Anderson, ABM. Turnbull AC (1977). Evidence for a local control of prostaglandins within the pregnant human uterus. Br J Obstet Gynaecol, 84: 35–38.

Miyazaki FS, Taylor NA (1983). Saline amnioinfusion for relief of variable or prolonged decelerations. Am J Obstet Gynecol, 146: 670–678.

Moberg LJ, Garite TJ, Freeman RK (1984). Fetal heart rate patterns and fetal distress in patients with preterm premature rupture of membranes. Obstet Gynecol, 64: 60–64.

Morales WJ, Diebel ND, Lazar AJ, Zadrozny D (1986). The effect of antenatal dexamethasone administration on the prevention of respiratory distress syndrome in preterm gestations with premature rupture of membranes. Am J Obstet Gynecol, 154: 591–595.

Munson LA, Graham A, Koos BJ, Valenzuela GJ (1985). Is there a need for digital examination in patients with spontaneous rupture of the membranes? Am J Obstet Gynecol, 153: 562–563.

Naeye RL, Blanc WA (1970). Relation of poverty and race to antenatal infection. New Engl J Med, 283: 555–560.

Naeye RL, Peters EC (1980). Causes and consequences of premature rupture of fetal membranes. Lancet, 1: 192–194.

Naeye RL, Ross SM (1982). Amniotic fluid infection syndrome. Clin Obstet Gynaecol, 9: 593–607.

Nageotte MP, Freeman RK, Garite TJ, Dorchester W (1985). Prophylactic intrapartum amnioinfusion in patients with preterm premature rupture of membranes. Am J Obstet Gynecol, 153: 557–562.

Nelson LH, Meis PJ, Hatjis CG, Ernest JM, Dillard R, Schey HM (1985). Premature rupture of membranes: A prospective, randomized evaluation of steroids, latent phase, and expectant management. Obstet Gynecol, 66: 55–58.

Nelson DM, Stempel LE, Zuspan FP (1986). Association of prolonged, preterm premature rupture of the membranes and abruptio placentae. J Reprod Med, 31: 429–432.

Nimrod C, Varela-Gittings F, Machin G, Campbell D, Wesenberg R (1984). The effect of very prolonged membrane rupture on fetal development. Am J Obstet Gynecol, 148: 540–543.

Ogita S, Imanaka M, Matsumoto M, Hatanaka K (1984). Premature rupture of the membranes managed with a new cervical catheter. Lancet, 1: 1330–1331.

Perkins RP (1982). The neonatal significance of selected perinatal events among infants of low birth weight. II. The influence of ruptured membranes. Am J Obstet Gynecol, 142: 7–16.

Reid DE (1970). The right and the responsibility. Am J Obstet Gynecol, 108: 825–832.

Rochelson BL, Rodke G, White R, Bracero L, Baker DA (1987). A rapid colorimetric AFP monoclonal antibody test for the diagnosis of preterm rupture of the membranes. Obstet Gynecol, 69: 163–166.

Romem Y, Artal R (1984). C-reactive protein as a predictor for chorioamnionitis in cases of premature rupture of the membranes. Am J Obstet Gynecol, 150: 546–550.

Romero R, Quintero R, Oyarzun E, Wu YK, Sabo V, Mazor M, Hobbins JC (1988). Intraamniotic infection and the onset of labor in preterm premature rupture of the membranes. Am J Obstet Gynecol, 159: 661–666.

Saling E (1979). Successes and problems with tocolysis and management of premature rupture of membranes. In: Recent Progress in Perinatal Medicine and Prevention of Congenital Anomaly. Tokyo: IYC Commemorative International Congress, pp 103–120.

Schmidt PL, Sims ME, Strassner HT, Paul RH, Mueller E, McCart D (1984). Effect of antepartum glucocorticoid administration upon neonatal respiratory distress syndrome and perinatal infection. Am J Obstet Gynecol, 148: 178–186.

Schutte MF, Treffers PE, Kloosterman GJ, Soepatmi S (1983a). Management of premature rupture of the membranes: The risk of vaginal examination to the infant. Am J Obstet Gynecol, 146: 395–400.

Schutte MF, Treffers PE, Koppe JG (1983b). Threatened preterm labor: the influence of time factors on the incidence of respiratory distress syndrome. Obstet Gynecol, 62: 287–293.

Simpson GF, Harbert GM (1985). Use of β-methasone in management of preterm gestation with premature rupture of membranes. Obstet Gynecol, 66: 168–175.

Smith RP (1976). A technique for the detection of rupture of the membranes. A review and preliminary report. Obstet Gynecol, 48: 172–176.

Sperling RS, Ramamurthy RS, Gibbs RS (1987). A comparison of intrapartum versus immediate postpartum treatment of intra-amniotic infection. Obstet Gynecol, 70: 861–856.

Spinnato JA, Shaver DC, Bray EM, Lipshitz J (1987). Preterm premature rupture of the membranes with fetal pulmonary maturity present: A prospective study. Obstet Gynecol, 69: 196–201.

Stedman CM, Crawford S, Staten E, Cherny WB (1981). Management of preterm premature rupture of the membranes: Assessing amniotic fluid in the vagina for phosphatidylglycerol. Am J Obstet Gynecol, 140: 34–38.

Tabor A, Philip J, Madsen M, Bang J, Obel EB, Nordgaard-Pedersen B (1986). Randomized controlled trial of genetic amniocentesis in 4066 low-risk women. Lancet, 1: 1287–1293.

Taylor J, Garite TJ (1984). Premature rupture of membranes before fetal viability. Obstet Gynecol, 64: 615–620.

Thibeault DW, Beatty EC, Hall RT, Bowen SK, O'Neill DH (1985). Neonatal pulmonary hypoplasia with premature rupture of fetal membranes and oligohydramnios. J Pediatr, 107: 273–277.

Trudinger BJ, Boshell L (1987). A survey of the management of premature labour by Australian obstetricians. Austral NZ J Obstet Gynaecol, 27: 188–195.

Van Kamp I, Kanhai HH, Keirse MJNC (1989). The changing pattern of preterm birth. In preparation.

Varner MW, Galask RP (1981). Conservative management of premature rupture of the membranes. Am J Obstet Gynecol, 140: 39–45.

Verloove-Vanhorick SP, Verwey RA (1987). Project on Preterm and Small for Gestational Age Infants in The Netherlands 1983: A Collaborative Survey. Leiden University: MD thesis.

Vintzileos AM, Campbell WA, Nochimson DJ, Connolly ME, Fuenfer MM, Hoehn GJ (1985a). The fetal biophysical profile in patients with premature rupture of the membranes—An early predictor of fetal infection. Am J Obstet Gynecol, 152: 510–516.

Vintzileos AM, Campbell WA, Nochimson DJ, Weinbaum PJ (1985b). Degree of oligohydramnios and pregnancy outcome in patients with premature rupture of the membranes. Obstet Gynecol, 66: 162–167.

Vintzileos AM, Campbell WA, Nochimson DJ, Weinbaum PJ (1986a). The use of the nonstress test in patients with premature rupture of the membranes. Am J Obstet Gynecol, 155: 149–153.

Vintzileos AM, Campbell WA, Nochimson DJ, Weinbaum PJ, Mirochnik MH, Escoto DT (1986b). Fetal biophysical profile versus amniocentesis in predicting infection in preterm premature rupture of the membranes. Obstet Gynecol, 68: 488–494.

Vintzileos AM, Campbell WA, Nochimson DJ, Weinbaum PJ (1986c). Fetal breathing as a predictor of infection in premature rupture of the membranes. Obstet Gynecol, 67: 813–817.

Vintzileos AM, Feinstein SJ, Lodeiro JG, Campbell WA, Weinbaum PJ, Nochimson DJ (1986d). Fetal biophysical profile and the effect of premature rupture of the membranes. Obstet Gynecol, 67: 818–823.

Vintzileos AM, Bors-Koefoed R, Pelegano JF, Campbell WA, Rodis JF, Nochimson DJ, Kontopoulos VG (1987a). The use of fetal biophysical profile improves pregnancy outcome in premature rupture of the membranes. Am J Obstet Gynecol, 157: 236–240.

Vintzileos AM, Campbell WA, Nochimson DJ, Weinbaum PJ (1987b). Preterm premature rupture of the membranes: A risk factor for the development of abruptio placentae. Am J Obstet Gynecol, 156: 1235–1238.

Vintzileos AM, Campbell WA, Nochimson DJ, Weinbaum PJ (1987c).The use and misuse of the fetal biophysical profile. Am J Obstet Gynecol, 156: 527–533.

Weiner CP, Renk K, Klugman M (1988). The therapeutic efficacy and cost-effectiveness of agressive tocolysis for premature labor associated with premature rupture of the membranes. Am J Obstet Gynecol, 159: 216–222.

Wennergren M, Krantz M, Hjalmarson O, Karlsson K (1986). Interval from rupture of the membranes to delivery and neonatal respiratory adaptation. Br J Obstet Gynaecol, 93: 799–803.

White DR, Hall MH, Campbell DM (1986). The aetiology of preterm labour. Br J Obstet Gynaecol 93: 733–738.

Wigglesworth JS, Desai R (1982). Is fetal respiratory function a major determinant of perinatal survival? Lancet, 1: 264–267.

Wigglesworth JS, Desai R, Guerrini P (1981). Fetal lung hypoplasia: Biochemical and structural variations and their possible significance. Arch Dis Childhood, 56: 606–615.

World Health Organization (1977). Recommended definitions, terminology and format for statistical tables related to the perinatal period and use of a new certificate for cause of perinatal deaths. Acta Obstet Gynecol Scand, 56: 247–253.

Yoon JJ, Harper RG (1973). Observations on the relationship between duration of rupture of the membranes and the development of idiopathic respiratory distress syndrome. Pediatrics, 52: 161–168.

44 Preterm labour

Marc J. N. C. Keirse, Adrian Grant, and James F. King

'Every article on the care of the preterm baby ends with a wish that preterm delivery could be prevented'

Lancet 1980

'The use of drugs to inhibit labour is usually unnecessary, frequently ineffective, and occasionally harmful'

British Medical Journal 1979

1 Introduction

Preterm labour differs little from labour at term, except in one crucial aspect: it occurs too early. In the absence of major complications that override physiological processes, the mechanism that initiates preterm labour is likely to be a precocious activation of the same events that cause labour at term. Whether that assumption is correct or not, it is of little help. The exact causal mechanism of labour is unknown and what triggers it remains a mystery.

Judging whether labour has started or not is no easier preterm than it is at term (see Chapter 53). Judging whether preterm labour will or will not lead to preterm delivery is even more difficult. This would not be so if one could adopt the same expectant attitude as at term and observe the steady progress in signs that foretell delivery. Signs of steady progress are useful to prepare for preterm delivery (see Chapter 74). They are not very helpful if preterm delivery needs to be averted and if preterm labour itself is undesirable and needs to be stopped. The more advanced labour is, the more difficult it is to stop.

Successful inhibition of preterm labour therefore depends on early diagnosis, but early diagnosis, particularly of uterine contractions, is notoriously inaccurate for predicting whether preterm delivery will occur or not. O'Driscoll (1977) has suggested that the woman's diagnosis of preterm labour is erroneous about 80 per cent of the time. No data were provided to substantiate that point, however. Kragt and Keirse (1990) found the woman's diagnosis to be far more accurate. Nevertheless, their one year study of all women admitted with threatened preterm labour revealed that as many as 33 per cent of women, whose primary complaint was preterm uterine contractions, could safely return home within 48 hours.

Several authors have attempted to improve upon the classical diagnostic criteria by measurement of hormone levels (Tamby Raja *et al.* 1974; Cousins *et al.* 1977), assessment of fetal breathing movements (Castle and Turnbull 1983; Agustsson and Patel 1987), measurement of prostaglandin metabolites (Fuchs *et al.* 1982), or assessment of thromboxane excretion (Noort *et al.* 1988). Some have attempted to forestall the problem by serial cervical examinations in pregnancy (Papiernik *et al.* 1986; Stubbs *et al.* 1986), by antenatal monitoring of uterine contractions (Anderson and Turnbull 1967; Bell 1983; Katz *et al.* 1986; Morrison *et al.* 1987), or by screening for the risk of preterm delivery (see Chapter 22). Some of these approaches have resulted in the administration of labour inhibiting drugs to more than 40 per cent of low risk pregnant women (Bréart *et al.* 1981), demonstrating how the best results of treatment can be obtained when there is nothing to be treated. Although some of these approaches have shown some merit in controlled comparisons (Morrison *et al.* 1987), it is fair to conclude that the diagnosis of preterm labour has remained as problematic as ever.

Over many years a wide variety of drugs and other interventions have been used in attempts to suppress uterine contractions. Many of these showed such high success rates in the initial reports documenting their use (Table 44.1), that at first glance one would have expected the problem of preterm labour to have been solved many years ago. This has not happened. Nor have these drugs disappeared from the obstetric armentarium. New drug treatments continue to capture the imagination of clinicians desiring to solve the issue of preterm labour once and for all. The introduction of new treatments also continues to follow a pattern, in which enthusiasm for the treatment seems to be at least as persuasive as evidence that it works.

When drug treatments appear to fail, they are not necessarily abandoned. Often other, and equally unvalidated drugs are added in the hope that two unvalidated treatments will be better than one. For example, in 1970, fenoterol was introduced in West Germany (Heilmann and Ludwig 1981), where it is considered to be 'the most used and best explored β-mimetic substance in Europe' (Jung 1982). Soon combinations with various calcium antagonists (Wiedinger and Wiest 1973; Neubüser 1974), beta receptor blockers (Trolp *et al.* 1980), magnesium (Spätling 1981; Wiedinger 1984) and various prostaglandin synthesis inhibitors (Halle and Hengst 1978; Wolff *et al.* 1981) were introduced to compensate for the perceived deficiencies of fenoterol. These combinations have flourished in West Germany

Table 44.1 Summary of approaches used to inhibit preterm labour in the past 35 years and their purported success rates in the first English language publication documenting their use

Agent	Year	Authors	No. of women	Criterion of success	Per cent success
Relaxin	1955	Abramson and Reid	5	delivery after 36 weeks	100
Isoxsuprine	1961	Bishop and Woutersz	120	contractions delayed 24 hours	82
Ethanol	1967	Fuchs *et al.*	52	delivery delayed 72 hours	67
Orciprenaline	1970	Baillie *et al.*	30	delivery after 36 weeks	70
Mesuprine	1971	Barden	17	delivery delayed 24 hours	53
Ritodrine	1971	Wesselius-De Casparis *et al.*	43	not delivered during treatment	80
Fenoterol	1972	Edelstein and Baillie	28	delivery delayed 1 week	71
Salbutamol	1973	Liggins and Vaughan	88	delivery delayed 24 hours	85
Indomethacin	1974	Zuckerman *et al.*	50	arrest of contractions	80
Sodium salicylate	1974	Györy *et al.*	50	diminished uterine activity	100
Buphenine	1975	Castrén *et al.*	43	birthweight ⩾2500 g	86
Terbutaline	1976	Ingemarsson	15	not delivered during treatment	80
Nifedipine	1977	Andersson	10	delivery delayed 3 days or more	100
Magnesium sulphate	1977	Steer and Petrie	31	contractions stopped 24 hours	77
Acupuncture	1977	Tsuie *et al.*	12	delivery after 36 weeks	92
Flufenamic acid	1978	Schwartz *et al.*	18	delivery delayed 24 hours	83
Diazoxide	1984	Adamsons and Wallach	118	complete cessation of contractions	94
Utrogestan	1986	Erny *et al.*	57	decrease in contraction frequency	76
Oxytocin analogue	1987	Akerlund *et al.*	13	inhibition of contractions	100

for years (Kubli 1977; Wiedinger 1977; Jung and Lamberti 1982; Wiedinger 1984), but in all these years fenoterol itself has never been evaluated against placebo in preterm labour.

Assessment of the effects of treatment in preterm labour is by no means easy. First, differentiation between true and false labour can be extremely difficult. In many instances, apparently progressive preterm labour stops, irrespective of whether any treatment is instituted. Second, the finding that uterine contractility is suppressed does not necessarily mean that delivery will be postponed to an extent that is clinically useful. Third, even if pregnancy is prolonged to an extent which is thought to be clinically useful, it does not necessarily follow that the outcome for the infant will be improved. Fourth, any drug or treatment that is powerful enough to suppress uterine contractions effectively, is bound to have other effects on the mother or the baby, some of them undesirable, that must be taken into account. Emphasizing the uterine relaxant effects of the treatment without considering the possible risks to both the baby and the mother is needlessly naïve.

Numerous criteria have been applied to describe 'successes' of one treatment or another. Some of the most commonly used relate to temporary arrest of uterine contractions, number of hours or days gained before delivery, number of deliveries delayed until 36 or 37 weeks of gestation, number of infants weighing more than 2500 g at birth, and increases in mean gestational age or mean birthweight at delivery. None of these, of themselves, is of great relevance to mother and baby, unless accompanied by an increase in the number of survivors or by an increase in the quality of life for the infants and their mothers.

2 Betamimetic drugs

Betamimetic agents are used more extensively than any of the other approaches that are employed to suppress uterine contractions (tocolysis) preterm (Table 44.2). Data from several European countries testify to the widespread use of several of these agents both for the inhibition of active preterm labour (Table 44.2) and in attempts to forestall uterine contractility preterm (Kubli 1977; Bréart *et al.* 1981; Keirse 1984b).

2.1 Range of drugs and their mechanism of action

Within 15 years of the first reports on the use of a betamimetic agent, isoxsuprine, in preterm labour (Bishop and Woutersz 1961; Hendricks *et al.* 1961), a great variety of betamimetic drugs was developed and applied to the inhibition of preterm labour. They have included, in addition to isoxsuprine, orciprenaline (Baillie *et al.* 1970), mesuprine (Barden 1971), ritodrine (Wesselius-De Casparis *et al.* 1971), fenoterol (Edelstein and Baillie 1972), salbutamol (Liggins and Vaughan 1973), buphenine (Gummerus 1975), hexoprenaline (Lipshitz *et al.* 1976), and terbutaline (Ingemarsson 1976). A number of them are also known under different names. Buphenine, for example, is encountered in the literature also as nylidrin, dilatol, arlidine, dihydrine, and rolidrine.

All of these drugs are chemically and pharmacologically related to the catecholamines, epinephrine (adrenalin) and norepinephrine (noradrenalin), and all stimulate the beta receptors that are present in the uterus and in other organs throughout the body. It is that stimulation which, by mediation of the adenyl cyclase system (Roberts 1981), is responsible for their uterine relaxant

Table 44.2 Tocolytic drugs that are reported to be normally used by obstetricians to arrest preterm labour in the United Kingdom (Lewis *et al.* 1980), in northern Belgium (Flanders) and in The Netherlands (Keirse 1984a)

Tocolytic drugs used to arrest preterm labour	Used by obstetricians (per cent) in:		
	Belgium ($n=154$)	Netherlands ($n=367$)	United Kingdom ($n=353$)
Ritodrine	61	63	43
Salbutamol	0	0	33
Fenoterol	34	30	–*
Isoxsuprine	3	2	20
Isoprenaline	0	0	1
Terbutaline	0	0	0
Orciprenaline	0	4	–*
Buphenine	0	0.3	–*
Indomethacin	2	0.3	–*
None of the drugs	0	0.3	3

* Drug not listed in the survey of Lewis *et al.* (1980)

(tocolytic) effect and for their influence on many other bodily functions (Eskes and Essed 1979).

Following the observations of Lands *et al.* (1967) on the presence of different populations of beta receptors, much effort has been directed at developing agents that would selectively stimulate the beta-2 and not the beta-1 receptors. These efforts have not been entirely successful, and all betamimetic agents available today stimulate, albeit to different degrees, both beta-1 and beta-2 receptors. The publicized beta-2 selectivity of betamimetic agents currently used in preterm labour only means that these agents will interact with beta-2 receptors at lower agonist concentrations than with beta-1 receptors. Stimulation of beta-1 receptors is responsible for actions such as an increase in heart rate and stroke volume, relaxation of intestinal smooth muscle and lipolysis. Beta-2 stimulation mediates glycogenolysis and relaxation of smooth muscle in the arterioles, the bronchi and the uterus. Other efforts have been directed at blocking the activation of beta-1 receptors while beta-2 stimulation is in progress. As discussed below, these efforts have been even less promising.

A wealth of literature is available on the pharmacological effects of the betamimetic drugs and on their application in preterm labour. Most of that literature consists of observational data and very little of it refers to controlled trials. Furthermore, many of the trials that have been conducted merely compared one drug with another, leaving unanswered the primary question as to whether any drug should be used.

2.2 Prophylaxis

Many clinicians rely on the use of betamimetic drugs to prevent uterine contractions in women who, for one reason or another, are considered to be at increased risk of preterm labour. More than 40 per cent of obstetricians in Belgium and The Netherlands were reported to prescribe betamimetic drugs for this purpose. An additional 30 per cent reported that they prescribed these agents for maintaining uterine quiescence after an acute episode of preterm uterine contractions had been overcome (Keirse 1984b). A study conducted in two maternity units in France indicated that in one unit 22 per cent of women, considered to be at low risk of preterm labour, were treated with progesterone or betamimetic preparations; in the other unit an astonishingly 46 per cent of low risk women were so 'treated' (Bréart *et al.* 1981). In women considered to be at average risk of preterm labour, these percentages rose respectively to 30 and 57 per cent (Bréart *et al.* 1981).

Several controlled trials on the prophylactic administration of betamimetic drugs for prevention of preterm labour have been reported in the literature. Five of these were conducted in women with multiple pregnancies (Cetrulo and Freeman 1976; Marivate et al. 1977; O'Connor *et al.* 1979; Skjaerris and Aberg 1982; Gummerus and Halonen 1987). One included women both with multiple and with singleton pregnancies (Mathews *et al.* 1967) and two included only singleton pregnancies (Briscoe 1966; Walters and Wood 1977). Data on two further, unpublished studies in singleton pregnancies were available from the Oxford Database of Perinatal Trials (Grant 1988; Varma 1988).

Trials in which oral betamimetics were administered to prevent uterine contractility after prelabour rupture of the membranes (Levy and Warsof 1985; Dunlop *et al.* 1986) are considered in Chapter 43.

Other trials in which betamimetic drugs or placebo were administered to women with threatened abortion (Bigby *et al.* 1969; Ruppin *et al.* 1981; Soltan 1986) have not been considered.

2.2.1 *Multiple pregnancies*

Multiple pregnancies are at much greater risk of preterm labour and delivery than singleton pregnancies (see Chapter 74). They are also readily identified and are therefore particularly susceptible to prophylactic measures, such as bed rest (see Chapter 39), cervical cerclage (see Chapter 40) or betamimetic drugs.

Of the 6 placebo controlled trials of betamimetic agents used prophylactically in multiple pregnancies, 2 dealt with isoxsuprine (Mathews *et al.* 1967), 2 used ritodrine (Cetrulo and Freeman 1976; O'Connor *et al.* 1979), 1 used terbutaline (Skjaerris and Aberg 1982), 1 salbutamol (Gummerus and Halonen 1987) and 1 fenoterol (Marivate *et al.* 1977). This wide variety of agents used renders it difficult to make meaningful comparisons across trials. Indeed, both the half-lives and the bioavailability after oral administration differ considerably from one agent to another, a problem that is not encountered when intravenous infusions are used, as in the treatment of active preterm labour. In the study of Marivate *et al.* (1977), for example, a daily dose of 5 mg fenoterol was administered to women in the treatment group. This drug has a half-life of a mere 22 minutes (Rominger 1977), which is much shorter than that of ritodrine or terbutaline (Leferink *et al.* 1977; Post 1977), and its bioavailability after oral administration is only 35 per cent of that after parenteral administration.

It is therefore not entirely surprising that the incidence of preterm delivery was nearly identical in both the treatment and the control groups across the trials (Table 44.3). Preterm delivery in the trial of Marivate *et al.* (1977) was considered to be present if delivery ocurred before 38 weeks, but the authors stated that both groups would still have had the same frequency of preterm labour if the dividing line had been put at 36 or 37 weeks instead of at 38 weeks. The typical odds for all 6 trials, taken together, was 0.93 with a confidence interval from 0.64 to 1.37 (Table 44.3).

Table 44.3 Effect of prophylactic oral betamimetics in twin pregnancies on preterm delivery

Study	EXPT		CTRL		Odds ratio	Graph of odds ratios and confidence intervals
	n	(%)	*n*	(%)	(95% CI)	0.01 0.1 0.5 1 2 10 100
Skjaerris and Aberg (1982)	7/25	(28.00)	10/25	(40.00)	0.59 (0.19–1.89)	
Mathews *et al.* (1967)	6/20	(30.00)	2/19	(10.53)	3.20 (0.69–14.86)	
O'Connor *et al.* (1979)	5/25	(20.00)	10/23	(43.48)	0.34 (0.10–1.15)	
Cetrulo and Freeman (1976)	15/42	(35.71)	13/42	(30.95)	1.24 (0.50–3.05)	
Marivate *et al.* (1977)	7/23	(30.43)	7/23	(30.43)	1.00 (0.29–3.46)	
Gummerus and Halonen (1987)	37/101	(36.63)	37/99	(37.37)	0.97 (0.55–1.72)	
Typical odds ratio (95% confidence interval)					0.93 (0.64–1.37)	

Table 44.4 Effect of prophylactic oral betamimetics in twin pregnancies on low birthweight

Study	EXPT		CTRL		Odds ratio	Graph of odds ratios and confidence intervals
	n	(%)	*n*	(%)	(95% CI)	0.01 0.1 0.5 1 2 10 100
Mathews *et al.* (1967)	21/40	(52.50)	27/38	(71.05)	0.46 (0.19–1.14)	
O'Connor *et al.* (1979)	33/50	(66.00)	22/44	(50.00)	1.92 (0.85–4.35)	
Cetrulo and Freeman (1976)	54/92	(58.70)	38/84	(45.24)	1.71 (0.95–3.09)	
Gummerus and Halonen (1987)	88/203	(43.35)	84/199	(42.21)	1.05 (0.71–1.55)	
Typical odds ratio (95% confidence interval)					1.17 (0.88–1.56)	

Data on the incidence of low birthweight were available for 4 of the trials (Mathews *et al.* 1967; Cetrulo and Freeman 1976; O'Connor *et al.* 1979 Gummerus and Halonen 1987). There is no indication that prophylactic betamimetic drug administration decreased the incidence of low birthweight in twin pregnancies. The combined typical odds ratio was 1.17, with a confidence interval from 0.88 to 1.56 (Table 44.4).

All except 1 trial, in which there were apparently no perinatal deaths (Skjaerris and Aberg 1982), provided data on the incidence of perinatal death. There were no statistically significant differences between the drug and placebo groups, with a typical odds of 0.79 and a confidence interval of 0.41 to 1.51 (Table 44.5). Data on the incidence of respiratory distress syndrome in the newborn were available from 4 trials (Cetrulo and Freeman 1976; O'Connor *et al.* 1979; Skjaerris and Aberg 1982; Gummerus and Halonen 1987). All 4 showed a lower incidence of respiratory distress syndrome after active than after placebo treatment, and the typical odds ratio across the trials was 0.45. This was statistically significant, with a 95 per cent confidence interval of 0.22 to 0.92 (Table 44.6).

2.2.2 Singleton pregnancies at increased risk

The placebo-controlled trials in singleton pregnancies have also dealt with different betamimetic agents. Two used isoxsuprine (Briscoe 1966; Mathews *et al.* 1967), 2 used ritodrine (Walters and Wood 1977; Varma 1988) and 1 used salbutamol (Grant 1988). The latter 2 trials were not mounted specifically to prevent preterm labour but intended to prevent low birthweight (Grant 1988) or treat intrauterine growth retardation (Varma 1988) in women considered to be at high risk of delivering an infant with these characteristics. The trial of Mathews *et al.* (1967) included women with a history of a previous preterm birth after the spontaneous onset of labour. Walters and Wood (1977) studied primigra-

Table 44.5 Effect of prophylactic oral betamimetics in twin pregnancies on perinatal death

Study	EXPT		CTRL		Odds ratio	Graph of odds ratios and confidence intervals
	n	(%)	*n*	(%)	(95% CI)	0.01 0.1 0.5 1 2 10 100
Mathews *et al.* (1967)	4/40	(10.00)	0/38	(0.00)	7.61 (1.03–56.21)	
O'Connor *et al.* (1979)	0/50	(0.00)	1/48	(2.08)	0.13 (0.00–6.55)	
Cetrulo and Freeman (1976)	6/96	(6.25)	11/96	(11.46)	0.53 (0.19–1.42)	
Marivate *et al.* (1977)	0/46	(0.00)	0/46	(0.00)	1.00 (1.00–1.00)	
Gummerus and Halonen (1987)	7/204	(3.43)	9/199	(4.52)	0.75 (0.28–2.04)	
Typical odds ratio (95% confidence interval)					0.79 (0.41–1.51)	

Table 44.6 Effect of prophylactic oral betamimetics in twin pregnancies on respiratory distress syndrome

Study	EXPT		CTRL		Odds ratio	Graph of odds ratios and confidence intervals
	n	(%)	*n*	(%)	(95% CI)	0.01 0.1 0.5 1 2 10 100
Skjaerris and Aberg (1982)	0/50	(0.00)	4/50	(8.00)	0.13 (0.02–0.93)	
O'Connor *et al.* (1979)	3/62	(4.84)	8/64	(12.50)	0.39 (0.11–1.32)	
Cetrulo and Freeman (1976)	5/94	(5.32)	6/92	(6.52)	0.81 (0.24–2.72)	
Gummerus and Halonen (1987)	2/204	(0.98)	4/199	(2.01)	0.50 (0.10–2.48)	
Typical odds ratio (95% confidence interval)					0.45 (0.22–0.92)	

Table 44.7 Effect of prophylactic oral betamimetics in singleton pregnancies on preterm delivery

Study	EXPT		CTRL		Odds ratio	Graph of odds ratios and confidence intervals
	n	(%)	*n*	(%)	(95% CI)	0.01 0.1 0.5 1 2 10 100
Mathews *et al.* (1967)	2/31	(6.45)	2/33	(6.06)	1.07 (0.14–7.97)	
Grant (1988)	4/32	(12.50)	2/31	(6.45)	2.00 (0.38–10.59)	
Walters and Wood (1977)	3/21	(14.29)	1/17	(5.88)	2.38 (0.31–18.63)	
Varma (1988)	5/43	(11.63)	2/47	(4.26)	2.76 (0.59–12.84)	
Briscoe (1966)	62/590	(10.51)	66/575	(11.48)	0.91 (0.63–1.31)	
Typical odds ratio (95% confidence interval)					1.02 (0.73–1.43)	

Table 44.8 Effect of prophylactic oral betamimetics in singleton pregnancies on birthweight <2500 g

Study	EXPT		CTRL		Odds ratio	Graph of odds ratios and confidence intervals
	n	(%)	*n*	(%)	(95% CI)	0.01 0.1 0.5 1 2 10 100
Mathews *et al.* (1967)	6/31	(19.35)	4/33	(12.12)	1.72 (0.45–6.55)	
Grant (1988)	5/28	(17.86)	5/26	(19.23)	0.91 (0.23–3.57)	
Walters and Wood (1977)	5/21	(23.81)	0/17	(0.00)	7.61 (1.18–49.18)	
Varma (1988)	15/43	(34.88)	13/47	(27.66)	1.40 (0.57–3.39)	
Briscoe (1966)	47/590	(7.97)	67/575	(11.65)	0.66 (0.45–0.97)	
Typical odds ratio (95% confidence interval)					0.85 (0.61–1.18)	

Table 44.9 Effect of prophylactic oral betamimetics in singleton pregnancies on perinatal death

Study	EXPT		CTRL		Odds ratio	Graph of odds ratios and confidence intervals
	n	(%)	*n*	(%)	(95% CI)	0.01 0.1 0.5 1 2 10 100
Mathews *et al.* (1967)	0/31	(0.00)	1/33	(3.03)	0.14 (0.00–7.26)	
Grant (1988)	1/32	(3.13)	0/31	(0.00)	7.16 (0.14–99.99)	
Walters and Wood (1977)	1/21	(4.76)	0/17	(0.00)	6.11 (0.12–99.99)	
Typical odds ratio (95% confidence interval)					1.84 (0.19–17.76)	

vid women in whom the cervix was found to be one or more fingerbreadths dilated at 28 to 32 weeks of pregnancy. The trial of Briscoe (1966), also the largest of the 5 trials, included all women registered for antenatal care, without any preselection.

The incidence of preterm delivery was similar with the active and the placebo treatment, the typical odds ratio being 1.02 (confidence interval 0.73–1.43; Table 44.8), as was the incidence of low birthweight infants (typical odds: 0.85; confidence interval: 0.61–1.18; Table 44.7).

Data on the incidence of perinatal death were available for only 3 of the trials (Mathews *et al.* 1967; Walters and Wood 1977; Grant 1988) and these deal with a total of only 165 women. Not surprisingly the confidence interval for this outcome was extremely wide from 0.19 to 17.8, thus providing no meaningful data on the effect of betamimetic prophylaxis on perinatal death (Table 44.9).

Only 3 trials reported the incidence of respiratory distress syndrome in the infants (Walters and Wood 1977; Grant 1988; Varma 1988). All 3 gave odds ratios above unity for this outcome, contrary to what was observed in twin pregnancies (see Table 44.6), suggesting that chance may be responsible for the observed differences. All 3 trials in singletons showed wide confidence intervals. Even the typical odds ratio, although greater than unity (2.36), still has a 95 per cent confidence interval that ranges from 0.76 to 7.36 (Table 44.10).

2.3 Inhibition of active preterm labour

2.3.1 Placebo-controlled trials

Only 3 of the many betamimetic agents available have ever been compared with a control group which received either no active treatment or placebo for inhibition of preterm labour (Table 44.11). Some of the drugs that are widely used, such as salbutamol or fenoterol (Table 44.2), have never been tested against no active treatment in preterm labour.

Eighteen studies have been published in which one or other betamimetic agent was reported to have been compared against no labour inhibiting drugs in preterm

Table 44.10 Effect of prophylactic oral betamimetics in singleton pregnancies on respiratory distress syndrome

Study	EXPT		CTRL		Odds ratio	Graph of odds ratios and confidence intervals
	n	(%)	*n*	(%)	(95% CI)	0.01 0.1 0.5 1 2 10 100
Grant (1988)	1/32	(3.13)	0/31	(0.00)	7.16 (0.14–99.99)	
Walters and Wood (1977)	2/21	(9.52)	0/17	(0.00)	6.42 (0.38–99.99)	
Varma (1988)	6/43	(13.95)	4/46	(8.70)	1.68 (0.45–6.24)	
Typical odds ratio (95% confidence interval)					2.36 (0.76–7.36)	

labour (Adam 1966; Das 1969; Wesselius-De Casparis *et al.* 1971; Sivasamboo 1972; Castrén *et al.* 1975; Ingemarsson 1976; Csapo and Herzeg 1977; Spellacy *et al.* 1979; Christensen *et al.* 1980; Larsen *et al.* 1980; Merkatz *et al.* 1980; Penney and Daniell 1980; Howard *et al.* 1982; Cotton *et al.* 1984; Calder and Patel 1985; Larsen *et al.* 1986; Leveno *et al.* 1986; Weiner *et al.* 1988). Six of these 18 studies (Das 1969; Castrén *et al.* 1975; Csapo and Herzeg 1977; Merkatz *et al.* 1980; Penney and Daniell 1980; Weiner *et al.* 1988) were either conducted or reported in a manner that precludes unbiased evaluation of the treatment given. Das (1969) gave no reassurance (confirmed by personal communication) that treatment allocation had been at random in his study, and there were inconsistencies in the methods by which the treatments had been given. Csapo and Herzeg (1977) included a substantial proportion of women, whose treatment had been decided by clinical opinion in the group allocated to betamimetic administration; it was impossible to separate these from the remaining women and the method of treatment allocation was also unclear. Castrén and his colleagues (1975) reported a study in which there were three women in the betamimetic group for every two in the control group, despite the use of 'alternate allocation'. Merkatz and his colleagues (1980) combined a number of trials in a way which made the results impossible to interpret. Women entered into trials of oral betamimetic maintenance therapy, all of whom had previously been 'successfully' treated with intramuscular ritodrine without randomization, were included in the treatment group. Furthermore, the control group contained some women treated not with placebo, but with ethanol. The report did, however, contain data from five centres in which intravenous ritodrine or placebo had been given randomly to women who were thought to be in preterm labour. Although the results from only one of these centres (Spellacy *et al.* 1979) had been published separately, it was possible to gain access to the original data collected at the other four centres (King *et al.* 1988) and these have been included in our analyses. Penney and Daniell (1980) reported on the use of a prolongation index for their trial, but provided no data on outcome by treatment allocation. Weiner *et al.* (1988) conducted a trial of tocolysis vs. no tocolysis in women with ruptured membranes before 34 weeks' gestation. Thirty-four of 109 women (31 per cent) entered into the trial were excluded from the analysis. Women receiving tocolysis were treated not only with betamimetic agents but also with magnesium sulphate. They received ritodrine, terbutaline, or magnesium sulphate, and 17 (23 per cent) of the women on whom results were reported received two agents.

Data are therefore available from 12 published and from the 4 unpublished trials, conducted by Barden, Hobel, Mariona and Scommegna and Bieniarz, and included in the report of Merkatz *et al.* (1980). These 16 trials (Table 44.11) involved a total of 484 betamimetic-treated women and 406 women treated with placebo or some 'standard treatment'. The imbalance in the numbers reflects one trial (Larsen *et al.* 1980) in which placebo was compared with more than one actively treated group. All but one (Cotton *et al.* 1984) of these trials involved the use of oral betamimetic maintenance therapy after acute tocolysis had been achieved (Table 44.11).

The large majority of the trials (12 of 16) dealt with ritodrine (Table 44.11). In 10 of these trials, ritodrine was initially given intravenously, in 1 (Larsen *et al.* 1986) it was given intramuscularly, and in 1 (Larsen *et al.* 1980) the allocation was to one of three different ritodrine regimes or to a 'standard' control management. All of these trials included oral maintenance treatment if and after contractions stopped. Three trials tested terbutaline (Ingemarsson 1976; Howard *et al.* 1982; Cotton *et al.* 1984), initially given intravenously, and followed by oral maintenance in 2 of the trials (Ingemarsson 1976; Howard *et al.* 1982). In the remaining and oldest trial (Adam 1966) the drug used was isoxsuprine, administered intramuscularly followed by oral maintenance.

As shown in Table 44.11, allocation to the treatment or control group was stated to have been 'blind' in 11 of the 16 trials. In the others the method of allocation was

Table 44.11 Description of the 16 trials comparing betamimetics with placebo or no active treatment for inhibition of preterm labour

Authors and date	Betamimetic treatment	Control treatment	Method of allocation	No. randomized: reported on	
				Allocated to betamimetic	Allocated to to control
Leveno *et al.* (1986)	Ritodrine (in saline) IV + oral maintenance	Saline IV	Random by envelopes	54:54	52:52
Calder and Patel (1985)	Ritodrine (in 5% dextrose) IV + oral maintenance	Dextrose IV	Hospital case note number	37:37	39:39
Larsen *et al.* (1986)	Ritodrine 10 mg IM 6 hourly + oral maintenance	Placebo IM 6 hourly + oral placebo	Random 'blind' at allocation	63:49	62:50
Larsen *et al.* (1980)	Ritodrine —IV long —IV short —IM + oral maintenance	'Standard' treatment 5% glucose IV, bedrest, occasional sedatives + placebo maintenance	Random method unstated	48:41 52:46 150:131 50:40	49:45
Christensen *et al.* (1980)	Ritodrine IV + oral maintenance (all ruptured membranes)	Placebo IV + placebo maintenance	Random 'blind' at allocation	14:14	16:16
Spellacy *et al.* (1979)	Ritodrine IV→IM→oral maintenance	Similar placebo regime	Random 'blind' at allocation	14:14	15:15
Barden (unpub*)	Ritodrine IV→IM→oral maintenance	Similar placebo regime	Random 'blind' at allocation	12:12	13:13
Hobel (unpub*)	Ritodrine IV→IM→oral maintenance	Similar placebo regime	Random 'blind' at allocation	16:16	15:15
Scommegna and Bieniarz (unpub*)	Ritodrine IV→IM→oral maintenance	Similar placebo regime	Random 'blind' at allocation	15:15	17:17
Mariona (unpub*)	Ritodrine IV→IM→oral maintenance	Similar placebo regime	Random 'blind' at allocation	5:4 Six other cases unreported—allocation unknown	6:5
Sivasamboo *et al.* (1972)	Ritodrine IV + oral maintenance	Librium IM	? Random 'blind selection'	33:33	32:32
Wesselius-de Casparis *et al.* (1971)	Ritodrine IV + oral maintenance	Similar placebo regime	Random 'blind' at allocation	33:33	30:30
Total number of women in ritodrine trials				446:412	346:329
Cotton *et al.* (1984)	Terbutaline IV	5% dextrose in lactated Ringer solution IV	Random method not stated	19:19	19:19
Howard *et al.* (1982)	Terbutaline IV→SC→oral maintenance	Similar placebo regime	Random 'blind' at allocation	16:16	21:21
Ingemarsson (1976)	Terbutaline IV→oral maintenance	Similar placebo regime	Random 'blind' at allocation	15:15	15:15
Total number of women in terbutaline trials				50:50	55:55
Adam (1966)	Isoxsuprine IM→oral maintenance	Similar placebo regime	Random 'blind' at allocation	24:22	24:22
Total number of women in all trials				520:484	425:406

* Data previously published in part in Merkatz *et al.* (1980)

either not described (Larsen *et al.* 1980; Cotton *et al.* 1984; Sivasamboo 1972) or was such that the investigators may have known in advance to which group the woman would be allocated (Calder and Patel 1985; Leveno *et al.* 1986). For 12 of the 16 trials, data were available on all women entered and for these trials there is no selection bias after entry (Table 44.11). Often that information had not been published in the original reports, but additional data were sought and obtained from the authors (King *et al.* 1988). This control for selection bias after entry into the trial, was not possible for the other trials, and unfortunately 2 of these (Larsen *et al.* 1980, 1986) were the two largest studies in the series (Table 44.11). In the second study of Larsen *et al.* (1986) as many as 26 of 125 women (21 per cent) were excluded after randomization. The authors' comment (Larsen and Lange 1987) that 'human bias cannot have influenced the exclusions' is difficult to accept without evidence to support it.

In at least 8 of the trials there was evidence that the investigators had tried hard to achieve blinding to the type of treatment given when assessing outcomes. Full blinding may be impossible to achieve in view of the marked cardiovascular effects of betamimetic drugs, although in one of the ritodrine trials 3 of the 4 women withdrawn because of unwanted side-effects were in receipt of placebo (Calder and Patel 1985).

Data on delivery within 24 hours and within 48 hours of trial entry were available for respectively 14 and 12 of the 16 studies. They are shown in Tables 44.12 and 44.13. In 13 of 14 studies there were fewer deliveries within the first 24 hours in the group allocated to betamimetic treatment than in the control group and in 6 trials this difference reached statistical significance. Although most of the studies dealt with ritodrine, the direction and magnitude of effect in delaying delivery for 24 hours or more were similar in the terbutaline trials (odds ratio 0.23; 95 per cent confidence interval 0.10–0.56) as in the ritodrine trials (odds ratio 0.31; 95 per cent confidence interval 0.21–0.45).

The effect on delaying delivery beyond the preterm period was less marked. In only three of the 15 studies,

Table 44.12 Effect of betamimetic tocolytics in preterm labour on delivery within 24 hours

Study	EXPT		CTRL		Odds ratio	Graph of odds ratios and confidence intervals
	n	(%)	*n*	(%)	(95% CI)	0.01 0.1 0.5 1 2 10 100
Christensen *et al.* (1980)	0/14	(0.00)	6/16	(37.50)	0.10 (0.02–0.60)	
Spellacy *et al.* (1979)	6/14	(42.86)	11/15	(73.33)	0.30 (0.07–1.27)	
Barden (unpub)	0/12	(0.00)	8/13	(61.54)	0.07 (0.01–0.34)	
Hobel (unpub)	2/16	(12.50)	3/15	(20.00)	0.58 (0.09–3.85)	
Cotton *et al.* (1984)	6/19	(31.58)	11/19	(57.89)	0.35 (0.10–1.25)	
Howard *et al.* (1982)	2/15	(13.33)	2/18	(11.11)	1.22 (0.15–9.68)	
Ingemarsson (1976)	0/15	(0.00)	10/15	(66.67)	0.06 (0.01–0.24)	
Larsen *et al.* (1986)	5/49	(10.20)	16/50	(32.00)	0.27 (0.11–0.72)	
Calder and Patel (1985)	4/37	(10.81)	9/39	(23.08)	0.43 (0.13–1.40)	
Scommegna (unpub)	1/15	(6.67)	5/17	(29.41)	0.24 (0.04–1.36)	
Mariona (unpub)	0/4	(0.00)	0/5	(0.00)	1.00 (1.00–1.00)	
Wesselius-De Casparis *et al.* (1971)	6/33	(18.18)	15/30	(50.00)	0.24 (0.09–0.69)	
Leveno *et al.* (1986)	15/54	(27.78)	25/52	(48.08)	0.42 (0.19–0.93)	
Larsen *et al.* (1980)	11/131	(8.40)	6/45	(13.33)	0.57 (0.18–1.79)	
Typical odds ratio (95% confidence interval)					0.30 (0.21–0.42)	

Table 44.13 Effect of betamimetic tocolytics in preterm labour on delivery within 48 hours

Study	EXPT		CTRL		Odds ratio	Graph of odds ratios and confidence intervals
	n	(%)	*n*	(%)	(95% CI)	0.01 0.1 0.5 1 2 10 100
Christensen *et al.* (1980)	7/14	(50.00)	9/16	(56.25)	0.78 (0.19–3.22)	
Spellacy *et al.* (1979)	8/14	(57.14)	11/15	(73.33)	0.50 (0.11–2.26)	
Barden (unpub)	2/12	(16.67)	9/13	(69.23)	0.13 (0.03–0.61)	
Hobel (unpub)	6/16	(37.50)	3/15	(20.00)	2.27 (0.49–10.47)	
Cotton *et al.* (1984)	9/19	(47.37)	12/19	(63.16)	0.54 (0.15–1.90)	
Howard *et al.* (1982)	2/15	(13.33)	2/18	(11.11)	1.22 (0.15–9.68)	
Larsen *et al.* (1986)	5/49	(10.20)	17/50	(34.00)	0.26 (0.10–0.66)	
Calder and Patel (1985)	10/37	(27.03)	12/39	(30.77)	0.84 (0.31–2.24)	
Scommegna (unpub)	6/15	(40.00)	7/17	(41.18)	0.95 (0.24–3.84)	
Mariona (unpub)	2/4	(50.00)	1/5	(20.00)	3.32 (0.24–46.04)	
Leveno *et al.* (1986)	17/54	(31.48)	29/52	(55.77)	0.38 (0.17–0.81)	
Larsen *et al.* (1980)	29/131	(22.14)	10/45	(22.22)	1.00 (0.44–2.24)	
Typical odds ratio (95% confidence interval)					0.59 (0.42–0.83)	

which provided that information, was the incidence of preterm delivery statistically significantly lower in the betamimetic-treated group than in the control group (Table 44.14). Overall, the data from these 15 studies convincingly demonstrate, however, that betamimetic drug treatment results in a lower incidence of preterm birth than observed without such treatment (Table 44.14). As mentioned earlier, in all but 1 of the trials (Cotton *et al.* 1984) acute tocolysis was followed by oral maintenance treatment (Table 44.11) and it is possible that this component of the betamimetic drug administration may have contributed to the overall gain in gestational age (see Section 2.4, below).

The data on the incidence of low birthweight from the 13 trials with usable data on this outcome suggest that this incidence is reduced by betamimetic therapy. This is consistent with the observed lengthening of gestation, but it does not reach conventional levels of statistical significance (Table 44.15).

The effects on delay of delivery, gestational duration and birthweight did not, however, result in a detectable decrease in the incidence of mortality or morbidity. The typical odds ratio for perinatal death not attributalbe to lethal malformations across the 15 trials, was 0.95 with a confidence interval from 0.55 to 1.67 (Table 44.16). Usable data on respiratory distress syndrome and severe respiratory disorders in the newborn were obtained for 12 trials, and the typical odds ratio across these trials was 1.07 with a confidence interval from 0.71 to 1.61 (Table 44.17).

This apparent lack of effect of betamimetic drug treatment on the serious adverse outcomes of mortality and respiratory morbidity may be due to a number of factors. It may be due to the inclusion in these trials of too large a proportion of women in whom postponement of delivery and prolongation of pregnancy were unlikely to confer any further benefit to the baby (Heyting 1980). A treatment that is effective in stopping preterm labour between 36 and 37 weeks may well reduce the likelihood of delivery within 24 hours, of delivery before 37 weeks, and of delivering a low birthweight infant; but at that gestational age it will have little potential for reducing perinatal mortality or serious morbidity (see Chapter 74). The lack of effect on infant mortality and respiratory morbidity may also be due to direct or indirect adverse effects of the drug treatment. These could include the prolongation of pregnancy when this is contrary to the best interests of the baby, as may be the case with clinically unrecognized placental abruption (see Chapter 37), severe

Table 44.14 Effect of betamimetic tocolytics in preterm labour on delivery before 37 completed weeks

Study	EXPT		CTRL		Odds ratio	Graph of odds ratios and confidence intervals
	n	(%)	*n*	(%)	(95% CI)	0.01 0.1 0.5 1 2 10 100
Christensen *et al.* (1980)	14/14	(100.0)	16/16	(100.0)	1.00 (1.00–1.00)	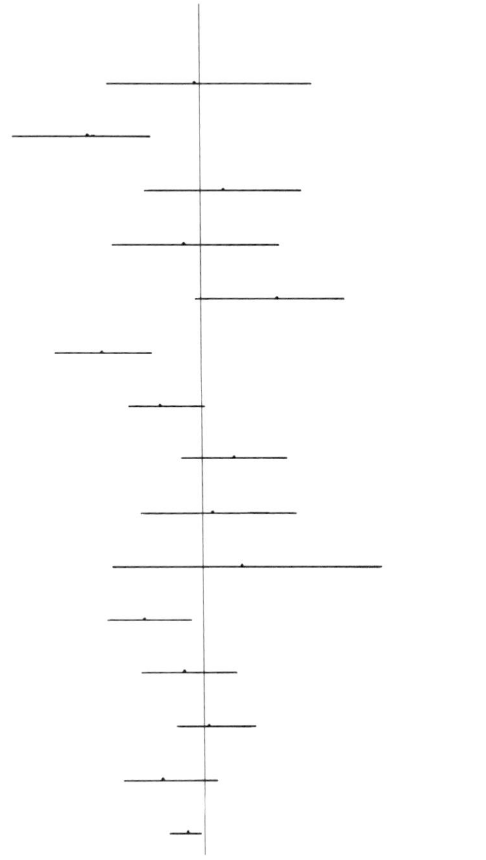
Spellacy *et al.* (1979)	12/14	(85.71)	13/15	(86.67)	0.93 (0.12–7.38)	
Barden (unpub)	6/12	(50.00)	13/13	(100.0)	0.07 (0.01–0.44)	
Hobel (unpub)	10/16	(62.50)	8/15	(53.33)	1.44 (0.35–5.86)	
Cotton *et al.* (1984)	15/19	(78.95)	16/19	(84.21)	0.71 (0.14–3.59)	
Howard *et al.* (1982)	9/15	(60.00)	5/18	(27.78)	3.59 (0.92–14.08)	
Ingemarsson (1976)	3/15	(20.00)	12/15	(80.00)	0.10 (0.02–0.40)	
Larsen *et al.* (1986)	14/49	(28.57)	23/50	(46.00)	0.48 (0.21–1.08)	
Calder and Patel (1985)	23/37	(62.16)	19/39	(48.72)	1.71 (0.70–4.20)	
Scommegna (unpub)	10/15	(66.67)	10/16	(62.50)	1.19 (0.28–5.08)	
Mariona (unpub)	3/4	(75.00)	3/5	(60.00)	1.82 (0.13–25.27)	
Wesselius-De Casparis *et al.* (1971)	13/33	(39.39)	21/30	(70.00)	0.30 (0.11–0.80)	
Leveno *et al.* (1986)	40/54	(74.07)	42/52	(80.77)	0.68 (0.28–1.69)	
Larsen *et al.* (1980)	65/131	(49.62)	21/45	(46.67)	1.12 (0.57–2.21)	
Sivasamboo (1972)	14/33	(42.42)	20/32	(62.50)	0.45 (0.17–1.19)	
Typical odds ratio (95% confidence interval)					0.71 (0.53–0.96)	

pregnancy-induced hypertension (see Chapter 33) or intrauterine growth retardation (see Chapter 26). It is also possible that too little use was made of the time gained by postponing delivery. Only 4 of the trial reports, for instance, indicated whether or not corticosteroids had been given before delivery. Nevertheless, the 2 reports that made it clear that at least some women had received corticosteroids yielded a comparable odds ratio for neonatal respiratory morbidity to that derived from all 12 trials (Table 44.17).

2.3.2 Controlled comparisons of different betamimetics

Several randomized trials have compared one betamimetic drug with another. Some of these studies were conducted in late pregnancy or during labour at term (Lipshitz and Baillie 1976; Lipshitz *et al.* 1976). Others were conducted more specifically in preterm labour (Richter *et al.* 1975; Richter 1977; Ryden 1977; Essed *et al.* 1978; Bréart *et al.* 1979; Richter and Hinselmann 1979; Karlsson *et al.* 1980; Gummerus 1983; Caritis *et al.* 1984; Beall *et al.* 1985; Kosasa *et al.* 1985). The interpretation of such studies is difficult as the authors of the studies themselves often recognize. Some of the studies, for example those conducted by Richter and his co-workers (Richter *et al.* 1975; Richter 1977; Richter and Hinselmann 1979), have been the subject of several reports, none of which gave clear assurance that the allocation to alternative treatments had been truly unbiased.

None of the studies has been large enough to have had a chance of detecting or excluding important differences in the outcomes that really matter. The drugs are administered primarily to reduce infant mortality and morbidity, and none of the studies showed dif-

Table 44.15 Effect of betamimetic tocolytics in preterm labour on birthweight <2500 g

Study	EXPT		CTRL		Odds ratio	Graph of odds ratios and confidence intervals
	n	(%)	*n*	(%)	(95% CI)	0.01 0.1 0.5 1 2 10 100
Christensen *et al.* (1980)	13/14	(92.86)	15/16	(93.75)	0.87 (0.05–14.71)	
Spellacy *et al.* (1979)	13/15	(86.67)	12/15	(80.00)	1.59 (0.24–10.51)	
Barden (unpub)	7/12	(58.33)	10/13	(76.92)	0.44 (0.08–2.29)	
Hobel (unpub)	10/17	(58.82)	8/16	(50.00)	1.41 (0.37–5.45)	
Cotton *et al.* (1984)	18/19	(94.74)	18/19	(94.74)	1.00 (0.06–16.61)	
Howard *et al.* (1982)	9/16	(56.25)	7/21	(33.33)	2.48 (0.68–9.06)	
Ingemarsson (1976)	4/15	(26.67)	10/15	(66.67)	0.21 (0.05–0.87)	
Larsen *et al.* (1986)	13/49	(26.53)	17/50	(34.00)	0.70 (0.30–1.65)	
Calder and Patel (1985)	24/37	(64.86)	15/39	(38.46)	2.84 (1.16–6.94)	
Scommegna (unpub)	5/16	(31.25)	11/17	(64.71)	0.27 (0.07–1.05)	
Mariona (unpub)	2/4	(50.00)	4/5	(80.00)	0.30 (0.02–4.18)	
Leveno *et al.* (1986)	41/56	(73.21)	46/55	(83.64)	0.54 (0.22–1.34)	
Larsen *et al.* (1980)	39/131	(29.77)	17/45	(37.78)	0.69 (0.34–1.43)	
Sivasamboo (1972)	12/32	(37.50)	21/32	(65.63)	0.33 (0.12–0.87)	
Typical odds ratio (95% confidence interval)					0.75 (0.55–1.02)	

ferences in this respect. This is hardly surprising since the placebo-controlled trials suggest that 'placebo treatment' performs just as well in this respect (Tables 44.16 and 44.17). Nor did the trials show clear differences in serious maternal outcomes, such as pulmonary oedema or other potentially life-threatening conditions. In addition, none of the trials showed that any one of the drugs tested was particularly free of maternal side-effects.

When differences in the incidence of less serious maternal side-effects or in average gain in gestational age were detected, it is never entirely clear whether the drugs were used in equipotent doses. The wide differences among betamimetic drugs in the ratio between drug weight and drug effect make this virtually impossible to assess. Without a clearer delineation of both benefit and harm, such small differences are difficult to interpret, irrespective of whether or not they reach statistical significance. None of the studies thus far has investigated the differential in the costs of treatment between one drug or another.

Taken together, the comparative trials of different betamimetic agents offer no justification for substituting betamimetic agents that have not been tested against placebo (or no treatment) for those that have been so tested. No other firm conclusions can be reached from these studies.

2.3.3 *Unwanted effects*

The randomized controlled trials discussed above provide sufficient evidence on the postponement of delivery and prolongation of pregnancy in order to ignore all data from uncontrolled observational studies. Unfortunately, the same does not apply in respect of the maternal and fetal hazards of betamimetic drug treatment in preterm labour.

A number of subjective maternal symptoms may occur as a result of betamimetic-induced changes in many bodily functions. The most frequently observed are palpitations, tremor, nausea, and vomiting. Headache, vague uneasiness, thirst, nervousness, and restlessness may occur. Chest discomfort and shortness of

Table 44.16 Effect of betamimetic tocolytics in preterm labour on perinatal death

Study	EXPT		CTRL		Odds ratio	Graph of odds ratios and confidence intervals
	n	(%)	*n*	(%)	(95% CI)	0.01 0.1 0.5 1 2 10 100
Christensen *et al.* (1980)	1/14	(7.14)	0/16	(0.00)	8.52 (0.17–99.99)	
Spellacy *et al.* (1979)	1/15	(6.67)	4/15	(26.67)	0.25 (0.04–1.64)	
Barden (unpub)	1/12	(8.33)	0/13	(0.00)	8.03 (0.16–99.99)	
Hobel (unpub)	2/17	(11.76)	0/16	(0.00)	7.42 (0.44–99.99)	
Cotton *et al.* (1984)	1/19	(5.26)	4/19	(21.05)	0.26 (0.04–1.67)	
Howard *et al.* (1982)	1/16	(6.25)	1/21	(4.76)	1.33 (0.08–22.65)	
Ingemarsson (1976)	0/15	(0.00)	0/15	(0.00)	1.00 (1.00–1.00)	
Larsen *et al.* (1986)	1/49	(2.04)	2/50	(4.00)	0.52 (0.05–5.09)	
Calder and Patel (1985)	0/37	(0.00)	1/39	(2.56)	0.14 (0.00–7.19)	
Scommegna (unpub)	0/16	(0.00)	1/17	(5.88)	0.14 (0.00–7.25)	
Mariona (unpub)	1/4	(25.00)	1/5	(20.00)	1.29 (0.07–25.50)	
Wesselius-De Casparis *et al.* (1971)	2/33	(6.06)	1/30	(3.33)	1.81 (0.18–18.08)	
Leveno *et al.* (1986)	2/56	(3.57)	3/55	(5.45)	0.65 (0.11–3.87)	
Larsen *et al.* (1980)	11/131	(8.40)	2/45	(4.44)	1.78 (0.49–6.46)	
Adam (1966)	9/28	(32.14)	7/24	(29.17)	1.15 (0.36–3.69)	
Typical odds ratio (95% confidence interval)					0.95 (0.55–1.67)	

breath should alert those providing care to the possibility of pulmonary congestion.

From the placebo-controlled trials discussed above there is little evidence that betamimetic drug treatment frequently poses great hazards to either mother or baby. But this 'negative' finding is not convincing, in view of the fact that all 16 trials taken together provided information on less than 500 betamimetic treated women (Table 44.11). This is probably less than 1 per cent of the number of women who annually receive treatment with one of these agents. The likelihood that rare but serious adverse effects of betamimetic drugs, if they exist, would have been uncovered by any one of these trials must be infinitely small. Yet, other data in the literature indicate that these drugs are not harmless.

2.3.3.1 Pulmonary oedema

Maternal hypotension, sometimes accompanied by fetal bradycardia, was a relatively common finding in the early observational studies of betamimetic drug administration. The betamimetic agent used in these studies was isoxsuprine, the selectivity for beta-2 over beta-1 receptors of which is much smaller than that of the newer substances, such as ritodrine and terbutaline. Clinical experience at the time taught that adequate filling of the vascular bed and the avoidance of supine positions greatly reduced the incidence of these worrying side-effects (Caritis *et al.* 1979). Thus liberal administration of crystalloid fluids became standard practice with betamimetic treatment. As much as 400 (Caritis *et al.* 1982) to 1000 ml (Cotton *et al.* 1984) of intravenous fluid was often administered routinely for 30 minutes before starting infusion with betamimetics. Probably this practice has caused more harm than it prevented.

In the late 1970s in West Germany, incidents of pulmonary oedema, congestive cardiac failure, and even maternal death started to be noticed in young

Table 44.17 Effect of betamimetic tocolytics in preterm labour on respiratory distress syndrome

Study	EXPT		CTRL		Odds ratio	Graph of odds ratios and confidence intervals
	n	(%)	*n*	(%)	(95% CI)	0.01 0.1 0.5 1 2 10 100
Christensen *et al.* (1980)	2/14	(14.29)	1/16	(6.25)	2.37 (0.23–24.88)	
Spellacy *et al.* (1979)	0/14	(0.00)	3/15	(20.00)	0.12 (0.01–1.31)	
Barden (unpub)	5/12	(41.67)	4/13	(30.77)	1.57 (0.32–7.81)	
Hobel (unpub)	9/17	(52.94)	5/16	(31.25)	2.37 (0.61–9.22)	
Cotton *et al.* (1984)	4/19	(21.05)	6/19	(31.58)	0.59 (0.14–2.45)	
Howard *et al.* (1982)	3/16	(18.75)	1/21	(4.76)	4.10 (0.52–32.38)	
Ingemarsson (1976)	0/15	(0.00)	3/15	(20.00)	0.12 (0.01–1.22)	
Larsen *et al.* (1986)	3/49	(6.12)	6/50	(12.00)	0.49 (0.13–1.93)	
Calder and Patel (1985)	4/37	(10.81)	3/39	(7.69)	1.44 (0.31–6.78)	
Scommegna (unpub)	0/16	(0.00)	3/17	(17.65)	0.13 (0.01–1.31)	
Leveno *et al.* (1986)	25/56	(44.64)	24/55	(43.64)	1.04 (0.49–2.20)	
Larsen *et al.* (1980)	15/131	(11.45)	1/45	(2.22)	3.04 (0.94–9.83)	
Typical odds ratio (95% confidence interval)					1.07 (0.71–1.61)	

women who had received the betamimetic drug fenoterol in combination with corticosteroids for preterm labour (Bender *et al.* 1977; Jonatha *et al.* 1977; Kubli 1977). Within a year a case of severe pulmonary oedema following administration of terbutaline and dexamethasone was reported from the United States (Stubblefield 1978) and by 1980 a large number of such reports had appeared in the medical literature (Daubert *et al.* 1978; Elliott *et al.* 1978; Babenerd and Flehr 1979; Rogge *et al.* 1979; Tinga and Aarnoudse 1979; Wolff *et al.* 1979; Abramovici *et al.* 1980; Barden *et al.* 1980; Davies and Robertson 1980; Jacobs *et al.* 1980; Milliez *et al.* 1980; Neibuhr-Jorgensen 1980).

Initially, much of the blame for this dreadful complication was directed either at corticosteroid administration, which had been the more recently introduced (Liggins and Howie 1972) of the two drug treatments, or at a cumulative and mutually potentiating effect of corticosteroids and betamimetic drugs. As more of these reports became available, pulmonary oedema was recognized to be a complication not only of the combination of betamimetics with corticosteroids, but also of the combination of magnesium sulphate with corticosteroids (Elliott *et al.* 1979; Morales *et al.* 1986), of diazoxide (Adamsons and Wallach 1984), and of betamimetics used alone (Katz *et al.* 1981) in preterm labour.

Many of the cases described have been secondary to fluid overload, and no instance of pulmonary oedema has been reported in women receiving betamimetics orally. Fluid overload during betamimetic treatment can occur by two mechanisms: by too vigorous administration of intravenous fluids and by decreased renal excretion of sodium, potassium and water as a direct result of high doses of betamimetics. This antidiuretic effect and the decrease in urinary output is most pronounced in the first 48 hours of tocolytic treatment. It normalizes slowly thereafter, even when tocolytic treatment is continued (Grospietsch 1981). Most cases of pulmonary oedema are also observed within the first two or three days of treatment. In experimental animals, the development of intravascular hypervolaemia during betamimetic administration has been directly correlated with increasing doses of the betamimetics and with increasing rates of crystalloid infusion (Grospietsch *et al.* 1982). Both of these concur when betamimetic drugs are administered in dilute solutions: the higher the dose, the larger the amount of fluid.

The frequency with which pulmonary oedema develops during betamimetic drug administration is difficult to estimate. Katz *et al.* (1981) observed clinical signs and symptoms of pulmonary oedema in 5 per cent of 160 women treated with terbutaline for preterm labour, but half of the women with this complication had twin pregnancies. If 5 per cent was a reasonable approximation of the frequency of this complication, it would have been observed and described much earlier than in the late 1970s and it would have been noted in several of the women who participated in the placebo-controlled trials. It is possible that the complication occurs more frequently with terbutaline than with other betamimetic drugs, as suggested by Robertson *et al.* (1981). Whether this is true and whether it relates specifically to this agent or to the way in which it is administered (Robertson *et al.* 1981) is not clear. Ingemarsson *et al.* (1985) remarked that 'very few cases' of pulmonary oedema have been observed in Sweden, where terbutaline has been used routinely since 1971. An association is commonly observed with underlying heart disease, multiple pregnancy, and the use of corticosteroids or multiple drugs in addition to the betamimetic agents.

In the absence of underlying disease, it is likely that most, if not virtually all cases of pulmonary oedema relate to aggressive intravenous hydration and to the neglect of signs of a positive fluid balance (Finley *et al.* 1984). The nature of the fluid that is administered may also be of influence.

Three trials have investigated the influence of using either saline or dextrose solutions (Philipsen *et al.* 1981; Lenz *et al.* 1985; Ferguson *et al.* 1984). Philipsen *et al.* (1981) randomly allocated 23 women in preterm labour to receive ritodrine in an infusion of either sodium chloride or glucose. They found that women receiving the saline infusion retained statistically significantly more fluid than those receiving the glucose infusion. Seven of 11 women in the saline group developed signs of pulmonary congestion as compared with none of the 12 women in the glucose group. A similar trial involving 36 women was conducted by Lenz and her colleagues (1985). None of the women receiving either isotonic dextrose or isotonic saline showed severe cardiodynamic changes and there were no cases of threatening pulmonary oedema. The authors found no difference in the rate of betamimetic induced acidosis between the saline and dextrose groups.

Ferguson *et al.* (1984) randomly allocated 50 women to six different groups. Twenty-two women received ritodrine and 28 received ritodrine in combination with magnesium sulphate; these two drug treatments were administered in either 5 per cent dextrose in water, 5 per cent dextrose in half normal saline (0.45 per cent), or lactated Ringer's solution. Five of the 22 women receiving ritodrine (22 per cent) were subsequently excluded from the analysis, so that results are reported on only 3 women who received the drug in dextrose, on 8 who received it in dextrose-saline and on 6 who had the Ringer's solution. Only 1 of these women experienced side-effects; she belonged to the group receiving the drug in Ringer's solution and the side-effects consisted of chest pain 'with associated electrocardiogram changes' (Ferguson *et al.* 1984).

Although the totality of the evidence derived from these trials is thus not very convincing and deals with only one of the betamimetic drugs, the consensus would seem to be in favour of dextrose as the preferred infusion fluid. Wiedinger (1977, 1984) has argued that, for various reasons, fructose is the best infusion fluid for the administration of betamimetic drugs, but this claim has not been assessed in controlled comparisons.

On the whole, it is much safer to administer betamimetic drugs in a small volume of fluid with the use of a perfusion pump, than to rely on intravenous infusion of dilute solutions of the drug. If the mother is allowed to drink freely, there should be no need for extra fluid and fluid overload is far less likely to occur. It still remains prudent to keep an accurate record of fluid intake and output. Betamimetic induced thirst may cause the woman to drink twice as much as she usually does, and the antidiuretic effect of these agents should not be underestimated. A simple measure such as weighing the woman twice daily during the first few days, when most cases of pulmonary oedema occur, will reveal excessive retention of fluid. Hypervolaemia is also readily diagnosed by the resulting haemodilution and decrease in haematocrit.

Incipient pulmonary oedema manifests itself by a number of clinical signs. The heart rate usually increases slowly but progressively to well above 130 beats per minute. This type of progressive increase should not be misinterpreted as a tachycardia response to betamimetics that is excessive, but of later onset. Women tend to develop a dry cough, feel more comfortable when sitting than when lying down, increase their respiration rate above 16 per minute, and may feel short of breath. When pO_2 is measured at that time, it will be found to be decreased, despite hyperventilation (Grospietsch 1981). Central venous pressure should be measured and treatment instituted with oxygen and diuretics, if necessary. The condition has a good prognosis if diagnosed early enough and reacted to swiftly (Katz *et al.* 1981; Benedetti *et al.* 1982). The two essential features of treatment are termination of the betamimetic drug infusion and administration of oxygen. When pulmonary congestion is diagnosed early enough, this should be adequate. Diuretics, with their known propensity to enhance hypokalaemia, should not be necessary. By the time pulmonary oedema becomes audible on auscultation it will usually be so massive as to require intubation and mechanical ventilation.

Many of the cases of pulmonary oedema have been observed in twin pregnancies (Robertson *et al.* 1981).

Not only does preterm labour occur more frequently in twin pregnancies, but plasma volume expansion is also much larger in twin pregnancies than in singleton pregnancies (Campbell and MacGillivray 1977). These women are therefore at greater risk of developing pulmonary oedema during treatment with betamimetics, although drug-induced cardiovascular changes appear to differ little between twin and singleton pregnancies (Rayburn *et al.* 1986). If an indication for caesarean section arises during labour, careful control of fluid input and output becomes even more important. The betamimetic-induced decrease in urinary output should certainly not be interpreted as a sign of hypovolaemia that requires aggressive hydration.

2.3.3.2 Myocardial ischaemia

Myocardial ischaemia has been described as the other main, but rare complication of betamimetic drug treatment (Dhainaut *et al.* 1978; Ries 1979; Eskes *et al.* 1980; Kubli 1980; Katz *et al.* 1981; Robertson *et al.* 1981; Ying and Tejani 1982; Benedetti 1983; Michalak *et al.* 1983; Hendricks *et al.* 1986). This complication is a separate entity from that of pulmonary oedema. Diffuse micronecrosis in the myocardium has been known since 1959, when it was induced in the rat by administration of isoproterenol (Rona *et al.* 1959). Similar lesions have been observed in the myocardium after 'betamimetic related' death. Unlike genuine myocardial infarcts, micronecrosis is not a direct result of hypoxia. It relates to the increasing energy and oxygen requirements of the beta-stimulated myocardial cell; if demand exceeds supply, ischaemia develops.

Not all electrocardiographic changes suggestive of myocardial ischaemia are clinically relevant, however. Most of the 'electrocardiographic pathology' is asymptomatic. Hendricks and her colleagues (1986) found that a majority of women treated with ritodrine in preterm labour developed electrocardiographic signs suggestive of myocardial ischaemia. The main changes were depression of the ST segment and flattening or inversion of the T wave; either or both occurred in 76 per cent of the women, but were not associated with symptoms. Hendricks *et al.* (1986) suggested that these electrocardiographic changes relate to a relative hypoperfusion of the subendocardium, which is a physiological adaptation to the induced tachycardia and has no known pathological significance. ST segment depression and T wave flattening or inversion were also observed in the majority of women treated with fenoterol for preterm labour and investigated by Wiest *et al.* (1979). These authors and others (Ying and Tejani 1982) found no changes in cardiac enzyme levels and concluded that the electrocardiographic changes do not represent significant myocardial damage. Whatever the clinical implications of these findings, betamimetic drugs should not be given to women with poor cardiac reserve.

2.3.3.3 Other cardiovascular effects

The most common and dose-related side-effect observed in all betamimetic-treated women is tachycardia. The heart rate response to a given concentration of the drug varies considerably from one woman to another and even in the same woman (Caritis *et al.* 1983). Only rarely will effective tocolysis be reached with maternal heart rates below 100 beats per minute. Heart rates of 130 to 140 beats per minute, on the other hand, should preclude further increases in the dose of betamimetics administered.

Clinically significant hypotension is rarely encountered with the newer betamimetic drugs such as ritodrine and terbutaline (Bieniarz *et al.* 1974; Brettes *et al.* 1976; Ingemarsson 1976; Wallace *et al.* 1978). Yet, others report hypotension in more than one-third of the women during initial treatment with these betamimetics (Caritis *et al.* 1983; Beall *et al.* 1985). In the trial of Beall and her colleagues (1985), for example, hypotension contributed to the decision to stop ritodrine in 16 per cent and terbutaline in 29 per cent of the women in whom treatment needed to be stopped because of side-effects.

Much of the argument as to whether or not betamimetic agents cause hypotension, relates to a question of definitions. When hypotension is defined in terms of the height of the diastolic blood pressure, there is no doubt that it does occur. Osler (1979) reported an average decrease in diastolic blood pressure of 16 mm Hg in the ritodrine-treated women and of 8 mm Hg in the control women who took part in the Danish multicentre trial of Larsen *et al.* (1980). All betamimetic agents show a clear tendency to lower diastolic blood pressure. However, hypotension will be noted rarely, when it is defined in terms of mean arterial pressure (see Chapter 24), because the decrease in diastolic pressure is usually accompanied by an increase in systolic blood pressure. Whatever definition is used, the net effect is an increase in pulse pressure. This is observed with all betamimetic agents that are currently employed (Bieniarz et al. 1974; Lipshitz and Baillie 1976; Osler 1979; Ross *et al.* 1983; Finley *et al.* 1984).

Betamimetic drug administration results in a marked increase in cardiac output in pregnancy, which is roughly of the same order as that observed during moderate exercise (Bieniarz *et al.* 1974; Finley *et al.* 1984). This increase is attributed to the combination of an increase in heart rate and a decrease in peripheral vascular resistance due to relaxation of vascular smooth muscle. In late pregnancy, cardiac output is already 40 per cent above prepregnancy values and the increase is even larger in twin pregnancies (De Swiet 1980). The additional work imposed on the myocardium by betamimetic drug treatment, may thus become too much for women with pre-existing, overt or hidden, cardiac disease (Eskes *et al.* 1980). These women should not be given betamimetics as the hazards for them are likely to be greater than any benefit that could be derived for their infants. For the same reason, it is wise to insist on a normal electrocardiogram before betamimetics are administered, although the likelihood of finding an abnormal electrocardiogram in a normal pregnant woman without symptoms or suggestive history must be small. It must not be implied, however, that a normal electrocardiogram before treatment will protect against subsequent development of pulmonary oedema (Katz *et al.* 1981; Hendricks *et al.* 1986).

2.3.3.4 Metabolic and biochemical changes

All betamimetic agents greatly influence carbohydrate metabolism (Eskes and Essed 1979; Grospietsch and Kuhn 1984). This is most marked at the beginning of tocolysis. Blood sugar levels increase by about 40 per cent and there is an increase in insulin secretion. The latter occurs both as a response to the elevated glucose levels and from beta receptor stimulation in the pancreas (Caldwell *et al.* 1987). In women with diabetes the rise in glucose levels is even more pronounced. It increases their insulin requirements. Thus, a woman with a well-regulated diabetes invariably becomes deregulated when betamimetics are administered (Lenz *et al.* 1979; Wager *et al.* 1981). This applies even more when betamimetics are combined with corticosteroids, which also have diabetogenic effects. Lipolysis induced by betamimetic drugs is manifested by an increase in acidic metabolites, and this may be accompanied by a slight metabolic acidosis. These effects too are more accentuated in diabetic women. All of these metabolic changes may lead to severe ketoacidosis in diabetic women treated with betamimetic drugs (Leslie and Coats 1977; Thomas *et al.* 1977; Schilthuis and Aarnoudse 1980).

A rapid drop in serum potassium levels is a universal finding at the beginning of betamimetic drug treatment (Schreyer *et al.* 1979; Grospietsch and Kuhn 1984). This is not due to loss of potassium from the body and it thus requires no substitution of such loss. It is due to a net flux of potassium from the extracellular to the intracellular space. This is considered to be a by-product of the combined glucose and insulin elevations, which induce accelerated transfer of potassium into the intracellular compartment. The resulting hypokalaemia is transient. Levels remain low for a few hours, but normalize within 24 hours even when tocolytic treatment is continued beyond that time (Kirkpatrick *et al.* 1980).

2.3.3.5 Fetal and neonatal effects

There is no doubt that betamimetic agents, probably all of them, cross the placenta (Gandar *et al.* 1980; Ingemarsson *et al.* 1981; Brazy *et al.* 1981; Van Lierde and Thomas 1982). Stimulation of beta receptors in the fetus evokes roughly the same effects as it does in the mother. The cardiovascular effects result in fetal tachycardia (Ingemarsson 1976), although this is not universally observed and usually far less pronounced than it is in the mother. Since the metabolic effects in mother and fetus may result in hypoglycaemia and hyperinsulinism after birth (Wiedinger *et al.* 1976; Epstein *et al.* 1979), assessment of blood sugar levels is essential in infants born during or shortly after tocolysis. Data from the placebo-controlled trials discussed above show no differences in either mortality or severe respiratory morbidity between infants born after treatment with betamimetics and those born after placebo treatment in preterm labour. Such data, however, are only available for three of the betamimetic agents that are used in obstetrical practice (Table 44.11).

A few studies have compared long term outcomes between infants whose mothers had received betamimetic drugs and infants whose mothers had not received such treatment (Freysz *et al.* 1977; Polowczyk *et al.* 1984; Hadders-Algra *et al.* 1986). All of these studies have been rather small, and the control groups have been variously constructed. No long term ill-effects were observed.

2.3.4 Supplementing betamimetic drugs with other tocolytic agents

A number of controlled comparisons have been conducted between a betamimetic drug used alone and in combination with other labour inhibiting drugs to enhance tocolytic activity (Gamissans *et al.* 1978; Gamissans *et al.* 1982; Katz *et al.* 1983; Gamissans and Balasch 1984; Ferguson *et al.* 1984). These will be discussed in the sections that pertain to these other drug treatments.

Other trials have addressed the question whether the combination of betamimetics with other treatments could reduce some of the unwanted effects of the betamimetic drugs. Some of these comparisons, involving alternative infusion fluids (Philipsen *et al.* 1981; Lenz *et al.* 1985; Ferguson *et al.* 1984), have been discussed above (see Section 2.3.3.1). All other attempts to reduce the systemic, and especially the cardiovascular, effects of betamimetic agents have centred on the use of calcium antagonists or beta-1 receptor blockers. Both categories of drugs, and often the same agents, have also been used for the treatment of hypertension in pregnancy (see Chapter 33).

Not many of the studies that reported on the combination of these agents with betamimetic drugs have included control groups. When they did, it has been either difficult or impossible to determine whether women were assigned to the different groups at random or by clinical selection. Most of these studies have been conducted in German-speaking countries and the specific method of allocation is usually not described. The evidence in favour of combining betamimetic agents with either calcium antagonists or beta-1 receptor blockers is so weak, however, that we have made no attempts to obtain unpublished information that might allow us to distinguish biased from unbiased allocation. Moreover, most of the studies that we reviewed dealt with fenoterol as the betamimetic agent. As mentioned above, this agent has never been tested against placebo (or no treatment) in preterm labour. Nor is there any evidence that it is more effective than any other labour-inhibiting drug either to delay delivery or to prolong pregnancy. Many reasons have been proposed for combining betamimetic agents with either calcium antagonists or beta-1 receptor blockers. To be of value, however, such combination treatments should be demonstrated to achieve at least one of the following three aims. First, infant outcome in terms of mortality and serious morbidity should be demonstrated to be better with the combined than with the single treatment. Second, it should be shown that the addition of these drugs decreases the incidence of serious maternal complications during betamimetic drug treatment. Third, the combined treatment should also be shown to result in a significant decrease in the incidence of less serious, but troublesome maternal side-effects. Our review of the studies, which appear to have included adequate control groups and which are therefore less likely to be biased, gave no indication that any of these goals has been adequately achieved.

Historically, the first approach has been to use a calcium antagonist, verapamil or isoptin, widely used for the treatment of ischaemic heart disease. The available data suggest that 'cardioprotection' was not the original aim. This goal appears to have been chosen after, contrary to expectations, the drug showed no tocolytic promise in preterm labour (Fleckenstein *et al.* 1971; Mosler and Rosenboom 1972). Impairment of cardiac atrioventricular conduction limited the use of doses that would be required for adequate tocolysis.

From the trials that have been conducted there is no evidence whatsoever that simultaneous use of calcium antagonists will protect the woman against the severe complications of betamimetic drug treatment. On the contrary, the alarming reports on cardiac complications often came from institutions where betamimetic drugs were routinely combined with a calcium antagonist, mostly verapamil, for treatment of preterm labour (Kubli 1977, 1980). Fendel *et al.* (1982) found that electrocardiogram changes during infusion of fenoterol occurred just as frequently with or without the addition of verapamil. Hofstetter *et al.* (1979) conducted extensive investigations in healthy volunteers and found that there were no differences in heart rate, blood pressure, and various parameters of cardiac ventricular function, as measured by echocardiography, between the administration of fenoterol with or without supplementary calcium antagonist 'treatment'. Differences in the degree of maternal tachycardia have been reported to be minimal, if detectable, in controlled studies (Fendel *et al.* 1982; Hiltman and Wiest 1982). Subjective maternal symptoms too have been reported to be as frequent with a combined calcium antagonist and betamimetic drug treatment as with the betamimetic drug alone (Trolp *et al.* 1982).

The lack of evidence for a protective effect of calcium antagonists appears to be clear. Nevertheless, it has been argued that cardioprotection does not need to be demonstrated, as it means 'a higher loading limit of the heart—which in fact cannot be measured with routine parameters' (Wiedinger 1984). Those, who follow that reasoning continue to feel that 'calcium antagonists certainly have a justification . . . during treatment with betamimetics' (Wiedinger 1984). More than anything else, this illustrates, first, how little evidence is required to introduce treatments that appear to be based on sound physiological principles and, second, how much evidence is needed to weed them out, when the application of these physiological principles does not appear to confer benefit to the mother or her baby.

Where calcium antagonists failed, blockers of beta-1 receptors stepped in. They too appeared to be a logical answer to the problem. If no betamimetic agents can be found that stimulate only beta-2 receptors, why not combine them with some other agent that will block the receptivity of the beta-1 receptors? Unfortunately, the solution has not been quite as simple as that. The property of the beta-2 agonists to stimulate mainly beta-2 receptors, but also, albeit to a lesser extent, beta-1 receptors, is shared by the beta-1 blockers. They not only block beta-1 receptors, but to a lesser extent also beta-2 receptors. The result ought to be predictable. This combined treatment is analogous to two persons on a bicycle, one of whom is constantly pedalling while the other constantly applies the brakes. Yet, this has not limited wide application of such combined treatments in some countries (Jung and Lamberti 1982), before the 'logical hypothesis' was subjected to controlled assessment in well-designed and well-executed clinical trials.

Several such agents, including bunitrolol, atenolol, and metoprolol were tried from the mid-1970s onwards, mostly in West Germany (Müller-Tyl *et al.* 1974). As mentioned above, these agents have also been tried for the treatment of hypertension in pregnancy (see Chapter 33). In preterm labour, the main aim apparently was to reduce the maternal tachycardia.

Reinold and Müller-Tyl (1977) succeeded in doing so with bunitrolol, but at the expense of abolishing the tocolytic effect of the betamimetic agent. Since 1977, most of the data have related to metoprolol. This apparently is because the drug itself, or the doses in which it is used, have less effect on the uterus (Trolp *et al.* 1980). Among many reports describing either experiences with or merits of concurrent blocking and stimulating of beta receptors, two randomized trials were uncovered.

One, stated to be a 'prospective randomized study', allocated three groups of 33 women to either fenoterol, fenoterol and verapamil, or fenoterol and metoprolol (Trolp *et al.* 1982). The method of randomization is not described, and another publication (Irmer *et al.* 1982) apparently refers to two, but not three of the three groups of 33 women. The other study (Ross *et al.* 1983) allocated 20 women double-blind to terbutaline and placebo or to terbutaline and metoprolol. Three women were subsequently excluded, one because she had given birth to a still born baby! As only 7 women remained in the metoprolol group and 10 in the placebo group, we assume that all exclusions, including fetal death, had been in the metoprolol group.

It has not been possible to combine the results of the two studies, since none of the outcomes is reported in a similar way. Both studies appear to indicate that the use of the beta-1 blocker reduces some of the beta-1 effects of the betamimetic agents. Both also appear to indicate that the drug diminishes some of the desired beta-2 effects on the uterus. In the 'trial' of Trolp *et al.* (1982) women in receipt of the metoprolol and fenoterol combination had a statistically significantly lower heart rate than women receiving either fenoterol alone or fenoterol plus verapamil. However, 16 of the 33 women in receipt of that treatment delivered 'prematurely', which in this report appears to refer to infants of less than 2500 g, as opposed to 11 of the 33 women in the fenoterol group. The doses of fenoterol in both groups were the same, averaging respectively 2.0 and 2.1 microgram per minute. In the trial of Ross *et al.* (1983), the mean delay of delivery was 8.7 days in women receiving terbutaline alone and only 1.9 days in women receiving the metoprolol as well.

Ross *et al.* (1983) concluded that metoprolol thus interfered with terbutaline stimulation of the beta-2 receptors in the uterus and that their study illustrated the lack of pure β_1- or β_2-specificity of either one of these agents. Trolp *et al.* (1982), on the other hand, concluded that 'it was possible to eliminate and normalize the systemic cardiac effects of tocolytic therapy by using a cardioselective beta-blocking agent'. It should be noted, however, that these authors started treatment with the beta blocker after uterine contractions were thought to have been arrested. They then maintained the maximal betamimetic drug dose for 4 days, while counteracting its effects with metoprolol (Trolp *et al.* 1982).

Beta-blockers, like betamimetics, cross the placenta, but their rates of placental transfer are not the same. Nor do they have the same half-lives. The assumed 'cardioprotection' in the mother could thus be accompanied by 'cardioviolation' in the fetus or neonate born during such treatment. Moreover, the use of this assumed cardioprotection in the mother has thus far not been shown to reduce the incidence of any of the serious cardiac complications associated with betamimetic drug treatment. From the uncontrolled studies, it appears that this treatment is used mainly in combination with excessive and prolonged use of betamimetics, mostly fenoterol, long after any threat of preterm delivery has subsided.

The data currently available do not justify routine combination of betamimetic agents with beta-blockers in the treatment of preterm labour. Other approaches to limit maternal side effects may be more deserving. For instance, Caritis and his colleagues (1983), who measured drug concentrations during ritodrine infusion, found that maternal side-effects occur mostly when concentrations of betamimetics are increasing. They suggested that the rate of change in drug concentrations is a more important determinant of the occurrence and severity of side-effects than the absolute levels reached. This claim is testable in adequate trials of different treatment regimens. It may be a more useful avenue to pursue in clinical practice than the continuation of unvalidated attempts to counteract one undesirable drug effect by administering another drug, with its own unwanted effects.

2.4 Maintenance of tocolysis

As mentioned above, all but one of the placebo-controlled trials of betamimetic drugs in preterm labour used oral maintenance treatment, after uterine contractions had been suitably arrested. The apparent success of these agents in prolonging the duration of pregnancy may have depended not only on their ability to stop uterine contractions. It may in part have depended on the ability of the oral treatment to prevent the recurrence of contractions.

Three placebo-controlled trials, in which betamimetic agents were administered orally to maintain uterine quiescence after an acute episode of preterm labour had been overcome by more aggressive treatment, have been reported in the literature (Creasy *et al.* 1980; Brown and Tejani 1981; Smit 1983). All 3 of these trials are small and they are rather heterogeneous. Creasy and his colleagues (1980) administered either oral ritodrine or placebo after preterm labour had been arrested with intramuscular ritodrine. Brown and Tejani (1981) administered either oral terbutaline or placebo after labour had been overcome with intravenous ethanol.

Smit (1983) used either oral ritodrine or placebo after intravenous ritodrine.

All 3 trials showed that oral betamimetic drug treatment will to some extent prevent a recurrence of preterm labour in the same pregnancy. Only 2 provided categorical data and these are shown in Table 44.18. Creasy and his colleagues (1980), however, reported that women in the ritodrine maintenance group had an average of 1.11 relapses of preterm labour as compared with an average of 2.71 in the control group, a difference that was statistically significant at the 0.5 per cent level. The evidence thus suggests that the incidence of recurrent preterm labour can be reduced by oral betamimetic administration.

The prevention of recurrences will not necessarily lead to a reduction in the incidence of preterm delivery. In Creasy's trial an equal number of women in both groups delivered preterm. In the trial of Smit (1980) there was a lower incidence of preterm delivery in the active treatment group, but this was not statistically significant. The report of Brown and Tejani (1981) contained no data on this outcome. The overall data available showed no reduction in the incidence of preterm delivery (Table 44.19).

Since all three trials combined included less than 250 women, it should not be surprising that the incidence of perinatal death not attributable to congenital malformations (Table 44.20) and the incidence of respiratory

Table 44.18 Effect of oral betamimetics for maintenance after preterm labour on recurrence of preterm labour

Study	EXPT		CTRL		Odds ratio	Graph of odds ratios and confidence intervals
	n	(%)	*n*	(%)	(95% CI)	0.01 0.1 0.5 1 2 10 100
Brown and Tejani (1981)	6/23	(26.09)	9/23	(39.13)	0.56 (0.17–1.89)	
Smit (1983)	18/44	(40.91)	25/45	(55.56)	0.56 (0.24–1.28)	
Typical odds ratio (95% confidence interval)					0.56 (0.28–1.11)	

Table 44.19 Effect of oral betamimetics for maintenance after preterm labour on delivery before 37 weeks

Study	EXPT		CTRL		Odds ratio	Graph of odds ratios and confidence intervals
	n	(%)	*n*	(%)	(95% CI)	0.01 0.1 0.5 1 2 10 100
Smit (1983)	21/44	(47.73)	30/45	(66.67)	0.47 (0.20–1.07)	
Creasy *et al.* (1980)	17/35	(48.57)	17/34	(50.00)	0.95 (0.37–2.41)	
Typical odds ratio (95% confidence interval)					0.64 (0.34–1.19)	

Table 44.20 Effect of oral betamimetics for maintenance after preterm labour on perinatal death (excluding lethal malformations)

Study	EXPT		CTRL		Odds ratio	Graph of odds ratios and confidence intervals
	n	(%)	*n*	(%)	(95% CI)	0.01 0.1 0.5 1 2 10 100
Smit (1983)	0/47	(0.00)	0/47	(0.00)	1.00 (1.00–1.00)	
Brown and Tejani (1981)	0/25	(0.00)	0/26	(0.00)	1.00 (1.00–1.00)	
Creasy *et al.* (1980)	2/36	(5.56)	2/38	(5.26)	1.06 (0.14–7.84)	
Typical odds ratio (95% confidence interval)					1.06 (0.14–7.84)	

Table 44.21 Effect of oral betamimetics for maintenance after preterm labour on respiratory distress syndrome

Study	EXPT		CTRL		Odds ratio	Graph of odds ratios and confidence intervals
	n	(%)	*n*	(%)	(95% CI)	0.01 0.1 0.5 1 2 10 100
Smit (1983)	2/47	(4.26)	1/47	(2.13)	1.98 (0.20–19.48)	
Brown and Tejani (1981)	1/25	(4.00)	6/26	(23.08)	0.21 (0.04–1.00)	
Creasy *et al.* (1980)	6/36	(16.67)	6/38	(15.79)	1.07 (0.31–3.64)	
Typical odds ratio (95% confidence interval)					0.69 (0.28–1.69)	

distress syndrome (Table 44.21) showed no differences between the active drug and placebo.

2.5 Conclusions

Powerful drugs are dangerous when used inappropriately. Attempts to prevent preterm labour by long term administration of oral betamimetic drugs during pregnancy have had no demonstrated benefit for either mother or baby. Chronic fetal exposure to these drugs has the potential for several, albeit equally undemonstrated, long term adverse effects. Use of these drugs prophylactically cannot be considered as appropriate in the light of current evidence.

Administration of betamimetic agents in preterm labour requires a valid indication and careful attention to maternal vital signs. For women with cardiac disease, hyperthyroidism, and diabetes mellitus the risks of betamimetic drug treatment nearly always outweigh its potential benefits. Women with multiple pregnancy, impaired renal function and with various other drug treatments, are at substantially greater risk of complications than women whose only problem is preterm labour.

Maternal side-effects are inevitable with betamimetic drug treatment. With good care serious complications are largely avoidable, however. There is no evidence that concurrent administration of calcium antagonists or beta-1 receptor blockers protects the mother against complications of betamimetic drug treatment. Nor is there any evidence that such combinations are of benefit to the baby. There is enough evidence, albeit observational, that vigorous hydration causes more harm than it avoids. It may be wise to insist that a normal electrocardiogram tracing be obtained before betamimetic drug treatment is started. There is no valid reason, however, for routine electrocardiograms at regular intervals in asymptomatic women during betamimetic drug treatment.

Betamimetics are highly effective for postponing delivery and also, albeit to a lesser extent, for prolonging pregnancy. By themselves they do not appear to have a beneficial effect on the fetus or the infant. No gain in reducing either mortality or morbidity has been demonstrated in the placebo-controlled trials that have been conducted thus far. This would imply that these drugs should only be used when something useful can be done in the time that is gained by their administration. Such useful measures might include administration of corticosteroids to promote pulmonary maturity (see Chapter 45), transfer of the mother to a centre with adequate facilities for preterm delivery (see Chapter 74), or judicious use of 'expectant management' in the period of gestation in which the infants chances of intact survival are poor.

3 Inhibitors of prostaglandin synthesis

There is substantial evidence that prostaglandins are of critical importance in the initiation and maintenance of human labour (Keirse 1985). Suppression of endogenous prostaglandin synthesis is therefore a logical approach to the inhibition of preterm labour. The first report on the application of this principle in preterm labour (Zuckerman *et al.* 1974) was published within a year of a retrospective study showing prolongation of pregnancy in chronic aspirin users (Lewis and Schulman 1973) and after an experimental study demonstrated that inhibitors of prostaglandin synthesis prolong the induction-abortion interval in women undergoing 2nd-trimester abortion by hypertonic saline (Waltman *et al.* 1973). The first review of the subject was published in 1979 (Wiqvist 1979) and many have followed since (Keirse 1981; Niebyl 1981; Wiqvist 1981; Gamissans and Balasch 1984; Witter and Niebyl 1986).

3.1 Range of drugs and their actions

Several agents with widely different chemical structures and pharmacokinetic properties (Keirse 1981) inhibit prostaglandin synthesis. They include acetylsalicylic acid (aspirin), indomethacin, naproxen and several fenamates. They are sometimes referred to as prostaglandin synthetase inhibitors. Since there is no such enzyme as prostaglandin synthetase, these drugs are more appropriately referred to as inhibitors of prostaglandin synthesis. Those that have been used to treat preterm labour include naproxen (Wiqvist 1979), flufenamic acid (Schwartz *et al.*, 1978) and acetylsalicylic acid (Győry *et al.* 1974; Dornhöfer and Mosler 1975), but the most widely used has been indomethacin (Witter and Niebyl 1986).

All of these drugs act by inhibiting the activity of prostaglandin endoperoxide synthase, an enzyme also known as cyclo-oxygenase. This enzyme converts fatty acids, arachidonic acid in particular, into prostaglandin endoperoxides. It is present in high concentrations in the myometrium of pregnant women (Moonen *et al.* 1984), but is found throughout the body both in and outside pregnancy. Inhibition of prostaglandin endoperoxide synthase does not only suppress prostaglandin synthesis; it also suppresses the formation of prostacyclin and thromboxane A_2, both of which may have a number of important, though largely unknown functions in pregnancy (Mitchell 1986; Keirse *et al.* 1987). Inhibition of the enzyme is not always achieved in the same way. Aspirin, for example, causes an irreversible inhibition of the enzyme, whereas indomethacin results in a competitive and reversible inhibition. This is because aspirin acetylates the enzyme, and thereby incapacitates it permanently. Indomethacin, on the other hand, competes with arachidonic acid for utilization by the enzyme; it leaves the enzyme itself intact and, when indomethacin levels decrease, the enzyme can resume activity.

In contrast to the betamimetic drugs, which all act in a similar way with regard to both their desired and their undesired effects, prostaglandin synthesis inhibitors show large differences from one compound to another. This implies that it is not justified to assume that effects which have been observed with one particular compound can be extrapolated to another compound simply because both are known to suppress prostaglandin synthesis.

All prostaglandin synthesis inhibitors are effective inhibitors of myometrial contractility, both during and outside pregnancy. There is also no doubt that they are more effective in this respect than any of the betamimetic drugs. No case has been reported in which a betamimetic drug resulted in suppression of uterine contractility after inhibition of prostaglandin synthesis had failed. The reverse has repeatedly been observed (Wiqvist *et al.* 1975; Halle and Hengst 1978; Van Kets *et al.* 1979; Suzanne *et al.* 1980; Keirse 1981), and a single dose of a suitable prostaglandin synthesis inhibitor can either stop or prolong labour in a large proportion of women labouring at term (Reiss *et al.* 1976).

3.2 Inhibition of active preterm labour

Only two studies have been reported that purported to compare a prostaglandin synthesis inhibitor with placebo in preterm labour (Niebyl *et al.* 1980; Zuckerman *et al.* 1984). Both used indomethacin as the active treatment, and both were stated to have been conducted in a double-blind manner. Neither of them was entirely placebo-controlled, however, since a number of women in whom treatment was considered to have failed received other tocolytic drugs (Table 44.22). In the study of Niebyl *et al.* (1980) other tocolytic drugs were given to 30 per cent of women in the placebo group and in the study of Zuckerman *et al.* (1984) to 44 per cent (Table 44.22).

Niebyl and her colleagues (Blake *et al.* 1980; Niebyl *et al.* 1980) did not report whether and to what extent delivery was postponed; information on the failure rate in their report only relates to whether or not cervical dilatation increased. Zuckerman *et al.* (1984) found statistically significant differences in the delay of delivery for 48 hours or more, in prolongation of pregnancy for more than 1 week, and in the incidences of preterm birth and of low birthweight. All of these outcomes were more favourable in the indomethacin treated group.

The only outcomes on which data are available in the reports of both Niebyl *et al.* (1980) and Zuckerman *et*

Table 44.22 Characteristics of 'placebo'-controlled trials of indomethacin for inhibition of preterm labour

	No. randomized:reported		Dose regimen	No. of failure and their treatment	
	Indomethacin	Placebo		Indomethacin	Placebo
Niebyl *et al.* (1980)	17:15	15:15	orally 50 mg→6 × 25 mg for 24 hours	1 failed during treatment 3 failed at 48 hours 2nd course of indomethacin (n=3)	9 failed during treatment 10 failed at 48 hours 2nd course of placebo (n=2) isoxsuprine (n=4) ethanol (n=1)
Zuckerman *et al.* (1984)	18:18	18:18	100 mg suppository→4 × 25 mg orally for 24 hours	1 failure –	14 failures ritodrine (n=8)

al. (1984) relate to perinatal mortality and respiratory distress syndrome. All of these data are shown in Tables 44.23 to 44.28, along with data from other controlled trials involving the use of indomethacin. It was reported by Niebyl and her colleagues (1980) that fewer infants in the treatment group had conditions that either caused death or were life-threatening (3 of 16; 0.2 per infant) than in the 'placebo' group (9 of 15; 0.6 per infant). In another publication by the same authors (Blake *et al.* 1980), however, it is stated that there were 2 infants who died and 3 others who had major life-threatening problems in each of the two groups. It is impossible to know which of these two reports is correct.

A few controlled studies have been conducted in which a prostaglandin synthesis inhibitor was either given or not given to women treated with other labour-inhibiting drugs. All of the trials used indomethacin and the other drug treatment was either ethanol or a betamimetic agent.

In the one study in which the standard treatment was ethanol, 42 women were assigned in sequence to a combined treatment with indomethacin and ethanol or to ethanol alone (Spearing 1979). Two rectal suppositories of 100 mg indomethacin were given 12 hours apart within the first 24 hours, and this was followed by 25 mg orally every 6 hours up to 48 hours after cessation of uterine contractions. Delivery within 48 hours occurred in 4 of 20 (20 per cent) indomethacin-treated women and in 10 of 22 women (45 per cent) who received only ethanol. The trial appears to indicate that the use of indomethacin in addition to ethanol is more likely to

Table 44.23 Effect of indomethacin in preterm labour on delivery within 48 hours

Study	EXPT		CTRL		Odds ratio	Graph of odds ratios and confidence intervals
	n	(%)	*n*	(%)	(95% CI)	0.01 0.1 0.5 1 2 10 100
Zuckerman *et al.* (1984)	1/18	(5.56)	14/18	(77.78)	0.06 (0.02–0.21)	
Spearing (1979)	4/20	(20.00)	10/22	(45.45)	0.33 (0.09–1.16)	
Typical odds ratio (95% confidence interval)					0.14 (0.06–0.34)	

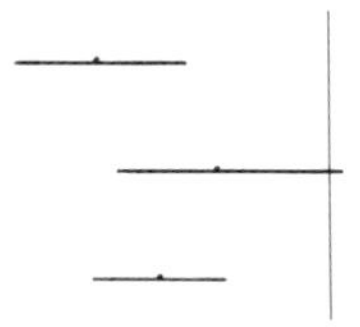

Table 44.24 Effect of indomethacin in preterm labour on delivery within 7–10 days

Study	EXPT		CTRL		Odds ratio	Graph of odds ratios and confidence intervals
	n	(%)	*n*	(%)	(95% CI)	0.01 0.1 0.5 1 2 10 100
Zuckerman *et al.* (1984)	3/18	(16.67)	15/18	(83.33)	0.07 (0.02–0.27)	
Gamissans and Balasch (1984)	33/148	(22.30)	55/149	(36.91)	0.50 (0.30–0.82)	
Typical odds ratio (95% confidence interval)					0.39 (0.24–0.62)	

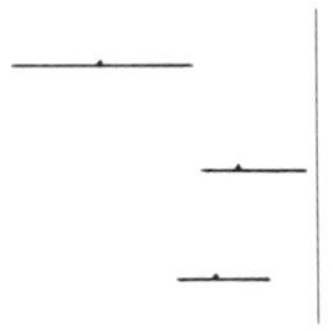

Table 44.25 Effect of indomethacin in preterm labour on delivery before 37 weeks

Study	EXPT		CTRL		Odds ratio	Graph of odds ratios and confidence intervals
	n	(%)	*n*	(%)	(95% CI)	0.01 0.1 0.5 1 2 10 100
Zuckerman *et al.* (1984)	3/18	(16.67)	14/18	(77.78)	0.09 (0.03–0.34)	
Gamissans and Balasch (1984)	69/148	(46.62)	94/149	(63.09)	0.52 (0.33–0.81)	
Typical odds ratio (95% confidence interval)					0.43 (0.28–0.65)	

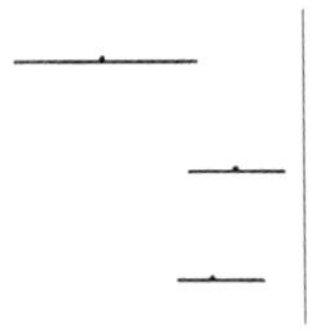

Table 44.26 Effect of indomethacin in preterm labour on birthweight <2500 g.

Study	EXPT		CTRL		Odds ratio	Graph of odds ratios and confidence intervals
	n	(%)	*n*	(%)	(95% CI)	0.01 0.1 0.5 1 2 10 100
Zuckerman *et al.* (1984)	3/18	(16.67)	14/18	(77.78)	0.09 (0.03–0.34)	
Gamissans and Balasch (1984)	56/148	(37.84)	78/149	(52.35)	0.56 (0.35–0.88)	
Katz *et al.* (1983)	15/60	(25.00)	22/60	(36.67)	0.58 (0.27–1.26)	
Spearing (1979)	10/20	(50.00)	13/23	(56.52)	0.77 (0.24–2.54)	
Typical odds ratio (95% confidence interval)					0.50 (0.35–0.72)	

Table 44.27 Effect of indomethacin in preterm labour on fetal and neonatal death

Study	EXPT		CTRL		Odds ratio	Graph of odds ratios and confidence intervals
	n	(%)	*n*	(%)	(95% CI)	0.01 0.1 0.5 1 2 10 100
Zuckerman *et al.* (1984)	1/18	(5.56)	2/18	(11.11)	0.49 (0.05–5.07)	
Gamissans *et al.* (1984)	11/148	(7.43)	20/149	(13.42)	0.53 (0.25–1.11)	
Niebyl *et al.* (1980)	2/16	(12.50)	2/15	(13.33)	0.93 (0.12–7.35)	
Katz *et al.* (1983)	0/60	(0.00)	0/60	(0.00)	1.00 (1.00–1.00)	
Spearing (1979)	4/20	(20.00)	5/23	(21.74)	0.90 (0.21–3.87)	
Typical odds ratio (95% confidence interval)					0.61 (0.33–1.11)	

delay delivery than ethanol alone. In view of evidence discussed below, this is hardly surprising. The data available from this report (Spearing 1979) have been combined with those of other indomethacin trials in Tables 44.23, 44.26 and 44.27.

Three trials have been reported in which a prostaglandin synthesis inhibitor was either added or not added to treatment with a betamimetic drug. All three trials dealt with indomethacin for inhibition of prostaglandin synthesis and all used ritodrine as the betamimetic agent. One was conducted by Katz *et al.* (1983). These authors alternately assigned 120 women treated with ritodrine for preterm labour before 35 weeks of gestation to receive, in addition, either 200 mg indomethacin (as a 100 mg suppository followed by 4 oral 25 mg capsules at 6-hourly intervals), or no indomethacin. All women received ritodrine intravenously, followed by oral maintenance treatment up to 35 weeks of gestation. The other two trials, one in women with intact membranes and one in women with ruptured membranes, were conducted double-blind by Gamissans and his colleagues (Gamissans *et al.* 1978, 1982; Gamissans and Balasch 1984). Ritodrine was given intravenously to obtain uterine relaxation and then continued intramuscularly or orally until 35 weeks of pregnancy, if the membranes were ruptured, or until 38 weeks, if they were intact. Placebo or 50 mg indomethacin suppositories were added to the treatment and administered every 8 hours for 2 weeks. Women were entered in these trials up to 34 weeks of gestation if they had ruptured membranes, and up to 36 weeks if the membranes were intact.

Gamissans and his colleagues produced several interim reports on their 2 trials (Gamissans *et al.* 1978, 1982; Gamissans and Balasch 1984). Unfortunately, there are a number of internal inconsistencies, which make one wary about drawing conclusions from these trials. For example, in the first report on women with ruptured membranes (Gamissans *et al.* 1982) only 12 of 55 women reached a gestational age of 37 weeks or more at delivery. At the time of the second report (Gamissans and Balasch 1984), a further 19 women had been

Table 44.28 Effect of indomethacin in preterm labour on respiratory distress syndrome

Study	EXPT		CTRL		Odds ratio	Graph of odds ratios and confidence intervals
	n	(%)	*n*	(%)	(95% CI)	0.01 0.1 0.5 1 2 10 100
Zuckerman *et al.* (1984)	1/18	(5.56)	4/18	(22.22)	0.26 (0.04–1.66)	
Gamissans and Balasch (1984)	3/148	(2.03)	5/149	(3.36)	0.60 (0.15–2.45)	
Niebyl *et al.* (1980)	4/16	(25.00)	3/15	(20.00)	1.32 (0.25–6.92)	
Katz *et al.* (1983)	0/60	(0.00)	0/60	(0.00)	1.00 (1.00–1.00)	
Typical odds ratio (95% confidence interval)					0.62 (0.25–1.58)	

entered, but an additional 42 women (54 of 74) had now reached 37 weeks or more at delivery. There are other aspects in these trials that are difficult to comprehend. For instance, there is also a three-times lower incidence of delivery within 10 days in women entered into the intact membranes' trial between the second and the third report (13 per cent; Gamissans and Balasch 1984) than that documented in the second report (37 per cent; Gamissans *et al.* 1982).

Despite our reservations about the heterogeneous nature of these trials and potential bias in many of them, the data that could be reliably extracted from the reports (Spearing 1979; Blake *et al.* 1980; Niebyl *et al.* 1980; Katz *et al.* 1983; Gamissans *et al.* 1978, 1982; Gamissans and Balasch 1984; Zuckerman *et al.* 1984) have been combined in Tables 44.23 to 44.28. Extreme caution is necessary, however, in the interpretation of these data.

Thus, the three studies that provide data on delay of delivery showed indomethacin to be more effective than 'placebo' in delaying delivery for 48 hours and for 7–10 days. The typical odds ratio for delivery within 48 hours was 0.14 with a 95 per cent confidence interval of 0.06 to 0.34 (Table 44.23). For delivery within 7 to 10 days it was 0.39 with a confidence interval of 0.24 to 0.62 (Table 24). The incidence of preterm delivery was similarly reduced in the indomethacin-treated group with a typical odds ratio of 0.43 and a confidence interval of 0.28 to 0.65 (Table 44.25). Data on the incidence of low birthweight were available from 4 trials. They showed a statistically significant reduction in the incidence of low birthweight in the indomethacin-treated group across trials (typical odds ratio: 0.50, confidence interval 0.35–0.72; Table 44.26).

All reports on the indomethacin trials provided data on fetal and neonatal death (Table 44.27). Overall, the data suggest that the use of indomethacin in preterm labour may reduce the incidence of fetal and neonatal death. The typical odds ratio of 0.61 had a confidence interval 0.33–1.11 (Table 44.27), but nearly all of this trend was due to the difference in mortality in the two trials of Gamissans and his colleagues (1978, 1982, 1984). The incidence of respiratory distress syndrome, on the other hand, showed even less evidence of a difference between the indomethacin and the control groups across trials, with a typical odds ratio of 0.62 and a wide confidence interval from 0.25 to 1.58 (Table 44.28).

Only a few reports on the use of naproxen (Wiqvist 1979), flufenamic acid (Schwartz *et al.* 1978), and acetyl salicylate (Győry *et al.* 1974; Dornhöfer and Mosler 1975; Wolff *et al.* 1981), have appeared in the literature. These drugs have not been used as widely as indomethacin (Gamissans and Balasch 1984; Witter and Niebyl 1986), and none of them has been subjected to controlled trials.

The doses of prostaglandin synthesis inhibitors that have been used in uncontrolled studies have varied considerably and some of these have been clearly excessive. Doses of indomethacin have ranged from 100 mg a day to as much as 500 mg a day (Csaba *et al.* 1978), and duration of treatment has been from 1 day to 3 weeks or more (Van Kets *et al.* 1979). Acetylsalicylic acid has been used in doses of up to 6 g orally (Dornhöfer and Mosler 1975) and up to 10 g intravenously (Wolff *et al.* 1981) per day. Often the large doses have resulted from lack of knowledge on the half-life of these drugs. For example, a total of 150 mg indomethacin, administered as 25 mg suppositories every 4 hours, is more likely to maintain inhibition of uterine prostaglandin synthesis for 24 hours than the larger dose of 200 mg administered in 2 suppositories of 100 mg, 12 hours apart (Keirse 1981). Unfortunately, there are no controlled data to indicate what doses of what drugs will most effectively suppress uterine contractions in preterm labour.

3.3 Unwanted effects

None of the trials discussed above have indicated that the use of inhibitors of prostaglandin synthesis is associated with an increased incidence of major problems for either mother or baby. On the other hand, none of these trials were truly placebo-controlled, and the number of women included in these trials has not been large enough to stand a chance of uncovering rare adverse effects.

Inhibitors of prostaglandin synthesis are not innocuous. Three points need to be considered. First, there are numerous potential side-effects because of the ubiquitous nature of the prostaglandins. Second, the drugs and doses that are used for inhibition of preterm labour, also suppress prostacyclin and thromboxane synthesis. Third, the drugs are both chemically and pharmacologically so different from each other that they should not be considered as interchangeable. They may roughly fulfil the same function, but this does not mean that they will all have the same effects and ill-effects.

The most serious potential side-effects are peptic ulceration, gastrointestinal and other bleeding, thrombocytopenia, and allergic reactions. Gastrointestinal irritation is common with the use of prostaglandin synthesis inhibitors, and it can occur irrespective of the route of administration. With indomethacin it is less frequent with rectal than with oral administration and, as the bioavailability of the drug is identical with both routes of administration (Alvan *et al.* 1975; Wallusch *et al.* 1978), the rectal route offers some advantage. Nausea, vomiting, dyspepsia, diarrhoea, and allergic rashes have all been observed in women treated, even briefly, with prostaglandin synthesis inhibitors in preterm labour. Headache and dizziness may occur at the very start of treatment. Gamissans and his associates reported systematically on the incidence of headache, maternal tachycardia above 120 beats per minute, vomiting, epigastric pain, and rectal intolerance in their trials (Gamissans *et al.* 1978, 1982; Gamissans and Balasch 1984), comparing indomethacin with placebo in association with ritodrine treatment. Only 2 of these side-effects were observed more frequently in the indomethacin-treated group. Epigastric pain was observed in 6 (4 per cent) and rectal intolerance in 7 (5 per cent) of 148 indomethacin treated women; these symptoms occurred in only 2 of 149 women in the control group (Gamissans and Balasch 1984).

It is generally believed that signs of infection may be masked by administration of prostaglandin synthesis inhibitors. It is not known, however, whether this also hampers or postpones the diagnosis of incipient intrauterine infection if it occurs. The effects of prostaglandin synthesis inhibitors in prolonging bleeding time are well-known; this is an important consideration when the prospects of care for labour and delivery include epidural anaesthesia.

Prostaglandin synthesis inhibitors cross from the mother to the fetus (Traeger *et al.* 1973; Turner and Collins 1975; Wilkinson 1980) and may influence several fetal functions. A great deal of information has been gathered on the fetal effects of these drugs in experimental animals. The results are not always easy to interpret, however, because of the variety of species studied, differences in the type of drug used and in the dose, route and duration of administration. Apart from a prolonged bleeding time, which is a constant feature in infants born with detectable levels of such drugs, effects in human fetuses and neonates are mostly based on anecdotal reports. The most consistent observations relate to the cardiopulmonary circulation and to renal and haemostatic functions (Keirse 1981).

The major worries about the use of such drugs for the inhibition of preterm labour have resulted from their influence on the ductus arteriosus. Closure of the ductus after birth consists of an initial functional closure by muscular contraction followed by definitive anatomical closure, which is a much slower process and rarely accomplished within the first week of life (Gittenberger-de Groot 1977). Prostaglandin synthesis inhibitors cause constriction of the ductus arteriosus in the neonate, an effect that has been conclusively demonstrated in placebo-controlled trials of neonatal indomethacin administration (Mahony *et al.* 1982; Gersony *et al.* 1983). Autopsy and cardiac catheterization data from infants who presented with congestive heart failure at or after birth, have suggested that severe constriction of the ductus may also occur before birth in association with inhibition of prostaglandin synthesis (Arcilla *et al.* 1969; Kohler 1978; Levin 1980).

Constriction of the ductus during fetal life probably has little effect on fetal oxygenation in the short term, as effective shunting can be maintained through the foramen ovale. In experimental animals even complete surgical ligation is compatible with intrauterine survival for a considerable length of time (Haller *et al.* 1967). Levin and his co-workers (Levin et al. 1978b; Levin *et al.* 1979; Levin 1980) showed experimentally that constriction of the ductus arteriosus *in utero* causes a marked increase in pulmonary arterial pressure, which results in increased smooth muscle development in the wall of pulmonary arterial resistance vessels. These morphological changes, which were also observed in human fetuses (Levin *et al.* 1978a), are similar to those seen in the clinical syndrome of persistent pulmonary hypertension of the newborn. Further experimental evidence has indicated that the increase in both pulmonary and ductal vascular resistance could, by increasing right ventricular and diastolic pressure, produce subendothelial ischaemia, particularly in the papillary muscles of the tricuspid valve (Levin 1980).

Prolonged prenatal constriction of the ductus arteriosus could thus lead to both persistent pulmonary hypertension and tricuspid insufficiency in the newborn.

Several other reports have linked the syndrome of persistent pulmonary hypertension, also known as persistent fetal circulation, progressive pulmonary hypertension and persistent transitional circulation, to the prenatal use of prostaglandin synthesis inhibitors. Only two cases of persistent pulmonary hypertension have been reported in the controlled trials that we reviewed. Both of these, one in the placebo group and one in the indomethacin treated group, occurred in Gamissans' trial on ruptured membranes (Gamissans *et al.* 1982; Gamissans and Balasch 1984). No cases was reported in an uncontrolled study of Van Kets *et al.* (1979) who reported on 51 women who had received indomethacin 25 mg three to four times a day for up to 3 weeks or more.

Wiqvist (1981) compiled reports from controlled and uncontrolled clinical studies in which careful paediatric examination of the newborn had been carried out. For a total of 730 mothers included in these studies he found 17 infants with persistent pulmonary hypertension (2.3 per cent); 14 of these infants recovered within a few days and 3 died. A similar approach was followed by Gamissans and Balasch (1984), who found 19 cases (1.5 per cent) among a total of 1235 women who received prostaglandin synthesis inhibitors in preterm labour; 16 of the infants survived and 3 died. Whether or not this incidence is higher than it would have been without inhibition of prostaglandin synthesis is impossible to determine from such data.

Data both from experimental animals and human neonates suggest that the responsiveness of the ductus arteriosus to indomethacin is lower at lower gestational ages. If such a difference in responsiveness exists *in utero*, it would imply that the risk of ductus constriction and its potential sequelae would be smallest when most gain can be expected from arresting preterm labour, and largest at gestational ages at which inhibition of labour is probably not justified. It is also probable, although not detected in the available data from controlled and uncontrolled studies, in preterm labour, that the duration of treatment is of influence. The longer prostaglandin synthesis inhibition is continued, the greater the risk is likely to be.

Indomethacin treatment may alter both fetal and neonatal renal function. Renal dysfunction and reduced urinary output has repeatedly been noted in infants treated with indomethacin to close a patent ductus arteriosus (Heymann *et al.* 1976; Betkerur *et al.* 1981; Gleason 1987). The effect is apparently dose related and transient. Renal function usually returns toward pretreatment values within 24 hours after stopping the treatment (Gleason 1987). Several reports have indicated impaired renal function in fetuses and in the neonates at birth following administration of prostaglandin synthesis inhibitors to the mother (Cantor *et al.* 1980; Itskovitz *et al.* 1980; Veersema *et al.* 1983). Long term maternal treatment may influence fetal urine output enough to alter amniotic fluid volume, although other mechanisms may also be involved in the reduction of amniotic fluid volume occasionally seen during indomethacin treatment (De Wit *et al.* 1988). There is no evidence from either maternal or neonatal indomethacin treatment that the use of this drug in preterm labour would lead to permanent impairment of renal function in the infant (Gleason 1987).

Inhibitors of the cyclo-oxygenase enzyme all inhibit platelet aggregation and prolong bleeding time. They do so in the mother, in the fetus and in the neonate at birth (Friedman *et al.* 1980; Wilkinson 1980). Since neonates, and particularly preterm neonates, eliminate these drugs far less efficiently than their mothers (Keirse 1981), these effects will be of longer duration in the baby than in the mother. There are major differences in this respect between different inhibitors of prostaglandin synthesis. Salicylates are particularly troublesome. As mentioned earlier, they acetylate the cyclo-oxygenase enzyme and incapacitate it permanently. Unlike most cells in the body, blood platelets cannot manufacture new enzyme. This implies that not only the cyclo-oxygenase enzyme, but that also the platelets themselves are rendered permanently non-functional. They cannot restore normal haemostasis; for this to occur they must be replaced by new platelets.

3.4 Conclusions

The overall quality of the controlled trials of inhibitors of prostaglandin synthesis is not high. Nevertheless, it appears that indomethacin can be a useful drug for obtaining sufficient delay of delivery to institute measures that may improve infant outcome. More, and better controlled data will be needed, however, before the usefulness of prostaglandin synthesis inhibition in preterm labour can be adequately assessed.

The lasting effect of salicylates on platelet function and the fact that these substances are less efficient prostaglandin synthesis inhibitors than some of the other drugs, and thus require very high doses, provide a strong case for not using them in the treatment of preterm labour.

4 Ethanol

Ethanol, for a long time one of the main labour inhibiting drugs, particularly in the United States where no betamimetic drugs were approved for use in preterm labour until 1980 (Barden *et al.* 1980), is now only of historical interest. In a survey among British obstetricians, Lewis *et al.* (1980) found that only 2 per cent of the obstetricians would use ethanol in attempts to stop preterm labour. Keirse (1984a) found that it was used by none of 521 obstetricians and trainee obstetricians questioned about their use of tocolytic drugs in The Netherlands and Belgium (Table 44.2). The use of ethanol in preterm labour was propagated mainly by Fuchs and his associates. They were the first to apply ethanol, which had previously been used as an obstetric analgesic (Belinkoff and Hall 1950), to the treatment of preterm labour (Fuchs 1965; Fuchs *et al.* 1967), and they have reviewed the subject on a number of occasions (Fuchs 1976; Fuchs and Fuchs 1981, 1984).

The effect of ethanol on myometrial contractility is probably indirect. It is generally attributed to the inhibition of oxytocin release from the neurohypophysis (Fuchs and Fuchs 1981). There may also be some direct effect on the myometrium (Mantell and Liggins 1970), but this is likely to be small (Fuchs and Fuchs 1984).

4.1 Inhibition of active preterm labour

Two placebo-controlled trials have been reported in the literature (Zlatnik and Fuchs 1972; Watring *et al.* 1976). Zlatnik and Fuchs (1972), using sealed envelopes, assigned 21 women to a 9.5 per cent intravenous ethanol infusion and 21 to a glucose infusion. They reported a lower incidence of delivery within 3 days in the alcohol-treated group (Table 44.29) and this difference was statistically significant. No other outcomes were reported except for 'median' birthweight, which was 2080 g in the ethanol-treated and 1900 g in the control group. Their findings were not supported by those of Watring *et al.* (1976), who used a system of cards drawn by a disinterested third party to allocate 35 women to ethanol, in doses equivalent to those used by Zlatnik and Fuchs (1972), or to dextrose infusion. Six of 17 (35 per cent) ethanol-treated women and 8 of 18 (44 per cent) control women delivered within 24 hours, and an equal number of women in both groups delivered within 3 days (Table 44.29). The data on the preterm delivery rates and on infant outcomes in the trial of Watring *et al.* (1976) are summarized in Table 44.30. There is no indication that ethanol favourably influenced any of these outcomes.

A number of uncontrolled studies were reviewed by Fuchs and Fuchs (1984), who concluded that such studies show 'success' rates varying from 50 to 73 per cent when the membranes are intact. With ruptured membranes the reported 'success' is very poor; mere arrest of contractions is usually achieved in less than 25 per cent of cases (Fuchs and Fuchs 1984).

4.2 Controlled comparisons between ethanol and other agents

Several controlled trials have been conducted to compare ethanol with other drug treatments for the inhibition of preterm labour. There are 8 reports of trials in which ethanol was compared with a betamimetic drug (Castrén *et al.* 1975; Fuchs 1976; Lauersen *et al.* 1977; Reynolds 1978; Sims *et al.* 1978; Spearing 1979; Merkatz *et al.* 1980; Caritis *et al.* 1982). Castrén *et al.* (1975) reported a study in which 'every other patient' was allocated to buphenine and the others to ethanol, but this 'alternate' allocation resulted in 43 buphenine- and 50 ethanol-treated women. The report of Merkatz *et al.* (1980) contained no usable data on the 153 women who had been randomized to ethanol or ritodrine, but 150 of these women had been included in a previous report by Lauersen *et al.* (1977) and some of these had also been reported on by Fuchs (1976).

The characteristics of the other trials and the betamimetic agent used in them are summarized in Table 44.31. Although the 3 largest trials all excluded some women after randomization, we have not attempted to obtain unpublished data from the authors. Several outcomes could be assessed in only a few of these reports. For instance, only 1 trial provided data on delivery within 24 hours after treatment allocation (Sims *et al.* 1978). Two reports provided information on the number of deliveries within 48 hours (Sims *et al.* 1978; Spearing 1979), one on the number delivered within 3 days (Lauersen *et al.* 1977), and 1 on the number delivered too early for a full 36 hours' course of corticosteroids to be given (Caritis *et al.* 1982). The data from these 4 reports have been combined in Table 44.32. All 4 trials suggested an advantage for the betamimetic agent, and in 2 of them (Lauersen *et al.*

Table 44.29 Effect of ethanol in preterm labour on delivery within 72 hours

Study	EXPT		CTRL		Odds ratio	Graph of odds ratios and confidence intervals
	n	(%)	*n*	(%)	(95% CI)	0.01 0.1 0.5 1 2 10 100
Zlatnik and Fuchs (1972)	4/21	(19.05)	13/21	(61.90)	0.18 (0.05–0.60)	
Watring *et al.* (1976)	8/17	(47.06)	8/18	(44.44)	1.11 (0.30–4.11)	
Typical odds ratio (95% confidence interval)					0.41 (0.17–1.01)	

Table 44.30 Effect of ethanol in preterm labour on delivery before 37 weeks

Study	EXPT *n*	EXPT (%)	CTRL *n*	CTRL (%)	Odds ratio (95% CI)	Graph of odds ratios and confidence intervals
Watring *et al.* (1976)	10/17	(58.82)	9/18	(50.00)	1.41 (0.38–5.24)	
Typical odds ratio (95% confidence interval)					1.41 (0.38–5.24)	

Effect of ethanol in preterm labour on birthweight <2500 g.

Study	EXPT *n*	EXPT (%)	CTRL *n*	CTRL (%)	Odds ratio (95% CI)	Graph of odds ratios and confidence intervals
Watring *et al.* (1976)	12/17	(70.59)	9/18	(50.00)	2.30 (0.61–8.73)	
Typical odds ratio (95% confidence interval)					2.30 (0.61–8.73)	

Effect of ethanol in preterm labour on respiratory distress syndrome

Study	EXPT *n*	EXPT (%)	CTRL *n*	CTRL (%)	Odds ratio (95% CI)	Graph of odds ratios and confidence intervals
Watring *et al.* (1976)	4/17	(23.53)	5/18	(27.78)	0.81 (0.18–3.59)	
Typical odds ratio (95% confidence interval)					0.81 (0.18–3.59)	

Effect of ethanol in preterm labour on fetal and neonatal death

Study	EXPT *n*	EXPT (%)	CTRL *n*	CTRL (%)	Odds ratio (95% CI)	Graph of odds ratios and confidence intervals
Watring *et al.* (1976)	4/17	(23.53)	3/18	(16.67)	1.52 (0.30–7.77)	
Typical odds ratio (95% confidence interval)					1.52 (0.30–7.77)	

Graph scale: 0.01, 0.1, 0.5, 1, 2, 10, 100

Table 44.31 Characteristics of the trials comparing ethanol with betamimetics for inhibition of preterm labour

Authors and date	Betamimetic treatment	Method of allocation	No. randomized: reported on — Allocated to ethanol	No. randomized: reported on — Allocated to betamimetic	Other details
Caritis *et al.* (1982)	Terbutaline IV→oral maintenance for 5 days if membranes intact	random by sealed envelopes	92:85 (total) ?:40	?:45	corticosteroids were generally given magnesium sulphate given if assigned treatment failed ruptured and intact membranes reported separately
Spearing (1979)	Salbutamol IV→oral for 48 hours after contractions	alternate	22:22	22:20	salbutamol was given if ethanol failed and vice versa
Reynolds (1978)	Salbutamol IV + 200 mg sodium phenobarbitone	alternate	42:42	42:42	all ethanol-treated women received 500 mg methyl prednisolone IV
Sims *et al.* (1978)	Salbutamol IV no maintenance	random by open list	100:88 (total) ?:46	?:42	all women randomized to betamethasone vs. placebo 5 women ethanol→betamimetic; 2 betamimetic→ethanol
Lauersen *et al.* (1977)	Ritodrine IV→oral maintenance for 4 weeks or until term	random by sealed envelopes	150:135 (total) ?:67	?:68	
Fuchs (1976)	—all women are also included in the report of Lauersen *et al.* (1977)—				

Table 44.32 Effect of betamimetics vs. ethanol in preterm labour on delivery within 48 or 72 hours

Study	EXPT		CTRL		Odds ratio	Graph of odds ratios and confidence intervals
	n	(%)	*n*	(%)	(95% CI)	0.01 0.1 0.5 1 2 10 100
Caritis *et al.* (1982)	5/28	(17.86)	15/28	(53.57)	0.22 (0.07–0.64)	
Spearing (1979)	7/22	(31.82)	10/22	(45.45)	0.57 (0.17–1.89)	
Sims *et al.* (1978)	7/42	(16.67)	12/46	(26.09)	0.58 (0.21–1.59)	
Lauersen *et al.* (1977)	7/68	(10.29)	18/67	(26.87)	0.34 (0.14–0.80)	
Typical odds ratio (95% confidence interval)					0.38 (0.23–0.64)	

Table 44.33 Effect of betamimetics vs. ethanol in preterm labour on delivery before 36 or 37 weeks

Study	EXPT		CTRL		Odds ratio	Graph of odds ratios and confidence intervals
	n	(%)	*n*	(%)	(95% CI)	0.01 0.1 0.5 1 2 10 100
Caritis *et al.* (1982)	23/28	(82.14)	23/28	(82.14)	1.00 (0.26–3.88)	
Sims *et al.* (1978)	32/42	(76.19)	32/46	(69.57)	1.39 (0.55–3.54)	
Lauersen *et al.* (1977)	19/68	(27.94)	31/67	(46.27)	0.46 (0.23–0.92)	
Typical odds ratio (95% confidence interval)					0.72 (0.43–1.21)	

1977; Caritis *et al.* 1982) this reached statistical significance.The typical odds of 0.38, with a confidence interval from 0.23 to 0.64 (Table 44.32), convincingly showed the betamimetic agents to be far superior to ethanol for delaying delivery.

Data on the incidence of preterm delivery, which in 2 reports related to delivery before 36 weeks (Lauersen *et al.* 1977; Caritis *et al.* 1982) and in 1 to delivery before 37 weeks (Sims *et al.* 1978), are shown in Table 44.33. Only one of the trials (Lauersen *et al.* 1977) showed a lower incidence of preterm delivery in betamimetic-treated than in ethanol-treated women; in the other two the incidence was either identical or tended to be higher. The overall data, with a typical odds ratio of 0.72 (95 per cent confidence interval 0.43–1.21), although tending to support the greater efficacy of betamimetics in delaying delivery, showed no statistically significant difference between the groups (Table 44.33).

The incidence of low birthweight, available for only 3 of the trials (Table 44.34), was lower in the betamimetic than in the ethanol group, and the difference reached statistical significance with a typical odds of 0.54 (confidence interval 0.32–0.91).

Data on the incidence of fetal and neonatal death were available for all trials (Table 44.35), but only 2 provided data on the incidence of respiratory distress syndrome (Table 44.36). Neither of these two outcomes showed a statistically significant difference between the two groups, although the incidence of respiratory distress syndrome tended to be lower in babies whose mothers had received a betamimetic agent than in those whose mothers had received ethanol (typical odds ratio 0.57; confidence interval 0.31–1.07).

Two of the studies in which salbutamol was the betamimetic agent reported fewer side-effects with this drug than with ethanol (Reynolds 1978; Spearing 1979), but one reported the reverse to be the case (Sims *et al.* 1978). Sims *et al.* (1978) found side-effects in 52 per cent of salbutamol- and in 24 per cent of ethanol-treated women. Reynolds (1978), on the other hand, noted side-effects in 29 per cent of salbutamol- and in 74 per cent of ethanol-treated women, while Spearing (1979) commented that in comparison to ethanol 'salbutamol was more acceptable to both patients and staff'. The trials in which ritodrine or terbutaline were used both reported a statistically significantly higher incidence of vomiting in ethanol-treated women

Table 44.34 Effect of betamimetics vs. ethanol in preterm labour on birthweight <2500 g.

Study	EXPT		CTRL		Odds ratio	Graph of odds ratios and confidence intervals
	n	(%)	*n*	(%)	(95% CI)	0.01 0.1 0.5 1 2 10 100
Spearing (1979)	10/21	(47.62)	13/23	(56.52)	0.71 (0.22–2.28)	
Lauersen *et al.* (1977)	25/73	(34.25)	44/76	(57.89)	0.39 (0.20–0.74)	
Typical odds ratio (95% confidence interval)					0.45 (0.25–0.78)	

Table 44.35 Effect of betamimetics vs. ethanol in preterm labour on fetal and neonatal death

Study	EXPT		CTRL		Odds ratio	Graph of odds ratios and confidence intervals
	n	(%)	*n*	(%)	(95% CI)	0.01 0.1 0.5 1 2 10 100
Caritis *et al.* (1982)	10/50	(20.00)	7/43	(16.28)	1.28 (0.45–3.65)	
Reynolds (1978)	6/42	(14.29)	4/42	(9.52)	1.57 (0.42–5.82)	
Spearing (1979)	2/21	(9.52)	5/23	(21.74)	0.41 (0.08–2.03)	
Sims *et al.* (1978)	4/42	(9.52)	10/46	(21.74)	0.41 (0.13–1.26)	
Lauersen *et al.* (1977)	3/73	(4.11)	6/76	(7.89)	0.52 (0.13–1.98)	
Typical odds ratio (95% confidence interval)					0.75 (0.43–1.31)	

(Lauersen *et al.* 1977; Caritis *et al.* 1982). Lauersen *et al.* (1977) reported an increase in maternal and fetal heart rate and in systolic blood pressure with both ethanol and ritodrine. Both treatments also resulted in a decrease in diastolic blood pressure. The average size of each of these effects was greater with ritodrine than with ethanol, however.

There has been only one trial comparing ethanol with magnesium sulphate. Steer and Petrie (1977) assigned 31 women to ethanol and 31 to magnesium sulphate on the basis of their hospital number. In ethanol-treated women, labour was less likely to be suppressed for more than 24 hours and pregnancy less likely to be prolonged for a week or more than in magnesium-sulphate-treated women (Table 44.37). Data on infant outcome, on the rate of preterm delivery and on maternal side-effects are not available in the report (Steer and Petrie 1977).

4.3 Unwanted effects

Blood alcohol levels during a single course of labour inhibition have been reported to range from 0.4 to 2.8 g per litre depending on its duration (Fuchs 1976; Watring *et al.* 1976). The upper end of this range corresponds to anaesthetic doses and levels above 3.5 g per litre are likely to result in coma. Fuchs and Fuchs (1981) report that the desired concentration for labour inhibition is between 1.2 and 1.8 g per litre, and that it takes, on average, 10 hours to eliminate the ethanol after a standard infusion. At the doses that are commonly employed, all women reach alcohol levels above legal intoxication limits. They are often overtly inebriated due to the drug's effect on the brain. Emotional instability and restlessness are not uncommon. Euphoric effects are rarely seen during ethanol treatment for preterm labour; on the contrary, women often become depressed (Fuchs and Fuchs 1981).

As oral intake is frequently limited, these women are prone to develop hypoglycaemia and lactacidaemia. Lactic acidosis, although usually mild, may become severe and life-threatening if multiple courses of ethanol are given over a short period of time (Ott *et al.* 1976). Headache is the most frequent side-effect, followed by nausea and vomiting. The latter can be hazardous in women with an altered level of consciousness, and may result in aspiration pneumonia (Greenhouse *et al.* 1969). Fuchs and Fuchs (1981) therefore recommended routine prophylaxis with an antiemetic

Table 44.36 Effect of betamimetics vs. ethanol in preterm labour on respiratory distress syndrome

Study	EXPT *n*	(%)	CTRL *n*	(%)	Odds ratio (95% CI)	Graph of odds ratios and confidence intervals
Caritis *et al.* (1982)	16/50	(32.00)	16/43	(37.21)	0.80 (0.34–1.87)	
Lauersen *et al.* (1977)	6/73	(8.22)	15/76	(19.74)	0.39 (0.15–0.98)	
Typical odds ratio (95% confidence interval)					0.57 (0.31–1.07)	

Table 44.37 Effect of Mg SO4 vs. ethanol for inhibition of preterm labour on delivery within 24 hours

Study	EXPT *n*	(%)	CTRL *n*	(%)	Odds ratio (95% CI)	Graph of odds ratios and confidence intervals
Steer and Petrie (1977)	9/31	(29.03)	17/31	(54.84)	0.35 (0.13–0.96)	
Typical odds ratio (95% confidence interval)					0.35 (0.13–0.96)	
Effect of Mg SO4 vs. ethanol for inhibition of preterm labour on delivery within 7 days						
Steer and Petrie (1977)	8/31	(25.81)	18/31	(58.06)	0.27 (0.10–0.74)	
Typical odds ratio (95% confidence interval)					0.27 (0.10–0.74)	

Table 44.38 Characteristics of the placebo controlled trials of 17α-hydroxyprogesterone caproate for the prevention of preterm labour

Authors	Entry criteria	Treatment characteristics: Dose	Started	Stopped	No. treated: reported — Active drug	Placebo
LeVine (1964)	history ⩾3 miscarriages	500 mg weekly	booking at <16 weeks	36 weeks	– 56 entered – ?:15	?:15
Papiernik (1970)	high preterm risk score	250 mg every 3 days (8 doses)	28–32 weeks	after 8 doses	50:50	49:49
Johnson *et al.* (1975)	history ⩾2 miscarriages/ preterm births	250 mg weekly	at booking	37 weeks	23:18	27:25
Hartikainen-Sorri *et al.* (1980)	twin pregnancy	250 mg weekly	28–33 weeks	37 weeks	39:39	38:38
Hauth *et al.* (1983)	non-selected women (active duty military personnel)	1000 mg weekly	16–20 weeks	36 weeks	80:80	88:88
Yemini *et al.* (1985)	history ⩾2 miscarriages/ preterm births + viable fetus on ultrasound	250 mg weekly (all women also had cervical suture inserted)	at booking	37 weeks	40:39	40:40

drug when administering ethanol for preterm labour.

Some degree of respiratory depression is to be expected with high doses of alcohol and instances have been reported in which respiratory depression assumed life-threatening proportions (Hendricks 1981). Alcohol is a well-known diuretic agent and dehydration may occur both during and after treatment. The increased diuresis may be accompanied by urinary incontinence, and it has been recommended that women should wear diapers during ethanol treatment (Fuchs and Fuchs 1981).

Ethanol crosses the placenta freely, and blood levels in the fetus are approximately the same as those in the mother (Idänpään-Heikkilä *et al.* 1972). If the treatment is not successful, and the infant is born during or shortly after the treatment, the infant will be intoxicated. The ability of the neonate to eliminate ethanol is much less than that of the mother (Wagner *et al.* 1970; Idänpään-Heikkilä *et al.* 1972) and depression of the nervous system may thus last much longer.

In a study, in which liveborn infants of ethanol-treated mothers were carefully matched with controls, Zervoudakis *et al.* (1980) found the neonatal mortality rate (8.4 vs. 4.2 per cent) and the incidence of respiratory distress (20 vs. 12 per cent) to be higher with ethanol treatment than in the matched controls. A breakdown of the groups revealed that the statistically significantly higher incidence of respiratory distress syndrome in the ethanol-treated group, could mainly be attributed to infants delivered less than 12 hours after stopping the ethanol infusion. In 31 infants born within 12 hours after stopping ethanol infusion, the incidence of respiratory distress syndrome was as high as 48 per cent (Zervoudakis *et al.* 1980).

Sisenwein *et al.* (1983), in a follow-up study at 4 to 7 years of age, compared 25 children whose mothers had been given ethanol to arrest preterm labour with controls matched for gestational age and weight at birth. The testers, who were unaware of the group to which the children belonged, found 'major pathology', consisting of hyperactivity and 'significant problems in performance intelligence quotient and visual-motor integration and achievement tests', in 4 of 7 children born within 15 hours of terminating the ethanol infusion.

4.4 Conclusions

From the evidence available it can be concluded that ethanol should no longer be regarded as a useful therapy for preterm labour. Irrespective of its effect on uterine contractions, it is less efficacious than other drug treatments and has serious side-effects in both mothers and babies.

5 Progesterone

Progestational agents have been widely used to prolong pregnancy in women who were judged to be at increased risk of miscarriage or preterm birth, or who had experienced a threat of miscarriage (see Chapter 38).

5.1 Prophylaxis

Six placebo-controlled trials have been reported on the use of a progestational agent to prevent preterm labour (LeVine 1964; Papiernik 1970; Johnson *et al.* 1975; Hartikainen-Sorri *et al.* 1980; Hauth *et al.* 1983; Yemini *et al.* 1985). The active drug in all of these trials was 17α-hydoxyprogesterone caproate administered by intramuscular injections (Table 44.38).

Only two trials provided information on the incidence of preterm labour, but they showed a statistically significant difference in favour of the active drug (Table 44.39). Although all of this effect was due to one trial (Yemini *et al.* 1985), the typical odds ratio was 0.43 with a confidence interval of 0.20 to 0.89.

As far as preterm delivery is concerned, of the 5 studies from which data are available only the study conducted in twin pregnancies (Hartikainen-Sorri *et al.* 1980) showed a higher incidence of preterm delivery with the active treatment than with placebo (Table 44.40). Taken together, the trials showed a statistically significant reduction in the incidence of preterm delivery with a typical odds ratio of 0.50 and a 95 per cent confidence interval between 0.30 and 0.85 A similar

Table 44.39 Effect of prophylactic 17α-hydroxyprogesterone caproate in pregnancy on preterm labour

Study	EXPT		CTRL		Odds ratio	Graph of odds ratios and confidence intervals
	n	(%)	*n*	(%)	(95% CI)	0.01 0.1 0.5 1 2 10 100
Hauth *et al.* (1983)	5/80	(6.25)	5/88	(5.68)	1.11 (0.31–3.96)	
Yemini *et al.* (1985)	9/39	(23.08)	22/40	(55.00)	0.27 (0.11–0.65)	
Typical odds ratio (95% confidence interval)					0.43 (0.20–0.89)	

Table 44.40 Effect of prophylactic 17α-hydroxyprogesterone caproate in pregnancy on preterm birth

Study	EXPT		CTRL		Odds ratio	Graph of odds ratios and confidence intervals
	n	(%)	*n*	(%)	(95% CI)	0.01 0.1 0.5 1 2 10 100
Papiernik (1970)	2/50	(4.00)	9/49	(18.37)	0.24 (0.07–0.82)	
Hartikainen-Sorri *et al.* (1980)	15/39	(38.46)	9/38	(23.68)	1.97 (0.76–5.15)	
Yemini *et al.* (1985)	5/39	(12.82)	14/40	(35.00)	0.30 (0.11–0.84)	
LeVine (1964)	2/15	(13.33)	3/15	(20.00)	0.63 (0.10–4.15)	
Johnson *et al.* (1975)	2/18	(11.11)	12/25	(48.00)	0.19 (0.05–0.70)	
Typical odds ratio (95% confidence interval)					0.50 (0.30–0.85)	

Table 44.41 Effect of prophylactic 17α-hydroxyprogesterone caproate in pregnancy on birth weight <2500 g

Study	EXPT		CTRL		Odds ratio	Graph of odds ratios and confidence intervals
	n	(%)	*n*	(%)	(95% CI)	0.01 0.1 0.5 1 2 10 100
Hauth *et al.* (1983)	6/80	(7.50)	8/88	(9.09)	0.81 (0.27–2.42)	
Papiernik (1970)	2/50	(4.00)	8/49	(16.33)	0.26 (0.07–0.96)	
Yemini *et al.* (1985)	5/39	(12.82)	14/40	(35.00)	0.30 (0.11–0.84)	
LeVine (1964)	3/15	(20.00)	2/15	(13.33)	1.59 (0.24–10.51)	
Johnson *et al.* (1975)	4/18	(22.22)	11/26	(42.31)	0.42 (0.12–1.46)	
Typical odds ratio (95% confidence interval)					0.46 (0.27–0.80)	

reduction was noted in the incidence of low birthweight between the active drug and placebo across trials, with a typical odds ratio of 0.46 (confidence interval 0.27–0.80; Table 44.41).

These effects on the incidence of preterm delivery and low birthweight were not accompanied by a detectable difference in the incidence of perinatal death, excluding that due to lethal malformations, between the drug and placebo groups. The typical odds ratio of 0.76 showed a confidence interval from 0.31 to 1.90 (Table 44.42). Neither was there a statistically significant difference in the incidence of respiratory distress syndrome between the drug and placebo groups. Only 2 of the trial reports provided data on this outcome and there was thus a wide confidence interval from 0.54 to 3.54 (typical odds ratio 1.39; Table 44.43).

5.2 Inhibition of active preterm labour

The first and only controlled trial of progesterone in preterm labour was reported by Fuchs and Stakemann in 1960. It is not clear how many women participated in the trial. The authors report the number to be 'approximately 150' and report data on 126 women, after excluding women who delivered elsewhere or who were still pregnant at the time of writing. These women had received either progesterone in oil or inactive oil intramuscularly in a double-blind fashion. The doses of progesterone were 200 mg daily for 3 days, 150 mg daily for 2 days, and then 100 mg per day up to a week after disappearance of the symptoms.

As shown in Table 44.44, equal numbers of women delivered within 48 hours. Equal numbers in both groups gave birth to an infant below 2500 g, which was the internationally accepted definition of 'prematurity' at that time (see Chapter 74). Data on perinatal mortality or infant outcomes were not reported, except for the fact that no virilization of infants was observed. While the treatment apparently did no good, it caused tender

Table 44.42 Effect of prophylactic 17α-hydroxyprogesterone caproate in pregnancy on perinatal death excluding malformation)

Study	EXPT		CTRL		Odds ratio	Graph of odds ratios and confidence intervals
	n	(%)	*n*	(%)	(95% CI)	0.01 0.1 0.5 1 2 10 100
Hauth *et al.* (1983)	3/80	(3.75)	3/88	(3.41)	1.10 (0.22–5.61)	
Papiernik (1970)	0/39	(0.00)	0/40	(0.00)	1.00 (1.00–1.00)	
Hartikainen-Sorri *et al.* (1980)	4/78	(5.13)	2/76	(2.63)	1.94 (0.38–9.87)	
Yemini *et al.* (1985)	0/39	(0.00)	0/40	(0.00)	1.00 (1.00–1.00)	
LeVine (1964)	1/15	(6.67)	0/15	(0.00)	7.39 (0.15–99.99)	
Johnson *et al.* (1975)	0/18	(0.00)	7/26	(26.92)	0.14 (0.03–0.71)	
Typical odds ratio (95% confidence interval)					0.76 (0.31–1.90)	

Table 44.43 Effect of prophylactic 17α-hydroxyprogesterone caproate in pregnancy on respiratory distress syndrome

Study	EXPT		CTRL		Odds ratio	Graph of odds ratios and confidence intervals
	n	(%)	*n*	(%)	(95% CI)	0.01 0.1 0.5 1 2 10 100
Hartikainen-Sorri *et al.* (1980)	10/78	(12.82)	4/76	(5.26)	2.48 (0.83–7.42)	
Yemini *et al.* (1985)	1/39	(2.56)	4/40	(10.00)	0.29 (0.05–1.75)	
Typical odds ratio (95% confidence interval)					1.39 (0.54–3.54)	

infiltrations on the injection site 'in some patients'.

More than 25 years ago it was observed that intravenous progesterone in doses up to 90 mg per hour had no demonstrable effect on uterine contractility in labour (Taubert and Haskins 1963). Nevertheless, Erny and his colleagues (1986), in two hospitals in Marseilles and Paris, treated 57 women believed to be in preterm labour, each with four identical-looking capsules containing either 100 mg oral progesterone, or placebo. This treatment resulted in a decrease in the frequency of contractions 1 hour after the treatment in 22 of 29 (76 per cent) progesterone-treated women and in 12 of 28 (43 per cent) placebo-treated women. The remaining 23 women in whom the frequency of contractions increased or remained the same were then given intravenous ritodrine. This supplementary treatment with ritodrine is stated to have 'permitted tocolysis each time', except in 4 women who had failed to respond to the 400 mg progesterone treatment. Apparently, all 4 had ruptured membranes, whereas all of the placebo-treated women had intact membranes.

The authors therefore concluded that, if they 'consider these cases as inaccessible to medical treatment and exclude them from the analysis, the percentage of efficacy with oral progesterone rises from a mean of 75.8 per cent to 88 per cent' (Erny *et al.* 1986). Applying the same criteria, however, the success rate of the betamimetic treatment would have been 100 per cent, and considerably higher than anything shown thus far.

Other outcomes in that study (Erny *et al.* 1986) cannot be interpreted. The authors suddenly refer only to the 37 women in the Marseilles' part of the trial, in which 23 women (14 progesterone- and 9 placebo-treated) in whom the contractions had decreased during the 1 hour of observation were subsequently all continued on oral progesterone treatment up to 36 weeks of gestation. The authors' conclusion that this 'oral progesterone, at least in specific galenic formulation', named Utrogestan (Table 44.1), 'permits a sufficient beneficial effect in 9 of 10 cases' is clearly unjustified.

Table 44.44 Effect of intramuscular progesterone in preterm labour on delivery within 48 hours

Study	EXPT *n*	(%)	CTRL *n*	(%)	Odds ratio (95% CI)	Graph of odds ratios and confidence intervals (0.01 0.1 0.5 1 2 10 100)
Fuchs and Stakemann (1960)	13/63	(20.63)	13/63	(20.63)	1.00 (0.42–2.36)	
Typical odds ratio (95% confidence interval)					1.00 (0.42–2.36)	

Effect of intramuscular progesterone in preterm labour on delivery within 1 week

Study	EXPT *n*	(%)	CTRL *n*	(%)	Odds ratio (95% CI)	Graph of odds ratios and confidence intervals
Fuchs and Stakemann (1960)	19/63	(30.16)	23/63	(36.51)	0.75 (0.36–1.58)	
Typical odds ratio (95% confidence interval)					0.75 (0.36–1.58)	

Effect of intramuscular progesterone in preterm labour on birthweight <2500 g.

Study	EXPT *n*	(%)	CTRL *n*	(%)	Odds ratio (95% CI)	Graph of odds ratios and confidence intervals
Fuchs and Stakemann (1960)	35/63	(55.56)	35/63	(55.56)	1.00 (0.50–2.01)	
Typical odds ratio (95% confidence interval)					1.00 (0.50–2.01)	

5.3 Conclusions

The trials on prophylaxis, discussed above, provide strong evidence that the incidence of preterm delivery and of delivery of a low birthweight infant may be reduced with regular administration of 17α-hydroxyprogesterone caproate. The one trial dealing with twin pregnancies (Hartikainen-Sorri *et al.* 1980) did not show this effect, but it is unclear whether this is due to the play of chance or to inherent differences between singleton and multiple pregnancies in this respect.

By contrast the evidence available about the effects of progesterone in active preterm labour, does not suggest that it is effective in the inhibition of uterine contractions.

6 Magnesium sulphate

Magnesium has long been recognized to have the potential to decrease uterine contractility (Hall *et al.* 1959), but it is uncertain when it was first suggested as a possible means to achieve tocolysis in preterm labour. The first report in the English language literature (Steer and Petrie 1977) was certainly preceded by reports in other languages (Dumont 1965; Kiss and Szöke 1975) and it has been reported that magnesium sulphate to arrest preterm labour has been used routinely in some centres in the United States from 1969 onwards (Petrie 1981).

The mechanism by which magnesium sulphate interferes with myometrial contractility is not known. It can suppress both spontaneous and oxytocin-induced uterine contractions (Kumar *et al.* 1963). It is almost certain that magnesium acts by substituting for calcium at the level of the myometrial cell, but how this is achieved is unknown (Carsten and Miller 1987).

6.1 Prophylaxis

Only one trial has examined whether administration of magnesium could prevent preterm labour (Spätling and Spätling 1988). The trial was initiated by Spätling, who had found that oral magnesium supplementation apparently reduced the dose of betamimetics needed for tocolysis in preterm labour (Spätling 1981). The trial also addressed several other hypotheses, including effects of magnesium supplementation on the incidence of pre-eclampsia and fetal growth. A total of 568 women were allocated to receive either 15 mmol magnesium-aspartate-hydrochloride, or 13.5 mmol aspartic acid. In an earlier publication, one of the authors (Spätling 1981) had described the trial as 'double blind', but the allocation was based on odd or even date of birth. For this and other reasons mentioned below, it is very unlikely that the investigators did not know which women were receiving magnesium. Deciding treatment allocation based on date of birth is notoriously prone to selection bias, because the type of treatment is predictable prior to formal trial entry (Keirse 1989). Furthermore, there are major worries about medically or psychologically mediated differential effects as a consequence of differences in other components of care, and about 'non-blind' assessment of outcome (see Chapter 1).

Table 44.45 Effect of magnesium supplementation in pregnancy on hospital admission during pregnancy

Study	EXPT n	EXPT (%)	CTRL n	CTRL (%)	Odds ratio (95% CI)	Graph of odds ratios and confidence intervals (0.01, 0.1, 0.5, 1, 2, 10, 100)
Spätling and Spätling (1988)	44/278	(15.83)	65/290	(22.41)	0.65 (0.43–0.99)	
Typical odds ratio (95% confidence interval)					0.65 (0.43–0.99)	

Effect of magnesium supplementation in pregnancy on hospital admission for antepartum haemorrhage

Study	EXPT n	EXPT (%)	CTRL n	CTRL (%)	Odds ratio (95% CI)	Graph
Spätling and Spätling (1988)	4/278	(1.44)	17/290	(5.86)	0.29 (0.12–0.69)	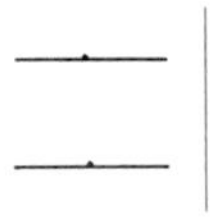
Typical odds ratio (95% confidence interval)					0.29 (0.12–0.69)	

Effect of magnesium supplementation in pregnancy on hospital admission for preterm labour

Study	EXPT n	EXPT (%)	CTRL n	CTRL (%)	Odds ratio (95% CI)	Graph
Spätling and Spätling (1988)	12/278	(4.32)	26/290	(8.97)	0.48 (0.25–0.92)	
Typical odds ratio (95% confidence interval)					0.48 (0.25–0.92)	

Effect of magnesium supplementation in pregnancy on hospital admission for incompetent cervix

Study	EXPT n	EXPT (%)	CTRL n	CTRL (%)	Odds ratio (95% CI)	Graph
Spätling and Spätling (1988)	8/278	(2.88)	17/290	(5.86)	0.49 (0.22–1.10)	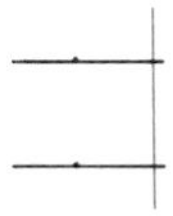
Typical odds ratio (95% confidence interval)					0.49 (0.22–1.10)	

Effect of magnesium supplementation in pregnancy on admission to special care nursery

Study	EXPT n	EXPT (%)	CTRL n	CTRL (%)	Odds ratio (95% CI)	Graph
Spätling and Spätling (1988)	20/278	(7.19)	36/290	(12.41)	0.56 (0.32–0.97)	
Typical odds ratio (95% confidence interval)					0.56 (0.32–0.97)	

Effect of magnesium supplementation in pregnancy on miscarriage

Study	EXPT n	EXPT (%)	CTRL n	CTRL (%)	Odds ratio (95% CI)	Graph
Spätling and Spätling (1988)	5/278	(1.80)	3/290	(1.03)	1.73 (0.43–6.99)	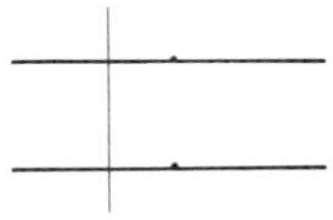
Typical odds ratio (95% confidence interval)					1.73 (0.43–6.99)	

Effect of magnesium supplementation in pregnancy on preterm delivery

Study	EXPT n	EXPT (%)	CTRL n	CTRL (%)	Odds ratio (95% CI)	Graph
Spätling and Spätling (1988)	7/278	(2.52)	14/290	(4.83)	0.52 (0.22–1.25)	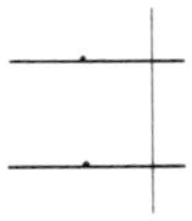
Typical odds ratio (95% confidence interval)					0.52 (0.22–1.25)	

Effect of magnesium supplementation in pregnancy on birthweight <2500 g

Study	EXPT n	EXPT (%)	CTRL n	CTRL (%)	Odds ratio (95% CI)	Graph
Spätling and Spätling (1988)	12/278	(4.32)	19/290	(6.55)	0.65 (0.31–1.34)	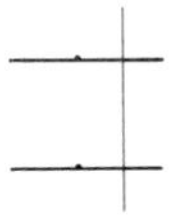
Typical odds ratio (95% confidence interval)					0.65 (0.31–1.34)	

Effect of magnesium supplementation in pregnancy on birthweight <1500 g

Study	EXPT		CTRL		Odds ratio	Graph of odds ratios and confidence intervals
	n	(%)	*n*	(%)	(95% CI)	0.01 0.1 0.5 1 2 10 100
Spätling and Spätling (1988)	3/278	(1.08)	6/290	(2.07)	0.53 (0.14–1.98)	
Typical odds ratio (95% confidence interval)					0.53 (0.14–1.98)	

The treatment was instituted as early in pregnancy as possible, but always before 16 weeks of gestation, and women were required to take 6 tablets a day. The results of the trial suggest a statistically significant reduction in the incidence of preterm labour, but this was defined as '*hospitalization* for preterm labour'. Various other outcomes that might have been influenced by the caregivers' knowledge of the type of treatment given, also occurred less frequently in the magnesium-treated group (Table 44.45). Among these were hospitalizations for 'incompetent cervix'. As many as 4.4 per cent of this 'unselected' group of women were hospitalized for that reason. It is interesting to note that one of the authors had, in a previous publication, referred to his belief that magnesium supplementation might prevent cervical incompetence (Spätling 1981).

No statistically significant differences were observed in any of the outcomes (such as the incidence of preterm delivery or of delivery of a low birthweight infant) that are less likely to be influenced by prior knowledge of treatment allocation (Table 44.45), although they tend to favour the supplemented group. Such outcomes can, of course, still be influenced by the incidence of elective preterm delivery in both groups, but these data are not available in the report. The authors did report, however, that after excluding women 'who did not take their tablets regularly', significant differences at the 5 per cent level appeared in birthweights below 2500 and below 1500 g, in infants' length and head circumference, in 10 minutes' Apgar scores, and in oedema graded as 1+. The median length of gestation was also reported to be statistically significantly longer in women who had received magnesium, but the difference between these medians consisted of 1 day.

6.2 Inhibition of active preterm labour

No placebo-controlled trials of magnesium sulphate in preterm labour have been reported. Four controlled trials have compared this drug with an alternative tocolytic agent in preterm labour, however. One of these, which has been discussed above, compared magnesium sulphate with ethanol (Steer and Petrie 1977). Two others compared magnesium sulphate with a betamimetic agent, either ritodrine (Tchilinguirian *et al.* 1984) or terbutaline (Parsons *et al.* 1987). The fourth, conducted by Ferguson *et al.* (1984), compared a combination of magnesium sulphate and ritodrine with a treatment consisting of ritodrine alone.

Parsons *et al.* (1987) randomly allocated 72 women to intravenous terbutaline or magnesium sulphate. They reported that women receiving magnesium sulphate were more likely to experience hypothermia. This difference was statistically significant, but 20 women had been excluded after randomization, and no other outcomes were reported. Tchilinguirian *et al.* (1984) randomly assigned 48 women with intact membranes and 19 women with ruptured membranes to either ritodrine or magnesium sulphate. The method of randomization is not mentioned; and oral ritodrine was used for maintenance treatment in both groups. The authors reported both treatments to be equally effective in that there were no statistically significant differences in either the failure rate (defined as 'inability to control labour for at least 24 hours'), or in long term success (defined as labour suppressed for more than 7 days). Data were not reported on the incidence of preterm delivery or on infant outcomes.

Ferguson *et al.* (1984) compared a combination of magnesium sulphate and ritodrine with a treatment consisting of ritodrine alone in a trial, which was designed to investigate the influence of various intravenous solutions as well. Fifty women were randomized to 6 different groups: two drug treatments and three different intravenous solutions. Nine of these women (18 per cent) were subsequently excluded from the analysis. The data thus refer to 41 women in 6 different groups, which contain from 3 to 11 women each. Despite the 18 per cent exclusions after randomization and the small groups, two conclusions can be drawn from this study. First, the combination of ritodrine and magnesium sulphate resulted in a higher incidence of serious side effects than ritodrine alone. Treatment was discontinued because of severe side-effects in 11 of 24 women (46 per cent) assigned to the combined therapy, but in only 1 of 17 (6 per cent) assigned to ritodrine alone. These side-effects included an adult respiratory distress syndrome in 1 woman receiving the combined treatment, and chest pain in the remaining 11 women, 7 of whom had electrocardiographic changes 'consisting chiefly of pathologic ST segment depression' (Ferguson *et al.* 1984). Even if we assume that all excluded women in receipt of the combined therapy were free of side-effects and that all those excluded from the ritodrine group had side-effects, the difference would become 11 of 28 (39 per cent) vs. 6 of 22 (27 per cent) and would still favour treatment with the single agent. Second, the combination therapy was less likely to delay delivery for more than 48 hours than ritodrine alone. This may in part have related to the more frequent discontinuation of treatment (because of side-effects) in the combined treatment group, or to the fact that further treatment after discontinuation consisted not of ritodrine alone but of magnesium sulphate alone.

There is little other evidence on the use of magnesium sulphate in preterm labour (Petrie 1981; Spisso *et al.* 1982). Kiss and Szöke (1975), who were among the first to report on this treatment for preterm labour, referred to a closed cervix as one of the criteria for instituting treatment. In the trial of Steer and Petrie (1977), 22 of the 24 successes (defined as arrest of contractions for one day) were in women with no more than 1 cm cervical dilatation. In an uncontrolled observational series reported by Spisso *et al.* (1982), only 14 of 38 women (37 per cent) with intact membranes and a cervical dilatation of 2 cm or more had delivery delayed for at least 48 hours. The authors considered magnesium sulphate to be an 'effective tocolytic agent' offering 'comparable success' to other agents (Spisso *et al.* 1982). Even advocates of the drug, however, admit that 'once labor has brought about cervical dilatation, the drug is reasonably ineffective' (Petrie 1981).

6.3 Unwanted effects

Pulmonary oedema has been reported in association with magnesium sulphate and corticosteroid administration in preterm labour (Elliott *et al.* 1979; Morales *et al.* 1986). Goodlin (1980), who reported on this complication in relation to the use of magnesium sulphate for treatment of hypertension in pregnancy (see Chapter 33), suggested that it bears more resemblance to the adult respiratory distress syndrome than to typical pulmonary oedema. Magnesium is primarily excreted by the kidney. Hypermagnesaemia can occur if renal function is impaired. This may lead to impaired reflexes, respiratory depression, alteration in myocardial conduction, cardiac arrest and death (Caritis *et al.* 1979). Regular examination of the knee-jerk reflex is said to offer protection against such complications, since these reflexes disappear at less elevated magnesium levels than those that cause respiratory depression and cardiac conduction defects (Caritis *et al.* 1979; Petrie 1981).

Magnesium levels in the fetus closely parallel those in the mother (Lipsitz 1971). Infants born during or shortly after treatment are reported to be drowsy; they have reduced muscle tone, low calcium levels, and may need 3 or 4 days to eliminate the excess magnesium (Petrie 1981).

6.4 Conclusions

The only trial on the prophylactic use of magnesium offers no clear-cut evidence for a beneficial effect of magnesium supplementation. The observed differences between the groups may well reflect selection bias, co-intervention bias, assessment bias, or a combination of all three. A better-designed trial, free of such bias, is needed to clarify whether the suggested benefits are real before magnesium supplementation is introduced into clinical practice.

The available evidence about the effects of the drug for 'preterm labour' suggests, first, that magnesium sulphate may be efficacious for arresting uterine contractions in women who are not actually in preterm labour, and, second, that the drug can have serious side-effects. Where it is still in use for the inhibition of preterm labour, it should be phased out. If this were to occur in the context of a well-designed and well-reported placebo-controlled trial, later generations of women and babies might be saved from a 'rediscovery' of this treatment on the basis of observational associations. This and the tiny chance that it might still do more good than harm in active preterm labor, would seem to be a justification for such a trial in centres where the treatment is currently being used.

7 Calcium antagonists

All agents that cause relaxation of the uterus ultimately do so by lowering the concentration of free calcium available to the contractile proteins in the myometrial cell. This can be accomplished in many ways that are not, as was once thought, mutually exclusive (Huszar and Roberts 1982; Carsten and Miller 1987). Basically, however, there are two mechanisms to regulate the intracellular availability of free calcium. One consists of regulating the influx of calcium ions through the cell membrane; the other relates to the uptake and release of calcium from the sarcoplasmic reticulum.

Some agents have been found to achieve a direct block of entry of calcium into the cell. They are called 'calcium channel blockers', 'calcium entry blockers', or simply 'calcium antagonists'. They include a wide range of different, and apparently unrelated compounds such as diltiazeme, fendiline, nicardipine, nifedipine, nitrendipine, perhexiline, prenylamine, terodiline, verapamil, and compound D600. Like the betamimetic drugs, some of these agents are known under a variety of different names. For example, verapamil is also known as iproveratril and under the trade name Isoptin (Fleckenstein *et al.* 1971). Some of these drugs, verapamil and nifedipine in particular, have been used for some years in the treatment of ischaemic heart disease and arterial hypertension (Pedersen and Mikkilsen 1978; Forman 1984), and have also been used for the treatment of hypertension in pregnancy (see Chapter 33).

The first report on the use of one of these agents in preterm labour apparently dates from 1972 (Mosler and Rosenboom 1972). The drug used was verapamil and no definite effects were registered, because the dosage had to be limited due to impairment of atrioventricular conduction in the heart. Instead of being applied to achieve tocolysis, it was soon being used for so-named 'cardioprotection' during treatment with betamimetic drugs (see Section 2.3.4). As nifedipine has less effect on atrioventricular conduction, it has been applied to the inhibition of preterm labour (Andersson 1977; Ulmsten *et al.* 1980).

Apart from trials in which calcium antagonists were used mainly to supplement tocolytic treatment with betamimetic drugs, there has been only one other trial on the use of one of these agents in preterm labour. Read and Welby (1986) randomly allocated 40 women to treatment with nifedipine or intravenous ritodrine and concluded that 'nifedipine was considerably more successful in halting labour than ritodrine'. The method of randomization was not described; a 'control' group of 20 women who received no treatment was added for comparison with the 20 nifedipine- and 20 ritodrine-treated women; and women in whom nifedipine 'was deemed to have failed' received intravenous ritodrine. This occurred in 5 (25 per cent) of the 20 nifedipine-treated women; none of the women in whom ritodrine failed were given nifedipine. The study appears to have been conducted in two cities. The authors stated that, when contractions recurred after completion of the course of treatment, 'the case was discussed with the appropriate consultant as to whether further treatment was to be given', but they also added that 'in this series no additional treatment was considered necessary'. All of this casts some doubt on the absence of selection bias. The description of side-effects does not suggest that assessment bias can be ruled out either. The authors (Read and Welby 1986) reported that 'troublesome side-effects were common with ritodrine therapy, and 13 women complained of palpitations and feelings of anxiety. In women receiving nifedipine, some 90 per cent experienced flushing, mainly of the face, neck, and chest but this was troublesome in only one woman, and one other woman experienced marked nausea.' They summarize their findings, however, by saying that 'nifedipine was found to be significantly more effective ... and was almost devoid of side-effects'. Nifedipine may have been devoid of side-effects, 90 per cent of the women apparently were not.

Thus far, there are not enough data on any of these agents to justify their use outside the context of well-designed and carefully monitored randomized trials.

8 Other drug treatments

8.1 Diazoxide

Diazoxide is a powerful antihypertensive agent. Its use in women in labour was found to be associated with a marked inhibition of uterine contractions and it was thus applied to the treatment of preterm labour (Barden and Keenan 1971). Structurally it is related to the thiazide diuretics, but it has no diuretic effects and instead reduces urinary output (Caritis *et al.* 1979). Its effects on the uterus are thought to be mediated in the same way as for the betamimetic drugs, through the adenyl cyclase system (Adamsons and Wallach 1984). In fact, it shares a large number of the properties of the betamimetic drugs both on the cardiovascular system (decreased peripheral resistance, increased heart rate and increased cardiac output) and in increasing glycaemia. It is thus non-selective in its action.

No controlled trials of this drug in preterm labour have been reported, although it is said to be the principal tocolytic agent in at least a few centres in North America (Adamsons and Wallach 1984). Adamsons and Wallach (1984) reported to have been 'randomizing cases between diazoxide and β-adrenergic agents', but to have found it difficult to justify continuation of that study because 'their experience with diazoxide over a period of more than 5 years has been so satisfactory' (Adamsons and Wallach 1984). No data nor results of that randomized experience were reported, however.

Also observational data on the use of this drug in preterm labour are few and not particularly encouraging. Barden and Keenan (1971) reported, in a meeting abstract, its use in 15 women in spontaneous preterm labour. They stated that diazoxide is 'an effective inhibitor of uterine motility', but no outcomes were reported. Adamsons and Wallach (1984) concluded that 'the potency of the drug compares favorably with that of other agents used to inhibit uterine activity'. They 'found diazoxide to be an effective and safe tocolytic agent with negligible side effects'. Yet, their account of their initial series of 118 women, who received this treatment, includes 3 cases of 'transient' pulmonary oedema (2.5 per cent). They further reported on 2 hypertensive women in whom the administration of diazoxide to arrest preterm labour was associated with partial separation of the placenta, and on the occurrence of hyperglycaemia in infants born shortly after treatment.

The available evidence does not justify the use of diazoxide for the inhibition of preterm labour.

8.2 Antimicrobial agents

There have been numerous suggestions that subclinical infection and bacterial colonization are important causes of preterm labour with or without prior rupture of the membranes (Minkoff 1983; Harvey *et al.* 1985; McGregor 1988; see also Chapter 34). A wealth of data in support of these suggestions has, for many years, been described in various epidemiological, microbiological, and histological associations between preterm birth and reproductive tract infections (McGregor 1988). In recent years, these have been supplemented with experimental data on pathogenetic mechanisms, by which microbial factors could lead to preterm uterine activity (McGregor 1988). This has led some to explore whether antimicrobial treatment would be effective in delaying delivery in women in preterm labour.

McGregor and his associates (McGregor *et al.* 1986) conducted a placebo-controlled trial in which enteric-coated erythromycin was given orally for 7 days to women who were in preterm labour before 34 weeks of gestation, and who also were being treated with terbutaline or magnesium sulphate. From their trial the authors concluded that the addition of erythromycin to their standard tocolytic treatment resulted in a greater prolongation of pregnancy and a lower rate of preterm delivery. They also observed, however, that these beneficial effects occurred only in women with cervical dilatation at the beginning of treatment and not in all women (McGregor *et al.* 1986).

These conclusions were based on a subanalysis of no more than 17 (29 per cent) of the 58 women entered into trial. These 17 were obtained as follows. First, the authors excluded 21 (36 per cent) of the 58 women for various reasons. Among the remaining 37 women, they then selected those 17 whose cervix was at least 1 cm dilated on admission. Moreover, from the long list of parameters assessed in these women, it would appear that some of them also received oral terbutaline for many days. It is not clear how many of them received that treatment nor whether they were in receipt of erythromycin or placebo.

The potential for bias in the selection of the subgroup that apparently benefited from the erythromycin treatment is so large that this study (McGregor *et al.* 1986) can only be seen as hypothesis-generating. In provides no clear evidence on potential harm or benefit of the treatment, particularly since, as the authors themselves pointed out, there were no differences in outcome between erythromycin or placebo treatment in the total group of women.

8.3 Relaxin

In 1955, Abramson and Reid reported the first experience with relaxin administered in various doses to 5 women in threatened preterm labour. In all 5 women they were able to control the uterine contractions and to prolong pregnancy to 36 weeks or longer. As Decker and his associates pointed out in 1958, 'this study had two obvious defects, too few cases and no controls'; but it aroused interest in the potential of this hormone for preventing preterm birth.

McCarthy *et al.* (1957) alternately allocated 15 women to intravenous relaxin, followed by maintenance doses given intramuscularly 'at periodic intervals' for 48 to 72 hours after labour had ceased, and 15 women to the standard treatment, which at their institution consisted of 'innumerable hormone and analgesic agents in various amounts at the discretion of the attending physician'. Delivery was postponed for more than a week in 8 of the relaxin-treated women (53 per cent) and in only 1 of the control women (7 per cent). Prolongation of pregnancy until the babies attained a weight of 2500 g or more at birth was achieved in 4 women in the relaxin-treated (27 per cent) and in 2 in the control group (13 per cent). There were 5 perinatal deaths in the relaxin-treated group and 6 in the control group. Whether the difference in delaying delivery was due to selection bias, to a relaxin effect, to the 2-hourly administration of 50 mg meperidine (pethidine), that the relaxin-treated women were allowed to receive 'if necessary', or to harmful effects of the 'innumerable hormone and analgesic agents' administered to the control group at the discretion of the physician, is impossible to tell.

One year later, Decker *et al.* (1958) reported a trial in which women, who were believed to be in preterm labour, received either relaxin intramuscularly and intravenously in doses ranging from 20 to 1000 mg, or the standard treatment, usually sedation and bed rest, depending on the day of admission to hospital. Labour was 'uninfluenced' by the treatment in 31 of 37 relaxin-treated women (84 per cent) and in 31 of 32 control women (97 per cent). Thirty-three women in the relaxin-treated (89 per cent) and 31 in the control group (97 per cent) delivered preterm. The authors concluded that the effect of relaxin 'is probably infrequent and inconsistent' and that 'the only effect demonstrable is a reflection of the vagaries of a motile uterus in the later stages of pregnancy' (Decker *et al.* 1958).

8.4 Oxytocin analogues

Some 30 years later, the introduction of new labour-inhibiting drugs still appears to follow the pattern set by relaxin in the 1950s: 'too few cases and no controls' (Decker *et al.* 1958).

Recently, Akerlund and his colleagues (1987) reported on the use of an oxytocin analogue, 1-de-amino-2-D-Tyr-(OEt)-4-Thr-8-Orn-oxytocin, which blocks uterine contractility, apparently through competitive binding to oxytocin receptors (Akerlund *et al.* 1985; Melin *et al.* 1986). The study contained no controls and the authors stated that 'only open trials and only one infusion session of limited size and duration per patient were permitted' (Akerlund *et al.* 1987). They reported an inhibition of uterine activity in every one of a total of 13 women treated in two different countries. Ten of the 13 women received subsequent treatment with betamimetics; 7 of them had additional treatment with terbutaline and the 3 others received 'prophylactic' oral ritodrine treatment. Despite the apparent 'success' of the oxytocin analogue (Table 44.1) and the additional betamimetic drug treatment, at least 3 women (23 per cent) delivered preterm; of the remaining 10 (77 per cent), it is only known that pregnancy proceeded to at least 36 weeks of gestation. No infant outcomes for any of the babies whose mothers had been treated are reported. An editorial commentary in the journal in which the study was published rightly pointed out that without controls such results cannot be interpreted, and that for all we know 'treatment might have had no effect at all' (Turnbull 1987).

Nevertheless, there is some rationale for the use of oxytocin receptor blockers in the treatment of preterm labour. Fuchs and her colleagues (1982) have shown that labour at term is associated with an increase in myometrial oxytocin receptors and that preterm labour is associated with an oxytocin receptor concentration in the myometrium which is as high as that found in early term labour (Fuchs *et al.* 1984). It remains to be seen, however, whether agents that block these receptors will, on the one hand, arrest preterm labour and, on the other, be as selective and as free of undesirable side-effects as Akerlund *et al.* (1987) have claimed. It would be deplorable if further studies were to be conducted without appropriate controls and without data on infant outcomes.

9 Conclusions

9.1 Implications for current practice

There is currently no evidence that the prophylactic use of oral betamimetic agents does more good than harm. Because long term treatment with these agents cannot be assumed to be free from adverse effects on the baby, they should currently not be used outside the context of controlled trials. There is some evidence, however, that oral maintenance treatment after inhibition of active preterm labour reduces the frequency of recurrent preterm labour. In as much as maintenance treatment is able to prevent recurrences of hospitalization and intravenous treatment with betamimetic agents, it would seem to have some merit.

At present, only two categories of drugs merit consideration for the inhibition of preterm labour: betamimetic agents and inhibitors of prostaglandin synthesis. All the others are either obsolete or in an experimental stage. There is no longer a place for ethanol, relaxin, or progesterone in the treatment of preterm labour. Oxytocin analogues and calcium antagonists have been insufficiently studied to assess whether they have any beneficial effect. Other drugs, such as magnesium sulphate or diazoxide, should not be used in attempts to inhibit preterm labour. Their use should, if at all, be permitted only within the context of adequately controlled trials to determine whether their claimed benefits both exist and outweigh their known adverse effects.

This does not imply that the evidence in favour of either the betamimetic agents or the inhibitors of prostaglandin synthesis is beyond reproach. On the contrary, there are many flaws in the evidence available, particularly with regard to prostaglandin synthesis inhibitors. Among these two categories of drugs, there are many compounds with widely different effects. This applies more to prostaglandin synthesis inhibitors than to the betamimetic drugs, but the basic recommendations are the same. It is worth remembering that there are, in these wide classes of agents, drugs that have never been evaluated against 'placebo treatment' in preterm labour, have never been shown to be superior to other, more validated drug treatments, and, yet, have caused serious complications including maternal death. Specific agents that have never been tested against placebo (or no treatment), or have not been shown conclusively to be superior to others, should be dropped from clinical practice. The only acceptable alternative would be to subject their use to properly controlled experimentation, involving both adequate methodology and a sufficiently large number of women. There is something to be said for firmly convincing the pharmaceutical companies that propagate such agents that uncontrolled exploitation of women in preterm labour is no longer on.

Both betamimetics and prostaglandin synthesis inhibitors are effective in postponing delivery. There is no evidence that the use of these drugs, *per se*, reduces infant morbidity. They are useful, however, when the time that is gained before delivery is used to implement effective measures. Such measures could include transfer of the mother to a centre with adequate facilities for intensive perinatal and neonatal care, the administration of corticosteroids to reduce perinatal mortality and morbidity, or judicious use of 'expectant management' in the period of gestation in which the infant's chances of intact survival are very poor.

Treatment with these powerful drugs may be dangerous for the mother and can occasionally result in maternal death. As far as betamimetics are concerned, the potential benefit weighed against the risk of adverse effects does not justify their use in women with cardiac disease, hyperthyroidism, or diabetes. If labour needs to be inhibited in these women, prostaglandin synthesis inhibitors are the logical choice. In all other women, betamimetic drugs are currently the drugs of choice, since the available data on prostaglandin synthesis inhibitors are not yet sufficient.

On the whole, prostaglandin synthesis inhibitors are more powerful inhibitors of uterine contractions than the betamimetic agents. Nevertheless, there are too few data from controlled comparisons, either with no treatment or with other drug treatments, to recommend prostaglandin synthesis inhibitors as a first-line approach in the inhibition of preterm labour. Their potential hazards, weighed against potential benefits, do not justify the use of these agents in the doses that are necessary to inhibit uterine contractions for any longer than is necessary (2 or 3 days). The available evidence does not justify the use of aspirin and other salicylates (in the large doses that are required) for inhibition of preterm labour.

9.2 Implications for future research

There is an indication from placebo-controlled trials that regular intramuscular injections of 17α-hydroxyprogesterone caproate may reduce the incidence of preterm labour and preterm delivery in women considered to be at high risk of preterm labour. Thus far, these effects have not been accompanied by a detectable decrease in either perinatal mortality or morbidity. The findings are encouraging enough, however, to warrant further study. It would probably be useful if further studies would be directed at evaluating a form of administration that does not require intramuscular administration.

The placebo-controlled trials of tocolytic agents in active preterm labour have clearly demonstrated that many women treated with labour-inhibiting drugs do not require such treatment. The trials have also demonstrated that, in many other women, these drugs are ineffective in delaying delivery to a clinically significant extent. Future research should focus on methods of distinguishing more clearly these two categories of women, so that women need not be exposed to treatments which are unlikely to benefit them or their babies.

References

Abramovici H, Lewin A, Lissak A, Palant A (1980). Maternal pulmonary edema occurring after therapy with ritodrine for premature uterine contractions. Acta Obstet Gynecol Scand, 59: 555.

Abramson D, Reid DE (1955). Use of relaxin in treatment of threatened premature labor. J Clin Endocrinol, 15: 206–209.

Adam GS (1966). Isoxuprine and premature labour. Austral NZ J Obstet Gynaecol, 6: 294–298.

Adamsons K, Wallach RC (1984). Diazoxide and calcium antagonists in preterm labor. In: Preterm Birth: Causes, Prevention and Management. Fuchs F, Stubblefield PG (eds). New York: Macmillan, pp 249–263.

Agustsson P, Patel NB (1987). The predictive value of fetal breathing movements in the diagnosis of preterm labour. Br J Obstet Gynaecol, 94: 860–863.

Akerlund M, Carlsson AM, Melin P, Trojnar J (1985). The effect on the human uterus of two newly developed competitive inhibitors of oxytocin and vasopressin. Acta Obstet Gynecol, 64: 499–504.

Akerlund M, Strömberg P, Hauksson A, Andersen LF, Lyndrup J, Trojnar J, Melin P (1987). Inhibition of uterine contractions of premature labour with an oxytocin analogue. Results from a pilot study. Br J Obstet Gynaecol, 94: 1040–1044.

Alvan G, Orme M, Bertillson L, Strand REK, Palmèr L (1975). Pharmacokinetics of indomethacin. Clin Pharmacol Ther, 18: 364–373.

Anderson ABM, Turnbull AC (1969). Relationship between length of gestation and cervical dilatation, uterine contractility and other factors during pregnancy. Am J Obstet Gynecol, 105: 1207–1214.

Andersson KE (1977). Inhibition of uterine activity by the calcium antagonist nifedipine. In: Pre-term Labour. Proceedings of the Fifth Study Group of the Royal College of Obstetricians and Gynaecologists. Anderson A, Beard R, Brudenell JM, Dunn PM (eds). London: Royal College of Obstetricians and Gynaecologists, pp 101–114.

Arcilla RA, Thilenius OG, Ranniger K (1969). Congestive heart failure from suspected ductal closure *in utero*. J Pediatr, 75: 74–78.

Babenerd J, Flehr I (1979). Mütterliche Zwischenfalle unter der Tokolyse mit Fenoterol. Med Welt, 30: 537–541.

Baillie P, Meehan FP, Tyack AJ (1970). Treatment of premature labor with orciprenaline. Br Med J, 4: 154–155.

Barden TP (1971). Inhibition of human premature labor by mesuprine hydrochloride. Obstet Gynecol, 37: 98–105.

Barden TP (unpublished). Unpublished data included in the reports of Merkatz *et al.* (1980) and King *et al.* (1988).

Barden TP, Keenan WJ (1971). Effects of diazoxide in human labor and the fetus-neonate. Obstet Gynecol, 37: 631–632.

Barden TP, Peter JB, Merkatz IR (1980). Ritodrine hydrochloride: a betamimetic agent for use in preterm labor. I. Pharmacology, clinical history, administration, side effects, and safety. Obstet Gynecol, 56: 1–6.

Beall MH, Edgar BW, Paul RH, Smith-Wallace T (1985). A comparison of ritodrine, terbutaline, and magnesium sulfate for the suppression of preterm labor. Am J Obstet Gynecol, 153: 854–859.

Belinkoff S, Hall OW (1950). Alcohol during labor. Am J Obstet Gynecol, 59: 429–432.

Bell R (1983). The prediction of preterm labour by recording spontaneous antenatal uterine activity. Br J Obstet Gynaecol, 90: 884–887.

Bender HG, Goeckenjan G, Meger C, Müntefering H (1977). Zum mutterlichen Risiko der medikamentösen Tokolyse mit Fenoterol (Partusisten). Geburtshilfe Frauenheilk, 37: 665–674.

Benedetti TJ (1983). Maternal complications of parenteral β-sympathomimetic therapy for premature labor. Am J Obstet Gynecol, 145: 1–6.

Benedetti T, Hardgrove J, Rosene K (1982). Maternal pulmonary edema during premature labor inhibition. Obstet Gynecol, 59: 33S-37S.

Betkerur MV, Yeh TF, Miller K, Glasser RJ, Pildes RS (1981). Indomethacin and its effect on renal function and urinary kallikrein excretion in premature infants with patent ductus arteriosus. Pediatrics, 68: 99–102.

Bieniarz J (unpublished). Unpublished data included in the reports of Merkatz *et al.* (1980) and King *et al.* (1988).

Bieniarz J, Ivankovich A, Scommegna A (1974). Cardiac output during ritodrine treatment in premature labor. Am J Obstet Gynecol, 118: 910–919.

Bigby MAM, Barnard EE, Chatterji S (1969). A clinical trial of isoxsuprine in the treatment of threatened abortion. J Obstet Gynaecol Br Commnwlth, 76: 934–935.

Bishop EH, Woutersz TB (1961). Isoxsuprine, a myometrial relaxant—a preliminary report. Obstet Gynecol, 17: 442–446.

Blake DA, Niebyl JR, White RD, Kumor KM, Dubin NH, Robinson JC, Egner EG (1980). Treatment of premature labor with indomethacin. Adv Prostaglandin Thromboxane Res, 8: 1466–1467.

Brazy JE, Little V, Grimm J (1981). Isoxsuprine in the perinatal period. II. Relationships between neonatal symptoms, drug exposure and drug concentrations at birth. J Pediatr, 98: 146–151.

Bréart G, Sureau C, Rumeau-Rouquette C (1979). Etude de l'efficacité comparée de l'ifenprodil et de la ritodrine pour le traitement de la menace d'accouchement prématuré. J Gynécol Obstét Biol Réprod, 8: 261–263.

Bréart G, Goujard J, Blondel B, Maillard F, Chavigny C, Sureau C, Rumeau-Rouquette C (1981). A comparison of two policies of antenatal supervision for the prevention of prematurity. Int J Epidemiol, 10: 241–244.

Brettes JP, Renaud R, Gandar R (1976). A double-blind investigation into the effects of ritodrine on uterine blood flow during the third trimester of pregnancy. Am J Obstet Gynecol, 124: 164–168.

Briscoe CC (1966). Failure of oral isoxsuprine to prevent prematurity. Am J Obstet Gynecol, 95: 885–886.

British Medical Journal (1979). Leading article: Drugs in threatened preterm labour. Br Med J, 1: 71.

Brown SM, Tejani NA (1981). Terbutaline sulfate in the prevention of recurrence of premature labor. Obstet Gynecol, 57: 22–25.

Calder AA, Patel NB (1985). Are betamimetics worthwhile in preterm labour? In: Pre-term Labour and Its Consequences. Proceedings of the Thirteenth Study Group of the Royal College of Obstetricians and Gynaecologists. Beard RW, Sharp F (eds). London: Royal College of Obstetricians and Gynaecologists, pp 209–218.

Caldwell G, Scougall I, Boddy K, Toft AD (1987). Fasting hyperinsulinemic hypoglycemia after ritodrine therapy for premature labor. Obstet Gynecol, 70: 478–480.

Campbell DM, MacGillivray I (1977). Maternal physiological responses and birthweight in singleton and twin pregnancies by parity. Eur J Obstet Gynecol Reprod Biol, 7: 17–24.

Cantor B, Tyler T, Nelson RM, Stein GH (1980). Oligohydramnios and transient neonatal anuria. A possible association with the maternal use of prostaglandin synthetase inhibitors. J Reprod Med, 24: 220–223.

Caritis SN, Edelstone DI, Mueller-Heubach E (1979). Pharmacologic inhibition of preterm labor. Am J Obstet Gynecol, 133: 557–578.

Caritis SN, Carson D, Greebon D, McCormick M, Edelstone DI, Mueller-Heubach E (1982). A comparison of terbutaline and ethanol in the treatment of preterm labor. Am J Obstet Gynecol, 142: 183–190.

Caritis SN, Lin LS, Toig G, Wong LK (1983). Pharmacodynamics of ritodrine in pregnant women during preterm labor. Am J Obstet Gynecol, 147: 752–759.

Caritis SN, Toig G, Heddinger LA, Ashmead G (1984). A double-blind study comparing ritodrine and terbutaline in the treatment of preterm labor. Am J Obstet Gynecol, 150: 7–14.

Carsten ME, Miller JD (1987). A new look at uterine muscle contraction. Am J Obstet Gynecol, 157: 1303–1315.

Castle BM, Turnbull AC (1983). The presence or absence of fetal breathing movements predicts the outcome of preterm labour. Lancet, 2: 471–473.

Castrén O, Gummerus M, Saarikoski S (1975). Treatment of imminent premature labour. A comparison between the effects of nylidrin chloride and isoxuprine chloride as well as of ethanol. Acta Obstet Gynecol Scand, 54: 95–100.

Cetrulo CL, Freeman RK (1976). Ritodrine HCL for the prevention of premature labor in twin pregnancies. Acta Genet Med Gemellol, 25: 321–324.

Christensen KK, Ingemarsson I, Leideman T, Solum H, Svenningsen N (1980). Effect of ritodrine on labor after premature rupture of the membranes. Obstet Gynecol, 55: 187–190.

Collins E, Turner G (1975). Maternal effects of regular salicylate ingestion in pregnancy. Lancet, 2: 335–338.

Cotton DB, Strassner HT, Hill LM, Schifrin BS, Paul RH

(1984). Comparison of magnesium sulfate, terbutaline and a placebo for inhibition of preterm labor. A randomized study. J Reprod Med, 29: 92–97.

Cousins LM, Hobel CJ, Chang RJ, Okada DM, Marshall JR (1977). Serum progesterone and estradiol-17-beta levels in premature and term labor. Am J Obstet Gynecol, 127: 612–615.

Creasy RK, Golbus MS, Laros RK, Parer JT, Roberts JM (1980). Oral ritodrine maintenance in the treatment of preterm labor. Am J Obstet Gynecol, 137: 212–219.

Csaba IF, Sulyok E, Ertl T (1978). Relationship of maternal treatment with indomethacin to persistence of fetal circulation syndrome. J Pediatr, 92: 484.

Csapo AI, Herczeg J (1977). Arrest of premature labor by isoxsuprine. Am J Obstet Gynecol, 129: 482–491.

Das R (1969). Isoxsuprine in premature labour. J Obstet Gynaecol India, 566–570.

Daubert JC, Gosse P, Rio M, Grall JY, Bourdonnec C, Pony JC, Gouffault J (1978). Myocardiopathies en cours de grossesse. Rôle possible des bêtamimétiques. Arch Mal Coeur, 71: 1283–1290.

Davies AE, Robertson MJS (1980). Pulmonary oedema after the administration of intravenous salbutamol and ergometrine. Case report. Br J Obstet Gynaecol, 87: 539–541.

De Swiet M (1980). The cardiovascular system. In: Clinical Physiology in Pregnancy. Hytten FE, Chamberlain G (eds). Oxford: Blackwell Scientific Publications, pp 3–42.

De Wit W, Van Mourik I, Wiesenhaan P (1988). Prolonged maternal indomethacin therapy associated with oligohydramnios. Case reports. Br J Obstet Gynaecol, 95: 303–305.

Decker WH, Thwaite W, Bordat S, Kayser R, Harami T, Campbell J (1958). Some effects of relaxin in obstetrics. Obstet Gynecol 12: 37–46.

Dhainaut J, Boutonnet G, Weber S, Degeorges M (1978). Responsabilité des bêta-2-mimétiques dans la genèse d'une cardiomyopathie du postpartum. Nouv Presse Méd, 7: 4058.

Dornhöfer W, Mosler KH (1975). Prostaglandine und β-Stimulatoren. In: Th 1165a (Partusisten) bei der Behandlung in der Geburtshilfe und Perinatologie. Jung H, Klöck FK (eds). Stuttgart: Georg Thieme, pp 196–202.

Dumont MM (1965). Traitement des douleurs utérines gravidiques par le lactate de magnésium. Lyon Méd, 213: 1571–1582.

Dunlop PDM, Crowley PA, Lamont RF, Hawkins DF (1986). Preterm ruptured membranes, no contractions. J Obstet Gynaecol, 7: 92–96.

Edelstein H, Baillie P (1972). The use of fenoterol (Berotec) as compared with orciprenaline (Alupent) in the treatment of premature labour. A comparative study. Med Proc, 18: 92–96.

Elliott HR, Abdulla U, Hayes PJ (1978). Pulmonary oedema associated with ritodrine infusion and betamethasone administration in premature labour. Br Med J, 2: 799–800.

Elliott JP, O'Keeffe DF, Greenberg P, Freeman RK (1979). Pulmonary edema associated with magnesium sulphate and betamethasone administration. Am J Obstet Gynecol, 134: 717–719.

Epstein MF, Nicholls E, Stubblefield PG (1979). Neonatal hypoglycemia after betasympathomimetic tocolytic therapy. J Pediatr, 94: 449–453.

Erny R, Pigne A, Prouvost C, Gamerre M, Malet C, Serment H, Barrat J (1986). The effects of oral administration of progesterone for premature labor. Am J Obstet Gynecol, 154: 525–529.

Eskes TKAB, Essed GGM (1979). Inhibition of uterine contractility with β-mimetic drugs. In: Human Parturition. Keirse MJNC, Anderson ABM, Bennebroek Gravenhorst J (eds). The Hague: Leiden University Press, pp 165–187.

Eskes TKAB, Kornman JJCM, Bots RSGM, Hein PR, Gimbrère JSF, Vonk JTC (1980). Maternal morbidity due to beta-adrenergic therapy. Pre-existing cardiomyopathy aggravated by fenoterol. Eur J Obstet Gynecol Reprod Biol, 10: 41–44.

Essed GGM, Eskes TKAB, Jongsma HW (1978). A randomized trial of two beta-mimetic drugs for the treatment of threatening early labor. Clinical results in a prospective comparative study with ritodrine and fenoterol. Eur J Obstet Gynecol Reprod Biol, 8: 341–348.

Fendel H, Drabe-Eikmann M, Meyer J, Jung H (1982). The time-relationship of the effect of Verapamil on the cardiac side-effects of intravenous tocolytic therapy with fenoterol. In: Beta-mimetic Drugs in Obstetrics and Perinatology. Jung H, Lamberti G (eds). Stuttgart: Georg Thieme, pp 148–150.

Ferguson JE, Hensleigh PA, Kredenster D (1984). Adjunctive use of magnesium sulfate with ritodrine for preterm labor tocolysis. Am J Obstet Gynecol, 148: 166–171.

Finley J, Katz M, Rojas-Perez M, Roberts JM, Creasy RK, Schiller NB (1984). Cardiovascular consequences of β-agonist tocolysis: an echocardiographic study. Obstet Gynecol, 64: 787–791.

Fleckenstein A, Grün G, Tritthart H, Byon K, Harding P (1971). Uterus-Relaxation durch hochaktive Ca^{++}-antagonistische Hemmstoffe der elektro-mechanischen Koppelung wie Isoptin (Verapamil, Iproveratril), Substanz D600 und Segontin (Prenylamin). Versuchen am isolierten Uterus virginellen Ratten. Klin Wochenschr, 49: 32–41.

Forman A (1984). Calcium entry blockade as a therapeutic principle in the female urogenital tract. Acta Obstet Gynecol Scand (Suppl), 121: 1–26.

Freysz H, Willard D, Lehr A, Messer J, Boog G (1977). A long term evaluation of infants who received a beta-mimetic drug while in utero. J Perinat Med, 5: 94–99.

Friedman Z, Whitman V, Maisels MJ, Berman W Jr, Marks KH, Vesell ES (1978). Indomethacin disposition and indomethacin-induced platelet dysfunction in premature infants. J Clin Pharmacol, 18: 272–279.

Fuchs A-R, Fuchs F (1981). Ethanol for prevention of preterm birth. Seminars Perinatol, 5: 236–251.

Fuchs F (1965). Treatment of threatened premature labour with alcohol. J Obstet Gynaecol Br Commnwlth, 72: 1011–1013.

Fuchs F (1976). Prevention of prematurity. Am J Obstet Gynecol, 126: 809–820.

Fuchs F, Fuchs A-R (1984). Ethanol for the prevention of preterm birth. In: Preterm Birth: Causes, Prevention and Management. Fuchs F, Stubblefield PG (eds). New York: Macmillan, pp 207–222.

Fuchs F, Stakemann G (1960). Treatment of threatened premature labor with large doses of progesterone. Am J Obstet Gynecol, 79: 172–176.

Fuchs F, Fuchs A-R, Poblete VG, Risk A (1967). Effect of

alcohol on threatened premature labor. Am J Obstet Gynecol, 99: 627–637.

Fuchs F, Fuchs A-R, Lauersen NH, Zervoudakis IA (1979). Treatment of pre-term labour with ethanol. Danish Med Bull, 26: 123–124.

Fuchs A-R, Fuchs F, Husslein P, Soloff MS, Fernström MJ (1982a). Oxytocin receptors and human parturition: A dual role for oxytocin in the initiation of labor. Science, 215: 1396–1398.

Fuchs A-R, Husslein P, Sumulong L, Micha JP, Yusoff Dawood M, Fuchs F (1982b). Plasma levels of oxytocin and 13,14-dihydro-15-keto-prostaglandin $F_{2\alpha}$ in preterm labor and the effect of ethanol and ritodrine. Am J Obstet Gynecol, 144: 753–759.

Fuchs A-R, Fuchs F, Husslein P, Soloff MS (1984). Oxytocin receptors in the human uterus during pregnancy and parturition. Am J Obstet Gynecol, 150: 734–741.

Gamissans O, Balasch J (1984). Prostaglandin synthetase inhibitors in the treatment of preterm labor. In: Preterm Birth: Causes, Prevention and Management. Fuchs F, Stubblefield PG (eds). New York: Macmillan, pp 223–248.

Gamissans O, Canas E, Cararach V, Ribas J, Puerto B, Edo A (1978). A study of indomethacin combined with ritodrine in threatened preterm labor. Eur J Obstet Gynecol Reprod Biol, 8: 123–128.

Gamissans O, Cararach V, Serra J (1982). The role of prostaglandin-inhibitors, beta-adrenergic drugs and glucocorticoids in the management of threatened preterm labor. In: Beta-mimetic Drugs in Obstetrics and Perinatology. Jung H, Lamberti G (eds). Stuttgart: Georg Thieme, pp 71–84.

Gandar R, de Zoeten LW, van der Schoot JB (1980). Serum level of ritodrine in man. Eur J Clin Pharmacol, 17: 117–122.

Gersony WM, Peckham GJ, Ellison RC, Miettinen OS, Nadas AS (1983). Effects of indomethacin in premature infants with patent ductus arteriosus: results of a national collaborative study. J Pediatr, 102: 895–905.

Gittenberger-de Groot AC (1977). Persistent ductus arteriosus: most problably a primary congenital malformation. Br Heart J, 39: 610–618.

Gleason CA (1987). Prostaglandins and the developing kidney. Seminars Perinatol, 11: 12–21.

Gonik B, Creasy RK (1986). Preterm labor: its diagnosis and management. Am J Obstet Gynecol, 154: 3–8.

Goodlin RC (1980). Pulmonary edema in pregnant patients treated for hypertension. Am J Obstet Gynecol, 136: 1087–1088.

Grant AM (1988). Oral salbutamol in the prevention of low birthweight. Unpublished trial. In: Oxford Database of Perinatal Trials. Oxford: Oxford University Press.

Greenhouse BS, Hook R, Hehre FW (1969). Aspiration pneumonia following intravenous administration of alcohol during labor. J Am Med Assoc, 210: 2393–2395.

Grospietsch G (1981). Lungenkomplikationen bei der Tokolyse. In: Indikationen und Gefahren der Tokolyse. Heilmann L, Ludwig H (eds). Ingelheim: Boehringer, pp 39–61.

Grospietsch G, Kuhn W (1984). Effects of β-mimetics on maternal physiology. In: Preterm Birth: Causes, Prevention and Management. Fuchs F, Stubblefield PG (eds). New York: Macmillan, pp 171–196.

Grospietsch G, Fenske M, Dietrich B, Ensink FBM (1982). Effect of the tocolytic agent fenoterol on body weight, urine excretion. blood hematocrit, hemoglobin, serum protein, and electrolyte levels in non-pregnant rabbits. Am J Obstet Gynecol, 143: 667–672.

Gummerus M (1975). Hemmung der drohenden Frühgeburt mit Nylidrin und Verapamil. Z Geburtsh Perinatol, 179: 261–266.

Gummerus M (1983). Tocolysis with hexoprenalin and salbutamol in clinical comparison. Geburtshilfe Frauenheilkd, 43: 151–155.

Gummerus M, Halonen O (1987). Prophylactic long-term oral tocolysis of multiple pregnancies. Br J Obstet Gynaecol, 94: 249–251.

Györy G, Kiss C, Benyo T, Bagdany S, Szalay J, Kurcz M, Virag S (1974). Inhibition of labour by prostaglandin antagonist in impending abortion and preterm and term labour. Lancet, 2: 293.

Hadders-Algra M, Touwen BCL, Huisjes HJ (1986). Long-term follow-up of children prenatally exposed to ritodrine. Br J Obstet Gynaecol, 93: 156–161.

Hall DG, McGaughey HS, Corey EL, Thornton WN (1959). The effects of magnesium sulfate therapy on the duration of labor. Am J Obstet Gynecol 78: 27–32.

Halle H, Hengst P (1978). Zusatztokolyse durch Prostaglandinsythetasehemmung mit Indometacin. Z Geburtsh Perinatol, 182: 367–370.

Haller JA, Morgan W, Rodgers B, Gengos D, Margulies S (1967). Chronic hemodynamic effects of occluding the fetal ductus arteriosus. J Thorac Cardiovasc Surg, 54: 770–776.

Hartikainen-Sorri AL, Kauppila A, Tuimala R (1980). Inefficacy of 17α-hydroxyprogesterone caproate in the prevention of prematurity in twin pregnancy. Obstet Gynecol, 56: 692–695.

Harvey J, Agustsson P, Patel N, Anderson J (1985). The role of infection in the aetiology of preterm labour. In: Pre-term Labour and Its Consequences. Proceedings of the Thirteenth Study Group of the Royal College of Obstetricians and Gynaecologists. Beard RW, Sharp F (eds). London: Royal College of Obstetricians and Gynaecologists, pp 249–258.

Hauth JC, Gilstrap LC, Brekken AL, Hauth JM (1983). The effect of 17α-hydroxyprogesterone caproate on pregnancy outcome in an active-duty military population. Am J Obstet Gynecol, 146: 187–190.

Heilmann L, Ludwig H (1981). Indikationen und Gefahren der Tokolyse. Ingelheim: Boehringer.

Hendricks CH (1981). The case for nonintervention in preterm labor. In: Preterm Labor. Elder MG, Hendricks CH (eds). London: Butterworths, pp 93–123.

Hendricks CH, Cibils LA, Pose SV, Eskes TKAB (1961). The pharmacologic control of excessive uterine activity with isoxsuprine. Am J Obstet Gynecol, 82: 1064–1078.

Hendricks SK, Keroes J, Katz M (1986). Electrocardiographic changes associated with ritodrine-induced maternal tachycardia and hypokalemia. Am J Obstet Gynecol, 154: 921–923.

Heymann MA, Rudolph AM, Silverman NH (1976). Closure of the ductus arteriosus in premature infants by inhibition of prostaglandin synthesis. New Engl J Med, 295: 530–533.

Heyting A (1980). Correspondence. Br J Obstet Gynaecol, 87: 1056.

Hiltmann WD, Wiest W (1982). Counteracting the effects of

tocolysis on the maternal cardiovascular system. In: Beta-mimetic Drugs in Obstetrics and Perinatology. Jung H, Lamberti G (eds). Stuttgart: Georg Thieme, pp 222–226.

Hobel CJ (unpublished). Unpublished data included in the reports of Merkatz *et al.* (1980) and King *et al.* (1988).

Hofstetter R, Schmidt HP, Krebs W, Lang D, Bernuth GV (1979). Kardiale Wirkung von Fenoterol allein oder in Kombination mit Verapamil. Z Geburtsh Perinatol, 183: 335–338.

Howard TE, Killam AP, Penney LL, Daniell WC (1982). A double blind randomized study of terbutaline in premature labor. Milit Med, 147: 305–307.

Huszar G, Roberts JM (1982). Biochemistry and pharmacology of the myometrium and labor: regulation at the cellular and molecular levels. Am J Obstet Gynecol, 142: 225–237.

Idänpään-Heikkilä J, Jouppila P, Akerblom HK, Isoaho R, Kauppila E, Koivisto M (1972). Elimination and metabolic effects of ethanol in mother, fetus and newborn infant. Am J Obstet Gynecol, 112: 387–393.

Ingemarsson I (1976). Effect of terbutaline on premature labor. A double-blind placebo-controlled study. Am J Obstet Gynecol, 125: 520–524.

Ingemarsson I, Westgren M, Lindberg C, Ahren B, Lundquist I, Carlsson C (1981). Single injection of terbutaline in term labor: placental transfer and effects on maternal and fetal carbohydrate mechanism. Am J Obstet Gynecol, 139: 697–701.

Ingemarsson I, Azulkumaran S, Kottegoda SR (1985). Complications of beta-mimetic therapy in preterm labour. Austral NZ J Obstet Gynaecol, 25: 182–189.

Irmer M, Trolp R, Steim H, Hillemans HG (1982). Cardiovascular effects of adrenergic β_2-receptor stimulation and imultaneous β_1-blockade in pregnant women in premature labor. In: Beta-mimetic Drugs in Obstetrics and Perinatology. Jung H, Lamberti G (eds). Stuttgart: Georg Thieme, pp 217–222.

Itskovitz J, Abramovice H, Brandes JM (1980). Oligohydramnion, meconium and perinatal death concurrent with indomethacin treatment in human pregnancy. J Reprod Med, 24: 137–140.

Jacobs MM, Knight AB, Arias F (1980). Maternal pulmonary edema resulting from betamimetic and glucocorticoid therapy. Obstet Gynecol, 56: 56–59.

Johnson JWC, Austin KL, Jones GS, Davis GH, King TM (1975). Efficacy of 17α-hydroxyprogesterone caproate in the prevention of premature labor. New Engl J Med, 293: 675–680.

Jonatha W, Goessens L, Traub E, Dick W (1977). Pulmonale Komplikationen während der Tokolyse. In: Fenoterol (Partusisten) bei der Behandlung in der Geburtshilfe und Perinatologie. Jung H, Friedrich E (eds). Stuttgart: Georg Thieme, pp 165–168.

Jung H (1982). General remarks on treatment with beta-mimetics. In: Beta-mimetic Drugs in Obstetrics and Perinatology. Jung H, Lamberti G (eds). Stuttgart: Georg Thieme.

Jung H, Lamberti G (1982). Beta-mimetic Drugs in Obstetrics and Perinatology. Stuttgart: Georg Thieme.

Karlsson K, Krantz M, Hamberger L (1980). Comparison of various betamimetics on preterm labor survival and development of the child. J Perinat Med, 8: 19–26.

Katz M, Robertson PA, Creasy RK (1981). Cardiovascular complications associated with terbutaline treatment for preterm labor. Am J Obstet Gynecol, 139: 605–608.

Katz Z, Lancet M, Yemini M, Mogilner BM, Feigl A, Ben-Hur H (1983). Treatment of premature labor contractions with combined ritodrine and indomethacine. Int J Gynaecol Obstet, 21: 337–342.

Katz M, Newman RB, Gill PJ (1986). Assessment of uterine activity in ambulatory patients at high risk of preterm labor and delivery. Am J Obstet Gynecol, 154: 44–47.

Keirse MJNC (1979). Epidemiology of pre-term labour. In: Human Parturition. Keirse MJNC, Anderson ABM, Bennebroek Gravenhorst J (eds). The Hague: Leiden University Press, pp 219–234.

Keirse MJNC (1981). Potential hazards of prostaglandin synthetase inhibitors for management of pre-term labour. J Drug Res, 6: 915–919.

Keirse MJNC (1984a). A survey of tocolytic drug treatment in preterm labour. Br J Obstet Gynaecol, 91: 424–430.

Keirse MJNC (1984b). Betamimetic drugs in the prophylaxis of preterm labour: extent and rationale of their use. Br J Obstet Gynaecol, 91: 431–437.

Keirse MJNC (1985): Biosynthesis and metabolism of prostaglandins within the human uterus in early and late pregnancy. In: The role of Prostaglandins in Labour. Wood C (ed). London: Royal Society of Medicine, pp 25–38.

Keirse MJNC (1989). Amniotomy or oxytocin for induction of labor: re-analysis of a randomized controlled trial. Acta Obstet Gynecol Scand, 67: 731–735.

Keirse MJNC, Noort W, Erwich JJHM (1987): The role of prostaglandins and prostaglandin synthesis in the pregnant uterus. In: Priming and Induction of Labour by Prostaglandins 'a state of the art'. Keirse MJNC, de Koning Gans HJ (eds). Leiden: Boerhaave Committee for Postacademic Medical Education, pp 1–25.

King JF, Grant A, Keirse MJNC, Chalmers I (1988). Beta-mimetics in preterm labour: an overview of the randomized controlled trials. Br J Obstet Gynaecol, 95: 211–222.

Kirkpatrick C, Quenon M, Desir D (1980). Blood anions and electrolytes during ritodrine infusion in preterm labor. Am J Obstet Gynecol, 138: 523–527.

Kiss VC, Szöke B (1975). Rolle des Magnesiums bei der Verhütung der Frühgeburt. Zbl Gynäkol, 97: 924–927.

Kohler HG (1978). Premature closure of the ductus arteriosus (P.C.D.A.): a possible cause of intrauterine circulatory failure. Early Hum Dev, 2: 15–23.

Kosasa TS, Nakayama RT, Hale RW, Rinzler GS, Freitas CA (1985). Ritodrine and terbutaline compared for the treatment of preterm labor. Acta Obstet Gynecol Scand, 64: 421–426.

Kragt H, Keirse MJNC (1990). How accurate is a woman's diagnosis of threatened preterm delivery? Br J Obstet Gynaecol, 97: 317–323.

Kubli F (1977). Discussion. In: Pre-term Labour. Proceedings of the Fifth Study Group of the Royal College of Obstetricians and Gynaecologists. Anderson A, Beard R, Brudenell JM, Dunn PM (eds). London: Royal College of Obstetricians and Gynaecologists, pp 218–220.

Kubli F (1980). Commentary on maternal morbidity due to beta-adrenergic therapy. Eur J Obstet Gynecol Reprod Biol, 10: 44–45.

Kumar D, Zourlas PA, Barnes AC (1963). *In vitro* and *in vivo* effects of magnesium sulfate on human uterine contractility. Am J Obstet Gynecol, 86: 1036–1040.

Lancet (1980). The fate of the baby under 1501 g at birth (Editorial). Lancet, 1: 461–463.

Lands AM, Arnold A, McAuliff JP, Luduena FP, Brown TG (1967). Differentiation of receptor systems activated by sympathomimetic amines. Nature, 214: 597–598.

Larsen JF, Lange AP (1987). Ritodrine in the treatment of preterm labor: second Danish multicenter study. Obstet Gynecol, 69: 282–283.

Larsen JF, Kern Hansen M, Hesseldahl H, Kristoffersen K, Larsen PK, Osler M, Weber J, Eldon K, Lange A (1980). Ritodrine in the treatment of preterm labour. A clinical trial to compare a standard treatment with three regimens involving the use of ritodrine. Br J Obstet Gynaecol, 87: 949–957.

Larsen JF, Eldon K, Lange AP, Leegaard M, Osler M, Sederberg Olsen J, Permin M (1986). Ritodrine in the treatment of preterm labor: second Danish multicenter study. Obstet Gynecol, 67: 607–613.

Lauersen NH, Merkatz IR, Tejani N, Wilson KH, Roberson A, Mann LI, Fuchs F (1977). Inhibition of premature labor: A multicenter comparison of ritodrine and ethanol. Am J Obstet Gynecol, 127: 837–845.

Leferink JG, Wagemaker-Engels L, Maes RAA, Lamont H, Pauwels R, Van der Straeten M (1977). Quantitative analysis of terbutaline in serum and urine at therapeutic levels using gas chromatography–mass spectrometry. J Chromatogr, 143: 299–305.

Lenz S, Kühl C, Wang P, Molsted-Pedersen L, Orskov L, Faber OK (1979). The effect of ritodrine on carbohydrate and lipid metabolism in normal and diabetic pregnant women. Acta Endocrinol, 92: 669–679.

Lenz S, Detlefsen G, Rygaard C, Vejerslev L (1985). Isotonic dextrose and isotonic saline as solvents for intravenous treatment of premature labour with ritodrine. J Obstet Gynaecol, 5: 151–154.

Leslie D, Coats PM (1977). Salbutamol-induced diabetic ketoacidosis. Br Med J, 2: 768.

Leveno KJ, Guzick DS, Hankins GDV, Klein VR, Young DC, Williams M Lynne (1986). Single-centre randomised trial of ritodrine hydrochloride for preterm labour. Lancet, 1: 1293–1296.

Levin DL (1980). Effects of inhibition of prostaglandin synthesis on fetal development, oxygenation, and the fetal circulation. Seminars Perinatol, 4: 35–44.

Levin DL, Fixler DE, Morriss FC, Tyson J (1978a). Morphologic analysis of the pulmonary vascular bed in infants exposed in utero to prostaglandin synthetase inhibitors. J Pediatr, 92: 478–483.

Levin DL, Hyman AI, Heymann MA, Rudolph AM (1978b). Fetal hypertension and the development of increased pulmonary vascular smooth muscle: a possible mechanism for persistent pulmonary hypertension of the newborn. J Pediatr, 92: 265–269.

Levin DL, Mills LJ, Parkey M, Garriott J, Campbell W (1979). Constriction of the fetal ductus arteriosus after administration of indomethacin to the pregnant ewe. J Pediatr, 94: 647–650.

LeVine L (1964). Habitual abortion. A controlled clinical study of progestational therapy. West J Surg, 72: 30–36.

Levy DL, Warsof SL (1985). Oral ritodrine and preterm premature rupture of membranes. Obstet Gynecol, 66: 621–623.

Lewis PJ, de Swiet M, Boylan P, Bulpitt CJ (1980). How obstetricians in the United Kingdom manage preterm labour. Br J Obstet Gynaecol, 87: 574–577.

Lewis RB Schulman JD (1973). Influence of acetylsalicylic acid, an inhibitor of prostaglandin synthesis, on the duration of human gestation and labour. Lancet, 2: 1159–1161.

Liggins GC, Howie RN (1972). A controlled trial of antepartum glucorticoid treatment for prevention of the respiratory distress syndrome in premature infants. Pediatrics, 50: 515–525.

Liggins GC, Vaughan GS (1973). Intravenous infusion of salbutamol in the management of premature labor. J Obstet Gynaecol Br Commnwlth, 80: 29–33.

Lipshitz J, Baillie P (1976). Uterine and cardiovascular effects of $beta_2$-selective sympathomimetic drugs administered as an intravenous infusion. S Afr Med J, 50: 1973–1977.

Lipshitz J, Baillie P, Davey DA (1976). A comparison of the uterine $beta_2$-adrenoreceptor selectivity of fenoterol, hexoprenaline, ritodrine and salbutamol. S Afr Med J, 50: 1969–1972.

Lipshitz PJ (1971). The clinical and biochemical effects of excess magnesium in the newborn. Pediatrics, 47: 501–509.

Mahony L, Carnero V, Brett C, Heymann MA, Clyman RI (1982). Prophylactic indomethacin therapy for patent ductus arteriosus in very-low-birth-weight infants. New Engl J Med, 306: 506–510.

Mantell CD, Liggins GC (1970). The effect of ethanol on the myometrial response to oxytocin in women at term. J Obstet Gynaecol Br Commnwlth, 77: 976–981.

Mariona FG, Scommegna A (unpublished). Unpublished data included in the reports of Merkatz *et al.* (1980) and King *et al.* (1988).

Marivate M, De Villiers KQ, Fairbrother P (1977). Effect of prophylactic outpatient administration of fenoterol on the time and onset of spontaneous labor and fetal growth rate in twin pregnancy. Am J Obstet Gynecol, 128: 707–708.

Mathews DD, Friend JB, Michael CA (1967). A double-blind trial of oral isoxuprine in the prevention of premature labour. J Obstet Gynaecol Br Commnwlth, 74: 68–70.

McCarthy JJ, Erving HW, Laufe LE (1957). Preliminary report on the use of relaxin in the management of threatened premature labor. Am J Obstet Gynecol 74: 134–138.

McGregor JA (1988). Prevention of preterm birth: new initiatives based on microbial-host interactions. Obstet Gynecol Survey, 43: 1–14.

McGregor JA, French JI, Reller LB, Todd JK, Makowski EL (1986). Adjunctive erythromycin treatment for idiopathic preterm labor: results of a randomized, double-blinded, placebo-controlled trial. Am J Obstet Gynecol, 154: 98–103.

Melin P, Trojnar J, Johansson B, Vilhardt H, Akerlund M (1986). Synthetic antagonists of the myometrial response to oxytocin and vasopressin. J Endocrinol, 111: 125–131.

Merkatz IR, Peter JB, Barden TP (1980). Ritodrine hydrochloride: a betamimetic agent for use in preterm labor. II. Evidence of efficacy. Obstet Gynecol, 56: 7–12.

Michalak D, Klein V, Marquette GP (1983). Myocardial ischemia: a complication of ritodrine tocolysis. Am J Obstet Gynecol, 146: 861–862.

Milliez J, Blot P, Sureau C (1980). A case report of maternal death associated with betamimetics and betamethasone administration in premature labour. Eur J Obstet Gynecol Reprod Biol, 11: 95–100.

Minkoff H (1983). Prematurity: infection as an etiologic factor. Obstet Gynecol, 62: 137–144.

Mitchell MD (1986). Pathways of arachidonic acid metabolism with specific application to the fetus and mother. Seminars Perinatol, 10: 242–254.

Moonen P, Klok G, Keirse MJNC (1984). Increase in concentrations of prostaglandin endoperoxide synthase and prostacyclin synthase in human myometrium in late pregnancy. Prostaglandins, 28: 309–322.

Morales WJ, Diebel ND, Lazar AJ, Zadrozny D (1986). The effect of antenatal dexamethasone on the prevention of respiratory distress syndrome in preterm gestations with premature rupture of membranes. Am J Obstet Gynecol, 154: 591–595.

Morrison JC, Martin JN, Maryin RW, Gookin KS, Wiser WL (1987). Prevention of preterm birth by ambulatory assessment of uterine activity. A randomized study. Am J Obstet Gynecol, 156: 536–543.

Mosler KH, Rosenboom HG (1972). Neuere Möglichkeiten einer tokolitischen Behandlung in der Geburtshilfe. Z Geburtsh Perinatol, 176: 85–96.

Müller-Tyl E. Reinold E, Hermuss P (1974). Gleichzeitige Anwendung einer betamimetischen und beta-rezeptoren blockierenden Substanz bei der Wehenhemmung. Z Geburtsh Perinatol, 178: 128–130.

Neibuhr-Jorgensen U (1980). Pulmonary oedema following treatment with ritodrine and betamethasone in premature labour. Danish Med Bull 27: 99–100.

Neubüser D (1974). Uber die Wirkung der Kalzium-inhibitoren Verapamil (Isoptin) und D600 auf die Nebenwirkungen der klinischen Tokolyse mit dem Beta-Stimulator Th 1165a (Partusisten). Geburtshilfe Frauenheilk, 34: 782–787.

Niebyl JR (1981). Prostaglandin synthetase inhibtors. Seminars Perinatol, 5: 274–287.

Niebyl JR, Blake DA, White RD, Kumor KM, Dubin NH, Robinson JC, Egner PG (1980). The inhibition of premature labor with indomethacin. Am J Obstet Gynecol, 136: 1014–1019.

Noort WA, Kragt H, De Zwart FA, Keirse MJNC (1988). Can urinary thromboxane excretion predict preterm delivery? Eicosanoids Fatty Acids, 4: 121.

O'Connor MC, Murphy H, Dalrymple IJ (1979). Double blind trial of ritodrine and placebo in twin pregnancy. Br J Obstet Gynaecol, 86: 706–709.

O'Driscoll M (1977). Discussion. In: Pre-term Labour. Proceedings of the Fifth Study Group of the Royal College of Obstetricians and Gynaecologists. Anderson A, Beard R, Brudenell JM, Dunn PM (eds). London: Royal College of Obstetricians and Gynaecologists, pp 369–370.

Osler M (1979). Side effects and metabolic changes during treatment with betamimetics (Ritodrine). Danish Med Bull, 26: 119–120.

Ott A, Hayes J, Polin J (1976). Severe lactic acidosis associated with intravenous alcohol for premature labor. Obstet Gynecol, 48: 362–364.

Papiernik E (1970). Etude en double aveugle d'un médicament prevenant la survenue prématurée de l'accouchement chez les femmes 'à risque élevé' d'accouchement prématuré. In: Edition Schering, Serie IV, fiche 3, pp 65–68.

Papiernik E, Bouyer J, Collin D, Winisdoerffer G, Dreyfus J (1986). Precocious cervical ripening and preterm labor. Obstet Gynecol, 67: 238–242.

Parsons MT, Owens CA, Spellacy WN (1987). Thermic effects of tocolytic agents: decreased temperature with magnesium sulfate. Obstet Gynecol, 69: 88–90.

Pedersen OL, Mikkelsen E (1978). Acute and chronic effects of nifedipine in arterial hypertension. Eur J Clin Pharmacol, 14: 375–381.

Penney LL, Daniell WC (1980). Estimation of success in treatment of premature labor: applicability of prolongation index in a double-blind, controlled, randomized trial. Am J Obstet Gynecol, 138: 345–346.

Petrie RH (1981). Tocolysis using magnesium sulfate. Seminars Perinatol, 5: 266–273.

Philipsen T, Eriksen PS, Lynggard F (1981). Pulmonary edema following ritodrine-saline infusion in premature labor. Obstet Gynecol, 58: 304–308.

Polowczyk D, Tejani N, Lauersen N, Siddiq F (1984). Evaluation of seven- to nine-year-old children exposed to ritodrine in utero. Obstet Gynecol, 64: 485–488.

Post LC (1977). Pharmacokinetics of beta-adrenergic agonists. In: Pre-term Labour. Proceedings of the Fifth Study Group of the Royal College of Obstetricians and Gynaecologists. Anderson A, Beard R, Brudenell JM, Dunn PM (eds). London: Royal College of Obstetricians and Gynaecologists, pp 134–148.

Rayburn W, Piehl E, Schork MA, Kirscht J (1986). Intravenous ritodrine therapy: a comparison between twin and singleton gestations. Obstet Gynecol, 67: 243–248.

Read MD, Wellby DE (1986). The use of a calcium antagonist (nifedipine) to suppress preterm labour. Br J Obstet Gynaecol, 93: 933–937.

Reinold E, Müller-Tyl E (1977). Tocolysis with betamimetics and beta-blockers. In: Labour Inhibition, Betamimetic Drugs in Obstetrics. Wiedinger H (ed.) Stuttgart: Gustav Fischer, pp 135–138.

Reiss U, Atad J, Rubinstein I, Zuckerman H (1976). The effect of indomethacin in labour at term. Int J Gynaecol Obstet, 14: 369–374.

Reynolds JW (1978). A comparison of salbutamol and ethanol in the treatment of premature labour. Austral NZ J Obstet Gynaecol, 18: 107–109.

Richter R (1977). Evaluation of success in treatment of threatening premature labor by betamimetic drugs. Am J Obstet Gynecol, 127: 482–486.

Richter R, Hinselmann MJ (1979). The treatment of threatened premature labor by betamimetic drugs: a comparison of fenoterol and ritodrine. Obstet Gynecol, 53: 81–87.

Richter R, Hammacher K, Hinselmann M (1975). Die Prophylaxe der drohenden Frühgeburt. Klinische Ergebnisse einer prospektiven Vergleichstudie mit Ritodrine und Buphenin. Gynäkol Rundsch, 15: 58–59.

Ries GH (1979). Kasuistische Mitteilung über das Auftreten einer Myokardischämie unter medikamentöser Tokolyse mit Ritodrin (Pre-Par). Geburtshilfe Frauenheilk, 39: 33–37.

Roberts JM (1981). Receptors and transfer of information into cells. Seminar Perinatol, 5: 203–215.

Robertson PA, Herron M, Katz M, Creasy RK (1981).

Maternal morbidity associated with isoxsuprine and terbutaline tocolysis. Eur J Obstet Gynecol Reprod Biol, 11: 371–378.

Rogge P, Young S, Goodlin R (1979). Post-partum pulmonary oedema associated with preventive therapy for premature labour. Lancet, 1: 1026–1027.

Rominger KL (1977). Zur Pharmakokinetik von Partusisten. In: Fenoterol (Partusisten) bei der Behandlung in der Geburtshilfe und Perinatologie. Jung H, Friedrich E (eds). Stuttgart: Georg Thieme, pp 15–20.

Rona G, Chappel CI, Balazs T, Ghaudry R (1959). An infarct-like myocardial lesion and other toxic manifestations produced by isoproterenol in the rat. Arch Pathol, 67: 443–455.

Ross MG, Nicolls E, Stubblefield PG, Kitzmiller JL (1983). Intravenous terbutaline and simultaneous β_1-blockade for advanced premature labor. Am J Obstet Gynecol, 147: 897–902.

Ruppin E, Ruppin J, Chelius HH (1981). A double blind study of the treatment of threatened abortion with fenoterol hydrobromide. Geburtshilfe Frauenheilk, 41: 218–221.

Ryden G (1977). The effect of salbutamol and terbutaline in the management of premature labour. Acta Obstet Gynecol Scand, 56: 293–296.

Schilthuis MS, Aarnoudse JG (1980). Fetal death associated with severe ritodrine-induced keto-acidosis, Lancet, 1: 1145.

Schreyer P, Caspi E, Ariely S, Herzianu I, User P, Gilboa Y, Zaidman JL (1979). Metabolic effects of intravenous ritrodrine infusion during pregnancy. Eur J Obstet Gynecol Reprod Biol, 9: 97–103.

Schwartz A, Brook I, Insler V, Kohen F, Zor U, Lindner H (1978). R. Effect of flufenamic acid on uterine contractions and plasma levels of 15-keto-13,14-dihydro-prostaglandin $F_{2\alpha}$ in preterm labor. Gynecol Obstet Invest, 9: 139–149.

Sims CD, Chamberlain GVP, Boyd IE, Lewis PJ (1978). A comparison of salbutamol and ethanol in the treatment of preterm labour. Br J Obstet Gynaecol, 85: 761–766.

Sisenwein FE, Tejani NA, Boxer HS, Di Giuseppe R (1983). Effects of maternal ethanol infusion during pregnancy on the growth and development of children at four to seven years of age. Am J Obstet Gynecol, 147: 52–56.

Sivasamboo R (1972). Premature labour. In: Proceedings of the International Symposium on the Treatment of Fetal Risks. Baden, Austria. Baumgarten K, Wesselius-De Casparis A (eds). Vienna: University of Vienna Medical School, pp 16–20.

Skjaerris J, Aberg A (1982). Prevention of prematurity in twin pregnancy by orally administered terbutaline. Acta Obstet Gynecol Scand, 108: 39–40.

Smit DA (1983). Efficacy of Orally Administered Ritodrine after Initial Intravenous Therapy. MD thesis, University of Limburg, The Netherlands.

Soltan MH (1986). Buphenine and threatened abortion. Eur J Obstet Gynecol Reprod Biol, 22: 319–324.

Spätling L (1981). Orale Magnesium-Zusatztherapie bei vorzeitiger Wehentätigkeit. Geburtshilfe Frauenheilk, 41: 101–102.

Spätling L, Spätling G (1988). Magnesium supplementation in pregnancy. A double-blind study. Br J Obstet Gynaecol, 95: 120–125.

Spearing G (1979). Alcohol, indomethacin and salbutamol. A comparative trial of their use in preterm labor. Obstet Gynecol, 53: 171–174.

Spellacy WN, Cruz AC, Birk SA, Buhi WC (1979). Treatment of premature labor with ritodrine: a randomized controlled study. Obstet Gynecol, 54: 220–223.

Spisso KR, Harbert GM Jr, Thiagarajah S (1982). The use of magnesium sulfate as a primary tocolytic agent to prevent premature delivery. Am J Obstet Gynecol, 142: 840–845.

Steer CM, Petrie RH (1977). A comparison of magnesium sulfate and alcohol for the prevention of premature labor. Am J Obstet Gynecol, 129: 1–4.

Stubblefield PG (1978). Pulmonary edema occurring after therapy with dexamethasone and terbutaline for premature labor: a case report. Am J Obstet Gynecol, 132: 341–342.

Stubbs TM, Van Dorsten JP, Miller MC (1986). The preterm cervix and preterm labor: relative risks, predictive values, and change over time. Am J Obstet Gynecol, 155: 829–834.

Suzanne F, Fresne JJ, Portal B, Baudon J (1980). Essai thérapeutique de l'indométacine dans les menaces d'accouchement prématuré. Thérapie 35: 751–760.

Tamby Raja RL, Anderson ABM, Turnbull AC (1974). Endocrine changes in premature labour. Br Med J, 4: 67–71.

Taubert HD, Haskins HL (1963). Intravenous infusion of progesterone in human females: blood levels obtained and effect in labor. Obstet Gynecol, 22: 405–408.

Tchilinguirian NG, Najem R, Sullivan GB, Craparo FJ (1984). The use of ritodrine and magnesium sulfate in the arrest of premature labor. Int J Gynaecol Obstet, 22: 117–123.

Thomas DJB, Gill B, Brown P, Stubbs WA (1977). Salbutamol-induced diabetic ketoacidosis. Br Med J, 2: 438.

Tinga DJ, Aarnoudse JG (1979). Post-partum pulmonary oedema associated with preventive therapy for premature labour. Lancet, 1: 1026.

Traeger A, Nöschel H, Zaumseil J (1973). Zur Pharmakokinetik von Indomethazin bei Schwangeren, Kreissenden und deren Neugeborenen. Zbl Gynäkol, 95: 635–641.

Trolp R, Irmer M, Bernius U, Pohl C, Stein H, Hillemans HG (1980). Tokolyseerfolge unter Fenoterol-Monotherapie und Fenoterol in Kombination mit einem kardioselektiven β-Blocker. Geburtshilfe Frauenheilk, 40: 602–609.

Trolp R, Irmer M, Bernius U, Pohl C, Hillemans HG (1982). Comparative investigations into the results of tocolysis with fenoterol, combination therapy with fenoterol/verapamil and combination therapy with fenoterol/metoprolol. In: Beta-mimetic Drugs in Obstetrics and Perinatology. Jung H, Lamberti G (eds). Stuttgart: Georg Thieme, pp 239–245.

Tsuie JJ, Lai YF, Sharma SD (1977). The influence of acupuncture stimulation during pregnancy. Obstet Gynecol, 50: 479–488.

Turnbull AC (1987). Commentary: an oxytocin inhibitor for suppressing preterm labour. Br J Obstet Gynaecol, 94: 1009–1013.

Turner G, Collins E (1975). Fetal effects of regular salicylate ingestion in pregnancy. Lancet, 2: 338–339.

Ulmsten U, Andersson KE, Wingerup L (1980). Treatment of premature labor with the calcium antagonist nifedipine. Arch Gynecol, 229: 1–5.

Van Kets H, Thiery M, Derom R, Van Egmond H, Baele G (1979). Perinatal hazards of chronic antenatal tocolysis with indomethacin. Prostaglandins, 18: 893–907.

Van Lierde M, Thomas K (1982). Ritodrine concentration in maternal and fetal serum and amniotic fluid. J Perinat Med, 10: 119–124.

Varma TR (1988). A randomised double-blind comparison of ritodrine versus placebo in the treatment of intrauterine growth retardation. Unpublished trial. In: Oxford Database of Perinatal Trials. Oxford: Oxford University Press.

Veersema D, deJong PA, VanWijck JAM (1983). Indomethacin and the fetal renal nonfunction syndrome. Eur J Obstet Gynecol Reprod Biol, 16: 113–121.

Wager J, Fredholm BB, Lunell N-O, Persson B (1981). Metabolic and circulatory effects of oral salbutamol in the third trimester of pregnancy in diabetic and non-diabetic women. Br J Obstet Gynaecol, 88: 352–361.

Wagner L, Wagner G, Guerrero J (1970). Effect of alcohol on premature newborn infants. Am J Obstet Gynecol, 108: 308–315.

Wallace RL, Caldwell DL, Ansbachter R, Otterson WN (1978). Inhibition of premature labor by terbutaline. Obstet Gynecol, 51: 387–392.

Wallusch WW, Novak H, Leopold G, Netter KJ (1978). Comparative bioavailability: influence of various diets on the bioavailability of indomethacin. Int Clin Pharmacol, 16: 40–44.

Walters WAW, Wood C (1977). A trial of oral ritodrine for the prevention of premature labour. Br J Obstet Gynaecol, 84: 26–30.

Waltman R, Tricomi V, Palav A (1973). Aspirin and indomethacin: Effect on installation/abortion time of mid-trimester hypertonic saline induced abortion. Prostaglandins, 3: 47–58.

Watring WG, Benson WL, Wiebe RA, Vaughn DL (1976). Intravenous alcohol a single blind study in the prevention of premature delivery: a preliminary report. J Reprod Med, 16: 35–38.

Weiner CP, Renk K, Klugman M (1988). The therapeutic efficacy and cost-effectiveness of aggressive tocolysis for premature labor associated with premature rupture of the membranes. Am J Obstet Gynecol, 159: 216–222.

Wesselius-De Casparis A, Thiery M, Yo Le Sian A, Baumgarten K, Brosens I, Gamissans O, Stolk JG, Vivier W (1971). Results of double-blind, multicentre study with ritodrine in premature labour. Br Med J, 3: 144–147.

Wiedinger H (1977). Labour Inhibition, Betamimetic Drugs in Obstetrics. Stuttgart: Gustav Fischer.

Wiedinger H (1984). The European experience with β-mimetic agents. In: Preterm Birth: Causes, Prevention and Management. Fuchs F, Stubblefield PG (eds). New York: Macmillan, pp 131–149.

Wiedinger H, Wiest W (1973). Die Behandlung des Spätabortes und der drohenden Frühgeburt mit Th 1165a in Kombination mit Isoptin. Z Geburtsh Perinatol, 177: 233–237.

Wiedinger H, Mohr D, Haller K, Hiltmann WD, Vogel M (1976). Zeitlicher Verlauf der Blutglukose, des immunoreaktiven Insulins und der Kaliumionen beim Neugeborenen nach langzeitiger und akuter Gabe von Partusisten mit und ohne Isoptin. Z Geburtsh Perinatol, 180: 258–265.

Wiest W, Hiltman WD, Eifler A, Stosiek U, Wiedinger H, Knab G, Pohl R (1979). Einfluss von Partusisten und Isoptin auf das mütterliche EKG und herzspezifische Serumenzyme. Arch Gynäkol, 228: 134–135.

Wilkinson AR (1980). Naproxen levels in preterm infants after maternal treatment. Lancet, 2: 591–592.

Wiqvist N (1979). The use of inhibitors of prostaglandin synthesis in obstetrics. In: Human Parturition. Keirse MJNC, Anderson ABM, Bennebroek Gravenhorst J (eds). The Hague: Leiden University Press, pp 189–200.

Wiqvist N (1981). Preterm labour: other drug possibilities including drugs not to use. In: Preterm Labor. Elder MG, Hendricks CH (eds). London: Butterworths, pp 148–175.

Witter FR, Niebyl JR (1986). Inhibition of arachidonic acid metabolism in the perinatal period: pharmacology, clinical application, and potential adverse effects. Seminars Perinatol, 10: 316–333.

Wolff F, Meier U, Bolte A (1979). Untersuchungen zum Pathomechanismus schwerer kardiopulmonaler Komplikationen unter tokolytischer Behandlung mit β-adrenergen Substanzen und Betamethason. Z Geburtsh Perinatol, 183: 343–347.

Wolff F, Berg R, Bolte A (1981). Klinische Untersuchungen zur wehenhemmenden Wirkung der Azetylsalizylsäure (ASS) und ihre Nebenwirkungen. Geburtshilfe Frauenheilk, 41 : 96–100.

Yemini M, Borenstein R, Dreazen E, Apelman Z, Mogilner BM, Kessler I, Lancet M (1985). Prevention of premature labor by 17α-hydroxyprogesterone caproate. Am J Obstet Gynecol, 151: 574–577.

Ying YK, Tejani NA (1982). Angina pectoris as a complication of ritodrine hydrochloride therapy in premature labor. Obstet Gynecol, 60: 385–388.

Zervoudakis IA, Krauss A, Fuchs F (1980). Infants of mothers treated with ethanol for premature labor. Am J Obstet Gynecol, 137: 713–718.

Zlatnik FJ, Fuchs F (1972). A controlled study of ethanol in threatened premature labour. Am J Obstet Gynecol, 112: 610–612.

Zuckerman H, Reiss U, Rubinstein I (1974). Inhibition of human premature labor by indomethacin. Obstet Gynecol, 44: 787–792.

Zuckerman H, Shalev E, Gilad G, Katzuni E (1984). Further study of the inhibition of premature labor by indomethacin. Part II. Double-blind study. J Perinat Med, 12: 25–29.

45 Promoting pulmonary maturity

Patricia Crowley

1 Introduction

Respiratory distress syndrome is the commonest complication of preterm birth, affecting over 50 per cent of babies born before 34 weeks' gestation (Roberton 1982). It is a significant adverse prognostic factor for the survival of very low birthweight infants (Stanley and Alberman 1978; Bajuk *et al.* 1981), and accounts for 1500 deaths per year in England and Wales (Roberton 1982). Furthermore, it is a risk factor for long term impairments in very low birthweight infants who survive. Mechanical ventilation improves survival, but treatment of neonatal respiratory distress constitutes exacting, time-consuming, and expensive medical care (Avery 1984).

In the late 1960s, while studying the initiation of labour in sheep, Liggins observed that prematurely delivered lambs exposed prenatally to corticosteroids survived longer than their placebo-treated control animals (Liggins 1969). Liggins subsequently mounted a randomized, placebo-controlled trial of antenatal betamethasone administration in women and demonstrated statistically significant reductions in the incidence both of respiratory distress in babies born before 32 weeks' gestation and of neonatal mortality in the total group of betamethasone-treated babies delivered before 37 weeks' gestation (Liggins and Howie 1972).

Since this classic study, numerous further investigations have indicated benefit from antenatal administration of those corticosteroids that cross the placental barrier. This chapter reviews the evidence from randomized trials for the efficacy of corticosteroids in preventing respiratory distress and other forms of neonatal morbidity. Trials in which only the influence on laboratory test results was examined have not been included in this analysis (Farrell *et al.* 1983; Gunston and Davey 1978a,b; Whitt *et al.* 1976). Four 'trials' which on closer analysis proved not to be randomized controlled trials have been excluded (Baillie *et al.* 1976; Dluholucky *et al.* 1976; Kleinschmidt *et al.* 1977; Szabo *et al.* 1977). Data presented in multiple reports of the same trial have been amalgamated (the New Zealand trial: Liggins and Howie 1972, 1973; Howie and Liggins 1973; Liggins and Howie 1974; Liggins 1976; Howie and Liggins 1980, 1982; the United States Collaborative Group on Antenatal Steroid Therapy 1981, 1984; Bauer *et al.* 1984; Burkett *et al.* 1986; and the Amsterdam trial: Schutte *et al.* 1979, 1980, 1983). A total of 12 trials, involving over 3000 women, were thus available for analysis. Table 45.1 lists their entry and exclusion criteria; treatment and diagnostic regimens; and completeness of reporting.

2 Evidence of efficacy

2.1 Neonatal respiratory distress

The incidence of respiratory distress is the principal outcome variable reported in the 12 trials, and the data

Table 45.1

Trial	Entry criteria	Exclusion criteria	Treatment regimen	Diagnostic criteria for RDS	Number randomized	Randomization unknown	No. unreported / No. randomized
Liggins and Howie (1972) Howie and Liggins (1977)	Threatened or planned preterm delivery >24 weeks >37 weeks.	Imminent delivery. 'Clinical decision not to randomize'.	Betamethasone 12 mg IM × 2 doses 24 hours apart.	Yes	1135	65 (Cases with lethal congenital abnormality)	0
Block *et al.* (1977)	Patient judged to be in preterm labour.	Not stated.	Betamethasone 12 mg IM × 2 doses 24 hours apart.	Yes	175	0	$\frac{20}{175}$
Morales *et al.* (1986)	Patient with premature rupture of the membranes 28 to 33 weeks.	Patients in labour on admission, with foul-smelling liquor, intrauterine growth retardation, fetal lung maturity confirmed by the presence of phos-phatidylglycerol	Dexamethsaone 6 mg IM × 4 doses at 12-hour intervals.	Yes	250	5	$\frac{5^*}{250}$
Morrison *et al.* (1978)	Threatened or planned preterm delivery <34 weeks or immature L/S ratio + above.	Mature L/S ratio even if <34 weeks; medical contraindication to corticosteroids. Imminent delivery.	Hydrocortisone 500 mg IV × 4 daily doses 12-hourly.	No	196	$\frac{70}{196}$	$\frac{70}{196}$
Papageorgiou *et al.* (1979)	Patients >25 weeks and <34 weeks in preterm labour or with premature rupture of membranes.	Diabetes, pre-eclampsia, hypertension, Rhesus disease, retarded intrauterine growth.	Betamethasone 12 mg IM × 2 doses 12 hours apart.	Yes	146	0	$\frac{15}{146}$
Schutte *et al.* (1979)	Threatened preterm labour >26 weeks <32 weeks 'if it seemed possible to postpone labour × 12 hours'.	Diabetes, hyperthyroidism, infection, severe hypertension, cardiac disease, fetal growth retardation, fetal distress.	Betamethasone phosphat 8 mg and betamethasone, acetate 6 mg × 2 doses at 24-hour intervals.	No	122	0	$\frac{0}{122}$
Taeusch *et al.* (1979)	Premature labour or premature rupture of membranes in patients either <34 weeks pregnant or with immature L/S ratio, or with a previous infant with RDS.	Cervix 5 cm dilated, severe bleeding, chorio-amnionitis, severe pre-eclampsia, pre-existing glucocorticoid therapy.	Dexamathasone 4 mg IM 8-hourly × 6 doses.	Yes	127	0	$\frac{0}{127}$
Doran *et al.* (1980)	Unplanned preterm labour, spontaneous premature rupture of membranes, planned preterm delivery >24 weeks <34 weeks.	Pre-eclampsia. medical contraindication to corticosteroid therapy.	Betamethasone 6 mg × 4 doses at 12-hour intervals.	Yes	144	$\frac{0}{144}$	$\frac{0}{144}$

Table 45.1 *continued*

Trial	Entry criteria	Exclusion criteria	Treatment regimen	Diagnostic criteria for RDS	Number randomized	Randomization unknown	No. unreported / No. randomized
Teramo *et al.* (1980)	Patient admitted in preterm labour. Gestation >28 weeks <36 weeks. Cervical dilatation <4 cm. No precipitous progression of labour after 12 hours' observation.	Pre-eclampsia, diabetes, mellitus.	Betamethasone 12 mg IM × 2 doses at 24-hour intervals.	Yes	80 (babies)	0	0
Collaborative Group (1981)	Patients >26 weeks <34 weeks at high risk for premature delivery. Patients >34 weeks at high risk for premature delivery with L/S ratio 2.0 or less.	Cervix 5 cm dilated. Delivery anticipated in <24 hours or >7 days. Intrauterine infection. Previous corticosteroid therapy during pregnancy. Medical contraindications to corticosteroid therapy. Infant unavailable for follow-up.	Dexamethasone 5 mg IM × 4 doses.	Yes	757	12	$\frac{18}{757}$
Schmidt *et al.* (1984)	Preterm labour or premature rupture of membranes at either >24 and <34 weeks or with estimated fetal weight 750 g.	Cervix >5 cm dilated. Medical contraindications to corticosteroids. 'Deemed unsafe to delay delivery >24 hours'.	Hydrocortisone 250 mg × 2 doses at 24-hour intervals. Methyl-prednisolone 125 mg × 2 doses at 24-hour intervals. Betamethasone 12 mg × 2 doses at 24-hour intervals.	Yes	149	$\frac{52}{149}$	$\frac{52}{149}$
Gamsu *et al.* (1989)	Patient less than 34 weeks pregnant in spontaneous labour or requiring elective induction.	Patients in whom corticosteroids were contraindicated. Those in whom a delay of 24 hours before delivery was not in the interests of mother or baby. Patients with diabetes and chorio-amnionitis.	Betamethasone 4 mg 8-hourly × 6 doses over 48 hours.	Yes	251 mothers 268 babies	0	0

Table 45.2 Effect of corticosteroids prior to preterm delivery on respiratory distress, overall

Study	EXPT		CTRL		Odds ratio	Graph of odds ratios and confidence intervals
	n	(%)	*n*	(%)	(95% CI)	0.01 0.1 0.5 1 2 10 100
Liggins and Howie (1972)	49/532	(9.21)	84/538	(15.61)	0.56 (0.39–0.80)	
Block *et al.* (1977)	5/69	(7.25)	12/61	(19.67)	0.34 (0.12–0.94)	
Schutte *et al.* (1979)	11/64	(17.19)	17/58	(29.31)	0.51 (0.22–1.18)	
Taeusch *et al.* (1979)	7/56	(12.50)	14/71	(19.72)	0.60 (0.23–1.52)	
Doran *et al.* (1980)	4/81	(4.94)	10/63	(15.87)	0.29 (0.10–0.88)	
Teramo *et al.* (1980)	3/38	(7.89)	3/42	(7.14)	1.11 (0.21–5.83)	
Gamsu *et al.* (1989)	7/131	(5.34)	16/137	(11.68)	0.45 (0.19–1.05)	
Collaborative Group (1981)	42/371	(11.32)	59/372	(15.86)	0.68 (0.45–1.03)	
Morales *et al.* (1986)	30/121	(24.79)	63/124	(50.81)	0.33 (0.20–0.56)	
Papageorgiou *et al.* (1979)	7/71	(9.86)	23/75	(30.67)	0.28 (0.13–0.63)	
Morrison *et al.* (1978)	6/67	(8.96)	20/59	(33.90)	0.22 (0.09–0.52)	
Schmidt *et al.* (1984)	9/34	(26.47)	10/31	(32.26)	0.76 (0.26–2.20)	
Typical odds ratio (95% confidence interval)					0.48 (0.40–0.58)	

presented in Table 45.2 indicate that antenatal corticosteroid administration is associated with a valuable reduction in the incidence of this form of morbidity.

In the first randomized trial of antenatal corticosteroid administration to be reported, Liggins and Howie (1972) showed that a statistically significant reduction in the incidence of respiratory distress syndrome was detected only if more than 24 hours and less than 7 days had elapsed between commencement of treatment and delivery. Forty per cent of the babies fell into this category and Table 45.3 shows the effect of corticosteroids on respiratory distress in this subgroup. As expected, the typical odds ratio of 0.31 (95 per cent confidence interval 0.23–0.42) suggests a more marked effect than that seen in the group taken as a whole (typical odds ratio 0.48; 95 per cent confidence interval 0.40–0.58). Analyses based on all the available data show that among babies born within 24 hours of starting corticosteroid treatment (Table 45.4) and among those delivered more than 7 days after starting treatment (Table 45.5), there were also reductions in the incidence of respiratory distress, but these did not reach conventional levels of statistical significance.

The majority of babies randomized in these trials were born between 30 and 34 weeks' gestation. Although there is a widespread view that corticosteroids are ineffective at gestational ages below 30 weeks (Roberton 1982), data available in 6 of the trials provides a better estimate of the effects of corticosteroid administration in these very immature babies. Among babies born at less than 31 weeks' gestation, corticosteroid administration is followed by a more dramatic reduction (typical odds ratio 0.38; 95 per cent confidence interval 0.24–0.60) in the risk of respiratory distress than observed for preterm babies as a whole (Table 45.6).

Respiratory distress is such a rare condition among babies born after 34 weeks' gestation that large numbers are required to assess any protective effects of corticosteroids that may exist at this gestational age. The available data yielded only 29 cases of respiratory distress from eight trials (Table 45.7). Although the point estimate of the typical odds ratio (0.62) is consistent with those derived from other subgroups, the confidence interval (0.29–1.30) includes unity, so it fails to prove or disprove the view that corticosteroid therapy is pointless in pregnancies of more than 34 weeks' gestation. Nevertheless, the available evidence does not

Table 45.3 Effect of corticosteroids prior to preterm delivery on respiratory distress following optimal treatment

Study	EXPT		CTRL		Odds ratio	Graph of odds ratios and confidence intervals
	n	(%)	*n*	(%)	(95% CI)	0.01 0.1 0.5 1 2 10 100
Liggins and Howie (1972)	16/182	(8.79)	37/156	(23.72)	0.32 (0.18–0.58)	
Block *et al.* (1977)	4/36	(11.11)	6/29	(20.69)	0.48 (0.13–1.86)	
Schutte *et al.* (1979)	0/22	(0.00)	6/25	(24.00)	0.12 (0.02–0.66)	
Taeusch *et al.* (1979)	2/15	(13.33)	7/28	(25.00)	0.50 (0.11–2.30)	
Doran *et al.* (1980)	1/18	(5.56)	1/13	(7.69)	0.71 (0.04–12.35)	
Teramo *et al.* (1980)	1/38	(2.63)	1/42	(2.38)	1.11 (0.07–18.08)	
Gamsu *et al.* (1989)	1/131	(0.76)	2/137	(1.46)	0.53 (0.06–5.18)	
Collaborative Group (1981)	14/151	(9.27)	29/144	(20.14)	0.42 (0.22–0.80)	
Morales *et al.* (1986)	16/64	(25.00)	31/48	(64.58)	0.20 (0.09–0.42)	
Papageorgiou *et al.* (1979)	6/29	(20.69)	19/32	(59.38)	0.21 (0.08–0.57)	
Morrison *et al.* (1978)	3/49	(6.12)	8/45	(17.78)	0.33 (0.09–1.15)	
Schmidt *et al.* (1984)	4/26	(15.38)	8/19	(42.11)	0.26 (0.07–0.99)	
Typical odds ratio (95% confidence interval)					0.31 (0.23–0.42)	

Table 45.4 Effect of corticosteroids prior to preterm delivery on respiratory distress following delivery <24 hours after treatment

Study	EXPT		CTRL		Odds ratio	Graph of odds ratios and confidence intervals
	n	(%)	*n*	(%)	(95% CI)	0.01 0.1 0.5 1 2 10 100
Liggins and Howie (1972)	19/96	(19.79)	25/107	(23.36)	0.81 (0.42–1.58)	
Block *et al.* (1977)	1/13	(7.69)	6/15	(40.00)	0.19 (0.04–1.02)	
Schutte *et al.* (1979)	5/10	(50.00)	6/12	(50.00)	1.00 (0.19–5.15)	
Taeusch *et al.* (1979)	5/19	(26.32)	5/19	(26.32)	1.00 (0.24–4.16)	
Doran *et al.* (1980)	3/26	(11.54)	5/20	(25.00)	0.40 (0.09–1.83)	
Teramo *et al.* (1980)	2/11	(18.18)	2/11	(18.18)	1.00 (0.12–8.31)	
Collaborative Group (1981)	11/56	(19.64)	8/50	(16.00)	1.28 (0.48–3.44)	
Morales *et al.* (1986)	7/27	(25.93)	19/35	(54.29)	0.32 (0.12–0.87)	
Morrison *et al.* (1978)	3/18	(16.67)	6/14	(42.86)	0.29 (0.06–1.32)	
Schmidt *et al.* (1984)	5/7	(71.43)	2/12	(16.67)	9.30 (1.42–60.98)	
Typical odds ratio (95% confidence interval)					0.72 (0.49–1.06)	

Table 45.5 Effect of corticosteroids prior to preterm delivery on respiratory distress following delivery >7 days after treatment

Study	EXPT		CTRL		Odds ratio	Graph of odds ratios and confidence intervals
	n	(%)	*n*	(%)	(95% CI)	0.01 0.1 0.5 1 2 10 100
Liggins and Howie (1972)	8/180	(4.44)	4/188	(2.13)	2.08 (0.66–6.56)	
Schutte *et al.* (1979)	6/17	(35.29)	5/9	(55.56)	0.45 (0.09–2.24)	
Doran *et al.* (1980)	0/30	(0.00)	3/28	(10.71)	0.12 (0.01–1.17)	
Teramo *et al.* (1980)	0/6	(0.00)	0/12	(0.00)	1.00 (1.00–1.00)	
Collaborative Group (1981)	6/102	(5.88)	11/105	(10.48)	0.55 (0.20–1.47)	
Morales et al. (1986)	7/30	(23.33)	13/30	(43.33)	0.41 (0.14–1.20)	
Typical odds ratio (95% confidence interval)					0.62 (0.35–1.08)	

Table 45.6 Effect of corticosteroids prior to preterm delivery on respiratory distress in babies <31 weeks' gestation

Study	EXPT		CTRL		Odds ratio	Graph of odds ratios and confidence intervals
	n	(%)	*n*	(%)	(95% CI)	0.01 0.1 0.5 1 2 10 100
Liggins and Howie (1972)	10/36	(27.78)	15/26	(57.69)	0.29 (0.11–0.82)	
Taeusch *et al.* (1979)	1/3	(33.33)	4/6	(66.67)	0.30 (0.02–4.18)	
Gamsu *et al.* (1989)	4/29	(13.79)	7/39	(17.95)	0.74 (0.20–2.70)	
Collaborative Group (1981)	6/10	(60.00)	7/16	(43.75)	1.87 (0.40–8.80)	
Morales *et al.* (1986)	17/53	(32.08)	32/52	(61.54)	0.31 (0.14–0.66)	
Papageorgiou *et al.* (1979)	2/5	(40.00)	11/12	(91.67)	0.07 (0.01–0.73)	
Morrison *et al.* (1978)	6/36	(16.67)	11/28	(39.29)	0.32 (0.11–0.97)	
Typical odds ratio (95% confidence interval)					0.38 (0.24–0.60)	

justify Keirse's (1984) condemnation of corticosteroid therapy in pregnancies of more than 34 weeks' maturity.

The results of the Collaborative Group (1981) suggested to the investigators that corticosteroid administration dramatically reduced the incidence of respiratory distress syndrome in female infants (odds ratio 0.25; 95 per cent confidence interval 0.12–0.53) but that it was without effect in male infants (odds ratio 1.07; 95 per cent confidence interval 0.58–1.96). Fortunately, Howie (1986) has provided data from the Auckland trial (Liggins *et al.* 1972) suggesting quite the reverse: male babies in that trial appeared to benefit substantially from antenatal corticosteroid administration (odds ratio 0.18; 95 per cent confidence interval 0.08–0.38), whereas no statistically significant advantage was detected in female infants (odds ratio 0.76; 95 per cent confidence interval 0.30–1.89)! Analyses based on all the available data on outcome by infant gender make it clear that this variable does not modify the effects of antenatal corticosteroid administration (Tables 45.8 and 45.9).

2.2 Other neonatal morbidity

Corticosteroid treatment reduces the risk not only of respiratory morbidity but also of other serious forms of

Table 45.7 Effect of corticosteroids prior to preterm delivery on respiratory distress in babies >34 weeks' gestation

Study	EXPT *n*	(%)	CTRL *n*	(%)	Odds ratio (95% CI)	Graph of odds ratios and confidence intervals (0.01 0.1 0.5 1 2 10 100)
Liggins and Howie (1972)	4/73	(5.48)	4/74	(5.41)	1.01 (0.25–4.20)	
Block *et al.* (1977)	1/36	(2.78)	3/25	(12.00)	0.23 (0.03–1.76)	
Schutte *et al.* (1979)	0/13	(0.00)	0/12	(0.00)	1.00 (1.00–1.00)	
Taeusch *et al.* (1979)	1/23	(4.35)	0/25	(0.00)	8.06 (0.16–99.99)	
Doran *et al.* (1980)	0/44	(0.00)	1/26	(3.85)	0.07 (0.00–3.91)	
Collaborative Group (1981)	5/183	(2.73)	8/166	(4.82)	0.56 (0.18–1.69)	
Papageorgiou *et al.* (1979)	0/25	(0.00)	0/17	(0.00)	1.00 (1.00–1.00)	
Schmidt *et al.* (1984)	1/77	(1.30)	1/67	(1.49)	0.87 (0.05–14.12)	
Typical odds ratio (95% confidence interval)					0.62 (0.29–1.30)	

Table 45.8 Effect of corticosteroids prior to preterm delivery on respiratory distress in male babies

Study	EXPT *n*	(%)	CTRL *n*	(%)	Odds ratio (95% CI)	Graph of odds ratios and confidence intervals (0.01 0.1 0.5 1 2 10 100)
Liggins and Howie (1972)	6/95	(6.32)	26/81	(32.10)	0.18 (0.08–0.38)	
Collaborative Group (1981)	24/161	(14.91)	24/170	(14.12)	1.07 (0.58–1.96)	
Morales *et al.* (1986)	19/63	(30.16)	36/57	(63.16)	0.27 (0.13–0.55)	
Typical odds ratio (95% confidence interval)					0.43 (0.29–0.64)	

Table 45.9 Effect of corticosteroids prior to preterm delivery on respiratory distress in female babies

Study	EXPT *n*	(%)	CTRL *n*	(%)	Odds ratio (95% CI)	Graph of odds ratios and confidence intervals (0.01 0.1 0.5 1 2 10 100)
Liggins and Howie (1972)	10/87	(11.49)	11/75	(14.67)	0.76 (0.30–1.89)	
Collaborative Group (1981)	7/146	(4.79)	24/128	(18.75)	0.25 (0.12–0.53)	
Morales *et al.* (1986)	11/58	(18.97)	27/61	(44.26)	0.32 (0.15–0.68)	
Typical odds ratio (95% confidence interval)					0.36 (0.23–0.57)	

Table 45.10 Effect of corticosteroids prior to preterm delivery on periventricular haemorrhage

Study	EXPT		CTRL		Odds ratio	Graph of odds ratios and confidence intervals
	n	(%)	*n*	(%)	(95% CI)	0.01 0.1 0.5 1 2 10 100
Liggins and Howie (1972)	6/532	(1.13)	14/538	(2.60)	0.45 (0.18–1.08)	
Doran *et al.* (1980)	1/81	(1.23)	3/63	(4.76)	0.27 (0.04–2.01)	
Gamsu *et al.* (1989)	2/131	(1.53)	4/137	(2.92)	0.53 (0.11–2.67)	
Morales *et al.* (1986)	1/121	(0.83)	2/124	(1.61)	0.52 (0.05–5.08)	
Typical odds ratio (95% confidence interval)					0.44 (0.22–0.88)	

Table 45.11 Effect of corticosteroids prior to preterm delivery on necrotizing enterocolitis

Study	EXPT		CTRL		Odds ratio	Graph of odds ratios and confidence intervals
	n	(%)	*n*	(%)	(95% CI)	0.01 0.1 0.5 1 2 10 100
Bauer *et al.* (1984)	6/307	(1.95)	21/297	(7.07)	0.30 (0.14–0.65)	
Morales *et al.* (1986)	1/121	(0.83)	4/124	(3.23)	0.30 (0.05–1.77)	
Morrison *et al.* (1978)	1/67	(1.49)	1/59	(1.69)	0.88 (0.05–14.30)	
Typical odds ratio (95% confidence interval)					0.32 (0.16–0.64)	

neonatal morbidity. Four of the randomized trials recorded information on periventricular haemorrhage (Table 45.10) indicating that antenatal corticosteroid therapy reduces the risk of this serious complication (odds ratio 0.44; 95 per cent confidence interval 0.22–0.88). This effect is likely to be related to the reduced risk of respiratory distress, although it might also reflect an effect of corticosteroids on the periventricular vasculature.

Three of the randomized trials also documented the incidence of necrotizing enterocolitis by treatment allocation (Table 45.11). Again, there appears to be a significant benefit. As with periventricular haemorrhage, this benefit probably arises secondarily to the reduction in respiratory distress syndrome and the need for mechanical ventilation. However, a more direct drug effect on the gastrointestinal tract or its vasculature may also be involved.

2.3 Mortality

Not surprisingly these marked effects on serious forms of neonatal morbidity are reflected in a substantial reduction (odds ratio 0.59; 95 per cent confidence interval 0.47–0.75) in the risk of early neonatal mortality (Table 45.12). It is also important to note that this reduction in neonatal mortality was not accompanied by an increased risk of fetal death. Stillbirth occurred with almost identical frequency in the two groups (Table 45.13).

2.4 Duration of hospital stay and cost of neonatal care

Further important evidence on the secondary benefits of a reduction in neonatal morbidity is provided by the data on the duration of hospital stay reported in two trials from the United States (Collaborative Group 1981; Morales *et al.* 1986) (Table 45.14). The significant reduction in the duration of neonatal hospitalization has obvious social and economic implications. Avery (1984) estimated that in the Collaborative Group trial the use of corticosteroids was associated with a saving of $1,197,000 and that appropriate use of antenatal corticosteroids could save $35 million per year in intensive care costs in the United States. Morales *et al.* (1986) reported an average saving of $17,300 per woman treated.

Table 45.12 Effect of corticosteroids prior to preterm delivery on early neonatal deaths

Study	EXPT		CTRL		Odds ratio
	n	(%)	*n*	(%)	(95% CI)
Liggins and Howie (1972)	36/532	(6.77)	60/538	(11.15)	0.58 (0.38–0.89)
Block *et al.* (1977)	1/69	(1.45)	5/61	(8.20)	0.22 (0.04–1.12)
Schutte *et al.* (1979)	3/64	(4.69)	12/58	(20.69)	0.23 (0.08–0.67)
Taeusch *et al.* (1979)	5/56	(8.93)	7/71	(9.86)	0.90 (0.27–2.96)
Doran *et al.* (1980)	2/81	(2.47)	10/63	(15.87)	0.18 (0.05–0.57)
Teramo *et al.* (1980)	0/38	(0.00)	0/42	(0.00)	1.00 (1.00–1.00)
Gamsu *et al.* (1989)	14/131	(10.69)	20/137	(14.60)	0.70 (0.34–1.44)
Collaborative Group (1981)	36/371	(9.70)	37/372	(9.95)	0.97 (0.60–1.58)
Morales *et al.* (1986)	7/121	(5.79)	13/124	(10.48)	0.54 (0.22–1.33)
Papageorgiou *et al.* (1979)	1/71	(1.41)	5/75	(6.67)	0.27 (0.05–1.36)
Morrison *et al.* (1978)	2/67	(2.99)	7/59	(11.86)	0.26 (0.07–1.03)
Schmidt *et al.* (1984)	5/34	(14.71)	5/31	(16.13)	0.90 (0.24–3.42)
Typical odds ratio (95% confidence interval)					0.59 (0.47–0.75)

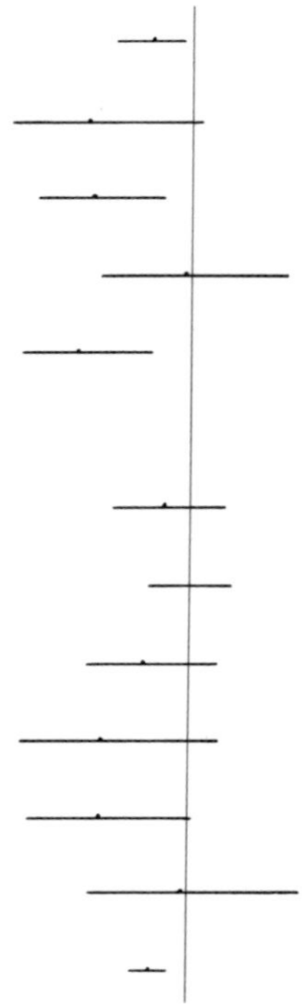

Graph of odds ratios and confidence intervals (scale: 0.01, 0.1, 0.5, 1, 2, 10, 100)

Table 45.13 Effect of corticosteroids prior to preterm delivery on stillbirths without lethal malformation

Study	EXPT		CTRL		Odds ratio
	n	(%)	*n*	(%)	(95% CI)
Liggins and Howie (1972)	31/532	(5.83)	28/538	(5.20)	1.13 (0.67–1.90)
Block *et al.* (1977)	3/69	(4.35)	0/61	(0.00)	6.78 (0.69–66.62)
Schutte *et al.* (1979)	2/64	(3.13)	0/58	(0.00)	6.84 (0.42–99.99)
Taeusch *et al.* (1979)	2/56	(3.57)	2/71	(2.82)	1.28 (0.17–9.42)
Doran *et al.* (1980)	1/81	(1.23)	3/63	(4.76)	0.27 (0.04–2.01)
Teramo *et al.* (1980)	0/38	(0.00)	0/42	(0.00)	1.00 (1.00–1.00)
Gamsu *et al.* (1989)	4/131	(3.05)	5/137	(3.65)	0.83 (0.22–3.14)
Collaborative Group (1981)	6/371	(1.62)	8/372	(2.15)	0.75 (0.26–2.16)
Morales *et al.* (1986)	0/121	(0.00)	0/124	(0.00)	1.00 (1.00–1.00)
Papageorgiou *et al.* (1979)	0/71	(0.00)	2/75	(2.67)	0.14 (0.01–2.28)
Typical odds ratio (95% confidence interval)					1.03 (0.68–1.54)

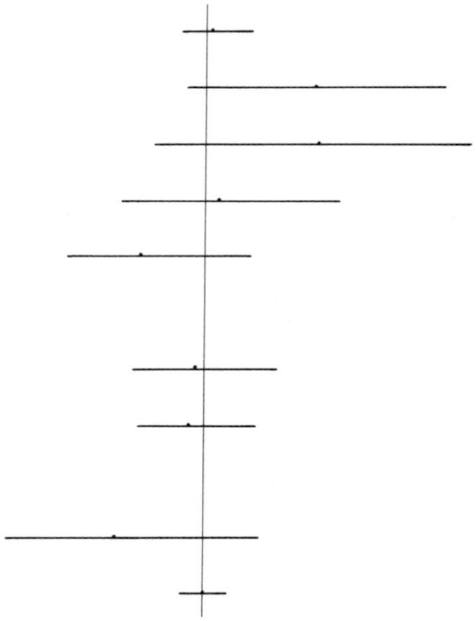

Graph of odds ratios and confidence intervals (scale: 0.01, 0.1, 0.5, 1, 2, 10, 100)

Table 45.14

Mean neonatal hospital days			
	Corticosteroid	Placebo	
Collaborative Group	21	25	$p = 0.03$
Morales *et al.*	22	38	$p < 0.05$

Estimated annual savings in USA assuming 10,000 babies at risk of RDS = $35,000,000 (Avery 1984)

3 Potential risks of antenatal corticosteroid administration

The valuable benefits of antenatal corticosteroid administration set out in Tables 45.2–45.14 must be weighed against potential maternal and fetal risks.

3.1 Potential risks to the mother

Instances of pulmonary oedema have been reported in pregnant women receiving a combination of corticosteroids and tocolytic drugs (Stubblefield and Kitzmiller 1980). In the trial of Morales *et al.* (1986), there were two cases of pulmonary oedema among women treated with corticosteroids and magnesium sulphate. Pulmonary oedema was not reported by the authors of the other randomized trials, so that it is difficult to estimate the magnitude of this risk (see Chapter 44). Other pharmacological effects of glucocorticoid therapy in adults are well known. Most of these side-effects relate to long term treatment and they provide little ground for concern when glucocorticoids are used for a period of 24–48 hours to promote fetal maturation, although even such short term treatment may carry a risk of gastrointestinal haemorrhage (Brown *et al.* 1975). The potential risks of glucocorticoid treatment in women with ruptured membranes, hypertensive diseases, and diabetes mellitus will be considered below.

An increased risk of infection is another theoretical adverse effect of antenatal corticosteroid therapy. In the reports on confidential enquiries into maternal deaths in England and Wales covering the period 1973 to 1981 (Department of Health and Social Security 1979, 1982, 1986), use of corticosteroids in association with preterm labour was mentioned in only two of the maternal deaths from septicaemia. Seven trials cited the incidence of maternal infection as a measure of outcome, using a wide-ranging series of criteria for this diagnosis. The confidence intervals around the point estimate of the effect on maternal infection are wide; they are compatible with either an increase or a decrease in the risk of infection (Table 45.15).

3.2 Potential risks to the baby

Many of the potential risks of steroid therapy are likely to be common to all infants delivered following corticosteroid administration, although the maturity of the infant and the dose and duration of exposure may influence the response. Evidence concerning such effects is available from four sources: animal studies; glucocorticoid treatment for maternal disease; glucocorticoid treatment in the neonate; and follow-up data from the trials of antenatal glucocorticoid administration for the prevention of neonatal morbidity and mortality (the studies on which this chapter focuses).

3.2.1 Evidence from animal studies

Glucocorticoids injected into mammalian fetuses pro-

Table 45.15 Effect of corticosteroids prior to preterm delivery on maternal infection

Study	EXPT *n*	EXPT (%)	CTRL *n*	CTRL (%)	Odds ratio (95% CI)	Graph of odds ratios and confidence intervals (0.01 0.1 0.5 1 2 10 100)
Liggins and Howie (1972)	5/108	(4.63)	6/91	(6.59)	0.69 (0.20–2.32)	
Taeusch *et al.* (1979)	14/56	(25.00)	8/71	(11.27)	2.59 (1.03–6.51)	
Gamsu *et al.* (1989)	6/126	(4.76)	6/125	(4.80)	0.99 (0.31–3.16)	
Collaborative Group (1981)	27/349	(7.74)	29/347	(8.36)	0.92 (0.53–1.59)	
Morales *et al.* (1986)	16/121	(13.22)	18/124	(14.52)	0.90 (0.44–1.85)	
Papageorgiou *et al.* (1979)	9/71	(12.68)	9/75	(12.00)	1.06 (0.40–2.85)	
Morrison *et al.* (1978)	4/67	(5.97)	2/59	(3.39)	1.76 (0.34–9.03)	
Schmidt *et al.* (1984)	13/32	(40.63)	9/29	(31.03)	1.51 (0.53–4.25)	
Typical odds ratio (95% confidence interval)					1.11 (0.81–1.51)	

duce impaired somatic and lung growth (Motoyama *et al.* 1971; Kotas *et al.* 1974). Since rapid glial cell proliferation, which normally occurs during the third trimester in the human fetus, occurs during early postnatal life in the rat (Cotterell *et al.* 1972), neonatal rats have been used to assess the effects of corticosteroids on the brain. The data indicate impairment of brain growth, myelinization, and subsequent neurological development (Howard and Granoff 1968; Schapiro *et al.* 1970; De Souza and Adlard 1973). Administration of 2 mg of betamethasone daily from day 120 to day 133 to pregnant Rhesus monkeys was associated with lower weights of fetal brain ($p < 0.01$), liver, pancreas, and heart ($p < 0.05$), compared with controls (Johnson *et al.* 1981).

The effect of corticosteroids on fetal lung growth has also been examined in animal models. Increased surfactant production appears to be achieved at the expense of a decrease in lung DNA and total weight (Kotas and Avery 1971). By 20 days of postnatal life, catch-up growth occurs in the neonatal lung (Kotas *et al.* 1974). Johnson *et al.* (1981) also found smaller lungs ($p < 0.005$) in treated neonatal Rhesus monkeys than in controls.

Most of the experimental studies in animals have been extensively reviewed by Taeusch (1975). These studies, however, while worrisome, do not reflect the doses and conditions of human antenatal glucocorticoid therapy. For instance, the dose of cortisol per kilogram of body weight that caused depression of cell division in the neonatal rat (Cotterell *et al.* 1972) is 25 times greater than the 12 mg betamethasone recommended by Howie and Liggins (1977). The dose of cortisol administered by Schapiro *et al.* (1970) to neonatal rats is comparable to a dose of 200 mg betamethasone given to a pregnant woman. These studies do, however, indicate areas that should be examined very carefully in humans.

3.2.2 Evidence from glucocorticoid therapy for maternal disease

Human fetuses may be exposed to exogenous glucocorticoids throughout pregnancy if their mothers are receiving long term steroid therapy for ulcerative colitis, asthma, rheumatoid arthritis, or other conditions. In a review of the literature, Bongiovanni and McPadden (1960) reported on 260 women who were given glucocorticoids for maternal disease during pregnancy. There were 15 'premature' infants, 8 stillbirths and 1 miscarriage—not a striking excess over expectation for any of these adverse outcomes. Two babies had cleft palates and one showed adrenocortical insufficiency. Walsh and Clark (1967) examined children between 1 and 6 years of age whose mothers had been treated with glucocorticoids during pregnancy and found no abnormalities. In a retrospective study, Koppe *et al.* (1979) identified 17 women who were treated with glucocorticoids during a total of 25 pregnancies. There was an increased incidence of fetal growth retardation, but at follow-up the children exhibited catch-up growth. With the exception of one child who had mental retardation, all children were developmentally normal when examined at various ages between 2 and 13 years.

3.2.3 Evidence from glucocorticoid therapy in human neonates

Human neonates have been exposed to glucocorticoid therapy in unsuccessful attempts to prevent retrolental fibroplasia and to treat respiratory distress syndrome substantially. In one of the three relevant trials (Silverman *et al.* 1951) infection was more common in the infants exposed to steroids; in the other two trials (Baden *et al.* 1972; Taeusch *et al.* 1979; Fitzhardinge *et al.* 1974) infection was more common among those who had received placebo. None of the observed differences was statistically significant.

Silverman and his colleagues (1951) observed cessation of growth during the treatment period, and catch-up growth occurred after completing therapy. This is consistent with the findings of Fitzhardinge *et al.* (1974) who found no differences in the growth of corticosteroid- and placebo-treated babies 1 year after exposure. Fitzhardinge *et al.* (1974), in a developmental assessment of infants treated with corticosteroids and untreated controls at 1 year of age, failed to detect any statistically significant differences in social development, speech, hearing, and fine motor skills. However, glucocorticoid-treated infants did show an excess of minor electroencephalographic abnormalities and poorer gross motor skills compared with controls.

It should be emphasized that the doses of glucocorticoid used in these attempts to prevent retrolental fibroplasia and to treat respiratory distress syndrome were up to five times higher than the equivalent dose of betamethasone recommended by Howie and Liggins (1977) for antenatal use. These differences in dose of glucocorticoids between human neonatal and antenatal therapy make it impossible to reach firm conclusions on the long term effects of antenatal therapy on the basis of data from neonatal treatments.

3.2.4 Evidence from the randomized trials of antenatal corticosteroid administration

The immunosuppressive effects of corticosteroid therapy could result in an increased susceptibility to infection or to a delay in its recognition. Table 45.16 presents an overview of the incidence of fetal or neonatal infection in the 8 trials which reported this information. There is no evidence that corticosteroid therapy results in an increased risk of perinatal infection (typical odds ratio 0.83; 95 per cent confidence interval 0.54–1.26), although the confidence interval is wide. A further analysis examining the incidence of perinatal

Table 45.16 Effect of corticosteroids prior to preterm delivery on fetal or neonatal infection

Study	EXPT		CTRL		Odds ratio	Graph of odds ratios and confidence intervals
	n	(%)	*n*	(%)	(95% CI)	0.01 0.1 0.5 1 2 10 100
Howie and Liggins (1977)	5/532	(0.94)	6/538	(1.12)	0.84 (0.26–2.76)	
Taeusch *et al.* (1979)	7/56	(12.50)	4/71	(5.63)	2.37 (0.68–8.18)	
Doran *et al.* (1980)	1/81	(1.23)	3/63	(4.76)	0.27 (0.04–2.01)	
Gamsu *et al.* (1989)	4/126	(3.17)	7/125	(5.60)	0.56 (0.17–1.88)	
Collaborative Group (1981)	4/371	(1.08)	10/372	(2.69)	0.42 (0.15–1.21)	
Morales *et al.* (1986)	11/121	(9.09)	11/124	(8.87)	1.03 (0.43–2.46)	
Papageorgiou *et al.* (1979)	4/71	(5.63)	4/75	(5.33)	1.06 (0.26–4.39)	
Schmidt *et al.* (1984)	5/34	(14.71)	5/31	(16.13)	0.90 (0.24–3.42)	
Typical odds ratio (95% confidence interval)					0.83 (0.54–1.26)	

Table 45.17 Effect of corticosteroids prior to preterm delivery on fetal or neonatal infection after rupture of membranes

Study	EXPT		CTRL		Odds ratio	Graph of odds ratios and confidence intervals
	n	(%)	*n*	(%)	(95% CI)	0.01 0.1 0.5 1 2 10 100
Taeusch *et al.* (1979)	4/19	(21.05)	3/24	(12.50)	1.85 (0.37–9.25)	
Morales *et al.* (1986)	11/121	(9.09)	11/124	(8.87)	1.03 (0.43–2.46)	
Papageorgiou *et al.* (1979)	4/17	(23.53)	2/19	(10.53)	2.48 (0.44–14.03)	
Schmidt *et al.* (1984)	4/24	(16.67)	3/17	(17.65)	0.93 (0.18–4.78)	
Typical odds ratio (95% confidence interval)					1.26 (0.66–2.40)	

infection in cases with prolonged rupture of the membranes revealed no increased risk of infection, although, once again, the confidence interval is wide (typical odds ratio 1.26; 95 per cent confidence interval 0.66–2.40) (Table 45.17) (see Chapter 43). Unfortunately, this information is not available for the two largest trials (Howie and Liggins 1977; Collaborative Group 1981). However, 44 per cent of women in each arm of the Collaborative Group had ruptured membranes for more than 1 hour before the onset of uterine contractions, and there was no increase in the incidence of infection among women who had received corticosteroids. In fact, there was a lower incidence of positive cultures in the first 72 hours of life in the corticosteroid-treated group than among the controls.

The most reliable evidence about the long term effects of antenatal corticosteroid therapy comes from follow-up of children whose mothers had been treated in the randomized trials. Three follow-up studies have been published (Butterfill and Harvey 1979; MacArthur *et al.* 1981, 1982; Collaborative Group 1984). Butterfill and Harvey's (1979) follow-up study, however, incorporated non-randomized with randomized cohorts, and unfortunately it is not now possible to disaggregate the data to allow unbiased comparisons (Harvey, personal communication).

MacArthur and his colleagues (1981, 1982) followed 318 children of mothers with unplanned preterm labour who entered the Auckland trial between October 1969 and April 1972. Because of the reduced neonatal mortal-

Table 45.18 Effect of corticosteroids prior to preterm delivery on neurological abnormality at follow-up

Study	EXPT		CTRL		Odds ratio	Graph of odds ratios and confidence intervals
	n	(%)	*n*	(%)	(95% CI)	0.01 0.1 0.5 1 2 10 100
MacArthur *et al.* (1982)	12/139	(8.63)	15/111	(13.51)	0.60 (0.27–1.35)	
Collaborative Group (1984)	9/200	(4.50)	15/206	(7.28)	0.61 (0.27–1.38)	
Typical odds ratio (95% confidence interval)					0.61 (0.34–1.08)	

Table 45.19 Effect of corticosteroids prior to preterm delivery on fetal death with maternal hypertension

Study	EXPT		CTRL		Odds ratio	Graph of odds ratios and confidence intervals
	n	(%)	*n*	(%)	(95% CI)	0.01 0.1 0.5 1 2 10 100
Liggins and Howie (1972)	12/47	(25.53)	3/43	(6.98)	3.75 (1.24–11.30)	
Gamsu *et al.* (1989)	0/12	(0.00)	0/6	(0.00)	1.00 (1.00–1.00)	
Collaborative Group (1981)	0/40	(0.00)	0/43	(0.00)	1.00 (1.00–1.00)	
Typical odds ratio (95% confidence interval)					3.75 (1.24–11.30)	

ity rate in corticosteroid-treated babies in this trial (Liggins and Howie 1972; Howie and Liggins 1977) (see Table 45.12), survivors from the corticosteroid arm had a lower mean gestational age at delivery than survivors from the control group. Thus one might expect the corticosteroid-treated group to be more likely to show impaired function. The follow-up studies, however, suggest that neurological and intellectual functions, if anything, are better in the corticosteroid-treated group than in the controls (Table 45.18). This is plausible in the light of the complications that sometimes accompany both respiratory distress and its treatment.

4 Special circumstances

The foregoing has dealt with the use of corticosteroids to promote pulmonary maturity in all situations in which preterm birth is anticipated. There are, however, certain situations in which its use could confer special benefits or involve special hazards. Most of these involve elective delivery.

Elective preterm delivery differs from spontaneous preterm birth in at least four main ways. First, in contrast to spontaneous preterm labour, the timing of elective preterm delivery is under the control of the obstetrician, thus facilitating the interval required to gain maximum benefit from corticosteroid administration.

Second, caesarean section with its increased risk of respiratory distress (Usher *et al.* 1971; Fedrick and Butler 1972; Farrell and Avery 1975) (see Chapter 70), is the most common route of delivery in this group of babies (Rush *et al.* 1976; Boylan and O'Driscoll 1983).

Third, elective preterm delivery usually takes place somewhat later in gestation than spontaneous preterm delivery (Rush *et al.* 1976) and consequently the absolute risk of respiratory distress is usually lower.

Fourth, elective preterm delivery is often undertaken for conditions such as severe hypertension, Rhesus isoimmunization, or diabetes (Kanhai and Keirse 1982) which give rise to concern when corticosteroid administration is contemplated.

Although most of these situations are addressed in more detail in other chapters in this book (see Chapters 33, 35, and 36), their relation to the use of corticosteroids will be dealt with in this section.

4.1 Hypertensive disease

Hypertensive disorders in pregnancy constitute one of the major indications for elective preterm delivery (Keirse and Kanhai 1981). Four of the trials (Howie and Liggins 1977; Morrison *et al.* 1978; Collaborative Group 1981; Gamsu *et al.* 1989, and unpublished data) included women with hypertensive disease. Three groups of investigators responded to requests for additional information about these women, however. Table 45.19 shows that there was a statistically significantly increased risk of fetal death associated with corticosteroid use in the 90 women with pre-eclampsia studied in the Auckland trial (Howie and Liggins 1977). Detailed analysis of these deaths subsequently showed that all 12 deaths occurred in women with proteinuria of more than 2 g per day for more than 14 days, a severity of disease that was not found in any of the placebo treated women. There were no fetal deaths of babies of a similar number of hypertensive women in the two other trials from which data are available to address this issue. A consistent adverse effect of corticosteroids would have resulted in an increased incidence of stillbirth overall, but as shown previously (Table 45.13) this did not occur.

Even in the absence of any adverse effect of corticosteroids in women with pre-eclampsia, the clinician is faced with the possible risks of postponing delivery for the amount of time required to achieve a useful effect of corticosteroid administration. In some cases the delay involved may constitute an unacceptable risk of eclampsia or cerebral haemorrhage in the mother.

4.2 Intrauterine growth retardation

Intrauterine growth retardation, like hypertensive disease in pregnancy, is a common indication for elective preterm delivery. Moreover, the two conditions often coexist. Fetuses with growth retardation in the absence of maternal hypertension may have accelerated pulmonary maturation (Gluck and Kulovich 1973). This does not of necessity imply that there would not be benefit from corticosteroid administration in these fetuses.

A potential disadvantage of antenatal glucocorticoid therapy in this situation is the risk of neonatal hypoglycaemia, which is an important complication in growth-retarded infants. One trial (Papageorgiou *et al.* 1979) reported 11 cases of neonatal hypoglycaemia among 75 corticosteroid-treated babies compared with 5 in 71 controls. Without information from other trials it is difficult to know whether this is anything more than a chance difference.

4.3 Diabetes mellitus

Maternal diabetes mellitus may predispose to the development of respiratory distress syndrome (see Chapter 36). Infants of mothers with diabetes mellitus had 5.6 times the risk of developing respiratory distress syndrome when compared with infants of non-diabetic mothers, matched for gestational age and mode of delivery (Robert *et al.* 1976). The results of the 12 randomized trials reviewed here do not clarify whether or not the use of corticosteroids is of benefit in preterm delivery of diabetic women as only 35 such women were included in the trials.

While the efficacy of antenatal glucocorticoids in pregnancies complicated by diabetes mellitus is unknown, the potential side-effects should be a source of concern. Fetal hyperinsulinism may or may not cause cortisol resistance in the fetal lung. There can be little argument that administration of glucocorticoids will cause insulin resistance in the diabetic. Loss of diabetic control is to be expected with the doses of glucocorticoids administered to promote pulmonary maturation. Therefore, antenatal corticosteroid therapy in the diabetic woman would require exceptionally close supervision, possibly with continuous intravenous insulin and frequent blood glucose estimation. Failure to maintain control can result in either ketoacidosis which carries a high perinatal mortality rate (Drury *et al.* 1976) or in a state of fetal hyperinsulinism which would increase the likelihood of failure to respond to glucocorticoid therapy. Corticosteroid administration, if used at all in diabetic women, should be used with great caution, as it may well do more harm than good.

4.4 Rhesus isoimmunization

Elective preterm delivery plays an important role in the management of Rhesus isoimmunization (Ogborn *et al.* 1977) (see Chapter 35). Unlike other conditions associated with chronic intrauterine stress, Rhesus disease is not thought to provoke an acceleration of pulmonary maturation (Gluck and Kulovich 1973). In fact, there is some evidence that the lecithin/sphingomyelin ratio in the 3rd trimester may be lower in Rhesus-sensitized infants than in normal pregnancy (Aubry *et al.* 1976), and may actually fall in response to an acute haemolytic crisis in the fetus (Whitfield 1976). However, it is not clear whether this is a true reflection of lung maturity in those circumstances.

Fifty-nine women with Rhesus sensitization were included in the trials conducted by Liggins and Howie (1972) and 3 in the trial conducted by Morrison *et al.* (1978). While there is a trend towards a reduction in perinatal mortality and in the incidence of respiratory distress syndrome in betamethasone-treated infants compared with controls (Liggins and Howie 1972), the numbers are too small for separate analysis.

There are no specific contraindications to the administration of glucocorticoids in women with Rhesus isoimmunization. The fact that amniocentesis for bilirubin spectrophotometry is an essential part of the management of Rhesus isoimmunization, provides an opportunity for the estimation of lung maturity. When the lecithin/sphingomyelin ratio is less than 2.0 and there is a high risk of intrauterine death, early delivery, facilitated by the use of corticosteroids, may be worth considering as an alternative to intrauterine transfusions (see Chapter 35). As corticosteroids may result in an artefactual drop in optical density (Caritis *et al.* 1977) they should not be administered until a commitment to delivery has been made.

Table 45.20

Authors	Entry criteria	Exclusion criteria	Treatment regimen	Diagnostic criteria for RDS	No. randomized	Randomization unknown	No. unreported
Wauer *et al.* (1982)	Premature rupture of membranes. Progressive dilatation of cervix. Estimated gestation 24–36 weeks.	Delivery expected within 24 hours.	Ambroxol 1 g daily for 5 days or placebo.	Yes	246	0	130
Klink (1984)	Women in premature labour 29–36 weeks.	Not stated	Ambroxol 1 g daily of Intralipid 60 ml intra-amniotically.	No	37	0	0
Luerti *et al.* (1987)	Women with threatened or planned premature delivery 27–34 weeks.	Severe hypertension. Uncertain dates. Diabetes. Hyperthyroidism. Drug addition with heroin.	Ambroxol 1 g daily for 5 days or 1 g 12-hourly × 4 or betamethasone 12 g in 2 doses.	Yes	315	0	38
Wolff *et al.* (1987)	Premature contractions or induced labour 28–36 weeks.	Results not reported for preterm delivery <72 hours after admission.	Ambroxol 1 g daily for 5 days; betamethasone 8 mg daily × 2 days.	Yes	133	10	$\frac{10}{133}$

4.5 Multiple pregnancies

Multiple pregnancies make an important contribution to the mortality and morbidity associated with preterm delivery. Data derived from the multiple pregnancies studied in the Collaborative Group trial (1981) analysed by Burkett *et al.* (1986) suggest that the benefits associated with steroids might be less in multiple than in singleton pregnancies. This apparent difference may simply reflect the play of chance, but it may also reflect a need for higher doses of the drug in these circumstances.

5 Other agents used to promote pulmonary maturity

There are strong theoretical reasons why other agents such as thyroxine, thyroid-releasing hormone, aminophylline, and caffeine should accelerate lung maturation (Gross 1979; Schellenberg *et al.* 1988). Table 45.20 summarizes the trials of Ambroxol (bromhexine metabolite VIII) reported by Wauer *et al.* (1982), Klink *et al.* (1984), Luerti *et al.* (1987) and Wolff *et al.* (1987). Wauer *et al.* (1982) compared Ambroxol with placebo. Only 116 of 246 patients appear to have delivered liveborn infants of less than 36 weeks' gestation. These are the only adequately reported cases in the trial. A reduction in the incidence of respiratory distress is seen in Ambroxol-treated cases (Table 45.21). The numbers in the Klink *et al.* (1984) trial do not permit firm conclusions to be drawn about Intralipid and Ambroxol. Luerti *et al.* (1987) and Wolff *et al.* (1987) reported a reduced incidence of respiratory distress syndrome in babies whose mothers were treated with Ambroxol compared with those treated with betamethasone (Table 45.22). However, the betamethasone-treated group contained 20 preterm twins, of whom 7 developed respiratory distress syndrome, while the Ambroxol group contained only 11 preterm twins, none of whom developed respiratory distress.

The main disadvantage of Ambroxol therapy appears to be the 5 days required to complete therapy. In the trial of Luerti *et al.* (1987), 18 per cent of cases allocated to Ambroxol did not complete the course of treatment, while all allocated to corticosteroid therapy did.

Preliminary evidence derived from trials assessing the effects of giving thyroid-releasing hormone in conjunction with corticosteroids are encouraging (Liggins *et al.* 1988; Morales *et al.* 1989). In the trial of Morales *et al.* (1989) maternal administration of thyroid releasing hormone with corticosteroids was associated with an important reduction in the need for artificial ventilation and in the incidence of bronchopulmonary dysplasia.

6 Conclusions

6.1 Implications for current practice

This overview of randomized trials provides ample evidence that antenatal treatment with 24 mg betamethasone, or 24 mg dexamethasone, or 2 g hydrocortisone is associated with a significant reduction in the risks of neonatal respiratory distress. This reduction is of the order of 40 to 60 per cent and is independent of

Table 45.21 Effect of antenatal ambroxol vs. placebo prior to preterm delivery on respiratory distress syndrome

Study	EXPT		CTRL		Odds ratio	Graph of odds ratios and confidence intervals
	n	(%)	*n*	(%)	(95% CI)	0.01 0.1 0.5 1 2 10 100
Wauer *et al.* (1982)	13/56	(23.21)	25/60	(41.67)	0.44 (0.20–0.94)	
Typical odds ratio (95% confidence interval)					0.44 (0.20–0.94)	

Table 45.22 Effect of maternal ambroxol vs. betamethasone for fetal lung maturation on respiratory distress syndrome

Study	EXPT		CTRL		Odds ratio	Graph of odds ratios and confidence intervals
	n	(%)	*n*	(%)	(95% CI)	0.01 0.1 0.5 1 2 10 100
Luerti *et al.* (1987)	11/171	(6.43)	27/144	(18.75)	0.31 (0.16–0.62)	
Wolff *et al.* (1987)	2/59	(3.39)	6/60	(10.00)	0.35 (0.08–1.47)	
Typical odds ratio (95% confidence interval)					0.32 (0.17–0.59)	

gender. Furthermore, the benefit of antenatal corticosteroids appears to apply to babies born at all gestational ages at which respiratory distress syndrome may occur. While the greatest benefits are seen in babies delivered more than 24 hours and less than 7 days after commencement of therapy, babies delivered before or after this optimum period also appear to benefit. This reduction in the risk of respiratory distress is accompanied by reductions in periventricular haemorrhage and necrotizing enterocolitis. This in turn results in a reduced mortality rate and in a reduction of the cost and duration of neonatal care.

These benefits are achieved without any detectable increase in the risk of maternal, fetal, or neonatal infection, even in the presence of prolonged rupture of the membranes. Antenatal corticosteroid therapy does not increase the risk of stillbirth.

6.2 Implications for future research

The benefits of antenatal corticosteroids have been established. No further trials are necessary with the exception of certain specific situations (such as pre-eclampsia), or to establish other dosages or routes of administration. Specifically, a trial to establish the correct dose of drugs to use in multiple pregnancy would be helpful. Although the 5-day interval required makes it impractical, the demonstrated efficacy of Ambroxol suggests that other agents as well as corticosteroids may accelerate pulmonary maturity. In particular, the currently recruiting randomized comparisons of corticosteroids and thyroid releasing hormone with corticosteroids used alone (Liggins *et al.* 1988; Gross, personal communication) should provide valuable information.

References

Aubry RH, Rourke JE, Almanza R, Cantor RM, Van Doren JE (1976). The lecithin–sphingomyelin ratio in a high risk obstetric population. J Obstet Gynaecol, 47: 21–27.

Avery ME (1984). The argument for prenatal administration of dexamethasone to prevent respiratory distress syndrome. J Pediatr, 104: 240.

Baden M, Bauer C, Colle E, Klein G, Taeusch HW, Stern L (1972). A controlled trial of hydrocortisone therapy in infants with respiratory distress syndrome. Pediatrics, 50: 526–534.

Baillie CR, Malan AF, Saunders MC, Davey DA (1976). The active management of preterm labour and its effects on fetal outcome. Austral NZ J Obstet Gynaecol, 16: 94–99.

Bajuk B, Kitchen WH, Lissenden JV, Yu VYH (1981). Perinatal factors affecting survival of very low birthweight infants—a study of two hospitals. Austral Paediatr J, 17: 277–280.

Bauer CR, Morrison JC, Poole WK, Korones SB, Boehm JJ, Rigatto H, Zachman RD (1984). A decreased incidence of necrotising enterocolitis after prenatal glucorticoid therapy. Pediatrics, 73: 682–688.

Block MF, Kling OR, Crosby WM (1977). Antenatal glucorticoid therapy for the prevention of respiratory distress syndrome in the premature infant. Obstet Gynecol, 50: 186–190.

Bongiovanni A, McPadden A (1960). Steroids during pregnancy and possible fetal consequences. Fertil Steril, 2: 181.

Boylan P, O'Driscoll K (1983). Improvement in perinatal rate attributed to spontaneous preterm labor without use of tocolytic agents. Am J Obstet Gynecol, 145: 781–783.

Brown G, Gabert H, Stenchever M (1975). Respiratory distress syndrome. Obstet Gynecol Surv, 30: 71–90.

Burkett G, Bauer CR, Morrison JC, Cuet LB (1986). Effect of prenatal dexamethasone administration on prevention of respiratory distress syndrome in twin pregnancies. J Perinatol, 6: 304–308.

Butterfill AM, Harvey DR (1979). Follow-up study of babies exposed to betamethasone before birth. Arch Dis Child, 54: 725.

Caritis SN, Mueller-Heubach E, Edelstone DJ (1977). Effect of betamethasone on analysis of amniotic fluid in rhesus sensitised pregnancy. Am J Obstet Gynecol, 127: 529–532.

Collaborative Group on Antenatal Steroid Therapy (1981). Effect of antenatal dexamethasone therapy on prevention of respiratory distress syndrome. Am J Obstet Gynecol, 141: 276–287.

Collaborative Group on Antenatal Steroid Therapy (1984). Effect of antenatal steroid administration on the infant: Long-term follow-up. J Pediatr, 104: 259–267.

Cotterell M, Balazs R, Johnson AL (1972). Effects of corticosteroids on the biochemical maturation of rat postnatal cell formation. J Neurochem, 19: 2151–2167.

Department of Health and Social Security (1979). Report on Confidential Enquiries into Maternal Deaths in England and Wales 1973–1975. Report on Health and Social Subjects No. 14. London: Her Majesty's Stationery Office.

Department of Health and Social Security (1982). Report on Confidential Enquiries into Maternal Deaths in England and Wales 1976–1978. Report on Health and Social Subjects No. 26. London: Her Majesty's Stationery Office.

Department of Health and Social Security (1986). Report on Confidential Enquiries into Maternal Deaths in England and Wales 1979–1981. Report on Health and Social Subjects No. 29. London: Her Majesty's Stationery Office.

De Souza S, Adlard B (1973). Growth of suckling rats after treatment with dexamethasone or cortisol. Arch Dis Child, 48: 519–522.

Dluholucky S, Babic J, Taufer J (1976). Reduction of incidence and mortality of respiratory distress syndrome by administration of hydrocortisone to the mother. Arch Dis Child, 51: 420–423.

Doran TA, Swyer P, MacMurray B, Mahon W, Enhorning G, Bernstein A, Falk M, Wood M (1980). Results of a double blind controlled study on the use of betamethasone in the prevention of respiratory distress syndrome. Am J Obstet Gynecol, 136: 313–320.

Drury MJ, Greene AT, Stronge JM (1976). Pregnancy complicated by diabetes mellitus. A study of 600 pregnancies. Obstet Gynecol, 49: 519–522.

Farrell PM, Avery ME (1975). Hyaline membrane disease. Am Rev Respir Dis, 3: 657–688.

Farrell PM, Engle MJ, Zachman RD, Curet LB, Morrison JC, Rao AV, Poole WK (1983). Amniotic fluid phosopholipids after maternal administration of dexamethasone. Am J Obstet Gynecol, 145: 484–490.

Fedrick J, Butler NR (1972). Hyaline membrane disease. Lancet, 2: 768–769.

Fitzhardinge PM, Eisen A, Letjenyi C, Metrakos K, Ramsay M (1974). Sequelae of early steroid administration to the newborn infant. Pediatrics, 53: 877–883.

Gamsu HR, Mullinger BM, Donnai P, Dash CH (1989). Antenatal administration of bethamethasone to prevent respiratory distress syndrome in preterm infants: report of a UK multicentre trial. Br J Obstet Gynaecol, in press.

Gluck L, Kulovich MV (1973). Lecithin sphingomyelin ratios in normal and abnormal pregnancy. Am J Obstet Gynecol, 115: 539–552.

Gross I (1979). The hormonal regulation of fetal lung maturation. Clin Perinatol, 6: 377–395.

Gunston KD, Davey DA (1978a). Effects of prenatal phenobarbitone, and dexamethasone administration on the total phospholipid concentration of amniotic fluid. S Afr Med J, 54: 1141–1143.

Gunston KD, Davey DA (1978b). Growth retarded fetuses and pulmonary maturity. S Afr Med J, 54: 493–494.

Howard E, Granoff DM (1968). Increased voluntary running and decreased motor coordination in mice after neonatal corticosterone implantation. Exp Neurol, 22: 661–673.

Howie RN (1986). Pharmacological acceleration of lung maturation In: Respiratory Distress Syndrome. Villee CA, Villee DB, Zuckerman J (eds). London: Academic Press, pp 385–396.

Howie RN, Liggins GC (1973). Prevention of respiratory distress syndrome in premature infants by antepartum glucocorticoid treatment. In: Respiratory Distress Syndrome. Villee CA, Villee DB, Zuckerman J (eds). London: Academic Press, pp 369–370.

Howie RN, Liggins GC (1977). Clinical trial of antepartum betamethasone therapy for prevention of respiratory distress in pre-term infants. In: Preterm Labour: Proceedings of the Fifth Study Group of the Royal College of Obstetricians and Gynaecologists. Anderson ABM, Beard R, Brudenell JM, Dunn P (eds). London: Royal College of Obsteticians and Gynaecologists, pp 281–289.

Howie RN, Liggins GC (1980). Corticosteroids can prevent neonatal respiratory distress syndrome. Drug Ther Bull, 18: 101.

Howie RN, Liggins GC (1982). The New Zealand study of antepartum glucocorticoid treatment. In: Lung development: Biological and Clinical Perspectives, II. Farrell PM (ed). London: Academic Press, pp 255–265.

Johnson JW, Mitzner W, Beck JC, London WT, Sly DL, Lee PA, Khouzami VA, Cavalieri RL (1981). Long-term effects of betamethasone on fetal development. Am J Obstet Gynecol, 141: 1053–1064.

Kanhai HHH, Keirse MJNC (1982). Perinatal hazards of elective versus spontaneous preterm birth. In: Abstracts of VIII European Congress of Perinatal Medicine, Brussels, 1982. Thiery M, Senterre J, Derom R (eds).

Keirse MJNC (1984). Obstetrical attitudes to glucocorticoid treatment for lung maturation: Time for a change? Eur J Obstet Gynecol Reprod Biol, 17: 247–255.

Keirse MJNC, Kanhai HHH (1981). An obstetrical viewpoint on preterm birth with particular reference to perinatal morbidity and mortality. In: Aspects of Perinatal Morbidity. Huisjes HJ (ed). Groningen: Universitaire Boekhandel Nederland, pp 1–35.

Kleinschmidt R, Schroeder M, Preibsch W, Mattheus R, Hofman D (1977). Induction of lung maturity in pending premature delivery and scheduled premature delivery. Zbl Gynäkol 99: 147–154.

Klink F, von Klitzing L, Oberhauser F (1984). A comparitive study between Ambroxol and Intralipid for respiratory distress prophylaxis in premature babies. J Perinat Med, 12: 42–43.

Koppe JG, Smolders De Haas H, Kloosterman GJ (1979). Effects of glucocorticoids during pregnancy on the outcome of the children directly after birth and in the long run. Eur J Obstet Gynecol Reprod Biol, 7: 293.

Kotas RV, Avery ME (1971). Accelerated appearance of pulmonary surfactant in the fetal rabbit. J Appl Physiol, 30: 358–361.

Kotas RV, Mims LC, Hart LK (1974). Reversible inhibition of lung cell number after glucorticoid injection into fetal rabbits to enhance surfactant appearance. Pediatrics, 53: 358–361.

Liggins GC (1969). Premature delivery of foetal lambs infused with glucorticoids. J Endocrinol, 45: 515–523.

Liggins GC (1976). Prenatal glucocorticoid treatment: Prevention of respiratory distress syndrome. In: Lung Maturation and the Prevention of Hyaline Membrane Disease: Report of the 70th Ross Conference on Paediatric Research. Moore TD (ed). Evanston: Ross Laboratories, pp 97–103.

Liggins GC, Howie RN (1972). A controlled trial of antepartum glucorticoid treatment for prevention of the respiratory distress syndrome in premature infants. Pediatrics, 50: 515–525.

Liggins GC, Howie RN (1973). Prevention of respiratory distress syndrome by antepartum corticosteroid therapy. Proceedings of Sir Joseph Barcroft Centenary Symposium, Fetal and Neonatal Physiology. Cambridge: Cambridge University Press, pp 613–617.

Liggins GC, Howie RN (1974). The prevention of RDS by maternal steroid therapy. In: Modern Perinatal Medicine. Gluck L (ed). Chicago: Yearbook Publishers, pp 415–424.

Liggins GC, Knight DB, Wealthall S, Howie RN (1988). A randomized, double-blind trial of antepartum TRH and steroids in the prevention of neonatal respiratory disease. In: Clinical Reproductive Medicine—The Liggins' Years. Aukland, New Zealand: 29–30 July.

Luerti M, Lazzarin A, Corbella E, Zavattini G (1987). An alternative to steroids for prevention of respiratory distress syndrome (RDS): Multicentre controlled study to compare ambroxol and betamethasone. J Perinat Med, 15: 227–238.

MacArthur BA, Howie RN, Dezoete JA, Elkins J (1981). Cognitive and psychosocial development of 4-year-old children whose mothers were treated antenatally with betamethasone. Pediatrics, 68: 638–643.

MacArthur BA, Howie RN, Dezoete JA, Elkins J (1982). School progress and cognitive development of 6-year-old children whose mothers were treated antenatally with betamethasone. Pediatrics, 70: 99–105.

Morales WJ, Diebel ND, Lazar AJ, Zadrozny D (1986). The effect of antenatal dexamethasone on the prevention of respiratory distress syndrome in preterm gestations with premature rupture of membranes. Am J Obstet Gynecol, 154: 591–595.

Morales WJ, O'Brien WF, Angel JL, Knuppel RA, Sawai S (1989). Fetal lung maturation: the combined use of corticosteroids and thyrotropin-releasing hormone. Obstet Gynecol, 73: 111–116.

Morrison JC, Whybrew WD, Bucovaz ET, Schneider JM (1978). Injection of corticosteroids into mother to prevent neonatal respiratory distress syndrome. Am J Obstet Gynecol, 13: 358–366.

Motoyama EK, Orzalezi MM, Kikkawa Y, Kibbara M, Low B, Zigas C, Cook C (1971). Effect of cortisol on the maturation of fetal lungs. Pediatrics, 48: 547–555.

Ogborn AD, Hunt KM, Gordon H (1977). Factors affecting fetal survival after intrauterine transfusion for rhesus isoimmunisation. Br J Obstet Gynaecol, 84: 665–668.

Papageorgiou AN, Desgranges MF, Masson M, Colle E, Shatz R, Gelfand MM (1979). The antenatal use of betamethasone in the prevention of respiratory distress syndrome. A controlled double-blind study. Pediatrics, 63: 73–79.

Robert MF, Neff RK, Hubell JP, Taeusch HW, Avery ME (1976). Association between maternal diabetes and the respiratory distress syndrome in the newborn. New Engl J Med, 294: 357–360.

Roberton NRC (1982). Advances in respiratory distress syndrome. Br Med J, 284: 917–918.

Rush RW, Keirse MJNC, Howatt P, Baum JD, Anderson ABM, Turnbull AC (1976). Contribution of preterm delivery to perinatal mortality. Br Med J, 2: 965–968.

Schapiro S, Salas M, Vukovich K (1970). Hormonal effects on ontogeny of swimming ability in the rat: Assessment of central nervous development. Science, 168: 147–151.

Schellenberg JC, Liggins GC, Manzai M, Kitterman JA, Lee CC (1988). Synergistic hormonal effects of lung maturation in fetal sheep. J Appl Physiol, 65: 94–100.

Schmidt PL, Sims ME, Strassner HT, Paul RH, Mueller E, McCart D (1984). Effect of antepartum glucocorticoid administration upon neonatal respiratory distress syndrome and perinatal infection. Am J Obstet Gynecol, 148: 178–186.

Schutte MF, Treffers PE, Koppe JG, Breur W, Filedt Kok JC (1979). The clinical use of corticosteroids for acceleration of foetal lung maturity. Ned Tijdschr Geneeskd, 123: 420–427.

Schutte MF, Treffers PE, Koppe JG, Breur W (1980). The influence of betamethasone and orciprenaline on the incidence of respiratory distress syndrome in the newborn after premature labour. Br J Obstet Gynaecol, 87: 127–131.

Schutte MF, Treffers PE, Koppe JG (1983). Threatened premature labour: The influence of time factors on the incidence of respiratory distress syndrome. Obstet Gynecol, 62: 287–293.

Silverman W, Day R, Blod F (1951). Inhibition of growth and other effects of ACTH in premature neonates. Pediatrics, 8: 177–190.

Stanley FJ, Alberman ED (1978). Infants of very low birthweight 1. Perinatal factors affecting survival. Dev Med Child Neurol, 20: 300–312.

Stubblefield PG, Kitzmiller JL (1980). Maternal pulmonary edema following combination treatment with betamimetics and high-dose steroids during pregnancy. A review. In: Betamimetic Drugs in Obstetrics and Perinatology. Third Symposium on Betamimetic Drugs. Jung H, Lamberti G (eds). New York: Thieme Stratton, p 144.

Szabo I, Csabo I, Novak P, Drozgynik I (1977). Single dose glucorticoid for prevention of respiratory distress syndrome Lancet, 2: 243.

Taeusch HW (1975). Glucocorticoid prophylaxis for respiratory distress syndrome. A review of potential toxicity. J Pediatr, 87: 617–623.

Taeusch HW, Frigoletto F, Kitzmiller J, Avery ME, Hehre A, Fromm B, Lawson E, Neff RK (1979). Risk of respiratory distress syndrome after prenatal dexamethasone treatment. Pediatrics, 63: 64–72.

Teramo K, Hallman M, Raivio KO (1980). Maternal glucorticoid in unplanned premature labor. Pediatr Res, 14: 326–329.

Usher RH, Allen AC, McLean FH (1971). Risk of respiratory distress syndrome related to gestational age, route of delivery and maternal diabetes. Am J Obstet Gynecol, 111: 826–831.

Walsh S, Clark F (1967). Pregnancy in patients with long term glucocorticoid therapy in pregnancy. Scott Med J, 12: 302–306.

Wauer RR, Schmalisch G, Menzel K, Schroder M, Muller K, Tiller R, Methfessel G, Sitka U, Koepke E, Plath C, Schlegel C, Bottcher M, Koppe I, Fricke U, Severin K, Jacobi R, Schmidt W (1982). The antenatal use of ambroxol (bromhexine metabolite VIII) to prevent hyaline membrane disease: A controlled double-blind study. Biol Res Pregnancy Perinatol, 3: 84–91.

Whitfield CR (1976). Amniotic fluid analysis. In: Fetal Physiology. Beard R, Nathanielsz P (eds). London: W B Saunders, p 337.

Whitt GG, Buster JE, Killam AP, Scragg WH (1976). A comparison of two glucocorticoid regimens for acceleration of fetal lung maturation in premature labor. Am J Obstet Gynecol, 124: 479–482.

Wolff F, Ponnath H, Wiest W (1987). Induction of fetal lung maturation with ambroxol and betamethasone—results of an open multicenter study. Geburtsh Frauenheilk, 47: 19–25.

46 Post-term pregnancy: magnitude of the problem

Leiv S. Bakketeig and Per Bergsjø

1 Introduction

A search through the literature on post-term pregnancy is a bewildering one. Not only do definitions vary, but the contradictory findings and conclusions with regard to the fetal risks lead to opposing views concerning management. In this chapter we shall start with a historical outline, with special emphasis on these contradictions. Many studies have been based on hospital materials and few have been true epidemiological, population based, surveys. Based on the medical birth registries in Norway and Sweden with complete nation wide notification of all births, we are privileged to present data from these sources, hoping to shed some new light on this clinical problem.

1.1 Definition

The expressions post-term pregnancy, prolonged pregnancy, post-dates pregnancy, and after-term pregnancy are used synonymously. The standard internationally recommended definition, endorsed by the World Health Organization (WHO) and the International Federation of Gynecology and Obstetrics (FIGO), is 'forty-two completed weeks or more (294 days or more)' (World Health Organization 1977a; FIGO 1986). However, the same two organizations phrased it differently in a 1980 proposal, which said 'pregnancy that is calculated to have proceeded beyond the end of the 42nd week (ie, more than 294 days from onset of the last menstrual period)' (FIGO 1980). By starting with day 295, this differs both from a previous WHO proposal, which included day 294 in the post-term period (World Health Organization 1972) from a later recommendation from WHO and FIGO (World Health Organization 1977b; FIGO 1976), and from the most recent one, quoted above. While a distinction of one day may seem trivial, it is important for statistical comparisons. Unfortunately, this one day is not the only point of confusion. An American compilation of obstetric/gynaecologic terms defines prolonged pregnancy as one that goes beyond 294 days, but a post-term infant as one born after day 287 (Hughes 1972). Forty-one completed weeks was also used by McKiddie (1949), while Clifford (1954) and Zwerdling (1967) used the other extreme, 43 completed weeks, as a dividing line.

For the new data from Norway and Sweden to be presented in this chapter, we have used the old WHO definition '294 days and beyond'.

'Post-term' and its synonyms are time-related, but neutral with regard to clinical phenomena. They should not be confused with the expressions 'hypermaturity' and 'post-maturity', which connote a clinical condition of the newborn in addition to prolonged gestation (Ballantyne 1902; Bøe 1950; Clifford 1954). Although both the time-related and the clinically-related concepts were introduced to indicate an added risk with regard to perinatal outcome, it is important to stick to the time-related definition in epidemiological studies aiming to quantify this condition and its associated risks.

1.2 Incidence

To compare incidence rates is not as straightforward as it may appear, even though the same definition of post-term labour is being used. The various study materials which have been presented in the past differ in many other respects which influence the proportion of pregnancies going beyond term. The ideal situation is one in which every pregnancy of the population is known from conception, none is lost to follow-up, every event is recorded, and there is no interference with the biological process. These conditions were almost met in the study from the Hawaiian island Kauai, where 14 per cent of 3000 pregnancies went beyond 42 weeks, and 6 per cent beyond 43 weeks (Bierman *et al.* 1965).

Studies from obstetrical departments, which seldom admit cases of less than 28 weeks, will have a relatively smaller denominator, thereby tending to increase the incidence rates, while a liberal policy of term elective deliveries will reduce them. In addition to such inevitable factors, some authors have excluded stillbirths, multiple births, malformations, and various other conditions of mothers and children from their study materials. Pregnancies with uncertain menstrual dates further tend to confound the picture.

Some of these selection criteria are summarily mentioned in Table 46.1, which shows that reported incidence rates for post-term pregnancy range from 4 to 14 per cent, with an average of about 10 per cent. Pregnancies going beyond 43 weeks range from 2 to 7 per cent. The difference of 2 per cent in incidence between two university hospitals of neighbouring Swedish cities (Lindell 1956) was thought to be due to different induction policies. It is also noteworthy that the incidence of post-term birth in Britain fell from 11.5 per cent in 1958 to 4.4 per cent in 1970 (Butler and Bonham 1963; Chamberlain *et al.* 1978). These two nation-wide studies were conducted in very similar ways. According to the reports, the rate of induction of labour rose from 13 to 26 per cent during the same period. The birth notification forms to the Swedish Birth Registry ask for the reliability of gestational dating, based on clinical impression. By excluding the 9.8 per cent with uncertain dates the frequency of post-term singleton births in Sweden 1981 was reduced from 13.7 per cent to 11.6 per cent (Bergsjø 1985).

Studies of differences within the single material may be more rewarding than the comparison between non-standardized groups. Concerning the sex of the child, a Finnish study found that the duration of pregnancy was significantly longer in para 0 mothers delivered of girls (Timonen *et al.* 1966), while other studies have found no such significant sex difference (Lindell 1956; Engström and Sterky 1966). Most materials show no significant effect of parity on the incidence of post-term pregnancy (Clayton 1941; Lindell 1956; Magram and Cavanagh 1960; Perlin 1960; Timonen *et al.* 1965), while Evans *et al.* (1963) found significantly more prolonged pregnancies among para 0 mothers. Lucas *et al.* (1965) found a 'relative increase' in para 0 mothers, and the British 1958 survey demonstrated a slightly higher incidence in para 0 and para 4 mothers compared to the intervening parities (Butler and Bonham 1963). Similar U-shaped curves for parity were found by Zwerdling (1967) both in Oakland, California, and in New York.

The reports on the influence of maternal age are somewhat conflicting. While Zwerdling (1967) and Butler and Bonham (1963) found a steady decrease in the incidence of post-term pregnancies with advancing age, Timonen *et al.* (1966) regarded prolongation of pregnancy with increasing age as highly significant. However, the Finnish group referred to the mean duration of pregnancy and not to post-term pregnancies. Obviously, different policies of elective delivery may obscure true biological effects both for age and parity.

Social factors have also been studied, with equally contradictory results. While more pregnancies were prolonged in the British lower social classes (Butler and Bonham 1963), the reverse was true in Finland (Timonen *et al.* 1965).

In the Finnish studies the duration of pregnancy was positively correlated with increasing prenatal maternal weight, resulting in higher post-term fractions in the heavier mothers (Timonen *et al.* 1965).

One interesting feature, which will be examined in greater detail below, is the tendency for some mothers to repeat post-term births, noted by Zwerdling (1967) and by Bakketeig *et al.* (1979). This indicates that in some women post-term births could be biologically determined and not a random event.

2 Assessment of gestational age

The problem of accurate menstrual dates is ever present. When the cycles are 4-weekly, regular, and the last menstrual period is recalled accurately, the calculated term must be considered certain for epidemiological purposes. In clinical practice the expected date of delivery is sometimes adjusted according to additional results, particularly of ultrasound examinations, but such individual corrections are impractical in large-scale studies.

The real difficulty arises with those whose cycles are irregular and those who have no last menstrual period to report. For example, in Amsterdam University Hospital the percentage of women with uncertain dates rose from about 3 in 1957–63 to 13 in 1974–76 because of increasing use of the contraceptive pill during that period (Kloosterman 1979). Thus the frequency of uncertain dates will vary both with time and place. Even with rigid criteria and constant use of the contraceptive pill, much depends on the interview technique of the person taking the case history. In Aberdeen, Hall *et al.* (1985) found that 73 per cent of the mothers had certain dates; 20 per cent approximate and 7 per cent

Table 46.1 Incidence of post-term pregnancy: literature review

Author(s) and year of publication	Material: H: One hospital HH: Two or more hospitals P: Population-based			Size	Selection criteria: E: Excluding I: Including		Incidence rates: 42+ weeks A: 294+ B: 295+	43+ weeks C: 300+ D: 301+	Induction
Waaler (1933)	Oslo	H	1919–30	10,325	E	Stillbirths	11.3%		Infrequent
Clayton (1941)	London	HH	1935–38	9649	E	'Doubtful' cases	7.3% A		1.2%
Clifford *et al.* (1951)	Boston	H	1940–50	2187				5.6% C	
Lindell (1956)	Stockholm Uppsala	H H	1943–52 1943–52	21,281 25,100	E	Twins and certain conditions	11.6% A 9.5% A	3.2% D 2.1% D	Infrequent 2.5% before week 43
Magram and Cavanagh (1960)	New York	H	1953–55	6235	E	Uncertain dates, twins, breech, deliveries <28 weeks		4.4% D	1.9%
Perlin (1960)	Halifax	H	1950–55	12,000	E	Irregular cycles	8.0%		Infrequent
Butler and Bonham (1963)	United Kingdom	P	1958	16,994	E	Uncertain dates	11.5% A	3.3% D	K13.0
Evans *et al.* (1963)	Ann Arbor, Mich.	H	1943–60	20,052			8.9%	3.2%	2.8%
Bierman *et al.* (1965)	Kauai, Hawaii	P	1954–56	3000	I	All pregnancies	14.0%	6.0%	
Lucas *et al.* (1965)	USA	HH	1960–62	63,370	I	Single, >500 g	10.4%		
Timonen *et al.* (1965)	Finland	HH	1957–58	57,089	E	Multiple births, diabetes	8.3% B		
Zwerdling (1967)	Oakland, Calif.		1959–64	9712	E	Multiple births		7.3%	
Bjerkedal and Bakketeig (1975)	Norway	P	1967–71	326,264	I	All pregnancies with registered dates	14.9% A		11.8%
Chamberlain *et al.* (1978)	United Kingdom	P	1970	16,815	I	Singleton pregnancies	4.4%		26.0%
Kloosterman (1979)	Amsterdam	HH	1947–77	57,976	E	Uncertain dates Multiple births	10.0% B		'Conservative attitude'
Hauth *et al.* (1980)	Texas	H	1976–79	4436	I	Reliable dates	6.8%		62.0% post-t.
Freeman *et al.* (1981)	Long Beach, Calif.	H	1976–79	10,083			6.7% A		21.0% post-t.
Bakketeig and Bergsjø: This chapter	Sweden	P	1978	93,156	I	All births in Sweden	12.2% A		
Bergsjø (1985)	Sweden	P	1981	82,889	E	Multiple births and uncertain dates	11.6% A		

uncertain dates. Uncertain dates were more prevalent in social classes IV and V, among mothers aged 14–19, in illegitimate pregnancies, in primiparae with minimum education, and among heavy smokers.

In addition to those mentioned above, reported figures for uncertain dates vary from 12 to 18 per cent (McKiddie 1949; Schildbach 1953; Magram and Cavanagh 1960; Timonen *et al.* 1965; Bergsjø *et al.* 1982). Timonen *et al.* (1965), who recorded the length and the regularity of the menstrual periods, found increasing frequencies of post-term births with increasing cycle length. Of gravidae with irregular cycles (9 per cent of all), 14.2 per cent went post-term, compared with 7.6 per cent of those with regular cycles. Similar Swedish figures for 1979 were quoted above. Unpublished data, to which we have been given access, show that the proportion of pregnancies with uncertain dates in Sweden is fairly constant over time, the figures being 9.9 per cent for 1976–77 and 9.5 per cent for 1979–80.

A reasonable explanation is that the interval between menstruation and ovulation in women with long or irregular periods is longer than presupposed in Naegele's rule. Some of the post-term pregnancies in this group therefore only reflect our inability to measure their true biological length.

Consequently, it is accepted that some pregnancies are falsely labelled post-term. Another confounding phenomenon with the opposite effect is post-conceptional bleeding interpreted as a true menstruation. Iffy *et al.* (1973) have convincingly demonstrated this for certain types of pathological pregnancy. We may assume that some cases in this way may be misclassified as being at term while in fact being post-term, but there are no available data on their frequency.

3 Causation

As long as the mechanism of the start of labour remains an enigma, the reason for some pregnancies to go beyond term is equally obscure. As with any biological process, a certain range of the normal variation is inevitable. The concept of post-term has its root in perinatal mortality, which, following a steady fall from 100 per cent at mid-pregnancy to a minimum at term, again tends to rise after the 42nd week. In the search for explanations, ageing has been the clue word. Walker (1954) examined the oxygen levels in umbilical cord blood and found that reduced oxygen content was a common denominator in post-term pregnancies. On the other hand, Bancroft-Livingston and Neill (1957) and Evans *et al.* (1963) found no correlation between oxygen saturation or tension in umbilical cord blood and the duration of pregnancy.

Clifford (1954), who described the postmaturity syndrome of the newborn, postulated a rapid decline of placental function in the post-term period, but admitted that histological examinations of post-term placentas up to that time had not supported his hypothesis. Neither Clayton (1941) nor Naeye (1978) were able to pinpoint any obvious features of the placenta as being particularly prevalent in the post-term period.

It would be presumptuous to postulate one single cause for the prolonged pregnancies. In the following discussion, and in our presentation of our own data we hope to clarify some points.

4 Coincidental phenomena

Several studies of birthweight show that the average weekly increase tends to slow down some time during the 3rd trimester towards a plateau which is reached near week 42. Examples are given by Gruenwald (1974) and by Naeye and Dixon (1978). National data from Norway even indicate a fall in mean birthweight after week 42 (Bjerkedal *et al.* 1973). This, as well as increasing variation of birthweights with advancing gestational age (Gruenwald 1974) may partly be an effect of uncertain menstrual dates. Studies with expected date of confinement based on ultrasonographic dating show no such slowing of fetal growth as the length of pregnancy passes 40 weeks (Eik-Nes *et al.* 1980).

A relative decrease in growth during the last weeks of pregnancy can also be expressed through the weight-to-length ratio. This ratio was shown by Gruenwald (1974) to increase up to term, but to fall thereafter. However, similar change of constitution from stout to slim children with advancing gestational age was not immediately apparent in a Finnish material (Timonen *et al.* 1966).

To explain the apparent reduction in growth rate, Gruenwald (1966) postulated a decreasing supply line to the fetus, near the end of pregnancy. Another intriguing hypothesis is that the flattening of the growth curve is a statistical misleader due to cross-sectional birth data, whereas the individual normal fetal weight follows a straight line. Support for this was given by Eik-Nes *et al.* (1980), who examined a number of pregnancies with intrauterine ultrasonic measurements after correcting for dates. If substantiated, this will alter our whole concept of fetal growth (see Chapter 26).

The most important aspect is that of perinatal morbidity and mortality. Again we must recall that there have been substantial changes in morbidity and mortality figures during the past 40 to 50 years, so that what was true in 1940 is not necessarily true today. Also, the influence of changing obstetric practice cannot easily be separated from the influence of the external environment.

Nearly all who have recorded perinatal mortality in large materials have found increasing rates for post-term births (Clifford 1954; Walker 1954; Kloosterman

1956; Lindell 1956; Butler and Bonham 1963; Evans *et al.* 1963; Lucas *et al.* 1965; Timonen *et al.* 1965; Zwerdling 1967; Chamberlain *et al.* 1978; Bjerkedal and Bakketeig 1972; Naeye 1978; Stubblefield and Berek 1980). Clayton (1941), who found no significant increase, only included birthweights over 7.5 lb in the post-term group. Bierman *et al.* (1965), who found almost the same mortality rates for post-term as for term births, had very accurate pregnancy dating, which resulted in a higher frequency of post-term cases than is usually reported; they claimed that post-term pregnancies in most reported series are selected high risk groups. As a corollary, Wenner and Young (1974) and Hall and Carr-Hill (1985) found that uncertain dates were strongly associated with high rates of unfavourable outcomes.

Taken as a whole, the perinatal mortality rate in post-term births appears to be about twice that of term births. In evaluating such figures, due consideration should be paid to the confounding influence of the inevitable fraction of pregnancies with uncertain dates. Although Lindell (1956) found no sex difference, other large materials have shown a preponderance of boys among post-term deaths (Butler and Bonham 1963; Bjerkedal and Bakketeig 1972; Kloosterman 1956).

Bøe (1950), Clifford (1954), Lindell (1956), Walker (1954), and Kloosterman (1956) all agreed that post-term perinatal death rates were highest among primigravidae. It is reasonable to link this phenomenon with the reported high incidences of prolonged labours (Bøe 1950; Evans *et al.* 1963; Lucas *et al.* 1965), resulting in higher rates of fetal distress and birth trauma in post-term para 0 births.

Contrary to these results, Timonen *et al.* (1965) found no parity difference in the post-term perinatal mortality rates. Kloosterman (1979), who had acted upon his own 1954 results with a conservative attitude towards multiparous but not towards nulliparous post-term pregnancy, found a reversal of the trend, with relatively more perinatal deaths among para 1+ mothers in his 1958–76 material.

Regardless of cause, the duration of labour in all parity groups is now apparently shorter than it used to be, and excessively long labours of the kind that caused intrapartum fetal death, are now seldom seen (Bergsjø *et al.* 1979).

The search for causes of post-term death is important, as it is the clue to possible intervention strategies. Few large scale investigations have been undertaken. Using the US Collaborative Perinatal Project of the National Institute of Neurological and Communicative Disorders and Stroke, comprising 53,158 pregnancies, Naeye (1978) found that the excess mortality post-term compared to term was due to severe congenital anomalies (26 per cent), amniotic fluid infections (19 per cent), abruptio placentae (10 per cent), Rh erythroblastosis fetalis (8 per cent), large placental infarcts (8 per cent), growth-retarded placentas (8 per cent), and the rest a variety of other disorders. Most of the congenital anomalies were marked adrenal hypoplasia and anencephaly. These results were largely substantiated by another US multicentre study (Lucal *et al.* 1965) in which various anoxic conditions, congenital anomalies and neonatal infections were the main causes of excess post-term deaths. Zwerdling (1967) showed that excess post-term mortality was not related to birthweight, and that significantly increased mortality rates persisted into the second year of life for children born after 43 completed gestational weeks.

An enigmatic clinical problem is that of unexplained antepartum death. Kloosterman (1979), after excluding all reasonably clear causes, remained with 6.9 unexplained deaths per 1000 pregnancies of all durations. These cases could also be labelled 'placental insufficiency'. Although more prevalent with advancing gestational age, such stillbirths occurred at any time past 28 weeks, and numerically, only 13 out of 208 came after day 296. One is reminded that Clifford's (1954) postmaturity syndrome of newborns did also include cases born before the magic 295 day limit. In fact, his description of the postmaturity syndrome is remarkably similar to that of the growth-retarded fetus, regardless of gestational age.

It is quite impossible to tell whether present-day induction policies have influenced the state of affairs beneficially. In the British 1970 survey (Chamberlain *et al.* 1978) the perinatal mortality rate following induced post-term labour was twice as high as that following spontaneous labour, but selection bias most likely operated, precluding further attempts at explanation. Three randomized studies of early versus late induction of labour around term were too limited in numbers to address the question of perinatal death rates (Breart *et al.* 1982; Cole *et al.* 1975; Martin *et al.* 1978).

5 Scandinavian data sets

Data presented in this chapter derive from two different sources; The Medical Birth Registry of Norway and the Swedish Medical Birth Registry.

Our data from the Medical Birth Registry of Norway cover all livebirths and fetal deaths of gestational age 16 weeks or more during a 10-year period, 1967–76, a total of 635,140 births. In the analyses presented, however, are included only mothers with successive births during this time period. Unique identification numbers are assigned to all births and their parents, and therefore linkage of successive births to the same mother is easily accomplished (Bakketeig *et al.* 1979). Similarly, information on infant survival as provided by the Central Bureau of Statistics of Norway has been linked to the birth information through use of the personal identification number (Bjerkedal and Bakketeig 1975).

The length of gestation is based on the date of the last menstrual period and the birth or expulsion of the fetus.

Post-term birth is defined as births of gestational age 42 completed weeks or more (294 days or more).

Induced as well as spontaneous births are included in the analyses.

Certainty of expected date of confinement in the Swedish data set was based on clinical judgement.

5.1 Frequency of post-term birth

Post-term birth occurred among 15.4 per cent of all births in Norway, 1967–76. There is reason to believe that for a substantial part of these pregnancies the expected date of confinement was uncertain. Therefore, as a result of this, some of these births were not really post-term.

The Norwegian data do not permit any distinction between pregnancies with certain and uncertain dates. However, the Swedish Medical Birth Registration includes such information. Table 46.2 shows the distribution of gestational age among Swedish births 1978, by certainty of expected date of confinement. A total of 12.2 per cent of the births were reported to be post-term. Among those with certain EDC 10.2 per cent were post-term, while as many as 22.3 per cent of the births were labelled as post-term among those where EDC was uncertain. Of all Swedish births 16.7 per cent were reported as having uncertain dates. The corresponding proportion was 15.3 per cent in a Norwegian Hospital material (Bergsjø *et al.* 1982). Judging from the Swedish data this should indicate that the true frequency of post-term birth among Norwegian births was approximately 13 per cent during the study period.

5.2 Time trends

The reported frequency of post-term birth was 14.2 per cent in Norway in 1967. In 1976 the frequency had increased to 15.9 per cent. Since decreasing parity is associated with increased frequency of post-term birth as shown below, the observed change in the frequency of post-term birth can partly be explained through the corresponding trend towards more para 0 births over the 10-year period.

5.3 Parity

In Table 46.3 the association between post-term birth and parity is examined within groups of mothers with different sibship sizes. It appears that in all groups there was a considerable drop (15–20 per cent) in the risk of post-term birth between para 0 and higher parities. If the data shown in Table 46.3 are analysed

Table 46.2 Proportion of post-term birth by certainty of expected date of delivery. Based on 93,156 births in Sweden, 1978

Expected date of confinement (EDC)	Total number of births	Of these with gestational age (weeks)— number and per cent						Post-term (42+) total
		40	41	42	43	44	45+	
Certain	77,638	22,084	15,926	6897	929	112	13	7933
		28.4	20.5	8.9	1.2	0.1	0.0	10.2
Uncertain	15,518	3085	2493	2114	902	305	134	3455
		19.9	16.1	13.6	5.8	2.0	0.9	22.3
Total	93,156	25,169	18,419	8993	1831	417	147	11,388
		27.0	19.8	9.7	2.0	0.4	0.2	12.2

Source: The Swedish Medical Birth Registry

Table 46.3 Proportion of post-term birth (GA 42+ weeks) by parity and sibship size. Based on 245,893 mothers with one, two, three, or four single births, Norway, 1967–76

Sibship size	Number of mothers	Proportion of post-term birth (per cent)			
		Para 0	Para 1	Para 2	Para 3
1	107,974	18.0			
2	107,495	17.4	14.3		
3	26,923	16.8	14.4	14.4	
4	3501	15.6	13.4	13.9	14.3

cross-sectionally, the post-term rates were 17.6, 14.3, 14.3, and 14.3 in para 0, para 1, para 2, and para 3 births, respectively. Thus in this case the two methods of analysis reveal similar results, which, however, is not always so (Bakketeig and Hoffman 1979).

5.4 Tendency to repeat post-term birth

If the first birth was not post-term the risk of the subsequent (second) birth being post-term was 12.2 per cent as shown in Table 46.4. If, however, the first birth was post-term then this risk increased to 27.4 per cent, which reveals a relative risk of 2.2. It appears from the table that the risk of repeating a post-term birth was cumulative. Thus, if a woman had two post-term births, then her risk of the subsequent birth being post-term increased to 39.1 per cent, or a relative risk of 3.2.

Conversely, if both of the two first births were not post-term, the risk of the third birth being post-term was reduced to 10.7 per cent (RR = 0.9).

5.5 Maternal complications and complications during delivery

Maternal complications during pregnancy were more frequently present in post-term compared to not post-term pregnancies. For example, among para 0 mothers with post-term birth 21.4 per cent were reported as having one or more complications during pregnancy, compared to 17.3 per cent among para 0 not post-term births. No particular condition or conditions accounted for this difference, rather the difference reflected a generally increased risk of complications.

Position anomalies did not occur more frequently among post-term births compared to not post-term births.

Instrumental delivery was slightly more frequently used among para 0 post-term births. This tendency did not exist among higher parity mothers.

5.6 Induction of labour

The frequency of induction was more than three times higher among post-term births than among not post-term births; 29.2 vs. 9.0 per cent, respectively. Induction of labour tended to be slightly more common among mothers who repeated post-term births, compared to mothers who only occasionally had a post-term birth. Over the period under study there was in general a marked increase in the use of induced labour. Thus, the overall induction rate in 1976 was 14.9 per cent compared to 11.1 per cent in 1967. This increased use of induction applies not only to post-term pregnancies, but to pregnancies of shorter duration as well.

5.7 Congenital malformations

In Table 46.5 the occurrence of congenital malformations is related to post-term birth. It appears as if congenital malformations were not more common among post-term births than among other births. Particularly it should be noted that central nervous system malformations were as common among births of mothers with no post-term births as among mothers with one or more post-term births. However, if post-term births had been contrasted with term births the picture might have been somewhat altered.

5.8 Perinatal mortality

In Table 46.6 shows the perinatal mortality rates (stillbirths plus first-week deaths per 1000 births) for Swedish term and post-term births. The data is here restricted to those births where the expected date of confinement was considered as certain.

As it appears, the total perinatal mortality was only slightly higher for 'early' post-term births (42 weeks of gestation), namely 3.0 per 1000 compared to 2.3 and 2.4 per 1000 for term births of 40 and 41 weeks of gestation,

Table 46.4 The risk of post-term birth (42 weeks or more) in successive births. Based on 27,677 mothers with their first three singleton births, Norway, 1967–76

First birth	Second birth	Number of mothers	Subsequent post-term birth		
			Numbers	Per cent	Relative risk
Not post-term		22,990	2808	12.2	1.0
Post-term		4687	1284	27.4	2.2
Not post-term	Not post-term	20,202	2170	10.7	0.9
Post-term	Not post-term	3403	722	21.2	1.7
Not post-term	Post-term	2788	688	24.7	2.0
Post-term	Post-term	1284	502	39.1	3.2

Table 46.5 Congenital malformations by number of post-term births. Based on 30,979 mothers with their first three singleton births, Norway, 1967–76

Number of post-term births	Total number of mothers	Total number of births	Congenital malformations per 1000 births				
			CNS	Cardio-vascular	Down's syndrome	Multiple	All other
0	18,032	54,096	3.1	2.4	1.1	1.1	22.1
1	6971	20,913	3.4	2.3	0.6	0.8	24.0
2	2172	6516	2.5	3.4	0.8	0.8	24.1
3	502	1506	2.0	2.0	0	2.0	23.9
Unknown	3302	9906	3.0	2.3	0.7	1.1	18.9
Total	30,979	92,937	3.0	2.4	0.9	1.0	22.5

Table 46.6 Perinatal mortality by gestational age for term and post-term births. Based on 157,677 births with certain expected date of delivery, Sweden, 1977 and 1978

Gestational age (weeks)	Number of births	Perinatal deaths per 1000 births
38	16,325	7.2
39	34,390	3.1
40	44,986	2.3
41	32,527	2.4
42	13,883	3.0
43 +	2227	4.0

Table 46.7 Perinatal mortality of post-term second births by gestational age of the elder sibling. Based on 138,861 mothers[1] with their first two singleton births, Norway, 1967–76

Gestational age of elder sibling (weeks)	Post-term second births (number of births and perinatal deaths per 1000) 42 +
36–38	1407 5.7
39–41	11,064 4.8
42 +	6336 4.4

[1] Mothers with unknown gestational ages or gestational age below 36 weeks for either one of their births are not included in the table.

respectively. However, for births with gestational age of 43 weeks or more, the mortality rate was nearly doubled (4.0 per 1000). These mortality differences were even greater when the associations were examined within birthweight groups. For example for births weighing 3625–3874 g the perinatal mortality increased from 0.9 to 1.3 to 3.4 and to 4.4 per 1000 as the gestational age increased from 40, through 41 and 42 to 43 weeks or more, respectively.

Perinatal mortality seems to be associated with the tendency to repeat post-term birth as shown in Table 46.7. The mortality tended to be lower among post-term births of mothers who repeated this condition compared to post-term births of mothers who only occasionally had a post-term birth. As shown in the table the perinatal mortality was 4.4 per 1000 among post-term births if the elder sibling was also post-term, compared to 4.8 and 5.7 per 1000 if the sibling was born at term or slightly pre-term, respectively.

6 Conclusions

This literature survey and our own data are based on materials in which the last menstrual period was used as starting point for the measurement of gestational length, which is the only practical yardstick for large-scale epidemiological studies. When correction was made for unreliable menstrual dates in the nationwide Swedish birth notifications, the incidence of post-term pregnancies was reduced from 12 to 10 per cent, as the present data show. These figures are consistent with other published results. Because of the uncertainty of the menstruation to ovulation interval, even in women with regular periods, the figures presented should not be mistaken for the biological truth concerning gestational length and the frequency of post-term births.

At this point it is pertinent to look into studies of gestational length using the rise of basal body temperature to indicate ovulation. Such materials are few and small in size, but the results are consistent, showing a much lower variation of pregnancy duration than in the menstruation-based groups (Stewart 1952; Döring 1962). In a similar French material (Boyce *et al.* 1976) the menstruation-to-ovulation interval was also measured, so that the incidence of 'true' and 'false' post-term cases could be estimated. Post-term according to menstrual dates occurred in 10.7 per cent of the pregnancies, whereas the 'true' rate based on temperature charts, was 4.7 per cent. Of the latter group, about one quarter was incorrectly labelled 'term pregnancies' by menstrual dates. By a different method of assessing the expected date of delivery, namely ultrasonic measurement of the biparietal diameter in the assumed 17th week of pregnancy, Eik-Nes *et al.* (1980) found that only 3.9 per cent of nearly 5000 pregnancies went post-term.

The implication of these studies is that a large fraction of the pregnancies which are post-term by current definition, are really mislabelled. However, assuming that ovulation or even ultrasonic dating on a large scale is not yet feasible, the clinical challenge is to recognize the few threatened cases among those which are truly post-term.

Returning, then, to our own data, the present study shows a rather strong association between parity and post-term birth. Thus, the risk of a post-term birth is 15–20 per cent higher among para 0 mothers compared to higher parity mothers. Even though young maternal age is associated with an increased risk of post-term birth, maternal age as a whole is not closely associated with post-term birth.

The study of successive births in the same mother in Norway shows that some mothers tend to repeat post-term births, and that the perinatal mortality rate in this group is lower than among babies of mothers whose previous birth was not post-term. This tendency is present also when the analysis is restricted to births with spontaneous onset only. Thus, the pattern is not affected by induction of labour and the tendency to repeat such procedures.

It should be stressed that the perinatal mortality in week 42 (day 295–301 inclusive) is only slightly higher than in weeks 40 and 41, and lower than in week 39, according to the Swedish 1977–78 data. Even in and following week 43 the perinatal mortality is quite modest, yet we must ask if these deaths can be prevented. Based on previously quoted lists of causes of excess post-term mortality, it should be possible to avoid some post-term deaths, at least in theory. To prevent unexplained intrauterine deaths by mass elective delivery before these fetuses die is hardly feasible. In Kloosterman's (1979) Amsterdam material there were 2.8 unexplained fetal deaths per 1000 pregnancies beyond day 290, a rather small number for such heroic measures, which may even do more harm than good (see Chapter 45).

The benefit of mass induction of pregnancies in week 42 remains to be proven and weighed against possible hazards. Use of randomized controlled trials would be the only valid evaluation of the effects of such induction. Two such trials have been reported (Cardozo *et al.* 1986; Augensen *et al.* 1987), neither of which showed any benefit of induction at 42 weeks compared to continued surveillance. Two other trials of similar design, one from Norway and the other from China, may go some way towards clarification. Preferably one should be able to establish a set of discriminatory rules based on case history, clinical examination and ultrasonic, electronic, and biochemical tests, to select the small percentage of pregnancies in immediate need of elective delivery. Then one could let nature run its course with the rest, which presumably would be to the benefit of mothers and their offspring. To arrive at such selection criteria is an important task for modern obstetrics.

References

Augensen K, Bergsjø P, Eikeland T, Askvik K, Carlsen J (1987). A randomised comparison of early versus late induction of labour in post term pregnancy. Br Med J, 294: 1192–1195.

Bakketeig LS, Hoffman HJ (1979). Perinatal mortality by birth order within cohorts based on sibship size. Br Med J, 2: 693–696.

Bakketeig LS, Hoffman HJ, Harley EE (1979). The tendency to repeat gestational age and birth weight in successive births. Am J Obstet Gynecol, 135: 1086–1103.

Ballantyne JW (1902). The problem of the postmature infant. J Obstet Gynaecol Br Empire, 2: 521–544.

Bancroft-Livingston G, Neill DW (1957). Studies in prolonged pregnancy. Part I—cord blood oxygen levels at delivery. J Obstet Gynaecol Br Empire, 64: 498–503.

Bergsjø P (1985). Post-term pregnancy 121–133. In: Progress in obstetrics and gynaecology, Volume 5. Studd J (ed). Edinburgh and London: Churchill Livingstone.

Bergsjø P, Bakketeig LS, Eikhom SN (1979). Duration of labour with spontaneous onset. Acta Obst Gynecol Scand, 58: 129–134.

Bergsjø P, Bakketeig LS, Eikhom SN (1982). Case-control analysis of post term induction of labour. Acta Obstet Gynecol Scand, 61: 317–324.

Bierman J, Siegel E, French FE, Simonian K (1965). Analysis of the outcome of all pregnancies in a community Kauai pregnancy study. Am J Obstet Gynecol, 91: 37–45.

Bjerkedal T, Bakketeig LS (1972). Medical registration of births in Norway 1967–68. Some descriptive and analytical aspects. University of Bergen, Institute of Hygiene and Social Medicine, Medical Birth Registry of Norway, Bergen, Norway, p 144.

Bjerkedal T, Bakketeig LS (1975). Medical registration of births in Norway during the 5-year period 1967–71. Time trends and differences between counties and between municipalities. Institute of Hygiene and Social Medicine, University of Bergen, Bergen, Norway, p 71.

Bjerkedal T, Bakketeig LS, Lehmann EH (1973). Percentiles of birth weights of single live births at different gestation periods. Based on 125,485 births in Norway, 1967 and 1968. Acta Paediatr Scand, 62: 449–457.

Bøe F (1950). Hypermature pregnancy. I. Clinical significance. Acta Obstet Gynecol Scand (Suppl), 30: 1–21.

Boyce A, Mayaux MJ, Schwartz D (1976). Classical and 'true' gestational postmaturity. Am J Obstet Gynecol, 125: 911–914.

Bréart G, Goujard J, Maillard F, Chavigny C, Rumeau-Rouquette C, Sureau C (1982). Comparaison de deux attitudes obstétricales vis-à-vis du déclenchement artificiel du travail à terme. Essai randomisé. J Gynécol Obstét Biol Réprod, 11: 107–112.

Butler NR, Bonham DG (1963). Perinatal mortality. The first report of the 1958 British perinatal mortality survey under the auspices of the National Birthday Trust Fund. Edinburgh and London: E & S Livingstone, p 304.

Cardozo L, Fysh J, Pearce J M (1986). Prolonged pregnancy: the management debate. Br Med J, 293: 1059–1063.

Chamberlain G. Phillip E, Howlett B, Masters K (1978). British Births 1970. Vol 2: Obstetric Care. London: Heinemann Medical Books, p 292.

Clayton SG (1941). Fetal mortality in post-maturity. J Obstet Gynaecol Br Empire, 48: 450–460.

Clifford SH (1954). Postmaturity—with placental dysfunction. Clinical syndrome and pathological findings. J Pediatrics, 44: 1–13.

Clifford SH, Reid DE, Worcester J (1951). Postmaturity. Am J Dis Children, 82: 232–233.

Cole RA, Howie PW, MacNaughton MC (1975). Elective induction of labour. A randomized prospective trial. Lancet, i: 767–770.

Döring GK (1962). Über die tragzeit post ovulationem. Geburtshilfe Frauenheilk, 22: 1191–1194.

Eik-Nes SH, Persson PH, Gröttum P (1980). Revaluation of standards for human fetal growth, 103–117. In Ultrasonic Assessment of Human Fetal Weight, Growth and Blood flow. Eik-Nes SH (ed). p 173. Department of Obstetrics and Gynecology, University of Lund, General Hospital, Malmö, Sweden, and Department of Obstetrics and Gynecology Department of Radiology, Ålesund Central Hospital, Ålesund, Norway. Thesis, University of Lund.

Engström L, Sterky G (1966). Standardkurvor för vikt och langd hos nyfödda barn. Läkartidningen, 63: 4922–4926.

Evans TN, Koeff S, Morley GW (1963). Fetal effects of prolonged pregnancy. Am J Obstet Gynecol, 85: 701–709.

FIGO (1976). FIGO news: List of gynecologic and obstetrical terms and definitions. Int J Gynaecol Obstet, 14: 570–576.

FIGO (1980). International classification of diseases: update. Int J Gynaecol Obstet, 17: 634–640.

FIGO (1986). Report of the FIGO subcommittee on perinatal epidemiology and health statistics following a workshop in Cairo, November 11–18, 1984, on the methodology of measurement and recording of infant growth in the perinatal period. Published by International Federation of Gynecology and Obstetrics (FIGO) Secretariat: 27 Sussex Place, Regent's Park, London NW1 UK, p 54.

Freeman RK, Garite TJ, Modanlou H, Dorchester W, Rommal C, Devaney M (1981). Postdate pregnancy: Utilization of contraction stress testing for primary fetal surveillance. Am J Obstet Gynecol, 140: 128–135.«1»

Gruenwald P (1966). Growth of the human fetus. I. Normal growth and its variation. Am J Obstet Gynecol, 94: 1112–1119.

Gruenwald P (1974). Pathology of the deprived fetus and its supply line. 3–26. In: Size at Birth, Ciba Foundation Symposium 27 (new series). Elsevier/Exerpta Medica, North-Holland, p 407.

Hall MH, Carr-Hill RA (1985). The significance of uncertain gestation for obstetric outcome. Br J Obstet Gynaecol, 92: 452–460.

Hall MH, Carr-Hill RA, Fraser C, Campbell D, Samphier MI (1985). The extent and antecedents of uncertain gestation. Br J Obstet Gynaecol, 92: 445–451.

Hauth JC, Goodman MT, Gilstrap LC, Gilstrap JER (1980). Post-term pregnancy. I. Obstet Gynecol, 56: 467–470.

Hughes EC (1972). Obstetric–gynecologic terminology with section on neonatology and glossary of congenital anomalies. Philadelphia: F A Davis, p 731.

Iffy LI, Chatterton RT, Jakobovits A (1973). The 'high weight for dates' fetus. Am J Obstet Gynecol, 115: 238–247.

Kloosterman GJ (1956). Prolonged pregnancy. Gynaecologia, 142: 373–388.

Kloosterman GJ (1979). Epidemiology of Postmaturity in Human Parturition. Keirse MJNC *et al.* (ed). The Hague: Martinus Nijhoff, pp 247–261.

Lindell A (1956). Prolonged pregnancy. Acta Obst Gynecol Scand, 35: 136–163.

Lucas WE, Anctil AO, Callagan DA (1965). The problem of post-term pregnancy. Am J Obstet Gynecol, 91: 241–250.

Magram HM, Cavanagh WV (1960). The problem of postmaturity. A statistical analysis. Am J Obstet Gynecol, 79: 216–223.

Martin DH, Thompson W, Pinkerton JHM, Watson JD (1978). A randomized controlled trial of selective planned delivery. Br J Obstet Gynaecol, 85: 109–113.

McKiddie JM (1949). Foetal mortality in postmaturity. Br J Obstet Gynaecol, 56: 386–392.

Naeye RL (1978). Causes of perinatal mortality excess in prolonged gestations. Am J Epidmiol, 108: 429–433.

Naeye RL, Dixon JB (1978). Distortions in fetal growth standards. Pediatr Res, 12: 987–991.

Perlin IA (1960). Postmaturity. Am J Obstet Gynecol, 80: 1–5.

Schildbach HR (1953). Neue erkenntnisse über die Dauer der Schwangerschaft beim Menschen mit Hilfe der Basaltemperaturmessung. Klin Wochenschr, 31: 654–656.

Stewart HL (1952). Duration of pregnancy and postmaturity. JAMA, 148: 1079–1083.

Stubblefield PG, Berek JS (1980). Perinatal mortality in term and post-term births. Obstet Gynecol, 56: 676–682.

Timonen S, Vara P, Lokki O, Hirvonen E (1965). Duration of pregnancy. Ann Chir Gynaecol Fenn Suppl, 54: p 33.

Timonen S, Uotila U, Kuusisto P, Vara P, Lokki O (1966). Effect of certain maternal foetal and geographical factors on the weight and length of the newborn and on the duration of pregnancy. Ann Chir Gynaecol Fenn, 55: 196–213.

Waaler GHM (1933). Über die normale Schwangerschaftsdauer und ihre Variationen sowie über die Länge und das Gewicht des Neugeborenen. Skrifter utgitt av Det Norske Videnskaps-Akademi i Oslo I Matem–Naturvid Klasse No. 7 Oslo, Norway, p 64.

Wenner WH, Young EB (1974). Nonspecific data of last menstrual period. Am J Obstet Gynecol, 120: 1071–1079.

Walker J (1954). Foetal anoxia A clinical and laboratory study. Br J Obstet Gynaecol, 61: 162–180.

World Health Organization (1972). The Prevention of Perinatal Morbidity and Mortality. Report on a seminar, Tours, 22–26 April 1969, Geneva: World Health Organization.

World Health Organization (1977a). Manual of the Internat-

ional Statistical Classification of Diseases Injuries and Causes of Death. Based on the recommendations of the Ninth Revision Conference, 1975, and adopted by the 29th World Health Assembly, Vol 1. Geneva: World Health Organization, p 773.
World Health Organization (1977b). WHO: Recommended Definitions Terminology and Format for Statistical Tables related to the Perinatal Period and Rise of a New Certificate for Cause of Perinatal Deaths. Modifications recommended by FIGO as amended. October 14, 1976, Acta Obstet Gynecol Scand, 56: 247–253.
Zwerdling MA (1967). Factors pertaining to prolonged pregnancy and its outcome. Pediatrics, 40: 202–212.

47 Post-term pregnancy: induction or surveillance?

Patricia Crowley

'When I use a word,' Humpty Dumpty said in a scornful tone, 'it means just what I choose it to mean, neither more nor less.' 'The question is,' said Alice, 'if you can make a word do that'. 'The question is,' said Humpty Dumpty, 'which is to be master, that's all.'

Lewis Carroll, *Alice Through The Looking Glass*

1 Introduction

Post-term pregnancy is one of the commonest indications for elective delivery, and a source of much controversy in both the obstetric and the lay literature (Anonymous 1974; Robinson 1974).

The difficulty of determining the incidence of post-term pregnancy is compounded by variations in the way it is defined; these have ranged from 41 weeks (Racker *et al.* 1953) to 43 weeks (Zwerdling 1967) (see Chapter 46).

Semantic problems have also contributed to the confusion. The terms 'post-term', 'prolonged', 'post-dates', and 'post-mature' are all listed as synonymous in the International Classification of Diseases (World Health Organization 1978). Yet nuances of meaning remain, and the terms, while synonymous, are laden with different evaluative overtones.

The term 'post-mature' has also been applied to a clinical syndrome with variable characteristics. Clifford's (1954) 'post-maturity syndrome' refers to a hierarchy of features in the infant, ranging from evidence of loss of subcutaneous fat and dry cracked skin (Stage I, post-maturity), through Stage II, when meconium-staining and birth asphyxia are also present, to Stage III where respiratory distress, convulsions, and fetal death occur, in addition to the other features. The bias inherent in the use of the word 'post-mature' is reflected in its preferential use by those who regard post-term pregnancy as a pathological state. When a clearly pathological syndrome is described by a word which is also used to make a simple statement about the chronological duration of a pregnancy, confusion is bound to arise. Further confusion is caused by the inclusion of 'dry, cracked skin', both among the criteria used for diagnosing the 'post-maturity syndrome' and in some schemes for paediatric assessment of gestational age at delivery (Farr *et al.* 1966).

Kloosterman (1979) recognized that a semantic problem had arisen, and described 'statistical' and 'clinical' post-maturity as two separate entities. 'Statistical post-maturity' simply referred to pregnancies that were 42 weeks or more in duration. Like Vorherr (1975), Clifford (1954), and Callenbach and Hall (1979), Kloosterman's 'clinical post-maturity' carried a pathological connotation and added yet another definition to an overworked word. He described as post-mature 'every fetus that dies before or during labour or shows signs of severe fetal distress whereas its development and degree of maturity would have guaranteed survival had it been brought into the outer world at an earlier date'.

The *post hoc* judgement that earlier delivery would have guaranteed survival is based on a number of assumptions that underlie much of the care currently offered to women with post-term pregnancy. It assumes that the 'post-mature' fetus is merely a passive victim of a pregnancy that has gone on too long. It also assumes that those fetuses retrospectively identified as post-mature can be selected for delivery prospectively at some arbitrary earlier date.

Strict adherence to the statistical definitions of 'post-term', 'prolonged', or 'post-dates' for all pregnancies that exceed 42 weeks is also dangerous. Just as the use of the term 'post-maturity' strengthens the fallacy that all post-term pregnancies are pathological, strict adherence to statistical definitions may also invite an inappropriate uniformity of management.

2 Risks in post-term pregnancy

Evidence that the perinatal mortality rate is increased in post-term pregnancy has been presented intermittently for almost 60 years (Ballantyne and Browne 1922; Kloosterman 1979). Other case series of post-term pregnancies have presented no evidence of an increased perinatal mortality rate (Daichman and Gold 1954; Magram and Cavanah 1960; Perlin 1960; Evans *et al.* 1963; Bierman *et al.* 1965), but these series all tend to be smaller than those showing an increased risk. This merely underlines the rarity of perinatal death and the consequently large numbers required to show a statistically significant difference.

Post-term pregnancy is associated with an excess incidence of congenital malformation compared with delivery at term (Malpas 1933; Evans *et al.* 1963; Zwerdling 1967). About 25 per cent of the excess mortality risk in post-term pregnancy relates to congenital malformations (Naeye 1978). Failure to take account of perinatal mortality from congenital malformation results in an overestimation of the risk of potentially avoidable perinatal death after 42 weeks relative to the rate at term. For example, Butler and Bonham's (1963) much quoted analysis of the 1958 British Perinatal Mortality Survey showed that delivery at 42 weeks' gestation was associated with a doubling of the perinatal mortality rate compared with delivery at 39 to 41 weeks, but these risk estimates did not correct for deaths from congenital malformations.

Most observational studies on post-term pregnancy have compared the outcome of delivery at or beyond 42 weeks with that of delivery between 37 and 41 weeks. Twin pregnancy, Rhesus haemolytic disease, pre-eclamptic toxaemia, a previous history of perinatal death, and recurrent haemorrhage may all act as confounding variables in such comparisons. They increase the risk of perinatal death and reduce the likelihood of being delivered at 42 weeks or later. Just as the inclusion of infants with congenital malformations causes an overestimate of the risk of death associated with post-term delivery *per se*, the risk may be underestimated by the inclusion in the control group of women with such conditions.

Comparisons between term and post-term pregnancies often exclude from analysis those women who fail to satisfy strict criteria for certainty of gestational age (Hertz *et al.* 1978). If we subscribe to the view that post-term pregnancy carries an increased perinatal risk, we might expect a group of post-term pregnancies with certain dates to carry a higher perinatal mortality rate than a group with uncertain dates, in which the 'pathology' of post-term pregnancy would be diluted by the normality of pregnancies that were in reality at term. This is not the case. Data from the Cardiff Births Survey (Chalmers 1975) showed that at all gestational ages, pregnancies with uncertain dates had a higher perinatal mortality rate than those with certain dates, and this pattern persisted after 42 weeks of gestation. This persistent tendency for women with uncertain dates to experience an increased perinatal mortality risk has also been reported by Buekens *et al.* (1984) and Hall and Carr-Hill (1985). Confining the analysis of post-term pregnancy to women with certain dates thus ignores a group of pregnancies at increased perinatal risk. While inclusion of women with uncertain dates undoubtedly inflates the incidence of post-term pregnancy, it would give a more accurate reflection of the problem as it is encountered by obstetricians in clinical practice.

2.1 Nature of the mortality risk

In order to assess the potential place of elective delivery in the management of post-term pregnancy, it is necessary to examine the specific perinatal risks associated with it. In balance, one must also consider the risk of iatrogenic preterm delivery due to a miscalculation of dates.

A retrospective analysis was conducted of 62,804 births at the National Maternity Hospital Dublin between 1979 and 1986 inclusive. Babies born before 37 weeks and those with lethal malformation were excluded. There were 6301 post-term births (42 completed weeks or more) during this period, an incidence of 10 per cent. Perinatal mortality by time of death and gestational age is presented in Table 47.1.

Prolonged pregnancy was associated with an increased risk of intrapartum and neonatal death but not of antepartum death. The corrected perinatal mortality rate of 6.7 per 1000 is higher than that noted in the randomized trials of post-term pregnancy management discussed below. In these trials 6 deaths occurred in 1568 normally formed infants, a perinatal mortality rate of 3.8 per 1000.

Other authors have drawn attention to the increased risk of intrapartum death associated with prolonged pregnancy (Lanman 1968; Hasseljo and Anberg 1962). In Lindell's series (1956), 75 per cent of perinatal deaths in post-term pregnancy occurred during labour, compared with only 38 per cent in all births. We can conclude then, that the risk associated with post-term pregnancy appears to increase with the onset of labour, and this fact must be borne in mind when considering the role of elective delivery.

As the excess mortality in babies delivered after 42

Table 47.1 Perinatal mortality from causes other than congenital malformation among births at term and post-term, by time of death, National Maternity Hospital, Dublin, 1979–86

	Post-term births (>42 weeks)		Term births (37–42 weeks)		Odds ratio (95 per cent confidence interval)
	n	per 1000	*n*	per 1000	
Total births	6301		56,503		
Stillbirths	32	4.9	217	3.8	1.37 (0.90–2.07)
Antepartum	21	3.2	180	3.1	1.05 (0.66–1.66)
Intrapartum	11	1.7	37	0.7	4.17 (1.63–10.70)
Live births	6269		56,248		
Early neonatal deaths	10	1.6	40	0.7	3.05 (1.21–7.69)
Perinatal deaths	42	6.7	257	4.5	1.57 (1.08–2.30)

Table 47.2 Pathological cause of death in 21 babies born post-term and dying between the onset of labour and within seven days of delivery, National Maternity Hospital, Dublin, 1979–86

Cause of death	Time of death	
	Intrapartum	1st week of life
Asphyxia, with meconium	7	2
Asphyxia, clear liquor	1	2
Meconium aspiration	0	3
Trauma	0	3
Abruptio placentae	1	0
Cord accident	1	0
Asphyxia, secondary to uterine rupture	1	0

weeks in the Dublin study was due to an excess of intrapartum and neonatal deaths, these 21 cases were analysed separately (Table 47.2). All 21 babies had a post-mortem examination. Outstanding features were the high prevalence of meconium-stained amniotic fluid among the intrapartum and asphyxial neonatal deaths (9 of 11 deaths) and the high incidence of traumatic intracranial haemorrhage, which accounted for 3 of the 8 neonatal deaths.

In the comparison of intrapartum and neonatal events in post-term and term pregnancies presented in Table 47.3 there is a significantly higher rate of forceps delivery both for fetal distress and for prolonged second stage of labour. In view of the strong association between forceps delivery and lethal intracranial haemorrhage (O'Driscoll *et al.* 1981) an increase in the incidence of intracranial haemorrhage might be expected in post-term pregnancies. Given the incidence of forceps delivery presented in Table 47.3 and the case-fatality rate quoted by O'Driscoll and his colleagues (1981), 1 in 20,000 infants delivered post-term might be expected to die from this condition. The series in Table 47.2, however, indicated a higher incidence of 3 in 5353 births, a rate of 0.6 per 1000 births.

The data in Tables 47.1 and 47.2 date from a period when the duration of labour was limited to 12 hours, so the excess intrapartum mortality rate cannot be attributed to prolonged labour *per se*. In the comparative study (Table 47.3), the mean duration of labour appeared longer in the post-term pregnancies than in those delivered at term, but the difference was not statistically significant. Neither can the excess mortality be ascribed to increased fetal weight. Only one baby in our series of deaths weighed more than 4.5 kg. Bakketeig and Bergsjo (see Chapter 46) note that the differences in perinatal mortality rates before and after 42 weeks are even greater when rates are compared within birthweight groups. Zwerdling (1967) also found the risks to be independent of birthweight.

2.2 Morbidity risk

In 1982, Dennis and Chalmers proposed that the incidence of early neonatal convulsions in infants born at or after term might serve as an epidemiological indicator of the quality of perinatal care. In a case-control study of 54 cases of early neonatal seizures in Cardiff babies born during the years 1970 to 1979, 54 babies with convulsions were identified among 41,144 singleton babies delivered after 37 weeks. Twenty-six of the babies with convulsions were delivered after 41 completed weeks, giving an odds ratio of 2.7 (95 per cent

Table 47.3 Comparison of intrapartum and early neonatal events in post-term and term pregnancies, National Maternity Hospital, Dublin, 1979–86

Events	Index cases (>42 weeks) (*n* = 257)		Control cases (37–42 weeks) (*n* = 257)			Uncertain dates (>42 weeks) (*n* = 134)		
	n	per cent	*n*	per cent		*n*	per cent	
Meconium-stained liquor	78	30	44	17	$p<0.01$	29	22	NS
Fetal blood sampling	26	10	7	2.7	$p<0.01$	7	5.2	NS
Apgar 7 at 5 minutes	4	1.5	1	0.3	NS	4	3	NS
'Cerebral dysfunction'	3	1.2	0	0	NS	0	0	NS
Caesarean section in labour	15	5.8	8	3.1	NS	13	9.7	$p<0.01$
Forceps delivery	28	10.8	13	5.1	$p<0.05$	13	9.7	$p<0.05$
Mean ± SD duration of labour (min)	264.5 ± 43		223.7 ± 45		NS	235.1 ± 48		NS

NS = not significantly different from the control group

confidence interval: 1.6–4.8) for seizures after 41 weeks (Minchom *et al.* 1987). In a similar case-control study of 89 babies with 'asphyxial' seizures within 48 hours of birth (out of 101,829 liveborn infants delivered after 37 weeks' gestation between 1 January 1980 and 31 December 1984 in three Dublin Maternity Hospitals), 27 were delivered after 42 weeks compared with 6 of 89 controls (odds ratio: 4.73 (95 per cent confidence interval: 2.22–10.05)) (Curtis *et al.* 1988). Meconium-stained amniotic fluid had been noted in 40 of the births of babies with seizures, compared with only in 10 of the control births.

In the National Maternity Hospital Dublin from 1979 to 1985 inclusive, early neonatal seizures occurred in 20 out of 5353 babies born after 42 weeks (5.4 per 1000), and in 48 out of 50,283 babies born between 37 and 42 weeks (0.9 per 1000) (odds ratio: 9.76 (95 per cent confidence interval: 4.36–21.87)).

2.3 Redefining the population at risk

'The patient is the one with the disease'

Samuel Shem, *The House of God*

This analysis of the morbidity and mortality risks of post-term pregnancy leads to two important conclusions. The increased risks of post-term pregnancy are strongly associated with meconium-stained amniotic fluid and begin to have their impact only with the onset of labour.

This raises an interesting paradox. The release of clear liquor at induction of labour in post-term pregnancy could be interpreted as rendering the act of induction unnecessary. On the other hand, the initiation of labour in post-term pregnancy with meconium-stained liquor moves the fetus immediately from the relatively low risk antepartum period into the high risk state of labour. This paradox is largely an intellectual one. In practice, all post-term pregnancies must end, either spontaneously or electively.

A comparison of intrapartum and neonatal events in term and post-term pregnancies permitted an estimate of the number of women who were both 42 weeks pregnant and had meconium-stained amniotic fluid. After excluding women with diabetes, multiple pregnancy, and pre-eclampsia, information was recorded over a 6-month period on 257 women (5.4 per cent) who had definite post-term pregnancies, and 257 parity-matched controls delivered between 37 and 42 weeks' gestation. Data were also recorded on 134 women whose pregnancies were possibly post-term, but who had uncertain dates.

Using the purely statistical approach to post-term pregnancy, 381 women (9.4 per cent of the hospital population) over 6 months might have been defined as 'at risk'. However, only 78 (30 per cent) of those with certain dates and 29 (22 per cent) of those with uncertain dates had meconium-stained amniotic fluid in labour, i.e. 2.6 per cent of the total population. Unfortunately, there is no evidence that it is possible to confine elective delivery to this group alone and that to do so would abolish the increased risk of intrapartum and neonatal mortality and morbidity documented in association with prolonged pregnancy.

3 Implications of post-term birth

3.1 Possible reasons for post-term birth

The practice of elective delivery before 42 weeks' gestation is based on the idea that the post-term fetus differs from the term fetus only with respect to the duration of pregnancy and that any increased perinatal risk is due to this factor alone. Recent evidence suggests that in the minority of fetuses that are at increased risk, the long duration of pregnancy may be only one manifestation of a more fundamental difference.

Studies in experimental animals indicate that the

fetus plays a crucial role in initiating labour (Challis and Mitchell 1981). There are also some relevant data from experiments in women (Anderson *et al.* 1971). Mati *et al.* (1973) compared intra-amniotic injection of betamethasone with placebo in 11 women who were 41 weeks pregnant or more. Jennsen and Wright (1977) compared such dexamethasone therapy with no treatment in 120 women who were all beyond their expected date of delivery. Both of these trials showed a lower mean interval between admission to the trial and the onset of labour in women allocated to corticosteroid therapy than in the control group. Nwosu *et al.* (1975a) found lower plasma cortisol levels in post-term neonates with physical signs of post-maturity than in control infants delivered at term. The same investigators (Nwosu *et al.* 1975b) went on to compare plasma cortisol levels in neonates who had suffered fetal distress during labour at term and post-term with controls delivered at term following labour uncomplicated by fetal distress. Infants who had experienced fetal distress in labour had mean cortisol levels 80 per cent above those of the control group if they were born at term, but 39 per cent below those of the controls if they were born post-term. Post-term infants with 'sufficient intrapartum fetal distress to warrant emergency caesarean section' had levels that were as much as 63 per cent below those of the control infants.

Although the number of infants in this study is small and some of the 13 women described as post-term were less than 42 weeks pregnant, the results were accepted as evidence that post-term infants may not be able to respond to fetal distress in the same way as term infants. These observations tend to support the hypothesis of Vorherr (1975), that a relative adrenocortical insufficiency might contribute both to the delayed onset of labour and to an increased risk of intrapartum hypoxia or death in post-term pregnancy.

There are other possible differences between term and post-term pregnancies. For instance, it is now clearly established that prostaglandins play a crucial role in the onset and maintenance of human labour (Keirse *et al.* 1983). Thus, it is not inconceivable that suppression of endogenous prostaglandin synthesis may be involved in delaying the onset of labour. On the other hand, there is increasing evidence that formation of prostacyclin, and possibly thromboxane, may be of vital importance for placental function and fetal well-being (Keirse 1985). Some factor that influences the metabolic pathway of arachidonic acid and affects either prostaglandin synthesis, prostacyclin production, or both, could well be behind some of the variable manifestations of post-term pregnancy. Depending on the type and magnitude of the effect, it could then be envisaged as both delaying labour and jeopardizing efficient placental exchange mechanisms.

Further support for the theory that some infants may be born post-term due to an inherent biological defect comes from Zwerdling (1967), who found that infants delivered following post-term pregnancy had a significantly increased infant mortality rate from all causes up to 2 years of age. This large retrospective study was based on 19,662 births at more than 43 weeks' gestation in New York City and 705 equally post-term pregnancies in Oakland, California. No other studies reported on long term infant mortality rates in babies born post-term.

The hypothesis that at least some post-term fetuses are fundamentally different from term fetuses remains unsubstantiated. Nevertheless, the possibility that this is so casts doubt on the prescription of elective delivery to cope with all the problems associated with post-term pregnancy. Just as suppression of preterm labour may be inappropriate in some cases where there is an underlying fetal problem (see Chapter 44), so may elective delivery represent a crude approach to the management of a fetal condition which may be responsible both for delaying the onset of labour and for altering the fetal response to labour.

3.2 Effects of elective delivery

A policy of elective delivery to improve perinatal outcome in post-term pregnancy may operate in a number of ways. If all women are delivered electively on or before the 294th day of pregnancy, prolonged pregnancy as defined by the World Health Organization (1977) and Fédération Internationale de Gynécologie et d'Obstétrique (FIGO News 1980) will no longer exist. A policy of elective delivery on the 295th day will have no effect on the incidence of prolonged pregnancy.

Obstetricians have, for many years, expressed irreconcilably different opinions on the place of induction of labour (see, for example, Tipton and Lewis 1975; O'Driscoll *et al.* 1975). It is important to verify that any policy proposing to address the problem of post-term pregnancy is achieving what it sets out to do. The doubling of the induction rate seen in Britain between 1958 and 1970 was partly attributed to an attempt to reduce the incidence of post-term pregnancy (Chamberlain *et al.* 1978). Surprisingly, the recorded incidence of post-term pregnancy actually rose slightly from 11.5 per cent of all births after 28 weeks' gestation in 1958 to 11.9 per cent in 1970 (Butler and Bonham 1963; Chamberlain *et al.* 1978). When comparing data from the two national surveys, the incidence of perinatal death in post-term pregnancy also appears to have been unaffected by the change in intervention rates. In contrast, data from the Cardiff Births Survey showed that, as the rate of induction of labour rose from 7.5 per cent in 1965 to 27.5 per cent in 1974, the incidence of post-term birth dropped from 11.8 per cent of all births in the 1965–69 quinquennium to 6.3 per cent in the

1970–74 quinquennium. This major increase in intervention was associated with a decrease in the relative risk of perinatal death after 42 weeks' gestation. When compared with the risk of perinatal death between 37 and 42 weeks, the relative risk fell from 1.37 in 1965–69 to 1.16 in 1969–74 (Chalmers 1975).

Critical evaluation of the effects of obstetric intervention is often hampered by the persistent and welcome tendency of perinatal mortality rates to fall with time. This can lead to misleading assumptions of cause and effect. The fall in the perinatal mortality rate at 43 weeks' gestation or more from 28 per 1000 in 1958 (Butler and Bonham 1963) to 17.6 per 1000 in 1970 (Chamberlain *et al.* 1978) was described as 'very acceptable' and was attributed to the high induction rate at this stage of pregnancy (Chamberlain *et al.* 1978). Nevertheless, had the perinatal mortality rate at 43 weeks fallen at the same rate as that at 38–39 weeks, we would have expected a perinatal mortality rate of 15.2 per 1000 instead of the observed rate of 17.6. Thus, the relative position of pregnancies of more than 42 weeks worsened between 1958 and 1970 despite increasing intervention.

Changes in perinatal mortality rates with time may also alter the cost–benefit ratio of intervention. In 1958, the perinatal mortality rate was 14.6 per 1000 at 41 weeks and 21.6 per 1000 at 42 weeks. Induction of labour in 1000 women prior to 42 weeks might theoretically have prevented 5 perinatal deaths from causes other than lethal malformation. In 1979–86 at the National Maternity Hospital, Dublin, the perinatal mortality rate for normally formed term infants delivered before 42 weeks was 4.5 per thousand and after 42 weeks was 6.7 per 1000, and 2300 inductions of labour would have been required to prevent 5 perinatal deaths.

4 Trials in post-term pregnancy

Thirteen trials of elective delivery in post-term pregnancy have been reported (Table 47.4). These trials fall into three main categories. Six of them (Cole *et al.* 1975; Martin *et al.* 1978; Tylleskar *et al.* 1979; Bréart *et al.* 1982; Sande *et al.* 1983; Husslein *et al.* 1986) compare routine induction of labour at about 40 weeks with expectant management until 42 weeks, followed by induction of labour for women who remain undelivered. Six trials (Henry 1969; Katz *et al.* 1983; Cardozo *et al.* 1986; Dyson *et al.* 1987; Augensen *et al.* 1987; Witter and Weitz 1987) compare induction of labour at 292–294 days with expectant management. One trial (Knox *et al.* 1979) compares two methods of supervising post-term pregnancy, each of which was associated with different rates of induced labour.

The trials which examine the effects of induction at 40 weeks address the risks and benefits of pre-empting post-term pregnancy, while those which deal with management at 42 weeks address the risks and benefits of alternative ways of managing post-term pregnancy when it has already occurred. The trials also vary with respect to the methods of induction of labour employed and the state of cervical 'favourability' required for entry into the trials. Two trials (Katz *et al.* 1983; Dyson *et al.* 1987) deal with the very specific issue of the management of post-term pregnancy in women with a cervix unfavourable for induction of labour. Despite these variations in the entry criteria, the trials permit an evaluation of the risks and benefits of elective delivery.

4.1 Perinatal death

If we estimate that post-term pregnancy is associated with a risk of perinatal death of approximately five per 1000, a trial involving 70,000 subjects would be required to give an 80 per cent chance of showing a 25 per cent reduction in perinatal mortality. In the 12 trials, only 8 perinatal deaths were reported in 3422 women randomized, and 7 of these 8 deaths occurred in pregnancies of 290 days or more. Two perinatal deaths occurred in the 1841 women allocated to induction and 6 in the 1581 allocated to expectant management. These small numbers make any conclusion about the effect of active induction policies on the risk of perinatal death impossible. Since the risk of antepartum death ceases by definition at the onset of labour, induction of labour must be associated with a small but finite reduction in the risk of antepartum fetal death. This saving could be offset by an increased risk of intrapartum or neonatal death following induction of labour, but the available data do not permit us to draw any confident conclusions about this.

4.2 Perinatal morbidity

Our analysis of the nature of the increased risk in post-term pregnancy identified meconium-stained amniotic fluid as a marker for increased risk of intrapartum mortality and neonatal mortality and morbidity. The results of 8 trials indicate that elective delivery reduces the risk of meconium-stained fluid (Table 47.5). This effect was more marked in the trials of routine induction at term (Table 47.6) than in the trials of active management at 42 weeks (Table 47.7).

Six of the trials give the incidence of abnormalities of the fetal heart rate during labour as an outcome, but there is no evidence that active induction policies affect this, either when all trials are considered together (Table 47.8), or when routine induction at term (Table 47.9) and routine induction at 42 weeks are considered separately (Table 47.10). The incidence of depressed Apgar score does not appear to be affected by active induction policies (Table 47.11).

During the 1970s, there were several reports of elective induction of labour being associated with unintended preterm delivery followed by respiratory dis-

Table 47.4 Entry criteria and management regimens in trials of elective delivery

Trial	Entry criteria	Active regimen	Expectant regimen
Cardozo *et al.* (1986)	Women at 40 weeks' and 10 days' gestation who had booked for obstetric care before 20 weeks' gestation and had had gestational age confirmed by ultrasound examination.	Induction of labour with intravaginal Prostaglandin E followed by amniotomy and oxytocin infusion if necessary.	Ultrasound examination at 40 weeks and 12 days and again at 40 weeks and 16 days. Cardiotocography on alternate days. Induction of labour if asymmetric growth retardation diagnosed or abnormal cardiotography, premature rupture of membranes or hypertension.
Dyson *et al.* (1987)	Low-risk women with well-established gestational age of at least 287 days; a modified Bishop score of less than six, a reactive non-stress test and normal amniotic fluid on ultrasound.	Cervical ripening with prostaglandin gel followed by oxytocin induction.	Twice weekly non-stress tests and weekly amniotic fluid volumes. Induction if these were abnormal or if Bishop score >6.
Tylleskar *et al.* (1979)	Primiparae aged 18–30 and multiparae aged 18–35. Certain dates. Normal fundal height and weight gain. Previous normal pregnancies. Present pregnancy normal. Cephalic presentation. Normal pelvic outlet on clinical examination. Modified Bishop score 5 or more in primiparae and 4 or more in multipaeae.	Induction of labour on EDD ± 2 days with amniotomy and intravenous oxytocin.	Expectant management until term + 14 days then induction of labour.
Henry (1969)	Women in whom the sole reason for induction of labour was prolonged pregnancy.	Forewater amniotomy and intravenous Syntocinon (maturity unspecified).	Amnioscopy 3 times per week until spontaneous labour or liquor found to be scanty or meconium-stained.
Cole *et al.* (1975)	Primigravidae aged 18–30 or women of parity 1, 2, 3, aged 18–35 with normal pregnancy and certain gestational age.	Induction of labour between 39 and 40 weeks using forewater amniotomy and oxytocin administration with the Cardiff pump.	Expectant management until 41 weeks unless an obstetric complication supervened. Induction of labour at 41 weeks.
Martin *et al.* (1978)	Present and past pregnancies obstetrically normal. Certain gestational age.	Induction of labour with forewater amniotomy and intravenous oxytocin.	Expectant management until 42 weeks' gestation then induction of labour.

Knox *et al.* (1979)	Pregnancy of 42 weeks' gestation with a reliable menstrual history confirmed by either pelvic examination before 12 weeks, ultrasonic cephalometry between 20 and 30 weeks, or ausculatation of an amplified fetal heart for at least 22 weeks.	Amniocentesis at entry into the trial and repeated weekly until meconium-stained liquor or no fluid obtained or until spontaneous labour occurred.	Amniocentesis at entry into the trial then oxytocin challenge tests weekly until spontaneous labour occurred or oxytocin challenge positive.
Breărt *et al.* (1982)	Low-risk women between 37 and 39 weeks' gestation with no other indication for induction of labour and no contraindication to induction of labour.	Planned induction of labour at 40 weeks with intravenous oxytocin and amniotomy at 3–4 cm dilatation.	Fetal surveillance at 2–3-day intervals with amnioscopy and cardiotocography. Induction at 42 weeks if still undelivered.
Sande *et al.* (1983)	Normal pregnancy between 40 and 41 weeks, vertex presentation, singleton fetus, cervical score of 5 points of more.	Induction of labour with oxytocin infusion followed by artificial rupture of the membranes.	Expectant management until 42 weeks then induction of labour.
Katz *et al.* (1983)	Women with pregnancies of 292 days' duration with certain dates and a pelvic score of 4 or less, with a cephalic presentation, no previous delivery by caesarean section. Clear amniotic fluid non-stress test.	Induction of labour by amniotomy and oxytocin infusion.	Expectant management with fetal movement counting, oxytocin challenge tests and amnioscopy every 3 days. Induction if abnormal fetal surveillance tests or pelvic score >4.
Augensen *et al.* (1987)	Healthy women with normal pregnancies between 290 and 297 days from LMP, with a single fetus in cephalic presentation and reliable dates.	Induction with intravenous oxytocin and amniotomy when labour was established. If labour not established 6–8 hours after induction, management as in expectant regimen.	Cardiotocography at entry to trial and again 3–4 days later if undelivered. Induction at 303 days from LMP if undelivered.
Husslein *et al.* (1986)	Low-risk pregnancies with cephalic presentation dates confirmed by early ultrasound favourable cervix.	Induction at term with 3 mg vaginal Prostaglandin tablet with repeat dose of 3 mg 6 hours later if not in labour.	Cardiotocography at 2–3-day intervals while awaiting spontaneous labour. Induction at 42 weeks if undelivered.
Witter and Weitz (1987)	Healthy women with normal pregnancies at 41 completed weeks, reliable dates, fetal motion assessment by women $3\times$/day, 24-hr urinary oestriol between 42 and 43 weeks.	Induction at 42 completed weeks with IV oxytocin and amniotomy when labour established. Caesarean section if not in active phase of labour after 20 hours' regular contractions.	Two urinary oestriols between 42 and 43 weeks, and thrice weekly thereafter. If results <10th centile, oxytocin challenge tests $2\times$/week with daily oestriols. Induced if diagnosis of fetal compromise, or Bishop score of 9.

Table 47.5 Effect of elective induction of labour at or beyond term on meconium-stained amniotic fluid

Study	EXPT n	EXPT (%)	CTRL n	CTRL (%)	Odds ratio (95% CI)	Graph of odds ratios and confidence intervals
Augensen *et al.* (1986)	37/214	(17.29)	32/195	(16.41)	1.06 (0.63–1.79)	
Cardozo *et al.* (1986)	21/195	(10.77)	21/207	(10.14)	1.07 (0.56–2.02)	
Dyson *et al.* (1987)	29/152	(19.08)	70/150	(46.67)	0.29 (0.18–0.46)	
Cole *et al.* (1975)	1/118	(0.85)	13/119	(10.92)	0.16 (0.06–0.48)	
Martin *et al.* (1978)	3/131	(2.29)	13/133	(9.77)	0.27 (0.10–0.74)	
Witter and Weitz (1987)	35/103	(33.98)	38/97	(39.18)	0.80 (0.45–1.42)	
Knox *et al.* (1979)	42/90	(46.67)	37/90	(41.11)	1.25 (0.70–2.25)	
Katz *et al.* (1983)	11/78	(14.10)	12/78	(15.38)	0.90 (0.37–2.18)	
Husslein *et al.* (1986)	21/188	(11.17)	19/168	(11.31)	0.99 (0.51–1.90)	
Typical odds ratio (95% confidence interval)					0.69 (0.56–0.86)	

Graph scale: 0.01 0.1 0.5 1 2 10 100

Table 47.6 Effect of elective induction of labour at <42 weeks' gestation on meconium-stained amniotic fluid

Study	EXPT n	EXPT (%)	CTRL n	CTRL (%)	Odds ratio (95% CI)	Graph of odds ratios and confidence intervals
Cole *et al.* (1975)	1/118	(0.85)	13/119	(10.92)	0.16 (0.06–0.48)	
Martin *et al.* (1978)	3/131	(2.29)	13/133	(9.77)	0.27 (0.10–0.74)	
Husslein *et al.* (1986)	21/188	(11.17)	19/168	(11.31)	0.99 (0.51–1.90)	
Typical odds ratio (95% confidence interval)					0.50 (0.31–0.82)	

Graph scale: 0.01 0.1 0.5 1 2 10 100

Table 47.7 Effect of elective induction of labour at 42+ weeks' gestation on meconium-stained amniotic fluid

Study	EXPT n	EXPT (%)	CTRL n	CTRL (%)	Odds ratio (95% CI)	Graph of odds ratios and confidence intervals
Augensen *et al.* (1986)	37/214	(17.29)	32/195	(16.41)	1.06 (0.63–1.79)	
Cardozo *et al.* (1986)	21/195	(10.77)	21/207	(10.14)	1.07 (0.56–2.02)	
Dyson *et al.* (1987)	29/152	(19.08)	70/150	(46.67)	0.29 (0.18–0.46)	
Witter and Weitz (1987)	35/103	(33.98)	38/97	(39.18)	0.80 (0.45–1.42)	
Knox *et al.* (1979)	42/90	(46.67)	37/90	(41.11)	1.25 (0.70–2.25)	
Katz *et al.* (1983)	11/78	(14.10)	12/78	(15.38)	0.90 (0.37–2.18)	
Typical odds ratio (95% confidence interval)					0.75 (0.59–0.95)	

Graph scale: 0.01 0.1 0.5 1 2 10 100

Table 47.8 Effect of elective induction of labour at or beyond term on fetal heart rate abnormality in labour

Study	EXPT *n*	(%)	CTRL *n*	(%)	Odds ratio (95% CI)	Graph of odds ratios and confidence intervals (0.01 0.1 0.5 1 2 10 100)
Bréart *et al.* (1982)	53/481	(11.02)	28/235	(11.91)	0.91 (0.56–1.50)	
Cardozo *et al.* (1986)	27/195	(13.85)	17/207	(8.21)	1.78 (0.95–3.33)	
Dyson *et al.* (1987)	4/152	(2.63)	27/150	(18.00)	0.19 (0.09–0.40)	
Cole *et al.* (1975)	12/118	(10.17)	16/119	(13.45)	0.73 (0.33–1.61)	
Witter and Weitz (1987)	34/103	(33.01)	33/97	(34.02)	0.96 (0.53–1.72)	
Knox *et al.* (1979)	11/94	(11.70)	13/93	(13.98)	0.82 (0.35–1.92)	
Katz *et al.* (1983)	9/78	(11.54)	5/78	(6.41)	1.87 (0.62–5.58)	
Typical odds ratio (95% confidence interval)					0.86 (0.67–1.11)	

Table 47.9 Effect of elective induction of labour at <42 weeks' gestation on fetal heart rate abnormalities

Study	EXPT *n*	(%)	CTRL *n*	(%)	Odds ratio (95% CI)	Graph of odds ratios and confidence intervals (0.01 0.1 0.5 1 2 10 100)
Bréart *et al.* (1982)	53/481	(11.02)	28/235	(11.91)	0.91 (0.56–1.50)	
Cole *et al.* (1975)	12/118	(10.17)	16/119	(13.45)	0.73 (0.33–1.61)	
Typical odds ratio (95% confidence interval)					0.86 (0.57–1.30)	

Table 47.10 Effect of elective induction of labour at 42+ weeks' gestation on fetal heart rate abnormalities

Study	EXPT *n*	(%)	CTRL *n*	(%)	Odds ratio (95% CI)	Graph of odds ratios and confidence intervals (0.01 0.1 0.5 1 2 10 100)
Cardozo *et al.* (1986)	27/195	(13.85)	17/207	(8.21)	1.78 (0.95–3.33)	
Dyson *et al.* (1987)	4/152	(2.63)	27/150	(18.00)	0.19 (0.09–0.40)	
Witter and Weitz (1987)	34/103	(33.01)	33/97	(34.02)	0.96 (0.53–1.72)	
Knox *et al.* (1979)	11/94	(11.70)	13/93	(13.98)	0.82 (0.35–1.92)	
Katz *et al.* (1983)	9/78	(11.54)	5/78	(6.41)	1.87 (0.62–5.58)	
Typical odds ratio (95% confidence interval)					0.86 (0.62–1.19)	

Table 47.11 Effect of elective induction of labour at or beyond term on Apgar score <7 at 5 minutes

Study	EXPT		CTRL		Odds ratio	Graph of odds ratios and confidence intervals
	n	(%)	*n*	(%)	(95% CI)	0.01 0.1 0.5 1 2 10 100
Breárt *et al.* (1982)	5/481	(1.04)	2/235	(0.85)	1.21 (0.25–5.92)	
Cardozo *et al.* (1986)	2/195	(1.03)	4/207	(1.93)	0.54 (0.11–2.71)	
Dyson *et al.* (1987)	2/152	(1.32)	3/150	(2.00)	0.66 (0.11–3.84)	
Witter and Weitz (1987)	0/103	(0.00)	2/97	(2.06)	0.13 (0.01–2.03)	
Knox *et al.* (1979)	6/94	(6.38)	2/93	(2.15)	2.80 (0.68–11.48)	
Katz *et al.* (1983)	3/78	(3.85)	1/78	(1.28)	2.77 (0.38–20.07)	
Typical odds ratio (95% confidence interval)					1.11 (0.55–2.26)	

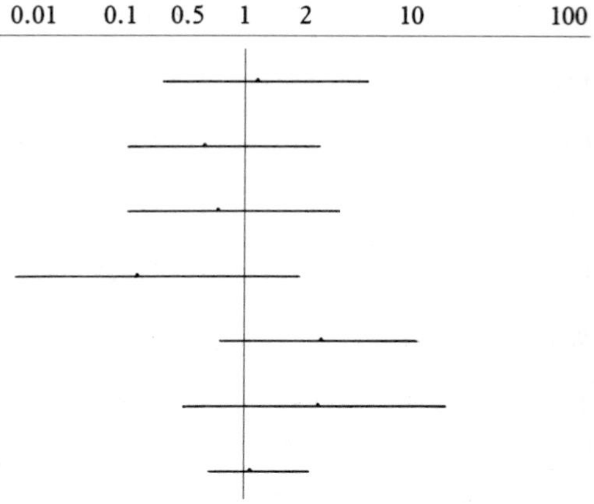

Table 47.12 Effect of elective induction of labour at or beyond term on neonatal jaundice

Study	EXPT		CTRL		Odds ratio	Graph of odds ratios and confidence intervals
	n	(%)	*n*	(%)	(95% CI)	0.01 0.1 0.5 1 2 10 100
Breárt *et al.* (1982)	6/481	(1.25)	9/235	(3.83)	0.28 (0.10–0.84)	
Augensen *et al.* (1986)	10/214	(4.67)	1/195	(0.51)	4.88 (1.47–16.18)	
Cole *et al.* (1975)	12/118	(10.17)	6/119	(5.04)	2.07 (0.79–5.40)	
Typical odds ratio (95% confidence interval)					1.37 (0.74–2.55)	

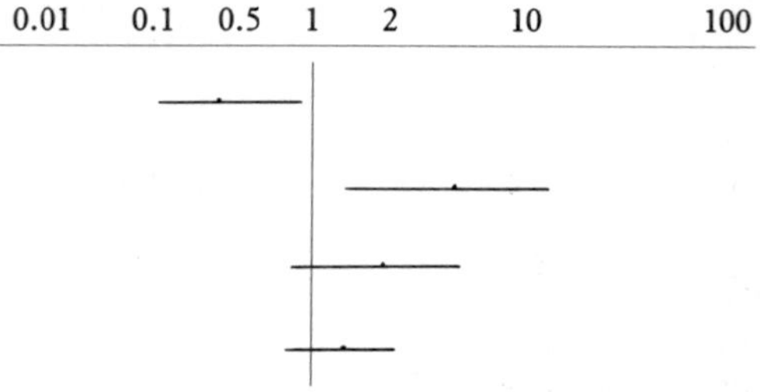

tress and other problems associated with this (Newcombe and Chalmers 1977; Chalmers *et al.* 1978; Clinch 1979). By the 1980s, there was evidence that this iatrogenic problem had become less (Newcombe 1983; Berkowitz *et al.* 1986), presumably because of greater awareness of the dangers of elective induction of labour without firm grounds for being certain about the duration of gestation. No cases of iatrogenic respiratory distress syndrome are reported in the randomized trials of elective delivery, but it must be remembered that well-documented fetal maturity was among the entry criteria for all of them (Table 47.4).

Data derived from the three trials which report on the incidence of neonatal jaundice show no consistent effect of elective induction on this outcome (Table 47.12).

None of the trials provide outcome data on the incidence of neonatal convulsions by trial allocation. In view of the apparent increase in the risk of early neonatal convulsions associated with prolonged pregnancy, this index of morbidity should be an outcome measure in all future randomized trials of alternative ways of managing post-term pregnancy.

Another more common outcome of great importance to parents is admission of their baby to special care nurseries in the postnatal period. This measure of outcome has only been reported by Cardozo *et al.* (1986) who showed that 6 out of 195 of babies born after a policy of active induction were admitted to paediatric special care compared with 3 out of 207 in the more conservatively managed group. As a number of conditions requiring admission to paediatric units might be altered by elective delivery, including suspected perinatal asphyxia, meconium inhalation, neonatal jaundice, and neonatal respiratory distress syndrome, this measure of outcome, too, should be incorporated in future trials.

4.3 Maternal outcomes

The 3 trials which give the incidence of epidural analgesia by allocation show no striking effect of active

Table 47.13 Effect of elective induction of labour at or beyond term on epidural anaesthesia

Study	EXPT *n*	(%)	CTRL *n*	(%)	Odds ratio (95% CI)	Graph of odds ratios and confidence intervals (0.01 0.1 0.5 1 2 10 100)
Bre͞art *et al.* (1982)	125/481	(25.99)	70/235	(29.79)	0.83 (0.58–1.17)	
Cardozo *et al.* (1986)	68/195	(34:87)	68/207	(32.85)	1.09 (0.72–1.65)	
Cole *et al.* (1975)	22/118	(18.64)	14/119	(11.76)	1.70 (0.84–3.45)	
Typical odds ratio (95% confidence interval)					1.00 (0.78–1.29)	

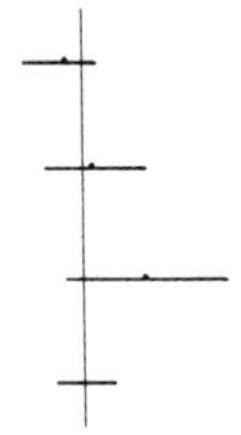

Table 47.14 Effect of elective induction of labour at or beyond term on instrumental vaginal delivery

Study	EXPT *n*	(%)	CTRL *n*	(%)	Odds ratio (95% CI)	Graph of odds ratios and confidence intervals (0.01 0.1 0.5 1 2 10 100)
Bre͞art *et al.* (1982)	125/481	(25.99)	35/235	(14.89)	1.89 (1.30–2.75)	
Augensen *et al.* (1986)	22/214	(10.28)	19/195	(9.74)	1.06 (0.56–2.02)	
Cardozo *et al.* (1986)	20/195	(10.26)	26/207	(12.56)	0.80 (0.43–1.47)	
Henry (1969)	8/55	(14.55)	7/57	(12.28)	1.21 (0.41–3.58)	
Cole *et al.* (1975)	34/118	(28.81)	26/119	(21.85)	1.44 (0.80–2.59)	
Martin *et al.* (1978)	17/131	(12.98)	23/133	(17.29)	0.72 (0.37–1.40)	
Tylleskar *et al.* (1979)	2/56	(3.57)	1/56	(1.79)	1.97 (0.20–19.35)	
Husslein *et al.* (1986)	4/188	(2.13)	3/168	(1.79)	1.19 (0.27–5.33)	
Typical odds ratio (95% confidence interval)					1.29 (1.03–1.63)	

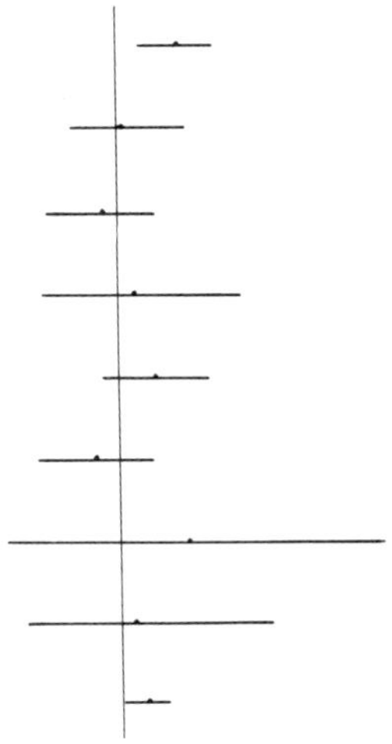

Table 47.15 Effect of elective induction of labour at <42 weeks' gestation on instrumental vaginal delivery

Study	EXPT *n*	(%)	CTRL *n*	(%)	Odds ratio (95% CI)	Graph of odds ratios and confidence intervals (0.01 0.1 0.5 1 2 10 100)
Bre͞art *et al.* (1982)	125/481	(25.99)	35/235	(14.89)	1.89 (1.30–2.75)	
Cole *et al.* (1975)	34/118	(28.81)	26/119	(21.85)	1.44 (0.80–2.59)	
Martin *et al.* (1978)	17/131	(12.98)	23/133	(17.29)	0.72 (0.37–1.40)	
Tylleskar *et al.* (1979)	2/56	(3.57)	1/56	(1.79)	1.97 (0.20–19.35)	
Husslein *et al.* (1986)	4/188	(2.13)	3/168	(1.79)	1.19 (0.27–5.33)	
Typical odds ratio (95% confidence interval)					1.48 (1.12–1.96)	

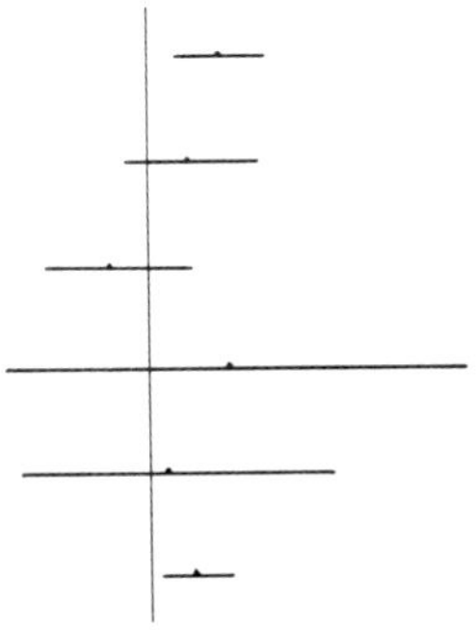

Table 47.16 Effect of elective induction of labour at 42+ weeks' gestation on instrumental vaginal delivery

Study	EXPT		CTRL		Odds ratio	Graph of odds ratios and confidence intervals
	n	(%)	*n*	(%)	(95% CI)	0.01 0.1 0.5 1 2 10 100
Augensen *et al.* (1986)	22/214	(10.28)	19/195	(9.74)	1.06 (0.56–2.02)	
Cardozo *et al.* (1986)	20/195	(10.26)	26/207	(12.56)	0.80 (0.43–1.47)	
Henry (1969)	8/55	(14.55)	7/57	(12.28)	1.21 (0.41–3.58)	
Typical odds ratio (95% confidence interval)					0.95 (0.63–1.44)	

Table 47.17 Effect of elective induction of labour at or beyond term on caesarean section

Study	EXPT		CTRL		Odds ratio	Graph of odds ratios and confidence intervals
	n	(%)	*n*	(%)	(95% CI)	0.01 0.1 0.5 1 2 10 100
Bréart *et al.* (1982)	21/481	(4.37)	17/235	(7.23)	0.57 (0.28–1.13)	
Augensen *et al.* (1986)	14/214	(6.54)	20/195	(10.26)	0.61 (0.30–1.24)	
Cardozo *et al.* (1986)	25/195	(12.82)	20/207	(9.66)	1.37 (0.74–2.55)	
Dyson *et al.* (1987)	22/152	(14.47)	41/150	(27.33)	0.46 (0.26–0.80)	
Henry (1969)	0/55	(0.00)	1/57	(1.75)	0.14 (0.00–7.07)	
Cole *et al.* (1975)	5/118	(4.24)	9/119	(7.56)	0.55 (0.19–1.62)	
Martin *et al.* (1978)	4/131	(3.05)	1/133	(0.75)	3.43 (0.59–20.10)	
Tylleskar *et al.* (1979)	1/59	(1.69)	1/55	(1.82)	0.93 (0.06–15.11)	
Witter and Weitz (1987)	30/103	(29.13)	27/97	(27.84)	1.07 (0.58–1.97)	
Knox *et al.* (1979)	11/94	(11.70)	8/93	(8.60)	1.40 (0.54–3.61)	
Katz *et al.* (1983)	16/78	(20.51)	7/78	(8.97)	2.49 (1.03–6.02)	
Husslein *et al.* (1986)	2/188	(1.06)	3/168	(1.79)	0.59 (0.10–3.48)	
Typical odds ratio (95% confidence interval)					0.86 (0.67–1.10)	

induction policies on the use of epidural analgesia (Table 47.13). This may be surprising in view of the fact that women who have labour induced are in the labour ward throughout labour, and during daylight hours—both factors increasing their opportunity to avail themselves of an epidural service. The 3 trials that report mean doses of pethidine used (Cole *et al.* 1975; Martin *et al.* 1978; Cardozo *et al.* 1986) showed no consistent direction of effect.

The trials which provide data on the use of instrumental delivery indicate that an active induction policy may increase the incidence of it (Table 47.14). The results of 5 trials of routine induction at term suggest that this effect is mediated by this policy (Table 47.15), for there is no evidence of an increased use in association with routine induction at 42 weeks' gestation (Table 47.16).

Eleven of the 12 studies in which induction was part of the intervention provide data on caesarean section rates, and the results suggest that active induction

Table 47.18 Effect of elective induction of labour at <42 weeks' gestation on non-compliance with allocated treatment

Study	EXPT		CTRL		Odds ratio	Graph of odds ratios and confidence intervals
	n	(%)	*n*	(%)	(95% CI)	0.01 0.1 0.5 1 2 10 100
Bréart *et al.* (1982)	51/481	(10.60)	0/235	(0.00)	4.96 (2.70–9.08)	
Cole *et al.* (1975)	1/118	(0.85)	0/119	(0.00)	7.45 (0.15–99.99)	
Martin *et al.* (1978)	10/131	(7.63)	0/134	(0.00)	8.12 (2.30–28.66)	
Tylleskar *et al.* (1979)	0/59	(0.00)	0/55	(0.00)	1.00 (1.00–1.00)	
Husslein *et al.* (1986)	8/188	(4.26)	3/168	(1.79)	2.28 (0.68–7.56)	
Typical odds ratio (95% confidence interval)					4.72 (2.88–7.73)	

policies are not associated with an increased use of caesarean delivery (Table 47.17). These results challenge a widely held belief (see, for example, Smith *et al.* 1984) that there is an inherent association between elective delivery and an increased risk of caesarean section, and they confirm the findings of Chalmers *et al.* (1976a,b) in their comparison of two obstetric teams with contrasting induction policies.

4.4 Women's views

The trials which reported on refusal of allocated treatment following randomization were analysed to obtain information on women's views with regard to post-term pregnancy. At term, women were much more likely to refuse the policy of routine induction than the alternative policy (Table 47.18). The available information does not permit analysis of where women's preferences lie at 290 days or later. Cardozo *et al.* (1986) included an assessment of women's satisfaction among the reported outcomes in their trial of elective delivery at 290 days. They found that the level of satisfaction related more to the outcome of labour than to the allocation.

5 Conclusions

Prolonged pregnancy is rare, with a true incidence of 4 to 6 per cent in pregnancies of 28 weeks or more. In the majority of cases, it probably represents a variant of normal and is associated with a good outcome, regardless of management. In a minority of cases there is an increased risk of perinatal death and early neonatal convulsions. These cases have a high incidence of meconium-stained amniotic fluid. It is possible that the delayed onset of labour and the increased risk of perinatal hypoxia have a common aetiology.

Confronted with this evidence, obstetricians can respond in a number of ways. They can adopt a policy of elective delivery at 290–294 days. This is a justifiable response to the risks of post-term pregnancy. Such a policy should probably be allied to one of routine ultrasound examination in early pregnancy in order to reduce the false-positive diagnosis of post-term pregnancy (see Chapter 27). Alternatively, they can manage post-term pregnancy conservatively on the basis that the risks are low. Finally, they can deliver babies electively at any time after 280 days in order to prevent post-term pregnancy altogether.

There is no justification for the last of these approaches. The randomized trials showed one useful benefit in association with this strategy—a significant reduction in the incidence of meconium-stained amniotic fluid. No other benefits or hazards emerged in association with this method of management. However, a significant number of women found elective delivery at 40 weeks unacceptable. Assuming that about 50 per cent of babies are undelivered at 280 days and only about 5 per cent are undelivered at 294 days, 10 women would be subjected to intervention in order to prevent 1 case of post-term pregnancy.

The two remaining options of elective versus selective delivery at 290–294 days must be assessed in the light of available evidence from the randomized trials and women's views. The central issue of perinatal mortality and neonatal seizures remains unanswered because insufficient numbers of pregnancies have been studied. Contrary to a large amount of evidence from retrospective studies, elective delivery does not increase the likelihood of caesarean section. At 42 weeks, the increased risk of instrumental delivery seen at term is no longer apparent. Against these hazards we can weigh some benefits in terms of a reduced risk of meconium-stained amniotic fluid and fetal heart rate abnormalities in labour. In view of the association between meconium-staining and poor perinatal outcomes already discussed, this must be seen as a useful benefit. The limited evidence available suggests that at 42 weeks an equal proportion of women request and refuse elective delivery.

In all of the randomized trials of elective delivery at 42 weeks, the participating obstetricians found it necessary to provide some form of fetal surveillance for the conservatively managed arm of the trial. This probably reflects the practice of obstetricians who manage post-term pregnancy conservatively outside the context of randomized trials. Most of these tests involve consultations at 2– to 3– day intervals after 42 weeks' and vary from the mildly intrusive use of ultrasound or cardiotocography, to the highly invasive procedures of amnioscopy or amniocentesis. There is some evidence that these tests can detect pregnancies in which there is 'something wrong', but less evidence that their use improves the outcome.

Faced with such finely balanced evidence, there are only two ways of managing post-term pregnancy that can be classified as truly effective care. The first is to enrol all cases of prolonged pregnancy in a large multicentre trial of elective versus selective delivery. The combined incidence of perinatal death and early neonatal convulsions forms the major adverse outcome to be measured in such a trial. Subordinate hypotheses to be tested relate to the effect of induction on the incidence of caesarean section, instrumental delivery, and neonatal jaundice. Further evidence of women's views on elective delivery may be sought either through the use of questionnaires or by incorporating into the trial an arm in which women make their own choice between elective and selective induction. The alternative option is to discuss the currently available evidence with the woman and allow her to decide between elective and selective induction.

References

Anderson ABM, Laurence KM, Davies K, Campbell H, Turnbull AC (1971). Fetal adrenal weight and the cause of premature delivery in human pregnancy. J Obstet Gynaecol Br Commnwlth, 78: 481–488.

Anonymous (1974). A time to be born. Lancet, 2: 1183.

Augensen K, Bergsjo P, Eikeland T, Ashnik K, Carlsen J (1987). A randomised trial of early versus late induction of labour in prolonged pregnancy. Br Med J, 294: 1192–1195.

Ballantyne JW, Browne FJ (1922). The problems of postmaturity and prolongation of pregnancy. J Obstet Gynaecol Br Empire, 19: 177.

Berkowitz G, Chang F, Chervenak F, Krouskop R, Wilkins I (1986). Decreasing frequency of iatrogenic neonatal respiratory distress syndrome. Am J Perinatol, 3: 205–208.

Bierman J, Siegel E, French F, Simonian K (1965). Analysis of the outcome of all pregnancies in a community. Am J Obstet Gynecol, 91: 37–45.

Bréart G, Goujard J, Maillard F, Chavieny C, Rumeau-Rouquette C, Sureau C (1982). Comparison of two obstetric policies with regard to artificial induction of labour at term. A randomised trial. J Gynecol Obstet Biol Reprod, 11: 107–112.

Buekens P, Delvoie P, Woolast E, Robyn C (1984). Epidemiology of pregnancies with unknown last menstrual period. J Epidemiol Community Health, 38: 79–80.

Butler NR, Bonham DG (1963). Perinatal Mortality. Edinburgh: Churchill Livingstone.

Callenbach JC, Hall TT (1979). Morbidity and mortality of advanced gestational age. Post-term or post-mature? Obstet Gynecol, 53: 721–724.

Cardozo L, Fysh J, Pearce JM (1986). Prolonged pregnancy: The management debate. Br Med J, 293: 1059–1063.

Challis JRG, Mitchell BF (1981). Hormonal control of preterm and term parturition. Seminars Perinatol, 5: 192–202.

Chalmers I (1975). Description and Evaluation of Different Approaches to the Management of Pregnancy and Labour 1965–1973. MSc thesis, University of London.

Chalmers I, Lawson JG, Turnbull AC (1976a). Evaluation of different approaches to obstetric care I. Br J Obstet Gynaecol, 83: 921–929.

Chalmers I, Lawson JG, Turnbull AC (1976b). Evaluation of different approaches to obstetric care II. Br J Obstet Gynaecol, 83: 930–933.

Chalmers I, Dauncey ME, Verrier-Jones ER, Dodge JA, Gray OP (1978). Respiratory distress syndrome in infants of Cardiff residents during 1965–1975. Br Med J, 2: 1119–1121.

Chamberlain R, Chamberlain G, Howlett B, Masters K (1978). British Births 1970, Vol. 2. Obstetric Care. London: Heinemann Medical.

Clifford SH (1954). Postmaturity with placental dysfunction. J Pediatr, 44: 1–13.

Clinch J (1979). Induction of labour—a six year review. Br J Obstet Gynaecol, 86: 340–342.

Cole RA, Howie PW, Macnaughton MC (1975). Elective induction of labour. Lancet, 1: 767–770.

Curtis P, Matthews T, Crowley P, Griffin E, O'Connell P, Gorman W, O'Brien N, O'Herlihy C, Clarke T, Darling M, O'Regan M (1988) (in press). The Dublin Collaborative Seizure Study: Do early neonatal seizures indicate quality of perinatal care? Arch Dis Child.

Daichman I, Gold EM (1954). Postdate labor: Effects on mother and fetus. Am J Obstet Gynecol, 68: 1129–1135.

Dennis J, Chalmers I (1982). Very early neonatal seizure rate: A possible epidemiological indicator of the quality of perinatal care. Br J Obstet Gynaecol, 89: 418–426.

Dyson DC, Miller PD, Armstrong MA (1987). Management of prolonged pregnancy—induction of labor versus antepartum fetal testing. Am J Obstet Gynecol, 156: 928–934.

Evans TN, Koeff ST, Morley GW (1963). Fetal effects of prolonged pregnancy. Am J Obstet Gynecol, 85: 701–712.

Farr V, Mitchell RG, Neligan GA, Parkin JM (1966). The definition of some external characteristics used in the assessment of gestational age in the newborn infant. Dev Med Child Neurol, 8: 507–511.

FIGO News (1980). International Classification of Diseases: Update. Int J Obstet Gynaecol, 17: 634–640.

Hasseljo R, Anberg AC (1962). Prolonged pregnancy. Acta Obstet Gynecol Scand, 61 (Suppl) 5: 23–29.

Hall MH, Carr-Hill RA (1985). The significance of uncertain gestation for obstetric outcome. Br J Obstet Gynaecol, 92: 452–460.

Henry G (1969). A controlled trial of surgical induction of labour and amnioscopy in the management of prolonged pregnancy. J Obstet Gynaecol Br Commnwlth, 76: 795–798.

Hertz RH, Sokol RJ, Knoke JD, Rosen MG, Chik L, Hirsch VJ (1978). Clinical estimation of gestational age: Rules for avoiding preterm delivery. Am J Obstet Gynecol, 131: 395–402.

Husslein P, Egarter C, Sevelda P, Genger H, Salzer H, Kofler E (1986). Induction of labour with prostaglandin E_2 vaginal tablets: A revival of elective induction. Results of a randomized trial. Geburtsh Frauenheilkd, 46: 83–87.

Jennsen H, Wright PB (1977). The effect of dexamethasone therapy in prolonged pregnancy. Acta Obstet Gynecol Scand, 56: 467–473.

Katz Z, Yemini M, Lancet M, Mogilner BM, Ben-hur H, Caspi B (1983). Non-aggressive management of post-date pregnancies. Eur J Obstet Gynecol Reprod Biol, 15: 71–79.

Keirse MJNC (1985). Biosynthesis and metabolism of prostaglandins within the human uterus in early and late pregnancy. In: The Role of Prostaglandins in Labour. Wood C (ed). London: Royal Society of Medicine, pp 25–38.

Keirse MJNC, Thiery M, Parewijck W, Mitchell MD (1983). Chronic stimulation of uterine prostaglandin synthesis during cervical ripening before the onset of labor. Prostaglandins, 25: 671–682.

Kloosterman GJ (1979). Epidemiology of postmaturity. In: Human Parturition. Keirse MJNC, Anderson ABM, Bennebroek Gravenhorst J (eds). The Hague: Leiden University Press, pp 247–261.

Knox E, Huddleston JF, Flowers CE, Eubanks A, Sutliff G (1979). Management of prolonged pregnancy: Results of a prospective randomized trial. Am J Obstet Gynecol, 134: 376–384.

Lanman JT (1968). Delays during reproduction and their effects on the embryo and fetus. New Engl J Med, 278: 1092–1099.

Leijon I, Finnstrom O, Hedenskop S, Ryden G, Tylleskar J (1980). Spontaneous labour and elective induction—a prospective randomized study. II. Bilirubin levels in the neonatal period. Acta Obstet Gynecol Scand, 59: 103–106.

Lindell A (1956). Prolonged pregnancy. Acta Obstet Gynecol Scand, 35: 136–163.

Magram HT, Cavanah WV (1960). The problem of postmaturity. A statistical analysis. Am J Obstet Gynecol, 79: 216–223.

Malpas P (1933). Postmaturity and malformations of the foetus. J Obstet Gynaecol Br Empire, 40: 1046–1053.

Martin DH, Thompson W, Pinkerton JHM, Watson JD (1978). A randomized controlled trial of selective planned delivery. Br J Obstet Gynaecol, 85: 109–113.

Mati JKB, Horrobin DF, Bramley PS (1973). Induction of labour in sheep and in humans by single doses of corticosteroids. Br Med J, 2: 149–151.

Minchom P, Niswander K, Chalmers I, Dauncey M, Newcombe R, Elbourne D, Mutch L, Andrews J, Williams G (1987). Antecedents and outcome of very early neonatal seizures in infants born at or after term. Br J Obstet Gynaecol, 94: 431–439.

Naeye R (1978). Causes of perinatal mortality excess in prolonged gestations. Am J Epidemiol, 108: 429–433.

Newcombe R (1983). Reversal of changes in distribution of gestational age and birthweight among firstborn infants of Cardiff residents. Br Med J, 287: 1095–1097.

Newcombe R, Chalmers I (1977). Changes in distribution of gestational age and birthweight among firstborn infants of Cardiff residents. Br Med J, 2: 925–926.

Nwosu U, Wallach EE, Boggs TR, Nemiroff C, Bongiovanni AM (1975a). Possible role of fetal adrenal glands in the etiology of postmaturity. Am J Obstet Gynecol, 121: 366–370.

Nwosu U, Wallach EE, Boggs TR, Bongiovanni AM (1975b). Possible adrenocortical insufficiency in postmature neonates. Am J Obstet Gynecol, 122: 969–974.

O'Driscoll K, Carroll C, Coughlan M (1975). Selective induction of labour. Br Med J, 4: 727–729.

O'Driscoll K, Meagher D, MacDonald D, Geoghegan F (1981). Traumatic intracranial haemorrhage in first born infants and delivery with obstetric forceps. Br J Obstet Gynaecol, 88: 577–581.

Perlin IA (1960). Postmaturity. Am J Obstet Gynecol, 80: 1–5.

Racker D, Burgess GH, Manly G (1953). The management of post-maturity. Lancet, 2: 953–956.

Robinson J (1974). The Times, 12 August.

Sande HA, Tuveng J, Fontstelien T (1983). A prospective randomized study of induction of labour. Int J Gynaecol Obstet, 21: 333–336.

Smith LP, Nagourney BA, McLean FH, Usher RH (1984). Hazards and benefits of elective induction of labour. Am J Obstet Gynecol, 148: 579–585.

Tipton RH, Lewis BV (1975). Induction of labour and perinatal mortality. Br Med J, 1: 391.

Tylleskar J, Finnstrom O, Leijon I, Hedenskop S, Ryden G (1979). Spontaneous labour and elective induction—a prospective randomized study. 1: Effect on mother and fetus. Acta Obstet Gynecol Scand, 58: 513–518.

Vorherr H (1975). Placental insufficiency in relation to post-term pregnancy and fetal postmaturity. Am J Obstet Gynecol, 123: 67–103.

Witter FR, Weitz CM (1987). A randomised trial of induction versus expectant management for postdates pregnancies. Am J Perinatol, 4: 206–211.

World Health Organization (1977). Recommended definitions, terminology and format for statistical tables related to the perinatal period and use of a new certificate for cause of perinatal deaths. Acta Obstet Gynecol Scand, 56: 247–253.

World Health Organization (1978). International Classification of Diseases. Geneva: World Health Organization.

Zwerdling M (1967). Factors pertaining to prolonged pregnancy and its outcome. Pediatrics, 40: 202–209.